DEVELOPMENTAL NEUROPSYCHIATRY

Volume II

DEVELOPMENTAL NEUROPSYCHIATRY

Assessment, Diagnosis, and Treatment of Developmental Disorders

VOLUME II

James C. Harris, M.D.

Director of Developmental Neuropsychiatry
Associate Professor of Psychiatry and Behavioral Sciences,
Pediatrics, and Mental Hygiene
Johns Hopkins University School of Medicine

New York Oxford
OXFORD UNIVERSITY PRESS
1995

OXFORD UNIVERSITY PRESS

Oxford New York
Athens Auckland Bangkok Bombay
Calcutta Cape Town Dar es Salaam Delhi
Florence Hong Kong Istanbul Karachi
Kuala Lumpur Madras Madrid Melbourne
Mexico City Nairobi Paris Singapore
Taipei Tokyo Toronto

and associated companies in
Berlin Ibadan

Published by Oxford University Press, Inc.,
198 Madison Avenue, New York, New York 10016

Library of Congress Cataloging-in-Publication Data
Harris, James C.
Developmental neuropsychiatry / James C. Harris.
p. cm. Includes bibliographical references and index.
Contents: v. 1. Fundamentals — v. 2. Assessment, diagnosis, and
treatment of development disorders.
ISBN 0-19-509849-3 (v. 2)
1. Developmentally disabled children—Psychology. 2. Pediatric
neuropsychiatry. 3. Developmental neurology. I. Title.
[DNLM: 1. Child Psychiatry. 2. Child Development. 3. Child Development
Disorders. 4. Child Behavior Disorders. WS 350 H314d 1995]
RJ506.D47H37 1995
618.92′8—dc20
DNLM/DLC for Library of Congress 94-42699

Credits for copyrighted materials appear on page 579.

9 8 7 6 5 4 3 2 1

Printed in the United States of America
on acid-free paper

To Mary, Cathy, and Joan
Who made it all possible
and
To the memory of Leo Kanner
Scholar, Teacher, and Advocate
For all children with disabilities

FOREWORD

Although developmental concepts have held a prominent place in American psychiatry for over 50 years because of the dominance of psychodynamic theory, it is only in recent years that advances in neuroscience have begun to have an impact on developmental psychiatry. Two major factors have served as impediments to the incorporation of fruits of brain research in the understanding of the developmental aspects of psychopathology. First, the roots of child psychiatry in the United States can be traced back early in this century to the child guidance movement, which established free-standing community clinics that focused primarily on the psychosocial needs of youth. Thus, with a few exceptions, the primary sites for treatment and training in child psychiatry were isolated from medical school–affiliated departments of psychiatry where biobehavioral research began to flourish. Second, with the ascendance of psychoanalytic theory, the child guidance clinics were predisposed to embrace it as a coherent explanation of child psychopathology. This geographic segregation and the emphasis on psychosocial concepts of etiology rendered child psychiatry poorly prepared to incorporate neuroscientific advances that began to transform psychiatry in the 1970s.

Other barriers have impeded the comprehensive involvement of psychiatry in developmental disorders and mental retardation. The cognitive and communicational limitations of these patients rendered them poorly suited for psychodynamic psychotherapy, the main treatment modality of psychiatry in the past. Thus the management of the psychiatric and behavioral concomitants of these disorders was largely ceded to behavioral psychologists. Furthermore, parents and advocates for the developmentally disabled strongly objected to the indiscriminate mixing of the developmentally disabled and the severely mentally ill in state psychiatric institutions. Thus state and federal policy, anger over stigmatization, and the lack of clinical interest on the part of psychiatry resulted in a wide gulf between psychiatry and the clinical services for the developmentally disabled.

Against this background, a number of advances commencing in the 1970s provided a climate in which academic psychiatry could reestablish its linkages to child psychiatry and to the behavioral complications of developmental disorders. The movement to utilize an atheoretical, phenomenologic strategy to construct a diagnostic schema for psychiatry (*The Diagnostic and Statistical Manual,* or DSM-III) that would provide predictability about course and treatment uncoupled diagnosis from psychodynamic theory. Clinicians began to apply these diagnostic criteria more widely, leading to the identification of psychiatric syndromes in populations such as children and the developmentally disabled, who were previously thought to be unaffected. For example, clinical studies indicated that depressed children often satisfied the diagnostic criteria for major depressive disorder; these observations, at variance with accepted theory of the time, led to the use of treatments for depression found to be effective in adults. With the advances in psychopharmacology, clinicians began to examine whether drugs effective for specific psychiatric disorders might have efficacy in the symptomatic management of psychiatric symptoms in special populations. For example, the use of the serotonin uptake inhibitor chlorimipramine, a drug effective in obsessive-compulsive disorder, was examined in developmentally disabled children with compulsive self-injurious behavior. Finally, the cytogenetic teasing out of different causes for mental retardation began to reveal behavioral phenotypes unique to specific syndromes such as Down syndrome, Prader-Willi syndrome, and Fragile X syndrome. The link between developmental brain disorders caused by specific genetic abnormalities and particular behavioral problems rekindled interest both in clinical research and psychiatric management of developmental disorders.

The rapid advances in brain research over the last two and a half decades, moreover, provided the foundation for the understanding of nervous system development and function that has now permitted the rise of a new and meaningful discipline of developmental neuropsychiatry. The application of the methods of molecular biology to developmental brain research is disclosing the laws dictating the formation of the brain and its neuronal circuitry. Furthermore, animal models to elucidate the role of specific genes through the creation of mice transgenic for normal or mutant genes now allow investigators to track the consequences of abnormal gene expression on brain development and function. At a clinical level, powerful imaging methods provide windows into the human brain to determine quantitatively abnormalities in structure and function in specific disorders. The findings from neuroscience research have undermined the traditional classification of disorders simply on the basis of their age of symptomatic onset and have revealed that the seeds of psychopathology in disorders such as schizophrenia and Alzheimer's disease are sown early in brain development.

Against this background, Dr. Harris's two-volume work on developmental neuropsychiatry sets the agenda for this emerging clinical specialty. Written by an individual with the developmental expertise of a pediatrician, the behavioral sophistication of an adult and child psychiatrist, and a deep appreciation of neuroscience, his two books offer an integrated yet comprehensive conceptual approach to developmental neuropsychiatry. Grounded in neuroscience but enriched by clinical realities, the first volume provides the unified vision of the "new" psychiatry, which places the brain at the epicenter of psychopathology and recognizes the essential interplay between intrinsic vulnerabilities and life experience. The second volume translates this unifying neuroscientific perspective into the practical clinical issues of the diagnosis, assessment, and management of specific developmental disorders. Dr. Harris's *Developmental Neuropsychiatry* continues the tradition of Leo Kanner's *Child Psychiatry*, first published 60 years ago, in defining the field of developmental psychopathology in a way that will have significance for years to come. Thus this two-volume set will be an essential resource not only for physicians but for all professionals involved in the treatment of developmental disorders.

Joseph T. Coyle, M.D.
Eben S. Draper Professor of
Psychiatry and Neuroscience
Chairman, Consolidated
Department of Psychiatry
Harvard Medical School

PREFACE

Anomalies when rightly studied yield rare instruction; they witness and attract attention to the operation of hidden laws or of known laws under new and unknown conditions; and so set the inquirer on new and fruitful paths of research.

—H. Maudsley, 1880

An appreciation of recent advances in developmental and cognitive psychology, an understanding of basic brain mechanisms, knowledge about recent approaches to modeling in the cognitive neurosciences, and an awareness of descriptive psychopathology are essential background for professionals who are working with children and adolescents with neurodevelopmental disorders. This book provides a resource and a critical appraisal for both the student and the practitioner on the central topics related to developmental neuropsychiatry. It is an effort to bring together in one place background material in these many areas and to offer a developmental perspective that addresses maturation of the brain, the facilitating psychosocial environment, and competence in the mastery of developmental tasks by the disabled person. This approach considers that developmental impairment may magnify brain mechanisms, thereby providing a window on developmental processes that may be difficult to isolate when studied in the normally maturing person in an average expectable environment, the standard situation in which Gesell sought to establish landmarks of development.

The co-occurrence of mental events and neural events has long been recognized. For the experiencing person, subcortical events are cortically reconstructed and influence behavior; the latter is most evident in the case of traumatic life events. Developmental changes take place from infancy throughout the life span. Determining how they occur is a major challenge to current research.

The book is intended to provide a synthesis of recent developments in basic neurobiology, cognitive neuroscience, ethology, child development, and developmental psychopathology and apply them to children and adolescents with neuropsychiatric conditions. Specific conditions occurring during the developmental period are reviewed to examine the potential basis for differences among them, and methods of assessment and effective means of intervention are discussed. Included are conditions involving brain disorder or dysfunction whose origins are genetic, metabolic, traumatic, toxic, or psychosocial. Their effects on developing persons and their families are central to the discussion. Although both sexes are affected, these conditions occur most commonly in males. For convenience in reading, the pronoun "he" is used to denote both sexes throughout the text.

Developmental Neuropsychiatry: Assessment, Diagnosis, and Treatment of Develop-

mental Disorders begins with an introduction that traces the historical background and societal attitudes toward neuropsychiatric conditions beginning in childhood. Part I discusses methods of assessment and investigation, includindg the cytogenetic history, which is particularly important in the developmental disorders. Emphasis is placed on neuropsychological testing rather than on traditional psychological tests, because such testing is critical in the evaluation of specific developmental disorders. Part I also discusses brain imaging techniques (CT, MRI, SPECT, PET) and electrophysiologic measures.

Part II focuses on neurodevelopmental disorders and brain injury that occurs during the developmental period. The general categories of developmental disability are included—that is, mental retardation, cerebral palsy, learning disorders, and pervasive developmental disorders along with traumatic brain injury occurring in early childhood.

Part III discusses behavioral phenotypes (patterns of behavior characteristic of a syndrome) that occur in cytogenetic disorders, cytometabolic conditions, and gestational substance abuse syndromes. The occurrence of both physical and behavioral consequences of gestational substance use has become a major public health concern. There is a growing interest in the study of behavioral phenotypes as evidenced by the establishment of the international Society for the Study of Behavioural Phenotypes (SSBP). The last two international conferences had as their themes "From Genes to Behavior" and "Brain and Behaviour: The Mechanisms of Expression of Behavioural Phenotypes."

Part IV describes child developmental psychopathology. Since these syndromes may be linked to brain dysfunction, they are considered together in this part. Sleep disorders are included because they occur commonly both as specific conditions (e.g., night terrors) and as complications of a developmental disorder. Problems in sleep often exact a heavy toll on family members. Aggressive behavior and self-injury are the most common co-occurring disorders in developmentally disabled persons. Throughout Part IV the DSM-IV term "disorder" is used for consistency, although several conditions, such as Tourette's, are more commonly referred to as syndromes.

Part V deals with treatment for developmental disorders, the most widely used being behavioral, psychoeducational, and pharmacological approaches. Yet attention to individual, interpersonal, and family therapy is essential. The establishment of self-regulation and self-control for the child and the full acknowledgment of the disability by the parents are critical to long-term outcome. In regard to the correction of developmental disabilities, some of the most exciting prospects are in the realm of gene therapy, an approach that is still in its infancy. The final chapter in this section discusses genetic counseling and reviews recent advances in gene therapy.

Part VI brings together the legal decisions that have been critical in establishing the rights of developmentally disabled persons. The process of deinstitutionalization is discussed along with the various public laws that guarantee the rights of the developmentally disabled. The issue of legal competency is considered. Finally, legal aspects of psychopharmacology are reviewed.

The goal of the book is to assist the professional working with developmental disorders to facilitate the mental growth and social adaptation of children and adolescents with neurodevelopmental disorders. It provides psychiatric background information and reviews treatment approaches that will help professionals facilitate change in these children and their families. The intended audience includes child and adolescent psychiatrists, developmental pediatricians, child neurologists, physicians in training (fellows, residents, and medical students), nurses, educators, psychologists, and other nonmedical professionals who treat these conditions and neuroscientists who wish to learn more about child and adolescent neuropsychiatric disorders.

Baltimore, Maryland J.C.H.
August 1995

ACKNOWLEDGMENTS

Developmental Neuropsychiatry provides a comprehensive summary of knowledge acquired and literature consulted as a result of my work with children and adolescents with developmental disorders and their families. It is the outcome of many interactions and discussions with faculty members, residents, medical students, and nonmedical professionals over the past two decades at the Johns Hopkins Medical Institutions. Dr. Paul McHugh, Chairman of the Department of Psychiatry, the Johns Hopkins University School of Medicine, was instrumental in stimulating me to consider writing a textbook and has provided ongoing guidance. Dr. Joseph Coyle, Director of the Division of Child and Adolescent Psychiatry at the Johns Hopkins University School of Medicine from 1982 to 1991, enthusiastically supported the book and offered his expertise in developmental neuroscience. Dr. Hugo Moser, Director of the Johns Hopkins Center for Research in Mental Retardation and Related Aspects of Human Development, encouraged me in the early stages of manuscript development and provided the primary setting for me, as the director of developmental neuropsychiatry, to evaluate and treat children and adolescents with developmental disorders.

Dr. Paul MacLean, Chief, Laboratory of Brain Evolution and Behavior at NIH, stimulated my interest in comparative neuroanatomy, established a position for me as guest worker in his laboratory (1978–1984), and made me as excited as he is about the prospects of evolutionary neurobiology. Dr. Edward Edinger, analytic psychologist and former Chairman of the Jung Training Center in New York, encouraged me to think about the psychology of developmental disorders and how the self system might emerge in those with disabling conditions. Dr. Edinger provided an important and greatly appreciated stimulus in looking at the developmental perspective on the pervasive developmental disorders and its interface with psychological theory.

Dr. Roland Fisher, formerly at Johns Hopkins and now Professor at the University of the Balearics in Mallorca, stimulated my interest in the brain/mind interface, particularly as to how experience may shape the brain. Ralph Harper, Adjunct Professor at Johns Hopkins in the history of ideas program, and an existential theologian, reflected with me on the nature of the life experiences of the family of the disabled person. Most important, he provided ongoing support which sustained me throughout the preparation of the manuscript and its final stage of completion. Finally, my wife, Dr. Catherine DeAngelis, reminded me of the importance of completing what I had begun and in all ways provided the environment that made this book possible. Simply put, without her this book could not have been written.

A number of colleagues have been instrumental in reading and critiquing the various parts of these books. A single-authored textbook is now uncommon, and its completion would not have been possible without the assistance of colleagues at the Johns Hopkins University School of Medicine and the NIH Laboratory of Comparative Ethology. Dr. M. Christine Zink, D.V.M., Ph.D., Associate Professor of Comparative Medicine and Pathology at the Johns Hopkins University School of Medicine, reviewed the initial chapter on molecular neurobiology and provided a comprehensive critique. The chapter on the development of neurotransmitter systems is an expansion of an earlier chapter on this subject, which I prepared with Dr. Joseph Coyle, now Professor of Psychiatry and Neuroscience and Chair of the Consolidated Department of Psychiatry at Harvard University School of Medicine. His expertise in this area was invaluable.

Dr. Paul Wender, Professor, Department of Psychiatry, University of Utah School of Medicine, reviewed the entire section on basic neural science. Dr. Wender had stimulated my interest in developmental neuropsychiatry during my child and adolescent psychiatry residence in 1973 as we discussed minimal brain dysfunction (now AD/HD), its diagnosis and treatment, each Friday morning. Drs. Stephen Suomi and Dee Higley, NIH Laboratory of Comparative Ethology, provided helpful critiques of Chapters 12 through 17 dealing with ethology and the developmental perspective. Dr. Suomi generously arranged for me to become a guest worker in the Laboratory of Comparative Ethology (1984–1992), where I conducted behavioral research on separation vocalizations in squirrel monkeys with Dr. John Newman.

The chapters of Part I, Volume II, on assessment and rating scales were reviewed by Dr. Ludwik Szymanski, Director of the Diagnostic Evaluation Clinic, the Children's Hospital Medical Center, Harvard University. I am particularly appreciative of Dr. Szymanski's help. He and I have worked closely for many years on the Mental Retardation and Developmental Disability Committee of the American Academy of Child and Adolescent Psychiatry. The chapter on neuropsychological testing was reviewed extensively with Dr. Martha Denckla, Professor of Neurology and Director of Developmental Cognitive Neurology, Kennedy Krieger Institute, the Johns Hopkins University School of Medicine. This chapter underwent multiple revisions under her guidance. The chapter on the evaluation of brain structure and functions, which deals with the various neuroimaging techniques, was reviewed by Dr. Nick Bryan, Director of Neuroradiology, Johns Hopkins University School of Medicine. Dr. Bryan provided a comprehensive critique, and his suggestions were readily incorporated into this chapter. Dr. Ludwik Szymanski was also the reviewer of Chapters 5 through 9 of Part II, Volume II, on developmental disorders, an area in which he is eminently qualified. He pointed out the relevance of these chapters to both physicians and nonphysicians who work with the developmental disorders.

Part III, Volume II, on behavioral phenotypes, was reviewed by Dr. Hugo Moser, who made many valuable comments and suggestions, particularly relating to the metabolic disorders. This section was revised extensively in keeping with his suggestions. His help was particularly appreciated in the section on adrenoleukodystrophy, an area in which he and I have worked together for many years.

Dr. Paul Wender reviewed Chapters 13 through 17 of Part IV, Volume II, on developmental psychopathology and commented on their usefulness to physicians and nonphysicians working with these types of problems. Dr. Ludwik Szymanski reviewed Chapters 18 through 21 on the treatment of children with developmental disorders as well as Chapter 22 on public law and the rights of the disabled. Final thanks are to Dr. Frank Oski, Chairman, Department of Pediatrics, the Johns Hopkins University School of Medicine, who reviewed the overall structure of the manuscript.

The works of Sir Michael Rutter, C.B.E., M.D., provided the foundation for the establishment of this specialty area. I have benefited from my contacts with him over the years and have sought to follow his lead in the further development of this specialty. Contacts with many other individuals have enriched my experiences with children with developmental disorders and contributed in great part to my thinking and perspective. Among them are Leo Kanner, Alejandro Rodriguez, Dennis Whitehouse, Arnold Capute, Sakkubai Naidu, Fred Palmer, Bruce Shapiro, Susan Hyman, Joan Gerring, Allan Reiss, Wayne Fisher, Rebecca Landa, Richard Allen, Paula Tallal, Susan Harriman, Eileen Atkins, Jean Patz, Georgette Evler, and a host of others whose professional association has made our mutual interest in the care of children exciting and worthwhile.

Gratitude is expressed particularly to the many authors whose publications I have summarized in this textbook. Their efforts have led to a better understanding of developmental disorders. I bear full responsibility for the synthesis of their work.

Finally, I express my appreciation to the administration of the Department of Psychiatry at the Johns Hopkins University School of Medicine and the Kennedy Krieger Institute for providing support for a one-year, full-time sabbatical to allow me to integrate the disparate elements of the field of developmental neuropsychiatry and frame them into what I hope is a comprehensive and coherent textbook that may be used by both physicians and nonphysicians who devote their efforts to working with children, adolescents, and their families as they compensate and struggle with disorders of development.

Special thanks are due Joan Bossert, my editor at Oxford University Press. From our initial meeting in 1988 at the Society of Neuroscience meeting through the completion of my manuscript she has provided unfailing support, been a sounding board, offered insightful suggestions, and demonstrated her expertise in navigating these books through the production process. For all this, I am especially grateful.

Baltimore, Maryland J.C.H.
August 1995

CONTENTS

INTRODUCTION: HISTORICAL LANDMARKS IN DEVELOPMENTAL NEUROPSYCHIATRY

Although recognized since antiquity, explanations of the nature, causes, and treatment of mental retardation and developmental disabilities have varied considerably. Historically, the earliest reference and discussion of developmental retardation may be in the Egyptian Papyrus of Thebes (1552 B.C.) (Bryan, 1930). Over the intervening centuries, there has been considerable confusion about the nature of developmental retardation. Approaches to intervention have ranged from infanticide to exorcism and removal of evil spirits to humane education. In Greek and Roman culture, infanticide was practiced and trephining may have been used in Europe, Central, and South America as a treatment, presumably to allow spirits to escape. Some of the mentally retarded may have become slaves and others court jesters. In the Middle Ages, demon possession continued to be suspected, but adequate care of the retarded was practiced as well, for example, in the famous Hospice in Gheel, Belgium. A retarded child might also have been regarded as a changeling—an unusual child who was substituted at birth for a normal child by the fairies. In some instances, retarded people were regarded as "children of God" or harmless innocents who were allowed to wander at will. Based on this more benign view, Henry II of England promulgated legislation to provide for their protection. "Natural fools" were made wards of the king (Deitz and Repp, 1989).

Despite this early recognition and a historical distinction between the mentally retarded, abnormal from birth, and the demented whose difficulties began later in life, an emphasis on child development and on education of the mentally retarded did not begin until the 19th century. Although the French and American revolutions were accompanied by humane treatment and reforms in care and their aftermath saw the appearance of schools for deaf-mutes and for the blind, there was little specific study of child development. For this to occur, a new orientation toward children was required that began toward the end of the 18th century (Kanner, 1964). It was stimulated by the philosophy of Rousseau who had emphasized the development of the child's natural, but latent abilities, through education. He viewed the child's nature as essentially good and suggested these qualities are capable of development, which was in contrast to the prevailing view that children lack innate qualities of goodness and require a rigid form of education. With a shift to considering the child's nature as essentially good, free individual expression was encouraged. The publication in 1762 of *Emile* by Rousseau stimulated considerable interest in Europe among educators. By emphasizing the role of the child as an active participant in learning, Rousseau's philosophy provided an orientation to the child that is one aspect of current developmental theory.

In the 19th century, an interest in child development was further stimulated by a theory posed to the French Academy of Sciences by Etienne Bonnet, Abbé de Condillac, in his essay on the *Origin of Human Knowledge* and his *Treatise on the Sensations* (Crutcher, 1943). He taught that "all knowledge is gained through the senses," which suggests the child's mind is a blank slate at birth. A person without language, he maintained, utilizes sight, sound, and his or her sensing experience of events or objects, which evoke ideas corresponding to their sensory input. He speculated that the human being first acquires the sense of smell, and later on acquires the other senses. Through sensory experience intellectual abilities and knowledge of the world are established. This question of the nature of humans was the central question during the period known as the Enlightenment. Was the difference between human and animal one of kind or degree? How should wild children be classified, as human or animal? The nature of human beings and how they gain knowledge led to experiments with feral children; the most famous of these was Victor, the wild boy of Aveyron, France. Apparently, he was a boy who was found in the forest living among animals. He had lacked human contact for many years and was unable to talk.

A classic study was initiated by Itard in 1800 to educate Victor (Itard, 1806). Itard was a student of Pinel, who had supervised the freeing of the insane from their chains in Paris and was the preeminent psychiatrist of that time. Despite Pinel's conclusion that Victor was mentally retarded, Itard, following Condillac's approach, denied this. His task was to test Condillac's theory that all knowledge is acquired through the senses. Itard, under the auspices of the French Academy of Sciences, worked with Victor for 5 years. Although he made progress, Itard was not able to educate him successfully and finally concluded that Victor was mentally retarded. Yet the gains he had made with Victor were encouraging. This was the first systematic, scientific attempt to train a mentally retarded person which demonstrated that benefits could come from education. Often neglected and an object of ridicule, it became apparent that something could be done to help a mentally handicapped person make progress. This case has been reviewed in detail by Harlan Lane (1976), who suggests that Victor was not originally either autistic or severely mentally retarded.

Likewise, in the 19th century, the view of demon possession and the view of retarded persons as harmless innocents was replaced by early attempts to educate and house them. In 1837 Seguin, a pupil of Itard, began private instruction for mentally retarded persons, and in 1846 he published *Idiocy and Treatment,* an approach to intervention that was the standard text for many years (Seguin, 1846, 1866). Itard's investigations led to the establishment of the first residential European center for young mentally defectives by Guggenbuhl in 1841 (Kanner, 1960). The first state school in the United States was established in Massachusetts in 1848, but it was not until 1875 that the need for care became generally recognized. Initially, the interventions were in designated educational institutions, but later it became clear that some custodial care was also needed.

During the same time period in England, J. Langdon Down described and classified mental retardation syndromes. He is credited with providing the first major separate classification and complete description of a specific mental retardation syndrome. His general classification included congenital, accidental, and developmental categories. In 1866 he published his observations of congenitally mentally retarded persons in the London Hospital Reports as *An Ethnic Classification of Idiots* (Down, 1866) and subsequently expanded them (Down, 1887). His classification was based on a then current biological theory of recapitulation; he assumed ontogeny recapitulates phylogeny. According to this theory, in higher animals embryonic development follows stages or sequences so the adult forms of lower creatures are successively passed through, one after the other, in development. Normal traits of infant life are considered more primitive, but arrested, ancestral adult forms. Traits and abilities of an abnormal adult are considered throwbacks or arrests in development at the level of one of the lower races. Down included Ethiopian, Malay, Negroid, Aztec, and Mongolian as less developed forms in classifying mentally retarded children and adults. Among these, the term "Mongolian idiot" or "mongolism" persisted for many years without reference to its racial origins. It was finally abandoned after the 21 chromosomal anomaly was demonstrated. The term "Down syndrome" is now in current usage. With Down's classification, earlier fanciful explanations were replaced by new ideas but couched in what is now an antiquated scientific theory.

Several decades later, intelligence testing was introduced. This was also an outgrowth of efforts at education of developmentally disabled persons and led to the establishment of measures to determine ability. In France, Binet and Simon (1905, 1916) evaluated methods to deal with backward school children by developing a series of tests with progressively more difficult questions and subsequently arranging them by age level. Terman (1916) in the United States standardized these tests for American children as the Stanford-Binet test, whose revision was published in 1916 based on assessment of 1,000 American children. Subsequently, tests were developed by Kuhlman for younger children who could not speak.

Not only intelligence but also other areas of child development began to be investigated in the 19th century. In 1872 Darwin published *The Expression of the Emotions in Man and Animals,* the product of 40 years of reflection on the inheritance of behavioral patterns (Darwin, 1965). Stages of development also had been considered by Darwin, and in 1877 he completed *A Biographical Sketch of an Infant* (Darwin, 1877). This study was based on notes Darwin had made on his son William's development beginning in 1839 (Bowlby, 1991). He was particularly interested in behavior that occurs without being learned, such as the infant's smile. He wondered how such patterns of behavior were inherited and considered their survival value. Darwin studied emotional expression and postures as well as vocalizations. He noted how social awareness begins to focus on others and reported on the gradual differentiation of the infant cry. His studies signaled the beginning of a socioemotional approach to development.

An emphasis on child development brought to an end the view that children are miniature adults who were to be given adult responsibilities as soon as possible (Arles, 1962). In 1891 Stanley Hall began the first systematic application of the scientific method to the study of the child. Hall analyzed several thousand parent questionnaires on child development and published his results. He subsequently established the first journal of child psychology, *The Pedagogical Seminary* (Crutcher, 1943). The concept of adolescence was established as a developmental stage that follows the onset of puberty and was subsequently studied by Hall (1904).

During the same period in which an interest had emerged in child development, mental disorders in children were formally described. According to Parry-Jones (1989), a discussion of mental disorders in children was provided by West in 1852 and 1871. Griesinger (1867) suggested that mania and melancholia do occur in children but that hallucinations and delusions are much less common than in adults. Maudsley (1867), in his *The Physiology and Pathology of Mind,* included a chapter entitled "Insanity of Early Life." After this, insanity in children gradually became differentiated from idiocy, epilepsy, and other neurological disorders. Maudsley suggested that "Anomalies, when rightly studied, yield rare instruction." His focus was on the chronicity of these conditions. Subsequently, Emminghaus, Moreau, and Manheimer applied adult psychiatric diagnostic terms to children (Kanner, 1959). During this period, the idea of hereditary transmission became popular as did the view that the developing brain is vulnerable to infections, disease, head injury, frightening experiences, and bereavement (Parry-Jones, 1989). Beach (1898) spoke of both organic and psychological causative factors. Puberty began to be recognized as a physiologic cause of disturbance and pubertal, or adolescent, insanity was recognized (Maudsley, 1895).

With these 19th-century origins in the education of mentally handicapped persons, the early attempts at classification, an emerging interest in socioemotional development, and the recognition of mental disorders in children, the foundation was laid for the emergence of developmental neuropsychiatry as a specialty focus in the 20th century. Moreover, during the first two decades of the 20th century, there was a dramatic change in attitude toward mental retardation. Earlier views of amorality and incorrigibility, necessitating lifelong support, were replaced by an understanding that education and community support are effective interventions.

The beginning of the 20th century saw an

increased focus on behavior and juvenile delinquency. Still (1902), in the Coulstonian lectures, described disorders of volition or moral self-control. In 1909 Healey introduced child psychiatry into the juvenile court through the Illinois Institute of Juvenile Research. The juvenile court had previously been established in 1899 in the United States and several years earlier in Australia. Both social work assessment and psychological testing to establish the level of intelligence were introduced into the juvenile court. In 1915 his book, *The Individual Delinquent,* which presented case histories of children as distinct persons, was published (Healey, 1915). That same year, the National Committee for Mental Hygiene, inspired by Clifford Beers's book, *A Mind That Found Itself* (Beers, 1908), was established.

Adolph Meyer introduced objective psychology, or psychobiology, as a pragmatic approach to psychiatry in which the central focus was on the person whose total life history must be studied along with his or her mental and physical capacities (Meyer, 1915). A stimulus to Meyer's efforts was Kraeplin's psychiatric classification, which clearly described mental disorders but did not specify a treatment. According to Meyer, this emphasis on classification introduced an element of hopelessness once a diagnosis was made (Meyer, 1910). He had earlier taught that intervention in the schools and in the social environment through interpersonal experiences could alleviate hopelessness (Meyer, 1895). Meyer's psychobiology emphasized the contribution of life events to the development of a psychiatric disorder.

By 1920 the Commonwealth Foundation established fellowships for psychiatrists to study difficult predelinquent and delinquent children in the schools and, through the juvenile courts, to develop sounder methods of treatment (Stevenson and Smith, 1934). In 1928 Leo Kanner, an earlier recipient of a Commonwealth Foundation University Fellowship, came to Johns Hopkins to work under Adolph Meyer. In 1930 he established the first Child Psychiatry/Pediatric Liaison Service in a University Hospital in the Johns Hopkins Harriet Lane Home. The Children's Neuropsychiatric Hospital opened in 1931 for the treatment of children with problems in behavior. In 1935 Kanner completed the first English language textbook of child and adolescent psychiatry based on the first several hundred referrals seen in his pediatric consultation clinic. Many of the first cases referred to him were mentally retarded children. A 1938 referral subsequently became the first case of a new syndrome, described a few years later as infantile autism (Kanner, 1943). The recognition of variability in intelligence in the autistic child and that interpersonal disorders could have infantile onset led to more careful scrutiny of early emotional development. It became apparent that mentally retarded persons require careful examination, have widely differing personalities, and can become emotionally disturbed.

The involvement of the parent in child development was increasingly emphasized, and both parental overprotection and parental rejection were recognized. The focus on the negative aspects of the parental role in development became so much emphasized that Kanner felt compelled to write a response, *In Defense of Mothers* (1941). Parents of disabled children established their own support groups to help one another cope with their child's disability. The earliest of these was the Council for the Retarded Child, which began in 1933 in Ohio, the Washington Association for Retarded Children (1936), and the Welfare League for Retarded Children. Once initiated, these groups eventually became nation-wide organizations.

By 1940 most states had abandoned practices of restricted marriage, sterilization, and institutionalization as ways to prevent future generations of mentally retarded persons (Scheerenberger, 1983). Yet during World War II, mentally retarded and developmentally retarded adults were designated as undesirable and exterminated in Germany. The aftermath of World War II was an enhanced awareness of human rights, and efforts were extended to provide better treatment for mentally retarded and mentally ill persons. With these efforts, mentally retarded persons became a more highly visible social responsibility. The National Mental Health Act, passed in 1946, included funds for training and research in mental retardation.

With the expansion of child guidance clinics after World War II, the treatment emphasis began to focus specifically on psychodynamic techniques, and mentally retarded persons were increasingly excluded from guidance clinic care. When new major tranquilizers became available, they were initially touted as effective in managing maladaptive behavior and eventually were used extensively with mentally retarded persons. With many false starts, efforts also were made to find drugs that would cure mental retardation.

In the 1940s and 1950s, there was new impetus to clarify the definition of mental retardation and to develop training for mental retardation specialists. In 1958 the first categorical mental retardation legislation was passed (P.L. 85–926), which provided funds to universities for training. Social competence, in addition to cognitive level, was introduced into the classification of mental retardation and measured initially by Doll's Vineland Social Maturity Scale. In 1952 the American Association on Mental Deficiency formed a committee to establish a new nomenclature. The new classification was announced in 1959 and included both adaptive and cognitive components and replaced the terms previously used in classification—idiot, imbecile, and moron—with the current designations of profound, severe, moderate, and mild mental retardation. In the schools, programs for the mentally retarded were extended from serving educable (mildly retarded) to serving trainable children (moderately retarded). Difficulties with the brain-injured mentally retarded child began to receive increasing interest during this period. Strauss and Lehtinen (1947) published *Psychopathology of the Brain Injured Child* in which they emphasized that disturbances in perception, thinking, and emotional behavior, alone or in combination, may impede learning. Increasingly, special education programs were developed. During this era, institutions for the mentally retarded grew in size and number. Often unable to recruit and maintain well-trained staff, they frequently provided inadequate care and, in many instances, relied extensively on the use of medications for behavior management. Overcrowding, inadequate programming, high turnover rates, and inadequate community services set the stage for reform in the next decade.

In the 1960s and 1970s, stimulated by the report of the President's Panel on Mental Retardation (1962), substantial changes in the care of developmentally disabled persons were initiated. During these years, the rights and needs of the handicapped were clearly delineated and were highlighted by President Kennedy's address to the U.S. Congress (Kennedy, 1963). He announced we must act to "bestow the full benefits of society on those who suffer from mental disabilities; to prevent the occurrence of mental illness and mental retardation wherever and whenever possible; to provide for early diagnosis and continuous and comprehensive care, in the community, for those suffering from these disorders . . ." The United Nations General Assembly passed the "Declaration of General and Special Rights of the Mentally Retarded," which designated that "the mentally retarded person has the same basic rights as other citizens of the same country and same age" (United Nations, 1971).

From 1950 to 1970, the number of residents in state-administered institutions increased from 125,000 to 190,000. Concern about their care led to over 100 legal decisions that eventually resulted in the deinstitutionalization movement of the 1970s. As a result, from 1970 to 1979, the number of residents in state-administered institutions decreased by 50,000. Accompanying these reductions in institutional placement came a critical review of treatment approaches, both behavioral and pharmacological. New guidelines have been established for therapeutic interventions. The main emphasis for community and school programming has been to provide normalization for the mentally retarded person (Wolfensberger, 1972). With extensive efforts at community programming, maladaptive behavior is now recognized as a major limiting factor in community placement. This recognition has led to a new emphasis on the dually diagnosed individual, the child with both a developmental disability and a mental disorder. Psychiatrists who were initially actively involved in working with mentally retarded and developmentally disabled children are now returning to their care with new tools and understanding based on advances in diagnosis, neurobiology, new imaging techniques, new pharmacotherapies, and a better understanding of the natural history and course of developmental disorders.

The strongest statement in regard to the right to education in the United States was the

Education for All Handicapped Children Act of 1975, which mandated free and appropriate education for all mentally retarded youngsters up to age 21 years. These guarantees have now been extended to preschool children. Concurrently, new emphasis has been placed on the developmental psychopathology of attention deficit/hyperactivity disorder, schizophrenia, Tourette's disorder, and behavioral disturbance in mentally retarded persons. Both training and research activities have been instituted, leading to the publication of an increasing number of research articles. New journals have been introduced, including the *Journal of Autism and Developmental Disorders* in 1979 (with Leo Kanner as the founding editor) and *Development and Psychopathology* in 1989.

Tracing the origins of a developmental perspective on childhood disorders demonstrates how attitudes toward children with developmental psychopathology have changed in the past two centuries as new knowledge has been acquired. In the chapters that follow, an integrated approach to developmental neuropsychiatric disorders will be provided. The emphasis is on the child or adolescent as an experiencing person who is actively adapting to an impairment.

REFERENCES

Arles, P. (1962). *Centuries of childhood.* Jonathan Cope, London.

Beach, F. (1898). Insanity in children. *Journal of Mental Science,* 44:459–474.

Beers, C.W. (1981). *A mind that found itself: An autobiography.* University of Pittsburgh Press, Pittsburgh. (Original work published 1908)

Binet, A., and Simon, T. (1905). Méthodes nouvelles pour le diagnostic du niveau intellectuel des anormaux. *L'Année Psychologique,* 11:191–244.

______, and ______. (1916). *The development of intelligence in children.* Williams and Wilkins, Baltimore, MD.

Bowlby, J. (1991). *Charles Darwin: A new life.* W. W. Norton, New York.

Bryan, C. (1930). *The papyrus Ebers.* D. Appleton and Co., New York.

Crutcher, R. (1943). Child psychiatry: A history of its development. *Psychiatry: Journal of the Biology and Pathology of Interpersonal Relationships,* 6:191–201.

Darwin, C. (1965). *The expression of the emotions in man and animals.* University of Chicago Press, Chicago. (Original work published 1872)

______. (1877). A biographical sketch of an infant. *Mind,* 2:285–294.

Deitz, D.E.D., and Repp, A.C. (1989). Mental retardation. In T.H. Ollendick and M. Hersen (eds.), *Handbook of child psychopathology,* pp. 75–77. Plenum Press, New York.

Down, J.H.L. (1866). Ethnic classification of idiots. *Clinical Lecture Reports, London Hospital 3,* p. 259.

______. (1887). *On some of the mental affections of childhood and youth.* J. and A. Churchill, London.

Griesinger, W. (1867). *Mental pathology and therapeutics.* New Sydenham Society, London.

Hall, S. (1904). *Adolescence.* D. Appleton and Co., New York.

Healey, W. (1915). *The individual delinquent.* Little, Brown and Co., Boston.

Itard, J.M.G. (1806). *The wild boy of Aveyron.* (G. Humphrey and M. Humphrey, trans). Appleton-Century-Crofts, New York.

Kanner, L. (1941). *In defense of mothers.* Charles C. Thomas, Springfield, IL.

______. (1943). Autistic disorders of affective contact. *Nervous Child,* 2:217–250.

______. (1959). The thirty-third Maudsley lecture: Trends in child psychiatry. *Journal of Mental Science,* 105:581–593.

______. (1960). Itard, Seguin, Howe: Three pioneers in the education of retarded children. *American Journal of Mental Deficiency,* 65:2–10.

______. (1964). *A history of the care and study of the mentally retarded.* Charles C. Thomas, Springfield, IL.

Kennedy, J.F. (1963). *Message from the President of the United States.* House of Representatives, Washington, DC (88th Congress), Document no. 58.

Lane, H. (1976). *The wild boy of Aveyron, p. 177.* Harvard University Press, Cambridge.

Maudsley, H. (1867). *The physiology and pathology of the mind.* Macmillan, London.

______. (1895). *The pathology of mind. A study of its distempers, deformities and disorder.* Macmillan, London.

Meyer, A. (1895). *Mental abnormalities in children during primary education.* Transactions of the Illinois Society for Child Study.

______. (1910). The dynamic interpretation of dementia praecox. *American Journal of Psychology,* 21:385.

______. (1915). Objective psychology or psychobiology: With subordination of the medically useless contrast of mental and physical. *Journal of the Medical Association,* 65:860.

Parry-Jones, W.L. (1989). The history of child and adolescent psychiatry: Its present day relevance. *Journal of Child Psychology and Psychiatry,* 30:3–11.

Rousseau, J. (1911). *Emile.* (B. Foxley, trans.) E. P. Dutton, New York.

Scheerenberger, R.C. (1983). *A history of mental retardation.* Brookes Publishing Co., Baltimore, MD.

Séguin, E. (1846). *Traitement moral, hygiène, et éducation des idiots et des autres enfants arrières.* J. B. Baillière, Paris.

______. (1866). *Idiocy and its treatment by the physiological method.* William Wood, New York.

Stevenson, G.S., and Smith, G. (1934). *Child guidance clinics. A quarter century of development.* The Commonwealth Fund, New York.

Still, G.F. (1902). The Coulstonian lectures on some abnormal psychical conditions in children. *Lancet,* i:1008–1012, 1077–1082, 1163–1168.

Strauss, A.A., and Lehtinen, L. (1947). *Psychopathology and education of the brain-injured child.* Grune & Stratton, New York.

Terman, L.M. (1916). *The measurement of intelligence.* Houghton Mifflin, Boston.

United Nations. (1971). *Declaration of general and special rights of the mentally retarded.* United Nations, New York.

West, C. (1852). *Lectures on the Diseases of Infancy and Childhood.* Longman, Brown, Green and Longmans, London.

______. (1871). *On Some Disorders of the Nervous System in Childhood:* Being the Lumleian Lectures Delivered at the Royal College of Physicians of London in March 1871.

Wolfensberger, W. (1972). *The principle of normalization in human services.* National Institute on Mental Retardation, Toronto, Ontario.

PART I

METHODS OF ASSESSMENT AND INVESTIGATION

The assessment process in developmental neuropsychiatry involves the evaluation of the individual child and his family. The family unit is the focus for both assessment and intervention. Part I consists of four chapters. Chapter 1 addresses the assessment process and discusses diagnostic and therapeutic interviewing, behavior rating scales, and case formulation. It outlines the assessment process in detail and explains how clinical interviewing functions as the main tool for gathering information from children, parents, and other informants. The interview also provides an opportunity to acquire information for diagnostic purposes, serves as a standard situation to assess emotions and attitudes, and enables the interviewer to establish a therapeutic alliance with family members. The interview process includes full family interviews, interviews with parents individually, and interview, mental status examination, and observations of the child or adolescent. The clinical interview is supplemented with specific behavior rating scales from the parents, teacher, or supervisor in a work program. The formulation of the case is the means of synthesizing the information from these various sources. It includes a discussion of the diagnosis along with a description of predisposing, precipitating, and protective factors that are important in treatment planning.

Chapter 2 focuses on the genetic history. A detailed family history of developmental and mental disorders is an essential part of the psychiatric assessment and is critical for genetic counseling. The chapter also includes commonly used symbols for pedigree charts, which are useful for genetic analysis. The information gathered from the family genetic assessment is then used for genetic counseling, an essential part of treatment.

Chapter 3 focuses specifically on neuropsychological testing. It describes how neuropsychological testing assesses the mechanisms for cognition and complex behavioral functioning. It discusses neuropsychological and clinical psychological approaches, reviews current issues in the application of tests and instrument development, describes a theoretical neuropsychological model to utilize in planning neuropsychological testing, reviews the indications for such testing, describes assessment strategies for particular neuropsychological capacities, and outlines the most commonly used tests and offers a rationale for their use. Finally, it discusses how to coordinate neuropsychological testing with information gathered from the mental status examination.

Chapter 4 reviews the evaluation of brain structure and function. Brain imaging techniques are assuming particular importance in assessing children with developmental neuropsychiatric disorders. It describes the specific techniques now available, including computerized (axial) tomography (CT), magnetic resonance imaging (MRI), functional MRI (fMRI), positron emission tomography (PET), and single photon emission computed tomography (SPECT). In addition, non-invasive electrophysiologic techniques, such as computerized electroencephalography (CEEG) and event-related potentials (ERPs) are included. Background information is provided on each of these methodologies, and their application to the study of developmental neuropsychiatric disorders is discussed. Line diagrams provide schematics for the various imaging methodologies.

CHAPTER 1

ASSESSMENT, INTERVIEW, AND BEHAVIORAL RATING SCALES

ASSESSMENT IN DEVELOPMENTAL NEUROPSYCHIATRY

The assessment process in developmental neuropsychiatry requires a comprehensive evaluation of the individual child and his family. Three approaches are involved: (1) clinical assessment, which include the history, individual and family clinical interviews, and mental status examination of the child; (2) structured interviews, questionnaires, behavior checklists, and rating scales; and (3) stardardized tests including psychological and neurological examinations. Background knowledge in normal child development, child psychopathology, diagnostic classification, and the specific tests used is a prerequisite. In dealing with developmental psychopathology, knowledge of the specific syndromes and their natural history is essential. The establishment of a diagnosis based on clinical assessment is complicated by difficulties in adapting the mental disorders classification system to children with developmental disorders and acquired neurological dysfunction. Because of the complexities of each case, familiarity with a variety of assessment approaches and instruments is important.

This chapter discusses the rationale for the clinical interview and procedures involved in psychiatric interviewing and reviews the psychiatric history, the psychiatric examination, behavior rating scales, and the clinical formulation.

THE CLINICAL INTERVIEW: RATIONALE

The interview is the main tool of investigation used with parents, other informants, and the child or adolescent. With children, adaptations of the interview process are necessary to facilitate establishing emotional contact with them. The psychiatric interview and behavioral observations that accompany it are specialized techniques. Skilled interviewing includes each of the following considerations (Russell et al., 1987):

1. *The interview is a method to acquire information.*

   The primary goal is to establish an accurate account of the child or adolescent's behavior, emotions, and interpersonal relationships, background facts and significant life events, and to obtain an understanding of his past experiences and attitudes toward others.

   Both factual and emotional information is gathered during the interview process. When gathering factual information, specific questions are necessary that provide the structural component to the interview. However, the elicitation of emotional information requires an open-ended, nonstructured approach. Therefore, because the first goal of the interview is to establish contact with the patient to facilitate both parent and child openly discussing their difficulties, it is best to begin the interview in an unstructured way so as to elicit feelings and concerns before moving on to specific questions to establish diagnostic categories. Questions asked must be presented in a way that the patient can readily understand them and be posed sensitively and tactfully. The aim of the interviewer is to maintain professional objectivity while establishing empathetic contact with the parent (or guardian) or the child.

2. *The interview is a standard situation to assess emotions and attitudes.*
   In working with children and adolescents, the interviewer maintains an active role from the beginning of the interview; stereotyped questions must be avoided. In whole-family interviewing, family members are engaged with one another and interactions are promoted among them to demonstrate that everyone's communications, including those of siblings, are valued.

   In the whole-family interview and in the individual interview, the interviewer must be aware of facial expressions, tone of voice, gestures, and the type of comments made. Throughout the interview process, family members and the patient will reveal a great deal about themselves as they describe their attitudes and their reactions to others. Moreover, the examiner reflects on his own reactions to the patient, and this also provides useful information in the context of the interview as a standard situation. The total interaction between the interviewer and the family member or child, then, provides an important source of information about personality and mental state. In some instances, a parent or disturbed child may elicit fear of harm in the interviewer. If this happens, the interview may have to be terminated if the interviewer feels it cannot be conducted safely and objectively. A patient who detects fear potentially could feel more out of control and could react violently.

3. *The interview provides an opportunity to offer support and to establish an understanding with the child and family, which may be the basis of a subsequent working relationship.*
   A valuable supportive role may be established during the interview that becomes the basis of subsequent work together. An understanding comment may increase confidence, but predetermined structured questioning or ill-timed interruptions can interfere with the therapeutic alliance and have the opposite effect.

   In conducting the interview, the examiner should be interactive—warm, engaging, empathetic, and responsive. Nonverbal facial expression, tone of voice, and gestures can facilitate positive contact. Those patients who are anxious, hostile, or suspicious may be unable to provide comprehensive factual information in their initial interview. In these instances, empathetic listening is particularly important to facilitate understanding and compliance. Because of the importance of establishing the relationship in the first interview, the examiner should not attempt to obtain information too quickly if it impedes this process.

   In summary, the clinical interview has several aspects. It is a technique to establish an account of the present illness and to acquire information about events, experiences, and behavior. Further, it provides a setting for the recording of expressed feelings, emotions, and attitudes about these events, or those who were involved in them. The interview also provides an opportunity to initiate a therapeutic relationship with both the child and his family. By keeping in mind that both factual material and feelings are important, the elicitation of emotional and attitudinal information should be encouraged. Although specific diagnostic information is needed, the interview is approached in terms of the patient's present needs.

THE PSYCHIATRIC INTERVIEW

Informants

Children and adolescents with neuropsychiatric problems are most often referred because of parental concerns about their development and behavior. The assessment aims at establishing a clear account of the child or adolescent's behavior and its effects on others. Because children do not live alone and uniformly attend school programs, their development is substantially influenced by interpersonal relationships and the attitudes of those with whom they come in contact both at home and in school. The assessment, then, involves not only the child but also the attitudes and behavior of others (parents, siblings, teachers, peers, and other significant adults) that are directed toward the child in the context of the developmental disorder. Moreover, because of limitations in the child's ability to provide a detailed account of his behavioral difficulties, informants who can describe behavior at home, at school, and in the community are essential in the assessment process. One may then compare accounts of the child's behavior in each of these settings to clarify whether the behavioral problem is situational, i.e., only occurring at home, at school, or in the community, or pervasive, i.e., occurring in each of these settings. It is not uncommon for there to be major differences in reports that come from school, home, and community.

The assessment process must take into account that children and adolescents are continually developing so their expressed behavior and psychological symptoms must be evaluated in the context of their developmental phase. To do so, it is best to consider the child and family together as a unit. Background information about the family will assist in understanding how development has proceeded for this particular child. In addition, an understanding of the strengths and weaknesses of the family unit is essential for treatment planning. The response of parents and siblings, peers, and teachers to the child's difficulties, i.e., the impact of the behavior on others, must always be considered.

In conducting the assessment, observations of the child both alone and in his interactions with family members must be arranged. The examiner observes the child in both structured and unstructured settings. The assessment begins in the waiting area, with observations of the child with parents and/or siblings together, and continues with observations of the manner of separation when the child is taken from the family to enter the examining room. Observation in structured settings, such as neuropsychological testing, is also important.

A flexible approach is most helpful whether the child is seen separately or as part of a family group. One approach is for the interviewer to see the child and family together to clarify the child's understanding of the reason for the consultation, to clarify whether the reason for the visit has been discussed between the parent and child, and to establish the confidential nature of the interviews with both parent and child.

A complete assessment includes a phase of interviewing the whole family that allows information to be gathered about hierarchical relationships within the family, communication patterns, affective tone among family members, and alliances among them. Individual interviews are then conducted with each parent to establish their perspective on the child's difficulties. While interviews with parents are conducted, the preschool and middle school child generally waits outside to be interviewed after the parents. An adolescent may be interviewed first prior to meeting with the parents.

Before leaving his parents, a child is informed about what will take place and then taken to a waiting section where there is adequate supervision and play facilities. While waiting, the child may be given tasks to perform, such as the production of a kinetic family drawing, or other drawing tasks, such as the "draw a person" and the "house-tree-person" task. Special arrangements may be necessary for preschool children who have difficulty separating from parents in a strange setting and for mentally retarded and brain-injured children who have severe behavioral problems.

Interview with Parents

It is always best to see both the mother and the father. The role of both parents in the life of the child is essential and, although the extent of involvement may differ between the parents and the child at different ages, each parent is intimately involved in the child's psychological experience whether they are physically present or not. For children with developmental disorders, involvement of both parents is of particular importance because it is not uncommon for one parent to have borne the burden of primary care, which may have precluded the other parent's developing a realistic attitude regarding the child's abilities. Moreover, an interview with both parents together often provides an excellent opportunity to observe parental interaction and their relationship. When parents are divorced or separated and the child spends time with each of them, it may be best and more appropriate to see each parent on a separate occasion.

Information from Other Sources

Parental consent must be obtained to contact agencies, primary physicians, and other referral sources. Permission to contact the school and other agencies is essential to establish a well-rounded view of the current life situation. The teacher's account of the child's behavior at school is critical. Knowledge about the type of classroom and the specific individualized educational program for developmentally disordered children must be reviewed as part of the assessment process. In addition, information on school attendance, particular academic strengths and weaknesses, nonacademic skills, such as artistic and musical ability, behavior in the classroom and during recess, relationships with peers and with teachers, and other teacher comments are important. Moreover, behavior rating scales completed by teachers are gathered at the time of the initial assessment and on an ongoing basis. If an older adolescent or young adult is enrolled in a workshop program, then information from the job coach or supervisor will be needed.

Developmental Aspects of Interviewing

Children are developing organisms so the diagnostic assessment must maintain a developmental perspective that considers the following: (1) children behave differently at different ages so a knowledge of age-appropriate behavior is necessary; (2) the disorder may interfere with the normal course of development; (3) different phases of development are associated with different stresses, thus a toddler is most likely to be affected by separation experiences and a stressed adolescent may exhibit frequent mood swings; and (4) specific developmental tasks to be mastered vary with age.

The interview with the child must take into account both the child's developmental level and the child's ability to communicate. The purpose of the initial interview is to make contact with the child and establish confidence and cooperation, to know the child, and to learn his responses to current difficulties and his perception of them and ability to cooperate in treatment. The child will experience anxiety in encountering the interviewer and will concurrently be sizing up the interviewer as the interviewer makes observations and talks to him.

When examining infants or severely and profoundly retarded children who have not established expressive language milestones, the initial observations must focus on social milestones. During the first year, the most important of these are the establishment of eye contact, attachment, stranger anxiety, and the reciprocal use of language in babbling and jargon. With infants, one uses the infantile form of language called "motherese," which involves extending vowel sounds and speaking more slowly. An infant responds to the adult's mood and gestures in an active and perceptive way, which emerges from his own experience with familiar caregivers. The response to change or newness is more intense after 6 months of age when selective attachments and stranger anxiety have emerged as developmental milestones.

In examining an infant, the approach is indirect, almost casual. The interviewer should be still and quiet but close enough to observe. Initially, he makes no gesture or movement and does not use direct eye contact until the infant has looked the interviewer over from a safe and comfortable distance. In approaching an infant or a withdrawn mentally retarded child, an outstretched hand may be offered to encourage the child to reach out. For infants and nonverbal mentally retarded children, it is generally best for them to make the first move. In making infant observations, it is important to observe the parents' preferred holding posture and imitate it.

With toddlers and many mentally retarded children, one should keep in mind that although they may not be speaking, their receptive language may be adequate to understand what is said about them. Because language comprehension precedes verbal expression, words they hear may be misinterpreted by them.

For children between ages 2 and 4 who are able to talk and have a better understanding of what is said to them, the interviewer may proceed verbally and with the use of play materials. Children at this age are very literal in their understanding of the words they use and those they hear from others. Because thinking is concrete, actions may be understood in a concrete way. Descriptions to young children should avoid the use of analogies, and it is important to be aware that abstractions should be used cautiously when discussing problems with the child. Learning to speak at the child's language level will facilitate communication in future visits. In addition to literalness, children between 2 and 4 may use transductive reasoning to give inanimate objects human attributes. The child may attribute feelings and motives to household objects or at least speak as if they have them. For example, a child may say a machine that has stopped has gone to sleep and may practice putting toys to sleep and waking them up. During this age period, children tend to be active and may be difficult to please or satisfy in a new office setting. Feelings such as sadness, anger, fearfulness, and jealousy are poorly modulated. Moreover, the child may have difficulty controlling anger and show unpredictability in behavior related to emotions.

During an examination, an initial period of warming up and talking to a child about personal interests and successes may alleviate this initial anxiety. Younger children communicate their feelings through their behavior or through imaginary play. During play interviews, the child may show themes that are conflictual in home or in preschool settings.

By middle childhood, from age 7 on, children are better able to express fears and feelings verbally but may be unclear about the nature of their concerns. They may ask questions in a veiled fashion, so it is essential to clarify the meaning of their questions before responding to them. A frequent and persistent question may indicate a hidden concern.

Children who are in middle childhood and adolescence may be interviewed more directly about their concerns and life experiences. For the older child, the interview is semistructured, as is described in the following section.

Interview with the Child

The child is the most important source of information, and during the assessment must be seen separately unless severe separation anxiety or the extent of behavioral difficulty does not allow this. The child's view of the presenting problem should be sought out, although the quality of his report will vary according to developmental age. For children who are nonverbal, specific adaptations of the interview are necessary and specific devices, such as letter boards and speech aids, may be necessary to facilitate communication.

In the past, there has been reluctance to use a formalized mental status examination with younger children because of concerns about the reliability of verbal information from children and a sense that the language and thought of the child are too elusive for clinical description. Concerns have been expressed regarding the child's developmental level, the age when verbal approaches could be used, and the possible transient nature of psychopathology. There have been concerns that an adult-type interview would lead to anxiety and hostility, and questions have been raised about phenomenology, psychodynamics, and their usefulness in determining etiology in younger children. Because of these considerations, interview behavior has varied, with some interviewers using direct questioning and observation and others less formal approaches, such as play, drawings, and other imaginative methods. Yet both approaches are needed—the formal direct interview to elicit symptoms needed to make a diagnosis and the imaginal methods to establish contact and conduct treatment.

Because of past concerns about the nature of the mental status examination in the child, considerable effort has gone into improving psychiatric interviewing procedures for children and adolescents. The establishment of structured and semistructured interviews has been motivated by dissatisfaction with reliability and validity of traditional child and adolescent diagnostic procedures (Edelbrock and Costello, 1988). The development of structured interview schedules for children followed the development of such interview schedules for adults that have been found to increase diagnostic reliability substantially (Endicott and Spitzer, 1978; Robins et al., 1981). Moreover, the development of a more comprehensive classification of child and adolescent disorders with more explicit diagnostic criteria has required a more standardized approach to the assessment of child and adolescent symptoms (APA, 1987, 1994; WHO, 1992).

Face-to-face interviews are important to establish rapport with the child or adolescent, and by focusing on symptoms of concern, help maintain the child's interest during the interview. Such interviews help to clarify misunderstandings about the parents' interpretation of the child's behavior and provide an opportunity to document the context and chronicity of a child's symptoms. Although the assessment of child psychopathology requires data from parents and other informants, children are essential informants regarding their own feelings, behaviors, and social relationships. Symptom-oriented interviews are effective means for establishing diagnoses in children who may be too young to complete verbal self-reports.

The earliest structured and semistructured interviews for children are those of Lapouse and Monk (1958) and Rutter and Graham (1968). The most detailed evaluation of structured and semistructured interviewing took place in the late 1970s and 1980s. These interviews are used for both clinical and research purposes and have encountered conceptual, methodological, and technical problems in their development. All of these instruments provide a list of target behaviors, symptoms, and life events that must be covered, together with guidelines for conducting the interview and recording the child or adolescent's responses. The degree of structure imposed on the interview varies from the semistructured approach, where only general and flexible guidelines for conducting the interviewing and recording the information are given, to highly structured interviews that specify the exact order, wording, and coding of each item. Because they can be individualized to the child and provide greater range in phrasing questions and following alternative lines of inquiry and interpreting responses, semistructured interviews are usually conducted by clinically sophisticated interviewers. The highly structured interview, which is used most commonly in epidemiologic studies, reduces the role of clinical inference made by a more experienced examiner and can be administered by lay interviewers.

Although there are differences in the type of information gained from structured and semistructured interviews, the majority produce information about the presence, absence, severity, onset, and/or duration of specific symptoms. Some interviews produce a quantitative score regarding symptom profiles or a global index of psychopathology. Generally, assessment interview schedules are designed for parents with parallel formats for children, but some are developed specifically for children (Costello, Edelbrock, and Costello, 1985; Chambers, Puig-Antich, and Hirsh, 1985; Herjanic and Reich, 1982; Hodges et al., 1982a, and 1982b; Puig-Antich and Chambers, 1978). Herjanic and Campbell (1977) have reviewed the basis of use of structured interviews, and Herjanic et al. (1975) have demonstrated that children can be reliable reporters. Herjanic and Reich (1982) initially pointed out the importance of interviewing both child and parents by establishing that there may be differences in the child's and parents' reports of individual symptoms depending, to some extent, on whether the symptoms are externalizing or internalizing.

Development of other structured interviews has led to more precise recognition of disorders, such as depression in childhood, in epidemiologic studies. However, the use of semistructured approaches to elicit the nature and extent of abnormalities of emotions, behavior, and interpersonal relationships is the most appropriate method in a clinical setting. Specific probes related to particular diagnostic criteria are incorporated into the clinical interview.

THE PSYCHIATRIC HISTORY

After establishing demographic and other background information and clarifying the reliability of the parents or other informants, the parents are asked about their specific concerns. The reason for referral is elicited as well as a statement about the onset of the current difficulties and the family life situation at the time the difficulties began. The interviewer specifically asks about why the child is being referred at this particular time. Precipitating stressful events that may contribute to the behavioral, emotional, or interpersonal problem are reviewed and the parents' specific concerns are addressed. Among the specific concerns to be considered are academic and school problems, antisocial behavior, emotional conflicts, regressive behavior, and interpersonal difficulties with others. The child's previous treatment should be reviewed, and the effects of the child's current behavior on family functioning addressed and clarified. Following these questions, a reclarification of the parents' goals in seeking help at this time is elicited.

The family history is reviewed, clarifying what the child's current status is in regard to stepparenting, adoption, foster care, or other family-related issues. Specific questions include who has custody of the child, who the child is like in personality, and who the child is named after? The family background for both parents is obtained, including information about their own childhood, with particular emphasis on the family atmosphere in their homes as they grew up, stresses related to emotional and economic issues, and deaths or separation from close relatives. Information about the grandparents and others closely affiliated with the child is elicited along with a developmental family history of how the parents' marriage evolved. The quality of relatedness in the current marriage, including frequency of disagreements and how disagreements are expressed, coping mechanisms, how conflict is dealt with in the family, and the relationship to the family of origin are reviewed. The child's siblings are described in regard to age, school placement, history of significant illness, personality, and relationship to other family members.

The family history should include specific questions about developmental disorders, alcoholism, abnormal personality, suicide/homicide, mood disorders, and schizophrenia. A family history of executive dysfunction in parents and extended family members is also sought, as is parental difficulty in learning and in school achievement.

A review of past and personal history should include the date and place of birth, birth weight, attitude of both parents toward the pregnancy, and whether the pregnancy was planned or unplanned. If there were difficulties with the pregnancy or delivery, the emotional response of the parents to those events should be included.

Developmental milestones should emphasize the social developmental milestones, which include eye contact, social smile, language communication, and interpersonal attachment. Quality of the parent–child (diadic) relationship and the child–mother–father (triadic) relationship are discussed. Interpersonal issues that relate to feeding and illness must be considered along with the parents' attitudes toward child rearing. Child-rearing practices and attitudes about permissiveness and limit setting are reviewed.

A behavioral review of systems is then carried out that includes information on temperament, early development, emotional responsiveness, antisocial behavior, attentional difficulties, self-stimulation, and play behavior.

This is followed by an assessment of school activities including the age of beginning school, the current grade, schools attended, types of class placement, and emotional adjustment to beginning school. Separation problems at the time of entry into preschool or elementary school are discussed. If there were prolonged absences from school or if school years were repeated, this information along with specific difficulties in reading, writing, math, and spelling are noted. Study habits and academic goals for the child are discussed, and the child's peer relationships are clarified. If the child is teased or is a bully, this information is included, as is information about particular friendships. Attitudes toward teachers, peers, and schoolwork are obtained.

An assessment is made of the child's awareness of sexual identity, which includes questions regarding curiosity about his own body and about reproduction as well as sexual interest and activities. For the adolescent, the interview includes information regarding the mastery of adolescent developmental tasks and the young person's attitude toward entry into adolescence. One looks for mature versus pseudomature behavior, attitudes toward peers, family members, and those in authority. Rebelliousness, drug taking, periods of depression and withdrawal, and the adolescent's fantasy life are discussed with the parents. Questions about how the young person has responded to puberty with accompanying voice changes, hair growth, and menarche, as well as masturbation and sexual concerns, are issues that are discussed.

Previous mental health history is gathered, which includes details of any disturbances for which treatment was received and the type of treatment that was carried out. This is followed by a description of the life situation at present, which includes current housing, social situation, parents' work and financial circumstances, the composition of the household, the relationship with neighbors, recent stresses, bereavement, losses or disappointments and how both parents and child have reacted to them. A typical day in the child's life is described, which includes getting off to school, activities during the school day, returning home, and evening activities.

In the parent interview, questions about the child or adolescent's particular personality are addressed. This includes habitual attitudes and patterns of behavior that distinguish him as an individual. Among the personality characteristics reviewed are attitudes toward others, including ability to trust others and to make and sustain a relationship with them. Whether the child is secure or insecure in interpersonal relationships, a leader or a follower, is established. The attitude toward interpersonal relationships, whether it is friendly, warm, and demonstrative or reserved, cold, or indifferent is considered. Other characteristics discussed include aggressiveness, quarrelsomeness, sensitivity, and suspiciousness. The interviewer asks about the child's attitude toward himself, including self-dramatizing behavior, egocentric behavior, self-consciousness, and ambition. Moreover, attitudes of the child or adolescent to his own health and bodily functions are included in the assessment to establish whether or not the child's self-appraisal is realistic.

An assessment of personality also includes moral and religious attitudes, an assessment of whether the individual is easygoing or permissive, overconscientious, perfectionistic, or conforming. Mood is considered in regard to lability and general attitude and whether the child is optimistic or pessimistic. The presence of anxiety, irritability, excessive worrying, and apathy are noted. The ability to express and control feelings of anger, sadness, pleasure, and disappointment is reviewed.

Leisure time activities and interests, including interest in books, pictures, music, sports, and creative activities, are noted. Determining how the child or adolescent spends leisure time is essential, including descriptions of whether the child is alone or with others during free time.

Finally, questions are asked about daydreams, nightmares, and reactions to stress. This involves the ability to tolerate frustration, loss, or disappointment and includes a description of circumstances that arouse anger, anxiety, or depression. Evidence of excessive use of particular psychological defenses, such as denial, rationalization, and projection, are obtained.

Because executive dysfunction (see Chapter 3) interferes with adaptive behavior both at home and at school, the parent interview asks about both settings; however, teacher interviews may be necessary to cover school matters (since parents may not know). Children with executive dysfunction have difficulty regulating or organizing their behavior in relation to their schoolwork and their interpersonal activities. To clarify these problems, the history identifies the frequency and severity of target symptoms in each of these settings.

THE PSYCHIATRIC EXAMINATION (MENTAL STATE EXAMINATION)

Appearance

The first part of the interview relies on the interviewer's powers of observation. In many ways, it is the easiest part of the examination because one needs primarily to be alert and observant; however, it takes skill and experience to understand the implications of what has been observed.

The child's appearance, stature, and nutritional status are observed to determine his medical well-being. The examiner should note personal reactions to the child, i.e., whether he is appealing. Extremes in height and weight have implications metabolically and in regard to emotional development. The examiner observes whether the child is clumsy or ataxic, shows disinhibited movements, has strabismus, or shows rigid or floppy muscle tone. Skin coarseness or rash and hair abnormalities, which might suggest metabolic disorders, may be easily visible. Bruises should prompt thinking regarding child abuse, accident proneness, or clumsiness.

Behavior

Relatedness

How does the child relate to parents and to the interviewer? Does he maintain reserve with the interviewer and only gradually warm up, or never warm up? Is he overly friendly? Does the child make eye contact with the interviewer and show turn taking as the dialogue progresses? Is he sullen, angry, oppositional, aggressive, or totally withdrawn and preoccupied by his own thoughts and actions? The extent of relatedness varies from the child with autistic disorder who may constantly ignore others, including parents, or only make fleeting glances at them, to the shy child who may show no initial eye contact but gradually warms up over time, to the disinhibited child who hugs total strangers.

Motor Behavior

How active and impulsive is the child? Is he moving all over the room and getting into everything? Responding to every passing stimulus? Maintaining interest in a task or toy or losing interest quickly? Will the child pay attention and inhibit his disruptiveness when verbal limits are imposed? Does he squirm and fidget in the chair, stay immobile, or move normally in response to what is said to him ? Does the child have nervous tics or repetitious behaviors? Are movements graceful and coordinated? Because different degrees of activity may be appropriate at different ages, a 4-year-old and a 10-year-old may show the same activity level with very different implications.

Speech and Language

The assessment of speech and language is based not only on what is said but how it is said. The quality of speech gives some clues about the child's mood. Does the child speak clearly, slur words, stutter, substitute letters (e.g., *w* for *r*)? How verbal is the child? Does he become frustrated trying to communicate ideas, knows words but has difficulty with conceptual communication? Is the rate of speech fast or slow? Does he whine, whisper, or shout? Does the child speak spontaneously or in monosyllabic grunts? Is the rate, rhythm and prosody of speech appropriate? Is the volume loud or soft? Finally, can the child hear what is said and understand at a normal conversational tone? Hearing deficits for certain frequencies may make words virtually unintelligible to the listener.

Thought Process and Content

How a child thinks and what he thinks about can be assessed both indirectly and directly. The first part of the interview entails getting to know the child—his likes or dislikes, his friends, what they do together, what school is like, how he does in school, how he gets along with parents and sibs, what he wants to be when he grows up and why. What are the child's preoccupations? Are there intrusive thoughts? What does the child talk about with interest and affective investment? Telling a joke or a favorite story may clarify how the child organizes his thoughts.

The second part of the interview is specifically related to why the child is being evaluated, what his parents said about coming, what he sees the problems to be, and how he feels about the problems presented and about family relationships. In a child over age 5, thought content as it relates to mood, fears, somatic problems, hallucinations, and delusions is elicited.

For adolescents, the mental status examination is similar to the adult mental status examination. Content items also focus on drug and alcohol use, difficulties with antisocial behavior, attitudes toward dating, peers, sex, menarche, growing up, and parents.

From interchanges in the interview, the interviewer assesses the coherence of the child or adolescent's thought process and whether his concerns are age, sex, and situation appropriate.

Mood and Self-Concept (Emotional Feeling Tone and Its Outward Manifestations)

Mood and self-concept are ascertained directly and indirectly. Does the child look happy, sad, tense, or angry? Smile or seem tearful? Speak dejectedly or assertively or with excess bravado? How does the child respond to questions about feelings like "When were you the most angry, happy, frightened or sad?" And what does the child do when he feels those ways? What are his specific fears and worries? Does he like himself, or is he self-blaming? Does he think others like him? Does he feel picked on, does he "fight back"? Is he comfortable with his gender identity? Does he blame himself or others for his problems? Is he dramatic in talking about his problems, or does he minimize them? Is he guarded and suspicious, irritable, and volatile? Does he see himself as evil, bad tempered? What has he done that he is proud of doing? How does he feel about his future?

Abnormal Beliefs and Interpretation of Events

Are there ideas of persecution or special treatment? Are there delusional beliefs? Does the child believe others can read his mind?

Abnormal Experiences Referring to the Environment, Body, or Self

Does the child report sensory or somatic hallucinations or recurrent dreams? These areas may be addressed indirectly by asking the child if his eyes or ears ever play tricks on him causing him to see things that others do not see or hear things others do not hear. Are there feelings of depersonalization?

Cognition (Orientation, Memory, Attention and Concentration, General Intelligence)

How alert is the child? Is he oriented to time, place, and person in an age-appropriate manner? Does he seem to know what is happening around him, or does he appear distracted or inattentive? How does his historical account compare to that of his parents in regard to past significant events? Does he know colors and body parts? Depending on the child's age, he should be able to copy the Gesell figures (circle, square, diamond, Maltese cross, cylinder) or draw a human figure in some detail. The interviewer observes how the child draws, how he holds the pencil, how he plans the task. How is his memory? Does the child know where he lives and how he got to the site where the interview is taking place? Are there problems with attention and concentration? Can the child perform basic arithmetic (addition, subtraction, multiplication, division)? Can he carry out subtraction of serial 3s from 20 and serial 7s from 100? How is his reading comprehension? What is his level of intelligence? In play, what is his choice of toys, how does he approach them and use them in imaginative ways? Does he show curiosity about how things work?

Insight and Judgment

Does he appreciate his role in the current difficulties? Does he take responsibility for his behavior? What is his capacity to reflect on his behavior? Does he link current difficulties with life stresses?

BEHAVIOR RATING SCALES AND CHECKLISTS

Behavior rating scales and checklists are commonly used in both clinical and research settings. The items rated vary from highly specific behaviors to more abstract qualities of personal and social functioning. In some scales, particular constructs, such as activity level, are used and, in others, broad categories of psychopathology, such as internalizing or externalizing dimensions, are included. The major rating scales utilize parents or teachers to assess the various dimensions of child psychopathology. In addition to these scales, self-reports are also available, which are completed by the child or adolescent. For children with developmental neuropsychiatric problems, the self-rating scales will often have to be read to the child because reading difficulty is commonly associated with these conditions. Reliable rating scales are based on the assumption that the parent or teacher shares a common understanding of the behavior or attribute to be rated. If the area to be rated is more abstract, a discrepancy may exist between the informant's rating and the information the therapist wishes to have rated. Raters must be able to extract information from their experiences and observations of the child that coincide with the item to be rated. Moreover, the informant and interviewer must share a common understanding about which behaviors actually represent the item requested on the scale. Some behaviors that may be relevant to a particular scale item might vary depending on situational or developmental issues. Finally, the raters and the interviewer must share common views about the reference points for scaling the behavior along the lines required by the particular instrument. If there are differences in understanding the base rates of the behavior, then making judgments, such as the behavior occurs "just a little," or "very much," may be problematic (Barkley, 1988; Cairns and Green, 1979).

Completion of the behavior rating scale may be affected by the educational level, intelligence, and emotional status of the informant at the time the rating is conducted, so the report may vary and not simply represent only the actual behavior of the child being rated. There also may be variability in the instrument itself in regard to how the scales are constructed, the specificity of the weighting used in questions, the time period over which ratings are made, and variations in the child's behavior from one situation to the next.

Rating scales differ from specific behavioral observations in that rating scales require the rater to make observations over longer time periods—sometimes weeks or months—and in various situations at home or in the community (in camp, for example). Behavioral observations generally focus on highly specific time periods and very specific situations and make observations over short time intervals. Consequently, ratings and direct observational measures may not be highly correlated. There are a number of reasons for this, including the fact that ratings are less clearly defined than observations, are more influenced by characteristics of the informant who, in research settings, tend not to be trained to the same extent as those who use direct observational methods. However, each of these approaches offers unique sources of information not attained by the other. So although complete agreement between these two approaches is not expected, both make contributions to the assessment process.

Although there are problems inherent in the use and interpretation of rating scales, there are also advantages over other methods (Barkley, 1988; Edelbrock and Rancurello, 1985; Mash and Terdal, 1981). Among the advantages of behavior rating scales (Barkley, 1988) are the following: (1) the capability of getting information from informants with many years of experience with the child in multiple settings; (2) an opportunity to collect information on behaviors that occur extremely infrequently and may be missed in short, intense observation periods; (3) the fact that they are inexpensive and efficient in regard to time needed for completion; (4) the availability of normative value when used for screening nonpsychiatric populations; (5) their availability in various forms, which allows for a variety of dimensions in child psychopathology; (6) incorporation of the views of significant people in the child's natural environment who are involved in management, care, and therapeutic interventions; (7) provision of an account for situational variation to achieve more stable ratings of the child; and (8) allowance for quantitative distinctions to be made, which are often difficult to establish using the qualitative direct observational method.

Rating scales are used in various situations, including epidemiologic research, for subgrouping of children into homogeneous clusters to determine the prognosis of clinical groups followed over longer time intervals and to allow further exploration of hypotheses related to etiology. Moreover, rating scales demonstrate sensitivity to change that may be used in treatment outcome studies for a particular condition. Some scales cover a sufficient range of child psychopathology to allow them to be used to develop a classification system for psychopathological disorders through profile analysis (Barkley, 1988).

The most commonly used parent rating scales for children with learning and behavioral problems are the Conners Parent Rating Scale (Conners, 1985), the Child Behavior Checklist-Parent Form (Achenbach and Edelbrock, 1981), and the Personality Inventory for Children (Wirt et al., 1984). Commonly used teacher rating scales include the Conners Teacher Rating Scale (Conners, 1969, 1973) and the Child Behavior Checklist-Teacher Form (Edelbrock and Achenbach, 1984). In addition to these two teacher rating scales, there are a variety of other scales, such as the ADHD Comprehensive Teacher Rating Scale (ACTeRS) (Ullmann, Sleator, and Sprague, 1984). Besides individual parent and teacher ratings, other rating scales have been devised to be used by multiple informants. Moreover, rating scales are available to rate preschool behavior, affective behavior (fears and anxieties), and self-control. Finally, Rapoport, Conners, and Reatig (1985) provide a comprehensive listing of rating scales and assessment instruments for use in monitoring pharmacological interventions.

THE CLINICAL CASE FORMULATION

The clinical case formulation is a concise summary that takes into account all of the information available from the assessment process. It should begin with a brief statement of the current problem and be followed by a description of how the clinician understands the case. It is a synthesis of the assessment rather than a restatement of facts. The formulation provides an integration of the known biological, psychological, and social factors that contribute to the development of the current problem. It includes a discussion of the diagnosis and of the etiological factors and conditions that are deemed important from a review of the course of the condition. It takes into account both the patient's current life situation and background. Cleghorn, Bellissimo and Will (1983) suggest that the formulation (1) supplements the formal diagnosis; (2) enriches the clinical database by providing a synthesis that leads to hypotheses which are testable in part by clinical observation; and (3) provides an understanding of the case that is crucial to planning treatment.

Barker (1988) specifies consideration of predisposing factors, precipitating factors, perpetuating factors, and protective factors in preparing a case formulation. Predisposing factors include factors in the child or family that may predispose to the disorder. These include genetic and constitutional predispositions, temperament, physical abnormalities, and traumatic life events. Precipitating factors refer to experiences that may have precipitated the onset of the current problem. Precipitants interact with predisposing factors in the genesis of the disorder. Perpetuating factors are those that maintain the condition once it has become established. Finally, protective factors relate to strengths in the child and parent. Protective factors limit the severity of the disorder and assist in healthy functioning.

In considering the various factors that have led to and maintain the current condition, psychodynamic aspects are important to a clinical case formulation. These include three broad categories of experience (Cleghorn, Bellissimo, and Will, 1983): (1) key relationships, their history, and their representation in memory; (2) conflict (the type of anxiety, the coping strategy mobilized, and the solution); and (3) the experience of the self, i.e., the modulation of self-concept.

Cameron et al. (1978) suggest the method outlined below for recording the formulation.

Introduction

In one or two sentences, describe the patient, the illness or problem, and why the person or family seeks assistance at this time.

Biological Considerations

Biological considerations should be divided, when possible, into predisposing, precipitating, or perpetuating, as noted earlier. If no specific neurobiological factors have been identified, this should be recorded.

Psychosocial Considerations

Psychodynamic Issues

Key relationships, conflict, and experience of the self are included in this section. The emphasis is on psychological and/or intellectual problems within the child.

Social Considerations

Important family and peer relationships, family diagnostic issues, and significant social influences on the family are discussed. One takes into account the problems of the child within the family, the problems of the child with parents and with peers, problems that occur at school, and the effects of sociocultural/religious factors on the child.

Phenomenological

In this section of the formulation, one extracts the important findings from the mental status examination. Attempts are made to link these with underlying biological, psychodynamic, and social factors elicited in the general clinical history.

Protective Factors

Protective factors are those that limit the disorder and facilitate adaptation and are recorded with an emphasis on the child and family strengths.

Hypothesis Construction

Having synthesized each of these areas of concern, hypotheses are generated about internal connections between psychosocial and biological events. These associations are linked to the developmental life task important for a child at this particular age. In hypothesis construction, findings are arranged in an attempt to understand how the child and family have developed their current difficulties.

In summary, the clinical case formulation is not a list of difficulties but is a synthesis that describes the interplay and relative importance of various issues. It should be a clearly written dynamic explanation that leads to a plan of treatment and a suggested prognosis.

TREATMENT PLANNING

Treatment planning involves determining the appropriate intervention for the child and family's problems based on the clinical formulation; this takes into account the multiple conditions that influence psychological disturbances. Because of the unique presentation of symptoms involved for each child and family, two patients with the same Diagnostic and Statistical Manual-IV (DSM-IV) diagnosis may require different treatment approaches. This is the case because life circumstances will vary from one child to the next and treatment needs are influenced by the child or adolescent's developmental stage.

The Group for the Advancement of Psychiatry (GAP, 1973) suggested that treatment planning involves the selection of curative, corrective, ameliorative, or paliative approaches for the child or adolescent patient and his family. A properly developed formulation suggests guides for appropriate intervention. The treatment modalities chosen should be the most efficacious, the least restrictive, and the most cost effective. Although treatment planning must take into account the problem areas identified in the clinical case formulation, it must also consider the patient's and family's strengths. It addresses problems in the individual (both psychological and physical), problems in the family, problems with peers, problems at school, and problems in the sociocultural environment (Looney, 1984). Treatment goals are developed for the individual child and his family, utilizing individual psychodynamic, family systems, behavioral, pharmacological, and group treatment and environmental approaches, i.e., multimodal intervention. Treatment planning for the child or adolescent with mental retardation, using the new American Association on Mental Retardation (AAMR) definition, is described in Chapter 5.

REFERENCES

Achenbach, T.M., and Edelbrock, C.S. (1981). Behavioral problems and competencies reported by parents of normal and disturbed children aged four through sixteen. *Monographs of the Society for Research in Child Development,* 46(1).

American Psychiatric Association, Committee on Nomenclature and Statistics. (1987). *Diagnostic and Statistical Manual of Mental Disorders,* 3rd ed., revised. Author, Washington, DC.

______. (1994). *Diagnostic and Statistical Manual of Mental Disorders,* 4th ed. Author, Washington, DC.

Barker, P. (1988). *Basic child psychiatry,* 5th ed. University Park Press, Baltimore, MD.

Barkley, R.A. (1988). Child behavior ratings and checklists. In M. Rutter, A.H. Tuma, and I.S. Lann (eds.), *Assessment and diagnosis in child psychopathology,* pp. 113–155. The Guilford Press, New York.

Cairns, R.B., and Green, J.A. (1979). How to assess personality and social patterns: Observations or ratings? In R.B. Cairns (ed.), *The analysis of social interactions,* pp. 209–226. Erlbaum, Hillsdale, NJ.

Cameron, P.M., Kline, S., Korenblum, M., Seltzer, A. and Small, F. (1978). A method of reporting formulation. *Canadian Psychiatric Association Journal,* 23:43–50.

Chambers, W.J., Puig-Antich, J, and Hirsh, M. (1985). The assessment of affective disorders in children and adolescents by semi-structured interview. *Archives of General Psychiatry,* 42:696–702.

Cleghorn, J.M., Bellissimo, A., and Will, D. (1983). Teaching some principles of individual psychodynamics through an introductory guide to formulations. *Canadian Journal of Psychiatry,* 28:162–172.

Conners, C.K. (1969). A teacher rating scale for use in drug studies with children. *American Journal of Psychiatry,* 126:884–888.

______. (1973). Rating scales for use in drug studies with children. *Psychopharmacology Bulletin: Special Issue, Pharmacotherapy with Children,* pp. 24–84.

______. (1985). *The Conners rating scales: Instruments for the assessment of child psychopathology.* Unpublished manuscript, Washington, DC.

Costello, A.J., Edelbrock, C., and Costello, A.J. (1985). The validity of the NIMH Diagnostic Interview for Children: A comparison between pediatric and psychiatric referrals. *Journal of Abnormal Child Psychology,* 13:579–595.

Edelbrock, C., and Achenbach, T.A. (1984). The teacher version of the Child Behavior Profile: I.

Boys aged 6–11. *Journal of Consulting and Clinical Psychology,* 52:207–217.

______, and Rancurello, M.D. (1985). Childhood hyperactivity: An overview of rating scales and their applications. *Clinical Psychology Review,* 5:429–445.

______, and Costello, A.J. (1988). Structured psychiatric interviews for children. In M. Rutter, A.H. Tuma, and I.S. Lann (eds.), *Assessment and diagnosis in child psychopathology,* pp. 87–112. The Guilford Press, New York.

Endicott, J., and Spitzer, R.L. (1978). A diagnostic interview: The schedule for affective disorders and schizophrenia. *Archives of General Psychiatry,* 35:837–844.

Group for the Advancement of Psychiatry. (1973). *From diagnosis to treatment: An approach to treatment planning for the emotionally disturbed child,* Vol. 8, Report No. 87, September.

Herjanic, B., and Campbell, W. (1977). Differentiating psychiatrically disturbed children on the basis of a structured interview. *Journal of Abnormal Child Psychology,* 5:127–134.

______, and Reich, W. (1982). Development of a structured psychiatric interview for children: Agreement between child and parent on individual symptoms. *Journal of Abnormal Child Psychology,* 10:307–324.

______, Herjanic, M., Brown, F., and Wheatt, T. (1975). Are children reliable reporters? *Journal of Abnormal Child Psychology,* 3:41–48.

Hodges, K., Kline, J., Stern, L., Cytryn, L., and McKnew, D. (1982a). The development of a child assessment interview for research and clinical use. *Journal of Abnormal Child Psychology,* 10:173–189.

______, McKnew, D., Cytryn, L., Stern, L., and Kline, J. (1982b). The child assessment schedule (CAS) diagnostic interview: A report on reliability and validity. *Journal of the American Academy of Child Psychiatry,* 21:468–473.

Lapouse, R., and Monk, M.A. (1958). An epidemiologic study of behavior characteristics of children. *American Journal of Public Health,* 48:1134–1144.

Looney, J.G. (1984). Treatment planning in child psychiatry. *Journal of the American Academy of Child Psychiatry,* 23:529–536.

Mash, E.J., and Terdal, L.G. (eds.) (1981). *Behavioral assessment of childhood disorders.* The Guilford Press, New York.

Puig-Antich, J., and Chambers, W. (1978). *The schedule for affective disorders and schizophrenia for school-aged children.* Unpublished interview schedule, New York State Psychiatric Institute.

Rapoport, J., Conners, C.K., and Reatig, N. (1985). Rating scales and assessment instruments for use in pediatric psychopharmacology research. *Psychopharmacology Bulletin* 21:713–1125. DHHS Publication No. (ADM) 86-173.

Robins, L., Helzer, J.E., Croughan, J., and Ratcliff, K.S. (1981). National Institute of Mental Health Diagnostic Interview Schedule: Its history, characteristics, and validity. *Archives of General Psychiatry,* 38:381–389.

Russell, G.F.M., Jacoby, R.J., Campbell, L.B., Isaacs, A.D., Farmer, A.E., Gunn, M., Prendergast, M., Holden, N.L., and Taylor, E. (1987). Psychiatric examination: Notes on eliciting and recording clinical information in psychiatric patients. *Departments of Psychiatry and Child Psychiatry. The Institute of Psychiatry and the Maudsley Hospital,* London, 2nd ed. Oxford University Press, Oxford, England.

Rutter, M., and Graham, P. (1968). The reliability and validity of the psychiatric assessment of the child: Interview with the child. *British Journal of Psychiatry,* 11:563–579.

Ullmann, R.K., Sleator, E.K., and Sprague, R.L. (1984). A new rating scale for diagnosis and monitoring of ADD children. *Psychopharmacology Bulletin,* 20:160–164.

Wirt, R.D., Lachar, D., Klinedinst, J.K., and Seat, P.D. (1984). *Multidimensional description of child personality: A manual for the Personality Inventory for Children Revised 1984.* Western Psychological Services, Los Angeles.

World Health Organization. (1992). *The ICD-10 Classification of Mental and Behavioural Disorders: Clinical descriptions and diagnostic guidelines.* Author, Geneva.

CHAPTER 2

GENETIC HISTORY

A detailed family history of developmental and mental disorders is an essential part of a psychiatric assessment and is critical for genetic counseling. Not all disorders that affect more than one member of the family are genetic, and not all genetic disorders affect more than one member of a family. The genetic history begins with the establishment of the diagnosis. Because many genetic disorders lack specific diagnostic tests, the diagnosis is made on clinical grounds. For some neuropsychiatric conditions, such as Lesch-Nyhan disease, phenylketonuria (PKU), Turner's syndrome, and fragile X syndrome, diagnostic tests are available. Other disorders, such as schizophrenia, affective disorder, and attention deficit disorder, do not have such tests available. Regardless of whether a specific test is available, once a diagnosis is made, it is important to clarify the recurrence risk. Many families are unaware that, in any pregnancy, there is a risk for an unfavorable outcome. For example, the risk for a congenital abnormality in any child from any parents is about 1 in 30 (Thompson, McGinnes, and Willard, 1991). Moreover, the risk for specific genetic defects in relatives of identified patients is higher. It may be based on the pattern of inheritance or may simply be an empirical risk based on experience with a particular disorder (Levithan, 1988).

A comprehensive family history is the essential first step in the analysis of any disorder whether or not it is known to be genetic. The family history is important in diagnosis because it may indicate a disorder is genetic, provide information about the natural history of a disease and variations in its expression, and help clarify the pattern of inheritance so the recurrence risk in other family members can be estimated. The assessment includes information that may be relevant to single-gene disorders, multifactorial disorders, chromosomal disorders, abnormal traits or carrier states, consanguinity, and exposure to teratogens.

Single-gene disorders have characteristic pedigree patterns. However, single-gene inheritance may be simulated by other mechanisms, including multifactorial inheritance, chromosome rearrangement, or prenatal exposure of more than one child in a family to a neurotoxic agent used by the mother. Therefore, a careful history is needed to clarify the genetic pattern. Although cytogenetic disorders ordinarily do not recur, when they do, the basis of recurrence must be studied; recurrence may be based on structural chromosomal abnormalities or undetected mosaicism in parents. The multifactorial disorders show less characteristic genetic patterns, but most multifactorial traits can be distinguished from single-gene traits if a larger population is studied, although the mechanism may not be as apparent as in an individual pedigree.

A comprehensive family history includes information about the patient's relatives, including at least the grandparents and their siblings, the parents and their siblings, and the patient's first cousins. When information is collected, names, dates of birth and death, medical or psychiatric condition, early infant deaths, stillbirths, and spontaneous abortions must be recorded. In addition, consanguinity of the parents and geographic and ethnic backgrounds must be documented. Moreover, the mother's pregnancy history, particularly in regard to early events, and very importantly drug exposure, must be recorded. This pedigree must include unaffected family members as well as affected family members.

To establish the pattern of transmission, the family history is summarized in the form of a pedigree. Standard symbols for the pedigree are shown in Figure 2–1.

An analysis of the pedigree is particularly helpful because there is always the possibility that a particular family member will prove to be an exception. For example, a genetic defect generally considered to be autosomal recessive may, in some cases, be passed on as an autosomal dominant characteristic. This would suggest the same clinical disease may have separate genetic causes.

The rules used in drawing a pedigree are straightforward, but it is essential they be followed (Fuhrman and Vogel, 1983). The pedigree record must show all of the children of a sibship, whether normal or abnormal. If the informant cannot definitely state the number of children or their sexes, this should be indicated. Various births should be shown in proper order, and if the information provided is ambiguous,

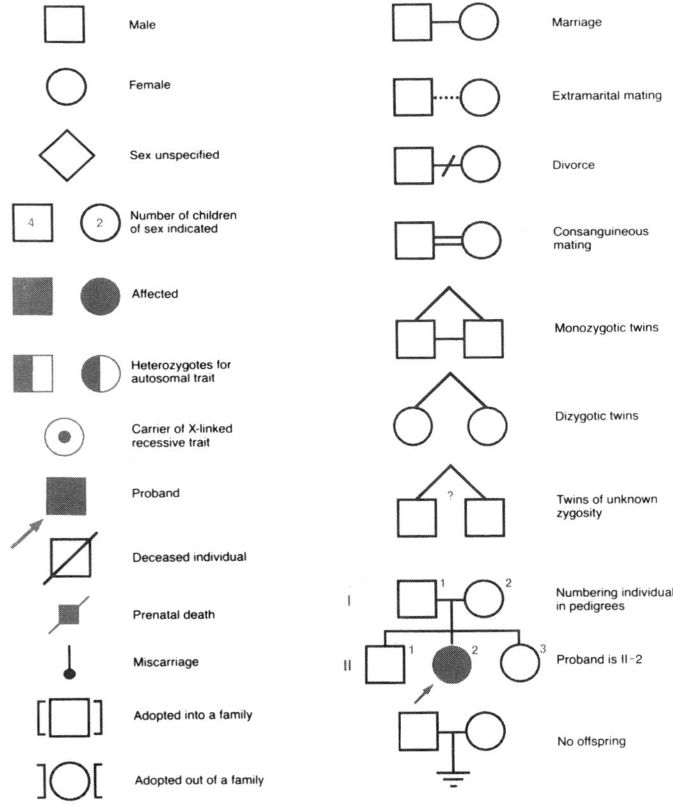

Figure 2–1. Symbols commonly used in pedigree charts (from Thompson, McInnes, and Willard, 1991).

then the ambiguity should be demonstrated in the chart. Stillbirths and miscarriages should be listed as correctly as possible.

It is desirable to arrange the pedigree with the paternal line on the left side and the maternal line on the right. It may also simplify matters to place the father at the end of his sibship outside the proper place in the birth order. Following the same reasoning, the mother should be placed at the beginning of hers. However, the actual place should be indicated as well. For the sake of subsequent discussion, the name and date of birth of the person appears on either side of the symbol referring to him or her.

In numbering the pedigree, the most common practice is to indicate successive generations with Roman numerals in descending order and designate the order within a generation with Arabic numbers from left to right. When there are conflicting reports of past events during the initial family sessions, the actual numbering is only possible when all information is available.

For accurate pedigree analysis, it is advisable to list all details for each family member separately. The information, then, must be verified and expanded or qualified by questioning other members of the family. The sources of information should be recorded and older family members from past generations should be included as informants. Both spouses are interviewed.

Although the parents involved in the consultation may supply accurate information to the best of their knowledge, the same may not be necessarily true of relatives. Consequently, information should be verified from several sources. The requirements of the particular case determine how many generations back one should go. The extent of genetic defect, the mode of inheritance, and how definitely the mode of inheritance has been established must be evaluated.

Often it is not possible to obtain and verify all necessary information. When this is the case, final counseling is usually based on restricted information furnished by the identified patient and the parents. When restricted information is used, subsequent genetic counseling must be considered provisional. The validity of the evaluation ultimately depends on the accuracy of the information received and the assumptions that are made about the presence of disorders in other family members. For multifactorial disorders, there may be variable expression among other family members, as in schizophrenia. In these instances, inquiry must be made about the milder symptom patterns rather than asking specifically and only about the full and severe manifestation. When a psychiatric disorder has been diagnosed in another family member, the medications used in its treatment should also be listed in the pedigree.

Information used from the family genetic assessment is used in genetic counseling. When a clinical disorder is diagnosed, the affected individual family members need assistance to understand and to come to terms with the nature and consequences of the disorder as well as the available treatment approaches. When the disorder is heritable, there is the need to know the genetic risk as well as the means available to prevent transmission. The genetic counseling session provides such information to the family.

Genetic counseling techniques are described in Part V, Treatment. When information about a genetic disorder is obtained from the assessment, the physician has the responsibility to make sure genetic counseling takes place and to make sure it is accurate.

REFERENCES

Fuhrman, W., and Vogel, F. (1983). *Genetic counseling,* pp. 14–18. Springer-Verlag, New York.

Levithan, M. (1988). *Textbook of human genetics,* pp. 410–421. Oxford University Press, New York.

Thompson, M.W., McInnes, R.R., and Willard, H.F. (1991). *Genetics in medicine,* pp. 395–410. W.B. Saunders, Philadelphia.

CHAPTER 3

NEUROPSYCHOLOGICAL TESTING: ASSESSING THE MECHANISMS OF COGNITION AND COMPLEX BEHAVIORAL FUNCTIONING

The developmental neuropsychiatric assessment requires the concurrent measurement of cognitive, emotional, social, and global adaptive functioning. Because problems in each of these areas may arise from brain dysfunction, developmental neuropsychological testing contributes a systematic way to evaluate several of these components. Neuropsychological testing integrates psychiatric and psychological information on behavior and the mind with neurological information on the brain and nervous system (Denckla, 1989). The neuropsychological examination uses psychological tests to measure cognition and complex behavioral functioning. An appreciation of neuropsychological testing will encourage the clinician to consider more carefully the relationship of brain and behavior than in the standard psychiatric mental status examination, which addresses the same areas in less depth and less systematically.

The neuropsychological assessment is similar to the clinical psychological examination in using some of the same tests; however, the neuropsychological approach uses a different conceptual/interpretive perspective. The child neuropsychological assessment of mental status is particularly important in developmental disorders where advances in neuropsychological testing make possible the specific evaluation of functions that are not addressed in standardized intelligence, achievement, and language assessment protocols. For example, test approaches are available to assess certain cognitive mechanisms in greater depth, such as executive functions associated with frontal lobe systems. It is hoped that through developmental neuropsychological assessment the basic processes that underlie brain growth and maturation will be better understood and that psycholinguistic development, emotion regulation, and models of cognitive memory will be more specifically elucidated (Rapin and Segalowitz, 1992).

The terminology introduced in this chapter should be particularly helpful in appreciating those mental status items that deal with speech/linguistic functions, memory, attention, executive functions (vigilance, set maintenance, planning, and inhibitory motor control), praxis (learned motor behavior), and visuomotor and visuospatial functions. In addition, the processing/production of social-emotional signals (including vocal tone, facial expression, and "body language," or gesture) is tested, although this is an area of ongoing research and new approaches are needed. Even though neuropsychological tests are increasingly available to test these and other specific capacities, these tests will account for only a proportion of the variance in the evaluation of an individual case and must be integrated into a total clinical case formulation that addresses the multiple facets of the child's life. The linking of test findings to adaptive function is crucial because children may compensate for their brain dysfunction in a way that their overall functioning is "better than they look" on the tests applied.

This chapter provides an orientation to using

developmental neuropsychological testing in assessing mental functioning. It (1) discusses a neuropsychological model of functional domains and modules; (2) reviews current issues in the application of tests and instrument development; (3) provides a comparison of neuropsychological and clinical psychological approaches; (4) considers the differences in brain–behavior relationships between adults and children on neuropsychological testing; (5) reviews indications for neuropsychological testing; (6) discusses assessment strategies for the neuropsychological capacities tested; (7) provides an outline of the types of tests used and a rationale for their use; and (8) discusses how these new approaches can be used to supplement and refine the mental status examination.

NEUROPSYCHOLOGICAL MODEL OF FUNCTIONAL DOMAINS AND MODULES

Domains of Function and Modular Organization

Neuropsychologists generally consider development to be "domain-specific." A distinction is sometimes made between domain and module, in that the term "module" is commonly used when speaking specifically about the modular organization of brain systems that are involved with specific functional domains. However, these terms have also been used interchangeably. A *domain* may be defined as a set of representations sustaining a particular area of knowledge (e.g., language). A *brain module* is an information processing unit which encapsulates that knowledge and the computations on it (Karmiloff-Smith, 1992). "Domain-specific" is the preferred general term, and "module" is the more specific term used to refer to microdomains or brain modules; for example, the language domain might include a phonological module.

The approach to assessing clinical brain–behavioral relationships in developmental neuropsychology increasingly emphasizes these domains of function and the hypothesized modular organization of the brain/mind within functional domains (Edelman and Mountcastle, 1978; Fodor, 1983; Pennington, 1991; Young, 1965) to designate brain regions involved. Domain-specificity refers to innately specified differences in how information is processed in relatively discrete brain systems that are organized to process a particular content, although there are constraints and restrictions on the type of information processed. Domain-specificity can be contrasted to behavioral associationism where the association of stimulus to response occurs in the same way for any kind of stimulus or response (Maratsos, 1992). Deficits in particular domains (e.g., visual/perceptual functioning, verbal memory) are significant at a neuropsychological level.

Emphasizing the modular organization of the brain derives from Fodor (1983), who argued that brain systems are specialized to process certain kinds of information and are autonomous in both function and neural representation. Fodor suggested the mind is made up of genetically specified, independently functioning, specific-purpose input systems. These are domain-specific, encapsulated, innately specified, hard wired (not assembled from more primitive processes), of fixed neuronal architecture, stimulus driven, and insensitive to central cognitive goals. Other parts of the mind can neither influence nor access the internal working of a module; only its output can be manipulated. He postulates that environmental information passes through sensory transducers that transform data into formats processed by special-purpose input systems. An output system provides information in a common format for central, domain-general processing.

These modules are designed to provide rapid processing of information. However, the idea of a hard-wired maturational model has been challenged; studies of language development by Karmiloff-Smith (1992) and Johnson and Karmiloff-Smith (1992) suggest an ontogenesis of modularity in higher brain functions. In their model, innate modules of mind are present but become specifically designated through life experience. Pennington (1991) suggests that modules are differentially vulnerable which is in keeping with the Johnson/Karmiloff-Smith (1992) proposal.

Fodor's definition of modularity contains two assumptions. First, the systems that handle output (control systems) are not modular and, second, they do not have access to the working of modules. Pennington (1991) questions this view when he characterizes executive function as an important component of control systems and describes executive function as an overarching yet dissociable module itself. Moreover, he suggests that the integrity of executive functions may affect how well other modules work and emphasizes the integration of the modular brain systems as being essential for function. For example, executive systems might modulate attention, which may be applied to modify behavior through self-monitoring.

CURRENT ISSUES IN THE APPLICATION OF TESTS AND INSTRUMENT DEVELOPMENT

Neuropsychological testing uses standardized means for clarifying deficits or impairments and in identifying strengths and capacities that may be used adaptively. Normative referencing is essential because capacities such as intellect, memory, and various functional domains are variable in the normal population. Peer group normative data is required and includes average levels of performance and the variability (standard deviation) of those performances. Although an extensive array of instruments with normative data is available for use in individuals for classical psychometric and achievement testing, normative data is not as well developed for developmental neuropsychological tests. However, new data is being collected and critically scrutinized on interrater reliability and test-retest reliability for neuropsychological tests. Among the variables that need to be considered are gender, age, educational experience, and sociocultural setting. In the assessment of the effects of illness or trauma, premorbid abilities also must be considered.

Several considerations arise uniquely in developmental neuropsychological instrument development and testing (Spreen, 1988). These include problems of reliability, developmental changes in cognition over time, special applications to learning disorders, appropriately designated domains for study, and concurrent testing for emotional disturbance and adaptive functioning (Denckla, 1989; Tramontana and Hooper, 1988). These are as follows:

1. *Use of assessment techniques originally developed for adults.*
   Are tests originally developed for adults to evaluate the mature nervous system reliable for testing children? The use of these adult tests may be acceptable for certain age ranges and for some functional areas. But many of these techniques bottom out for preschool children (up to age 5 or 6) who are not yet equipped with the test-taking attitudes required for school, and for learning-disordered children who may have certain forms of brain dysfunction which, in themselves, markedly affect the consistency of their performance (e.g., attention deficits).
2. *The problem of developmental change.*
   A major issue is the problem of developmental change or developmental sensitivity. The child development literature documents changing skills with increasing age as the child gradually attains complex adult skills. Existing neuropsychological measures need to be operationalized and adapted according to developmental level. When new age-appropriate measures are developed, they need to be linked to neuropsychological theory (Welsh and Pennington, 1988; Welsh, Pennington, and Groisser, 1991).
3. *Limited behavioral repertoire.*
   Because infants and preschool children show limited behavioral responses, testing may be less reliable than in older children and adolescents. Observations must replace more formal testing for the youngest children. Yet, despite their limited responsiveness, cognitive processing can be tested in infants (Diamond, 1990, 1991).

COMPARISON OF NEUROPSYCHOLOGICAL AND CLINICAL PSYCHOLOGICAL APPROACHES

Although the neuropsychological evaluation resembles the clinical psychological examination in some of the instruments that are used, in sharing some of the same goals, and in using the same testing environment, there are differences in the concepts that underlie the objectives of various tests, in the way tests are grouped, and in how the test data is analyzed. When a clinical psychologist performs a test of intelligence, the goal is to determine an individual's overall functional capacity. The IQ tests given have been constructed to avoid an emphasis on specific cognitive components. The neuropsychologist, however, is specifically interested in the various psychological and neurological components that form the basis for the individual's ability or inability to perform. Therefore, neuropsychological testing may be required in addition to, but not instead of, clinical psychological assessment. When viewed in this way, neuropsychological testing is needed along with clinical psychological measurement and both supplements and complements the typical psychoeducational evaluation. General intelligence (IQ) is of limited validity in children or adolescents with brain dysfunction; the summary IQ score has limited meaning when there is substantial subtest variability.

Neuropsychology utilizes knowledge gained from psychological, psychiatric, and neurological research to understand psychological deficits. Developmental neuropsychological testing differs from standardized clinical psychological batteries that tend to be more general in their approach and place their primary emphasis on intellectual and personality tests, or educational test batteries that generally include intelligence and educational testing. Although aspects of cognitive processing may be addressed in some of these batteries, such as in sections of the Woodcock-Johnson (1984), the focus of these tests is not primarily on establishing domains of brain function with implications for brain organization. However, adaptations of components of these tests may be used in neuropsychological contexts.

INTERPRETATIONS OF BRAIN–BEHAVIOR RELATIONSHIPS IN ADULTS AND CHILDREN

Child neuropsychology differs from adult neuropsychology just as developmental psychology differs from adult psychology. The major brain dysfunction responsible for neuropsychological dysfunction in children differs from that found in adults. The two major considerations in studying impaired brain systems in children and adults are (1) the differences in the effects of brain injury when it occurs in the developmental period in children in contrast to effects on the mature brain in adulthood, and (2) the differences between acquired versus developmental disorders regardless of the age when they are seen by the clinician.

The adult neuropsychological database was largely established through the evaluation of adults with known brain damage (strokes, seizures, tumors, penetrating wounds, head trauma). These adult studies with acquired disorders have contributed substantially to our understanding of the parts or systems of the brain that are involved in a number of psychological functions. Therefore, adult neuropsychology has focused on the impact of documented focal and diffuse acquired brain lesions on behavior and findings from experimental brain lesions in animals. Although experiments in immature animals have yielded useful information in pediatric neuropsychology, only some of the information available from adult brain dysfunction assessment may be useful in studying children. The types of lesions seen in adults, such as strokes and penetrating wounds, occur far less commonly in children where congenital malformations related to pre- and postnatal insults (prematurity, intraventricular hemorrhage, and ischemia/anoxia) are more common. A majority of the neuropsychological dysfunctions of early life are not then associated with known brain insults, nor are they associated with lesions demonstrable on routine neuroimaging studies. Moreover, in childhood, acquired pathologies, such as trauma, tumors, and infarctions, when they do occur, may have different neuropsychological presentations when they impact on an immature brain.

Traumatic brain injury is the most classic category to which anatomically based neuropsychological testing has been applied (Dennis, 1991; Dennis and Barnes, 1990; Levin et al., 1982). Developmental neuropsychological testing evaluates changes associated with injuries that occur during the developmental period and is also used to monitor progress in rehabilitation programs. When injury does occur at any age, recovery involves reversible changes in the affected regions. In addition, recovery also may involve compensatory processes because the accomplishment of complex behavior depends on the contributions of multiple and widely distributed brain systems that may be spared following injury. Noninvolved regions may be activated and provide flexibility in task performance and lead to demonstrable resiliency in the face of focal damage when lesions occur during the developmental period. New developmental acquisitions may involve undamaged functional units that may not be available in the more mature, differentiated, and committed adult brain. Plasticity in the immature brain is essential and its understanding is important in rehabilitation programs. It is possible that children who sustain major lesions in one hemisphere during development may compensate by involvement of the other hemisphere, using uncommitted "circuits." If such compensation does take place, these brain regions are now lost and may not establish their usual developmental function; in a sense, they have been crowded out. For example, Rapin and Segalowitz (1992) point out that large lesions of the left perisylvian cortex are compensated by language development taking place in the right hemisphere so that potential visuospatial skill deficits may occur. However, the lesion may remain silent after damage and emerge at a later time during development when that particular function is normally expected to arise, e.g., greater insight and initiative is expected during adolescence and may be influenced by brain damage earlier in life. Neuropsychological testing may address such possibilities and clarify whether or not they do occur.

The study of acquired disorders in adults and children only indirectly serves to provide a framework to study developmental disorders. This is the case for most children with mental retardation, autistic disorder, attention deficit/hyperactivity disorder, and learning disability. In these conditions, rather than acquired damage, the assessment evaluates differences in the formation and integration of the brain systems themselves.

Developmental neuropsychological testing is increasingly available to designate patterns of performance that may be used in diagnosis, patient management, habilitation, and rehabilitation planning in developmental disorders. Mental retardation syndromes and other learning disorders have been recognized since the 19th century, but it is only recently that developmental neuropsychologists have emphasized them. This focus has received increased attention with the introduction of brain-imaging techniques (neuroimaging), CT in the 1970s, and MRI and PET in the 1980s. Neuroimaging technology attempts to correlate specific aspects of information processing with specific brain regions. Structural imaging methods are used to link damage in particular brain regions with behavioral deficits; functional brain imaging investigates physiological changes associated with brain activity. Links to brain structure or physiology may validate neuropsychological assumptions for the developmental disorders.

The role of genetic abnormalities in the development of various brain systems is also a major area of focus in developmental neuroscience and developmental neuropsychology. In chromosomal abnormalities, e.g., single-gene defects that are associated with systemic disorders, and in progressive neurological degeneration syndromes, the neuropsychological investigation may be used to establish their profound effects on brain development. Neuropsychological test procedures have been applied both to learning disorders of unknown etiology and to those occurring with specific mental retardation and neurogenetic syndromes, such as Turner's syndrome, fragile X syndrome, Down syndrome, and Williams syndrome.

INDICATIONS FOR NEUROPSYCHOLOGICAL TESTING

There are numerous indications for neuropsychological tests. The list here follows suggestions by Tranel (1992):

1. *Diagnostic evaluation of developmental disorders.*
   Neuropsychological assessment is important in identifying domains of dysfunction that may be related to an individual's cognitive or behavior disorder, such as specific learning disabilities, attention deficit/hyperactivity disorder, and nonverbal learning disability. Among these, nonverbal learning disabilities present a particular challenge because these children have only subtle signs of neurological dysfunction (e.g., psychiatric symptoms including behavioral and

mood disturbance), as well as focal neuropsychological findings (e.g., visuospatial disturbance).

2. *Detection of conditions not demonstrated on standard neurodiagnostic testing.* Disorders may be suspected on clinical examination that are not revealed on routine clinical psychological testing. For example, the characterization of specific learning disorders is ultimately defined in terms of neuropsychology. Moreover, mild or subtle sequelae of traumatic brain injury may not be recognized with routine testing and requires neuropsychological testing.
3. *Monitoring the neuropsychological status of patients.* Baseline and subsequent neuropsychological testing is needed to follow up head trauma, to monitor behavioral change related to drug treatment, and to document any cognitive or behavioral change following other injury or toxic exposure. Baseline test data is collected at the time of presentation and the individual's progress is followed over time. For example, the neuropsychologist might monitor changes related to drug treatment for complex partial seizures or changes following surgery for a brain tumor.
4. *Characterization of the cognitive capacities in planning rehabilitation programs.* Full characterization of cognitive capacities is particularly important in patients with brain injuries to determine rehabilitation needs and to help find an appropriate school setting and placement. The assessment is carried out to evaluate cognitive strengths and weaknesses. Tranel (1992) suggests acute epoch assessments performed as soon as the patient is alert enough to cooperate and chronic epoch assessments (3 or more months after the event). These assessments are used to evaluate recovery, assess therapies, and determine suitability of educational or vocational programs.
5. *Medicolegal situations.* Neuropsychological testing may be an important component in forensic assessment. Executive function testing, evaluation of memory, assessment for learning disorder, and assessment of cognitive ability may be important in establishing the individual's culpability in legal cases. Dysfunction in any of these areas may furnish mitigating circumstances. Brain injury and associated cognitive impairment may be grounds for a legal suit, and damages may be claimed by the family on behalf of the child. In some instances, hard neurological signs (weakness, sensory loss, paralysis) may be absent and neuroimaging findings may be questionable. In these instances, a comprehensive neuropsychological profile assumes particular importance to clarify the nature of the injury. Neuropsychological testing may provide the objective evidence needed to support the plaintiff's claim.
6. *Research.* Neuropsychological testing has become an integral part of many research programs. Those test procedures linked to newly developed neuroimaging techniques are assuming increasing importance in child and adolescent neuropsychiatry.

DOMAINS LINKED TO PRIMARY LEARNING DISABILITIES

Pennington (1991) proposes five potential domains with associated modular brain functions to correspond to the primary learning disabilities as shown in Table 3–1. These are phonological processing (reading disability), social cognition (social understanding/autistic spectrum disorders), spatial cognition (specific math and handwriting disorder), executive function (attention deficit disorder), and long-term memory (amnesia). Of these, the proposed executive function domain is most likely made up of several modules or is considered to be an overarching module. Pennington's proposal considers the earlier formulation by Gardner (1983) about multiple intelligences but points out that, when specifically drawing parallels with brain function, the modular model may be more useful than one focusing on domains as proposed by Gardner.

Of the various modules, some seem more vulnerable to variation or to developmental insult than others. Pennington suggests that the prefrontal cortex and the left hemispheric language systems are most vulnerable to insult.

Table 3–1. Modular Brain Functions and Learning Disorders

Function	Localization	Disorder
Phonological processing	Left perisylvian	Dyslexia
Executive function	Prefrontal	ADD
Spatial cognition	Posterior right hemisphere	Writing/Math
Social cognition	Limbic, orbital, right hemisphere	PDD
Long-term memory	Hippocampus, amygdala	Amnesia

From Pennington, 1991.

These are the brain regions involving modular brain functions associated with aspects of executive function and phonological processing. These systems are of most recent evolutionary origin, which may account for their vulnerability. Models such as Pennington's provide an orientation to developmental neuropsychological testing that is critical for progress in this area.

ASSESSMENT STRATEGIES

Neuropsychological testing uses several strategies including the fixed test battery, a more flexible hypothesis-driven approach that uses tests chosen based on the particular referral question, and a combination fixed/flexible test battery approach.

PSYCHOLOGICAL CAPACITIES TESTED

Assessment of Intelligence, Adaptive Function, and Personality

Tests involving the assessment of intelligence, adaptive function, and personality are used by neuropsychologists but are not a core part of the neuropsychological assessment.

In intelligence testing, several obstacles may interfere with obtaining an accurate picture of the child's overall functioning. These include choice of available instruments for children with brain disorders and the high prevalence of associated problems in attention, concentration, motivation, and behavior in children with learning disorders and mental retardation. Available intelligence tests vary in their applicability to children with developmental disorders. Existing medical conditions, particularly neurological disorders, may influence the assessment process. The selection of appropriate instruments can be difficult, and consideration must be given to the variety of instruments available because several tests assess similar aspects of function. Attention must be given to the child's reported developmental level and behavioral difficulties and the range and complexity of the child's presenting problems. The referral questions and the goal of the assessment and awareness of the limitations of existing instruments are taken into account in choosing the test instrument used. Table 3–2 lists some of the existing instruments.

To assess the probability that an individual has a learning disorder or mental retardation, several screening strategies have been recommended. One strategy is to include a robust verbal and nonverbal measure of cognitive ability, such as the vocabulary and block design subtests from the WISC-III (Sparrow and Carter, 1992). In addition, a measure of adaptive behavior is needed, as described in the next section.

One limitation of available measures of intellectual functioning is that no instruments are available that provide a reliable diagnosis of mental retardation for children under 3 or 4 years. Thus, many professional psychologists withhold a diagnosis of mental retardation until a child is mature enough and old enough to be reliably assessed. Consequently, younger children may be grouped within the broader category of "developmental delay," which includes some children who eventually will be found not to be mentally retarded. Assessment is also difficult because of the limited repertoire of behaviors in children below a mental age of 2 to 3 years. The relationship between cognitive and sensorimotor functions in infancy and later intellectual ability is still unclear. Those tests designed for infants below 18 months primarily assess sensorimotor functions, but above this

Table 3–2. Tests of Cognitive, Intellectual, and Adaptive Behavior Skills

Test Name/Publisher	Age Range (Years)
Tests of cognitive and intellectual functioning	
Wechsler Intelligence Scale for Children-III (WISC-III) (The Psychological Corporation) IQ (verbal IQ, performance IQ, full scale IQ); yields subtest scores enabling specific skill assessment as well as overall IQ and percentiles. One caution is that with mentally retarded children below the age of 10, floor effects may restrict the range of scores obtained.	6–16
Wechsler Preschool and Primary Scale of Intelligence-Revised (WPPSI-R) (The Psychological Corporation) Recently revised; yields the same IQ scores as the WISC-R.	4–6½
Stanford-Binet, 4th Ed. (Riverside Publishing Company) Recently revised; provides scores for verbal reasoning, abstract/visual reasoning, quantitative reasoning, and short-term memory; IQ score, standard age score, percentiles. The use of this instrument with the mentally retarded does not appear to be as useful as the previous version of the Stanford-Binet L-M, in part because of floor effects.	2½–adult
Kaufman Assessment Battery for Children (K-ABC) (American Guidance Service) Based on a theoretical model of information processing; separates problem solving from acquired knowledge; scaled scores, mental processing composite (IQ equivalent); standard scores for sequential and simultaneous processing, achievement standard score, age equivalents, percentiles. Children who are mentally retarded tend to score higher on sequential as opposed to simultaneous processing.	2½–12½
Hiskey-Nebraska Test of Learning Aptitude (H-NTLA) (Hiskey, 1966) A nonverbal measure of intelligence that assesses verbal labeling, categorization, concept formation, and rehearsal; can be administered through pantomimed instruction; standard scores; norm sample of hearing-impaired and non-hearing-impaired children.	3–17
Adaptive behavior scales	
AAMR Adaptive Behavior Scales: Residential/Community and School Versions (American Association on Mental Retardation) Personal independence and maladaptive behavior; percentiles; norms are based on institutionalized mentally retarded. Based on information provided by a primary caregiver.	3–69
Vineland Adaptive Behavior Scales (American Guidance Service) Global adaptive behavior, communication, daily living skills, socialization, motor (below age 5), and maladaptive (above age 5); standard scores, percentiles, age equivalents, developmental scaled scores; normed for normal, visually handicapped, learning impaired, emotionally disturbed, and retarded. Based on an interview with primary caregiver.	Normal: 0–19 Retarded: All ages

Adapted from Sparrow and Carter, 1992.

age, more cognitively oriented functions may be evaluated. Because there is limited correspondence between performance on infancy measures and those in school-aged children in longitudinal studies, it is not appropriate to make long-term predictions on the basis of assessments in infancy. Besides qualitative changes in cognitive function, the lack of continuity in assessed intelligence from infancy to later childhood may also reflect that behavior in very young children is less predictable because of rapid developmental spurts and lags. Children who test in the severe and profound ranges of mental retardation will often show inadequate attention and concentration which also affects the reliability of tests. Yet infants who score in the severely mentally retarded range during the first years of life are likely to obtain scores in the mentally retarded range during the school years. However, developmental problems in testing preclude the diagnosis of mental retardation on the basis of a single test score in infancy. In contrast reliability problems do not interfere with adequate assessment of adaptive functioning for infants and young children (Sparrow and Carter, 1992). Therefore, results of assessment of adaptive behavior at very young ages may be more informative than results of the cognitive assessment.

In children who are over age 2, there continues to be difficulty in interpretating psychological testing. For the younger mental ages, tests do not provide enough items to allow sufficient variability to clarify how delayed a child is. On a practical level, we may only be able to say from a test that the child is unable to succeed on tasks in a given area. An adequate test must have items that are appropriate for at least 1 year below the child's mental age; therefore, to assess a moderately retarded 5-year-old child with a mental age of approximately 2½ years, an adequate testing instrument must have items at the 18-month level of functioning. Similar problems are involved in assessing variability across various domains of functioning (i.e., subtest scores) because of floor effects. In this instance, a paucity of items occurs at the child's baseline ability of several subscales within an assessment instrument. As an example of this difficulty, Sparrow and Carter point out that a child could obtain an IQ of 46 by answering one item on one of the 12 subtests of the WISC-R and not demonstrate any of the complexities of his behavioral and cognitive profile.

Another difficulty with intellectual assessment instruments is their reliance on individual verbal capacities. Because of the high correlation between language functioning and intelligence, ordinarily it is true that the lower an individual's IQ, the poorer his language ability. This makes it difficult to select an appropriate intelligence test for a child with limited expressive language skills. However, certain instruments have been devised for children with severe deficits in language. They include the Leiter International Performance Scale (Leiter, 1948) and the nonverbal scale of the Kaufman Assessment Battery for Children (Kaufman and Kaufman, 1983). Unfortunately, the Leiter International Performance Scale has serious shortcomings because it does not provide standard scores; the age equivalents were developed on a small nonrepresentative sample of children. Moreover, several items on the Leiter are outdated (Sparrow and Carter, 1992).

For the child with learning disabilities, neuropsychological testing can be conducted effectively if the child's cognitive level is high enough for the tests that are used. Of the tests that are available, the WISC-III, which has verbal and performance scales, is the most commonly used and has been investigated the most carefully in regard to neuropsychological testing.

Intellectual Abilities

Intelligence tests were originally constructed to measure, by multiple methods, a general intelligence, or G factor, that would predict future adaptive capacity. These tests were not developed as tests of specific brain functions. Despite this, a standardized IQ test is included as part of most neuropsychological test batteries. Tests, such as the Wechsler Intelligence Scales for Children (WISC-III), are standardized for ages 6 to 16 and have the advantage of broad-based, large-scale normative data, which make them useful for neuropsychological assessment. The IQ tests are very helpful in establishing the likelihood of success in a conventional school program.

The Wechsler scales are made up of two major subscales, verbal and performance; each of these subscales includes different subtests. The verbal IQ includes six subtests: information (the fund of general knowledge); vocabulary (word definition); comprehension (proverbs, practical reasoning); similarities (verbal abstract reasoning); digit span (immediate repetition of strings of digits forward and backward); and arithmetic (mental calculations performed as a response to orally presented problems). The performance IQ is made up of five subtests including block design (the timed construction of designs with colored blocks); picture arrangement (sequential arrangement of cartoon scenes to depict a theme); picture completion (identification of a detail missing in drawings of various entities); digit symbol substitution (a timed coding test in which symbols are matched to numbers); and object assembly (timed puzzle constructions).

Several difficulties arise in the neuropsychological interpretation of intelligence tests of this kind.

The Use of Verbal and Performance Scores as Indicators of Specific Hemispheric Dysfunction

Although verbal and performance subtests have been used to infer differential dysfunction of the cerebral hemisphere, verbal (left hemisphere), performance (right hemisphere), the test patterns do not occur regularly enough for clinical reliability (Lezak, 1983). Furthermore, although subtest scatter has been used as an indicator of dysfunction, scatter also occurs in the normal population, so it is not a reliable indicator. Still, the verbal and performance subtests may serve as a useful rule of thumb in regard to dysfunction and suggest more detailed assessment for differential hemispheric function. Any scatter, if it suggests dysfunction, can be used to point the way for further detailed neuropsychological testing.

Excessive Reliance on the Overall Summary Score (i.e., the Full Scale IQ) to Characterize a Patient

Although the subtests evaluate intellectual functions, many of these capacities have little in common in regard to cognitive demands or underlying neurological mechanisms. Therefore, for purposes of neuropsychological assessment, the summary score (full scale IQ) is not an adequate or appropriate description. However, the subtest results may be beneficial if they are broken down according to various subareas of function, such as attention/concentration, verbal reasoning, and visuospatial analysis (Lezak, 1988).

In general, standardized IQ tests contribute to the neuropsychological battery in that they provide an overall ability level score, provide a basis for more specific neuropsychological testing, and offer extensive normative information for certain subtests that may be relevant for the neuropsychological assessment.

Scores on intelligence tests are used to separate children with generalized learning impairment (e.g., mental retardation) from those with isolated forms of learning disability. Definitions of learning disability used for making placement decisions include intelligence as an indicator of learning potential. Discrepancy between cognitive ability (IQ) and academic achievement is often used in diagnosing learning disabilities. However, there are conceptual problems in using the IQ test scores to predict the future performance and learning potential of children with learning disabilities because the IQ score is a summary of several aspects of cognitive functioning. For example, although some aspects of the test are relevant to reading ability, others have little relationship to reading skill (e.g., puzzle assembly). Also, although the IQ scores may correlate with the severity of the reading disorder (the median correlation is 0.70), a child's reading level may be higher than predicted on the intelligence test. The IQ test per se does not measure a skill related to reading proficiency. For example, no IQ test measures phonological segmentation skills that are strongly correlated with decoding ability in reading.

Adaptive Functioning and Personality

The assessment of personality is an important accompaniment of neuropsychological assessment. The temperamental response style, sociability, affective status, activity level, and motivation to cooperate are not only important in the interpretation of test results, but also may provide cues regarding the presence of a developmental neuropsychiatric disorder. Aman (1991) provides detailed descriptions of personality inventories for use in developmentally disabled individuals.

Adaptive Behavior and Personality Tests

The primary focus of neuropsychological testing is to establish an accurate description of a child's abilities based on test results that are then used in the diagnostic and rehabilitation process. However, from these tests little can be inferred about the child's ability to function in daily living situations at home and in new situations or in school and residential settings (Spreen and Strauss, 1991). Specific tests for adaptive function (Lambert, Nihiri, and Leland, 1993) to assess such abilities as self-care and tests of personality function, which include personality features, must be utilized.

Personality

The assessment of personality and temperament is of particular importance, but no generally accepted instruments are available for all types of problems that present in childhood. For children, one inventory available is the Personality Inventory for Children, which is described in Appendix 2.

MENTAL STATUS EVALUATION

Neuropsychological testing is organized to evaluate certain functional domains; the goal of testing is to evaluate these domains adequately. The tests used for these evaluations are continually being refined. Because assessment of domains of function is sought, the specific tests used will vary, so no specific core battery is recommended for neuropsychological testing. Instead, commonly used tests are discussed in the text and listed in Appendix 2. Standard texts, such as Spreen and Strauss's (1991) *A Compendium of Neuropsychological Tests*, should be consulted for a more detailed description of tests. *The Handbook of Neuropsychology*, Volume 6, provides a detailed description of the nature and scope of child neuropsychology (Rapin and Segalowitz, 1992).

Attention/Inhibition

Wakefulness and attention are essential to all other mental faculties. Neuropsychological evaluation assesses selective attention and the ability to inhibit perceptions that are irrelevant to the task demands. Dennis (1991) emphasizes the role of attention in information processing and highlights the following as basic regulatory operations of frontal lobe systems: vigilance, focusing attention, anticipating, maintaining psychological set, and exercising interference control. Difficulty with attention is most commonly linked to anxiety and personal preoccupations. Developmentally, problems in attention and concentration are most apparent in young children and in children who are mentally retarded throughout their life span. Disorders in attention are most commonly associated with sleep deprivation, posttraumatic brain injury, substance abuse, and attention deficit/hyperactivity disorder. Mentally retarded children and adolescents may meet diagnostic criteria for attention deficit/hyperactivity disorder more often than mental age- or chronologically age-matched peers. The neuropsychological assessment of attention/inhibition is increasingly utilized for the assessment of children with attention deficit/hyperactivity disorder along with the more commonly used parent and teacher behavior rating scales (Conners, 1985a, 1985b). One of the most frequently used measures of inattention and impulsivity is the Continuous Performance Test (CPT), which was originally developed as a measure of vigilance (Rosvold et al., 1956). Many versions of the CPT have been developed, but the basic methodology is the same as the original. Subjects are presented with a variety of stimuli that are displayed on a screen for a short duration and are instructed to respond to a predefined "target stimulus." A number of indices are recorded including omission errors (failures to detect the target) and commission errors (responses to nontargeted stimuli). In addition, response times for correct detections and for various commission errors and variability may be recorded. Commonly used CPT tests, such as the Conners CPT (1994) and the TOVA, are described in Appendix 2. Greenberg and Waldman (1993) have published developmental normative data for the TOVA.

Attentional problems may interfere with the neuropsychological assessment process and make it difficult to determine if an incorrect test response reflects lack of attention or lack of knowledge (Sparrow and Carter, 1992). Fluctuations in attention occurring over a 45- to 90-minute testing session may influence the results; moreover, reduced attention is a common sign of fatigue during testing. When demands are placed that require attention during the testing procedure, motor overflow may become apparent (Waber, Mann and Merola, 1985). Denckla (1985) has developed a neurological examination to measure such subtle signs in individuals with attention deficit/hyperactivity disorder.

Mood and Motivation

Mood and motivation underlie the capacity to participate fully in neuropsychological testing. Tests of attention are sensitive to disturbances in mood and motivation.

The extent of motivation is evaluated through observation and in monitoring participation in the testing procedure. The ability to cooperate, to sustain effort, and the extent of encouragement needed to complete a task are all observed (Weintraub and Mesulam, 1985). Motivation and task persistence overlap so those with poor motivation may do poorly on tasks that require perseverance. Specific disturbances in motivation are referred to as apathy and may be signaled by "I don't know" responses or delays in beginning a task. Encouragement and prompting may be necessary to obtain a correct estimate of ability in the apathetic child.

Mood and affect may be clinically observed during the interview or may be specifically assessed using visual analog scales, which show little verbal mediation, and through self-reports, such as the Children's Depression Inventory (CDI) (Kovacs, 1985) for children 8 and over who can read. The Children's Depression Rating Scale-Revised (Poznanski, Freeman, and Moqros, 1985), a clinician-rated instrument designed to measure the presence and severity of depression in children age 6 to 12 years, may also be used. In the assessment of affect, apathy must be distinguished from depression. Moreover, the experience of emotion must be clarified because in some conditions, such as certain right hemispheric dysfunction presentations or in pseudobulbar palsy, the physical expression of affect (e.g., facial expression, voice tone) may be impaired although inner experience may remain intact. Finally, with some frontal lobe lesions and in some metabolic encephalopathies, severe apathy may be noted in the absence of depression.

Orientation and Memory

Orientation

No standardized instrument to test orientation is available for children and adolescents. The clinical interview provides the best guide to the child or adolescent's orientation.

Memory

Severe amnesia in children is rare although it may occur with acute encephalitis and head trauma. Problems with new learning following encephalitis and traumatic brain injury more commonly present as mental retardation rather than as a focal deficit, although they may present as a specific learning disability.

Memory disturbance may involve deficits in registration and retrieval. Considerable advances have been made in understanding memory and metamemory skills in children. The examination of memory should include immediate and short-term retention, the pattern and rate of acquisition of new information, the efficacy of retrieval of remote and recently learned information, and the ability to make inferences based on memory (Spreen and Strauss, 1991). Each of the components should be assessed in both verbal and nonverbal modalities, using both recall and recognition techniques. Verbal and nonverbal memory can be assessed in any modality. Verbal memory is most conveniently studied, utilizing tests that use auditory input and require verbal output. Verbal memory tests ordinarily present the child with a list of words or a paragraph and ask for verbal recall at a later time. These tests include measures of long-term recall and recognition and also demonstrate learning ability.

The most commonly used tests for recent memory are variants of the Selective Reminding Test. Measures of selective reminding are available in both verbal (Buschke, 1973) and nonverbal areas (Benton, 1974). These techniques allow simultaneous analysis of a child's storage, retention, and retrieval abilities. Poor performance may relate to processing problems in the modality involved (e.g., language) and may not be caused by memory difficulty.

Visual Memory

Among the nonverbal memory tasks, several instruments are available for use in school-aged children. In these tests, children are shown geometric figures and then asked to reproduce them from memory. Two commonly used tests listed in Appendix 2 are the Benton Test of Visual Retention and the Rey-Osterrieth Complex Figure. For example, Prior and Hoffman (1990) used the complex figure to compare children with autistic disorder with matched mental age and chronological age control groups. They found that the group with autistic disorder had no particular problems in copying the figure; however, they performed significantly worse in producing the figure from memory, which suggested to the authors they had difficulty storing information in a coherent way.

Speech and Linguistic Function

Receptive Language

The assessment of receptive language skills involves an evaluation of the child's abilities to sustain attention to verbal stimuli, to comprehend conversation, requests, and instructions, to immediately recall verbal information, to interpret a speaker's intent within a social context, and to demonstrate sensitivity to social cues present in the social milieu.

Assessment of Language Structure

In linguistic theory, the major components of language or linguistic features include phonology, syntax, morphology and semantics. The assessment of language structure includes phonological assessment (phonic and phonetic skills), lexical and semantic skills, and syntactic skills. Instruments for assessment of language structure are well characterized (see Table 3–3). Assessments of language use, i.e., pragmatic language, also shown in the table, are of increasing importance but are less well characterized.

Phonological Skills (Phonetics and Phonics)

Phonology refers to the sound system of language. The most important aspect of phonology is phonemes, the study of significant speech sounds. Phonemes are significant if they alter the meaning of words, e.g., in the sounds *best* and *rest,* the "b" and "r" sounds change the meaning of the words. A second phonological category is phonetics, which refers to specific and discrete sounds called phonemes, e.g., the "a" in *art* and the "a" in *above* sound different but do not change the meaning of words. Phonological skills are assessed in the areas of phonetics (articulation, the output side), and phonemic segmentation (recognition of phonic patterns, the input side). Phonological assessment is necessary to evaluate children with reading disorders. A screening of an individual's articulation can be made based on language samples that are collected as part of a language assessment battery. For example, phonemic awareness might be assessed by evaluating phonemic segmentation tasks (Vellutino and Scanlon, 1987b), testing of phonological memory (Vellutino and Scanlon, 1987b), and assessing visual recognition of phonic patterns (Richardson and DiBenedetto, 1985). Tests evaluating these areas may be used to distinguish normal readers from reading-disabled children. Core tests are shown in Table 3–3. The CELF-R and TLC-E are commonly used.

Lexical and Semantic Skills (Primarily Naming and Word Retrieval)

The term "semantics" refers to the study of meaning in language. Semantics involves attaching meaning to phonological forms and prescribes the rules that determine how meaning is conveyed in sentences. Lexical and semantic skills are used in many studies that compare various learning-disabled groups with controls (Donahue, 1986). Semantic tests are frequently used with reading-disabled groups. Study results show that reading-disabled subjects perform at a lower level on these tests than do controls (Denckla and Rudel, 1976a; Eakin and Douglas, 1971; Stanovich, Nathan, and Vala-Rossi, 1986; Stanovich, Nathan, and Zolman, 1988; Vellutino and Scanlon, 1987a). These tests are good predictors of reading disability (Blackman, 1984; Vellutino and Scanlon, 1987b; Wolf, 1984). Core tests shown in Table 3–3 include the Boston Naming Test (Kaplan, Goodglass, and Weintraub 1978, 1983); the Rapid Automatized Naming Test (picture naming) (Denckla and Rudel, 1974, 1976a, 1976b); and the Test of Language Competence (Expanded) (Wiig and Secord, 1985, 1989). The best predictions come from tests that involve visual confrontational naming.

Syntactic Skills

Syntax refers to skills involved in forming and understanding sentences. It applies to sentence

Table 3–3. Language Assessment Tests

Instrument	Age Range in Years
Assessment of Language Structure	
Phonological Skills	
Articulation Screening Tests	Any age
Phonemic Segmentation	5–13
Arizona Articulation Proficiency Scale-Revised	3–11 years, 11 months
Goldman-Fristoe-Woodcock Test of Auditory Discrimination	4–adult
Lexical and Semantic Skills	
Boston Naming Test	6–adult
Rapid "Automatized" Naming Test	5–12
Test of Language Competence (TLC-E) (semantic)	9–11
Syntactic Skills	
Token Test for Children (Part V)	3–12½
Clinical Evaluation of Language Fundamentals-R (CELF-R)	K–12
General Assessment of Language	
Test of Language Competence (TLC-E)	9–11
Clinical Evaluation of Language Fundamentals-R (CELF-R)	K–12
Spoken Narrative Analysis Procedure	Used for all ages
Pragmatic Analysis	Used for all ages

From Denckla, 1993.

structure, i.e., the correct sequencing of words and inflections to make a sentence. Both expressive and receptive syntax should be assessed (see Table 3–3).

Pragmatic Language

Although the knowledge of the rules of phonology, semantics, and syntax is very important to listeners or speakers of any language, effective language communication also requires knowledge of the pragmatic rules of language. Methods for investigating this aspect of language are not as fully developed as those for phonology, semantics, and syntax. Language-related skills thought to be processed in the right hemisphere may be important in the study of pragmatic language, particularly as it relates to social skills.

The establishment of social language use begins in early life, and some pragmatic skills are acquired during infancy before the child learns to speak. These precursors include establishing eye contact, social smiling, engaging in vocal turn taking, and the use of anticipatory gestures.

During development, children learn the pragmatic rules that govern linguistic behavior in a social context. These rules include mastery of the following abilities: first, to express a variety of communicative intentions and use appropriate sentence structure. Examples include requesting, persuading, informing, and protesting. Second, to understand and produce intentions that are directly expressed, such as "Give me something to eat," or indirectly expressed, such as "I'm hungry." Third, to take turns in conversation in a reciprocal manner. Fourth, to keep the conversational interaction going and to recognize when one's turn to speak ends. Fifth, to change and maintain a conversational topic. Sixth, to understand and take into consideration the social context of the conversation. In this instance, the social status of the speaker and listener must be considered, the individual's familiarity with the listener, and language conceptual skills of the conversational partner are part of pragmatic understanding. One uses an understanding of the social context to decide how to express an intention, for example, when to use colloquial language or more formal language. Seventh, to judge the amount and type of information that the communicative partner needs to understand and then communicate to meet the partner's informational needs. Eighth, to recognize times when a communicative breakdown has occurred and how to repair that breakdown.

Pragmatic language disorders are assessed based on these pragmatic rules. The most common examples of pragmatic failures are inappropriate interpretation of indirect communicative expressions of intent. Children with language disorders may fail to communicate intentions effectively if they do not use semantic and grammatical rules appropriately. Such children may resort to simple behavioral patterns or gestures to communicate intentions. Language-disordered children may have difficulty formulating requests and in utilizing the range of linguistic strategies and devices used by normal children. Moreover, they may fail to develop the range of communicative intentions that are expected for their age. Classically, children with autistic disorder fail to display communicative intentions and interests such as commenting on their observations and spontaneously informing others about their experiences.

In addition, the inability to maintain topics and elaborate them over time with multiple conversational turns may be apparent in language-disordered children. Abnormalities in topic maintenance are seen when children exhibit limited knowledge of the topic and show attention deficits, reticence, echolalia, or perseveration. Failure to maintain the topic may also occur because the child is unable to identify the information in the speaker's utterance that pertains to the main topic so the child may focus on inappropriate and insignificant details of what is being said to them. Such behavior puts the burden on the conversational partner to decide how to modulate or shift the intended topic or redirect the child to the original topic that led to the exchange.

Limited topic maintenance can be characteristic of children who have difficulty with memory. These children may have problems integrating information that is presented to them and establishing its context to what was previously said. When this occurs, the main conversational points may not be understood. Moreover, a language-disordered child may have difficulty inferring the underlying message of an utterance which is presented if that message is not clearly and concretely stated. Difficulty recognizing implicit links that relate one idea to the other may make it difficult to maintain a conversational topic and lead to communication breakdown.

Finally, the ability to recognize and repair communicative breakdown may be impaired in language-disordered children. The repair, then, may be accomplished, if at all, in a simplistic manner, for example, through repetition of the original message. The basic reasons for the breakdown usually include failure to supply background information, unclear articulation, production of words in combination that lead to ambiguous messages, and failure to establish the referent pronoun.

Selected subtest scores from a standardized test that aims to assess the subject's ability to comprehend and use language beyond the literal level, to make inferences and understand metaphoric expressions (e.g., Test of Language Competence-E, Wiig and Secord, 1989) should be conducted to provide background for evaluating pragmatic skills.

Story Narration

Narrating a story and its analysis focus on how well the subject can produce an extended and cohesive sequence of sentences to express a meaningful story. These approaches currently have limited use clinically, but may be important in the research assessment of children with developmental disorders. Narrative abilities have been assessed in children with attention deficit disorder, learning disability, autistic disorder, and genetic syndromes such as Down syndrome and Williams syndrome. For example, Tannock, Purvis, and Schachar (1993) found that boys with attention deficit/hyperactivity disorder (AD/HD) produced stories that supplied less overall information, were poorly organized, less cohesive, and contained more inaccuracies. These same authors (Purvis, Schachar, and Tannock, in press) suggest that boys with AD/HD may be distinguishable from boys with learning disability. Narrative production before and after stimulant treatment for AD/HD is an area of ongoing investigation.

Narrative analysis is a means to assess language in mildly to moderately language-impaired children and can be an important aspect of the assessment. Story generation and story retelling have been used to assess language in older children. Both techniques can be effective ways to measure narrative ability and may activate the cognitive organizations involved with the schema of the story. Merritt and Liles (1989) suggest that story retelling is more clinically useful with older children in assessing their story grammar ability than is story generation. Retold stories tend to be longer and to contain more story grammar components and more complete episodes. Because of their length, retold stories facilitate more complete assessment of impaired language use including grammatical usage, syntax, and story cohesion. Standard story retelling/comprehension test measures based on large samples of children are not currently available. However, norms within individual groups for screening purposes are being developed.

Story grammar is a specific type of narrative analysis that is characterized by a formal set of rules describing stories as being joined together in predictable ways. These rules identify patterns of temporally and causally related information. Both comprehension and production of story grammar are directed by a cognitive organization referred to as "story schema" (Mandler and Johnson, 1977; Stein and Glenn, 1982).

Even though stories may vary in their presentation, a well-formed narrative uses these story grammar components, either directly or inferentially, and they are both temporally and causally linked. A complete episode contains the initiating event or internal response motivating a character to formulate a goal-directed plan, an action or attempt at resolving the situation, and a direct consequence marking attainment or lack of attainment of the goal (Stein and Glenn, 1979).

The narrative analysis takes into account three specific elements of the story grammar. These include an overall description of the child's story schema in regard to frequency of the use of the story grammar components, the story hierarchy, which represents the child's use of the story grammar components in regard to their importance in communicating the narrative, and the episode complexity in regard to how the story content develops within complete or incomplete episode structures. Language-disordered children make less effective use of story grammar components and episode units when they produce narratives and also show poor comprehension of the causal relations linking the parts of the story.

Visuospatial

Visuospatial tests evaluate right hemispheric function, especially the right occipitoparietal and occipitotemporal regions. There are separate visual, perceptual, and memory systems in the brain for places and things. Moreover, visual item perception should not be confused with visuospatial processing. Visual item perception refers to visual recognition of a stimulus, whereas the visuospatial processing addresses the relative position, the configuration, and the spatial orientation of visually presented items. These tests are sensitive to a variety of perceptual abilities. Typically, tests of visual/spatial functioning require no physical manipulation of test material or verbal labeling of responses. Although they do demand a significant contribution from the right hemisphere, they cannot strictly be dichotomized as free from left hemisphere involvement.

The examiner may have difficulty interpreting the results if verbal mediation has influenced performance on these "perceptual tests." However, by using a multiple-choice format and choosing configurational stimulus material that has been reported to be most specifically sensitive to right hemisphere damage, the examiner addresses this issue by shifting the balance toward nonverbal and motor-free visual processing (Benton et al., 1983a).

Visual-Motor Functioning

Visual-motor functioning is closely related to visual item perception and visuospatial processing, but adds a manipulation or graphomotor component to the perceptual function tasks. The Block Design and Object Assembly subtests from the WISC-III require visual-motor ability. Visual-motor functioning is a necessary but not a sufficient condition for successful performance of these subtests. Visuographomotor ability requires visual processing, motor control, and possibly the mediation of selective attention and sequential organizing capacities. Some of the more advanced copy tasks involve preplanning; earlier simple designs may be highly overlearned.

Social-Emotional Function Testing

Tests of social-emotional functioning are particularly important to evaluate nonverbal learning disabilities. However, instruments for neuropsycholgical testing of social-emotional functioning are not well developed, and extensive additional research is needed. Tests that are being evaluated (see Appendix 2) include tests of nonverbal affect (Facial and Vocal Affect Recognition Test) and the Test of Facial Affect Recognition. In the first of these tests, nonverbal perceptual capabilities are presented to the child through the visual and auditory channels. In the second, the subject is asked to describe the affective status of faces that show happy, sad, angry, or neutral expressions. All of these are research instruments.

Social-emotional functions are difficult to evaluate clinically because it is not only the capacity to recognize affect but the interpretation of the context in which the affect occurs and the capacity to modulate as well as recognize affective expression that is clinically important. An alternative approach in younger children and those who are severely cognitively impaired is the use of the Strange Situation Paradigm to evaluate attachment status. Moreover, studies of affect sharing in the context of joint attentional interactions in autistic and mentally retarded persons (Kasari et al., 1990) may be pertinent. It should be borne in mind that the measurement of neuropsychological competencies are essential to joint attention. In any assessment, the clinical history will provide anecdotes that testify to social obtuseness.

Executive Functions

The term "executive function" applies to capacities that include attending in a selective and focused manner, inhibition of off-task responding, self-monitoring, flexible concept formation, planning, judgment, and decision making. They are linked to the frontal lobe but involve other brain regions connected to the frontal lobe, e.g., the basal ganglia. To evaluate executive dysfunction in children, the neuropsychiatric interview of the child is tailored to gather data from parents on particular behaviors that require executive function, and the child is tested directly. Because executive dysfunction interferes with adaptive behavior both at home and at school, the parent interview should cover both settings, but teacher interviews may be necessary to cover school matters, as indicated earlier. Children with executive dysfunction have difficulty regulating their behavior as it pertains to their schoolwork and their interpersonal activities. To clarify these adaptive problems, the history specifies and clarifies the frequency and severity of target symptoms of executive dysfunction in each setting. In addition, the presence of associated neurological and psychological findings that are related to executive function is assessed. The presence of executive dysfunction symptoms, how these symptoms manifest in everyday life, their developmental history in regard to time of initial symptom onset, and the presence of associated difficulties are evaluated.

Neuropsychological Testing of Executive Function

The assessment of executive function is carried out in parallel with all of the psychoeducational and neuropsychological tests that are administered for the various cognitive content areas. Executive function status affects and impinges on content-based assessment. But executive function cannot be evaluated without the cognitive challenge of the test contents, which affect executive function processes. In assessing executive function, the examiner must focus on the processes the child follows in responding to the items presented. Because of the structured nature of routine assessment procedure, the deficiency (an absence of expected behavior) that one seeks to demonstrate in executive function may be compensated for, as the examiner, in a one-to-one situation, works to maintain the child's focused attention and helps the child organize the time for completing the test. Consequently, the "command and control" module of the neuropsychological repertoire of executive function is difficult to assess in structured one-to-one situations.

Only in more severe cases is obvious off-task behavior, inattentiveness, and disinhibition clearly enough seen in a one-to-one testing setting to diagnose executive dysfunction. Therefore, a period of unstructured observation around testing is essential when evaluating executive dysfunction. The examiner observes how the child approaches the content of the test information and makes clinical observations regarding the child's attention to test tasks and observes how well the child organizes his performance. It may be difficult to distinguish overall executive dysfunction from a child's cognitive difficulty as he struggles with the task itself. Therefore, qualitative data (for example, the types of errors produced) are helpful to differentiate context-related processing problems from executive function problems. One may compare the level of performance on tasks that address similar content but place different demands for executive functional abilities.

Tasks that make demands on executive function processes are those that challenge the ability to tolerate boredom, to operate independently, and to generate active plans to solve problems. These tasks focus on the subprocesses of executive function, such as task initiation (focused attention, organized problem solving), sustained effort, inhibition of off-task or unsuccessful behaviors, flexible shifts of attention, or the consideration of alternative strategies. Consequently, the examiner looks at the child's ability to initiate the task, sustain attention to it, inhibit impulses that may interfere with task completion, and shift attention to the next task.

Description of Executive Function Tests

Executive functioning refers to the underlying neuropsychological abilities necessary for higher-order "frontal lobe" related behavior. As stated earlier, it is primarily concerned with goal formulation, planning, implementation and execution, as well as the self-regulation necessary for efficient attainment of these goals. Executive functioning refers to the individual's ability to conceptualize long-term goals, develop possible alternatives for goal attainment, choose among the alternatives in a logical manner, organize the specific steps necessary for goal attainment, and evaluate the extent to which these steps are efficient in reaching the goal. Executive function refers to the self-regulatory process whereby the individual is constantly attending, evaluating the extent to which his thoughts or actions are fitting the demands of the situation, as well as the ability to shift and self-correct when confronted with negative feedback from the situation. It is dependent not only on the individual's ability to conceptualize, organize, attend, apply rules, and reason inductively and deductively, but also on his capacity for selective attention and inhibition of task-irrelevant perception, thoughts, and/or action described earlier under "attention/inhibition." Table 3–4 presents a list of tests and the major executive functions assessed in a test battery developed by Denckla. Executive function tests are described in Appendix 2.

EVALUATION OF TEST RESULTS

Three stages of analysis are involved in evaluating neuropsychological test results (Denckla, 1989). At the first level of analysis, the individual's level of performance is established in a similar manner to the calculation of results that might be performed by a clinical psychologist. This aspect of the evaluation establishes whether or not a particular behavioral function is at the level expected for age. The individual level of performance is determined, and raw scores obtained from the test are converted into an age or grade equivalent, a percentile rank or a scale score, to judge whether the individual's performance is below, at, or above average.

The second stage in evaluating neuropsychological test findings is the analysis of the constituent skills that are required to perform the particular function being tested. Can the

Table 3–4. Tests Measuring Executive Functions

Name of Test	Initiate	Sustain	Inhibit	Shift
	(Plan) (Organize)	(Concentrate) (Be Vigilant)	(Self-Control) (Self-Monitor)	(Cognitive Flexibility)
Continuous Performance		*		
Stroop Color Word Interference		*	*	*
Word Fluency	*	*	*	

From Denckla, 1993.

child or adolescent recognize the figure he is asked to describe, or is he capable of writing out an answer? Because many test results require graphomotor activity, they must be interpreted according to the child's capacity to perform the function. For example, failure on a test of copying designs might be the result of faulty perception of the designs so visual perception would need to be evaluated.

The third stage in neuropsychological evaluation is the interpretation of results and establishment of the underlying neuropsychological profile once it is clear the individual does possess the skills to complete the test successfully. This is an essential analysis from a neuropsychological perspective because it qualitatively assesses how an individual carries out a task and determines whether errors that emerge suggest a particular disorder. For example, errors on a memory test could be related to attentional drift, impulsivity, or poor planning.

Several tests may contribute to the construct being assessed. For example, if the construct vocabulary is being evaluated, how should the interpretation about vocabulary differ when comparing the capacity to name a picture, tell about a word, or point to a word picture equivalent (Denckla, 1989)? Analysis of results at these three stages may be used to demonstrate whether or not a subject can perform the task and to detect patterns of response that might indicate psychological dysfunction. Findings may be used for hypotheses regarding an imbalance between brain systems that may be contributing to specific brain dysfunction. A case illustration demonstrating a neuropsychological test profile of an 8-year-old with a neurodevelopmental disorder is provided in Appendix 1 on pages 44–45.

SUMMARY

Differences in ability may be better understood by using neuropsychological testing techniques than standard IQ tests. For example, some abilities are more stable in their functional organization than others. In some instances, following injury, the behavioral deficits seen in children are similar to those that occur in adults who were injured in similar brain regions, and their recovery from injury will be incomplete. In other instances, lesions involving some brain areas in children do not cause permanent deficits. These differences, according to the site and kind of lesion occurring in children, point to limitations in the functional capacity of the brain and provide evidence for reorganization of some regions, leading to limited recovery linked to some areas and better recovery when lesions occur in other areas. Neuropsychological testing assumes particular importance in developmental disorders where deviations may occur in the development of the brain and the integration of cognitive modules.

Longitudinal studies of the neuropsychological development of both normal and developmentally disordered children may potentially help in the understanding of the consequences of the early experiences that shape the development of later child, adolescent, and adult abilities and talents. The early detection of differences among children may lead to better understanding of the roots of adult personality traits and adult psychopathologies, such as antisocial behavior, substance abuse, depressive disorder, and other illnesses. Moreover, differences in the potential to recover from acquired head injury in children and adults of different ages lead to better understanding of neural plasticity in the recovery process as the brain reorganizes following injury.

Cognitive Neuropsychology and Cognitive Neuropsychiatry

In this chapter, the focus on cognitive neuropsychology complements psychiatric research into epidemiology and neuroscience. The neuropsychological assessment in the developmental disorders focuses on modular brain functions and learning disorders and, following brain injury, it addresses specific deficits that are gross and may be fixed. In contrast, the major mental disorders assessed in psychiatry use a different approach involving the use of observation, interaction, interview, and the use of rating scales and questionnaires. The neuropsychological approach tends to emphasize the underlying deficit or the discrepancy between an unusual ability and other deficiencies (David, 1993; Pennington, Johnson, and Welsh, 1987). However, major mental illnesses ordinarily present cognitively as aberrant behaviors or excessive activities, possibly as the consequence of the loss of inhibition. For example, hallucinations are not failures to perceive sensory input, but represent the perception or internal generation of images that are reported in the absence of external stimulation.

The neuropsychologist ordinarily evaluates deficits but, in some instances, may investigate hyperfunctions (for example, hyperlexia). Hyperfunctions have been studied in the description of hyperlalia (Yamdori et al., 1990) and in the evaluation of exceptional artistic ability in children with autistic disorder where highly developed access to brain modules, such as that for visual memory, have been postulated (O'Connor and Hermelin, 1987). There are also studies addressing a "hyperconnection" model of behavioral disturbance in association with temporal lobe epilepsy. Here, Bear (1979) has suggested that certain beliefs may attract strong affects due to the extent of increased linkage between cortical and limbic brain areas. He refers to this as a syndrome of sensory-limbic hyperconnection.

Cognitive neuropsychology and cognitive neuropsychiatry differ in that the psychiatrist tends to focus on mental disorders (syndromes) that are not psychological constructs whereas the neuropsychologist focuses on specific impairments, such as phonological abnormalities in reading disability and impairments in semantic memory. The neuropsychologist addresses solitary disturbances of function that may emerge from a variety of pathological disorders and assume a final, common path. Neuropsychology may demonstrate a deficit but not explain the phenomenology of the disorder, such as seen in psychosis that represents anomalous functioning. For the child neuropsychiatrist, the importance of developmental testing is broader than that used by general psychiatrists because the types of disorder differ; the child neuropsychiatrist works closely to incorporate findings from neuropsychology in his or her final formulation and is involved in close collaboration with the child neuropsychologist.

Note: This chapter was written in consultation with Martha B. Denckla, M.D., Professor of Neurology and Pediatrics, Johns Hopkins Medical Institutions, Director of Developmental Cognitive Neurology, Kennedy-Krieger Institute, Baltimore, MD.

REFERENCES

Aman, M.G. (1991). *Assessing psychopathology and behavior problems in persons with mental retardation: A review of available instruments* DHHS Publication No. (ADM) 91–1712. U.S. Department of Health and Human Services, Rockville, MD.

Army Individual Test Battery (1944). *Manual of directions and scoring.* War Department, Adjutant General's Office, Washington, D.C.

Barkley, R. A. (1977). A review of stimulant drug research with hyperactive children. *Journal of Child Psychology and Psychiatry,* 18:137–165.

Bear, D.M. (1979). Temporal lobe epilepsy—a syndrome of sensory limbic hyperconnection. *Cortex,* 15:357–384.

Beery, K.E. (1967). *Developmental Test of Visual-Motor Integration.* Follett Publishing Co., Chicago.

______. (1982). *Revised Manual for the Developmental Test of Visual-Motor Integration.* Modern Curriculum Press, Cleveland.

Benton, A.L. (1974). *The Revised Visual Retention Test,* 4th ed. Psychological Corporation, San Antonio, TX.

______, Hamsher, K.D., Varney, N.R., and Spreen, O. (1983a). Judgment of line orientation. In *Contributions to neuropsychological assessment: A clinical manual.* Oxford University Press, New York.

______, ______, ______, and ______. (1983b). Facial recognition. In *Contributions to neuropsychological assessment: A clinical manual.* Oxford University Press, New York.

Berg, E.A. (1948). A simple objective technique for measuring flexibility in thinking. *Journal of General Psychology,* 39:15–22.

Blackman, B.A. (1984). Relationship of rapid naming ability and language analysis skills to kindergarten and first-grade reading achievement. *Journal of Educational Psychology,* 76:610–622.

Buschke, H. (1973). Selective reminding for analysis of memory and learning. *Journal of Verbal Learning and Verbal Behavior,* 12:543–550.

______, and Fuld, P.A. (1974). Evaluating storage, retention and retrieval in disordered memory and learning. *Neurology,* 11:1019–1025.

Cairns, E., and Cammock, T. (1978). Development of a more reliable version of the matching familiar figures test. *Developmental Psychology,* 14:555–560.

Conners, C.K. (1985a). Parent Symptom Questionnaire. In J. Rapoport, C.K. Conners, and N. Reatig (eds.), Rating scales and assessment instruments for use in pediatric psychopharmacological research. *Psychopharmacology Bulletin,* 21:816–822.

______. (1985b). Teacher Questionnaire. In J. Rapoport, C.K. Conners, and N. Reatig, (eds.),

Rating scales and assessment instruments for use in pediatric psychopharmacological research. *Psychopharmacology Bulletin,* 21:823–831.

______. (1994) *Connors Continuous Performance Test.* Multi-Health Systems, Inc., Toronto, Canada.

David, A.S. (1992). Frontal lobology—psychiatry's new pseudoscience. *British Journal of Psychiatry,* 161:244–248.

______. (1993). Editorial: Cognitive neuropsychiatry? *Psychological Medicine,* 23:1–5.

Delis, D.C., Kramer, J.H., Kaplan, E., and Ober, B.A. (1987). *The California Verbal Learning Test.* Psychological Corporation, New York.

Denckla, M.B. (1985). Revised neurological examination for subtle signs. *Psychopharmacological Bulletin,* 21:773–800.

______. (1989). Neuropsychology and its role in the diagnosis of learning disabilities. In M.B. Denckla (ed.), *Attention deficit disorders, hyperactivity, and learning disabilities: Current theory and practical approaches,* p. 31. CIBA-Geigy Corp., Summit, NJ.

______. (1993). Neurodevelopmental pathways to learning disabilities, P50 HD 25806, a grant from NINCDS, National Institutes of Health, Bethesda, MD.

______, and Rudel, R. (1974). Rapid "automatized" naming of pictured objects, colors, letters, and numbers by normal children. *Cortex,* 10:186–202.

______, and ______. (1976a). Naming of pictured objects by dyslexic and other learning disabled children. *Brain and Language,* 39:1–15.

______, and ______. (1976b). Rapid "automatized" naming (R.A.N.): Dyslexia differentiated from other learning disabilities. *Neuropsychologia,* 14:471–479.

Dennis, M. (1991). Frontal lobe function in childhood and adolescence: A heuristic for assessing attention regulation, executive control, and the intentional states important for social discourse. *Developmental Neuropsychology,* 7:327–358.

______, and Barnes, M.A. (1990). Knowing the meaning, getting the point, bridging the gap, and carrying the message: Aspects of discourse following closed head injury in childhood and adolescence. *Brain and Language,* 39:428–446.

Diamond, A. (1990). Developmental time course in human infants and infant monkeys, and the neural bases of inhibitory control in reaching. *Annals of the New York Academy of Sciences,* 608:637–676.

______. (1991). Guidelines for the study of brain executive function during development. In H.S. Levin, H.M. Eisenberg, and A.L. Benton, (eds.), *Frontal lobe function and dysfunction,* pp. 338–380. Oxford University Press, New York.

DiSimoni, F. (1978). *The token test for children.* Teaching Resources, Highman, MA.

Donahue, M. (1986). Linguistic and communicative development in learning disabled children. In S.J. Ceci (ed.), *Handbook of cognitive, social and neuropsychological aspects of learning disabilities,* pp. 262–289. Erlbaum, Hillsdale, NJ.

Douglas, V.I. (1983). Attention and cognitive problems: In M. Rutter (ed.), *Developmental neuropsychiatry,* pp. 280–329. The Guilford Press, New York.

Drewe, E.A. (1974). The effect of type and area of brain lesion on Wisconsin Card Sorting Test performance. *Cortex,* 10:159–170.

Dupuy, T.R., McCarney, D., and Greenberg, L.M. (1990). *T.O.V.A. Manual. Test of variables of attention computer program.* Universal Attention Disorders (U.A.D.), Los Alamitos, CA.

Eakin, S., and Douglas, V.I. (1971). "Automatization" and oral reading problems in children. *Journal of Learning Disabilities,* 4:31–38.

Edelman, G.M., and Mountcastle, V.B. (1978). *The mindful brain.* MIT Press, Cambridge, MA.

Eslinger, P.J., and Damasio, A.R. (1985). Severe disturbance of higher cognition after bilateral frontal ablation: Patient EVR. *Neurology,* 35:1731–1741.

Fodor, G. (1983). *The modularity of the mind: An essay on faculty psychology.* Bradford/MIT Press, Cambridge, MA.

Gardner, H.G. (1983). *Frames of mind: The theory of multiple intelligences.* Basic Books, New York.

Golden, C.J. (1975). The measurement of creativity by the Stroop Color and Word Test. *Journal of Personality Assessment,* 39:386–388.

______. (1976). Identification of brain disorders by the Stroop Color and Word Test. *Journal of Clinical Psychology,* 32:621.

______. (1978). *Manual for the Stroop Color and Word Test.* Stoetling, Chicago.

Goldman, R., Fristoe, M., and Woodcock, R. (1970). *Goldman-Fristoe-Woodcock Test of Auditory Discrimination.* American Guidance Service, Circle Pines, MN.

______, ______, and ______. (1974). *Goldman-Fristoe-Woodcock Auditory Memory Tests.* American Guidance Service, Circle Pines, MN.

Gordon Diagnostic System. (1988). *Model III instruction manual.* Author, DeWitt, New York.

Grant, D., and Berg, E. (1948). A behavioral analysis of degree of impairment and ease of shifting to new responses in a Weigl-type card sorting problem. *Journal of Experimental Psychology,* 39:404–411.

Greenberg, L.M. (1987). An objective measure of

methylphenidate response: Clinical use of the M.C.A. (Minnesota Computer Assessment). *Psychopharmacology Bulletin,* 23:279–282.

______, and Waldman, I.D. (1993). Developmental normative data on the Test of Variables of Attention (T.O.V.A.). *Journal of Child Psychology and Psychiatry,* 34:1019–1030.

Hooper, H.E. (1958). *The Hooper Visual Organization Test: Manual.* Western Psychological Services, Beverly Hills, CA.

Johnson, M. H., and Karmiloff-Smith, A. (1992). Can neural selectionism be applied to cognitive developmental disorders? *New Ideas in Psychology,* 10:35–46.

Kagan, J. (1966). Reflection-impulsivity: The generality and dynamics of conceptual tempo. *Journal of Abnormal Psychology,* 71:17–24.

Kaplan, E.F., Goodglass, H., and Weintraub, S. (1978). *The Boston Naming Test: Experimental edition.* Lea and Febiger, Philadelphia.

______, ______, and ______. (1983). *The Boston Naming Test (2nd ed.)* Lea and Febiger, Philadelphia.

Karmiloff-Smith, A. (1992). *Beyond modularity: A developmental perspective on cognitive science.* MIT Press, Cambridge, MA.

Kasari, C., Sigman, M., Mundy, P., and Yirmiya, N. (1990). Affect sharing in the context of joint attention interactions of normal, autistic and mentally retarded children. *Journal of Autism and Developmental Disorders,* 20:87–100.

Kaufman, A.S., and Kaufman, N.L. (1983). *Kaufman Assessment Battery for Children.* American Guidance Service, Circle Pines, MN.

Kovacs, M. (1985). The Children's Depression Inventory. In J. Rapoport, C.K. Conners, and N. Reatig (eds.), Rating scales and assessment instruments for use in pediatric psychopharmacology research. *Psychopharmacology Bulletin,* 21:995–998.

Lambert, N., Nihiri, K., and Leland, H. (1993). *AAMR Adaptive Behavior Scales—School.* PRO-ED, Austin, TX.

Leiter, R.G. (1948). *Leiter International Performance Scale.* Stoelting Co., Chicago.

Levin, H.S., Benton, A.L., and Grossman, R.G. (1982). *Neurobehavioral consequences of closed head injury.* Oxford University Press, New York.

______, Culhane, K.A., Hartmann, J., Evankovich, K., and Mattson, A.J. (1991). Developmental changes in performance on tests of purported frontal lobe functioning. *Developmental Neuropsychology,* 7:377–395.

Lezak, M.D. (1983). *Neuropsychological assessment,* 2nd ed. Oxford University Press, New York.

______. (1988). IQ R.I.P. *Journal of Clinical and Experimental Neuropsychology,* 10:351–361.

Mandler, J.M., and Johnson, N.S. (1977). Remembrance of things parsed: Story structure and recall. *Cognitive Psychology,* 9:111–151.

Maratsos, M. (1992). Constraints, modules, and domain specificity. In M.R. Gunnar and M. Maratsos (eds.), *Modularity and constraints in language and cognition.* Erlbaum, Hillsdale, NJ.

Mattis, S. (1992). Neuropsychological assessment of school-aged children. In I. Rapin and S.J. Segalowitz (eds.), *Handbook of neuropsychology,* Vol. 6. Elsevier Science Publishers B.V., Holland.

Mercer, J.R. (1977). *System of multicultural pluralistic assessment.* Psychological Corp., New York.

Merritt, D.D., and Liles, B.Z. (1989). Narrative analysis: Clinical applications of story generation and story retelling. *Journal of Speech and Hearing Disorders,* 54:429–438.

Milner, B. (1963). Effects of different brain lesions on card sorting. *Archives of Neurology,* 9:90–100.

______. (1964). Some effects of frontal lobectomy in man. In J.M. Warren and K. Akert (eds.), *The frontal granular cortex and behavior,* pp. 313–334. McGraw-Hill, New York.

Nelson, K. (1986). *Event knowledge: Structure and function in development.* Erlbaum, Hillsdale, NJ.

Nihiri, K., Leland, H., and Lambert, N. (1993). *AAMR Adaptive Behavior Scales—Residential and Community.* PRO-ED, Austin, TX.

O'Connor, N., and Hermelin, B. (1987). Visual and graphic abilities of the idiot savant artist. *Psychological Medicine,* 17:79–90.

Osterrieth, P.A. (1944). Le test de copie d'une figure complexe (Rey). *Archives de Psychologie,* 30:206–356.

Ozonoff, S., Pennington, B.F., and Rogers, S.J. (1991). Executive function deficits in high functioning autistic children: Relationship to theory of mind. *Journal of Child Psychology and Psychiatry,* 32:1081–1105.

Passler, M.A., Isaac, W., and Hynd, G.W. (1985). Neuropsychological development of behavior attributed to frontal lobe functioning in children. *Developmental Neuropsychology,* 1:349–371.

Pennington, B.F. (1991). *Diagnosing learning disorders,* pp. 3–22. The Guilford Press, New York.

______, Johnson, C., and Welsh, M.C. (1987). Unexpected reading precocity in a normal preschooler: Implications for hyperlexia. *Brain and Cognition,* 30:165–180.

Perret, E. (1974). The left frontal lobe of man and the suppression of habitual responses in verbal categorical behavior. *Neuropsychologia,* 12:323.

Poznanski, E.O., Freeman, L.N., and Moqros, H.B.

(1985). Children's Depression Rating Scale-Revised. In J. Rapoport, C.K. Conners, and N. Reatig (eds.), Rating scales and assessment instruments for use in pediatric psychopharmacological research. *Psychopharmacology Bulletin,* 21:979–989.

Prior, M., and Hoffman, W. (1990). Brief report: Neuropsychological testing of autistic children through an exploration of frontal lobe tests. *Journal of Autism and Developmental Disorders,* 20:581–589.

Prutting, C., and Kirchner, D. (1987). A clinical appraisal of the pragmatic aspects of language. *Journal of Speech and Hearing Disorders,* 52:105–119.

Purvis, K.L., Schachar, R., and Tannock, R. (in press). Comparative analysis of narrative language abilities in boys with attention deficit hyperactivity disorder and learning disabilities. *Journal of Abnormal Child Psychology.*

Rapin, I., and Segalowitz, S.J. (1992). Child neuropsychology: Nature and scope. In I. Rapin and S.J. Segalowitz (vol. eds.), *Handbook of neuropsychology: Vol. 6. Child Neuropsychology.* Elsevier Science Publishers, New York.

Reitan, R.M. (1958). Validity of the Trail Making Test as an indication of organic brain damage. *Perceptual and Motor Skills,* 8:271–276.

______, and Davidson, L.A. (eds.). (1974). *Clinical neuropsychology: Current status and applications.* Halstead, New York.

Rey, A. (1941). L'examen psychologique dans les cas d'encephalopathie traumatique. *Archives de Psychologie,* 28:286–340.

______. (1964). *L'examen clinique en psychologie.* Presse Universitaire de France, Paris.

Richardson, E., and DiBenedetto, B. (1985). *Decoding Skills Test.* York Press, Parkton, MD.

Robinson, A.L., Heaton, R.K., Lehman, R.A.W., and Stilson, D.W. (1980). The utility of the Wisconsin Card Sorting Test in detecting and localizing frontal lobe lesions. *Journal of Consulting and Clinical Psychology,* 48:605–614.

Ross, E.D. (1985). Modulation of affect and nonverbal communication by the right hemisphere. In M.M. Mesulam (ed.), *Principles of behavioral neurology.* F.A. Davis Co., Philadelphia.

Rosvold, H.E., Mirsky, A.T., Sarason, I., Bronsome, E.D., and Beck, L.H. (1956). A continuous performance test of brain damage. *Journal of Consulting Psychology,* 20:343–350.

Ruff, R., Light, R., and Evans, R. (1987). The Ruff Figural Fluency Test: A normative study with adults. *Developmental Neuropsychology,* 3:37–51.

Ryalls, J. (1988). Concerning right hemisphere dominance for affective language. *Archives of Neurology,* 45:337–339.

Salkind, N.J., and Nelson, C.F. (1980). A note on the nature of reflection-impulsivity. *Developmental Psychology,* 6:237–238.

Semel, E., Wiig, E., and Secord, W. (1987). *Clinical Evaluation of Language Fundamentals-Revised. Examiner's manual.* The Psychological Corporation, New York.

Sparrow, S.S., and Carter, A.S. (1992). Mental retardation: Current issues related to assessment. In I. Rapin and S.J. Segalowitz (vol. eds.), *Handbook of neuropsychology: Vol. 6. Child neuropsychology,* pp. 439–452. Elsevier Science Publishers, New York.

______, Balla, D.A., and Cicchetti, D.V. (1984). *Vineland Adaptive Behavior Scales.* American Guidance Service, Circle Pines, MN.

Spreen, O. (1988). Foreword. In M.G. Tramontana and S.R. Hooper (eds.), *Assessment issues in child neuropsychology.* Plenum Press, New York.

______, and Strauss, S. (1991). *A compendium of neuropsychological tests: Administration, norms, and commentary.* Oxford University Press, New York.

______, and ______. (1991). Trail-making Test. In *A compendium of neurological tests: Administration, norms, and commentary,* pp. 320–331. Oxford University Press, New York.

Stanovich, K.E., Nathan, R.G., and Vala-Rossi, M. (1986). Developmental changes in the cognitive correlates of reading ability and the developmental lag hypothesis. *Reading Research Quarterly,* 21:267–283.

______, ______, and Zolman, J.E. (1988). The developmental lag hypothesis in reading: Longitudinal and matched reading-level comparisons. *Child Development,* 59:71–86.

Stein, N.L., and Glenn, C.G. (1979). An analysis of story comprehension in elementary school children. In R.O. Freedle (ed.), *New directions in discourse processing,* pp. 53–120. Ablex, Norwood, NJ.

______, and ______. (1982). Children's concept of time: The development of a story schema. In W. Friedman (ed.), *The developmental psychology of time,* pp. 255–282. Academic Press, New York.

Stroop, J.R. (1935). Studies of inferences in serial verbal reaction. *Journal of Experimental Psychology,* 18:643–662.

Tannock, R., Purvis, K.L., and Schachar, R.J. (1993). Narrative abilities in children with attention deficit hyperactivity disorder and normal peers. *Journal of Abnormal Child Psychology,* 21:103–117.

Thorum, A.R. (1980). *The Fullerton Language Test*

of Adolescents. Consulting Psychological Press, Palo Alto, CA.

Tramontana, M.G., and Hooper, S.R. (eds.). (1988). *Assessment issues in child neuropsychology.* Plenum Press, New York.

Tranel, D. (1992). Neuropsychological assessment. *Psychiatric Clinics of North America,* 15:283–299.

Vellutino, F.R., and Scanlon, D.M. (1987a). Linguistic coding and reading ability. In S. Rosenberg (ed.), *Advances in applied psycholinguistics,* Vol. 2, pp. 1–6. Cambridge University Press, New York.

______, and ______. (1987b). Phonological coding, phonological awareness, and reading ability: Evidence from longitudinal and experimental studies. *Merrill-Palmer Quarterly,* 33:321–363.

Voeller, K.K.S. (1986). Right hemisphere deficit syndrome in children. *American Journal of Psychiatry,* 143:1006–1009.

Waber, D.P., and Holmes, J.M. (1985). Assessing children's copy productions of the Rey-Osterrieth complex figure. *Journal of Clinical and Experimental Neuropsychology,* 7:264–280.

______, Mann, M.B., and Merola, J. (1985). Motor overflow and attentional processes in normal school-age children. *Developmental Medicine and Child Neurology,* 27:491–497.

Wechsler, D. (1991). *Wechsler Intelligence Scale for Children (WISC-III).* The Psychological Corporation, San Antonio, TX.

Weintraub, S., and Mesulam, M.M. (1985). Mental state assessment of young and elderly adults in behavioral neurology. In M.M. Mesulam (ed.), *Principles of behavioral neurology,* pp. 71–123. F.A. Davis, Philadelphia.

Welsh, M.C., and Pennington, B.F. (1988). Assessing frontal lobe functioning in children: Views from developmental psychology. *Developmental Neuropsychology* 4:199–230.

______, and ______. (1992). A critical evaluation of the current and potential applications of disc-transfer tasks to clinical and experimental neuropsychology. *Journal of Clinical and Experimental Neuropsychology,* 14:84.

______, ______, and Groisser, D.B. (1991). A normative-developmental study of executive function: A window on prefrontal function in children: *Developmental Neuropsychology,* 7:131–149.

Wiig, E., and Secord, W. (1985). *Test of Language Competence.* The Psychological Corporation, San Antonio, TX.

______, and ______. (1989). *Test of Language Competence- Expanded Edition. Technical Manual, Level 1 and Level 2.* The Psychological Corporation, San Antonio, TX.

______, and Semel, E. (1987). *Word association subtest, Clinical Evaluation of Language Function-Revised (CELF-R).* Charles E. Merrill, Columbus, OH.

Wirt, R.D., Lachar, D. Klinedinst, J.K., and Seat, P.D. (1984). *Multidimensional Description of Child Personality: A Manual for the Personality Inventory for Children-Revised.* Western Psychological Services, Los Angeles, CA.

Wolf, M. (1984). Naming, reading, and the dyslexias: A longitudinal overview. *Annals of Dyslexia,* 34:87–115.

Woodcock, R.W. (1984). *Woodcock-Johnson Proficiency Battery.* D.L.M. Teaching Resources, Allen, TX.

______, and Mather, N. (1989). *Woodcock-Johnson Tests of Achievement.* D.L.M. Teaching Resources, Allen, TX.

Yamdori, A., Osumi, Y., Tabuchi, M., Mori, E., Yoshida, T., Ohkawa, S., and Yoneda, Y. (1990). Hyperlalia: A right hemisphere syndrome. *Behavioural Neurology,* 3:143–151.

Young, J.Z. (1965). Organization of a memory system. Croonian Lecture. *Proceedings of the Royal Society of London,* B163, 285–320.

APPENDIX 1

Neuropsychological Testing: Case Illustration

The following case illustrates how neuropsychological tests can be used to identify developmental cognitive problems in a school-aged child. Test findings may be utilized in establishing an intervention program. In this case, the neurodevelopmental examination was carried out, and visual memory, spatial orientation, visual perception, language function and word fluency, selective attention, and executive functions were assessed.

Statement of Concern

Consultation was requested by the patient's parents because of poor frustration tolerance, impulsivity, and boredom.

Present Illness

This is an 8-year-old boy who, at age 4, was noted to be inattentive, demanding, and impulsive. As he has grown older, these problems have persisted. The patient has problems following routines that include dressing in the morning and completing chores. In school, he has difficulty concentrating, completing tasks, remembering what to do and when, remaining seated and, in addition, has problems in handwriting. Although the oldest of three children, he is the nost demanding of his mother's time and requires continuous redirection. In a group setting, he shows poor attention to task and is not "tuned in" to games. He is currently described as a perfectionist who becomes frustrated with his own imperfections.

Past History

The patient is the product of a full-term pregnancy. His presentation was breach and required Cesarean section. Birth weight was 8 lbs. The Apgar score at 5 minutes was 9. There was some difficulty in nursing, and poor coordination was noted in the early years of life, but no particular concerns were raised until age 4. In the preschool years, he had difficulty in coordination when riding a tricycle and problems with cutting, pasting, and color recognition milestones in kindergarten. He was also noted to have delays in articulation and to drool.

Contacts with peers have been limited, and only at age 8 did he begin to make friends. He is said to be a poor role model for his younger siblings because he becomes overly activated when stressed and is noncompliant with demands.

Family History

The patient's mother indicates that she was easily distracted and overly talkative in school. She continues to have difficulty with organizational skills and reports problems in concentration. Because of her school-related problems, she did not go further than high school. The maternal grandfather has the diagnoses of Tourette's disorder, obsessive-compulsive disorder, and bipolar disorder. There is no history of learning or psychiatric problems on the paternal side of the family. Both parents were enuretic until elementary school.

Interview with the Child

When interviewed, this 8-year-old acknowledged trouble concentrating, restlessness, and poor self-control. He indicated he has difficulty managing angry feelings and is periodically anxious and sad about his parents' criticism of his behavior. He does not report any abnormal mental experiences.

Neurodevelopmental Examination

On the neurodevelopmental examination, he shows choreiform hand movements, slow finger sequencing, tremor, and developmental overflow on heel, toe, and tandem gait tasks. Drooling is noted when he is asked to move his tongue from side to side.

Clinical Correlation

The choreiform movements and slow finger sequencing may correlate to the motor skill aspects of handwriting. His problems in motoric movement may be correlated with poor control over mental processes.

Neuropsychological Testing

Visual Memory

Visual memory was tested using the Benton Visual Retention Test. Scoring was at the 11th percentile, which is average for a child between 6½ and 7. Performance was poor but may potentially have been contaminated by the attentional demands needed for this visual memory task.

Judgment of Spatial Orientation

The patient became fatigued on the Test of Spatial Orientation but was able to score in the low-average range within 1 standard deviation of the norms for age 8.

Visual Perception

On the Facial Recognition Test, he scored in the average range for his age.

Visuomotor Integration

On the Berry Test of Visuomotor Integration, he showed poor line quality, which may be linked to motor difficulties with sequencing and his tremor. Graphomotor problems were suggested by these findings. His best score was at the 7-year, 11-month level.

Visual Memory and Planning

The Rey-Osterrieth Complex Figure was used. In copying the figure, his organizational ability was less than the 5-year level. Immediate recall was below the 6-year level, and delayed recall was average for a 6-year-old. However, his organization for delayed recall was at age level, although the copy that was made was disorganized. His difficulty in organization was attributed to problems in attention and difficulty in planning. The details of the complex figure were apparently lost due to inattention.

Language

Language tests included the Clinical Evaluation of Language Function (CELF), syntax comprehension, naming pictured items, rapid automatized naming, and word fluency (animals/foods).

Listening was poor, but his overall language was a strength. Sentence syntax comprehension was at the 8-year level, which was age appropriate. His best language skills were demonstrated on the Boston Naming Test where he scored at the 12th-grade level. Word fluency was particularly good, with scoring at the 15-year level. Verbal learning was excellent, although problems in comprehension related to listening were a handicap.

Scores on receptive language were discrepantly poor but were most probably linked to poor listening skills.

Selective Attention

On the test of cancellation of targeted items, his visual search was poor. He approached the task in a disorganized and random way but was able to be successful within normal limits on two out of three challenges. When numbers were used, however, he vocalized the number he was searching for and had to be asked to stop the test after 6 minutes, yet he still made three errors.

On the Test of Variables of Attention (TOVA), he was slow but was able to perform at age level on the commission and omission sections; however, his variability score was in the clinical range.

Conclusion

The history, neurodevelopmental examination, and neuropsychological testing are consistent with a verbally gifted 8-year-old with attention deficit/hyperactivity disorder who has difficulty listening and visually attending. The testing is consistent with severe organizational problems in the visual domain. Moreover, he has graphomotor problems that require compensation. The use of a computer for any extended writing that involves more than simple one-word or one-number responses is recommended.

The testing demonstrates executive function difficulties in regard to selective attention, organization, and planning. His disorganization in following through on requests and completing tasks requires a structured behavioral program at home so he can didactically be taught the organization skills he lacks. In addition to behavior management, pharmacotherapy with stimulant medication is recommended. The recommended dose is 0.3 mg/kg. After he is stabilized on this dose of medication, the TOVA should be repeated to see if his variability score is normalized. An additional test that may be performed to assess his narrative ability is the story retelling task, which should also be completed on and off medication.

APPENDIX 2

COMMONLY USED TESTS AND INSTRUMENTS

Adaptive Behavior

A description of adaptive behavior is intrinsic to all definitions of mental retardation that require significantly subnormal functions in both intelligence and adaptive behavior to establish the diagnosis. For both mentally retarded and nonretarded children, the Revised Vineland Adaptive Behavior Scale (Sparrow, Balla, and Cicchetti, 1984) is most commonly used. For mentally retarded persons, the American Association of Mental Retardation (AAMR) Adaptive Behavior Scales (Lambert, Nihiri, and Leland, 1993; Nihiri, Leland, and Lambert, 1993) have been developed. Moreover, the System of Multicultural Pluralistic Assessment (SOMPA) (Mercer, 1977) includes an adaptive behavior inventory for children as part of a comprehensive assessment and stresses culture fairness.

Personality

Personality Inventory for Children (PIC). The Personality Inventory for Children (PIC) (Wirt et al., 1984) is a true-false statement questionnaire that is completed by parents and is similar to the Minnesota Multiphasic Personality Inventory (MMPI). In the full-range version, there are 600 statements, including items such as, "My child has little self-confidence." The revised format allows scoring of four broad factor dimensions of childhood psychopathology (externalizing behavior, internalizing behavior, social incompetence, and cognitive dysfunction) that are based on the first 131 items (Part I only). The first 280 items (Part I and II) allow scoring of abbreviations of the 4 dimensions and 12 clinical scales. The 12 clinical scales include achievement, intellectual skills, development, somatic concerns, depression, family relations, delinquency, withdrawal, anxiety, psychosis, hyperactivity, and social skills. The use of additional items for Part III allows scoring of all scales in full, whereas the entire 600 items are used when research scales are included.

It is recommended that the Personality Inventory for Children be filled out by both parents independently and that the 280-item or 421-item version be used. Computer scoring is available. If the full-length version is used (600 items), several research scales may be scored, including the Louisville Behavior Checklist (LBC) and the Piers-Harris Children's Self-Concept Scale (PHCSC). It is important to keep in mind that the Personality Inventory for Children is not designed to detect neurological impairment in children. It reflects the parents' perceptions of the child's problems and is not a direct measure of the child's difficulties. It should be used as a supplement to parent interviews and as a screening instrument to demonstrate areas of parental concern and potential emotional and behavior problems. A hyperactivity scale can be derived to assist in the diagnosis of attention deficit/hyperactivity disorder.

Attention/Inhibition

The WISC-III (Wechsler, 1991). Freedom from distractibility factor, or cluster, i.e., arithmetic, digit span, and coding subtests, may serve as measures of both span and variability of attention. This profile of subtests is used to determine if a child shows a consistent pattern of weakness because they are known to be sensitive to interference from attentional difficulties.

Specific tests designed to measure attention and concentration include the computer vigilance tests, discussed next.

Continuous Performance Tests (CPT). The CPT was first found to be a useful attentional measure in adults (Rosvold et al., 1956) and is now widely used for children because of the availability of personal computers. There are many continuous performance tests that use a variety of stimuli. CPTs are primarily regarded as a measure of sustained attention, although they are also sensitive to visual recognition and short-term memory. These tests are used extensively with children diagnosed with attention deficit disorder (ADD) and require about 20 minutes to complete. Such tests have been successful in discriminating children with ADD from normal controls (Douglas, 1983) and in detecting the effects of stimulant medications on children with ADD (Barkley, 1977). In a typical CPT test, the stimuli consist of alphabetic characters displayed for 50 msec and have an interstimulus interval of 1.0 seconds. In one version, the task consists of two segments: an "X" target and a "BX" target. The subject presses a hand-held reaction time button whenever he or she detects an "X." In the second phase, the button is pressed whenever he or she detects an "X" that has been preceded by a "B." Dependent variables consist of hits, errors of omission, errors of commission, and reaction time. However, there are many versions of the CPT, especially because computers have made administration and scoring easily available. For example, the Conners' (Conners, 1994) CPT program presents the CPT results on the computer screen directly after the administration. The user can print a report that includes a table of results, graphs, and interpretative guidelines. This program offers a unique mode where the respondent presses the key for any letter *except* the X. Some tests are not alphabetic.

Vigilance Subtest of the Gordon Diagnostic System. In this test (Gordon Diagnostic System, 1988), a series of numbers is shown on a video monitor and the child must press a button when certain numbers appear. The vigilance task performance is computed electronically over a series of trial blocks that allow a temporal dimension for performance; norms are available for 4- to 16-year-old children.

Test of Variables of Attention (TOVA) Computer Program (Dupuy, McCarney, and Greenberg, 1990). The TOVA is a visual continuous performance test that was specifically developed for use in screening and diagnosing the treatment of neurologically based attentional deficits and in monitoring treatment of attention deficits in children and adults. This is a nonlanguage-based 22½-minute fixed interval computerized test with no left-right discrimination that has negligible practice effects. In this test, two easily discriminated visual stimuli, i.e., a colored square containing a very small square adjacent to the top or bottom edge, are presented to the subject for 100 milliseconds every 2 seconds. The designated target stimulus is the inner square adjacent to the top edge. The target is presented on 22.5% and 77.5% of the trials during the first and second halves, respectively. The TOVA indices include omission and commission errors, response time means, and anticipatory reponses. An added feature of the TOVA is that it is an excellent "go/no go" test.

The first TOVA variable includes errors of omission. This refers to failure to respond to the target, and such failures are interpreted as a measure of inattention. The second variable is errors of commission. This refers to responding inappropriately to the nontarget, which is interpreted as a measure of impulsivity. The third variable is mean correct response times, which are interpreted to measure processing and response time. In addition, standard deviations of response times are interpreted as a measure of consistency or variability. Anticipatory responses, i.e., those made before the two stimuli can be differentiated, are used to determine whether or not instructions are being followed. Finally, postcommission mean correct response times, which refer to the mean times of correct responses immediately following a commission error, are calculated and may help to differentiate children with attention deficits from those with conduct disorder (TOVA Manual, Dupuy, McCarney, and Greenberg, 1990). The TOVA variables are reported to differentiate children with attention deficit disorders from normal individuals and to measure responses to methylphenidate (Greenberg, 1987). Greenberg and Waldman (1993) collected developmental normative data for 775 (377 boys, 398 girls) children aged 6 to 16 and found that attention and impulse control developed in a nonlinear manner, changing rapidly in the early years of childhood and leveling off during later childhood and adolescence. The percentage of anticipation errors, however, decreased linearly with age. Sex differences were present on TOVA indices, especially for younger children. Although sustained attention and impulse control may develop later in males than females, the developmental course for these capacities seemed similar for both sexes.

Memory

Verbal Memory

Woodcock-Johnson Psychoeducational Battery-Revised. This test includes subtests for short-term memory (memory for repeat sentences of increasing length and complexity) and long-term retrieval (visual-auditory learning). On this simulated reading test, the child is taught the labels for a series of symbols that are then arranged in sentences. Both visual and auditory cuing are provided during instruction and feedback is provided when errors are made. Subtests of the Stanford-Binet may also be used to assess short-term memory.

Recognition Memory Test (Goldman, Fristoe, and Woodcock, 1974). Working memory is a system for the temporary holding and manipulation of information while carrying out cognitive tasks. It involves simultaneous processing of incoming material and its integration with other information. One commonly used measure of working memory is the Recognition Memory Test, which requires judgments about the prior occurrence of target words. The subject indicates whether, in the current session, they have heard items on a word list.

In children, areas of memory undergoing research investigation include event memory and eyewitness memory (Nelson, 1986).

Selective Reminding Paradigm

Word List Learning. The Selective Reminding Paradigm developed by Buschke (Buschke and Fuld, 1974) can be employed both as a measure of semantic memory and a measure of executive functioning. The test takes 20 minutes to administer. Stimuli for this task are six concrete and six abstract words. At the outset of the task, the child is told he or she will hear a list of words and to try to remember them. There are 2-second intervals between words as they are presented during list presentation on all trials. The child is subsequently reminded (selective reminding) of only those words he or she forgot to say on the immediately preceding trial. Testing is discontinued if the child reaches a criterion of three completely correct trials. A variety of scores are derived from this task that are designed to contrast storage in versus retrieval from long-term memory and consistent versus random retrieval from long-term storage. Perseverations (repetitions of the same words recalled during free recall trials) and intrusions (words never said) are scored.

The Rey Auditory Verbal Learning Test (RAVLT) (Rey, 1964). This test is used to assess verbal learning and memory. The RAVLT is a brief paper-and-pencil measure used to assess immediate memory span, new learning, susceptibility to interference, and recognition memory. The test consists of 15 nouns that are read aloud with a 1-second interval between each word for five consecutive trials, and each trial is followed by a free recall test. At the end of trial 5, an interference list of 15 words is presented, followed by a free recall test of that list. Immediately afterward, delayed recall of the first list of words is tested without further presentation of the words. Following a 20-minute delay, the individual subject is again requested to recall the words from the first list. Finally, a story that includes all of the words from List A, the first list, is presented and the individual subject must identify the words recognized from the first list. An individual with a generalized memory deficit will perform poorly on both free recall and recognition trials. The time required for administration is 10 to 15 minutes. Information from the test may be used to differentiate clinically among different memory disorders.

The California Verbal Learning Test (CVLT) (Delis et al., 1987). This is a verbal memory process test that provides information on learning and memory by measuring encoding strategy, learning rate, error types (intrusions, perseverations), and other process data. It involves multitrial verbal (word list) learning. The CVLT is a five-trial learning of 15 items (all items spoken by the examiner and retrieved immediately thereafter per trial) followed by a distractor list presented in the same manner. This is followed by a short-delay free and cued recall, and 20 minutes later, by long-delay free and cued recall, and finally by a recognition trial. It provides mean scores for long- and short-term delay. Data analysis provides information on verbal memory, and through cluster analysis on performance, this test also provides information that is useful for evaluating executive functioning.

Visual Memory

Benton Test of Visual Retention–Administration A (Benton, 1974). In this test, there are ten cards, the first presents one figure, and the others present three geometric figures. Each card is presented for 10 seconds, removed, and the child is asked to reproduce the designs from memory. There are two recognition memory variants of this task; in one, a card is presented for 5 seconds and removed and the child is asked to select the target from among four alternatives. In the other variant, the target is presented for 10 seconds and removed and a 15-second delay is imposed before the child is asked to detect the target from among the alternatives. The 5-second exposure is more heavily loaded for attentional factors and the 15-second delay for memory processes (Mattis, 1992).

The Rey-Osterrieth Complex Figure Test. This task measures visual-constructional ability, visual nonverbal memory following delay, and planning strategy in the completion of a complex figure drawing task. It was developed by Rey (1941) and elaborated by Osterrieth (1944). This copying test was originally designed to evaluate perceptual organization and visual memory in brain-damaged subjects (Rey, 1941; Osterrieth, 1944). The procedure is to have the subject copy the complex design; the examiner provides the subject successively with 5 or 6 colored pencils to use as the examiner monitors the strategy used in completing the figure. The figure is structured around a base rectangle that is, in turn, divided into eight equal segments by a horizontal, a vertical, and two diagonal lines; it includes internal and external detailed features. By handing the child a different colored pencil each time he has completed a section of the drawing, the examiner can analyze each epoch of copying in sequence. Organization, style, perceptual accuracy, and motor planning quality can be evaluated (Waber and Holmes, 1985). After an interval where another task is given, recall (with a single standard pencil) is requested. The difference between copy and recall, by item and by placement, yields a score, and memory organization is scored. Immediate, 3-minute, or delayed (30 to 45 minutes) recall may be tested. Two scores are generally derived, the copy accuracy score and the percentage of total time required for the subject to complete the figure. A recall score and a constructional score are measured. There is no time limit on delayed recall. Both age and intellectual level contribute to performance so that recall scores increase with age until the adult levels are reached at approximately age 11.

Language

The Clinical Evaluation of Language Fundamentals-Revised (CELF-R) (Semel, Wiig, and Secord, 1987). This test focuses primarily on the acquisition of linguistic skills and rules and on the interface with auditory memory abilities. It samples circumscribed linguistic skills, such as knowledge and use of morphology, syntax, words, and concepts, and recalled spoken language. The CELF-R diagnostic battery is designed for use with children in kindergarten through grade 12. It is an individually administered battery of tests that is designed to provide measures of receptive (processing) and expressive (production) of language skills that are basic to mature language use in communication. These include word meanings (semantics), sentence structure (syntax), and recall and retrieval (memory). The CELF-R battery includes 11 subtests for measuring syntax, semantics, and memory. These subtests lead to a receptive language score and an expressive language score that vary at different ages. For 5- to 7-year-olds, the receptive language score includes the subtests of linguistic concepts, sentence structure, and oral directions, but for those 8 and over, this score is based on oral directions, word classes, and semantic relationships. Administration time for receptive language subtests is approximately 20 minutes. When there are difficulties in regard to reliability in one of these tests using these receptive language scores, an additional subtest, the Listening to Paragraphs test, can be used to replace the problematic test.

Test of Language Competence-Expanded (TLC-E) (Wiig and Secord, 1989). In contrast to the CELF-R, the TLC-E emphasizes the evaluation of linguistic and cognitive attainments that indicate growth in metalinguistic-metacognitive functions and abilities. It emphasizes the understanding of multiple meanings and intentions, the use of figurative language and context, and the creation of intentional communications based on linguistic and contextual constraints. The TLC-E subtests and other items were designed to introduce the context within which the metalinguistic abilities are applied. In testing, when auditory memory is involved, the emphasis is on evaluating the use of recall strategies rather than the interface among linguistic and memory skills.

The CELF-R and TLC-E complement each other in an assessment process. Using these tests together, an individual may perform normally on the CELF-R but be several standard deviations below the mean on the TLC-E. When this occurs, basic linguistic skills and rules, as measured by the CELF-R, are within the normal range. However, metalinguistic abilities and attainments, as measured by the TLC-E, may be reduced. In this instance, the child continues with the diagnosis of a language and learning disorder, but the focus for language services is to develop metalinguistic aspects of language and communication since the basic rules and skills are present.

Other tests that may be used to assess syntactic skills are the Token Test for Children (DiSimoni, 1978), the Grammaticality Judgment Test (Vellutino and Scanlon, 1987a), the Fullerton Language Test for Adolescents (Thorum, 1980), and Pragmatic Analysis testing (Prutting and Kirchner, 1987).

Boston Naming Test (BNT) (Kaplan et al., 1983). This test assesses the ability to name pictured objects. The examiner presents sixty line drawings that range from simple words with a high frequency of usage (e.g., tree) to rare words (e.g., abacus) one at a time on cards, and offers two prompting cues (phonemic, stimulus cue) if the child does not produce the word spontaneously. Credit is given for items identified correctly in 20 seconds. A total naming score is determined from adding the number of correct responses between the baseline item and the ceiling item, and then adding that total to the number of test items that precede the baseline. The tester begins with item 1 and discontinues after six consecutive failures.

Narrative

Narrative tests are not yet routinely used in clinical settings but are being actively investigated for clinical use.

In the Stein and Glenn (1979) Story Grammar, six story components are considered: (1) settings—characters' locations, or habitual context or states; (2) initiating events—actions, events, changes in the physical environment, or a character's internal perception of an event; (3) internal responses—a character's emotions, goals, desires, intentions, or thoughts leading to a planned sequence; (4) attempts—actions toward resolving a situation or achieving the goal; (5) direct consequences—actions, natural occurrences, or end states representing the character's attainment or nonattainment of a goal; and (6) reaction—how the character thinks, feels, or acts relative to the direct consequence.

Visuospatial

A comprehensive visuospatial evaluation includes the Facial Recognition Test (Benton et al., 1983b), which requires the perceptual discrimination of unfamiliar faces that are presented under different lighting conditions and at varying angles, and the Judgment of Line Orientation test (Benton et al., 1983a) where the subject identifies the angles and slopes of visually presented lines. Another test is the Hooper Visual Organization Test (Hooper, 1958) in which the subject is asked to mentally manipulate puzzle fragments to make a whole.

Facial Recognition Test (Benton et al., 1983b). This is a multiple-choice test that involves matching a sample photograph of an unfamiliar and unadorned (no hairdo, eyeglasses, facial hair) face to one of six same-sex faces; it is completed in 10 minutes. The more difficult half of the test requires more than one match to sample. This second half of the test demands matching to sample three-angled (e.g., frontal, profile) photos of the same person. Norms for a long form are available on 286 subjects, 16 to 17 years old, and on 366 children, ages 6 to 14 years. The short form product-moment correlation with the long form is r = .88 for controls. Percentile conversions are available from the long-form score and convertible by table to short-form scores. In nonaphasic patients with unilateral brain disease, right hemisphere dysfunction has been found to be associated with defective performance.

Judgment of Line Orientation (Benton et al., 1983a). On this test, the spatial relationship or angular displacement between two lines is judged in reference to a "protractorlike" half circle of lines. Thirty items (30 pairs of lines) are presented. Test time is 10 minutes. The raw score is the number of correctly judged pairs ("1 and 3," "6 and 10," etc.). Norms based on 221 children (7 years and older) are available. For child subjects, split-half reliability was reported to be 0.84 and test-retest reliability was .89. The correlation coefficient with Facial Recognition was reported to be 0.27, indicating little common variance in the perceptual capabilities assessed by these two tests. Defective performance is most highly correlated with right parietal lobe dysfunction.

Visuomotor Tests

Block Design. This WISC-III (Wechsler, 1991) subtest measures several nonverbal abilities including analytic and synthetic reasoning, nonverbal concept formation, visual-motor coordination, and visual perception of abstract stimuli. In this subtest, the child is required to manipulate red and white blocks so the top facade of the blocks form a design modeled into a two-dimensional picture. Younger or lower functioning older children form a model constructed by the examiner. Reliability for Block Design is quite high (r = .83) and is well correlated with both the Performance IQ (r = .82) and the Full Scale IQ (r = .75).

Object Assembly. This WISC-III subtest is a measure of perceptual or organizational ability, although its primary sensitivity is for abilities such as synthetic reasoning for meaningful stimuli and visual-motor coordination. This test requires the child to put together pieces of puzzles within a limited amount of time. Loading on the Perceptual Organization Factor is .65. Reliability is estimated to be r = .70 and its correlation with FSIQ is r = .77 and PIQ is r = .60.

Beery-Buktenica Test of Visual-Motor Integration (VMI). The VMI (Beery, 1967; 1982) is designed to evaluate the child's ability to produce accurately a series of simple figures after receiving conceptual assistance and practice in producing each of the figures. It measures visual/fine motor functioning while limiting any potential effects related to conceptual differences and previous learning. The child is given a chart of paper containing a long series of the three figures randomly ordered in three rows of ten figures each. Starting at the upper left-hand corner, the child is instructed to copy the series as quickly as possible and to continue until instructed to stop. The child is given as much practice and feedback as is necessary to bring him to the point where he can produce each of the figures after seeing an example. Once it is clear the child understands the task and can readily produce each of the figures correctly, the test is administered. A liberal time allotment is provided for this task so most children will finish. One point is awarded for each figure correctly produced.

Rey-Osterrieth Complex Figure. This copying test is described in detail under visual memory tests.

Social-Emotional Testing

Nonverbal Affect (Facial and Vocal Affect) Recognition Test. Nonverbal perceptual capabilities tests are presented to the child visually and auditorially (Ross, 1985; Ryalls, 1988; Voeller, 1986). Both abilities are associated with right hemisphere function and both have face validity for information processing relevant to the use and acquisition of social skills.

Test of Facial Affect Recognition (Denckla, 1993). This instrument tests the subject's ability to judge from facial expression the affective status of the face, "happy," "sad," "fearful" "angry" or "neutral." The stimuli consist of 24 black and white 8.3 × 11 cm pictures of children who are "posed" to show emotional expressions. Five pictures of the same child are displayed in a vertical row on a sheet of posterboard. The subject is asked to "point to the happy or sad/angry/frightened face." There are 24 trials, 6 for each affective state, in random order.

Executive Function Testing

Wisconsin Card Sort Test (WCST) (Berg, 1948; Grant and Berg, 1948). This is the most commonly used test for executive function in the school-aged population. It has been used for children with diagnoses of attention deficit disorder, learning disability, and pervasive developmental disorder (Ozonoff, Pennington, and Rogers, 1991). The WCST has sometimes been shown to discriminate between some samples of hyperactive children and normal control subjects. It is available for administration in both computerized and manual forms.

The WCST is a neuropsychological test that assesses the ability to form abstract concepts, sustain attention, and to shift cognitive set flexibly in response to changing conceptual rules while inhibiting inappropriate responses. It provides an assessment of organizational capacity, attention shifting, and sustained attention. The WCST is generally considered to be sensitive to frontal lobe dysfunction (Drewe, 1974; Milner, 1963, 1964). Yet its specificity for "frontal lobe" processing has been called into question (David, 1992; Eslinger and Damasio, 1985). Robinson et al. (1980) point out that executive function tests may be so complex in their task demands that they do not reflect frontal lobe dysfunction uniquely but rather the integrity of the brain as a whole.

The test consists of stimulus cards which differ on three dimensions: shape, color, and number. The subject is given a pack of cards on each of which are printed one to four of a single symbol (triangle, star, cross, or circle) in red, green, yellow, or blue. The subject is asked to sort the deck of 64 cards under one of four stimulus cards and is given feedback on accuracy after each card is placed. Correct performance is facilitated by deducing the rule of classification, which changes after every ten consecutive correct responses. Derived scores include number correct, number of errors, perseverative errors (failures to shift set in spite of "wrong" feedback), and number of categories achieved. The percentage of conceptual responses and set maintenance with the "right" feedback is also scored.

There are normative data for children between the ages of 7 and 12 (Levin et al., 1991). Test-retest reliability is problematic because once the structure of the test is understood, the awareness of the rules may be retained. Therefore, there is interest in developing alternative forms. This could lead to future use of the test as an outcome measure for interventions. Some aspects of this test, such as flexibility regarding mental models, can also be assessed in the Concept Formation Test, which is part of the Woodcock-Johnson Battery (1984). Welsh, Pennington, and Groisser (1991) report that perseverations on the WCST, under standard conditions of administration, are not correlated with intelligence scores.

Verbal Fluency. These tests consist of time-limited, category-specific retrieval of words. In one test, the Clinical Evaluation of Language Fundamentals-Revised (CELF-R) (Wiig and Semel, 1987), the task required of the child is to name as many words as he or she can think of that fit a given category (e.g., foods and animals) in a given time period. The Benton Controlled Word Association Test asks for words starting with each of three alphabet letters, and the child is given one minute to name words for each letter. The number of words the child produces in each category is totaled. The score may include an evaluation of the strategy the child uses for the test. Thus, for example, a count is made of the number of times the child names items from the same semantic category (e.g., farm animals) and how often these items occur contiguously. The number of words represented in the child's list may be divided by the number of distinct categories represented to provide an index of the tendency to use categories. Further, the Adjusted Ratio of Clustering may be used as another index of hierarchical structuring. This index evaluates the number of contiguous occurrences of examples from the same taxonomic category, relative to the number of the contiguous occurrences that would be expected by chance (based on the total number of items and the number of categories represented in output lists). Verbal fluency is developmentally sensitive; it may not be significantly correlated with verbal IQ.

Figural Fluency. In a test of figural fluency, children are asked to create as many nonsense designs as possible in a segment of 3 minutes, first under free conditions, and then fixed use conditions (4 lines). Perseverative errors as well as total correct productions are scored. Fixed condition figural fluency shows greater developmental sensitivity. The 7- to 8-year-old group has been reported to be less productive than all of the older age groups under unconstrained conditions (Levin et al., 1991). Figural fluency can be used along with verbal fluency tests because no correlation has been demonstrated with motor speed or verbal fluency (Ruff, Light, and Evans, 1987).

Disc/Ring Transfer Tasks: Tower of Hanoi (TOH). The Tower of Hanoi task involves the child in copying an observed sample of discs of different sizes and different colors that are arranged on a peg to form a tower. The planning and sequencing moves to create a matching tower must follow the rule that larger discs cannot be placed on top of smaller ones. There are six problems for the three-disc and three problems for the four-disc version (Welsh, Pennington, and Groisser, 1991). The scoring system gives points that are inversely related to the number of trials required for solution and provide a planning efficiency score. Welsh and Pennington (1992) provide a critical evaluation of the current and potential applications of disc-transfer tasks in clinical and experimental settings.

The Stroop Color and Word Test (Stroop, 1935). This is a test involving selective attention, inhibition, or interference control. "Interference control" is the term applied to the Stroop test's challenge to attend selectively while inhibiting a prepotent response. This test measures the subject's ability to shift perceptual set in response to changing demands and to concentrate selectively or attend in situations requiring inhibition of responses. Administration time is approximately 10 minutes. It has also been associated with automaticity of reading, rapid naming, and continuous performance (Golden, 1978). In the Stroop test, the material consists of three cards on which are five columns of 20 items each: (1) color names are printed in black; color names are printed in conflicting colors—i.e.,. colors other than the color names; and (2) colored "XXXX's" in four colors. For card 3, the child must name the color of the ink in which the words are printed and ignore the semantic meaning of the words (the order is critical). Separate scores are derived for reading color names, naming colors, and naming the color of ink in which a color word is printed. In addition, a "pure" interference score based on the score derived from the third trial may be computed. If children cannot read, no interference score can be derived. The test can be used for children ages 7 years and older (Diamond, 1991; Passler, Isaac, and Hynd, 1985).

The Stroop test has been found to be capable of discriminating between brain-damaged and normal controls (Golden, 1976). It is generally regarded as a useful tool in the detection of frontal lobe disorders (Perret, 1974). Reliability data with adult subjects is reported to be r = .85, .81, and .73 for each of the three stimulus cards (Golden, 1975) and r = .70 for the "pure" interference measure. Normative data also is available for the Stroop, although age corrections precede T-score calculations for subjects below the age of 17.

Trail Making Test, Forms A and B (Trails) (Army Individual Test Battery, 1944; Spreen and Strauss, 1991). The Trails Test is used to assess the ability to initiate, switch, and stop a sequence of complex intentional behavior, and attention and concentration skills. The subject is asked to draw lines to connect consecutively numbered circles on a worksheet (A) and then must connect consecutively numbered and lettered circles on a second worksheet (B) by alternating between the two sequences. Validity and reliability have been reported by Reitan (1958). Three meaures are used; number of errors on Trails B, time required to complete Trails B, and the time required to complete Trails B minus the time required to complete Trails A (Reitan and Davidson, 1974).

Matching Familiar Figures Test (MFFT). The MFFT (Kagan, 1966) is a measure of impulse control that has been used extensively in the cognitive and neuropsychological evaluation of children with attention deficit disorder. The administration time is approximately 10 minutes. In this task, the child is shown a page containing a sample picture, below which is shown six very similar pictures, only one of which is identical to the sample. The child's scores are (1) the mean time taken to the first response, and (2) the total number of incorrect responses. The procedure has been shown to discriminate children with attention deficit disorder from normal control children (Barkley, 1977). Normative data are available for ages 5 to 12 years based on a sample of more than 2,800 children (Salkind and Nelson, 1980). Golden (1978) reported that test-retest reliability coefficients for 1-week intervals ranged from r = .41 (kindergarten children) to r = .78 (fifth-grade children) for latency scores and from r = .27 (fifth-grade children) to r = .77 (second-grade children) for error scores. In a more recent version of the MFFT, test-retest reliability coefficients for a 5- week period were r = .85 and r = .77 for latency and number of errors, respectively (Cairns and Cammock, 1978). A separate research version is available for adolescents and adults.

Motor Tests (Motor Sequencing, Go/No-Go,

PANESS-R). Compromised speed and efficiency of information processing is a common manifestation of cerebral dysfunction. Tasks based on frontal lobe involvement in motor planning and response inhibition are used. Tests of motor sequencing or planning have been reviewed by Welsh, Pennington, and Groisser (1991). The motor sequencing test involves touching each of four fingers to the thumb in sequence without skipping a finger or repetitively touching a finger. The test is scored for the number of correct sequences over 10 seconds. Developmental differences were shown between 12-year-olds and adults.

CHAPTER 4

EVALUATION OF BRAIN STRUCTURE AND FUNCTIONS

The investigation of brain structure and function in the living child and adolescent is assuming increasing importance as new methods for *in vivo* imaging become available to study brain structure and function during the developmental period. In the past the study of brain pathology in childhood and adolescence required autopsy examination of the brain using macroscopic, microscopic, and biochemical methods. This approach was limited because the majority of childhood-onset disorders are not fatal and these methods of examination may be confounded by ongoing pharmacotherapy or developmental changes in the brain.

In vivo imaging studies may be complicated by the child's difficulty in cooperating with procedures that require remaining still for long periods of time, the lack of agreement on appropriate protocols for scanning children, and the potential risk of radioisotope use when carrying out *in vivo* nuclear imaging studies in the developmental period. However, advances are being made in solving these problems through the appropriate use of sedation, the establishment of protocols, and clarification of risk/benefit ratios.

The techniques that are available for *in vivo* investigations may focus on brain structure or anatomy, brain function (blood flow, metabolism, and neuroreceptors), and electrophysiologic methods. The specific techniques most commonly used include computerized transaxial tomography (CT), magnetic resonance imaging (MRI), single photon emission computerized tomography (SPECT), positron emission tomography (PET), computerized electroencephalography (CEEG) and evoked response potential (see Table 4–1).

The first part of this chapter describes each of these techniques and discusses their advantages and disadvantages. Their application to specific childhood and adolescent-onset disorders is discussed in the chapters that deal with specific conditions. The second part of the chapter deals with event-related potentials (ERPs). Applications of the ERP technique are described in more detail because this methodology has been applied extensively to study neurodevelopmental disorders.

COMPUTERIZED TRANSAXIAL TOMOGRAPHY (CT)

The discovery of X-rays by Roentgen in 1895 made it possible, for the first time, to visualize the interior of the body. However, the visualization of soft tissue overlaid by bone could not be accomplished until the 1970s when the computerized tomography scanner was introduced by Godfrey Hounsfield (1973). Computerized transaxial tomography (CT) technology makes it possible to examine the entire brain *in vivo*. Prior to that time, imaging of the brain was carried out with skull films and ventricular pneumoencephalography, methods that provide less clear resolution of brain structures. The first

Table 4–1. Brain-Imaging Techniques

1. Structural techniques (to study brain structure and anatomy)
   a. Computed tomography (CT)
   b. Magnetic resonance imaging (MRI) (Nuclear magnetic resonance, NMR)
2. Functional/dynamic techniques (to study brain metabolism and regional change in brain activity and neurotransmitter systems and reuptake sites)
   a. Single photon emission computerized tomography (SPECT)
   b. Positron emission tomography (PET)
   c. Quantitative electrophysiology (computerized mapping of the electrical activity of the brain)
   d. Evoked response potential

Adapted from Lewis, 1991.

images produced by Hounsfield in the 1960s required 9 days to acquire the data and 2.5 hours to construct the image (Primack, Chiles, and Putman, 1992). By 1972 the acquisition of a single slice from a head scanner took about 8 minutes. Currently, a single slice acquisition may take only 1 second.

CT scanning utilizes X-rays and is based on the fact that various types of tissue attenuate the passage of X-rays to different degrees. CT utilizes standard X-rays that are passed through the head in a narrow beam and are directed at many different angles. Special radiation sensors located within the CT scanner generate an electrical impulse that is proportional to the intensity of the X-ray at that particular detecting point. The intensity that is registered depends on penetrance and attenuation that is caused by different tissues, such as the white matter and gray matter, and by bony structures and fluids. The electrical impulses generated by these detectors are digitized using a computer. The digitization allows energy values to be coded as numbers that are used to reconstruct the image. CT is used to image one slice or section of the area studied at a time so that through a sequence of one-dimensional projections, two-dimensional cross-sectioned images are produced. The computer is used to back calculate the density of brain tissue and reconstruct an image that allows identification of gray and white matter, bone, blood, cerebral spinal fluid, and pathological lesion areas. The X-rays go through just the desired slice or section thickness, and neighboring anatomy is not shown. Sections may be as thin as 1.0 to 2.0 mm. The images produced by CT are serial, cross-sectional views of the brain. Contrast material may be injected intravenously to evaluate blood vessels and the blood-brain barrier. The most recent development in CT is three-dimensional (3D) CT, which is used to reconstruct data from very thin slices. A typical X-ray computed tomography scanner is shown in Figure 4–1.

As shown in the figure, the CT scanner has seven components: a sliding patient table, a gantry, an X-ray source and collimating assembly, a data acquisition/detector system, a computer system, and a display and analysis console. The collimator is used to focus the X-ray beam on the body area being studied.

The CT technique is used to study central

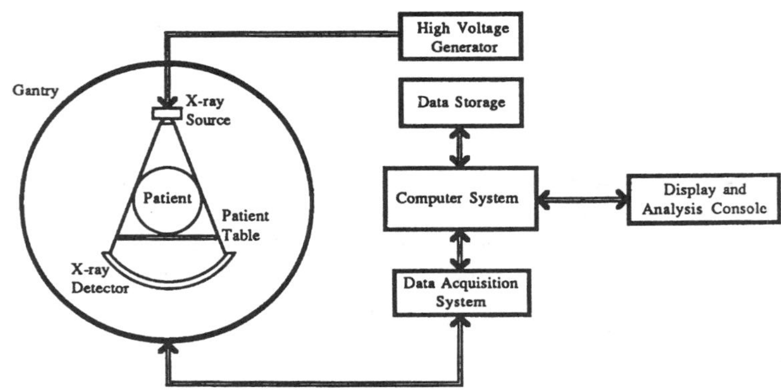

Figure 4–1. A typical X-ray computed tomographic scanner (from Stytz and Frieder, 1990).

Table 4–2. Computerized Transaxial Tomography (CT)

1. Advantages
   a. Widely available
   b. Low to moderate cost
   c. Relative simplicity
   d. Indicated for recognition of gross neuropathology
      - cortical atrophy
      - ventricular enlargement
      - tumors
      - strokes
      - calcified tissue
   e. Can visualize bony structures
   f. Alternative to MRI in the case of a pacemaker, neural stimulator, or claustrophobia
2. Disadvantages
   a. Uses ionizing radiation; however, the dosage is low
   b. Limited to visualization of structures in transverse (axial) plane. Therefore, capabilities for reconstructing three-dimensional anatomical images are limited
   c. Poor contrast between gray matter and white matter
   d. Soft tissue imaging adjacent to bone compromised by the beam-hardening artifact (especially in posterior fossa)
   e. Utility apparently limited to the determination of focal pathology, less useful for the imaging of more subtle, global brain abnormalities
   f. Possible allergic response to contrast material (intravenous iodine)
   g. No normal controls are available because radiation exposure does not permit epidemiologic studies in children

Adapted from Lewis, 1991.

nervous system abnormalities at a macroscopic level; its advantages and disadvantages are shown in Table 4–2.

CT does not provide the degree of soft tissue contrast of magnetic resonance imaging (MRI), but has some advantages when studying calcified tissue (Garber et al., 1988). It is less expensive to perform than magnetic resonance imaging and, unlike MRI, it may be used when the patient is utilizing a device, such as a pacemaker or a neural stimulator, that would be disturbed by the magnetic field. CT may also be utilized when fear of close spaces, or claustrophobia, is a factor in the individual's ability to participate in an MRI study.

The major disadvantages of the CT technique relate to the degree of radiation exposure and the risk of an allergic reaction to iodinated contrast material. Also, certain brain regions, such as the posterior fossa, may not be optimally visualized with the CT scanner because bony structures obscure them. A disadvantage in regard to research is that the developmental data available on using CT techniques has been gathered from medical populations because the radiation exposure from this technique has not made it ethically feasible to do systematic anatomical investigations of normal children and adolescents.

CT scan techniques have been used to investigate children and adolescents with a variety of neuropsychiatric conditions including autistic disorder (Chapter 9.1), attention deficit/hyperactivity disorder (Chapter 13), Tourette's disorder (Chapter 15), and schizophrenia (Chapter 14). In tuberous sclerosis complex (Chapter 10.7), tubers can be seen as calcified subependymal masses that do not enhance after the administration of contrast material. MRI shows the subependymal masses but is less sensitive in detecting calcifications; however, it is the preferred imaging technique because it shows superior tissue contrast differentiation to identify plaques in cortex and white matter that are difficult to identify on X-ray.

MAGNETIC RESONANCE IMAGING (MRI)

MRI uses nuclear magnetic resonance (NMR) approaches that have been utilized in physical chemistry for many years. The magnetic resonance image is produced when the body is stimulated to emit electromagnetic radiation, which is detected, interpreted, and organized to produce an image. The theoretical work that led to the development of magnetic resonance imaging is based on the research of Block and colleagues (1946) and Purcell and colleagues (1946), who were the first to carry out successful nuclear magnetic resonance experiments; the Block group detected proton NMR in liquid water, and the Purcell group detected it in solid paraffin. Block et al. essentially found that the atomic nucleus acts like a small magnet and developed a series of equations (Block equations) to describe this nuclear magnetism. These equations explain how a nucleus, because it spins on an imaginary axis, has an associated magnetic field, known as the magnetic moment.

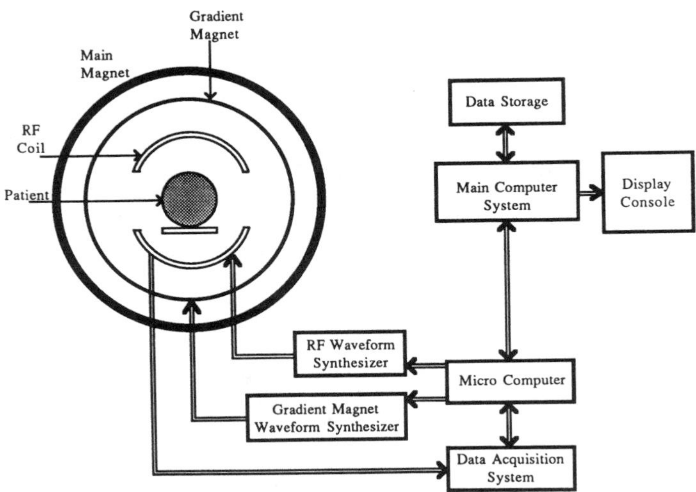

Figure 4–2. Diagram of a magnetic resonance imaging scanner (from Stytz and Frieder, 1990).

Block et al. (1946) showed that certain atoms, if placed in a magnetic field, can be made to resonate if a radio frequency pulse is applied. These atomic nuclei resonating in an external magnetic field induce an electromotive force in a surrounding recording coil. Atomic nuclei that have an odd number of protons or neutrons possess an aspect known as spin, so the nucleus, which is positively charged, generates a small magnetic field when it spins and moves about the axis of an externally applied magnetic field at a frequency that depends on the strength of that field. In the 1950s and 1960s Block's work was experimentally extended in the development of nuclear magnetic resonance (NMR) spectrometers, which allow the determination of the molecular configuration of a material from an analysis of its NMR spectrum. During this same period, Raymond Damadian (1971) found that malignant tissue has a different NMR spectrum than normal tissue. He went on to demonstrate that certain proton NMR parameters—spin density as well as T1 and T2 spin relaxation times—differ between normal and malignant tissue. In 1971 Damadian developed an NMR image of a rat tumor and in 1976 produced the first body image; this took 4 hr to construct (Bushong, 1988). The magnetic resonance image scanner is shown in Figure 4–2 (Stytz and Frieder, 1990).

A glossary of MRI terms that describes technical terms follows this chapter as an appendix.

MRI in humans is based on the interaction of atomic nuclei, protons (commonly hydrogen), and radio waves within a strong magnetic field. When the body, placed in a strong magnetic field, is exposed to a short burst of radio frequency (RF) energy at the resonance frequency of the moving or precessing nuclei, the nuclei become aligned and precess or move in phase and emit a detectable coherent radio frequency signal at the precession frequency, as shown in Figure 4–3.

The radio frequency signal that is emitted is directly related to the precession frequency. This, in turn, is related directly to the magnetic field strength. Because of these relationships, the location of objects within the body can be established by exposing the body to a strong, uniform magnetic field on which is superimposed a weak magnetic field. Nuclei located in different portions of the weak field precess at different frequencies and so respond to and emit different radio frequency signals. Because the magnitude of the weak magnetic field gradient is known, the location of nuclei that respond to a given frequency may be determined and processed by a computer to produce an image.

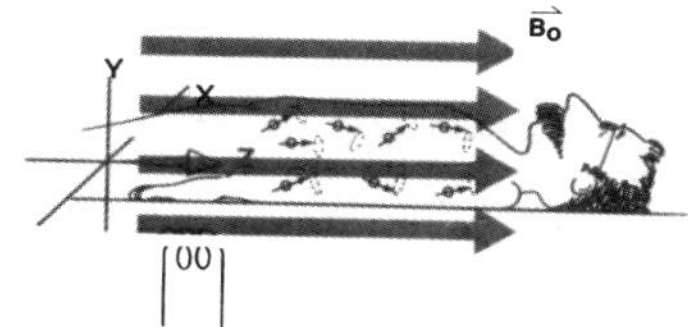

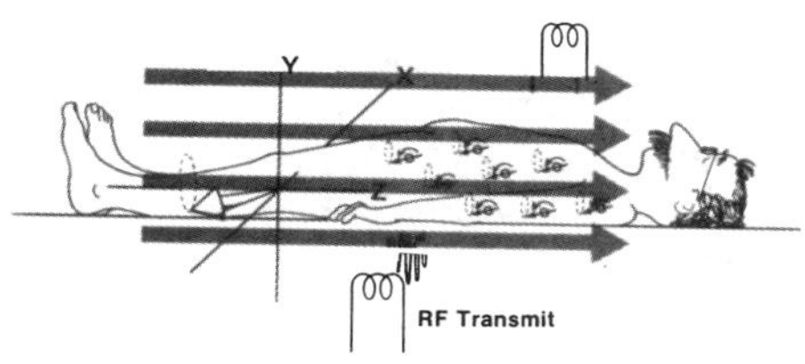

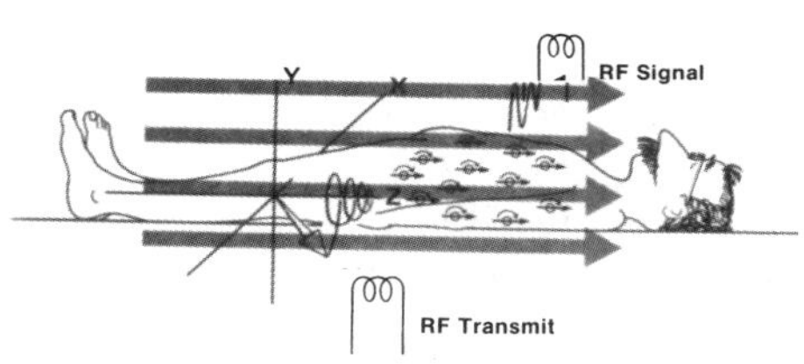

Figure 4–3. *Induction of a radio frequency (RF) signal into a receiving antenna.* In the top figure, placement in a strong magnetic field is shown to polarize the nuclear spins in the patient, as indicated by the arrow in the Z axis. Each proton dipole precesses randomly. In the middle figure, an appropriate radio frequency transmission changes net magnetization to the X-Y plane. Now the protons are in phase. In the lower figure, the net magnetization precesses around the Z axis and slowly returns (relaxes) to equilibrium. As the individual protons return to equilibrium, the precessing net magnetization induces an RF signal in the receiving antenna; this signal is called free induction decay (FID) and can be transformed into a nuclear magnetic resonance (NMR) spectrum and image. Multiple generations of such RF signals are needed to produce the spectrum and standard magnetic resonance image (from Bushong, 1988).

Gradually, the radio frequency signal emitted by the nuclei fades and is lost to detection. The response strength and the time involved until the signal fades are governed primarily by the spin density and by two physical properties, the T1 and T2 relaxation times, which are characteristic of the tissue. Each of these principal NMR parameters is fundamentally different and independent of the others.

Spin Density and Relaxation Times

One of the parameters that affects the strength of the NMR signal is the number of hydrogen nuclei in the volume of the sample. However, the signal not only depends on the presence or absence of hydrogen nuclei, but is also sensitive to the environment of the hydrogen nuclei. How strongly hydrogen is bound within a molecule determines the strength of the NMR signal. Tightly bound hydrogen does not create a usable signal; for example, hydrogen in bone does not emit a signal. The signal arises primarily from "mobile hydrogen" as is found in liquids.

The spin density (SD) is a measure of the amount of mobile hydrogen that is available in the tissues to generate an MRI signal. The higher the concentration of mobile hydrogen nuclei, the stronger the net magnetization and the more intense the MRI signal and the better the MRI image. Tissues with the highest spin density have the largest net magnetization values at equilibrium. However, at equilibrium the tissues emit no signal. A patient whose nuclei are at equilibrium in an external magnetic field creates no NMR signal. During an MRI imaging scan, the spin density is not manipulated; rather, it establishes the upper potential of signal strength. To obtain a signal, radio frequency pulse sequences are used in MRI in an attempt to tap this potential by aligning the nuclear magnetic moments of the individual protons so their vector sum leads to a net transverse magnetization vector of sufficient strength to be detected.

When a nucleus that is aligned in the external magnetic field of a magnetic resonance imager is excited by the radio frequency pulse at the proper frequency, the vector representing net magnetization of that nucleus is tipped out of alignment with the axis of the applied field. The nucleus is now in a relatively higher energy state and its vector of net magnetization gradually returns to the original magnitude and to a parallel position to the external field. This process is referred to as "relaxation."

Two general mechanisms are involved whereby an excited nucleus can dissipate the acquired energy from the applied RF pulse and return to equilibrium. One is the longitudinal, or spin-lattice, relaxation time that involves transfer of energy from the excited nucleus to surrounding molecules in the compound which contains the hydrogen (the molecular lattice) through the rotational, translational, and vibrational motion of the excited nucleus. It is longitudinal because it occurs along the axis of the external magnet field. The time constant characteristic of spin-lattice relaxation is called "T1." Energy is given up by an interaction between hydrogen nuclei (spin) and the surrounding molecule (lattice). In general, on T1-weighted images, tissue with short T1 will appear bright, and tissue with long T1 will appear dark. Ordinarily, T1 of diseased and damaged tissue is longer than that of healthy tissue. It takes about five times T1 for a spin system to return to equilibrium after it has been disturbed.

The other kind of relaxation is called transverse, or spin-spin, relaxation and is characterized by the T2 time constant; it involves loss of phase coherence between nuclear spins. T2 relaxation represents loss of magnetization in the XY plane. It shows loss of net magnetization in the plane perpendicular or transverse to that plane. The magnetic fields of adjacent nuclei in constant motion are interacting with each other. The constant interactions allow nuclear spins to transiently alter each other's frequency leading to loss of the XY component of net magnetization, hence the term "spin-spin relaxation." The radio frequency pulse sequence determines the degree of T2-related brightness of pixels. Ordinarily, on T2-weighted images, tissues with long T2 will appear bright, and tissue with short T2 will appear dark. The constants T1 and T2 play a role in an MRI that is analogous to the radioactive half-life and reflect the rate of decay of the components of the net magnetization vector; each is a fundamental property of tissue. A large value for T1 or T2 indicates a long, gradual decay; a small value suggests a rapid decay. For example, the T1 and T2 for tap water are approximately 2,000 milliseconds, suggesting that several seconds are required for decay. The process is analogous to a struck bell, which continues to sound for several seconds before the sound is no longer heard.

The measurement of T1 and T2 provides information on the local biophysical environment of the nuclei in magnetic resonance imaging and in magnet resonance spectroscopy (MRS), which is described later in this chapter. The comparison of T1 and T2 values in normal and diseased states may give clues to changes in the cellular environment in diseased tissue. In clinical studies, T1-weighted images are most often used to show normal anatomy and T2-weighted images to show pathology.

RF Pulse Sequences

The pulse sequence is essentially a set of instructions to the magnet telling it how to make an image. MRI pulse sequences specify the timing and magnitude of RF pulses and magnetic field gradients. RF pulses are important in establishing image contrast, and pulsed gradient magnetic fields influence spatial resolution of the image. The RF pulse sequence performs two tasks: It tells the imager how to collect data so that the origin of data, its pixel position, can be established, and it influences image contrast by specifying the timing and power of RF pulses. Two basic types of pulse sequences are in use: spin echo and gradient echo. There are many variations of each. Among the most common are partial saturation (saturation recovery), inversion recovery spin echo (Bushong, 1988). *Spin echo* refers to the reappearance of an NMR signal formed by a 180 degree pulse after the free induction decay (FID) has disappeared. It is the result of effective reversal of the dephasing of nuclear spins. Partial saturation spin echo refers to an excitation technique applying repeated 90 degree pulses at times on the order of or shorter than T1. When the 90 degree RF pulses are far enough apart in time that the return of nuclear spins to equilibrium is complete, the term "saturation recovery" is used. Inversion recovery spin echo refers to an RF pulse sequence wherein the net magnetization vector is inverted by a 180 degree pulse prior to spin echo. The other type of pulse sequence is *gradient echo*. Gradient echoes are formed by reversal of the gradients rather than by a 180 degree RF pulse. They are primarily used for 3D volumetric studies, MR angiography, and fast scans.

Multislice and multiecho techniques are used to decrease scan time. Multislice techniques are used because there is a waiting period while protons undergo some relaxation before the next excitation. One may take advantage of that time by energizing the RF transmitter, using a different frequency to excite a different slice. This pulse does not affect the other slices because the frequency is not appropriate for them. In this way, multiple slices can be performed in the same time it takes to complete a single slice. T2 relaxation times can be measured, using a spin-echo pulse sequence that involves multiple echoes. T1 relaxation time measurements require multiple inversion recovery or saturation recovery pulse sequences and require more time for completion.

It may be possible in the future to identify a suspicious region of interest with MRI and then retrieve the NMR spectrum from that area for analysis. Interpretation of the NMR spectrum might tell whether the tissue is normal or abnormal and, if abnormal, indicate the molecular structure of the abnormality. The hope of characterizing abnormalities in this way is an aspect of MRI/MRS that is continuing to develop.

Biological Effects of MRI

The energy fields used in clinical MRI are considered safe and harmless (Bushong, 1988). At very high intensities, transient magnetic fields and RF fields have been shown to induce responses in humans. However, there are no known effects from the static magnetic fields used in clinical studies and no known long-term effects of MRI fields. Acute effects of very high transient magnetic fields include induction of magnetic phosphenes (flashes of light with eyes closed), stimulation of healing in bones if a low-frequency coil is placed over a fracture, and ventricular fibrillation. Ventricular fibrillation has not been observed in humans in either clinical or experimental situations other than in those with pacemakers. Very high RF exposure has been implicated in excessive tissue heating, induction of nonspecific blood dyscrasias, and cataract formation, possibly through heating the avascular lens structure.

Maximum permissible operating MRI intensities have been prescribed. In the United States, the static magnetic field is not to exceed 2 Tesla (T) and transient magnetic fields are limited to 3 T. For RF exposure, the basic measure of dose of RF energy is the specific absorption rate (SAR), which is measured in ω/kg (ω refers to the Larmon frequency. See Appendix p. 84). It is a measure of the power absorbed per unit time per unit mass or power density (ω/M2). Specific absorption rate limitations are 0.4 ω/kg for whole-body exposure and 4.0 ω/kg for tissue exposure.

Acquisition Sequences: Recent Advances

The spin-echo acquisition sequence is most commonly used in brain imaging for tissue characteristics or abnormalities. A newer method (gradient echo) involves the three-dimensional acquisition of data. In this procedure, the data are collected as an entire image volume rather than two-dimensional slices of varying thickness. This approach shows superior image resolution relative to spin-echo images. Brain structures are displayed in three dimensions. The scan time is decreased because repetition time is less. Moreover, gradient reversal methods and partial flip angles are used to rephase spins instead of the 180 degree pulse used in spin-echo acquisition (Villafana, 1992). These are referred to as gradient-recalled echo techniques. Among them are FLASH (fast low-angle shots) and GRASS (gradient recalled acquisition in study state). Measurements made with these newer three-dimensional techniques are not directly comparable to those obtained using spin-echo techniques (Pearlson and Marsh, 1993); pixel intensity for a specific tissue may not be the same.

MRI Analysis Tools

The ability to identify three-dimensional volume sets and reformat them into a standardized stereotactic space allows MRI measures from subjects with brains of differing sizes and shapes to be referenced to a standardized system. Moreover, functional images from SPECT and PET (described in separate sections later in this chapter) can use the same coordinate system and be superimposed on structural images. Finally, stereotactic coordinates allow for statistical analysis of structure location.

Functional Magnetic Resonance Imaging (fMRI)

The most recent development in MRI is echo-planar imaging, fast "MRI" (Stehling, Turner, and Mansfield, 1991), which provides more rapid magnetic resonance image acquisition compared to conventional methods (i.e., milliseconds versus minutes). In this procedure, all echoes are produced in a single free induction decay (FID) that uses one nuclear spin excitation per image. This system potentially may lead to instantaneous image acquisition, higher quality images without motion artifact, and the ability to more rapidly acquire three-dimensional data sets (Pearlson and Marsh, 1993). Such vast increases in the speed of image formation makes functional MRI suitable for research in cognitive neuroscience. Physiologic imaging with magnetic resonance may allow a variety of brain functions to be studied, e.g., simultaneous measurement of molecular diffusion, temperature, or cerebral blood flow, and the use of echo-planar imaging to correlate brain structure and function. Of these, the measurement of cerebral blood flow is the most commonly studied. In physiologic studies, magnetic resonance contrast can be altered and often enhanced by injection of paramagnetic substances, such as gadolinium.

Functional brain imaging is possible with MRI mainly as a result of its ability to detect a signal related to brain function (Raichle, 1993). Specifically, it can be used to detect a change in blood flow via measurements related to hemoglobin oxygenation that occurs in an area of heightened neuronal activity; this measurement is possible due to the way oxygen is used by the brain. Essentially, the technique can distinguish between blood that is laden with oxygen and blood that is depleted of oxygen. This allows the use of functional MRI to measure brain blood flow and produce images of brain function (Belliveau et al., 1991).

The use of MRI for functional brain imaging was suggested by PET studies that demonstrated functionally induced increases in blood flow are accompanied by almost concurrent changes in the amount of brain glucose consumption, but not in the amount of brain oxygen used (Fox and Mintun, 1989; Fox and Raichle, 1986). This indicates the normal human brain resorts to anaerobic metabolism to provide the energy needed for the transient increases in neuronal activity that may accompany changes in behavior, even though there is abundant oxygen in the normal brain. The discovery that there is a functionally induced uncoupling of blood flow from oxidative metabolism has stimulated the evolution of new techniques of functional MRI brain imaging (Ogawa et al., 1990; Ogawa et al., 1992).

Hemoglobin carrying oxygen increases the magnetic field around it by a small amount whereas hemoglobin without oxygen does not. Those areas of the brain that are activated are engorged with oxygen-rich blood which flows to the area. This increase in blood flow that occurs in the brain without a concomitant increase in oxygen consumption in neurons results in a decrease in deoxyhemoglobin concentration in the cerebral venous blood which drains the activated brain areas being studied. This increased oxygenation of the hemoglobin in venous blood (decreased amount of deoxyhemoglobin) affects hemoglobin's magnetic properties; fMRI may be used to detect these small magnetic fluctuations in deoxyhemoglobin, which is weakly paramagnetic. In this way, fMRI can be used to measure blood flow for cognitive activation studies that in the past could only be carried out with SPECT or PET. The recognition of these functionally induced signals has led to increased interest in the use of functional MRI to study blood flow. For example, in brain activation studies, when a light is shined in a person's right eye, a small region of the left side of the brain is activated. When a person is asked to attach a verb like "drinks" to a noun like "man," a distinct area of the left frontal cortex lights up.

These new developments involving fMRI require standardization of procedures to guarantee reliability across the sites that carry out the procedures. Currently fMRI is being used in brain studies to investigate the organization of language, spatial organization, the creation of mental images, and memory (Raichle, 1994).

Advantages and Disadvantages of MRI

The principal advantage of MRI is its improved contrast resolution. Magnetic resonance imaging produces superior anatomical resolution and delineation (soft tissue contrast) when contrasted with computerized transaxial tomography; however, CT's spatial resolution continues to be superior in certain parts of the body. Therefore, spatial resolution is best with radiography, but the resolution of low-contrast objects is better with MRI. Spatial resolution refers to the ability to differentiate very small but dense objects, such as small calcifications, whereas contrast resolution emphasizes the visualization of low-density objects with similar soft tissue characteristics, such as white matter-gray matter.

Most MRI studies are done without contrast material; however, certain paramagnetic substances, such as manganese, gadolinium, and iron, have been utilized to change relaxation times for T1 and T2. These atoms can be incorporated into contrast material for MRI and injected intravenously (Imakita et al., 1988). They may pass the altered blood-brain barrier or diseased tissue. The amount of paramagnetic substance needed to induce changes in the MRI image is minimal so chemical toxicity is ordinarily of little concern in their use.

The MRI procedure provides considerable flexibility in scanning images and also allows one to vary the imaging plane according to previously set measurements. Its multiplanar capability has created greater possibilities for anatomical displays. A radiologist may select transverse or axial, coronal (transverse to the axis of the body) or sagittal (the anterior-posterior plane or section parallel to the long axis of the body). The radiologist may also zoom or cone in on areas that are questionable or of particular interest.

For studies in children, the MRI has considerable advantage over computerized transaxial tomography (CT). It does not involve ionizing radiation (Han et al., 1985), improved gray–white matter delineation is obtained (Steiner, 1985), and contrast injections are not necessary for quality images. Flexibility is possible in imaging and one does not have to be concerned about bone obscuring the posterior fossa in the imaging plane (Packer et al., 1984). The advantages and disadvantages of MRI scanning are shown in Table 4–3.

MRI may not be used in the presence of devices that may be affected by the procedure, such as a neural stimulator or a pacemaker, which may effectively act as an antenna and cause burns (neural stimulation) or cardiac arrhythmias (pacemaker). It should also not be used during pregnancy, unless clinically indicated, and may be problematic for patients with claustrophobia.

There are several additional advantages in conducting functional brain imaging with MRI (Table 4–4). First, the functional MRI technique is without known biological risk. Second, the signal is obtained directly from functionally induced changes in brain tissue, that is, change in venous deoxyhemoglobin concentration in a region of increased neuronal activity. Because no radioactive material is injected to obtain the signal, it can be carried out repeatedly in the same subject. Third, such fMRI studies can provide both anatomic and functional information that may lead to accurate anatomical identification of the regions of activation for the subject being stud-

Table 4–3. Magnetic Resonance Imaging (MRI)

1. Advantages
   a. Does not use ionizing radiation
   b. Visualization of structures in a variety of planes (transverse, coronal, sagittal)
   c. Excellent soft tissue resolution, particularly differentiation of gray and white matter
   d. High sensitivity for detection of white matter lesions (e.g., adrenoleukodystrophy)
   e. Optimal for imaging pathological lesions
   f. Capable of imaging brain structures adjacent to bone (particularly important for posterior fossa structures)
   g. Injection of contrast material not required
   h. Flexible imaging measurement parameters
2. Disadvantages
   a. More expensive and less available than CT scans
   b. Limited by conditions adversely affected by the MRI magnetic field or instrument (e.g., pacemaker, neural stimulator, claustrophobia, ferromagnetic foreign body)
   c. Possibility of toxicity if paramagnetic substances are injected as contrast material

Adapted from Lewis, 1991.

ied. Fourth, the spatial resolution is very good—approximately 2 to 5 millimeters. Fifth, when linked to very fast image acquisition (echoplanar capability), MRI can monitor the actual rate of change in the blood flow induced deoxyhemoglobin signal in real time. Sixth, the MRI systems are more widely available than PET systems and do not require special facilities for the production of radionuclides.

Yet problems remain to be worked out with fMRI technology. Although the functional MRI technique has been conducted, using standardized hospital instruments (1.5T MRI scanner) (Schneider, Noll, and Cohen, 1993), it is still unclear whether fully successful functional imaging will require MRI instruments with higher field strength (e.g., 3T or higher) and more rapid imaging capability. Because of the design of the typical MRI scanner as a long narrow tube, the delivery of stimuli for testing the subject is difficult and requires new innovative techniques. Although the functional MRI may show very high resolution, movement by the subject can render the scan data useless. Even verbal responses may be sufficient to prevent image production due to associated movement. Therefore, correction for movement artifact is a serious concern. Moreover, the exact nature of the functional MRI signal and its relationship to the task-induced changes in neuronal activity is still under study. Raichle (1993) suggests that additional study is needed regarding functional MRI in regard not only to evaluation of increases in blood flow to brain regions but also decreases in blood flow to brain regions and how functional brain activation is related to the basic physiology that leads to these shifts in metabolism. He indicates it is not known whether uncoupling of neuronal activity and oxidative metabolism during functional activation occurs under all circumstances and in all neuronal systems in the brain. In addition, he points out that PET can detect subtle chemical changes in the brain that would not result in enough change in blood flow to be demonstrated on fMRI. Although the applications of functional MRI are in an early phase of development, they do offer considerable promise.

Table 4–4. Functional MRI (fMRI)

1. Advantages
   a. No known biological risk—lack of ionizing radiation
   b. Signal directly obtained from functionally induced changes (venous oxygen concentration) in brain tissue
   c. Both anatomical and functional information obtained
   d. Spatial resolution is excellent; i.e., approximately 2 to 5 mm when signal to noise ratio is considered
   e. Fast image acquisition (echoplanar capability) allows monitoring of actual rate of change of blood flow
   f. More widely available than PET
2. Disadvantages
   a. Higher field strength and more rapid imaging capability beyond standard MRI capacity may be needed
   b. Due to long narrow tube, MRI housing and high magnetic field, delivery of test stimuli is complicated
   c. Movement artifact: Due to high resolution of MRI, any movement (including talk) limits any activation scan
   d. Nature of the fMRI signal to task-induced changes in neuronal activity is uncertain

Applications of MRI in Childhood and Adolescent Disorders

The examination of brain structure is important in developmental neuropsychiatry to (1) confirm a suspected diagnosis, (2) understand how an illness may be linked to brain pathology, and (3) "rule out" other diagnostic possibilities (Pearlson and Marsh, 1993). MRI has had a major impact on the imaging of congenital as well as developmental neuropsychiatric disorders in children and adolescents. The spatial resolution of magnetic resonance imaging (approximately 1.0 mm, much higher than that of PET scanning) and the absence of radioactivity have resulted in this method being commonly used. MRI is used in the evaluation of brain maturation (Barkovich et al., 1988) and in the localization of developmental abnormalities, tumors, and other lesions. In the leukodystrophic white matter disorders, MRI is very sensitive in the detection and demonstration of the extent of the abnormal areas of white matter (Chapter 11.5). In children with mucopolysaccharidosis who show central nervous system involvement, MRI shows nonspecific patterns of cerebral involvement. Hydrocephalus, atlantoaxial subluxation, and dural thickening also may be found. The application of volumetric MRI scans has demonstrated reduced volumes in whole brain in Rett's disorder and in the caudate nucleus in Lesch-Nyhan disease. MRI research studies have also been carried out in many childhood-onset disorders including autistic disorder (Chapter 9.1), fragile X syndrome (Chapter 10.3) and in learning disabilities (Chapter 7). Regarding functional MRI in children and adolescents with neuropsychiatric problems, the issue of movement artifact will be an important one. The advantages of not using ionizing radiation in the child and adolescent population to evaluate brain function are considerable.

MAGNETIC RESONANCE

In the 1940s NMR spectroscopy was introduced into chemistry. It is now being used for dedicated *in vivo* research where the NMR spectrum may be used to identify chemical substances. Magnet resonance spectroscopy (MRS), using combinations of radio frequency pulses and high strength magnetic fields, may make it possible to identify specific compounds *in vivo*. In MR spectroscopy the free induction decay (FID) obtained in an NMR study can undergo Fourier transformation into an NMR spectrum as well as an image. Quantification of energy metabolism can be carried out with ^{31}P because phosphorous is involved in metabolic processes. ^{31}P-spectroscopy has been used to study the brain in some developmental disorders (see Chapter 9.1, Autistic Disorder), making use of the fact that ^{31}P and ^{23}Na concentration varies with the functional state of the brain. However, because the concentration of these substances are less than hydrogen, adequate resolution is more difficult to obtain.

SINGLE PHOTON EMISSION COMPUTERIZED TOMOGRAPHY (SPECT)

SPECT is an established brain-imaging technique to study radioactive tracers introduced into the body, usually by I.V. injection or inhalation, to evaluate physiological activity, such as blood flow and oxygen transport and, more recently, to measure central nervous system neuroreceptors (dopamine, serotonin, and benzodiazepine) and presynaptic transporters. Its origins derive from early attempts to measure cerebral blood flow *in vivo*. In 1948 Kety and Schmidt initiated blood flow studies using nitrous oxide inhalation. During the 1950s and 1960s, inhaled nitrous oxide was replaced by inert gases, xenon and krypton, which were injected directly into the carotid artery. Single photon emission computerized tomography was suggested by Kuhl and Edwards (1963) in their paper describing emission tomographic radionuclide brain imaging. The further development of the technetium-99 mm generator and the Anger gamma camera (1967) in conjunction with enhanced computer power led to advances in these techniques in the 1970s. With the development of improved scintillation detectors and computer algorithms, a three-dimensional representation of regional blood flow became possible.

The primary goal of SPECT imaging is to produce a series of two-dimensional images that depict the three-dimensional distribution of a radioisotope in specific regions of interest as a function of time. SPECT is dependent on the gamma (γ) decay of radionuclides to stable states. Gamma decay results in the emission of a high-energy photon; γ rays are emitted by the nucleus as excess energy as it changes its energy states. The isolates are tagged to biologically active compounds and then injected into the body. This methodology involves the use of detectors—a rotating Anger camera that rotates around the subject's head, or a multidetector system. The detected radiation is processed by a computer that partially corrects for tissue absorption and generates the tomographic images. The subject is placed in a dimly lit room with eyes and ears open and a radionuclide is inhaled or injected. The radioisotopes used clinically are relatively long-lived γ emitters, such as ^{133}Xenon, ^{99m}Technetium, and ^{123}Iodine.

The term "single photon" refers to the fact that in SPECT the photons are detected by multiple discrete scintillation detectors, one at a time rather than in coincidence pairs, as in PET. Because the photons are detected one at a time, when many photons appear, they lack simple spatial correlation. Therefore, the origins of photons in SPECT must be traced by collimation (a process whereby electromagnetic radiation can be drawn into parallel beams). Lead structures are used that have specifically designed openings to allow photons from well-defined brain regions to enter. The tracers that are available to measure cerebral blood flow by SPECT are all lipid soluble (lipophilic) and diffuse easily from blood into brain tissue. There are two types of tracers, those that are chemically inert, which are not retained in the brain, and those that are chemically active, which are retained.

^{133}Xenon, an inert, diffusable gas that is administered by inhalation, is the most widely used of the chemically inert tracers. In a typical inhalation study, for the first minute the subject inhales ^{133}Xenon (Xe) as an air-oxygen mixture (wash-in). This is followed by a 3-minute wash-out phase in which the patient breathes room air. The arrival and cerebral wash-out is followed dynamically for 4 to 5 minutes with a series of four tomographic images per slice of brain tissue. Regional blood flow is calculated from variations in the count rate of the region in four images and from an arterial input function. The method is quantitative and lasts only 4½ minutes; the measurement can be repeated in 20 minutes. This procedure is limited by the requirement of a specialized dynamic SPECT system that rotates rapidly, spatial resolution is fairly poor, and various artifacts affect quantification (Lassen and Holm, 1992). Radioactivity in the lung is monitored by a scintillation probe placed on the patient's chest that correlates radioactivity in the lung with arterial blood concentration of ^{133}Xenon in the brain.

The limitations of current Xenon SPECT studies are being addressed by utilizing new lipid soluble radio pharmaceuticals that are injected intravenously. Although radiation exposure is somewhat higher using these substances, with these methods some investigators report images that are comparable to those obtained in PET (Andersen et al., 1988; Lassen et al., 1983; Yonekura et al., 1988). Intravenous SPECT ligands include ^{99m}Technetium-HMPAO and ^{123}IMP. ^{99m}Technetium-HMPAO, a commonly used compound, is described in detail here.

^{99m}Technetium-HMPAO is a lipophilic compound used to measure cerebral blood flow. HMPAO is a chemical microsphere (chemically active molecules that act as a microsphere) which freely crosses capillary walls. Once inside the brain, it is rapidly converted to another form that is hydrophilic and, thus, cannot leave the brain. Uptake and trapping of HMPAO is completed in about 10 minutes. HMPAO then remains fixed in the brain with a loss of approximately 0.4% per hour. This allows time for data acquisition over 20 minutes by a rotating gamma camera or a multidetector system. With a sensitive detector system and acceptable doses of radioactivity, a SPECT image can be recorded in 1 minute or less.

For blood flow studies, gender, age, handedness, and other physiologic factors need to be taken into account because they influence cerebral blood flow. Cerebral blood flow is inversely correlated with age, with decreases in males occurring 5 to 10 years earlier than in females (Devous et al., 1986; Gur et al., 1987a). Left-handed and right-handed individuals both have higher blood flows in the right hemisphere in contrast to the left, although the discrepancy is greater in the left-handed person (Gur et al., 1987b). Cerebral blood flow is affected by mild anxiety, REM sleep, and cognitive activity, each increasing blood flow. Extreme anxiety, slow wave or deep sleep, and habituation to test procedures are related to lower blood flow values. Blood flow will vary according to the brain region being evaluated. It is higher in the gray matter than in myelinated regions of the brain. Studies in normal subjects have indicated that, in adults, the visual cortex and parietal cortex receive higher blood flow than the temporal and frontal areas (Devous et al., 1986). However, others have noted the highest cerebral blood flow in the frontal regions in younger populations (Risberg, 1980).

Besides its use to measure cerebral blood flow, SPECT is also utilized to study neuroreceptors in the brain. For this purpose, ^{123}Iodine (physical half-life = 13.3 hours) has been found suitable; ^{99m}Technetium is difficult to incorporate into organic molecules. Although ^{123}I labeled compounds have been used for SPECT for both cerebral blood flow and neuroreceptor studies, it is their use in the examination of specific recognition sites for neuroreceptors that is particularly advantageous. That these compounds are good γ emitters and have high specific radioactivity facilitates their use for SPECT studies. ^{123}I compounds have been synthesized to study muscarinic cholinergic receptors, D_1 and D_2 receptors, serotonin 5-HT_2 receptors, and the presynaptic dopamine transporter.

The advantages of the SPECT, as shown in

Table 4–5, is that it is noninvasive, painless (except with intravenous injection), and relatively safe. It is also less expensive than PET scanning and does not take as much time or use as many personnel. It may have application in all age groups and can be used as a follow-up procedure, with minimal radiation exposure. For example, ^{133}Xenon data is acquired rapidly and the washout of a tracer allows repeated measurements within a short time period, which may be useful in studies that attempt to activate brain regions. Even though ^{133}Xenon studies show poorer image resolution compared to regional CBF techniques, such as SPECT HMPAO or IMP, ^{133}Xenon studies remain useful because absolute regional CBF can be noninvasively quantitated and studies may be repeated over short intervals.

Drawbacks to the SPECT are limited spatial resolution (although improving) and possible extracranial contamination from background radiation (Kuperman et al., 1990). Furthermore, regions of interest less than 3 millimeters in diameter may result in errors of measurement. Because clearance rates are slower in myelinated tissue, lesions in white matter may not be as easily demonstrated.

Table 4–5. Single-Photon Emission Computerized Tomography (SPECT)

1. Advantages
   a. Capable of monitoring a broad range of biochemical processes
   b. Monitors regional variations in brain blood flow
   c. Instrumentation widely available
   d. Relatively inexpensive in capital costs and recurring expenses
   e. Noninvasive and safe
   f. Minimal radiation exposure
   g. Good spatial resolution
   h. Good temporal resolution
   i. Repeated measures within a short period possible, e.g., using ^{133}Xe
   j. Examination of brain neurotransmitter systems is possible
   k. Indicates sites of action of psychoactive drugs and can be used to monitor treatment
   l. Indicates brain activity during behavioral and cognitive functioning
2. Disadvantages
   a. Limited spatial resolution when contrasted to PET
   b. Size of instrument and requirement for a dedicated scanner
   c. Does not measure glucose metabolic rates with available radioisotopes
   d. Quantification of radionuclide concentration less than PET
   e. Limited number of pharmaceuticals (primarily ^{123}I and ^{99m}Tc) that preserve the pharmacology of the natural substance.

Adapted in part from Lewis, 1991.

Applications of SPECT Scanning

SPECT studies may provide a better understanding of information processing in the brain through activation studies. Activation of brain regions in the performance of any task produces demands related to specific information processing. This leads to changes in neuronal activity in various functional areas of the brain; changes in neuronal activity lead to changes in blood flow that can be measured with SPECT. The functional areas involved in carrying out a particular task are distributed to several locations throughout the brain, each of which makes a specific contribution to the task performance. Studies of this brain activation are undertaken to understand functional localization. For example, with speech there is increased flow to the left precentral and midtemporal area, whereas calculation and arithmetic tasks increase profusion to the left and right suprasylvian regions. Sensory stimuli lead to increased flow in the contralateral sensory motor area, and spatial tasks increase flow to the right hemisphere (Gur et al., 1987a).

SPECT studies have been conducted with adult schizophrenics where activation tasks, such as a continuous performance test or the Wisconsin Card Sort test, are utilized; with adult depressed patients where reduced blood flow was demonstrated; in attention deficit/hyperactivity disorder where regional blood flow was assessed (Lou, Henriksen, and Bruhn, 1984, 1990; Lou et al., 1989); and in infants with perinatal ischemia. ^{123}I compounds are being used to study Alzheimer's disease and the major mental illnesses. Future applications will eventually focus on developmental neuropsychiatric disorders.

POSITRON EMISSION TOMOGRAPHY (PET)

Positron emission tomography (PET) uses radioisotope tracers to evaluate brain function. The use of positrons for coincidence detection, the basic imaging mechanism in PET, was initially suggested by Wren, Good, and Handler (1951), and later by Brownell and Sweet (1953). By 1962 (Robertson, Marr, and Rosenbloom, 1973), transverse section imaging had been accomplished using emitted positrons detected by arrays of sodium iodide detectors. Resolution was poor due to the large number of scattered X-rays that were included in the image, small number of angular views, and poor reconstruction algorithms. The first modern positron emission tomography (PET) machine was described in 1973 (Brownell and Burnham, 1973; Robertson, Mann, and Rosenbloom 1973). By 1975 Phelps and Ter-Pogossian (Phelps et al., 1975; Ter-Pogossian et al., 1975) had described their imaging procedure, which included the basic elements currently used for imaging studies today, i.e., Fourier reconstruction, high sampling rates, and attenuation correction. Positron emission tomography combines the imaging of positron emitting isotopes with transaxial tomography. It is a tool that can potentially detect functional abnormality before anatomic changes occur.

PET requires the use of a cyclotron, a special radio pharmaceutical laboratory, and detecting imaging equipment. In the cyclotron, charged particles, ordinarily protons and deuterons, are accelerated to high energy levels in a vacuum chamber. When acceleration is sufficient that the particles have reached an adequate energy state, a stream of the energized particles is extracted from the vacuum chamber. These energized particles are caused to collide with a purified nonradioactive isotope. The energized particle penetrates the field of electrons that surround the target atom, hits the nucleus, and is captured in the nucleus (electron capture), increasing the proton number. A diagram of a typical positron emission tomography (PET) scanner is shown in Figure 4–4.

In clinical studies, a cyclotron produces radioactive atoms with short half-lives, such as ^{11}C (20 min), ^{13}N (10 min), ^{15}O (2 min), and ^{18}F (110 min). A radioactive atom is then extracted from the cyclotron and in the radio pharmaceutical laboratory tagged into a molecule that will be utilized in the particular study. The process of tagging must be carried out immediately because of the short half-life (2 minutes to 110 minutes) of these isotopes. The newly created radioisotope tracer is injected intravenously, and rapid sequential images are obtained after the tracer has become localized to brain regions of interest. Blood samples are collected for quantification. The sequence of experimental procedures required for imaging neuroreceptors by PET is shown in Figure 4–5.

The injected tracer decays, yielding a positron (antimatter electron), $\beta+$, which is then ejected from the nucleus of the radioisotope. A $\beta+$ particle is identical to an electron except it has an electric charge of +1 instead of the electron's –1 charge, which makes the positron the antiparticle to the electron. In $\beta+$ decay, a proton in the nucleus is converted into a neutron and the excess energy is emitted from the nucleus as a positron and a neutrino. The neutrino passes through the body and the scanner

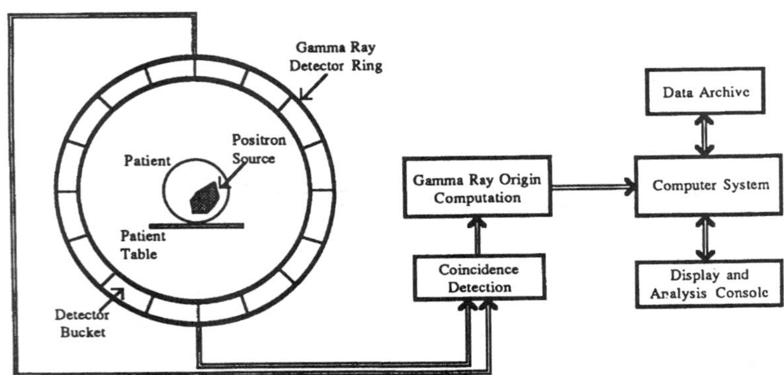

Figure 4–4. Diagram of a positron emission tomography (PET) scanner (from Stytz and Frieder, 1990).

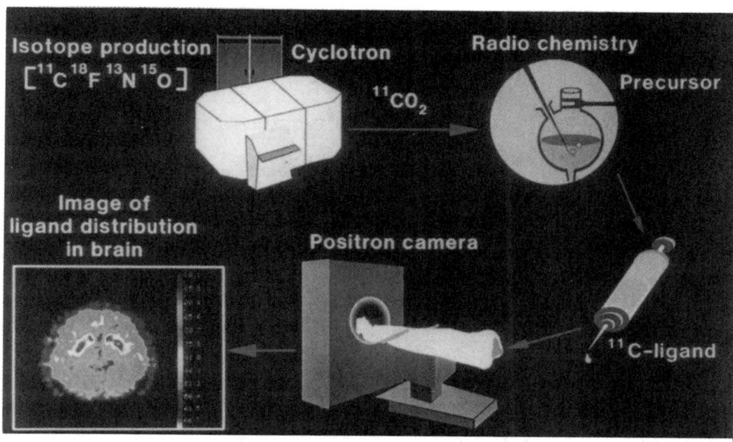

Figure 4–5. Sequence of experimental procedures required for imaging neuroreceptors by positron-emission tomography (from Sedvall et al., 1986).

without interaction and does not play a part in forming an image. The β+ particle is the major imaging element in β+ decay. After it is released from the nucleus, the β+ particle is decelerated by the drag that is exerted on it from the surrounding electrons. When the β+ particle has dissipated enough energy to be in equilibrium with its surroundings and essentially motionless, the attractive force between the positively charged β particle and local electrons cause the formation of an electron/positron pair. This electron/positron pair annihilates and converts all of its mass into energy. The liberated energy is realized as a pair of 511keV gamma rays that leave the site of the annihilation and travel in opposite or nearly opposite directions. The positron encounters an electron near its decay site, less than a millimeter away and a matter-antimatter reaction takes place. The two gamma photons are recorded by small gamma scintillation detectors on opposite sides (at 180°) of a ring of such detectors placed around the patient. Electronic circuitry recognizes the coincidence of the events in two detectors. A succession of such coincidences in different pairs of detectors enables the positron of the site of the bound tracer to be located, and an image is created. This methodology, which involves opposing detectors, has been particularly successful in increasing image resolution. The detected "event" is positron emission within the brain sample. The method for image reconstruction is by filtered back projection.

Because the location of the β+ decay is not the annihilation event, the resolution of a PET system is limited by the range of the β+ particle, approximately 0.15 cm in human tissue. Moreover, the resolution of the PET system is lowered because PET is also limited by the number of detectors and their size. Still, the production of the two gamma rays leads to increased resolution of PET over SPECT because coincidence detection can be used to more accurately locate the annihilation event and thereby the location of the decayed nucleus, through coincidence timing (Stytz and Frieder, 1990).

The two most common substances used for PET blood flow and metabolic studies are $H_2{}^{15}O$ and 2-[^{18}F]fluoro-2-deoxy-D-glucose (FDG). The short radioactive half-life of ^{15}O-labeled water, utilizing an equilibrium method, provides a useful tracer technique for the quantitative measurement of regional cerebral blood flow with PET. In this approach, a steady state is established between $H_2{}^{15}O$ delivered by arterial blood flow to tissue and removed by venous outflow along with the radioactive decay of the short-lived ^{15}O isotope. Metabolic activity is commonly studied, using the deoxyglucose model. The 2-deoxy-D-glucose

(DG) or the positron labeled 2-[^{18}F]fluoro-2-deoxy-D-glucose (FDG) are competitive substances that are analogs of glucose. The tracer kinetic model used in PET studies measures the local cerebral metabolic rate for glucose metabolism (LCMRGlc) based on the competitive kinetics of the compounds used. The FDG competes with glucose for carrier-mediated transport sites. Specifically, in cerebral tissue, FDG and glucose compete for hexokinase for phosphorylation to FDG-6-PO_4 and glucose-6-PO_4. The glucose-6-PO_4 is metabolized along the glycolytic pathway or it is converted to glycogen. The FDG-6-PO_4 is not significantly metabolized by either of these pathways, does not diffuse through membranes, is trapped, and accumulates within cells in proportion to the local cerebral metabolic rate for glucose. Having established the transport and metabolic rate of the brain for FDG, a correction term is applied to convert the FDG measure to the corresponding value for glucose (Phelps, 1992).

Table 4–6. Positron Emission Tomography (PET)

1. Advantages
   a. Capable of monitoring a broad range of biochemical processes
   b. Monitors brain metabolism and regional variations in brain activity
   c. Facilitates examination of brain neurotransmitter systems, particularly through postsynaptic receptor and presynaptic reuptake site mapping
   d. Indicates sites of action of psychoactive drugs and can be used to monitor treatment
   e. Indicates brain activity during behavioral and cognitive functioning
   f. Good temporal resolution (less than 1 minute)
   g. Good spatial resolution
   h. Sensitive to cellular dysfunction without structural pathology, so may be useful for differential diagnosis and identification of patients at risk
   i. Repeated measures within a short period of time, e.g., using ^{15}O
   j. Somewhat greater resolution and sensitivity than SPECT
   k. Theoretically better quantification of radionuclide concentration than SPECT
   l. Utilizes radioisotopes (i.e., ^{11}C, ^{15}O, and ^{18}F) that preserve the pharmacology of natural substances.
2. Disadvantages
   a. Difficult to establish a site for a cyclotron, especially in urban areas
   b. High capital investment expense
   c. High recurring costs
   d. Limited clinical availability
   e. Most applications in research phase

Adapted in part from Lewis, 1991.

Two commonly used PET techniques are activation scans and neuroreceptor/reuptake site scans (Frost and Wagner, 1990; Sedvall et al., 1986). PET studies, using blood flow and metabolic approaches, show us where and when an event is happening in the brain, but do not show how it occurs; neuroreceptor PET studies may shed light on how events occur. For activation scans, so called because the brain is activated, the subject must be imaged in areas where sound and light are controlled because brain regions may be activated by the ambient stimuli in the room. This is less important for receptor PET studies. In the activation method, adequacy of regional brain function is assessed and, in studies involving specific neurotransmitters, density and distribution of the neuroreceptors in brain areas are evaluated.

The advantages and disadvantages of PET are shown in Table 4–6. The advantage of PET scanning is that its spatial resolution tends to be better than SPECT scans, although the resolution is not as great as for CT or MRI scans. The spatial resolution for PET is approximately 5 to 10 mm, but the potential resolution is 2 to 3 mm. However, often both MRI and PET are performed concurrently, with the patient receiving an MRI scan prior to the PET scan. By combining these functional and structural methods, the information obtained may be more pertinent because both anatomical and physiologic information may be needed. The use of the cyclotron to create radiopharmaceuticals makes it possible to investigate receptors that may be affected by drug therapy and may permit better monitoring of drug therapy in the future. The disadvantages of PET are its cost, the difficulty of conducting studies in children because sedation or anesthesia is often necessary, and the fact that radiation exposure can be greater than in SPECT scans. The actual radiation exposure is comparable to the amount of radiation utilized in a renal scan.

Applications of PET Scanning

PET scanning can be utilized to study various perceptual and cognitive states. It provides an opportunity not previously available to investigate the living human brain.

Activation and Other Cerebral Flood Flow Studies

With PET, as is also the case with SPECT, uniquely human brain processes can be investigated. As described earlier, regional cerebral blood flow studies point to where metabolic demands are taking place. The half-lives and clearance times of injected ligands are such that several processes can be studied together, e.g., selective attention to somatosensory input. Specific PET studies allow assessment of higher brain functions including language. The approach has been used (Petersen, Fiez, and Corbetta, 1992) to demonstrate brain areas involved in reading single words and semantic tasks.

Blood flow and metabolic studies have been utilized in developmental studies of brain function and in studies of individuals with Down syndrome, pervasive developmental disorder (autistic disorder), attention deficit disorder, Tourette's disorder, and other neurodevelopmental disorders. These studies are described in the chapters dealing with the specific disorder.

PET scans may be used for seizure focus detection (Engel, 1981) and to study various perceptual and cognitive states. For seizure detection, PET scans may be used in conjunction with surface EEG. This approach has been utilized in children with refractory epilepsy but may also be of importance in disorders thought to involve neuronal migration (e.g., autistic disorder).

Developmental Studies

Kennedy and Sokoloff (1957) showed that the average cerebral blood flow in 9 normal children (ages 3 to 11) was 1.8 times that of a normal adult, and oxygen utilization was 1.3 times that of an adult. Chugani and colleagues (Chugani and Phelps, 1986; Chugani, Phelps, and Mazziotta, 1989; Chugani et al., 1991) have shown that local cerebral metabolic rates for glucose (LCMRGlc) in children undergo dynamic maturational trends before reaching adult values. Although the adult pattern of cerebral glucose utilization is reached at about 1 year of age, local changes occur in glucose metabolism over a more protracted period. The neonatal values are low, but by the second and third postnatal year they begin to exceed adult values. A plateau in glucose utilization is thought to occur by age 4 extending to age 9. This is followed by a gradual decline in LCMRGlc by the end of the second decade in comparison to adult values.

Most strikingly, the peak activity is pronounced in the neocortical brain regions, which peak at more than twice the adult value for local glucose utilization. The older structures of the brain phylogenetically, i.e., the brainstem and cerebellum, do not show a significant increase over adult values and are metabolically mature at birth. However, early increases over adult values do occur in subcortical structures, such as the basal ganglia and the thalamus. There is a hierarchical order of structures relating to the degree that maturation increases over the adult values.

It is thought that these changes are related to times of maximal brain plasticity during development, but their specific biological significance is not yet determined. An important issue here is to clarify the times of maximal plasticity in brain development.

Quantitative Studies

Another approach to PET scanning is the study of neurotransmitter receptors, utilizing ^{11}C and ^{18}F compounds. Among them are ^{11}C N-Methylspiperone and ^{11}C-Raclopride, which are used to study the postsynaptic dopamine system, ^{11}C-WIN 35,428 for the presynaptic dopamine system, and ^{11}C-Diprenorphine for the opiate system. These approaches have been utilized in the study of Tourette's disorder, Rett's disorder , and Lesch-Nyhan disease, among others, and are discussed in the chapters dealing with these disorders.

OVERVIEW OF MEDICAL IMAGING MODALITIES

In summary, the techniques of CT, MRI, SPECT, and PET provide various approaches to diagnostic medical imaging. The operation and imaging parameters related to these techniques are summarized in Table 4–7.

Each of these solutions to medical imaging requires the use of image reconstruction techniques to produce images that are based on the

Table 4–7. Medical Imaging Operation and Imaging Parameters

	CT	MRI	SPECT	PET
Imaging mechanism	Transmission X-rays	High-frequency radio frequency (RF) transmission and external magnetic fields	Emission γ rays	Coincidence timing of γ -ray pair produced by β+ annihilation
Physical measurement	X-ray linear attenuation	RF pulse stimulation. Emission of an RF signal from in-phase precessing proton	Uptake of radioactive nuclide labeled biochemical compounds	Uptake of biochemical compounds made from radioactive isotopes
Interpretation	Material density	Mobile hydrogen density contrast enhanced by T1 and T2 weightings	Biochemical activity	Biochemical activity
Resolution	0.5–2 mm	0.5–2 mm	7–10 mm or 3.5–9 mm	4–6 mm or 2.3–6.6 mm

From Stytz and Frieder, 1990.

body's response to different forms of energy. Although the interpretation of data and the physical processes involved vary from one modality to the next, the goal of each is to demonstrate the structure or function of the brain as clearly as possible. Each modality is useful because each provides different information and expands the armamentarium to choose from for an identified problem.

COMPUTERIZED ELECTROENCEPHALOGRAPHY (CEEG)

The electroencephalogram (EEG), first described in 1929 by a German psychiatrist, Hans Berger, provides a means to measure bioelectrical events in the brain (Berger, 1929). He hoped that progress in the quantification of EEG results would make them more meaningful to the diagnosis and treatment of mental disorders; however, the standard EEG did not demonstrate significant abnormalities in even the most severe mental disorders. This failure may relate not to the method itself but to the huge amount of information produced by the EEG; however, in the ensuing years, progress has been made with regard to the technical limitations and difficulty in establishing the neuronal sources that generate the electrical activity.

The standard EEG procedure utilizes the placement of electrodes following the International 10–20 System. Recordings are made on EEG paper of voltage-versus-time and this graph is then evaluated. The EEG is conducted during several standard situations including eyes closed, following hyperventilation, with photic stimulation, and during sleep. The EEG printout records voltage tracings representing 30 to 60 minutes of EEG recording. The EEG varies with age so brain maturation must be taken into account: slower waves, the delta waves (0 to 4 cps) are predominant in the newborn, faster posterior theta waves (4 to 8 cps), emerge in the first 12 months, and the alpha rhythmn gradually emerges in early childhood (Binnie and Boyd, 1994). Because the slower wave activity normally decreases with age, activity less than 7 cps, and especially less than 5 cps, is considered abnormal in waking adults. Because of a number of normal variants at each age, classification is more difficult in children with central nervous system pathology. Abnormalities include diffuse or sharp focal waves, spikes, and spike and wave formations as well as the paroxysmal appearance of areas with slower and sharper potentials.

More sophisticated assessment methods, using computers to collect and analyze data, have led to considerable advances in the field of electroencephalography, particularly regarding quantitative analysis, which allows for computerized tomographic mapping of brain electrical activity through electroencephalography (EEG). Quantitative electroencephalography uses conventional clinical EEG techniques including standard electrode placement; wave forms that result from electrical activity of the brain are amplified and recorded on magnetic tape or optical discs. Off-line computer processing is used for the removal of artifacts induced by movement, particularly eye movements, muscle activity, and 60 Hz interference. Specific computer algorithms are used for data analysis, and then an image or "map" is formed by assigning various shades of gray or colors. In this approach, the data can be depicted as a numerical array or shown as a topographical display of the head, viewed from various angles.

One approach, spectral analysis, involves the analysis of conventional frequency bands (alpha, beta, delta, theta), where short collections of EEG data are transformed by mathematical algorithms to measure the average power in each band. This method provides data on the relative local abundance of these frequency bands (Young et al., 1991).

The advantages and disadvantages of computerized EEG (CEEG) are shown in Table 4–8. The computerized EEG has several advantages as a method for functional analysis of brain activity in contrast to previous EEG methods and other methods of functional imaging. Although it is not inexpensive, it is easier and cheaper than other noninvasive techniques which require the use of radioactive isotopes. Because no radiation is used and it is not difficult for the patient, evaluation sessions may be of longer duration and may be repeated on multiple occasions. In contrast to other imaging methods, which are more static and reflect brain activity over a short period of time (several minutes), quantitative electrophysiologic methods make measurements in millisecond intervals and offer chronological resolution (i.e., over time), allowing recognition of specific phases of information processing. Data collected in this way may be quantified and compared among different groups of patients. However, there are disadvantages, too; because it is nonspecific, the brain electrical activity is not directly related to the part of the brain being recorded beneath the recording electrodes. An electrical signal recorded at the surface presents the average neuronal activity of millions of cells. This signal is also distorted because it must be conducted through scalp and bone, and muscle movement and other sources of noise may lead to artifactual interpretation. There may also be noncerebral electrical signals that provide artifacts. In addition, cognitive ability, handedness, sex, age, and other variables may lead to individual differences in response, making comparison with controls difficult. Finally, the clinical significance of computerized EEG findings must be interpreted. In mapping the quantitative results of EEG analysis, the values plotted at each site represent the difference between the electrode and a reference point rather than the central activity of that region. Temporal information is lost as the analysis presents a time average of some EEG feature over one or more epochs—often several seconds. Overall, there remains controversy in regard to the clinical utility of this method (Binnie and MacGillivray, 1992).

Table 4–8. Quantitative Electrophysiology

1. Advantages
   a. Monitors changing patterns and regional variations in brain electrical activity
   b. No radiation exposure
   c. Noninvasive and requires minimal cooperation from patients, even those who are retarded and noncommunicative, and can be repeated many times
   d. Relatively inexpensive
   e. Excellent time resolution
   f. Easily quantifiable data
2. Disadvantages
   a. The data do not necessarily bear a specific relation to any brain structure, and the neural generators are unknown
   b. Many electrical artifacts must be identified and filtered
   c. The effects of confounding variables, such as sex, age, and handedness, are not yet known in detail
   d. The use of computer programs for filtering and modeling makes assumptions and approximations that may be misleading
   e. It is controversial whether topographic mapping adds reliable scientific information beyond that of conventional EEG and evoked potential studies

Adapted from Lewis, 1991.

Computerized EEG techniques have been used widely in adult psychiatric patients. For children, two kinds of studies have been carried out (Kuperman et al., 1990). In one, children thought to be at high risk because their parent has a psychiatric disorder have been given computerized EEGs, and findings are compared with those of their parents. A second approach involves utilizing computerized EEG with specific psychiatric disorders in children. This technique has been applied in schizophrenia to study children thought to be at high risk, in alcoholics and their children, in autistic disorder, in attention deficit/hyperactivity disorder, in learning disability, and in Tourette's disorder.

EVENT-RELATED POTENTIALS

Event-related potentials (ERPs) are cortical electrical response patterns to sensory input recorded from the scalp; the ERP identifies the specific potential changes related to discrete external events and stimuli. Levels of brain function can be assessed in passive subjects, using ERP, without any task being performed, thereby making it an optimal tool to study children and those with developmental disorders. The event-related brain potential technique is used to record a person's neural responses, which are elicited by specific auditory, visual, or somatosensory stimuli. These techniques are being used for the neurobiological classification and diagnosis of developmental disorders of the nervous system. Event-related brain potentials indicate the "real time" neural activity taking place in motor, sensory, and cognitive systems as a response to information specifically presented to the patient. ERP methods provide an opportunity to measure the functioning of various neural systems in a noninvasive fashion for newborns, infants, and adolescents. These methods also provide a means to investigate the physiologic development of the human brain from the beginning of life in normal individuals and those with mental disorders.

ERP responses are tested in a variety of conditions in order to characterize normal and pathological responses at motor, sensory, and cognitive levels. Profiles of pathophysiologic responses may be compared among the developmental disorders to establish what are the most distinctive features of each disorder. Moreover, pathophysiologic responses are evaluated based on developmental norms to establish whether or not they are deviant or delayed.

ERP responses have been measured in a variety of developmental disorders, including autistic disorder, attention deficit disorder, specific learning disability (dyslexia), receptive developmental language disorder, and Down syndrome, among others. These studies have relied on the evaluation of sensory and cognitive ERP components because information is available on these components throughout the normal course of development. The ERP responses most commonly studied are auditory brainstem ERPs, A/Pcz/300, P3b, and Nc.

There is considerable interest in determining which neural systems generate ERP responses or components; however, there is more information available on the neural generators involved for some components than for others. The contingent negative variation (CNV) is most likely generated by neural responses to acetylcholine input to cortex from the nucleus basalis (Pirch et al., 1986). The A/Pcz/300 and possibly the P3b may at least, in part, depend on noradrenergic input to the cortex from the locus coeruleus (Foote et al., 1991). As information is gathered on the origins of the ERP responses, it will become increasingly possible to measure the functioning of the various neural systems during development.

This section reviews the types of event-related potentials, their clinical applications, strategies relating to them, and the clinical uses of cognitive event potentials.

Sensory (Exogenous) ERP Components

In general, ERP components have been divided into two classes: exogenous, or related to the character of the stimulus, and endogenous, or related to the reaction or attitude of the subject to the stimulus (Sutton et al., 1965). The exogenous ERPs are always elicited by external events, and their response characteristics (amplitude, latency) vary with the stimulus. The endogenous ERPs are nonobligatory responses and may occur in the absence of an expected stimulus (e.g., expectation, importance or relevance of the stimuli, recognition of novelty).

Among the sensory ERP components that are exogenous, the best studied is the auditory brainstem-evoked response. The auditory brainstem response pathways are evaluated by five ERP components generated by neural activity. The components are referred to as Waves I, II,

III, IV, and V; this series is triggered by a click stimulus. These components reflect some part of the neural activity that occurs during the first 8 milliseconds following the onset of the click, and each represents a different step in auditory-sensory processing. Latency (time of occurrence after stimulus onset) and amplitude of each component may be affected by stimulus intensity, the rate the stimulus is delivered, and into which ear the stimulus is delivered. Both body temperature and gender also influence these ERP responses (Stockard, Stockard, and Sharbrough, 1978).

Wave I is generated by the auditory nerve; however, the neurogenerators are not known with certainty for the other waves. They are likely to include neural activity in or near the cochlear nucleus, superior olive, lateral lemniscus, inferior colliculus, and acoustic radiations (Legatt, Arezzo, and Vaughan, 1986a, 1986b). Recording these sensory components provides reliable information to assess auditory brainstem sensory systems. These auditory brainstem responses are present at birth and mature rapidly during development so they are nearly fully mature before the end of the second year of life (Galambos, 1982).

Auditory brainstem-evoked responses have been studied in several developmental neuropsychiatric disorders; considerable research has been carried out in subjects with autistic disorder. Courchesne and Yeung-Courchesne (1988) tested subjects with autistic disorder under a variety of stimulus conditions, controlling for gender and body temperature. When testing subjects with autistic disorder who did not have complicated neurological diseases, every subject had normal auditory brainstem components. These authors concluded that although audiological abnormalities might be found in some individuals with autistic disorder, no evidence indicates a distinctive form of pathophysiology in the sensory pathways of all subjects with autistic disorder that is responsible for these ERP components. The same authors studied receptive developmental dysphasia but did not identify statistically significant differences between the receptive developmental dysphasic group and normal controls. Although one subject had conductive hearing loss and another sensorineural hearing loss, no distinctive form of pathophysiology was demonstrated. But Squires (1984) did demonstrate a distinctive pathology in auditory brainstem responses in Down syndrome and postulated it could lead to distorted acoustic perception. The abnormality consisted of a shortened time interval between the latencies of Wave I and II and between Waves III and IV. Moreover, the latency of Wave V did not increase, as expected, in response to increases in the rate of the auditory stimulus that was delivered. The latter effect raises questions about how well the initial stages of auditory-sensory processing in Down syndrome can temporally encode successive bits of information. The abnormal auditory brainstem response in Down syndrome is a developmental deviation rather than a delayed maturational response from normal ERP patterns.

Cognitive (Endogenous) ERP Components

Unlike the evoked potential, the event-related potential ordinarily requires mental activity on the part of the child and has been referred to as "the thinking person's evoked potential" (Barrett, 1993). Unlike the generalized EEG, cortical activity associated with a specific cognitive task or perceptual event can be assessed with the event-related potential. Both evoked potentials and event-related potentials have been used to investigate a number of disorders beginning in childhood, including disorders of attention and hyperactivity, autistic disorder, language disorder, schizophrenia, Down syndrome, depressive illness, exposure to lead, and children at risk of developing cognitive and psychiatric disorders.

Cognitive event-related potentials were first described in the mid-1960s. Walter et al. (1964) reported a slow, negative shift in potential that occurred between a warning stimulus (S1) and an imperative stimulus (S2). The potential had a maximum amplitude just prior to the imperative stimulus (S2) and was named "contingent negative variation" (CNV). The authors used a warning stimulus, a click, and an imperative stimulus, a series of light flashes. The light flashes had to be extinguished as rapidly as possible by a subject who pressed a button in response to them. These authors showed the potential was independent of the type of stimulus used at the first and second point by recording a contingent negative variation. Later, Sutton et al. (1965) provided a description of a large positive-going potential that varied in its amplitude depending on the subject's certainty in regard to the modality of the stimulus which was to be presented. When the patient was more uncertain, the amplitude was greater. This potential was found to peak at approximately 300 milliseconds and was later known as the "P300" or "P3." These authors also showed that if the individual guessed the stimulus modality, then P300 was smaller than if the individual guessed incorrectly.

Since these early studies, the type of tasks used to elicit a CNV has changed very little. However, at least two components are combined in a CNV. The first component is found to be distributed over the frontal scalp and is considered to be related to an orienting response to a warning stimulus (O wave). The second component (E wave) is considered to be analogous to the Bereitschaft's potential that is found immediately before voluntary self-paced movement.

The research on the P300 is considerable and involves reports of a variety of responses that contain both positive and negative-going potentials. Most of these have latencies that are different from 300 milliseconds and can be evoked through a series of experimental tasks. A specific ERP component is typically referred to in either spatial or temporal dimensions. Spatial reference specifies the first negative deflection of the ERP wave form as "N1"; a component labeled "P2" refers to the second positive inflection. Temporal reference specifies a negative wave occurring at 100 milliseconds after the stimulus onset as "N100"; a component labeled "P300" refers to a positive inflection of the wave form occurring at 300 milliseconds after stimulus onset.

A large number of cognitive ERP components are endogenous rather than exogenous. Among these, three represent different physiologic systems that are triggered by attention-getting information. These include the A/Pcz/300, P3b, and Nc (Courchesne, Elmasian, and Yeung-Courchesne, 1987). These ERP components are detected early in development and their maturational time course has been carefully studied. A valid investigation of these components requires comparison to experimental (e.g., designed) control studies for performance, cooperativeness, and general attention (Courchesne and Yeung-Courchesne, 1988). In order to carry out these tasks, the individual must understand the instructions for the procedure and be able to remain still and attentive for approximately a half hour at a time as well as perform specific behavioral tasks reliably during the ERP recording.

The maturation of exogenous ERPs has been extensively studied; overall, the response latency to auditory, visual, and somatosensory stimuli decreases rapidly during the first year of life and changes more slowly or not at all from early childhood to adolescence. In contrast, the endogenous ERP components have longer latencies and show changes throughout childhood, perhaps related to later myelination.

The A/Pcz/300 Component

The A/Pcz/300 component is elicited through the detection of novel, unexpected sounds. This component is located over the cortex and may possibly be specific to the auditory modality. It is large in amplitude at scalp electrode sites located over the central, superior-parietal, and frontal cortex. It is a positive peak and the peak latency is about 300 milliseconds following stimulation (Hillyard and Kutas, 1983). Lesion studies in squirrel monkeys suggest it may be dependent, at least in part, on noradrenergic input to the cortex from the locus coeruleus, as previously noted (Foote et al., 1991). It is present at all ages between 4 and 44 years (Courchesne, 1983) and may emerge during development. The amplitude of P300 increases with increasing relevance of a task associated with a stimulus and with decreasing probability that the stimulus will occur. This component is important in orienting to novelty and may be of major importance during development because detecting, paying attention to, and learning about new events are essential developmental acquisitions. A deficit in orienting to novelty might be reflected in the A/Pcz/300 response to novelty.

Testing procedure involves the administration of a monotonous, repetitive series of stimuli, with occasional presentation of a surprising novel sound that is unexpected. In these experiments, to control for attention, cooperation, and general arousal, participants press a button whenever they detect a specific target sound.

Cognitive ERP components have been studied in a variety of conditions, including autistic disorder, Down syndrome, attention deficit disorder, and specific learning disability, among others. Individuals with Down syndrome do not show normal orientation to novel stimuli. Courchesne et al. (1984) found that an abnormal A/Pcz/300 response to novelty in autistic disorder: The auditory A/Pcz/300 component is substantially smaller in persons with autistic disorder than in normal subjects. Still, it is larger to novel sounds than to monotonous, insignificant sounds, suggesting that individuals with autistic disorder detect and perceive novelty but may have a limited capacity to react to novelty when contrasted to normals of all ages. This abnormality is detected in individuals with autistic disorder who show a high level of function as well as those who show a low level of function. This abnormality of A/Pcz/300 response amplitude when found in autistic disorder is not a developmental delay, but represents a developmental deficit. Courchesne and Yeung-Courchesne (1988) suggest the smaller A/Pcz/300 may indicate defective automatic detection of auditory novelty and might involve the reticular formation, limbic structures, and prefrontal cortex. They point out that adults who have sustained lesions of the prefrontal cortex also have smaller A/Pcz/300 responses to auditory novelty (Knight, 1984).

In Down syndrome, the A/Pcz/300 amplitude is reported to be normal in 12-year-olds; however, this component is not completely normal. Lincoln et al. (1985) reported that the A/Pcz/300 latency was later in Down syndrome than in mental age-matched normal controls as well as in chronologically age-matched controls. In fact, it was later than it occurred in normal 4-year-olds, in children with autistic disorder, and in children with attention deficit disorder. Consequently, the neural reaction to auditory novelty in Down syndrome is slower than that seen in normals. However, when it does occur, the neural reaction which produces the A/Pcz/300 has a magnitude similar to that seen in normals.

In contrast to autistic disorder and Down syndrome, A/Pcz/300 has been found to be normal in a study of severe reading disorder and in attention deficit disorder (Holcomb, Ackerman, and Dykman, 1986). In both of these conditions, the amplitude and latency are normal. No ERP evidence of a deficit in alerting to auditory novelty is seen in these conditions.

The P3b Component

The most thoroughly studied of all human ERP components is P3b (Pritchard, 1981). It has a peak latency, ranging from 280 to 1,000 milliseconds following stimulation. It has been suggested that P3b is elicited when important information requires a cognitive updating or memory modification. When adult subjects are required to make two or more conscious decisions in fractions of a second about such information, the P3b amplitude elicited by each decision is substantially large, even when each decision is separated by only 300 to 500 milliseconds (Woods and Courchesne, 1986). The recovery cycle of P3b then is less than 300 to 500 milliseconds (the recovery cycle of a response is the minimum time interval that must exist between any two stimuli for the response to the second stimulus to be similar to that of the first stimulus). Courchesne and Yeung-Courchesne (1988) used the term "psychological recovery cycle" to describe the human capacity to make two or more conscious decisions in a row as long as they are separated by at least 300 to 500 milliseconds. Current research suggests that cortical synaptic potentials triggered by noradrenergic input from the locus coeruleus are involved in generating the P3b. Moreover, there may be a significant degree of independence of auditory P3b from visual P3b, and these responses may have different developmental origins (Courchesne and Yeung-Courchesne, 1988).

The visual P3b may be detected before age 2 and is distinct by age 3. Subsequently, the visual P3b is found in people of all ages (Mullis et al., 1985). The visual P3b latency in early childhood is approximately 600 to 800 milliseconds, but decreases until puberty when the latency is recorded at about 400 milliseconds.

The normal development of the auditory P3b has been interpreted as either developing in parallel to the visual P3b, which is consistent with there being only one P3b neural generator, or having a separate origin. The auditory P3b is a positivity with a latency of approximately 350 milliseconds at all ages, which grows in amplitude until preadolescence.

The auditory and visual P3b responses have been investigated in a number of developmental disorders including autistic disorder, receptive developmental language disorder, Down syndrome, attention deficit disorder, severe reading disorder, and schizophrenia with childhood onset. In autistic disorder, the auditory P3b is consistently smaller than normal when elicited by verbal, nonverbal, phonemic, and nonsensory information (Courchesne and Yeung-Courchesne, 1988). The small auditory P3b is increasingly thought to be intrinsic to the physiology of autistic disorder and is present regardless of the type of information used to elicit it or the rate that information is delivered. It occurs in individuals with autistic disorder, both when they show poor performance on a task or when they respond to a task as accurately as normals. However, in a specific context, such as attentional demands, normal amplitude auditory P3b responses can be produced.

Individuals with receptive developmental dysphasia may show P3b abnormalities opposite to that seen in autistic disorder. Courchesne et al. (1989) found that in nonretarded persons with autistic disorder P3b (recorded in response to auditory and visual stimuli and the omission of these stimuli) were smaller than normal, and Nc (described later) was small and often absent even when no auditory language or sensory processing was required. These findings were consistent with the hypothesis that nonretarded persons with autistic disorder have abnormal attentional and cognitive responses. In receptive developmental language disorder, P3b was found to be somewhat enlarged even under conditions when it was elicited by stimuli separated by 1 second and also when it was elicited by the omission of stimulation. Receptive language disorder has been associated with difficulties in processing sequences of auditory stimuli. Lincoln et al. (1993) have suggested that the small P3b may be significantly related to the difficulty that children with autistic disorder have in monitoring their expectancies to contextually relevant sequences of auditory information. In Down syndrome, auditory P3b latency is longer than in age-matched normal subjects, but is not as long as that seen in normal children matched to children with Down syndrome in mental age (Lincoln et al., 1985).

Children with attention deficit disorder and severe reading disorder may have abnormal P3b responses in both auditory and visual modalities. Auditory and visual P3b have been found to be smaller than normal when test conditions require the individual to focus attention for long periods of time during which they perform monotonous signal detection tasks (Holcomb, Ackerman, and Dykman, 1986).

The Nc Component

The Nc component is elicited through attention-getting and orienting stimuli whether they are novel, surprising, or significant. When it is recorded with scalp electrodes, Nc is largest in amplitude over the frontal and central cortex. It is a negative peak and its peak latency ranges from 350 to 1,000 milliseconds following stimulation. Nc may be generated by depolarizing potentials in the cortical synapses that are signaled through input from the intralaminar thalamic nuclei as one phase of the action of the reticular-thalamic-cortical activating system (Courchesne, Elmasian, and Yeung-Courchesne, 1987).

Nc appears to be an endogenous component as part of a neurophysiologic response initiated by internal attentional and cognitive mechanisms. Moreover, Nc may be present at birth. The normal recovery cycle for Nc is between 400 and 1,200 milliseconds, (Woods and Courchesne, 1986). The recovery cycle, then, is short for the endogenous cortical ERPs in contrast to the recovery cycle of the exogenous stimulus-dependent components; these may be up to 10 seconds or more.

Developmental changes in the Nc amplitude and latency occur in parallel to developmental changes in the number of cortical synapses and in the myelination of nonspecific thalamic radiations (Courchesne, Elmasian, and Yeung-Courchesne, 1987). Nc amplitude increases and decreases in parallel with the reduction in the number of cortical synapses in the frontal cortex that is reduced through synaptic pruning from infancy and early childhood through puberty (Courchesne, 1990). Moreover, Nc latency decreases from approximately 800 to 1,000 milliseconds for infants to about 350 to 500 milliseconds by 7 years of age. These changes occur in parallel to the time course of myelination of nonspecific thalamic radiations.

Increases in myelin with development enhance neuronal transmission speed and decrease response latencies.

The Nc response is abnormal in autistic disorder in both auditory and visual modalities. Courchesne and Yeung-Courchesne (1988) report that it is abnormally small and, under some conditions, a positive potential is present rather than the normal negative Nc potential. Interestingly, these authors found that when tested using auditory-visual stimuli and auditory and visual targets of various kinds, such as spoken words, tones, letters, and flashes of colored slides, the subjects with autistic disorder performed accurately in comparison to normals, although their ERPs showed they did so with an abnormal neurophysiology. In order to obtain near normal Nc amplitudes, extreme auditory stimulation, such as clanging or ringing, had to be presented. The authors concluded that this pathophysiology may reflect abnormal neural physiology rather than an absence or reduction in the normal physiologic response. Moreover, they suggest the aberrant Nc response, which is elicited by stimulus emissions in subjects with autistic disorder, indicates an impairment in the internal initiation of attentional mechanisms. Yet the presence of a small Nc in response to stimuli that are extreme may be consistent with the need for special external events to engage the attentional mechanisms which underlie Nc. One possible explanation for the abnormal Nc response is that it is involved with the initial depolarization in superficial layers of the cortex which occur as one phase of the action of the reticular activating system. Aberrant reticular activation function was one of the first neurobiological hypotheses suggested for autistic disorder because this system is essential for the activation, adjustment, and maintenance of attention and consciousness. The Nc findings may be consistent with earlier hypotheses regarding autistic disorder (Rimland, 1964).

In other disorders, such as receptive developmental aphasia and attention deficit disorder, Nc is normal. However, in Down syndrome, although the latency and amplitude of Nc is comparable to normal infants, the infant with Down syndrome appears to be nonselectively responsive to stimulus change. For older individuals with Down syndrome, Lincoln et al. (1985) found that 12-year-olds showed abnormally prolonged Nc latencies in response to target-presented events. Nc latency in the preadolescent Down children was found to be no earlier than that in Down syndrome babies. These findings may indicate a failure of the pathways that are involved in the generation of Nc to myelinate properly.

In summary, ERPs may be used to investigate developmental neuropsychiatric disorders, and distinctive patterns of pathophysiology may be identified. However, it is these patterns that characterize a disorder, so a single abnormality of an ERP component in isolation is not sufficient to diagnose a disorder. It is the overall pattern of normal and abnormal sensory and cognitive physiology and auditory, visual, and somatosensory modalities that differentiate one disorder from the other.

SUMMARY

Each of the techniques described in this chapter are leading to new understanding of developmental neuropsychiatric disorders. Refinements first in CT scanning, and then in MRI, have led to finding variability in brain structure in normal persons as well as abnormalities in individuals with a variety of disorders including schizophrenia, autistic disorder, Tourette's disorder, Rett's disorder and adrenoleukodystrophy. SPECT and PET scanning studies have been carried out in these disorders as well as in attention deficit/hyperactivity disorder and in metabolic disorders such as Lesch-Nyhan disease. Such investigations have established the importance of both structural and functional imaging in developmental neuropsychiatric disorders. Finally, advances in evoked potential research are leading to better understanding of electrophysiologic events in the brains of children and adolescents with developmental disorders. Application of these techniques may provide additional insight into the etiology of disease and its evolution over time.

In the future, these various techniques may be linked together. Currently coregistration of PET and MRI has been accomplished. Because PET and MRI provide spatial resolution but lack the temporal resolution sensitivity of electrical methods to monitor linked brain regions, combining PET and MRI and electrical recording could offer additional advantages. Combinations of PET and MRI might be applied to image the anatomy of the circuits underlying a behavior of interest. This, combined with electrical recording techniques, may reveal the time course of events in spatially defined circuits.

The images of brain activity provide massive amounts of information. As more data is collected on disorders beginning in the developmental period, advances in digitization may be used to create new systems for image management. These include the picture archiving and communication (PAC) system, which may be used to acquire, store, and display both digital images and text about patients (Huang et al., 1990). A PAC system allows immediate accessibility of radiographs at digital image-viewing stations. Such digital images can then be archived on magnetic and optical disks. These systems are providing rapid access to imaging information, remote image transmission, and offer the possibility of greater and better manipulation of digital information.

REFERENCES

Andersen, A.R., Friberg, H.H., Schmidt, J.F., and Hasselbalch, S.G. (1988). Quantitative measurements of cerebral blood flow using SPECT and [99mTc]-d, 1-Hm-PAO compared to Xenon-133. *Journal of Cerebral Blood Flow and Metabolism,* 8:S69-S81.

Barkovich, A.J., Kjos, B.O., Jackson, D.E., and Norman, D. (1988). Normal maturation of the neonatal and infant brain: MR imaging at 1.5T. *Radiology,* 166:173–180.

Barrett, G. (1993). Clinical applications of event-related potentials. In A.M. Halliday (ed.), *Evoked potentials in clinical testing,* 2nd ed. Churchill Livingstone, New York.

Belliveau, J.W., Kennedy, D.N, McKinstry, R.C., Buchbinder, B.R., Weisskiff, R.M., Cohen, M.S., Vevea, J.M., Brady, T.J., and Rosen, B.R. (1991). Functional mapping of the human visual cortex by magnetic resonance imaging. *Science,* 254:716–719.

Berger, H. (1929). Uber das Elekenkephalogram des Menschen 1. *Archives für Psychiatrie und Nervenkrankheiten,* 87:527–571.

Binnie, C.D., and MacGillivray, B.B. (1992). Brain mapping—a useful tool or a dangerous toy? *Journal of Neurology, Neurosurgery, and Psychiatry,* 55:527–529.

______ and Boyd, S. (1994). Clinical electrophysiology. In M. Rutter, E. Taylor, and L. Hersov (eds.). *Child and adolescent psychiatry: Modern approaches,* 3rd ed., p. 111. Blackwell Scientific Publications, Oxford.

Block, R., Hansen, W.W., and Packard, M.E. (1946). Nuclear induction. *Physical Review,* 69:127.

Brownell, G.L., and Burnham, C.A. (1973). MGH positron camera. In G.S. Freeman (ed.), *Tomographic imaging in nuclear medicine.* Society of Nuclear Medicine, New York.

______, and Sweet, W.H. (1953). Localization of brain tumors with positron emitters. *Nucleonics,* 11:40.

Bushong, S.C. (1988). *Magnetic resonance imaging: Physical and biological principles.* C.V. Mosby Company, St. Louis, MO.

Chugani, H.T., Houda, D.A., Villablanca, J.R., Phelps, M.E., and Xu, W. (1991). Metabolic maturation of the brain: A study of local cerebral glucose utilization in the developing cat. *Journal of Cerebral Blood Flow and Metabolism,* 1216:35–47.

______, and Phelps, M.E. (1986). Maturational changes in cerebral function in infants determined by 18FDG positron emission tomography. *Science,* 231:840–843.

______, ______, and Mazziotta, J.C. (1989). Positron emission tomography study of human brain functional development. *Annals of Neurology,* 22:487–497.

Courchesne, E. (1983). Cognitive components of the event-related brain potential: Changes associated with development. In A.W.K. Gaillard and W. Ritter (eds.), *Tutorials in ERP research: Endogenous components,* pp. 329–344. North-Holland, Amsterdam.

______. (1990). Chronology of postnatal human brain development: ERP, PET, myelinogenesis, and synaptogenesis studies. In J.W. Rohrbaugh, R. Parasuraman, and R. Johnson (eds.), *Event-related brain potentials: Basic issues and applications.* Oxford, New York.

______, Elmasian, R.O., and Yeung-Courchesne, R. (1987). Electrophysiological correlates of cognitive processing: P3b and Nc, basic, clinical and developmental research. In A.M. Halliday, S.R. Butler, and R. Paul (eds.), *A textbook of clinical neurophysiology,* pp. 645–676. Wiley, New York.

______, Lincoln, A.J., Yeung-Courchesne, R., Elmasian, R., and Grillon, C. (1989). Pathophysiologic findings in nonretarded autism and receptive language disorder. *Journal of Autism and Developmental Disorders,* 19:1–17.

______, Kilman, B.A., Galambos, R., and Lincoln, A.J. (1984). Autism: Processing of novel auditory information assessed by event-related brain potentials. *Electroencephalography and Clinical Neurophysiology: Evoked Potentials,* 59:238–248.

______, and Yeung-Courchesne, R. (1988). Event-related brain potentials. In M. Rutter, A.H. Tuma, and I.S. Lann (eds.), *Assessment and diagnosis in child psychopathology,* pp. 264–299. The Guilford Press, New York.

Damadian, R. (1971). Tumor detection by nuclear magnetic resonance. *Science,* 171:1151–1153.

Devous, M.D., Stockley, E.M., Chehabi, H.H., and Bonte, F.J. (1986). Normal distribution of regional cerebral blood flow measured by dynamic SPECT. *Journal of Cerebral Blood Flow and Metabolism,* 6:95–104.

Engel, J. (1981). The use of positron emission tomographic scanning in epilepsy. *Annals of Neurology,* 15:180–191.

Foote, S.L., Berridge, C.W., Adams, L.M., and Pineda, J.A. (1991). Electrophysiological evidence for the involvement of the locus coeruleus in alerting, orienting, and attending. *Progress in Brain Research,* 88:521–532.

Fox, P.T., and Mintun, M.A. (1989). Noninvasive functional brain mapping by change-distribution analysis of averaged PET images of $H_2{}^{15}O$. *Journal of Nuclear Medicine,* 30:141–149.

______, and Raichle, M.E. (1986). Focal physiological uncoupling of cerebral blood flow and oxidative metabolism during somatosensory stimulation in human subjects. *Proceedings of the National Academy of Sciences,* 83:140–144.

Frost, J.J., and Wagner, H.N. (1990). *Quantitative imaging: Neuroreceptors, neurotransmitters, and enzymes.* Raven Press, New York.

Galambos, R. (1982). Maturation of auditory evoked potentials. In G.A. Chiarenza and D. Papakostopoulos (eds.), *Clinical application of cerebral evoked potentials in pediatric medicine,* pp. 323–343. Excerpta Media, Amsterdam.

Garber, H.J., Weilburg, J.B., Bounanno, F.S., Manschreck, T.C., and New, P.F.J. (1988). Use of magnetic resonance imaging in psychiatry. *American Journal of Psychiatry,* 145:164–171.

Gur, R.C., Gur, R.E., Obrist, B.E., Skolnick, B.E., and Reivich, M. (1987a). Age and rCBF. *Archives of General Psychiatry,* 44:617–621.

______, ______, Resnick, S.M., Skolnick, B.E., Alavi, A., and Reivich, M. (1987b). The effect of anxiety on cortical CBF and metabolism. *Journal of Cerebral Blood Flow and Metabolism,* 7:173–177.

Han, J.S., Benson, J.E., Kaufman, B., Rekate, H.L., Alfidi, R.J., Huss, R.G., Sacco, D., Yoon, Y.S., and Morrison, S.C. (1985). MR imaging of pediatric cerebral abnormalities. *Journal of Computer Assisted Tomography,* 9:103–114.

Hillyard, S.A., and Kutas, M. (1983). Electrophysiology of cognitive processing. *Annual Review of Psychology,* 34:33–61.

Holcomb, P.J., Ackerman, P.T., and Dykman, R.A. (1986). Auditory event-related potentials in attention and reading disabled boys. *International Journal of Psychophysiology,* 3:263–273.

Hounsfield, G.N. (1973). Computerized transverse axial scanning (tomography): I. Description of the system. *British Journal of Radiology,* 46:1016–1022.

Huang, H.K., Aberle, D.R., Lufkin, R., Grant, E.G., Hanafee, W.N., and Kangarloo, H. (1990). Advances in medical imaging. *Annals of Internal Medicine,* 112:203–220.

Imakita, S., Nishimura, T., Yamada, N., Naito, H., Takamiya, M., Yamada, Y., Minamikawa, J., Kikuchi, H., Nakamura, M., Sawada, T., Choki, J., and Yamaguchi, T. (1988). Magnetic resonance imaging of cerebral infarction: Time course of Gd-DTPA enhancement and CT comparison. *Neuroradiology,* 30:372–378.

Kennedy, C., and Sokoloff, L. (1957). An adaptation of the nitrous oxide method to the study of the cerebral circulation in children: Normal values for cerebral blood flow and cerebral metabolic rate in childhood. *Journal of Clinical Investigation,* 36:1130–1137.

Knight, R. (1984). Decreased response to novel stimuli after prefrontal lesions in man. *Electroencephalography and Clinical Neurophysiology,* 59:9–20.

Kuhl, D.E., and Edwards, R.Q. (1963). Image separation radioisotope scanning. *Radiology,* 86:822.

Kuperman, S., Gaffney, R.R., Hamdan-Allen, G., Preston, D.F., and Venkatesh, L. (1990). Neuroimaging in child and adolescent psychiatry. *Journal of the American Academy of Child and Adolescent Psychiatry,* 29:159–172.

Lassen, N.A., Henriksen, L., Holm, S., Barry, D.L., Paulson, O.B., Vorstrup, S., Rapin, J., lePoncin, L., Moretti, J.L., Askienazy, S., and Raynaud, C. (1983). Cerebral blood flow tomography: Xenon-133 compared with isopropyl-amphetamine-iodine-123: Concise communication. *Journal of Nuclear Medicine,* 24:17–21.

______, and Holm, S. (1992). Single photon emission computed tomography (SPECT). In J.C. Mazziotta and S. Gilman (eds.), *Clinical brain imaging: Principles and applications,* pp. 108–134. F. A. Davis Company, Philadelphia.

Legatt, A.D., Arezzo, J.C., and Vaughan, H.G.,Jr. (1986a). Short latency auditory evoked potentials in the monkey: I. Wave shape and surface topography. *Electroencephalography and Clinical Neurophysiology,* 64:41–52.

______, ______, and ______. (1986b). Short latency auditory evoked potentials in the monkey: II.

Intracranial generators. *Electroencephalography and Clinical Neurophysiology,* 64:53–73.

Lincoln, A.J., Courchesne, E., Harms, L., and Allen, M. (1993). Contextual probability evaluation in autistic, receptive developmental language disorder, and control children: Event-related brain potential evidence. *Journal of Autism and Developmental Disorders,* 23:37–58.

______, ______, E., Kilman, B.A., and Galambos, R. (1985). Neurophysiological correlates of information processing in children with Down's syndrome. *American Journal of Mental Deficiency,* 89:403–414.

Lou, H.C., Henriksen, L., and Bruhn, P. (1984). Focal cerebral hypoperfusion in children with dysphasia and/or attention deficit disorder. *Archives of Neurology,* 41:825–829.

______, ______, and ______. (1990). Focal cerebral dysfunction in developmental learning disabilities. *Lancet,* 335:8–11.

______, ______, ______, Borner, H., and Nielsen, J.B. (1989). Striatal dysfunction in attention deficit and hyperkinetic disorder. *Archives of Neurology,* 46:48–52.

Mullis, R.J., Holcomb, P.J., Diner, B.C., and Dykman, R.A. (1985). The effects of aging on the P3 component of the visual event-related potential. *Electroencephalography and Clinical Neurophysiology,* 62:141–149.

Ogawa, S., Lee, L.M., Kay, A.R., and Tank, D.W. (1990). Brain magnetic resonance imaging with contrast dependent on blood oxygenation. *Proceedings of the National Academy of Sciences,* 87:9868–9872.

______, Tank, D.W., Menon, R., Ellermann, J.M., Kim, S-G, Merkle, H., and Ugurbil, K. (1992). Intrinsic signal changes accompanying sensory stimulation: Functional brain mapping with magnetic resonance imaging. *Proceedings of the National Academy of Sciences,* 89:5951–5955.

Packer, R.J., Zimmerman, R.A., Bilanuik, L.T., Leurssen, T.G., Sutton, L.N., Bruce, D.A., and Schut, L. (1984). Magnetic resonance imaging of lesions of the posterior fossa and upper cervical cord in childhood. *Pediatrics,* 76:84–90.

Pearlson, G.D., and Marsh, L. (1993). Magnetic resonance imaging in psychiatry. In J.M. Oldham, M.B. Riba, and A. Tasman (eds.), *Review of psychiatry,* pp. 337–379. American Psychiatric Press, Washington, DC.

Petersen, S.E., Fiez, J.A., and Corbetta, M. (1992). Neuroimaging. *Current Opinion in Neurobiology,* 2:217–222.

Phelps, M.E. (1992). Positron emission tomography (PET). In J.C. Mazziotta and S. Gilman (eds.), *Clinical brain imaging: Principles and applications,* pp.71–107. F. A. Davis Company, Philadelphia.

______, Hoffman, E.J., Mullani, N.A., and Ter-Pogossian, M.M. (1975). Application of annihilation coincidence detection to transaxial reconstruction tomography. *Journal of Nuclear Medicine,* 16:210.

Pirch, J.H., Corbus, M.J., Rigdon, G.C., and Lyness, W.H. (1986). Generation of cortical event-related slow potentials in the rat involves nucleus basalis cholinergic innervation. *Electroencephalography and Clinical Neurophysiology;* 63:464–475.

Primack, S.L., Chiles, C., and Putman, C.E. (1992). One hundred years of imaging: New benefits, new challenges. *Perspectives in Biology and Medicine,* 35:361–371.

Pritchard, W.S. (1981). Psychophysiology of P300. *Psychological Bulletin,* 89:506–540.

Purcell, E.M., Torrey, H.C., and Pound, R.V. (1946). Resonance absorption by nuclear magnetic moments in solids. Physical Review, 69:37–38.

Raichle, M.E. (1993, November). *New views of cognition: An introduction to functional brain imaging techniques.* Paper presented at the Society for Neuroscience Meeting, Washington, DC.

______. (1994). Visualizing the mind. *Scientific American,* 270:58–64.

Rimland, B. (1964). *Infantile autism.* Appleton-Century-Crofts, New York.

Risberg, J. (1980). RCBF measurements by Xe-133 inhalation. *Brain and Language,* 9:9–34.

Robertson, J.S., Marr, R.B., and Rosenbloom, B. (1973). Thirty-two crystal positron transverse section detector. In G.S. Freeman (ed.), *Tomographic imaging in nuclear medicine,* p. 141. Society of Nuclear Medicine, New York.

Schneider, W., Noll, D.C., and Cohen, J.D. (1993). Functional topographic mapping of the cortical ribbon in human vision with conventional MRI scanners. *Nature,* 365:150–153.

Sedvall, G., Farde, L., Persson, A., and Wiesel, F. (1986). Imaging of neurotransmitter receptors in the living human brain. *Archives of General Psychiatry,* 43:995–1005.

Squires, N.K. (1984). Auditory brainstem responses in aberrant development: The case for a different approach to ERP research. (*In* D. Otto, R. Karrer, R. Halliday, L. Horst, R. Klorman, N. Squires, W. Thatcher, B. Fenelon, and G. Lelord (eds), *Developmental aspects of event-related potentials: Aberrant development.) In* R. Karrer, J. Cohen, and P. Tueting (eds.), *Brain and information: Event-related potentials,* pp. 319–328. New York Academy of Sciences, New York.

Stehling, M.K., Turner, R., and Mansfield, P. (1991). Echo-planar imaging: Magnetic resonance imaging in a fraction of a second. *Science,* 254:43–50.

Steiner, R.E. (1985). Magnetic resonance imaging: Its impact on diagnostic radiology. *American Journal of Roentgenology,* 145:883–893.

Stockard, J.J., Stockard, J.E., and Sharbrough, F.W. (1978). Nonpathologic factors influencing brainstem auditory evoked potentials. *American Journal of EEG Technology,* 18:177–209.

Stytz, M.R., and Frieder, O. (1990). Three-dimensional medical imaging modalities: An overview. *Critical Reviews in Biomedical Engineering,* 18:1–25.

Sutton, S. Braren, M., Zubin, J., and John, E.R. (1965). Evoked potential correlates of stimulus uncertainty. *Science,* 150:1187–1188.

Ter-Pogossian, M.M., Phelps, M.E., Hoffman, E.J., and Mullani, N.A. (1975). A positron emission transaxial tomograph for nuclear medicine imaging (PETT), *Radiology,* 114:89.

Villafana, T. (1992). Physics and instrumentation: Magnetic resonance imaging. In F.H. Lee, K.C.V.G. Rao, and R.A. Zimmerman (eds.), *Cranial MRI and CT,* 3rd ed., pp. 39–62. McGraw-Hill, New York.

Walter, W.G., Cooper, R., Aldridge, V.J., McCallum, W.C., and Winter, A.L. (1964). Contingent negative variation: An electric sign of sensorimotor association and expectancy in the human brain. *Nature,* 203:380–384.

Woods, D.L., and Courchesne, E. (1986). The recovery functions of auditory event-related potentials during split-second discriminations. *Electroencephalography and Clinical Neurophysiology,* 65:304–315.

Wren, E.R., Good, M.L., and Handler, P. (1951). The use of positron emitting radioisotopes for the localization of brain tumors. *Science,* 113:525.

Yonekura, Y., Nishizawa, S., Mukai, T., Fujita, T., Fukuyama, H., Ishikawa, M., Kikuchi, H., Konishi, H., Lassen, N.A., and Andersen, A.R. (1988). SPECT with Tc-99m-(d,l)-hexamethyl-propyleneamine oxime (HM-PAO) compared with regional cerebral blood flow measured by PET: Effects of linearization. *Journal of Cerebral Blood Flow and Metabolism,* 9 (suppl.):S82-S89.

Young, J.G., Brasic, J.R., Kaplan, D., Golomb, J., Ostrer, H., Furman, J., and Biegon, A. (1991). Advances in research techniques. In M. Lewis (ed.), *Child and adolescent psychiatry,* pp. 1201–1224. Williams & Wilkins, Baltimore.

GLOSSARY OF MRI TERMS

Acquisition Process of detecting and storing NMR signals.

Antenna Device to send or receive electromagnetic radiation in the RF region of the spectrum.

B_o Conventional symbol for the main magnetic field in an MRI system. Measured in tesla (T).

Chemical shift Change in the Larmor frequency of a given nucleus when bound in different sites in a molecule, owing to the magnetic shielding effects of the electron orbitals.

Coil Single or multiple loops of wire designed either to produce a magnetic field from current flowing through the wire or to detect a changing magnetic field by voltage induced in the wire.

Contrast Relative difference of the MRI signal intensities and the associated image brightness in adjacent regions.

Detector Portion of the receiver that demodulates the RF NMR signal and converts it to a lower frequency signal. Most detectors now used are phase sensitive and also give phase information about the RF signal.

Filtered back projection Mathematical technique used in reconstruction from projections to create images from a set of multiple projection profiles.

Flip angle Amount of rotation of the net magnetization vector produced by an RF pulse, with respect to the direction of the static magnetic field B_o.

Fourier transform (FT) Mathematical procedure to separate the frequency components of a signal from its amplitudes as a function of time. The Fourier transform is used to generate the spectrum from the FID and is essential to most imaging techniques.

Fourier transform imaging MRI techniques in which at least one dimension is phase encoded by applying variable gradient pulses along that dimension. The Fourier transform is then used to reconstruct an image from the set of encoded MRI signals.

Free induction decay (FID) If transverse magnetization (M_{xy}) of the spins is produced, a transient NMR signal will result that will decay with a characteristic time constant T2 (or T2*); this decaying signal is the FID.

Gradient coils Current-carrying coils designed to produce a desired gradient magnetic field. Proper design of the size and configuration of the coils is necessary to produce a controlled and uniform gradient.

Gyromagnetic ratio (γ) Ratio of the magnetic moment to the angular momentum of a particle. This is a constant for a given nucleus (MHz/T).

Image acquisition time Time required to receive all

of the NMR signals necessary to produce an MR image. The additional image reconstruction time will also be important to determine how quickly the image can be viewed.

Inversion recovery (IR) RF pulse sequence for MRI wherein the net magnetization is inverted and returns to equilibrium with the emission of an NMR signal.

Inversion time (TI) Time between the 180° RF inversion pulse and the subsequent 90° RF pulse to bring net magnetization onto the X-Y plane.

Larmor frequency (ω) Frequency at which magnetic resonance can be excited; given by the Larmor equation. For hydrogen nuclei, the Larmor frequency is 42.6 MHz/T.

Lattice Magnetic environment with which nuclei exchange energy in longitudinal relaxation.

Longitudinal magnetization (M_z) Component of the net magnetization vector along the static magnetic field.

Longitudinal relaxation Return of longitudinal magnetization to its equilibrium value after excitation; requires exchange of energy between the nuclear spins and the lattice.

M_0 Equilibrium value of the net magnetization vector directed along the static magnetic field.

Magnetic dipole North and south magnetic poles separated by a finite distance.

Magnetic moment Measure of the net magnetic properties of an object or particle.

Magnetic resonance imaging Creation of images of patients by use of the nuclear magnetic resonance phenomenon. Image brightness in a given region usually depends on the spin density and the relaxation times.

Nuclear magnetic resonance (NMR) Absorption or emission of electromagnetic energy by nuclei in a static magnetic field, after excitation by a suitable RF magnetic field. The peak resonance frequency is proportional to the magnetic field and is given by the Larmor equation.

Paramagnetic Type of substance with a small but positive magnetic susceptibility. The addition of a small amount of paramagnetic substance may greatly reduce the relaxation times of a substance. Paramagnetic substances are considered promising for use as contrast agents in MRI.

Partial saturation (PS) Excitation technique applying repeated 90° RF pulses at times on the order of or shorter than T1. Although partial saturation is also commonly referred to as "saturation recovery," the latter term should properly be reserved for the particular case of partial saturation when the 90° RF pulses are far enough apart in time that the return of nuclear spins to equilibrium is complete.

Pixel Acronym for a picture element; the smallest discrete part of a digital image display.

Planar imaging Imaging technique in which image of a plane is built up from signals received from the whole plane.

Precession Comparatively slow gyration of the axis of a spinning body so as to trace out a cone, caused by the application of a torque tending to change the direction of the rotation axis.

Pulse, 90° RF pulse designed to rotate the net magnetization vector 90° to the main magnetic field. If the spins are initially aligned with the magnetic field, this pulse will produce transverse magnetization and an FID.

Pulse, 180° RF pulse designed to rotate the net magnetization vector 180°. If the spins are initially aligned with the magnetic field, this pulse will produce inversion. If the spins are initially in the X-Y plane, a spin echo will result.

Pulse sequences Set of RF or gradient magnetic field pulses and time spacings between these pulses.

Radio frequency (RF) Electromagnetic radiation just lower in energy than infrared. The RF used in MRI is commonly in the 10- to 100-MHz range.

Receiver coil Coil of the RF receiver; detects the NMR signal.

Reconstruction from projections MRI technique in which a set of projection profiles of the body is obtained by observing NMR signals in the presence of a suitable corresponding set of gradient magnetic fields. Images can then be reconstructed using techniques analogous to those used in computed tomography, such as filtered back projection.

Relaxation time After excitation, the nuclear spins will tend to return to their equilibrium position, in accordance with these time constants.

Resonance Large-amplitude vibration in a mechanical or electrical system caused by a relatively small periodic stimulus with a frequency at or close to a natural frequency of the system.

RF pulse Brief burst of RF electromagnetic energy delivered to patient by RF transmitter. If the RF frequency is at the Larmor frequency, the result is rotation of the net magnetization vector and phase coherence of the nuclear spins.

Saturation Nonequilibrium state in MRI in which equal numbers of spins are aligned against and with the B_0 magnetic field so there is no net magnetization.

Signal-to-noise ratio (SNR or S/N) Used to describe the relative contributions to a detected signal of the true signal and random superimposed signals or noise. The SNR can be improved by averaging several NMR signals, by sampling larger volumes, or by increasing the strength of the B_0 magnetic field.

Spatial resolution Ability of an imaging process to distinguish small adjacent high-contrast structures in the object.

Spin Intrinsic angular momentum of an elementary particle, or system of particles such as a nucleus, that is responsible for the magnetic moment.

Spin density (SD) Density of resonating nuclear spins in a given region; one of the principal determinants of the strength of the NMR signal from that region.

Spin echo Reappearance of an NMR signal after the FID has disappeared. The result of the effective reversal of the dephasing of the nuclear spins.

Spin echo imaging Any one of many MRI techniques in which the spin-echo NMR signal rather than the FID is used.

T1 Spin-lattice or longitudinal relaxation time; the characteristic time constant for spins to tend to align themselves with the external magnetic field.

T2 Spin-spin or transverse relaxation time; the characteristic time constant for loss of phase coherence among spins oriented at an angle to the main magnetic field owing to interactions between the spins. T2 never exceeds T1.

T2* Characteristic time constant for loss of phase coherence among spins oriented at an angle to the main magnetic field owing to a combination of magnetic field inhomogeneities and spin-spin relaxation. T2* is always much shorter than T2.

TE echo time Time between middle of 90° RF pulse and middle of spin echo.

Tesla (T) Preferred (SI) unit of magnetic flux density or magnetic field intensity. One tesla is equal to 10,000 gauss, the older (CSG) unit. One tesla also equals one newton/amp-m.

Thermal equilibrium State in which all parts of a system are at the same effective temperature at which time the relative alignment of the spins with the magnetic field is determined solely by the thermal energy of the system.

TI inversion time Time after middle of inverting RF pulse to middle of 90° pulse to detect amount of longitudinal magnetization.

Time reversal Technique of producing a spin echo by subjecting excited spins to a gradient magnetic field and then reversing the direction of the gradient field.

Transverse magnetization (M_{xy}) Component of the net magnetization vector at right angles to the main magnetic field, B_0.

TR repetition time Period between the beginning of a pulse sequence and the beginning of the succeeding and identical pulse sequence.

Tunnel Opening into MR imager for patient. Sometimes called the patient aperture.

Voxel Volume element; the element of three-dimensional space corresponding to a pixel for a given slice thickness.

From Bushong, 1988.

PART II

DEVELOPMENTAL DISORDERS

The developmental disorders are, for the most part, chronic conditions where there is a disturbance in the acquisition of cognitive, language, motor, or social skills (DSM-IV, 1994). Some signs of the disorder may persist in stable form into adult life, but, in less severe cases, full adaptation or full recovery is possible. In Part II, developmental disorders involving each of these systems will be reviewed. This part includes mental retardation (cognitive disorder); cerebral palsy (movement disorder); learning disorders (reading disorder, spelling disorder, mathematics disorder, disorder of written expression, social-emotional learning disabilities); traumatic brain injury; and pervasive developmental disorders (primarily language and social skills disorders). Four of these may have genetic and/or environmental bases; traumatic brain injury, described in Chapter 8, is an acquired condition whose course may be more complicated if the insult occurs in children with prior developmental disorders. Moreover, children with developmental disorders are more vulnerable to environmental insults.

For each disorder, the history, definition, epidemiology, etiology, developmental perspective, natural history, classification, associated disabling conditions, assessment process, vulnerability to mental illness, and interventions are described. In the ICD-10 classification, these conditions are classified under two sections: F70-F79, Mental Retardation, and F80-F89, Disorders of Psychological Development, as shown in Table II–1.

In the DSM-IV classification, the multiaxial classification has been maintained. To ensure that mental retardation is diagnosed along with the presenting psychiatric disorder, it is an Axis II diagnosis. Children and adolescents with these disorders are primarily seen by psychiatrists for associated behavior, emotional, and interpersonal disorders or concur-

Table II–1. Disorders of Psychological Development: ICD-10

F80 Specific developmental disorders of speech and language

F80.0	Specific speech articulation disorder
F80.1	Expressive language disorder
F80.2	Receptive language disorder
F80.3	Acquired aphasia with epilepsy (Landau-Kleffner syndrome)
F80.8	Other developmental disorders of speech and language
F80.9	Developmental disorder of speech and language, unspecified

F81 Specific developmental disorders of scholastic skills

F81.0	Specific reading disorder
F81.1	Specific spelling disorder
F81.2	Specific disorder of arithmetical skills
F81.3	Mixed disorder of scholastic skills
F81.8	Other developmental disorders of scholastic skills
F81.9	Developmental disorder of scholastic skills, unspecified

F82 Specific developmental disorder of motor function

F83 Mixed specific developmental disorders

F84 Pervasive developmental disorders

F84.0	Childhood autism
F84.1	Atypical autism
F84.2	Rett's syndrome
F84.3	Other childhood disintegrative disorder
F84.4	Overactive disorder associated with mental retardation and stereotyped movements
F84.5	Asperger's syndrome
F84.8	Other pervasive developmental disorders
F84.9	Pervasive developmental disorder, unspecified

F88 Other disorders of psychological development

F89 Unspecified disorder of psychological development

From WHO, 1992.

Table II–2. Disorders Usually First Diagnosed in Infancy, Childhood, or Adolescence: DSM-IV

Mental Retardation

317	Mild Mental Retardation
318.0	Moderate Mental Retardation
318.1	Severe Mental Retardation
318.2	Profound Mental Retardation
319	Mental Retardation, Severity Unspecified

Learning Disorders

315.00	Reading Disorder
315.1	Mathematics Disorder
315.2	Disorder of Written Expression
315.9	Learning Disorder NOS

Motor Skills Disorder

315.4	Developmental Coordination Disorder

Pervasive Developmental Disorders

299.00	Autistic Disorder
299.80	Rett's Disorder
299.10	Childhood Disintegrative Disorder
299.80	Asperger's Disorder
299.80	Pervasive Developmental Disorder NOS

From APA, 1994.

rent major mental disorder, with the possible exception of autistic disorders where a psychiatrist may make or confirm the initial diagnosis. Each of these conditions leads to increased vulnerability to mental disorder. In DSM-IV, the numbering system used in DSM-III has been retained (see Table II–2).

Each of these diagnostic categories is the generally accepted term for a disabling condition that has both psychological and social implications for families and for the provision of services. Each condition has multiple etiologies, and there are national associations and parent groups that advocate for services for all children with one of these designated developmental disorders. Furthermore, children and adolescents with developmental disorders and their families have problems in adapting to the specific diagnosis, leading to adjustment disorders and sometimes triggering more severe mental illness. Because of the nature of these disabling conditions, an interdisciplinary team is essential to provide comprehensive treatment. Early recognition, prevention, preventive interventions, and specific treatments are required. The approach to treatment is individualized for each child, following a careful evaluation. In each case, a developmental perspective is essential to understand the natural history of the disorder. In some instances, there are delays in development; in others, there are arrests in development after apparent normal development, and in still others, development is deviant from the beginning of life.

Recent developments in molecular genetics that are pertinent to mental retardation are described in Volume 1, Chapter 5. The mental retardation syndromes most commonly associated with behavioral phenotypes are described in Part III.

CHAPTER 5

MENTAL RETARDATION

Mental retardation is the currently accepted designation for an intellectual and adaptive behavior disability that begins in early life during the developmental period. Although "mental retardation" is the term used in both the International Classification of Diseases (ICD) and the Diagnostic and Statistical Manual (DSM) systems, the terms "mental deficiency" and "mental handicap" have been used in the past by national associations in the United States and in the United Kingdom, respectively. In the United Kingdom, the term "learning disability" is sometimes used in place of "mental handicap," but this term is applied primarily to academic skill disorders in the United States. The term "intellectual disability" is also used in the United Kingdom and has been incorporated into the title of a research journal. These variations in terminology derive from the long-standing concern about the stigma of a diagnosis of mental retardation and continuing efforts to deal with the social meaning of diagnostic labels as they apply to disabling conditions. This chapter retains the term "mental retardation" in keeping with the diagnostic terms used in the DSM-IV (APA, 1994) and the ICD-10 (WHO, 1992) classification systems and the recent name change of the American Association of Mental Deficiency to the American Association on Mental Retardation (AAMR).

Mental retardation is not a static disorder but rather a dynamic condition which has multiple etiologies that must be considered in treatment planning. It is not a disease or an illness in itself (Clarke, Clarke, and Berg, 1985). In mental retardation, thinking is not characteristically disordered and perception is not distorted unless there is a concurrent mental disorder. It is made up of a heterogeneous group of conditions that range from genetic and metabolic disorders to functional changes following trauma to the nervous system at birth or later in the developmental period. Because of its heterogeneity, each case must be considered independently according to whether or not there is an associated syndrome, for example, Down syndrome, or an associated etiology, for example, head trauma. There is no single cause, mechanism, clinical course, or prognosis.

Mentally retarded persons may be diagnosed with a full range of mental disorders. In fact, the prevalence of associated mental disorders is three to four times greater than in the general population. Furthermore, mentally retarded individuals are at greater risk for exploitation and physical or sexual abuse. Because adaptive behavior is, by definition, impaired, social stressors are particularly problematic. However, in protective social environments where adequate support is available, their impairments may not be obvious; this is particularly true of mildly retarded persons.

This chapter reviews history, diagnosis and classification, epidemiology, etiologies, developmental issues, assessment, psychopathology, and treatment. Institutional care and deinstitutionalization, public law and the right to education, and legal competency are discussed in Part VI, Public Law and the Rights of the Disabled.

HISTORY

Historically, the earliest reference to mental retardation may be in the Egyptian Papyrus of Thebes (1552 B.C.) (Bryan, 1930). Despite recognition since antiquity, there is little evidence of early medical interest in mental retardation. Religious references in the various traditions suggest mentally retarded people be treated with kindness. Despite these admonishments, humane education is a recent development. In Greek and Roman cultures, infanticide was practiced, and trephining may have been used in Europe and Central and South America as an intervention, presumably to release or remove evil spirits. Mentally retarded persons may have become slaves in some cultures or chosen for court jesters. In others, attitudes varied from humane concern to ostracism and abuse thoughout history. In some countries mentally retarded people were viewed as harmless innocents who were allowed to wander at will. Henry II of England showed a more enlightened view and promulgated legislation to provide for their protection, making them wards of the king.

It was not until around the end of the eighteenth century that a rising respect for the individual, which provided the impetus for the French and American revolutions, began to address the rights of not only slaves, the mentally ill, the blind and deaf, but also mentally retarded persons (Kanner, 1964). Early interventionists, such as Jean-Marc-Gaspard Itard, against the better judgment of the experts of the time, spent five years (1801–1806) (Lane, 1976) trying to teach Victor, the wild boy of Aveyron. Although Victor did not achieve normalization, the methods Itard developed were recognized as highly meritorious by the French Academy of Sciences, which closely followed his interventions. Subsequently, an organized effort to educate mentally retarded persons began in Switzerland and eventually moved from there to other parts of Europe and to the United States. Interest in mental retardation at the time was stimulated by new, more hopeful, ideas about development stimulated by the philosophy of Rousseau, the encyclopedists, and Pestalozzi. Itard's subsequent work in an institution for deaf-mutes encouraged Edouard Séguin to devote himself to the investigation and treatment of mentally retarded persons. Itard was influenced not only by his teachers, but also by his religious orientation. He was "striving for a social application of the principles of the gospel, for the most rapid evolution of the lowest and poorest by all means and institutions, mostly by free education (Kanner, 1960)."

Like Itard, Séguin began to work individually with a mentally retarded boy and, based on his success, began to work with more children at the Hospice for Incurables (Kanner, 1960). By 1844 Séguin was acknowledged by a commission of the Paris Academy of Sciences. His achievements were documented in his classical textbook (1846). He reported that his training of mentally retarded persons embraced "the muscular, imitative, nervous, and reflective functions." Later, Séguin came to the United States where he made contact with Samuel Gridley Howe, who was instrumental in establishing interventions for retarded persons there. In 1866, Séguin's text, *Idiocy and Its Treatment by the Physiological Method,* advocated an institution as an instrument for the treatment of children who were too severely mentally retarded to profit from normal classroom instruction (Séguin, 1866). In 1876 Séguin was selected as the first president of the Medical Officers of American Institutes for Idiotic and Feeble Minded Persons, which is now the American Association on Mental Retardation.

The first medical periodical devoted to mental retardation was published in 1850, and titled, *Observations on Cretinism.* Wilhelm Griesinger (1876) stated that although every cretin is retarded, every retarded person is not a cretin. In doing so, he insisted that mental retardation is a comprehensive category and not a single entity. The general trend at that time was to make no distinctions between the various types of mental retardation. Amentia or idiocy was considered to be a homogeneous category and both "idiocy" and "insanity" were regarded as homogeneous entities. Subsequently, a breakthrough was made in distinguishing the heterogeneous nature of mental retardation by John L.H. Down in his classical paper, *Observations on an Ethnic Classification of Idiots* (1866).

With the recognition that mental retardation was not a homogeneous category, a new interest developed in classification. However, Down was initially misled by the physical appearance of the individuals he examined. In the hope of absolving parents of self-blame by emphasizing a constitutional basis, he developed an ethnic classification, suggesting the various forms of mental retardation represented regressions to earlier racial forms. He subsequently abandoned this idea and proposed that the best classification is one based on etiology. He recognized three major groups: (1) congenital, which included microcephalic, macrocephalic, hydrocephalic, epileptic, and paralytic; (2) developmental, with a vulnerability to mental breakdown during a developmental crisis; and (3) accidental (caused by injury or illness). Subsequently, William Weatherspoon Ireland (1877), in his textbook *On Idiocy and Imbecility,* suggested 10 subdivisions, among which were genetous (congential), microcephalic, epileptic, eclamptic, hydrocephalic, paralytic, traumatic, inflammatory, cretinism, and idiocy by deprivation. The way was prepared to differentiate specific conditions that differed in both pathology and etiology but were characterized by mental retardation. Later tuberous sclerosis was identified in 1880 by Desire-Maglione Bourneville, and many degenerative diseases were recognized, such as Tay-Sach disease. These findings established the view that mental retardation is caused by brain pathology and is incurable. Thus began an era of searching for more clearly defined disorders, which were commonly named after their discoverers. It was an era when syndromes were recognized, but medicine had little to offer therapeutically. The only ameliorization that was offered was provided by educators. The recognition of brain pathology raised questions about the possibility of any medical habilitation.

With the discovery of intelligence testing and the establishment of an interest in eugenics, interest turned to the heredity of mental retardation. Psychometric tests were developed in France by two physicians, Alfred Binet and Théodore Simon, in 1905. They saw their test as a way to select children for specialized education, yet when introduced in the United States in 1908 by Henry Goddard, these tests were used specifically to diagnose mental retardation. Testing of large numbers of individuals at various ages was carried out in the United States. Intelligence quotients (IQs) which resulted from the tests were considered to be an adequate and accurate measure of intelligence. Intelligence was thought to be a constant feature that reflected a permanent and inherent level of mental ability. Because the tests were considered objective and scientific, they gradually replaced the individualized clinical evaluation. The tests were used in correctional institutions where drug abusers, prostitutes, and others showing antisocial behavior commonly tested in the mild range of mental retardation. Some considered mental retardation to be the source of their antisocial behavior rather than to consider fully the relationship of socially maladaptive behavior to neglect, poverty, and mistreatment.

Following the discovery of Gregor Mendel's principles of genetic inheritance, books such as Goddard's *The Kallikaks* sought to document that mental retardation and antisocial behavior were genetically rather than socially transmitted. Goddard's (1912) description of the Kallikaks pictured mentally retarded persons as a menace to society and a source of criminality, drug abuse, and the genetic source of more retarded persons. Subsequently, the eugenics movement picked up the idea that mildly retarded persons were a danger to society due to their "moral imbecility," indiscriminate sexual behavior, and excessive procreation. The eugenics movement suggested their indiscriminate sexual behavior would lead to an increase in mentally retarded persons and in delinquent populations. Eugenic considerations led to a movement to place mentally retarded persons in institutions and to sterilize them. Such views increased the size of the institutionalized population as well as the numbers admitted with emotional and behavior disorders.

The first preventive intervention for a mental retardation syndrome occurred when Ivar Folling (1934) recognized phenylketonuria (PKU) as a metabolic disturbance that could be reversed by proper diet. The recognition of a biochemically based syndrome led to the establishment of mental retardation research as a legitimate focus in the biological sciences. The medical profession began to look more carefully to identify the etiology of mental retardation syndromes (Kanner, 1967).

Following the Second World War, change in community attitudes reemphasized the possibility of remediation, analogous to what had taken place a century and a half before when Itard initiated the first remedial education program. This impetus for improved remediation developed from the response of parents to the needs of their children. In the 1950s parent groups were organized in the United States and other countries, culminating in the establishment of the National Association for Retarded Children in the United States. An advisory board drawn from representatives of the various specialties who might work for the study of prevention and care of mental retardation was established. This new thrust was most clearly demonstrated by U.S. President John F. Kennedy (February 5, 1963). In his congressional message on mental illness and mental retardation, he called for "a national program to combat mental retardation." This national program brought medicine, education, psychology, sociology, genetics, and the various specialties that are pertinent to the needs of a child who is mentally retarded together into special centers affiliated with universities to provide intervention. Through mental retardation research centers that are federally funded, mental retardation research began to grow. Finally, academic medicine had become fully involved with other specialties, community organizations, and parent groups to study the etiology of mental retardation syndromes, establish therapeutic interventions, and develop habilitation and prevention programs.

Neuropsychiatrists were frequently superintendents of the early institutions for mentally retarded persons. Later on, the child guidance clinics were involved in preventive care. However, with the expansion of psychoanalytic schools in the United States after the Second World War, psychiatric involvement with mental retardation declined as verbal, psychodynamically oriented treatment became the primary mode of treatment. Because of their cognitive deficiencies, mentally retarded persons seemed unable to benefit from a traditional psychoanalytic approach that was verbal, conceptual, and insight oriented. Advances in the neurosciences, developmental psychology, developmental psychopathology, phenomenology and classification, family, behavior, and drug treatments have led to a new perspective in psychiatry and a renewed commitment to mentally retarded/mentally ill persons. Recognition of the interface and the role of experience in brain development and a better understanding of the natural history of specific mental retardation syndromes has led to participation of psychiatrists with other professionals in the habilitation of mentally retarded/mentally ill individuals.

DIAGNOSIS AND CLASSIFICATION

Mental retardation is defined in the American Diagnostic and Statistical Manual for Mental Disorders (DSM-III-R and DSM-IV) (APA, 1987, 1994), the International Classification of Diseases (ICD-10) (WHO, 1992), and by the American Association on Mental Retardation (AAMR, 1992). Although all of the definitions include IQ and adaptive function, each provides a different emphasis, so it is important to be familiar with each of them. In applying the definitions, keep in mind that specific adaptive abilities often coexist with strengths in other adaptive skills or personal capabilities; therefore, adaptive strengths must be carefully considered. Because it focuses on function, the AAMR definition is described in detail.

DSM-IV Definition

Table 5–1 shows the DSM-IV diagnostic criteria (1994), and Table 5–2 compares these criteria with the previous DSM-III-R criteria (1987) and the AAMR criteria (1992), pointing out some differences among them.

It should be noted that persons under 18 who meet diagnostic criteria for dementia and whose IQ is below 70 are given both the diagnosis of dementia and mental retardation. However, an individual over 18 who develops multiple cognitive impairments, with a drop in IQ to below 70, receives only the diagnosis of dementia. The diagnosis of dementia can be made "any time after the IQ is fairly stable (usually by age 3 or 4)." Clarification of a diagnosis of dementia is important because mental retardation is a developmental disability.

Table 5–1. DSM-IV Diagnostic Criteria for Mental Retardation

A. Significantly subaverage intellectual function ıg: an IQ of approximately 70 or below on an individually administered IQ test (for infants, a clinical judgment of significantly subaverage intellectual functioning).
B. Concurrent deficits or impairments in present adaptive functioning (i.e., the person's effectiveness in meeting the standards expected for his or her age by his or her cultural group, in at least two of the following skill areas: communication, self-care, home living, social/interpersonal skills, use of community resources, self-direction, functional academic skills, work, leisure, health and safety).
C. Onset before the age of 18.

Code based on degree of severity reflecting level of intellectual impairment:

317	Mild Mental Retardation:	IQ level 50–55 to approximately 70
318.0	Moderate Retardation:	IQ level 35–40 to 50–55
318.1	Severe Mental Retardation:	IQ level 20–25 to 35–40
318.2	Profound Mental Retardation:	IQ level below 20 or 25
319	Mental Retardation, Severity Unspecified:	when there is a strong presumption of mental retardation but the person is untestable by standard intelligence tests.

From APA, 1994.

Table 5–2. Diagnostic Criteria for Mental Retardation

	DSM-III-R	DSM-IV	AAMR
Adaptive Function	Concurrent impairment in adaptive functioning.	Concurrent impairment in *present* adaptive functioning.	Limitations in *present* functioning.
	Does not specify extent of skills deficits.	Requires deficits in two or more skill areas (includes social/interpersonal).	Deficits in two or more skill areas. Same as DSM-IV but designates social skills rather than social/interpersonal skills.
Intelligence Quotient			
Child/Adolescent	IQ 70 or below on individually administered tests.	IQ of *approximately* 70 or below on individually administered tests.	IQ of approximately 70 to 75 on individually administered tests.
Infants	Clinical judgment of subaverage function.	Clinical judgment of subaverage function.	Level estimated as below the 3rd percentile by clinical judgment.
Levels of Mental Retardation	Mild, moderate, severe, profound.	Mild, moderate, severe, profound.	Rather than levels, categories of support needs are designated.

ICD-10 Definition

The International Classification of Diseases lists mental retardation as a disorder of psychological development and takes a somewhat different approach than the DSM-IV. The ICD-10 definition is as follows:

> Mental retardation is a condition of arrested or incomplete development of the mind, which is especially characterized by impairment of skills manifested during the developmental period, contributing to the overall level of intelligence, i.e., cognitive, language, motor, and social abilities.

This definition emphasizes that intelligence is not a unitary characteristic but is assessed on the basis of a large number of different but more or less specific skills. These skills generally develop to a similar degree in each individual; however, because mental retardation is a heterogeneous disorder, one may see large discrepancies among them. There may be severe impairments in one area, for example, language; in other instances, there may be an area of higher skill level that is maintained, often referred to as a splinter skill, such as better visuospatial abilities in a severely retarded person. This scatter in abilities presents difficulties in determining into which subgroup of mental retardation a person should be placed.

An assessment takes into account clinical findings, adaptive behavior (considered in relation to the individual's cultural background), and performance on psychometric tests. The category chosen should be based on global assessment and not on a single area or specific impairment. IQ levels are provided as a guide but should not be applied rigidly because they are divisions of a complex continuum that cannot be defined with absolute preciseness. The intelligence quotient should be determined utilizing standardized, individually administered tests, taking into account local cultural norms. The appropriate test must be selected based on the individual's level of functioning and any associated disabling conditions, such as expressive language difficulties, physical disabilities, and hearing or visual problems. In addition to cognitive tests, scales of adaptive function need to be completed by interviewing parents or care providers who are familiar with the individual's performance of daily activities required for personal and social sufficiency. If both intellectual level and social adaptation are not considered, then the assessment is simply a provisional estimate. Tests of adaptive behavior that are used together with intelligence tests include the AAMR Adaptive Behavior Scales (Lambert, Nihiri, and Leland, 1993; Nihiri, Leland, and Lambert, 1993) and the Vineland Adaptive Behavior Scales (Sparrow, Balla, and Cicchetti, 1984). With the development of these adaptive behavioral instruments, guidelines are being established to determine what constitutes a significant impairment in adaptive functioning. In some states, performance that falls below the third percentile (i.e., standard score below 70 to 75) in two of the following domains is used: communication, daily living skills/self-help, socialization/social functioning/interpersonal, and motor.

AAMR Definition

Although the DSM-IV definition is used in the standard classification, the American Association on Mental Retardation has proposed an extension of this definition that focuses more on the individual's needs, as shown later in Table 5–3, and what can be done to improve functioning. This revision replaces their 1983 definition (Grossman, 1983) and represents a major change in the way people with mental retardation are described for purposes of classification. The definition and detailed descriptions are provided in the manual *Mental Retardation: Definition, Classification, and Systems of Support* (AAMR, 1992). The AAMR definition of mental retardation provides a comprehensive orientation to the person with mental retardation but does not include specific levels of mental retardation. It emphasizes the risks of a unidimensional approach that focuses only on disability. In contrast, the ICD-10 and DSM-IV approaches maintain the levels of mental retardation as "mild, moderate, severe, and profound." It must be emphasized that, from a developmental perspective, the inclusion of levels of impairment is helpful.

The AAMR definition is as follows:

> Mental retardation refers to substantial limitations in present functioning. It is characterized by significantly subaverage intellectual functioning, existing concurrently with related limitations in two or more of the following applicable adaptive

> skills areas: communication, self-care, home living, social skills, community use, self-direction, health and safety, functional academics, leisure, and work. Mental retardation manifests before age 18.

This description emphasizes functional ability and considers the congruence of intellectual and adaptive abilities along with stressors that impact on adaptive functioning. The adaptive functioning assessment is essential because IQ tests alone are not an accurate measure of a mentally retarded person's ability although adaptive skills are closely related to intellectual limitations. Adaptive ability has been defined as "the effectiveness or degree with which an individual meets the standards of personal independence and social responsibility expected of his age and cultural group" (Grossman, 1983). This includes the areas of social/interpersonal skills and responsibility, communication, self-care, home living, use of community resources, self-direction, functional academic skills, work, leisure, health, and safety. As in DSM-IV, at least two of these areas must be involved to diagnose a generalized limitation. Because these skills vary with chronological age, the assessment must take age into account. The low intelligence score and limited adaptive ability must occur before 18 years of age, the age when adult roles are typically assumed.

The key elements of the AAMR approach are on: (1) instrumental competence (cognition and learning) and social competence (practical and social intelligence) that make up adaptive skills; (2) environments where an individual lives, works, and learns; and (3) overall functioning, which refers to the ability to cope with ordinary challenges of everyday living in the community. It is essential to remember that mental retardation is not a static condition; the developmental goal is to establish a "best fit match" of the person with environmental supports to maximize adaptive ability.

The AAMR definition is based on four assumptions (AAMR, 1992) that take into account cultural issues, communication, behavioral differences, and the expectation of improvement with appropriate supports because each person has unique strengths as well as limitations. These four assumptions also apply to the DSM-IV definition. The assumptions are as follows: (1) Valid assessment considers cultural and linguistic diversity, and differences in communication and behavioral factors. The language spoken at home, nonverbal language, and ethnicity may affect assessment results. (2) The existence of limitations in adaptive skills occurs within the context of community environments typical of the individual's age peers and is indexed to the person's individualized need for supports. The environments include the home, neighborhood, school, and work environments, and the peer group refers to those from a similar language and cultural background. (3) Specific adaptive limitations often coexist with strengths in other adaptive skills or other personal capabilities. There are personal strengths that are independent of the degree of mental retardation. These include physical and social capabilities and specific ability in one or more adaptive skills. (4) With appropriate supports over a sustained period, the life functioning of the person with mental retardation generally improves. Appropriate supports are matched to an individual's needs and include supportive individuals and services. Although mental retardation may not be lifelong, these supports may be needed for an extended period, and in some instances, throughout life. Improvement in function is expected for the majority but, for some, supports are needed to maintain a basic level of function or primarily to slow the regression process.

Levels of Mental Retardation

Mental retardation is divided into four levels of severity in DSM-IV (APA, 1994), reflecting the extent of intellectual impairment: mild, moderate, severe, or profound.

Mild Mental Retardation

Utilizing properly standardized intelligence tests, the mildly retarded range is 50 to 69. DSM-IV lists IQ level 50–55 to approximately 70. For mildly retarded persons, previously referred to as in the educable range, problems with the use of language and speech difficulties may limit independence in adult life. This group makes up about 85% of those who are classified as mentally retarded. These children often are not distinguishable from normal children in the early months of life and are recognized only at school or perhaps in preschool. During the preschool years (0 to 5), social and communication skills generally develop, although there may be minimal impairment in sensorimotor function. By their late teens, they may acquire academic skills up to the fifth- or sixth-grade level. During their adult years, mildly retarded persons may develop sufficient social and vocational abilities and only need a minimum of external support. Still, ongoing guidance will be needed under stressful social conditions or during economic hardship. Most individuals with mild retardation appear successful in the community and may live independently or in supervised apartments or group homes. Their developmental achievements allow them to hold conversations and participate in clinical interviews. Their learning difficulties may become evident in academic work. Socioculturally, when academic achievement is not required, their problems may be minimal. Yet there may be a noticeable degree of social and emotional immaturity leading to difficulties in coping. There may be an inability to cope with the demands of marriage or child rearing or to meet specific cultural expectations. For the most part, their behavioral, emotional, and social problems and their need for psychosocial and behavior treatment and support are similar to those of persons with normal intelligence. Brain abnormalities are identifiable in a minority of this group. Associated conditions include autistic disorder, other developmental disorders, epilepsy, conduct disorders, or physical disability.

Moderate Mental Retardation

The IQ range for moderate mental retardation is from 35 to 49. DSM-IV indicates IQ 35–40 to 50–55. However, the full-scale IQ score can be deceptive because variable cognitive profiles of abilities are common for this group, e.g., some individuals may have higher visuospatial skills than language skills. Moreover, some moderately retarded children may be thought to be functioning at a lower level due to motor incoordination, although they can be socially interactive and communicative with appropriate assistance. Language development is variable across this IQ range, spanning from the capacity to participate in simple conversations to simple language limited to communication of basic needs. Those who never learn language may understand simple instruction or learn to use sign language to compensate for speech difficulties. There are also limitations in their achievement of self-care and motor skills. School progress is limited, but the higher functioning individual may learn basic skills in reading, writing, and counting. As adults, moderately retarded individuals may participate in simple, practical work that is carefully structured, but generally need consistent supervision by others. Completely independent living is rarely achieved in adulthood. Moderately retarded individuals make up approximately 10% of the mentally retarded population.

In regard to etiology, brain abnormality can be identified in the majority. Seizure disorder and other neurological and physical disabilities also commonly occur. Autistic disorder and other pervasive developmental disorders may be associated, leading to problems in further social adaptation. Psychiatric diagnosis may be difficult because of their limited language development that often requires the use of other informants. In the past, the term "trainable" was used for moderately retarded persons, but it should be avoided because many individuals in this group can benefit from educational programs. Efforts should be made to identify appropriate sheltered workshops, group homes, and supportive employment programs.

Severe Mental Retardation

The IQ range for severe mental retardation is 20 to 35. In DSM-IV this is shown as 20–25 to 35–40. This group is similar to the moderately mentally retarded group in regard to their clinical picture and presence of brain abnormality. A significant number of severely retarded persons have marked motor impairment and other associated deficits.

During the preschool years, poor motor development and lack of communicative speech are readily recognized. During the school-age years, verbal language may emerge and elementary self-care skills may be taught. Depending on their cognitive ability, basic survival skills may be learned, including sight-reading of essential words, such as *stop, man,* and *woman.* In adulthood, supervision is needed to aid in task performance. Community programs and group homes are frequently needed or, in some cases, specific in-home assistance to families is required. Associated disabilities may require specialized nursing care. The severely mentally retarded group makes up 3% to 4% of the mentally retarded population.

Profound Mental Retardation

The IQ range for profound mental retardation is less than 20. DSM-IV suggests less than 20–25. Language comprehension and use is generally limited to understanding simple commands and making simple requests. Adaptive function is very variable although certain visuospatial skills, such as matching and sorting, may be acquired. With supervision and guidance, the child, and later the adult, may take part in practical tasks and domestic routines. As a result of their various disabilities, a highly structured environment with continual aid and supervision is necessary. Individualized relationships with caregivers are emphasized to facilitate optimal development. Self-care, communication skills, and motor abilities may require training in a structured setting. Living arrangements include small group homes in the community, intermediate care facilities, or living with their families along with day program support.

Brain abnormality can be identified in the majority of profoundly mentally retarded persons. Neurological and physical disabilities that affect mobility are common, as are associated seizure disorder and visual and hearing impairment. Pervasive developmental disorders, especially autistic-like behavior, is frequent. This group constitutes 1% to 2% of those diagnosed as mentally retarded.

Unspecified Mental Retardation

Overall, the younger the child, the more difficult it is to make a diagnosis of mental retardation, except for the most severe cases. The unspecified category is used when there is a presumption of mental retardation, but the person cannot be tested on standardized instruments. This may occur when children, adolescents, or adults are uncooperative or too impaired to participate in testing. This category may also be used for infants when available tests, such as the Catell or Bayley, do not provide IQ values. If intelligence is thought to be over 70, the category "unspecified mental retardation" should not be utilized. This category is most commonly used when an assessment of the degree of intellectual retardation, using the standard procedures, is difficult or impossible because of age and associated physical and sensory disabilities, for example, in blind, deaf, mute, and severely behaviorally disturbed, or physically disabled individuals.

Multiaxial Classification

One of the major advances in DSM-III (APA, 1980) was the establishment of the multiaxial classification system (Part V) to deal with complex cases. It is different than a multiple category system in that it provides for specific axes and rules for their use. This system was derivative of an earlier triaxial classification (Rutter et al., 1969) and of ongoing discussion about how mental retardation relates to psychiatric disorder (Tarjan et al., 1972). It provides a means to categorize both the intellectual and adaptive disability of mental retardation, associated psychiatric conditions, and associated brain disorder. Although, in general, the multiaxial classification system has been viewed from the perspective of the Axis I diagnosis, when dealing with developmental disorders its benefits become particularly clear because the major areas involved in treatment planning and predicting outcome can be designated on different axes. It provides a convenient format for organizing and communicating clinical information, and if all five axes are used, offers a far more comprehensive perspective than does a single diagnostic axis. For mental retardation, it highlights the need to plan for cognitive impairments.

In DSM-IV, the multiaxial system is maintained; however, it is not included in the ICD-10 classification. The diagnosis of mental retardation is on Axis II in DSM-IV, as was the case in DSM-III-R. Psychiatric diagnoses are placed on Axis I to emphasize the importance of making specific diagnoses for mentally retarded persons, rather than simply focusing on associated behaviors. If known, a particular mental retardation syndrome is coded on Axis III, general medical disorders. The Axis IV and V categories are domains that should be included for all mentally retarded persons. Axis IV refers to specific stressors, psychosocial and environmental problems, and Axis V to global assessment of functioning (GAF) scale, which provides an additional means to measure adaptive abilities. By using the multiaxial classification, factors that influence functioning can be better specified in the diagnostic system. Moreover, the complexity of a clinical situation can be demonstrated by describing comorbidity to highlight the heterogeneity of persons with a similar or the same diagnosis. The multiaxial system is of particular value in evaluating long-term prognosis because axes contribute to outcome risks.

In ICD-10, a different approach is taken. Provision is made for a fourth character to be added to the standard diagnostic code to specify the degree of behavioral impairment, if another ICD-10 mental disorder diagnosis is not appropriate. For example, mental retardation with a fourth character "0" indicates no or minimal behavioral impairment. The digit "1" indicates specific behavioral impairment requiring attention or treatment.

Table 5–3. AAMR Multidimensional Classification System

Dimension		Classification
Dimension I:	Intellectual Functioning and Adaptive Skills	• Cognitive • Adaptive • Develomental
Dimension II:	Psychological/ Emotional Considerations	• DSM-IV
Dimension III:	Physical/Health/ Etiology Considerations	• ICD-10 • Etiology
Dimension IV:	Environmental Considerations	• Ecological Analysis

From AAMR, 1992.

AAMR Multidimensional Approach

The AAMR classification provides its own multidimensional support systems approach, as shown in Table 5–3. Four dimensions are used to provide a more comprehensive picture of the individual: intellectual functioning and adaptive skills, psychological and emotional factors, general health and physical functioning, and environmental factors.

EPIDEMIOLOGY

Accurate estimates are needed on the number of mentally retarded individuals both for planning purposes and to gain better knowledge of the impact of interventions. Therefore, the prevalence and incidence of mental retardation has been studied extensively. Epidemiological research in mental retardation has a long history, going back at least to 1811 when Napoleon ordered a census of "cretins" to be made in one of the Swiss cantons (Kanner, 1964). Although little information is available about how this data was used, many surveys have been carried out since that time. In modern studies, there is wide variability in prevalence estimates. This variability stems from the heterogeneous nature of mental retardation and variation in ascertaining methodology. Because of this etiologic heterogeneity, IQ scores do not follow a normal distribution.

How mental retardation is defined and how the epidemiologic data is collected is critical to interpreting results (Munro, 1986). Both general population prevalence of mental retardation and separate prevalences for specific mental retardation syndromes are required. Screening for mental retardation in children who have very low birth weight or experience early trauma or illness is critical. Epidemiologic studies must be careful to consider the various terms used for mental retardation, i.e., mental deficiency, mental handicap, mental subnormality, intellectual retardation, developmental delay, and learning disability. When reviewing previous studies, the definition used in case findings must be carefully scrutinized.

At least three approaches have been used in epidemiologic research to define cases: statistical models, pathological models, and social systems models. Currently, the statistical model, which utilizes an IQ score 2 standard deviations below the mean along with an assessment of adaptive function to identify mental retardation, is the accepted system. Yet this statistical model implies a continuum of cognitive abilities that does not exist. Variability in cognitive profile and associated conditions that complicate assessment make it necessary to utilize general categories such as mild, moderate, severe, and profound.

The pathological model focuses on specific syndromes, such as Down syndrome, or a particular etiology, such as intraventricular hemorrhage. The social systems perspective designates individuals as mentally retarded if they are labeled by a social system, most commonly the school. For these purposes, children are not regarded as mentally retarded until they start school, and may no longer have the diagnosis after they leave school, if they are functioning adequately in society and have sufficient physical and social skills to work independently. The most pragmatic definitions are those provided by the statistical model, which considers psychometric scores, and the pathological model, which emphasizes adaptive functioning.

Despite the various approaches used in epidemiologic studies, there is general consistency in cross national studies of prevalence rates (Baird and Sadovnick, 1985; Koller et al., 1983). Overall population prevalence of mental retardation is less than 1% (fewer than 10 persons per 1,000 population). If the population in the United States is approximately 250 million, a 1% prevalence identifies 2.5 million people with mental retardation. Yet a 3% prevalence has often been chosen, using the statistical approach and basing the diagnosis on an IQ less than 70. The 3% rate assumes the mortality of mentally retarded individuals is similar to that of the general population, considers that mental retardation is routinely identified in infancy, and assumes the diagnosis does not change with increasing age. These assumptions cannot be supported. Because there are multiple etiologies, the survival rate is normal only for those with mild mental retardation, and mental retardation is not always diagnosed in preschool children. The prevalence may be higher during the school years due to the inclusion of mildly mentally retarded perons whose adaptive abilities may improve so the diagnosis may no longer apply after leaving school. Consequently, the diagnosis of mental retardation may change over time and, in this instance, is age dependent.

Furthermore, many factors influence the prevalence, such as normalization, mainstreaming, and improved interventions, for those who have been educationally and socially deprived. The reduction of poverty, improvement in nutrition, and more refined medical diagnoses also influence outcome. Greater availability of genetic counseling and abortion services for high-risk pregnancies also are factors, as are dietary/hormonal treatments for inborn errors of metabolism, such as galactosemia, phenylketonuria, and endocrine disorders like congenital hypothyroidism. Improved obstetrical techniques have lowered the incidence of brain damage at birth, yet improvements in care for the very small premature have led to an increased rate of mental retardation in this population.

Demographic considerations that influence prevalence include age, sex, socioeconomic level, race, and variations between urban and rural populations (Munro, 1986). In regard to age, most surveys show an increase in prevalence from the preschool years (0 to 4) to middle childhood (5 to 12). Prior to school entry, children with severe retardation are most likely to be identified. When performance expectations are greater on school entry, milder developmental disabilities become more apparent. In the mid-teen years, there may also be an apparent increase in rate when increasing demands are imposed by the school system. At this age, adaptive difficulties related to social judgment and behavior control may emerge. In young adulthood (22 to 34), prevalence rates generally decrease following the completion of school. Finally, in older persons, rates decrease when demands from vocational programs are reduced. Because of all these considerations, epidemiologic studies must look at age-specific rates for planning.

The rate of mental retardation has been reported to be higher in males than in females, perhaps because congenital anomalies are more prevalent in boys, as are prematurity, neonatal death, and stillbirth. Another important factor in males is the presence of X-linked mental retardation (see Chapter 10.3 on fragile X syndrome). Moreover, due to their aggressive behavior, boys may come to the attention of authorities more often than girls and may be more likely to be diagnosed. Still, not all studies show an increased prevalence among males, probably because both age and extent of mental retardation need to be considered. Higher rates among males have been reported in mildly retarded persons, but the gender difference is less apparent among persons who are more severely retarded.

Socioeconomic level is an important consideration as it relates to mental retardation regarding sensory and psychosocial deprivation, leading to the designation "retarded due to psychosocial disadvantage" (Grossman, 1983) or "cultural familial mental retardation" (Zigler, 1967). Psychosocial factors, such as poor living conditions, overcrowding, and lack of educational opportunity, may correlate with mental retardation, particularly in the mild range; however, genetic factors must be taken into account for these cases. For the more severe levels of mental retardation, clear-cut differences in socioeconomic status are less common. Prevalence rates have been reported to be higher among racial minorities, but may be linked to socioeconomic level rather than to race. Similarly, differences between urban and rural populations may be influenced by educational, occupational, and cultural opportunities. In some surveys, rates have been reported to be higher in rural areas, and in others, in inner-city populations.

Living arrangements vary, with the higher functioning groups tending to live in community residences or with family members. Individuals with moderate mental retardation are more often placed in foster and group homes, whereas the most severely and profoundly retarded individuals may be placed in institutional settings as well as in foster and group home settings. The percentage living with family members and in the communities is inversely related to the degree of intellectual deficit.

The life expectancy of mentally retarded persons is correlated with their level of intellectual functioning and the etiology of the disorder (Eyman et al., 1990). In a 1983 Canadian study, 98% of identified individuals with mild and moderate mental retardation and 92% in the severe range reached age 20. From ages 1 to 19, the death rate among individuals with mild and moderate retardation was twice that of the general population, whereas the rates for those with severe and profound mental retardation were 7 and 31 times as high, respectively (Herbst and Baird, 1983). Yet life expectancy among mentally retarded persons is increasing, particularly for those who survive beyond the first year of life.

Epidemiology of Associated Disabilities

Epidemiologic surveys of mental retardation usually consider associated physical disability, such as visual impairment, hearing loss, speech and language problems, seizure disorder, and cerebral palsy. Studies among the blind show 20% to 25% are also mentally retarded, with the highest rates of visual impairment occurring in those who are more severely retarded. Moreover, subtle problems in visual acuity and color blindness may be overlooked in mentally retarded individuals. The rate of visual disability, depending on the level of mental retardation, has been reported to be fifteen times greater than the general population rate.

Hearing impairment occurs at 3 to 4 times the general population rate and is present in approximately 10% of mentally retarded persons. Hearing problems in older individuals may be more common in certain syndromes, such as Down syndrome, where there is an increased risk of otosclerosis. Like blindness, hearing impairment is also greatest among severely and profoundly retarded persons. Rates are 5 to 8 times greater in severe to profoundly retarded individuals and may require special diagnostic tests, such as evoked response audiometry, because of their unreliability in responding to standard assessment techniques. Speech and language disorders are among the most common disabilities of mentally retarded persons, with rates of up to 80% in institutionalized severely and profoundly retarded individuals. Prevalence information on communication skills in nonverbal populations is limited. In noninstitutionalized mentally retarded persons, rates for speech problems are triple that of the general population prevalence.

Seizure disorders are commonly reported in mentally retarded persons. In institutional settings, approximately one third (generally, severely retarded individuals) have seizures. In noninstitutionalized groups, the rate of seizures is approximately 15% versus 1.5% for a control group. Rates in the mild to moderately retarded group range from 3%–6% to 12%–18%, depending on the population studied. For more severely retarded individuals, approximately 33% have seizures.

Static motor encephalopathy, or cerebral palsy (see Chapter 6), frequently co-occurs with mental retardation. Severely retarded persons have a rate of cerebral palsy ranging from 30% to 60%. Certain forms of cerebral palsy are more often related to mental retardation; for example, children with spastic quadriplegia and diplegia have a higher rate than those with the extrapyramidal forms.

ETIOLOGY

Etiology may be classified in several ways based either on identifying a causative agent or a specific mechanism. The American Association on Mental Retardation (1992) includes prenatal causes (chromosomal disorders, syndrome disorders, inborn errors of metabolism, developmental disorders of brain formation, environmental influences); perinatal causes (intrauterine disorders and neonatal disorders); and postnatal causes (head injuries, infections, demyelinating disorders, degenerative disorders, seizure disorders, toxic metabolic disorders, malnutrition, environmental deprivation, and hypoconnection syndrome). More than 500 genetic disorders are associated with mental retardation. Approximately 25% of known genetic conditions show their primary clinical effects on the brain, and others may lead to secondary effects to the central nervous system (Table 5–4).

Some disease categories involve abnormalities which, although occurring *in utero,* may not be evident until postnatal life. The best known of these include single-gene metabolic disorders (e.g., phenylketonuria) whose manifestations are not seen at birth. It has been estimated that between 30% and 50% of developmental disorders involve some temporal risk factors. Some chromosomal syndromes may increase susceptibility to perinatal trauma; e.g., inadequate central respiratory control may increase the risk of hypoxic-ischemic damage.

Advances in biomedical technology now allow identification of a neurobiological etiology for an increasing number of mental retardation syndromes. Neurobiological factors also play a significant etiological role in mild mental retardation and in borderline intellectual functioning. A variety of biomedical abnormalities, including subtle chromosomal abnormalities, perinatal trauma, and exposure to toxic substances, may be responsible for 30% to 45% of cases of mild mental retardation. These results have led to a reexamination of the etiological role of psychosocial disadvantage and polygenic inheritance.

A specific cause for mental retardation can be identified in about two thirds of cases. The more severe the degree of mental retardation, the greater the likelihood a specific cause will be uncovered. For example, an etiology can be identified for approximately 80% of those with severe mental retardation. A medical risk factor (perinatal trauma, genetic disorder) can be found in approximately 40% of those with mild mental retardation (Hagberg et al., 1981; Lamont and Dennis, 1988), but in only 25% to 30% of those with borderline intellectual functioning.

Multiple etiologies for mental retardation reflect a complex interaction involving genetic predisposition, environmental insults, developmental vulnerability, heredity, and environment. Genetic predisposition must take into account individual susceptibilities to the influence of environmental agents. Genetic damage is particularly likely when exposure occurs during periods of DNA replication or of gene expression. Multiple environmental factors may be involved that impinge on the developing organism, such as nutritional status, exposure to endogenous and exogenous toxins, microorganisms, radiation, and other psychosocial stressors. The developmental timing of exposure to potentially hazardous environmental agents is a crucial consideration. The severity of resulting mental retardation may be related to the timing of the insult to the central nervous system. Prenatal factors, which affect the developing fetal brain, are responsible for 55% to 75% of severe mental retardation cases, but only for 25% to 40% of mild mental retardation cases. Exposure of the fetus to the rubella virus during the first trimester of preg-

Table 5–4. Disorders Associated with Mental Retardation: Selected Examples

I. PRENATAL CAUSES

A. Chromosomal Disorders

1. Autosomes
   a. 4p-
   b. Ring 13
   c. Trisomy 18 (Edwards)
   d. Trisomy 21 (Down)
   e. Translocation 21 (Down)
2. X-Linked Mental Retardation
   a. Fragile X syndrome
   b. Glycerol kinase deficiency
   c. Juberg syndrome
   d. Renpenning syndrome
3. Other X Chromosome Disorders
   a. XO syndrome (Turner)
   b. XYY syndrome
   c. XXY syndrome (Klinefelter)
   d. XXXXX syndrome (penta-X)
4. Uniparental Disomy
   a. Prader-Willi syndrome
   b. Angelman's syndrome

B. Syndrome Disorders

1. Neurocutaneous Disorders
   a. Klippel-Trenauney syndrome
   b. Neurofibromatosis (Type 1)
   c. Sturge-Weber syndrome
   d. Tuberous sclerosis
   e. Xeroderma pigmentosum
2. Muscular Disorders
   a. Congenital muscular dystrophy
   b. Duchenne muscular dystrophy
   c. Myotonic muscular dystrophy
3. Ocular Disorders
   a. Aniridia-Wilm's tumor syndrome
   b. Anophthalmia syndrome (X-linked)
   c. Lowe syndrome
4. Craniofacial Disroders
   a. Acrocephalosyndactyly (e.g., Apert type)
   b. Craniofacial dysostosis (Crouzon)
   c. Multiple synostosis syndrome
5. Skeletal Disorders
   a. Hereditary osteodystrophy (Albright)
   b. Klippel-Feil syndrome
   c. Osteopetrosis (Albers-Schonberg)
   d. Radial hypoplasia-pancytopenia syndrome (Fanconi)

C. Inborn Errors of Metabolism

1. Amino Acid Disorders
   a. Phenylketonuria
   b. Histidinemia
   c. Branched-chain amino acid disorders
      1. Hyperleucine-isoleucinemia
      2. Maple-syrup urine disease
   d. Biotin-dependent disorder
   e. Propionic acidemia
   f. Methylmalonic acidemia
   g. Folate-dependent disorders
   h. Homocytinuria
   i. Hartnup disease
2. Carbohydrate Disorders
   a. Glycogen storage disorders
   b. Galactosemia
   c. Pyruvic acid disorders
3. Mucopolysaccharide Disorders
   a. Alpha-L-iduronidase deficiency (e.g., Hurler type)
   b. Iduronate sulfatase deficiency (Hunter type)
   c. Heparan N-sulfatase deficiency (San filippo 3A type)
4. Mucolipid Disorders
5. Urea Cycle Disorders
   a. Ornithine transcarbamylase deficiency
   b. Arginase deficiency (argininemia)
6. Nucleic Acid Disorders
   a. Lesch-Nyhan disease (HPRT deficiency)
   b. Orotic aciduria
7. Copper Metabolism Disorders
   a. Wilson disease
   b. Menkes disease
8. Mitochondrial Disorders
   a. Kearns-Sayre syndrome
9. Peroxisomal Disorders
   a. Zellweger syndrome
   b. Adrenoleukodystrophy

D. Developmental Disorders of Brain Formation

1. Neural Tube Closure Defects
   a. Anencephaly
   b. Spina bifida
2. Brain Formation Defects
   a. Hydrocephalus
   b. Lissencephaly
   c. Polymicrogyria
3. Cellular Migration Defects
   a. Abnormal layering of cortex
   b. Cortical microdysgenesis
4. Intraneuronal Defects
   a. Dendritic spine abnormalities
   b. Microtubule abnormalities
5. Acquired Brain Defects
   a. Hydranencephaly
   b. Porencephaly
6. Primary (Idiopathic) Microcephaly

E. Environmental Influences

1. Intrauterine Malnutrition
   a. Maternal malnutrition
   b. Placental insufficiency
2. Drugs, Toxins, and Teratogens
   a. Thalidomide
   b. Phenytoin (fetal hydantoin syndrome)
   c. Alcohol (fetal alcohol syndrome)
   d. Cocaine
   e. Methylmercury
3. Maternal Diseases
   a. Varicella
   b. Diabetes mellitus
   c. Hypothyroidism (fetal iodine deficiency)

d. Maternal phenylketonuria
4. Irradiation During Pregnancy

II. PERINATAL CAUSES

A. Intrauterine Disorders

1. Acute Placental Insufficiency
   a. Placenta previa/hemorrhage
   b. Toxemia/eclampsia
2. Chronic Placental Insufficiency (marginal reserve)
   a. Postmaturity (involution)
   b. Erythroblastosis (edema)
   c. Maternal diabetes
3. Abnormal Labor and Delivery
   a. Premature labor (prematurity)
   b. Premature rupture of membranes
   c. Abnormal presentation (especially breech)
   d. Obstetrical trauma
4. Multiple Gestation (smaller, later, or male infant)

B. Neonatal Disorders

1. Hypoxic-Ischemic Encephalopathy
2. Intracranial Hemorrhage
3. Posthemorrhagic Hydrocephalus
4. Periventricular Leukomalacia
5. Neonatal Seizures
6. Respiratory Disorders
   a. Hyaline membrane disease
7. Infections
   a. Septicemia
   b. Meningitis
   c. Encephalitis
8. Head Trauma at Birth
9. Metabolic Disorders
   a. Hyperbilirubinemia (kernicterus)
   b. Hypoglycemia
   c. Hypothyroidism
10. Nutritional Disorders
    a. Intestinal disorders
    b. Protein-calorie malnutrition

III. POSTNATAL CAUSES

A. Head Injuries

1. Cerebral concussion (diffuse axonal injury)
2. Cerebral contusion or laceration
3. Intracranial hemorrhage
4. Subarachnoid (with diffuse injury)

B. Infections

1. Encephalitis
   a. Herpes simplex
   b. Measles
   c. Human immunodeficiency virus
2. Meningitis
   a. Streptococcus pneumoniae
   b. Hemoophilus influenzae, type B
   c. Mycobacterium tuberculosis
3. Parasitic Infestations
   a. Malaria
4. Slow or Persistent Virus Infections
   a. Measles (Subacute sclerosing panencephalitis)
   b. Rubella (Progressive rubella panencephalitis)

C. Demyelinating Disorders

1. Postinfectious Disorders
2. Postimmunization Disorders
   a. Postpertussis encephalopathy

D. Degenerative Disorders

1. Syndromic Disorders (may be neurodevelopmental)
   a. Rett's disorder
   b. Childhood disintegrative disorder (Heller syndrome)
2. Poliodystrophies
   a. Friedreich ataxia
3. Basal Ganglia Disorders
   a. Hallervorden-Spatz disease
   b. Huntington disease (juvenile type)
   c. Parkinson disease (juvenile type)
   d. Dystonia musculorum deformans
4. Leukodystrophies
   a. Pelizaeus-Merzbacher disease
   b. Adrenoleukodystrophy
   c. Glactosylceramidase deficiency (Krabbe)
5. Sphingolipid Disorders
   a. Beta-galactosidase deficiency (GM1 gangliosidosis)
   b. Hexosaminidase A deficiency (Tay-Sachs)
6. Other Lipid Disorders
   a. Abetalipoproteinemia (Bassen-Kornzweig)

E. Seizure Disorders

1. Infantile Spasms
2. Myoclonic Epilepsy
3. Lennox-Gastaut Syndrome
4. Progressive Focal Epilepsy (Rasmussen)
5. Status epilepticus-induced brain injury

F. Toxic-Metabolic Disorders

1. Reye Syndrome
2. Intoxications
   a. Lead
   b. Mercury
3. Metabolic Disorders

G. Malnutrition

1. Protein-Calorie (PCM)
   a. Kwashiorkor
   b. Marasmus

H. Environmental Deprivation

1. Severe Psychosocial Deprivation
2. Child Abuse and Neglect
3. Chronic Social/Sensory Deprivation

I. Hypoconnection Syndrome

Adapted from AAMR, 1992.

nancy can lead to major congenital anomaly, and exposure to the same virus later in gestation or during the postnatal period leads to a milder disorder.

The search for an etiological diagnosis is essential because the effects of some progressive developmental disorders can be arrested or sometimes prevented through early diagnosis and treatment. For example, many of the clinical manifestations of several inborn errors of metabolism (e.g., PKU, galactosemia) can be prevented by recognition and dietary management. Accurate diagnosis can lead to important interventions, including genetic counseling, prenatal diagnosis, and possibly to corrective gene therapy in the future.

DEVELOPMENTAL ISSUES

Although Barbel Inhelder, in her *Diagnosis of Reasoning in the Retarded* (1968), suggested that arrests in Piaget's cognitive developmental stages (sensorimotor, preoperational, concrete operational) correspond to profound, severe, moderate, and mild mental retardation, and although Mary Woodward (1959, 1961) studied severely and profoundly retarded individuals using Piaget's approach, there has been a notable lack of emphasis on a developmental perspective in mentally retarded populations until recently. Developmental theorists have, for the most part, considered only familial mental retardation and normally intelligent persons in establishing developmental landmarks. Recently, the development of mentally retarded persons with brain dysfunction has begun to be evaluated systematically (Hodapp, Burack, and Zigler, 1990).

Currently, mental retardation researchers who study development consider mental retardation with or without brain damage. Those without brain damage are referred to as familial mental retardation and thought to be similar to nonretarded individuals in the developmental sequences they follow but to progress at a slower rate. Those with symptomatic brain dysfunction show atypical development. The traditional view has focused on both developmental delay and developmental difference hypotheses. Recently, developmentalists have proposed an expanded developmental approach and postulate that development theory may apply to both familial mental retardation and to symptomatic brain dysfunction. These authors present evidence suggesting that despite brain damage, there are universal sequences in development in several chromosomal disorder syndromes (Hodapp, Burack, and Zigler, 1990). Studies of developmental sequences carried out in mental retardation syndromes with different etiologies may clarify the degree that developmental processes might be altered in mental retardation. By acknowledging the heterogeneity of mental retardation, the developmental questions can be addressed more directly than by considering mentally retarded people as a homogeneous group. Difference in development may be studied among the various etiologic groups, such as Down syndrome, fragile X syndrome, and Prader-Willi syndrome. Moreover, subgroups may also be investigated within syndromes, such as Down syndrome, where there are potential genetic etiologies, e.g., trisomy 21, translocation, and mosaic groups.

In addition to developmental sequences, developmental rate must also be considered to understand fully the importance of maturational changes that may relate to neurological structures. In Down syndrome, the importance of developmental rate is demonstrated by studies that show a gradual decline in IQ with advancing age. During the first 2 years of life, infants with Down syndrome are noted to fall further and further behind nonretarded peers. This apparent slowing in development may be due to problems in moving qualitatively from one stage transition to another. In contrast, in the fragile X syndrome, little IQ change is noted until the early teens. At that point, mental age tends to plateau, but potentially there may be a decline in IQ here as well. In fragile X syndrome, endocrine changes associated with puberty might influence brain development and cause cognitive impairment, or test items requiring abstract reasoning may simply be too difficult.

Besides these maturational issues, the environment plays an important role in development, although it is unclear which aspects of the environment are most important and which times in development are most crucial. Environmental concerns have led to an emphasis on transactional intervention models that focus on language input and mother–child interaction. In these interventions, structure in both linguistic and nonlinguistic environments is needed to facilitate development. The development of social communication is particularly important. Most studies emphasize mother–child relationships, but, in mental retardation, it is particularly important to emphasize the role of the father. Environmental outcomes that must be monitored include not only intelligence but also the emergence of social competence and the management of aggression.

Children with Down syndrome, fragile X syndrome, autistic disorder, and those with multiple disabilities may differ from one another in their presentations, in their reactions to others, and in the behaviors of caregivers toward them.

Similar Sequences and Multiple Pathways

The expanded developmental approach highlights similar sequences and multiple pathways models (Hodapp, 1990). The similar sequence model suggests universal and invariant sequences in the development of cognition, morality, and language. In keeping with this model, Piaget (1952) studied the way children think and proposed that intelligence develops through a sequence of progressively complex patterns of action and thinking, with new patterns being organized from simpler ones that are present in earlier phases of development. Learning occurs through interaction with the material and the social environment. Piaget's approach has been documented as pertinent to the study of sensorimotor development in cross-cultural studies. Still, the speed of development and acquisition of Piaget's stages may be influenced by environmental experience. Other authors emphasize that rather than being universal and invariant, development may be variable and individualized multiple pathways.

One solution to the issue of universal development versus individualized development is to consider both approaches to be pertinent maturational or neurobiologically based developmental lines, such as sensorimotor development, and developmental lines that relate to higher cognitive ability. Neurobiologically-based development may follow a universal sequence if there is an average expectable environmental provision, so invariant sequences may be recognized for cognitive development or language development. However, later achievements, such as internalized language and social, cognitive, and moral development, may follow in time the establishment of higher cognitive function. These higher cognitive functions may be particularly dependent on interpersonal contact. If this approach is correct, then earlier cognitive development may be universal and neurobiologically based, but later, more sophisticated cognitive development may vary with cultural experiences (Hodapp, Burack, and Zigler, 1990).

The development of mentally retarded children may be used to study universal sequences of development and contrast them to deviant or idiosyncratic sequences of development. Biologically based developmental lines may be highly canalized and lead to development following a universal order. In contrast, other areas, such as moral development, might be considered to be culturally based, occur later, and be more dependent on life experiences.

Early investigations assumed there were universal defects in mental retardation in areas such as verbal mediation of thought and attentional dysfunction. As a result, mentally retarded children were thought to differ in their development from nonretarded children. Other authors emphasized the importance of normal development and hypothesized that development involves the same processes in mentally retarded persons as in the normal population but at a slower rate. From this debate, the issues raised focused on whether mentally retarded children show the same sequence or a similar sequence in development as nonretarded children. If so, they would be expected to show identical performance to that of nonretarded children of similar mental age on information processing tasks and other tasks measuring cognition. Comparable performance of mentally retarded persons and nonretarded persons on tests suggest that similar structures are involved in information processing. In these analyses, sequence indicates a constant and invariant order of acquisition of increasingly complex cognitive capabilities. Structure refers to how different behavioral manifestations show a developmental or stage like relationship to one another and may share common mechanisms.

Most research on the similar-sequence hypothesis focuses on sensorimotor development. Sensorimotor development addresses qualitative changes in psychological functioning in infants that takes place from birth to the beginning of symbolic and representational thought. The study of sensorimotor development derives from a psychobiological model of child development that emphasizes the infant's capacity to acquire, integrate, store, and act on information gained from nonsocial and social experiences.

Dunst (1990) indicates strong evidence for the ordinal acquisition of development in children with Down syndrome and children with mixed etiologies of mental retardation. He found that age-related changes do occur and that retarded children acquire more difficult test items in each of the six sensorimotor domains at later stages than they acquire items that are easier. Dunst demonstrated a strong relationship between the extent of sensorimotor acquisitions and increasing mental age and chronological age. He found that when the same retarded children were tested five to nine times over a span of years that sequential development could be demonstrated in individual cases. However, some groups of mentally retarded children may show variability across domains and regressions and spurts or lags at different phases in their development. Despite the unevenness of development, sequential acquisition of skills is supported in this study of Down syndrome.

However, investigations of moral development have not demonstrated sequential development so clearly. Although some evidence supports sequential moral development, Mahaney and Stephens (1974) found that results depended on the type of moral question asked. Moral development questions that dealt with a group's taking collective responsibility for the actions of group members did advance during a 2-year observation period. But when moral development questions were asked involving understanding the difference between the consequences of an action and the consequences of one's intent, the mentally retarded group did not progress and showed regression in some instances. For example, the mentally retarded subjects did not advance in their understanding and continued to interpret stealing and lying in terms of their consequences rather than considering the intention of the person. There was variability in regard to sequential acquisition of moral stages. The study of moral development is complicated because the stages of moral development described by Piaget may not be true stages. In summary, the issue of sequential stages of moral reasoning continues to be unsettled for mentally retarded persons. New studies on moral development should look to the stages outlined by Kohlberg (1969, 1974) and Hogan's measures of socialization, empathy, and autonomy (Hogan and Busch, 1984), which are better delineated. Overall, these findings are in keeping with the suggestion that the more neurobiologically related areas in infant development show invariant sequences across cultures, whereas later and more culture-determined achievements show variability.

The similar sequence hypothesis is relevant to the treatment of mentally retarded persons because it allows greater confidence in setting goals for the next steps in treatment. It confirms that prerequisite skills are necessary for later development in other domains. Similar sequence findings are also important in terms of the type of psychometric instruments used for testing. Severely and profoundly retarded children are often difficult to test and show variable profiles on Stanford-Binet and WISC III assessments. However, tests based on sensorimotor development, such as the Uzgiris and Hunt (1975), can be adapted to test mentally retarded and other disabled children. The sensorimotor approaches help clarify that the child has the ability to understand and make use of basic concepts which should be considered in intervention planning. Information about universal sequences in development is essential for both assessment procedures and the development of interventions.

Both sensory and motor disabilities influence developmental progress. Some children may be blind or deaf, and have absent limbs, yet their development proceeds in a universal manner if they are allowed to use other sensory modalities to compensate for impairments. Still, not all developmental achievements follow a universal sequence. For example, in language development, semantic relations and grammatic morphemes do develop in a set order, but pragmatic language functions may not follow fixed sequences. Children with autistic disorder show deviations in pragmatic language usage and may focus their attention on objects rather than on people in their early speech development. However, later in their development, higher-functioning children with autistic disorder may engage in pragmatic social communication directed specifically toward others. In autistic disorder, the development from object-related to quasi-social to fully social language may follow a different pattern than that seen in normal development. In contrast, in Down syndrome, social functions emerge in their earliest language communication. In both mentally retarded and nonretarded children, some behaviors have a lock-step sequence and others occur more flexibly.

A developmental approach to mental retardation emphasizes how development is organized even in those who are disabled. By studying different etiologic groups, there is an opportunity to make comparisons about developmental organization. Children with Down syndrome may have reduced affective responses and difficulties in language development, but may have relatively high levels of social skills whereas children with autistic disorder may have severe social skills deficits, echolalia, and a different profile of language development.

Behaviors may show relationships across developmental domains. The study of behavior across domains is important to help clarify how various behaviors fit together in development. In the final stage of Piaget's sensori-motor development sequence, one object is used to retrieve another object, a stage that can be demonstrated for nonretarded children and for children with autistic disorder. Another example of behaviors that cross domains is symbolic play, which may be important for early language development in some syndromes, such as Down syndrome. Specific deficits can be investigated across domains, as shown by the study of how sequential processing deficits in fragile X syndrome affect cognitive, linguistic, and adaptive functioning. Knowledge of cross-modal problems can be applied to an intervention program to assist the child in adapting to his specific impairments.

The individual study of the various etiologies of mental retardation takes into account the importance of individual impairments rather than simply targeting global differences in intelligence for intervention. Therefore, when asking about delay during an interview, questions should focus on which specific functions are delayed. Adaptive behaviors are best studied based on which behaviors are specific for a given mental age. The Vineland Adaptive Behavior Scales provide a means to assess adaptive functioning and contrast adaptive abilities with IQ level.

Normalization: The Developmental Model

Although mental retardation is a chronic condition and not curable, habilitation can be substantial. A developmental model of mental retardation acknowledges the capacity for growth and emphasizes independent living. The developmental model specifically emphasizes that adaptive behavior may improve with habilitation. The developmental model constitutes an important aspect of normalization in mental retardation. Normalization refers to retarded individuals' being entitled to services that are as culturally normative as possible to help them establish and maintain appropriate personal behavior (Wolfensberger, 1972). Normalization emphasizes that mentally retarded persons should live in community settings, attend regular schools, and seek competitive employment. Their behavior should be monitored to assist them to reach the standards for nonretarded persons at a comparable developmental age. They should be responsible for their behavior, and it should not be assumed their mental retardation precludes their ability to take on this responsibility.

In developmentally based normalization programs, communication skills, previous life experience, and any associated physical disorders are considered. Special efforts are needed to normalize communication, e.g., teaching sign language and utilizing facilitated communication. The nonverbal person with a physical disability, such as cerebral palsy and mental retardation, may require a speech synthesizer or communication board, or picture cards to assist in communication. Normalization attempts to provide the opportunity for decision making and exposure to varied life experiences.

Personality Development

Studies of mentally retarded persons have focused primarily on intellectual and cognitive functioning but have often neglected social and personality development. Problems associated with cognitive functioning have often overshadowed a needed focus on adaptive and maladaptive personality features, although personality variables and personal motivation are essential for predicting social and vocational adjustment. It is their behavior and social deficits that most commonly lead to psychiatric referral.

Investigations of personality dysfunction in children and adolescents which support the presence of characteristics, such as overdependency, low ideal self-image, limited levels of aspiration, and an outer-directed approach to problem solving (Zigler and Burack, 1989). These personality characteristics may have their origin in adverse psychosocial experiences, such as repeated failure and disapproval, leading to doubts about their capability to succeed. Experiences of rejection and the lack of consistent social support may lead to excessive reliance on others for feedback and guidance. Out of a need for recognition by others, they may suppress the desire to become more independent.

Operant behavior modification programs may not address these needs. Such programs do not emphasize making choices, but rather place primary emphasis on contingency management. As a result, the transition after completion of schooling to vocational programs may be difficult. During their adolescent years, parental restrictiveness and overprotection, peer rejection, and continuing low self-confidence often complicates mastery of developmental tasks involved in establishing the self-concept, sexual awareness, and identity. Mentally retarded adolescents may view their lives as being less fulfilling than that of their peers because they commonly experience dissatisfaction with their physical appearance and become frustrated by their difficulty in controlling their impulses, emotions, and behavior. These experiences may lead to social isolation, loneliness, and dysphoric mood. The failure to master developmental tasks is integral to producing maladaptive personality styles in adulthood. As many as one half of adults with mental retardation may have dysfunctional personalities. Even though the diagnosis of personality disorder in persons with mental retardation has been questioned, several personality disorder inventories that have adequate interrater and test-retest reliability have identified dysfunctional personality traits and personality disorders in adolescents and adults. The types of maladaptive personality characteristics most found on these inventories include affective instability, explosive and disruptive behaviors, and introverted personality patterns (Reid and Ballenger, 1987). Menolascino (1988) found that among 543 admissions for psychiatric care over a 5-year period, 13% of those age 16 and over had a diagnosis of personality disorder; passive-aggressive and antisocial types were the most common. It should also be kept in mind that the presence of a seizure disorder, especially one involving the temporal lobes, may increase the risk for a personality disorder among mentally retarded individuals.

Sexuality and Mental Retardation

Mentally retarded persons are commonly stereotyped in regard to their sexual behavior. These stereotypes include their being sexually uninhibited, sexually immature with sexual interests that correspond to their mental rather than chronological age, or lacking sexual interests altogether. Yet indiscriminate sexual behavior is not a characteristic feature in mentally retarded persons (Szymanski and Crocker, 1989). Based on stereotypes about uninhibited or indiscriminate sexual behavior, sterilization of mentally retarded persons was routinely practiced in the past, and some states in the United States continue to have such legislation on the books. Marriage between retarded persons has been prohibited in the past as a means of reducing the incidence of mental retardation. Because of these attitudes, a mentally retarded person might be denied the opportunity to socialize or develop an intimate relationship with someone of the opposite sex.

Sexual interest is ordinarily associated with the onset of puberty, so delays in puberty in mentally retarded individuals related to the particular etiology of the disorder will influence sexual interest. Regardless of the age of pubertal onset, the most severely and profoundly retarded individuals often show little interest in sexual activity with others. However, mildly retarded and many moderately retarded individuals may have normal pubertal development, demonstrate sexual interests, and establish sexual identities. If the expression of sexual interest is prohibited or prevented, inappropriate sexual activity may occur as a reaction. It may sometimes be used as a way to demonstrate self-importance. During adolescence, sexual behavior may also be part of an attempt to gain acceptance from others in a peer group, just as is the case in peer groups of nonretarded individuals. To facilitate the development of a normal sexual identity, encouragement of relationships with others and teaching appropriate social skills are prerequisites that should be emphasized before focusing specifically on instruction about sexual activity.

Mildly and moderately retarded adolescents often lack the most basic understanding of sexual anatomy, venereal disease, and contraceptive issues. Mentally retarded persons, particularly women, are at risk for sexual exploitation. Knowledge of sexuality is often not well established because the usual sources of information, namely, sex education in the schools, intimate peer discussions, and printed reading material, may be limited or unavailable. Family members may be reluctant to review or discuss sexual matters with their mentally retarded children or young adult family members. Most often knowledge of sexuality is based on life experience and sexual opportunity and not on systematic education.

PSYCHIATRIC ASSESSMENT

The psychiatric evaluation of persons with mild and moderate mental retardation includes the same areas that are covered with nonretarded individuals, with slight modifications. A comprehensive assessment includes a review of present concerns and symptoms, past and present developmental, medical, psychiatric, social, and family history, patient interview and physical examination, diagnostic formulation, treatment plan, informing conference, and follow-through (Szymanski, 1980). Both the patient and the caregivers who know the patient well are used as informants. Disorders of interpersonal functioning, communication, emotion, and behavior should be included. The interview must take into account the patient's cognitive and adaptive limitations. Interviews frequently need to be more structured, directive, and shorter than those conducted with nonretarded patients. After establishing rapport, the interview should provide overt support and social reinforcement so the patient does not react to the interview as a test he might fail. Care must be taken to avoid leading questions. Finally, interpretation about emotional and behavioral functioning should be presented within the context of the individual's overall developmental level.

The use of standardized assessment instruments and procedures have been introduced to improve the reliability and validity of psychiatric evaluation for mentally retarded persons. Because of variability in cognitive functioning and the use of multiple informants (physicians, psychologists, educators, direct care providers), it is harder to demonstrate reliability and validity for these instruments. Even so, several behavior checklists and semistructured interview schedules have been developed for use with mentally retarded patients and other informants (e.g., caregivers). Some instruments focus on making a specific diagnosis; others are used to assess the range and severity of affective and behavioral symptoms.

Aman (1991a, 1991b) reviewed instruments for assessing emotional and behavior disorders in individuals with mental retardation. The following items were reported most commonly among instruments reviewed, using factor analytic methodology: (1) aggressive, antisocial, self-injurious; (2) withdrawal; (3) stereotypic behavior; (4) hyperactivity; (5) repetitive verbalization; (6) anxious, tense, and fearful; and (7) self-injurious behavior. Rating scales for younger children are in the process of being validated. Although there is no one screening instrument that can be recommended for preschool children, the Reiss Scales for Children's Dual Diagnosis (Reiss and Valenti-Hein, 1990) should be considered for school-age children. For the assessment of broad behavioral dimensions in the age group, the Aberrant Behavior Checklist (ABC) (Aman, 1991a) and the Developmentally Delayed Child Behavior Checklist (DDCBCL) (Einfeld and Tonge,

Table 5–5. Instruments for Assessing Mentally Retarded Adolescents

Purpose	Instrument Name
Screening	Reiss Screen for Maladaptive Behavior
Broad Behavioral Dimensions	Aberrant Behavior Checklist
	Behaviour Disturbance Scale
	Strohmer-Prout Behaviour Rating Scale
Self-Ratings	Prout-Strohmer Personality Inventory
Psychiatric Classification	Clinical Interview Schedule
	Diagnostic Assessment for the Severely Handicapped
	Psychopathology Instrument for Mentally Retarded Adults

Adapted from Aman, 1991.

1990) should be considered. For the assessment of older adolescents, the instruments that are discussed next are recommended by Aman (Table 5–5):

The Aberrant Behavior Checklist (ABC) is an informant-based questionnaire that assesses the severity of 58 maladaptive behaviors. It is most appropriate for individuals with moderate to profound degrees of mental retardation. Extensive psychometric analyses have been carried out in several different countries, utilizing subjects of varying ages and IQ levels. Factor analysis identified five factors: irritability, lethargy/social withdrawal, stereotypic behavior, hyperactivity/noncompliance, and inappropriate speech, and the five-factor structure has been cross validated. The factors have high internal consistency, and the instrument itself possesses good reliability. Internal consistency has been found to be satisfactory but interrater reliabilities were relatively low.

The Psychopathology Instrument for Mentally Retarded Adults (PIMRA), developed by Matson (1988), is a 56-item scale with both self-report and informant versions that are designed to assess psychopathology among mildly and moderately mentally retarded persons. The individual items were derived from the symptom lists based on several DSM-III disorders and organized into seven clinical subscales. The subscales include the following diagnoses: schizophrenia, affective disorder, psychosexual disorder, adjustment disorder, anxiety disorder, somatoform disorder, and personality disorder. Factor analysis yielded two factors for the self-report version (termed "anxiety and social adjustment") and three factors for the informant version (termed "affective, somatoform, and psychosis"). The psychometric properties of the PIMRA have been evaluated in a number of studies. Initial analysis indicated high internal consistencies of the subscales and total scores, and good interrater and test-retest reliabilities. Yet follow-up analyses by several investigators have raised questions about this instrument's internal consistency and reliability. Other concerns raised about it include a low correspondence between the factor structure and the clinically derived scales and the limited number of disorders represented. Despite some shortcomings, the PIMRA is a useful instrument for the assessment of psychopathology in this population.

The Reiss Screen for Maladaptive Behavior (1988) is an informant-based rating scale that assesses the frequency, circumstances, and intensity associated with various symptoms of psychiatric disorders in mentally retarded persons. The instrument is organized into seven clinical scales, which include aggressive disorder, psychosis, paranoia, depression (behavioral signs), depression (physical signs), avoidant disorder, and dependent personality disorder. There are six maladaptive behaviors: drug abuse, overactivity, self-injury, sexual behavior, suicidal tendencies, and stealing. Factor analysis yields clinically meaningful results and its validity has been documented in conjunction with clinical psychiatric diagnosis. Other instruments where preliminary psychometric analyses are available are the Emotional Disorders Rating Scale for Developmental Disabilities (EDRSDD) (Feinstein, Kaminer, and Barrett, 1988) and the Diagnostic Assessment for the Severely Handicapped (DASH) Scale (Matson et al., 1990).

Assessment instruments developed for nonretarded children and adolescents have also been used to evaluate psychopathology among mentally retarded children and adults. These instruments generally have good test-retest reliability, yet vary in terms of their interrater reliability, internal consistency, and validity. Among them are the Child Behavior Checklist, the Rutter Behavioral Scales, the Beck Depression Inventory, the Zung Self-Rating Depression Inventory, and the Standardized Assessment of Personality. Further investigation is needed to provide information on their applicability to the mentally retarded population.

Basic Medical History

A comprehensive medical history and a careful physical examination are essential to uncovering the etiology of mental retardation. Following the history and physical examination, laboratory and diagnostic studies are chosen based on the clinical findings.

Brain imaging is playing an increasingly important role in the evaluation of children and adults with a variety of developmental disorders. These provide a noninvasive means to identify structural, and in some instances, functional abnormalities, such as abnormal metabolic activity, in mentally retarded persons. Computerized transaxial tomography (CT), magnetic resonance imaging (MRI), single photon emission computed tomography (SPECT), and positron emission tomography (PET) techniques may be used in the evaluation of mental retardation syndromes, to study structure–function relationships and to identify surgically correctable brain lesions associated with specific disorders. CT and MRI may be used to identify congenital malformations and/or brain changes related to infections of the central nervous system (CNS). Ventricular enlargement, cyst formation, cerebral asymmetry, neuronal migration disorders (e.g., polygyria, lissencephaly, schizencephaly), Chiari malformations, agenesis of the corpus callosum, and cerebral calcifications are among the abnormalities that may be demonstrated. CT is the preferred procedure for the visualization of calcifications, vascular lesions, and some tumors. MRI is superior to CT for specific identification of some structural anomalies (e.g., heterotopias), white matter abnormalities (e.g., demyelinating disorders), abnormality of the gray–white matter junction, and masses in the posterior fossa of the brain.

Diagnostic imaging is essential in the treatment of those neurocutaneous disorders where prognosis depends on the number, size, and location of associated neoplasms (e.g., neurofibromas, tubers, hamartomas, angiomas, malignancies). This is especially important in tuberous sclerosis, where CT and MRI may reveal tubers, subependymal calcified nodules, cortical hamartomas, and migration defects. The number and size of the tubers may be correlated with the degree of mental retardation and the severity of seizures. In Sturge-Weber syndrome, MRI is used to detect the extent and distribution of angiomatosis in the meninges, skull, and within the brain, but CT is best for detecting cortical calcifications.

PET and SPECT scans are being used to localize seizure foci prior to surgery, determine the extent of malignancy of certain neoplasms, identify tubers in tuberous sclerosis, evaluate the extent of intracranial hemorrhages in premature infants, and contribute to the early diagnosis of Huntington's disease and Sturge-Weber syndrome.

In the future functional imaging may be available to evaluate children with mental retardation. Newer techniques, such as fast MRI, may become available to conduct studies without the use of radioisotopes.

PSYCHOPATHOLOGY

Epidemiology of Mental Illness and Mental Retardation

For much of this century, mental retardation and mental illness have been regarded as mutually exclusive conditions. Affective and behavioral disturbances manifested by individuals with mental retardation generally have been regarded as manifestations of maladaptive learning profiles and adverse psychosocial experiences rather than as indications of psychiatric disorder. This view has been shared equally by mental retardation and mental health professionals. Recent studies have demonstrated that professionals typically fail to consider the diagnosis of a psychiatric disorder among mentally retarded individuals who exhibit signs and symptoms that are readily ascribed to psychiatric disturbance among individuals within the general population. This diagnostic bias is an outgrowth of several factors. First, the development of valid and reliable tests of intelligence and adaptive functioning early in this century enabled professionals to clearly distinguish mental retardation from mental illness for the first time (resulting in more specific and appropriate treatment interventions and remediation). Second, professionals wished to protect individuals with mental retardation from the stigma associated with the label of mental illness and ensure that their primary condition received appropriate intervention. Third, professionals believed the presence of cognitive impairment precluded the development of psychological structures and processes necessary for the development of most forms of psychopathology. Fourth, individuals with mental retardation were considered to be better candidates for educational and behavioral interventions than traditional methods of psychotherapy.

However, as systematic study has expanded, an appreciation for the true prevalence and complexity of psychopathology within this population has increased. Recent epidemiologic studies involving community samples indicate that children, adolescents, and adults with developmental disorders are at significant risk for the development of emotional and behavioral disturbance. Prevalence rates of psychiatric disorder range between approximately 30% and 70% depending on specific assessment procedures, diagnostic criteria, and the degree of mental retardation manifested by the subjects. These impressive figures represent a four- to five-fold increase over the prevalence of psychopathology in the general population.

Several studies are particularly noteworthy because of the representativeness of their samples and the systematic and reliable nature of their assessment procedures. Rutter, Tizard, and Whitmore (1970) reported that 30% to 40% of all 9- to 11-year-old mentally retarded children living on the Isle of Wight manifested a psychiatric disorder, a prevalence several times higher than that found among children of average intelligence. A representative birth cohort of mentally retarded Swedish adolescents was studied by Gillberg et al. (1986). Fifty-seven percent of the subjects with mild retardation and 64% of those with severe retardation met diagnostic criteria for a psychiatric disorder.

Lund (1985) identified an epidemiologic sample of 302 mentally retarded adults living in a region of Denmark. The demographics of the sample were representative of the country as a whole and included subjects with a wide age and IQ range. Comprehensive neuropsychiatric evaluations were conducted. Twenty-seven percent of the subjects received psychiatric diagnoses, using modified DSM-III criteria. A wide range of disorders were present, including affective, anxiety, schizophrenic, organic, and pervasive developmental disorders. Gostason (1985) applied a similar evaluation procedure to randomly selected groups of adults with and without mental retardation who were living in a representative region of Sweden. Psychiatric disorders were identified among three fourths of the severely retarded subjects, one third of the mildly retarded subjects, and one quarter of the nonretarded subjects. The severity of psychopathology also paralleled the degree of intellectual impairment.

Epidemiologic studies of mental disorders in mentally retarded persons are limited in number and scope. One issue that has influenced prevalence studies is referred to as "diagnostic overshadowing" (Reiss, Levitan, and Szysko, 1982). This term refers to situations where the presence of mental retardation is so blatant that the significance of an associated mental disorder is minimized; for example, mental retardation is given greater credence than concurrent emotional and behavior disorders. Moreover, in early pharmacological trials, mentally retarded persons were generally excluded because the diagnostic criteria for mental disorders were less well defined in mentally retarded persons.

Despite this lack of emphasis, overall, individuals with mental retardation have an increased vulnerability to emotional and behavioral disorders. Rates of psychiatric disorder are higher in individuals with mild to moderate mental retardation when compared to the general population, and are highest in those who test in the severe to profound range of mental retardation. Their vulnerabilities are primarily related to a reduced capacity to deal with complex social and cognitive demands, difficulty in problem-solving ability, especially in the resolution of conflicts, poor social judgment, and sensorimotor and language disorders that affect communication. Moreover, they may be further handicapped by the unwillingness of professionals to provide treatment for them.

Community surveys of noninstitutionalized persons show rates of 20% to 35% for behavioral and emotional disturbance in mentally retarded persons (Parsons, May, and Menolascino, 1984). Symptomatic forms of mental disorder related to associated brain dysfunction occur at high rates. Schizophrenia has been reported in 2% to 3% of mentally retarded persons (Reid, 1989), a prevalence that includes symptomatic forms. Both major depression and bipolar disorder may occur, but prevalence rates have not been determined. Anxiety disorders, obsessive compulsive, and repetitive behavior disorders and phobias may be diagnosed at higher rates than in the general population; however, there is no established evidence that persons with mental retardation have greater vulnerability to affective or anxiety disorders (Stark et al., 1988).

Because of concerns regarding increased criminality in mentally retarded persons, mental retardation has been regarded as a risk factor for criminal behavior. Even though a disproportionately higher number of adults with mental retardation are found in correctional facilities, criminal offenders account for only a small fraction of the entire mentally retarded population. Factors to consider are that those with mental retardation may be more likely to be apprehended when they are involved in antisocial behavior, and the mentally retarded person may lack the life experience to understand what is appropriate community behavior.

Suicidal behavior is not generally emphasized in mentally retarded persons, but suicides do occur and suicide threats must be taken seriously. Attempts are most likely to occur in mildly retarded individuals. As is the case with nonretarded persons, it is essential to look for an underlying psychiatric diagnosis. Suicidal behavior and deliberate self-harm may refer to a different group than self-injurious behavior, which occurs in severely mentally retarded persons.

In addition to these disorders, alcohol and substance abuse are problems identified in mildly retarded individuals. Of the two, alcoholism and alcohol misuse are the more common problems.

Self-injurious behavior is perhaps the most extreme and dangerous form of behavior seen in mentally retarded populations (NIH, 1990). Self-injury has been reported in 10% to 70% of institutionalized mentally retarded persons: The lower the IQ, the higher the prevalence rate. It occurs most often in severely and profoundly retarded individuals, and in younger children who have associated language disabilities, visual impairments, or seizures. In a community sample, Griffin et al. (1987) documented the prevalence of self-injury in 2,663 mentally retarded autistic or multiply-disabled children and adolescents in a large community metropolitan school district. They found 69 cases, or 2.6%, demonstrated self-injury during the 12-month period chosen for this study; 59% were male and 41% were female. The majority of this group (83%) were severely or profoundly retarded. The mean age of those surveyed was 10 years and the majority, three quarters of the group, demonstrated the behavior daily. For those 14 and above, prevalence was lower, perhaps related to community placement for older individuals. The most common symptoms were hand hitting, head hitting, and head banging. Other forms of self-injury include eye gouging, hair pulling, and nail picking, as well as multiple forms of self-injury in one individual (see Chapter 17).

The pattern of psychopathology seen in severely mentally retarded persons is different than that seen in mild and moderately mentally retarded persons. A particularly common association with mental retardation is social impairment. Wing and Gould (1979) conducted an epidemiologic study of severely retarded children in London and concluded that more than half were socially impaired. Social impairment in children with brain dysfunction consisted of a triad of impairments encompassing social interaction, nonverbal and verbal communication, and imaginative development, accompanied by an increase in repetitive and stereotyped behaviors. These problems are broadly grouped under the ICD-10 category of "pervasive developmental disorder." Although some children in the Wing and Gould study met diagnostic criteria for autistic disorder, the majority had less severe social impairments. Of these, three subgroups of social impairment were identified: (1) aloof and indifferent to others; (2) passive acceptance of social approaches; and (3) active, but odd and inappropriate, interaction. In other studies, the prevalence of social impairment has ranged from 25% to 42%. Depending on the population studied, the general prevalence of mental retardation in individuals with autistic disorder is approximately 85%.

When evaluating mentally retarded individuals, it is important to keep in mind that mentally retarded persons are generally multiply-disabled. Some are mobile and some are nonmobile. Community surveys will frequently demonstrate two or more additional disabilities. These disabilities are not simply additive but rather multiplicative in their effects. In regard to psychiatric presentations, persons with mental retardation experience the full range of psychiatric disorders; these usually present as maladaptive behavior. The origin of psychopathology is multiply determined. Moreover, acute psychiatric diagnosis may initially present as an increase in the rate of a previously established maladaptive behavior.

Spectrum of Psychiatric Disorders

There has been increasing study of the pattern of psychopathology manifested by children, adolescents, and adults with mental retardation. Systematic investigations indicate that the full spectrum of recognized psychiatric disorders can be identified among those with mental retardation. Chart reviews of clinical diagnoses, however, indicate that psychotic disturbances are overdiagnosed and anxiety, affective, and personality disorders are underrecognized.

Children and adults with mild to moderate mental retardation manifest a profile of psychiatric symptoms and disorders similar to what occurs within the nonretarded population. Studies using standardized methods of assessment reveal similar rates of attention deficit/hyperactivity disorder, conduct disorder, anxiety disorders (phobias, obsessive compulsive disorder, generalized anxiety), affective disorders, personality disorders, and schizophrenia. Some symptoms occur with particular frequency among community residents, including feelings of social inadequacy, dependency, and sensitivity to criticism (affecting one quarter to one half), anxiety (affecting one third), and aggressive behavior (affecting one fifth to one fourth).

Affective disorders (e.g., major depression, bipolar disorder, dysthymia) occur commonly and are responsible for a significant degree of morbidity. Approximately 2% to 10% of mentally retarded individuals manifest serious affective disorders; as many as 50% suffer from dysthymia. Preliminary investigations have reported the successful use of assessment instruments developed for the general population (e.g., Beck Inventory of Depression, Schedule for Affective Disorders and Schizophrenia, Children's Depression Inventory). However, studies are needed to confirm adequate reliability and validity with this population. Biological markers have been sought in an attempt to improve diagnostic accuracy. The dexamethasone suppression test (DST) has been piloted as an indicator of major depression in approximately 150 adults with mental retardation. Results are similar to those reported for the general population, including a sensitivity of 40% to 50% and a specificity of 75% to 85%. Further study may prove the DST to be useful as a corroborative tool in the diagnosis of major depression among mentally retarded individuals.

Schizophrenia occurs at a rate 2 to 3 times higher than that reported among the general population (Reid, 1982). Although schizophrenia was once a controversial diagnosis in mentally retarded persons, it is now well accepted. Careful studies have documented the presence of such symptoms as hallucinations, delusions, and thought disorder. The expression of these symptoms is generally more concrete and less elaborate than their occurrence in the general population. Comparisons of mentally retarded and nonretarded schizophrenic patients reveal that the former group has an earlier age of onset and a less favorable premorbid history. However, both groups exhibit a very similar profile of psychotic symptoms (e.g., hallucinations, delusions, thought disorder, etc.).

Among those with severe and profound mental retardation, a somewhat different profile of psychopathology is present. Certain symptoms occur less frequently, primarily because of limitations in cognitive and symbolic processes. These include delusions, hallucinations, referential ideation, obsessions, guilty ruminations, and so on. Other symptoms occur more frequently. For example, stereotyped behaviors, such as finger flicking and hand flapping, are present in 15% to 50% of individuals; self-injurious behaviors (SIB), such as eye gouging and head banging, are present in 10% to 20%. Several disorders are more common among children and adults with severe to profound mental retardation, including autistic disorder and related pervasive developmental disorders (PDD). As many as 4% to 8% of mentally retarded children meet criteria for autistic disorder, or approximately 10 to 20 times the general population prevalence. Conversely, approximately 75% of children and adults with autistic disorder are mentally retarded.

Specific Developmental Syndromes and Psychopathology

Personality profiles and behavioral patterns associated with individual disorders are described in Part III, Behavioral Phenotypes.

TREATMENT

Treatment for children and adults with mental retardation must address the complex interplay of neurobiological and psychosocial factors. A comprehensive interdisciplinary approach is essential, and consideration should be given to the full range of treatments used with nonretarded children. In most instances, multiple treatment modalities are needed. The AAMR (1992) multidimensional approach provides guidelines for intervention. Better environmental provision, cognitive and behavioral interventions, individual and family psychotherapy, and psychopharmacology are all applicable approaches. The efficacy of each of these interventions has been demonstrated when appropriately selected and implemented.

The Environmental Provision

Living conditions, vocational opportunities, and leisure time activities are essential environmental provisions for mentally retarded persons. It is equally important that they participate by expressing preferences and making personal choices about living conditions, work, and recreational activities. These issues have received increasing attention, and when handled well lead to an improved quality of life and a substantial reduction in maladaptive affective and behavioral symptoms. In those cases of a child with a mentally retarded parent, the parent requires particular support in providing for the child's needs (Accardo and Whitman, 1990). A home program includes increasing access to preferred activities, offering choices with regard to household tasks, and scheduling highly preferred tasks and activities immediately following nonpreferred (but essential) ones.

Educational Interventions/Skill Development

A fundamental challenge in the care and treatment of mentally retarded persons is to assist them in finding new ways to interact with others appropriately. Emotional and behavioral disturbances commonly result from a lack of self-monitoring and adaptive control over their inner lives and external environment. Communication deficits, learning difficulty, and limited educational experience often deprive them of the requisite skills needed for personal competence and social responsibility. Therefore, an educationally based program should emphasize social, communication, and vocational skills as a way to reduce maladaptive behavior by improving self-control. Essential elements of such a program include independence training (teaching self-help and leisure skills), communication training (enhancing speech and nonverbal communication—signing, gestures, picture/word boards), and self- management skill development (teaching strategies for self-monitoring and self-reinforcement). Social skills training provides concrete instructions, uses observation and modeling of effective behavior, offers reinforcement, and focuses on teaching through simple, observable behaviors. Social skills training procedures emphasize the enhancement of appropriate interpersonal behavior in a variety of social situations, such as being introduced to another person and properly responding, initiating and participating in social group activities, and learning to interpret and respond appropriately to verbal and nonverbal social cues. Successful social skills programs combine demonstration by instructors, modeling, role play, social practice, constructive feedback, and positive reinforcement. The training sequence might include initial instruction and practice in a therapeutic environment, followed by practice in natural community settings.

Behavioral Interventions

Behavioral approaches are the most widely used and best studied treatment interventions for behavioral disturbances in persons with mental retardation. Even though behavioral procedures are based on the principles of learning theory (which posits that maladaptive patterns of behavior are the result of faulty conditioning), they are effective for emotional and behavioral symptoms that result primarily from pathophysiological dysfunction. Behavioral procedures have been developed for improving adaptive behavior, reducing maladaptive behavior, and broadening skill development through direct training and education. Behavioral interventions may be specifically indicated for self-injurious behavior, self-stimulatory behavior, aggressive behavior, and habit training.

Behavioral approaches are generally grouped into those designed to enhance adaptive behavior and those designed to suppress maladaptive behavior. Behavior enhancement procedures are preferable because they reduce inappropriate behaviors by teaching adaptive solutions. This is accomplished by reinforcing appropriate behaviors and suppressing maladaptive ones.

Behavior enhancement procedures may be subdivided into several types of differential reinforcement strategies. The most commonly used method is the differential reinforcement of other behavior (DRO), where the individual is rewarded for not exhibiting the target behavior. If the undesirable behavior does not occur within a specified time interval, positive reinforcement is provided. The time interval for positive reinforcement is determined from the frequency of the target behavior. It should be long enough to require some effort, but short enough to promote success. When the procedure is successful, the frequency of target behaviors decreases as the frequency of the more adaptive, competing behaviors (those which are reinforced) increases. For maladaptive behaviors that occur very frequently, differential reinforcement of low rates of behavior (DRL) may be used. In this procedure, a predetermined frequency of the target behavior (lower than that occurring at baseline) is reinforced. This frequency is progressively lowered until the target behavior is eliminated. Another procedure, differential reinforcement of incompatible behavior (DRI), involves the direct reinforcement of preselected adaptive behaviors that compete with, and eventually replace, the target behaviors. The competing behaviors are chosen because they are incompatible with the target behaviors (e.g., using one's hand to shake another's hand rather than to slap another's face). These procedures are based on a careful determination of the characteristics of the maladaptive behaviors (frequency, duration, intensity, etc.) and through identification of a variety of motivating reinforcers. Negative reinforcement is sometimes used to enhance behavior. This procedure involves allowing the individual to avoid a predetermined punishment by engaging in desirable behavior.

Behavior reduction procedures involve the introduction of unpleasant consequences immediately following the occurrence of the target behavior. A wide variety of behavior reduction procedures have been used that range from nonexclusionary time-out to electric shock. Behavior reduction procedures include (1) extinction, the elimination of reinforcing consequences of maladaptive behavior; (2) time-out from positive reinforcement; (3) response cost, the loss of a previously earned reward; (4) overcorrection, restoring order after disrupting the environment or the repeated practice of an adaptive behavior (e.g., dressing); (5) physical or mechanical restraint; and (6) visual screening. Direct punishment procedures might include verbal reprimand, mild electric shock, ammonia capsules, and mist spray. Punishment procedures show short-term efficacy in suppressing maladaptive behaviors, at least under certain circumstances. However, the stability and generalization of these effects is questionable because punishment procedures primarily suppress behavior rather than teach adaptive solutions. The most intrusive procedures typically have been reserved for the most dangerous behaviors (e.g., serious aggression and self-injury).

Punishment procedures have been sharply criticized and are the source of considerable controversy. Many states have enacted regulations that either ban or seriously restrict the implementation of such procedures. These actions stem from ethical concerns but also because behavior suppression or punishment alone does not teach self-regulation or problem-solving skills that enhance future adaptive responses to stress. In 1989 the National Institutes of Health sponsored a Consensus Development Conference on Treatment of Destructive Behaviors in Persons with Developmental Disabilities. A panel of nationally recognized experts in the field of developmental disabilities reviewed the available research and heard testimony from investigators and clinicians working with behavior disorders in mentally retarded persons. The recommendations of the panel for the treatment of severely disruptive behavior included the following:

- Most successful approaches to treatment are likely to involve multiple elements of therapy (behavioral and psychopharmacologic), environmental change, and education.
- Treatment methods may require techniques for enhancing desired behaviors; for producing changes in social, physical, and educational environments; and for reducing or eliminating destructive behaviors.
- Treatments should be based on an analysis of medical and psychiatric conditions, environmental situations, consequences, and skill deficits. In the application of any of these treatments, an essential step involves a functional analysis of existing behavioral patterns.
- Behavior reduction procedures should be selected for their rapid effectiveness *only* if the exigencies of the clinical situation require such restrictive interventions and *only* after appropriate review. These interventions should *only* be used in the context of a comprehensive treatment package. (NIH, 1990).

Unfortunately, little systematic research has been conducted that identifies the specific behavioral interventions which are most efficacious for particular maladaptive behaviors. Most studies involve single-case designs with small sample sizes and rarely include clinical factors that might affect treatment outcome (e.g., clinical psychiatric syndromes and disorders, family history, psychosocial circumstances). Overall, positive behavioral interventions are useful for social skills deficits; mild punishment procedures (e.g., extinction, disapproval, overcorrection) for psychophysiologic symptoms (e.g., enuresis, encopresis); and more intrusive punishment procedures (e.g., restraint, time-out) for initial management of destructive behaviors (e.g., aggression, self-injurious behavior). Self-stimulatory behaviors, psychophysiologic symptoms, and noncompliance are the most responsive to behavioral treatment (65% to 75% success rate); destructive behaviors are next (45% to 65% success rate), and inappropriate social interactions are the least responsive (35% to 40% success rate).

Psychotherapy

Individuals with mild cognitive impairments have been shown to benefit from individual, family, and group psychotherapy. Psychotherapeutic interventions are most effective in the treatment of emotional and behavioral disturbances in individuals who have experienced traumatic psychosocial experiences that lead to internalized conflict and maladaptive personality functioning. Repeated failure, social rejection, frequent losses, and dependency on others often result in feelings of inferiority, ambivalence, anxiety, and anger, and each of these symptoms may be targeted. Family conflicts involving feelings of jealousy toward normally developing siblings and tension with parents regarding issues of emancipation and independence are other targets. Psychotherapeutic interventions tend to be underutilized, primarily because of misconceptions about their effectiveness for mentally retarded persons despite the fact that they are often good candidates for psychotherapy (Szymanski, 1980). They can be highly motivated to establish interpersonal relationships and often demonstrate a strong desire for enhancing their personal competence and independence.

The goals of psychotherapeutic treatment are similar to those for the general population and include the resolution of internalized conflict, improvement in self-esteem, and enhancement of personal competence and independence. Modifications of the usual treatment approaches may be necessary that take into account the developmental level of the patient. A supportive atmosphere, focused approaches by the therapist, and shorter, more frequent sessions may be needed.

Psychopharmacology

Psychopharmacological treatment is an important, but sometimes controversial, treatment modality for mentally retarded children and adults (Bregman, 1991). Psychotropic medications are effective in reducing the symptoms associated with a variety of psychiatric disorders and have been used quite extensively, particularly for the control of aggressive and destructive behavior. Surveys indicate that between one fifth and one half of mentally retarded individuals residing in institutions and one fourth to one third residing in community settings receive some type of psychotropic medication. There are significant interinstitutional and interagency differences in prescribing patterns, ranging from under 10% in some settings to more than 50% in others for patients with similar demographic and clinical characteristics. Overall, neuroleptics are prescribed most often and antidepressants and stimulants least often.

Despite the frequent use of psychopharmacologic interventions for mentally retarded individuals, relatively few studies include appropriate control groups. Single-case reports and nonblind, open clinical trials make up the majority of these reports. Clinical reports often show evidence of methodological problems, such as reporting bias (underreporting of negative findings), retrospective, anecdotal data, lack of interrated reliability, and the concurrent use of other psychotropic medications that may be changed during the course of the drug trial. Few studies fully adhere to the basic guidelines for clinical trials, namely, random assignment of an adequate number of subjects to treatment conditions, double-blind, placebo-controlled procedures, treatment phases of adequate length, and valid and reliable methods for assessment at baseline and throughout the study.

Drug Treatment for Specific Disorders

Attention Deficit/Hyperactivity Disorder

As many as 40% of children and adolescents with mental retardation exhibit a high activity level, impulsive behavior, and inattentiveness. Epidemiologic studies show that for 10% to 20%, these symptoms are severe enough to warrant the diagnosis of an attention deficit disorder (Gillberg et al., 1986). Therefore, central nervous system stimulants are among the most frequently prescribed psychotropic medications for mentally retarded children, with statistics showing that 6% to 8% of such children receive them. Yet systematic studies of efficacy in specific mental retardation syndromes are limited and the findings are mixed (Gadow, 1985). There is concurrence that the stimulants are useful for children and adolescents with mild mental retardation who meet diagnostic criteria for attention deficit/hyperactivity disorder. Approximately 50% to 75% of this group of children demonstrate a significant decrease in hyperactivity, impulsivity, and inattention and an increase in on-task behavior following drug treatment. Some studies have documented significant improvements on laboratory measures of attention, memory, and learning (e.g., continuous performance tasks, matching-to-sample tasks, and paired associate learning). In contrast, little evidence shows that the stimulants improve behavior, learning, or performance among mentally retarded children who either do not meet diagnostic criteria for attention deficit/hyperactivity disorder or whose behavioral symptoms are characteristic of other disorders (e.g., autistic disorder, anxiety disorders) (Aman, 1982). Additionally, side effects which occur at a greater frequency than that reported in the general population (especially among nonresponders) include irritability, lethargy, internal preoccupation, social withdrawal, increased motor stereotypy, and overinclusive attention.

Schizophrenia

Community epidemiologic studies indicate that schizophrenic disorders occur in 1% to 2% of the mentally retarded population. The available literature documents the usefulness of neuroleptic medication for psychotic symptoms manifested by affected mentally retarded patients. Treatment responsiveness is similar to that found in nonretarded persons (Menolascino et al., 1986).

Mood Disorders

Although major depression and dysthymic disorder commonly occur among mentally retarded individuals, the efficacy of antidepressant medication has not been investigated systematically. A number of case reports (one performed in blind fashion) have supported the efficacy of antidepressants (Bregman, 1991).

Mood stabilizing agents (e.g., lithium carbonate, valproate) have been studied for the treatment of bipolar disorder and the control of aggressive behavior. Several open trials and two controlled studies reported lithium to be effective in treating acute manic episodes and in reducing the frequency and duration of affective cycles (Bregman, 1991).

Aggressive and Self-Injurious Behavior

Most medication trials have focused on the treatment of destructive behaviors, such as aggression and self-injury. The neuroleptics have been most frequently used in clinical trials. Results are equivocal, particularly for the control of aggressive behavior. Although some studies have documented significant reductions in aggressive behavior, others have not. Findings for self-injurious behavior are more consistent. The potential involvement of dopaminergic mechanisms in self-injurious behavior is supported by studies of the adenosine system. Caffeine, theophylline, and clonidine are adenosine antagonists that act indirectly to increase dopamine activity; they are also known to exacerbate self-injurious behavior. Conversely, adenosine itself has been shown to block L-dopa-induced self-injurious behavior in an animal model. These data collectively indicate that self-injurious behavior might be successfully treated by medications which reduce dopamine transmission.

Findings regarding the efficacy of neuroleptics in the treatment of destructive behavior are equivocal; therefore, the use of these medications should be weighed against their potential adverse effects. Moreover, neuroleptics may cause tardive dyskinesia and, in some cases, may impair learning. Several studies have investigated the prevalence, clinical presentation, and risk factors associated with the development of tardive dyskinesia among mentally retarded individuals treated with neuroleptics. Prevalence figures range between 15% and 35% across studies. The clinical manifestations of the disorder are essentially identical to those manifested by nonretarded individuals, although orofacial dyskinesias may be more prevalent. Several potential risk factors have been identified, including advanced age, female gender, cumulative dose, and length of exposure. The severity of cognitive impairment and the presence of other neurological conditions may increase the risk of tardive dyskinesia according to some, but not all, studies.

Serotonergic dysfunction also has been hypothesized to underlie some forms of destructive behavior. Reduced central nervous system levels of serotonin have been reported in association with violent behavior. A number of case reports and several controlled studies have reported that lithium (which enhances serotonin synthesis) can reduce both aggressive and self-injurious behavior. These findings are supported by open clinical trials involving other medications that reportedly increase serotonergic activity, including buspirone, trazedone, and fluoxetine.

It has been suggested that the GABAergic

system may play a role in destructive behavior. However, medications that affect GABA functioning (e.g., benzodiazepines) do not appear to have consistent effects on aggression and self-injury. Some studies have reported that benzodiazepines reduce destructive behavior; others have reported an exacerbation of aggression and self-injurious behavior. Paradoxical excitement has also been reported.

Several lines of evidence implicate the endogenous opioid system (EOS) in the pathogenesis of destructive behavior, especially self-injurious behavior. Two major hypotheses have been offered to explain the potential role of the endogenous opioid system. Preliminary studies suggest that some patients have elevated peripheral (and perhaps central nervous system) levels of endogenous opioids, leading to a high pain threshold and a tendency to persist in self-injurious behavior. According to another line of reasoning, self-injurious injury itself causes endogenous opioid levels to rise resulting in stress-induced analgesia. Opioid antagonists have been recommended as treatment either to increase the perception of pain (thereby serving as a natural deterrent to self-injurious behavior) or to extinguish the theoretically pleasurable effects of self-injurious behavior-induced elevations in endogenous opioid levels. A number of studies (including several methodologically sound, controlled investigations) have assessed the efficacy of opioid antagonists (e.g., naloxone, naltrexone) in the treatment of mentally retarded individuals with self-injurious behavior. Although some of these studies have reported impressive beneficial effects, others have not. Additional investigations, employing larger subject samples, will be necessary in order to identify the types of patients likely to benefit from such treatment.

Finally, some evidence shows that increased noradrenergic activity may lead to aggressive behavior, perhaps secondary to anxiety or a state of heightened arousal. Several case reports and open clinical trials suggest that both centrally and peripherally acting beta-adrenergic blockers (e.g., propranolol, nadolol) may be helpful in reducing the frequency and intensity of explosive episodes of aggression.

Stereotypic Behavior

Study of the etiology and treatment of stereotypic behavior in children and adults with mental retardation has long been of interest. Both preclinical and clinical studies suggest involvement of the dopaminergic system (perhaps via postsynaptic DA supersensitivity) in the etiology of some forms of stereotypy. Dopamine agonists are known to induce stereotypic behavior, a response that can be blocked by treatment with DA antagonists. In addition, a relatively large number of studies indicate that neuroleptics may reduce stereotypic behavior among persons with mental retardation.

The initiation of psychotropic medication trials requires a thorough psychiatric evaluation to identify a medication-responsive psychiatric disorder or a specific target behavior that may be responsive to medication. A drug-free baseline period when the symptoms or behaviors identified for treatment are carefully defined and characterized (e.g., frequency, duration, intensity, etc.) is strongly recommended. Valid and reliable behavior rating scales should be selected and used at appropriate intervals during the medication trial in order to assess drug efficacy. Direct observational data and/or standardized rating scales should be used to monitor effects and potential side effects. The trial should include therapeutic doses of medication and should be conducted for an adequate length of time.

SUMMARY

This chapter traces the history and summarizes recent developments in the field of mental retardation. Epidemiologic studies have demonstrated the increased prevalence of mental and behavior disorders in this population. When considering the complexity of psychiatric diagnosis and treatment, old questions remain and new ones arise. Among them are the following: (1) With the establishment of a phenomenologic approach to the diagnosis of mental disorder, should clinical findings be clustered into diagnoses of neuropsychiatric disorders, or simply considered aspects of cognitive and adaptive impairment, or both, depending on the presentation? (2) How should diagnostic criteria be modified to take developmental issues into account? (3)

Is there an association of certain genetic syndromes and specific psychiatric disorders? (4) How should treatment be modified, based on the multiple etiologies of mental retardation?

Advances have been made in the treatment of both abnormal patterns of behavior and co-occurring neuropsychiatric disorders in individuals with mental retardation. Yet treatment programs are often fragmented and need to be pulled together in a comprehensive fashion, involving an interdisciplinary team. In the future, better methods of assessment are needed that highlight the interface between environmental and neurobiological mechanisms involved in both affective and behavioral disturbances. This additional information may lead to better focused treatment programs. Currently, full validation of specific treatment approaches for particular symptoms, or clusters of symptoms, is not available. In order to best determine the efficacy of a treatment approach, larger studies are needed with more subjects, greater homogeneity regarding symptoms, and the inclusion of neuropsychiatric diagnoses. In research, controlled procedures are necessary, which include randomization and double-blind designs, and standardized methods of assessment should be included. With a better understanding of the efficacy of treatment for established homogeneous clinical groups, the long-term outcome can be established more predictably. The clinical and research focus has shifted to a recognition of the occurrence of mental disorders in mentally retarded persons; in this area, we can anticipate future advances.

REFERENCES

American Association on Mental Retardation. (1992). *Mental retardation: Definition, classification, and systems of support,* special 9th ed. Author, Washington, DC.

Accardo, P.J., and Whitman, B.Y. (1990). Children of mentally retarded parents. *American Journal of Diseases of Children,* 144:69–70.

Aman, M.G. (1982). Stimulant drug effects in developmental disorders and hyperactivity—toward a resolution of disparate findings. *Journal of Autism and Developmental Disorders,* 12:385–398.

______. (1991a). *Assessing psychopathology and behavior problems in persons with mental retardation: A review of available instruments.* DHHS Publication No. (ADM) 91–1712. U.S. Department of Health and Human Services, Rockville, MD.

______. (1991b). Review and evaluation of instruments for assessing emotional and behavioural disorders. *Australia and New Zealand Journal of Developmental Disabilities,* 17(2):127–145.

American Psychiatric Association, Committee on Nomenclature and Statistics. (1980). *Diagnostic and statistical manual of mental disorders,* 3rd ed. Author, Washington, DC.

American Psychiatric Association, Committee on Nomenclature and Statistics. (1987). *Diagnostic and statistical manual of mental disorders,* 3rd ed, revised. Author, Washington, DC.

American Psychiatric Association, Committee on Nomenclature and Statistics. (1994). *Diagnostic and statistical manual of mental disorders,* 4th ed. Author, Washington, DC.

Baird, P.A., and Sadovnick, A.D. (1985). Mental retardation in over half-a-million consecutive live births: An epidemiologic study. *American Journal of Mental Deficiency,* 89:323.

Binet, A., and Simon, T. (1905). Méthodes nouvelles pour le diagnostic du niveau intellectuel des anormaux. *L'Année Psychologique,* 11:191–244.

Bourneville, D.M. (1880). Sclereuse tubereuse des convulsions cérébrales: Idiotie et épilepsie hémiplégique. *Archives of Neurology (Paris),* 1:81–91.

Bregman, J.D. (1991). Current developments in the understanding of mental retardation: II. Psychopathology. *Journal of the American Academy of Child and Adolescent Psychiatry,* 30:861–872.

Bregman, J.D., and Harris, J.C. (1995). *Mental retardation.* In Kaplan, H.I., and Sadock, B.J. (ed.), *Comprehensive textbook of psychiatry,* Vol. 2, 6th ed., Chap 35. Williams & Wilkins, Baltimore, MD.

Bryan, C. (1930). *The papyrus Ebers.* D. Appleton, New York.

Clarke, A.M., Clarke, D.B., and Berg, J.M. (1985). *Mental deficiency: The changing outlook,* 4th ed. Free Press, New York.

Cullinan, D., Gadow, K.D., and Epstein, M.H. (1987). Psychotropic drug treatment among learning-disabled, educable mentally retarded, and seriously emotionally disturbed students. *Journal of Abnormal Child Psychology,* 15:469–477.

Down, J.H.L. (1866). Ethnic classification of idiots. *Clinical Lecture Reports, London Hospital 3,* p. 259.

Dunst, C.J. (1990). Sensorimotor development of infants with Down syndrome. In D. Cicchetti and M. Beeghly (eds.), *Children with Down syndrome: A developmental perspective.* Cambridge University Press, New York.

Einfeld, S.L., and Tonge, B.J. (1990). *Development of an instrument to measure psychopathology in mentally retarded children and adolescents.* Unpublished manuscript. University of Sydney, Australia.

Eyman, R.F., Grossman, H.J., Choney, R.H., and Call, T.L. (1990). The life expectancy of profoundly handicapped people with mental retardation. *New England Journal of Medicine,* 323:584–589.

Feinstein, C., Kaminer, Y., and Barrett, R. (1988). *Emotional Disorders Rating Scale: Developmental Disabilities.* Unpublished document, Emma Pendleton Bradley Hospital, East Providence, RI.

Folling, A. (1934). Uber ausscheidung von Phenylbrenztraubensaure in den Harn als Stoffwechselanomalie in Verbindung mit imbezillitat. *Hoppe-Seyler's Zeitschrift füer physiologische chemie,* 227:169.

Gadow, K. (1985). Prevalence and efficacy of stimulant drug use with mentally retarded children and youth. *Psychopharmacology Bulletin,* 21:291–303.

Gillberg, C., Persson, E., Grufman, M., and Themner, U. (1986). Psychiatric disorders in mildly and severely mentally retarded urban children and adolescents: Epidemiological aspects. *British Journal of Psychiatry,* 149:68–74.

Goddard, H. (1912). *The Kallikak family: A study in the heredity of feeblemindedness.* Macmillan, New York.

Gostason, R. (1985). Psychiatric illness in the mentally retarded: A Swedish population study. *Acta Psychiatrica Scandinavia, Supplement (318),* 71:3–117.

Griesinger, W. (1876). *Die pathologie und therapie der psychischen krankheiten,* 4th ed. Braunschweight Vieweg. (quoted by Kanner, 1964)

Griffin, J.C., Ricketts, R.W., Williams, D.E., Locke, B.J., Altmeyer, B.K., and Stark, M.T. (1987). A community survey of self-injurious behavior among developmentally disabled children and adolescents. *Hospital and Community Psychiatry,* 38:959–963.

Grossman, H.J. (1983). *Manual on Terminology and Classification in Mental Retardation,* revised ed. American Association on Mental Deficiency, Washington, DC.

Hagberg, B., Hagberg, G., Leverth, A., and Lindberg, U. (1981). Mild mental retardation in Swedish school children. *Acta Pediatrica Scandinavia,* 70:444–452.

Herbst, D.S., and Baird, P.A. (1983). Nonspecific mental retardation in British Columbia as ascertained through a registry. *American Journal of Mental Deficiency,* 87:506–513.

Hodapp, R.M. (1990). One road or many? Issues in the similar-sequence hypothesis. In R.M. Hodapp, J.A. Burack, and E. Zigler (eds.), *Issues in the developmental approach to mental retardation.* Cambridge University Press, New York.

______, Burack, J.A., and Zigler, E. (1990). *Issues in the developmental approach to mental retardation.* Cambridge University Press, Cambridge.

Hogan, R., and Busch, C. (1984). Moral action as autointerpretation. In W.N. Kurtines and J.L. Gerwitz (eds), *Morality, Moral Behavior, and-Moral Development.* Wiley, New York.

Inhelder, B. (1968). *The diagnosis of reasoning in the mentally retarded.* Day, New York. (Original work published 1943)

Ireland, W.W. (1877). *On idiocy and imbecility.* Churchill, London.

Kanner, L. (1960). Itard, Séguin, Howe: Three pioneers in the education of retarded children. *American Journal of Mental Deficiency,* 65:2–10.

______. (1964). *A history of the care and study of the mentally retarded.* Charles C. Thomas, Springfield, IL.

______. (1967). Medicine in the history of mental retardation. *American Journal of Mental Deficiency,* 72:165–170.

Kohlberg, L. (1969). Stage and sequence: The cognitive-developmental approach to socialization. In D. Goslin (ed.), *Handbook of socialization theory and research.* Rand McNally, Chicago.

______. (1974). Discussion: Developmental gains in moral judgment. *American Journal of Mental Deficiency,* 79:142–146.

Koller, H., Richardson, S.W., Katz, M., and McLaren, J. (1983). Behavioral disturbance since childhood among a 5-year birth cohort of all mentally young adults in a city. *American Journal of Mental Deficiency,* 87:386.

Lambert, N., Nihiri, K., and Leland, H. (1993). *AAMR Adaptive Behavior Scales—School.* Pro-Ed, Austin, TX.

Lamont, M.A., and Dennis, N.R. (1988). Aetiology of mild mental retardation. *Archives of Diseases of Children,* 63:1032–1038.

Lane, H. (1976). *The wild boy of Aveyron.* Harvard University Press, Cambridge, MA.

Lund, J. (1985). The prevalence of psychiatric morbidity in mentally retarded adults. *Acta Psychiatrica Scandinavia,* 72:563–570.

Mahaney, E., and Stephens, B. (1974). Two-year gains in moral judgment by retarded and nonretarded persons. *Americal Journal of Mental Deficiency,* 79:134–141.

Matson, J.L. (1988). *The PIMRA manual.* International Diagnosti Systems, Inc., Orland Park, IL.

______, Gardner, W.J , Coe, D.A., and Sovner, R. (1990). *Diagnostic Assessment for the Severely Handicapped (DASH) Scale (User manual).* Unpublished manuscript, Louisiana State University, Baton Rouge.

Menolascino, F.J. (1988). Mental illness in the mentally retarded: Diagnostic and treatment issues. In J.A. Stark, F. J. Menolascino, M.H. Albarelli, and V.C. Gray (eds.), *Mental retardation and mental health: Classification, diagnosis, treatment, services.* Springer- Verlag, New York.

______, Wilson, J., Golden, C., and Ruedrich, S. (1986). Medication and treatment of schizophrenia in persons with mental retardation. *Mental Retardation,* 24:277–283.

Munro, J.D. (1986). Epidemiology and the extent of mental retardation. In C. Stavrakaki (ed.), Psychiatric perspectives on mental retardation. *Psychiatric Clinics of North America,* 9:591–624.

National Institute of Health. (1990). *Consensus conference on treatment of destructive behaviors in persons with developmental disabilities.* U.S. Government Printing Office, Washington, DC.

Nihiri, K., Leland, H., and Lambert, N. (1993). *AAMR Adaptive Behavior Scales—Residential and Community.* Pro-Ed, Austin, TX.

Parsons, J.A., May J.G., and Menolascino, F.J. (1984). The nature and incidence of mental illness in mentally retarded individuals. In F.J. Menolascino and J.A. Stark (eds.), *Handbook of mental illness in mentally retarded,* pp. 3–44. Plenum Press, New York.

Piaget, J. (1952). *The origins of intelligence in children.* Norton, New York.

Reid, A. (1982). *The psychiatry of mental handicap.* Blackwell Scientific Publications, Boston.

______. (1989). Schizophrenia in mental retardation: Clinical features. *Research in Developmental Disabilities,* 10:241–249.

______, and Ballenger, B.R. (1987). Personality disorder in mental handicap. *Psychological Medicine,* 17:983–987.

Reiss, S. (1988). *Test Manual for the Reiss Screen for Maladaptive Behavior.* International Diagnostic Systems, Orland Park, IL.

______, and Valenti-Hein, D. (1990). *Reiss Scales for Children's Dual Diagnosis: Test Manual.* International Diagnostic Systems, Orland Park, IL.

______, Levitan, G.W., and Szysko, J. (1982). Emotional disturbance and mental retardation: Diagnostic overshadowing. *American Journal of Mental Deficiency,* 86:567–574.

Rutter, M., Lebovici, S., Eisenberg, L., Sneznevskij, A.V., Sadoun, R., Brooke, E., and Lin, T-Y. (1969). A triaxial classification of mental disorders in childhood. *Journal of Child Psychology and Psychiatry,* 10:41–61.

______, Tizard, J., and Whitmore, K. (eds.). (1970). *Education, health and behaviour.* Longman, London.

Séguin, E. (1846). *Traitement moral, hygiène, et éducation des idiots et des autres enfants arrières.* J. B. Baillière, Paris.

______. (1866). *Idiocy and its treatment by the physiological method.* William Wood, New York.

Sparrow, S.S., Balla, D.A., and Cicchetti, D.V. (1984). *Interview edition. Expanded form manual. Vineland Adaptive Behavior Scales.* American Guidance Service, Circle Pines, MN.

______, and Carter, A.S. (1992). Mental retardation: Current issues related to assessment. In I. Rapon and S.J. Segalowitz (vol. eds.), *Handbook of Neuropsychology: Vol. 6. Child Psychology,* pp. 439–452. Elsevier, Amsterdam.

Stark, J.A., Menolascino, F.J., Albarelli, M.H., and Gray, V.C. (1988). *Mental retardation and mental health: Classification, diagnosis, treatment, services.* Springer-Verlag, New York.

Szymanski, L.S. (1980). Individual psychotherapy with retarded persons. In L.S. Szymanski and P.E. Tanguay (eds.), *Emotional disorders of mentally retarded persons.* University Park Press, Baltimore.

______, and Crocker, A. (1989). Mental retardaton. In H.I. Kaplan and B. J. Sadock (eds.), *Comprehensive textbook of psychiatry,* 4th ed. Williams & Wilkins, Baltimore.

______, and Grossman, H. (1984). Dual implications of dual diagnosis. *Mental Retardation,* 22:155.

Tarjan, M.D., Tizard, J., Rutter, M., Bergab, M., Brooke, E., de la Cruz, F., Lin, T-Y, Montenegro, H., Strotzka, H., and Sartorius, N. (1972). Classification and mental retardation: Issues arising in the Fifth WHO Seminar on Psychiatric Diagnosis, Classification and Statistics. *American Journal of Psychiatry,* 128(suppl.):34–35.

Uzgiris, I., and Hunt, J. McV. (1975). *Assessment in infancy: Affect, cognition, and communication.* University of Illinois Press, Urbana.

Wing, L., and Gould, J. (1979). Severe impairments of social interaction and associated abnormalities in children: Epidemiology and classification. *Journal of Autism and Developmental Disorders,* 9:11–30.

Wolfensberger, W. (1972). *The principle of normalization in human services.* National Institute on Mental Retardation, Toronto, Ontario.

Woodward, M. (1959). The behaviour of idiots interpreted by Piaget's theory of sensori-motor development. *British Journal of Educational Psychology,* 29:60–71.

______. (1961). Concepts of number of the mentally subnormal studied by Piaget's method. *Journal of Child Psychology and Psychiatry,* 2:249–259.

World Health Organization. (1992). *The ICD-10 classification of mental and behavioral disorders: Clinical descriptions and diagnostic guidelines.* Author, Geneva, Switzerland.

Zigler, E. (1967). Familial mental retardation: A continuing dilemma. *Science,* 155:292–298.

______, and Burack, J.A. (1989). Personality development and the dually diagnosed person. *Research in Developmental Disabilities,* 10:225–240.

CHAPTER 6

CEREBRAL PALSY

"Cerebral palsy" is the term used to describe a movement disorder thought to be the result of nonprogressive brain pathology caused by disordered development or due to brain damage incurred during pregnancy, delivery, or in early life. The term "cerebral palsy," per se, does not describe the severity or type of motoric deficit that is present. Like the terms "mental retardation," "learning disability," and "pervasive developmental disorder," it is the accepted general term for a disabling condition that has both psychological and social implications for families and for the provision of services. Because of this lack of specificity, neurologists often prefer the diagnostic term "static motor encephalopathy," and in their diagnosis list the specific motor impairment and other associated disabilities with it.

This chapter reviews the history, definition, epidemiology, etiology, classification, natural history, associated disabilities, developmental issues, the assessment process, family counseling, psychiatric disorders in individuals with cerebral palsy, and treatment of cerebral palsy.

HISTORY

Although recognized from antiquity, cerebral palsy was not distinguished from other motor disabilities until the 19th century when William John Little attributed spastic rigidity to obstetrical complications and perinatal anoxia (Accardo, 1989). In Little's classic report of 200 cases (1861–1862), *On the Influence of Abnormal Parturition, Difficult Labor, Premature Births, and Asphyxia Neonatorum, on the Mental and Physical Condition of the Child, Especially in Relation to Deformities,* he suggested specific etiologies for spastic diplegia and thereby offered an opportunity for preventive measures to be taken. Initially, the condition was referred to as "Little's disease" as a result of his work (Accardo, 1989). Later, William Osler introduced the term "cerebral palsy" (a contraction of the word "paralysis"), in his 1889 book, *The Cerebral Palsies of Children,* which was based on the neuropathological study of brains of affected children from the Elwyn School in Pennsylvania (Osler, 1989). Subsequently, in 1897, Sigmund Freud (Accardo, 1982; Freud, 1968), a child and adult neurologist before turning to psychoanalysis, introduced an early clinical classification in his *Infantile Cerebral Paralysis,* which provided a basis for the later classifications. In regard to etiology, Freud emphasized prenatal influences in suggesting that cerebral palsy might be linked to "symptoms of deeper lying influence which have dominated the development of the fetus." Modern refinements in classification were introduced and summarized in Crothers and Paine's *The Natural History of Cerebral Palsy* (1959). The current agreed upon classification of the clinical motor disorders was adopted by the American Academy of Cerebral Palsy in the 1950s (Minear, 1956). Efforts at prevention and early treatment of cerebral palsy were initiated at the beginning of the 20th century when programs in physical therapy were introduced. Extensive efforts have been focused on therapy, both for the movement disorder and for the psychological adaptation by the child and family.

DEFINITION

Cerebral palsy is a nonprogressive, but not unchanging, disorder of movement and posture that is the consequence of lesions or anomalies of the brain arising in the early stages of its development (Mutch et al., 1992). It becomes evident during the period of most rapid brain growth and is associated with sensory, behavioral, and cognitive manifestations. The term "cerebral palsy" along with these associated features designates a multiply-disabling condition which, depending on the extent of brain involvement, may be mild, moderate, or severe. It is a static motoric disability rather than a progressive neurological disorder. However, even though it is a static encephalopathy, changes do occur as the central nervous system matures. The cerebral lesion is static and nonprogressive, but the peripheral physical symptoms may change with brain development. For example, a hypotonic infant becomes a spastic or rigid child and a child who is originally diagnosed as choreoathetoid may subsequently become dystonic and develop contractures. In some instances, there is a gradual improvement, but other children reach a plateau where they remain. Many require bracing and surgery.

EPIDEMIOLOGY

The prevalence of moderately severe or severe cerebral palsy is estimated to be 1 to 2 per 1,000 live births (Stanley and Alberman, 1984). When milder cases are considered, prevalence may be as high as 1 to 6 per 1,000 live births. The incidence has not changed substantially in recent years despite better management of pregnancy, delivery, and care of the newborn (Stanley, 1987). There is disagreement regarding the age at which the cerebral palsy should be diagnosed because of the instability of the diagnosis when first detected in infancy. It has been suggested that brain damage occurring before the age of 3 should be used as a guideline. In this instance, children with acquired cerebral palsy as a result of infection or trauma may be included. The survival rate has remained high for children who live through the neonatal period and reached 88% in the 1940s and 1950s (Cohen and Mustacchi, 1966). Longer term survival offers challenges to both physical and psychological treatment.

Cerebral palsy is associated with a variety of risk factors occurring before pregnancy, during pregnancy, or during the perinatal period (Kuban and Leviton, 1994; Torfs et al., 1980). Factors occurring before pregnancy include long intervals between menses and a history of spontaneous abortion and stillbirth. Factors occurring during pregnancy include congenital malformation, fetal growth retardation, twin gestation, and abnormal fetal presentation. During labor and delivery, there is an association with premature separation of the placenta and nonvertex or face presentations. The abnormal presentation may be a marker for preexisting difficulties in developmental maturation rather than being a cause of cerebral palsy, i.e., a fetus with hypotonia or other anomalies may be less able to turn into a vertex position. During the early postnatal period, newborn encephalopathy may be linked to cerebral palsy.

Changes in care of the newborn have resulted in shifts in morbidity; for example, summaries of earlier research from the 1940s and 1950s and the monograph by Crothers and Paine (1959) suggested that birth injury and developmental problems accounted for approximately 50% of reported cases at that time. More recently, cerebral palsy associated with prematurity has been more commonly recognized as smaller, and smaller premature infants continue to survive. The rate of subsequent cerebral palsy is 25 to 31 times higher among infants with a birth weight less than 1,500 grams when contrasted to full-sized newborns. Those whose birth weight is less than 2,500 grams make up about one third of all infants who show signs of cerebral palsy later.

Spastic cerebral palsy is the most frequent type and accounts for approximately 50% of cases, followed by athetosis, 20%, and rigidity, ataxia tremor, and mixed forms (30%) (Stanley and Alberman, 1984). The incidence of the various forms is shown in Table 6–1, which

Table 6–1. Incidence of Various Forms of Cerebral Palsy

Symptom	% Occurrence
Pyramidal:	
Hemiplegia	25–40
Spastic Diplegia	10–33
Spastic Quadriplegia	9–43
Extrapyramidal:	
Athetoid, Ataxic, Dystonic	9–22
Mixed	9–22

From Nelson and Ellenberg, 1978.

includes composite data from various studies. One representative study that includes low birth weight premature infants is the California Cerebral Palsy Project (Grether, Cummins, and Nelson, 1992), which is a population-based study of 192 children born between 1983 and 1985 with moderate or severe congenital cerebral palsy; it includes both singleton and twin births. In the full sample, diplegia was the most common subtype, occurring in 33% of the cases. Quadriplegia was next, occurring in 29% of the total, followed by hemiplegia, which was found in 21%. Although there were no statistically significant differences between singletons and twins, spastic diplegia was found in 45% of the twin cases as contrasted with 32% of the singleton cases. Subtypes, which included dyskinesia and/or ataxia, occurred least commonly, occurring in 7% (dyskinesia/ataxia) and 10% (mixed) of the total cases. These findings indicate a high prevalence of pyramidal (83%) in contrast to extrapyramidal (17%) forms in a sample where 28% had a birth weight less than 1,500 grams.

ETIOLOGY

An analysis of The National Collaborative Perinatal Project (Nelson, 1988; Nelson and Ellenberg, 1986) concluded that the ability to recognize antecedents of cerebral palsy and predict the occurrence of the disorder failed to account for a substantial number of cases; a high rate of false positive identifications commonly occurred. They noted that for the mother–infant pairs in the 5% with the highest risk for cerebral palsy, only 2.8% produced a child with cerebral palsy. These authors found that the majority of cerebral palsy cases did not have specifically defined causes. Like etiologically unidentified mental retardation syndromes and congenital malformations, a specific etiology was lacking.

Cerebral palsy is not a single entity and the etiology of its various presentations is not the same. Developments in classification highlight how much there is to learn about its etiology. A legacy from early studies had been to place primary emphasis on perinatal asphyxia as causative, but later studies (Blair and Stanley, 1985) found asphyxia neonatorum in only 6% to 8% of cases. In the National Perinatal Collaborative study of NINCDS, 14% of quadriplegia was due to birth asphyxia. Therefore, the relative contributions of prenatal, perinatal, and genetic factors must all be considered in determining the etiology. Multiple brain regions are involved in the coordination of muscle activity so several sites may be involved.

The most common etiology is periventricular leukomalacia associated with prematurity (Kuban and Leviton, 1994). Yet in early childhood, encephalitis, meningitis, stroke, head injury, or poisoning also may be etiological factors. In 20% to 30% there is no known cause and unrecognized events during pregnancy or an unknown genetic abnormality is suspected. In one study of 1,048 low birth weight infants (Powell et al., 1988a, 1988b), 48 subjects with cerebral palsy were identified. Intrapartum events were most often associated with hemiplegia; however, factors involved in the rate of fetal development were more important in diplegia, which was more often associated with prematurity. Central nervous system infections in the first year have been reported to account for 6% of cases (Naeye et al., 1989) and about 2% are attributed to genetic factors (Hughes and Newton, 1992). Other inherited disorders may mimic a static encephalopathy in their early stages.

Brain damage in neonatal encephalopathy has been attributed to the excess production of excitatory amino acids during the first postnatal days (Espinoza and Parer, 1991; Ford, 1990; Riikonen, Kero, and Simell, 1992; Vannucci, 1990). However, N-methyl-D-aspartate

(NMDA) antagonists that block excitatory amino acids cannot be administered safely as a treatment for human subjects.

Caution is necessary before attributing the etiology to hypoxic-ischemic brain injury because a full-term infant with hypoxic-ischemic encephalopathy ordinarily will not only show abnormalities in tone but also signs, such as seizures, changes in alertness, and primitive reflex pattern. There may be systemic involvement of other organ systems as well. Moreover, fetal distress with meconium staining and reduced Apgar scores also may occur from nonasphyxial disorders.

Finally, disorders of neuronal migration may account for movement disorders and may lead to increased vulnerability to other kinds of injury. Immature neurons migrate to the cortical plate between 7 and 16 weeks of gestational age. Because the neocortex is laid down from inside to outside, newly developing neuronal terminals pass through layers that are already established. Abnormal migration may be associated with reduction in cell size, and early neuronal death may occur. Such abnormalities may subsequently affect the development of association pathways and lead to motor dysfunction, seizures, and learning and behavioral problems. Localized migrational problems have been described in cerebral palsy in addition to the more severe forms of migration disorders, such as polymicogyria and pachygyria. Environmental factors at sensitive developmental periods and genetic factors may affect neuronal migration.

CLASSIFICATIONS OF CEREBRAL PALSY

The multiaxial classification used to classify cerebral palsy includes the type of dysfunction (physiologic—pyramidal and extrapyramidal), the location of the dysfunction (topographic), and associated conditions (supplemental) (Bax, 1964; Minear, 1956). Because all cerebral palsy has an early hypotonic phase, initial classification must be tentative until the clear presentation of a syndrome can be identified. Cerebral palsy is then classified by the type of motor abnormality and the part of the body affected. The classification may be difficult because of subtle abnormalities and mixed features that may be demonstrated on the motor examination.

In regard to type of dysfunction (physiologic classification), there are two main groups: the pyramidal or spastic and the extrapyramidal or nonspastic types. The topographic classification is used only for the spastic types. It is ordinarily not used for the extrapyramidal types because they are classified according to their type of movement disorder.

Pyramidal (Spastic) Types

The spastic type of cerebral palsy is the most common and characterized by increased muscle tone in the involved muscle groups. Because of the increased tone, there is a state of constant muscle contraction. The neurological findings are persistent and vary little with movement, with emotion, or during sleep. Pathological reflexes are readily demonstrated in the spastic forms. The spastic subtypes are classified topographically depending on the number of limbs involved: monoplegia (1 limb), diplegia (2 limbs), triplegia (3 limbs), quadriplegia (4 limbs), and hemiplegia (an arm and a leg on the same side of the body). Infants with these various types are often described as floppy because of their hypotonicity. With increasing age, they show increased muscle tone and associated musculoskeletal deformities that may require orthopedic surgery. Furthermore, primitive reflexes, such as the tonic neck reflex, may persist, leading to problems in posture and movement. In hemiplegia, the upper limbs are generally more impaired than the lower ones. In diplegia, all four limbs may be involved, but the upper limbs may have only minimal involvement. In quadriplegia, the upper limbs may be less impaired, but there is generally severe dysfunction of all limbs. Monoplegia and triplegia are less common and are variations of hemiplegia and quadriplegia.

Extrapyramidal (Nonspastic) Types

Extrapyramidal forms are nonspastic types of cerebral palsy and are subdivided into choreoathetoid, ataxic, dystonic, and rigid forms. These groups are identified clinically, but are less clearly correlated with neuropathological findings. There is considerable variability in expression of extrapyramidal cerebral palsy. An increase in the movement disorder is associated with activity, with emotions, and when active muscle tension is necessary, but during sleep or relaxation, symptoms may be less intense. Abnormal involuntary movements increase with emotional stress and may be evident in a psychiatric interview. Primitive reflexes are more apparent in the extrapyramidal forms.

Individuals with athetosis have involuntary movements that involve various muscle groups. Consequently, they may appear contorted, stiff, or in continuous motion. Their speech may be dysarthric, and hearing impairment may be an associated finding. Chorea may occur with athetosis; the individual is then described as choreoathetoid. (Chorea consists of involuntary jerky movements involving the face, tongue, portions of the extremities, especially the distal portions, and, in some instances, the trunk.) These movements are rapid and irregular and are more pronounced during voluntary movement. The dystonic form involves extreme athetoid movements where the body and/or the extremities are forced into fixed postures by strong muscle contraction.

Individuals with extrapyramidal forms of cerebral palsy of the dyskinetic type are thought to have damage to the basal ganglia and to the cranial nerves. The cerebrum is usually not involved; therefore, in this form of cerebral palsy, there is less cognitive impairment than in the spastic types. Both extrapyramidal and pyramidal forms may be present in the same person. In addition, there are mixed types of the extrapyramidal forms.

Ataxic, Rigid, and Atonic Types

The other types, ataxic, rigid and atonic, are much less common. Ataxic cerebral palsy involves the cerebellum; therefore, problems with muscle tone are the primary manifestations. These children are hypotonic and show severe motor delays, but as they get older, functioning may improve. The rigid and the atonic types are very rare forms; there is very poor muscle tone and possibly associated bone deformities.

SUPPLEMENTAL CLASSIFICATION (ASSOCIATED DISABILITIES)

The associated nonmotoric disabilities that occur in children with cerebral palsy include mental retardation, sensory impairment of vision and hearing, learning disability, and language disorders. These associated disabilities along with psychological and psychiatric problems determine the extent that rehabilitation is possible.

Capute and Accardo (1991) note that certain associated features accompany particular types of cerebral palsy. For example, spastic hemiplegia is more often associated with seizures, hemianopsia, growth arrest, and cortical sensory deficits (including a visual field abnormality). Spastic diplegia may be associated with strabismus, and spastic quadriplegia is associated with epilepsy, mental retardation, dysarthria, and strabismus. Choreoathetosis is associated with mental retardation, auditory impairment, and dysarthria. Quadriplegia is more likely to be associated with seizures, extrapyramidal abnormalities, and severe cognitive impairment than hemiplegia or diplegia (Grether, Cummins, and Nelson, 1992).

Both mentally retarded and nonmentally retarded affected children are at risk for academic skills disorder or other cognitive impairments, visual and hearing deficits (6% to 16%), seizures (overall 20% to 30%; 70% in spastic and 20% in athetoid cases), strabismus (50%), sensory impairment (especially in hemiplegia), and social/emotional family dysfunction (Capute and Accardo, 1991). The increased prevalence of seizures, cognitive dysfunction, and perceptual disorders among those with cerebral palsy suggests these conditions may have common or related origins.

As the child matures, the problems associated with cerebral palsy may assume particular prominence. The most disabling problems for the child with cerebral palsy are the associated cognitive difficulties. In addition, speech and motor disability may become apparent in the preschool years and learning disabilities may be recognized at school entry. Associated difficulties that may influence learning include visual-perceptual problems, speech impairment, and hearing impairment. Communication disorder is particularly important to recognize; speech synthesizers and communication boards are essential for nonverbal children to facilitate interpersonal communication. For the family, recognition of the new difficulties as the child grows older is stressful, compounding problems already present that require the continuing need for surgery, bracing, and the use of other adaptive equipment.

Mental Retardation

Mental retardation is among the most important factors in vulnerability to environmental stressors and psychiatric disorder, occurring in 30% to 60% of those with cerebral palsy (Evans, Evans, and Alberman, 1990; Rumeau-Rouquette, et al., 1992). The extent of cognitive impairment varies considerably and determines the child's instructional level. Assessment of intelligence is a particular challenge due to the multiple physical disabilities that make cooperation with testing difficult. A variety of tests are needed to establish the extent of involvement. In their survey of 1,000 6-year-olds, Blair and Stanley (1985) found an average IQ of 68 with a broad and variable range, broader than in the general population. Those with ataxia showed the most variability, but those with athetoid and spastic types showed less impairment. The spastic group was more cognitively impaired than the athetoid group; the intellectual deficit was more severe in those with spastic quadriplegia than in those with paraplegia or spastic hemiparesis.

Learning Disorders

Associated learning disability is often a consequence of deficits in visual perception, in auditory processing, and in phonological sequencing. Neuropsychological testing is essential to identify strengths and weaknesses in learning.

NATURAL HISTORY

For children who experience lesions or anomalies of the brain arising in the early stages of its development and have subsequent involvement of the motor system, sequential changes have been documented as the motor disorder evolves over time (see Figure 6–1).

As the child grows older, early hypotonia (floppy baby) may progress to spasticity. The earliest motor changes observed are resistance to movement of the forearm, ankle, and knee as a result of an abnormal stretch reflex. For spastic diplegia, symptoms are first noted in the legs and may be associated with leg extension or scissoring when the child is vertically suspended, and increased tone is present when the child is placed down to walk. In spastic hemiplegia, symptoms are first noted in the arms and unequal muscle tone may be noted along with tight fists and an unequal response to the parachute maneuver. Furthermore, poor feeding may become apparent. The duration of hypotonia is variable and may last 6 to 17 months or even longer; the longer it lasts, the greater the severity of the disability. If it lasts longer than 3 years, the term "hypotonic cerebral palsy" is used.

Changes in muscle tone become apparent with ongoing development. The hypotonia may be followed by dystonia, e.g., when the infant holds up its head, extensor decerebrate rigidity may become apparent if the head is extended. Dystonic episodes may be present from 2 to 12 months of age, but eventually rigidity appears. In extrapyramidal cerebral palsy, persistent hypotonia is accompanied by immature (primitive) postural reflexes. With extrapyramidal forms, the asymmetric tonic neck reflex and the righting response persist longer than in those with spastic forms. The earliest signs of extrapyramidal dysfunction is finger posturing, which becomes apparent when the infant reaches for an object; finger/hand posturing may be seen by 9 months of age. In dyskinesis, dyskinetic postures are elicited by sudden changes in the position of the head, trunk, or limbs. In one study, one third of the group subsequently showed perceptual problems and hyperactivity.

With increasing age, the consequences of early birth injury are more variable, and cognitive, academic, and behavior problems become more apparent. The extent of disability varies considerably — from mild spasticity, where ambulation is possible in an individual who may be mentally retarded, to athetoid conditions or mixed athetoid and spastic conditions, where the individual may be essentially nonverbal and dependent on the family for care, yet have average or above intelligence and require special communication devices to interact with others.

DEVELOPMENTAL ISSUES

The normal phases of development are impacted by associated temperamental and

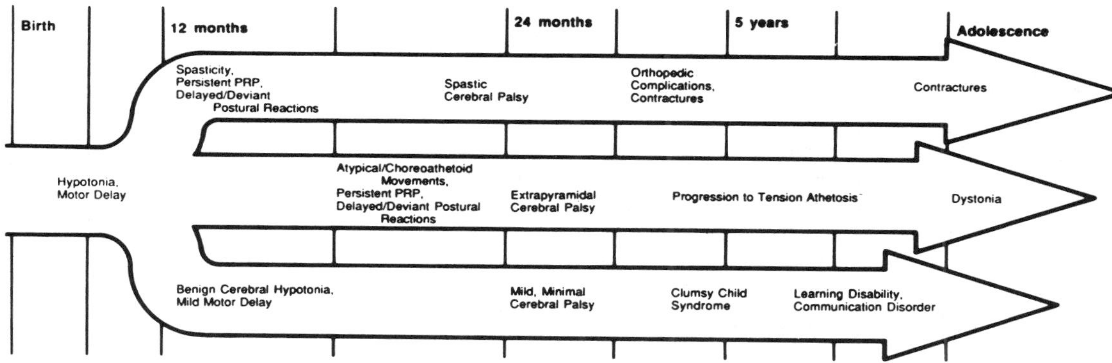

Figure 6–1. *Evolution of motor disorders.* Although the cerebral lesion remains stable and nonprogressive, the peripheral signs change as the brain matures. Thus hypotonia may evolve into spasticity or rigidity, and choreoathetosis may be transformed into dystonia (from Capute and Accardo, 1991).

physical features related to brain dysfunction, which may interfere with parent–infant attunement and attachment (Cox and Lambrenos, 1992). Attunement between child and parent is particularly affected by the cerebral palsy. Ordinary coordination of bodily movement with mother's voice may not occur due to the movement disorder. The early practicing subphase in the development of the self described in Mahler's theory of separation individuation is truncated by the inability to move away spontaneously from the parent and explore the environment. The child's limited ability to explore the environment and return to a secure base, along with parent–child communication problems, may affect bonding. Older children may benefit from environmental devices, such as motorized wheelchairs, to explore the environment.

Appropriate inhibition of primitive reflexes in the affected child is essential to help the family deal with developmental issues. The tonic neck reflex, which involves reflex arm extension when the head is turned, can be confusing to parents. Some mothers have interpreted the child's reflexive arm extension as an intentional movement to push them away. In other instances, the child may make a high-pitched cry, associated with opistotonic movements, which elicits anxiety in the parent and may interfere with the emergence of an attachment relationship. Effective holding and handling to inhibit these reflex activities may enhance attachment by normalizing the parent–child relationship.

The early phases of normal child development result in their internalization of "working models" of the caregivers. To facilitate the establishment of working models in children with cerebral palsy, the use of communication devices is of particular importance. Because younger children are unaware of their disabilities, positive internal working models are important to prepare them for the early school years. As children with cerebral palsy grow older, their motoric disability is readily apparent to other children, and good internal working models serve to help them cope with possible stigmatization. Identified as different by other children, the higher functioning group become increasingly aware of being different by the time they begin school. During each phase of development, there are potential developmental crises.

ASSESSMENT

Evaluation by the Interdisciplinary Team

Evaluating the child with cerebral palsy requires an integrated approach to the child's multiple disabilities by a physician-led interdisciplinary team. This team carries out pediatric, neurological, psychiatric, orthopedic, ophthalmologic, physiatric, dental, psychological, educational, physical therapy, occupational therapy, social work, and speech and language evaluations, as indicated. Cognitive ability may be difficult to assess due to the motor disability and the associated language disorder. Consequently, standardized testing needs to be adapted to reflect accurately the child's particular strengths and weaknesses. After completing their assessments, the team members meet to discuss treatment planning and the assignment of intervention tasks.

Establishing whether there is a permanent movement disorder can be difficult because early motor signs may improve or resolve. However, the recognition of motor delay is essential to the diagnosis of cerebral palsy. There is a reticence to diagnose cerebral palsy during the first 6 months of life before the disability is fully expressed. Motor delays will resolve with maturation in some children of this age as well as in children between 6 and 18 months. Follow-up for movement disorders should continue into the school-age years because one third to one half of very low birth weight infants may have some type of developmental disability.

In addition to the standard neurological examination, a neurodevelopmental examination is necessary to evaluate motor development. This examination includes testing for persisting primitive reflexes and postural reactions. The primitive reflexes include the asymmetric tonic neck reflex, the Moro Reflex, and the tonic labyrinthine reflex (Capute et al., 1984; Capute and Accardo, 1991). These reflexes are ordinarily inhibited by higher cortical regions by 6 months of age, as shown in Figure 6–2.

In normal development, following the disap-

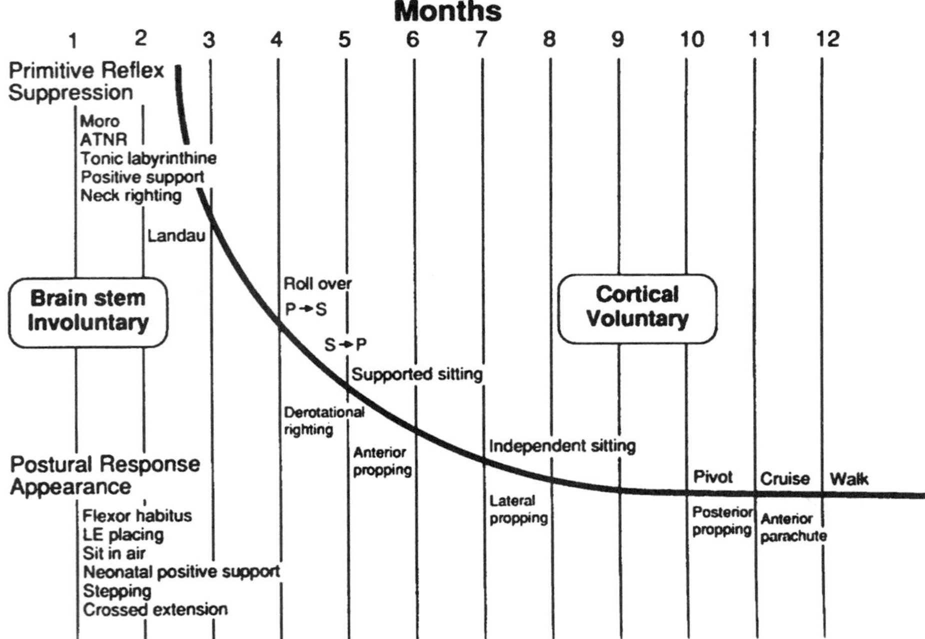

Figure 6–2. Evolution of motor development in infancy. Premature reflexes are a useful screening tool to aid in the detection of motor problems. The suppression of these premature reflexes is followed by the appearance of postural reactions as shown in the figure. These reactions can be useful in evaluating readiness for motor function (from Capute and Accardo, 1991).

pearance of the primitive reflexes, postural reactions emerge. These postural responses include head righting, the Landau reaction, and derotational righting. They are present before the child begins to roll over, sit, and crawl.

Brain-Imaging Studies

Advances in the use of noninvasive imaging techniques are now being utilized to improve and enhance assessment methods. Currently, ultrasound is used in the early diagnosis of periventricular leukomalacia in prematures. Cranial ultrasound through the open anterior fontanelle in premature babies makes it possible to identify hyperechoic and hypoechoic lesions and correlate them to later motor disability.

Computerized transaxial tomography (CT) and magnetic resonance imaging (MRI) may be utilized to evaluate structural changes in the brain (Volpe, 1992). For example, hemiplegic spastic cerebral palsy is associated with cerebral injury in the distribution of the middle cerebral artery based on both pathological findings and on CT and MRI scans. These assessments identify necrosis or atrophy with or without gliosis but do not identify when the ischemic or hemorrhagic insult occurred. Periventricular atrophy, suggesting white matter abnormalities and gross malformations of cerebral development, may be found. Menkes and Curran (1994) found MRI lesions in the putamen and thalamus in each of the 6 children with severe extrapyramidal cerebral palsy that they studied. However, the CT or MRI scan is normal in about one quarter of children with presumed congenital hemiplegia (Kuban and Leviton, 1994). The lack of identifiable abnormality provides support for the hypothesis that some cases of cerebral palsy are related to abnormalities of brain development at a microscopic level and have a developmental origin. In the future, assessments of metabolic activity and blood flow, using SPECT or positron emission tomography (PET) (Chugani, 1992), as shown in Figure 6–3, may become more generally available.

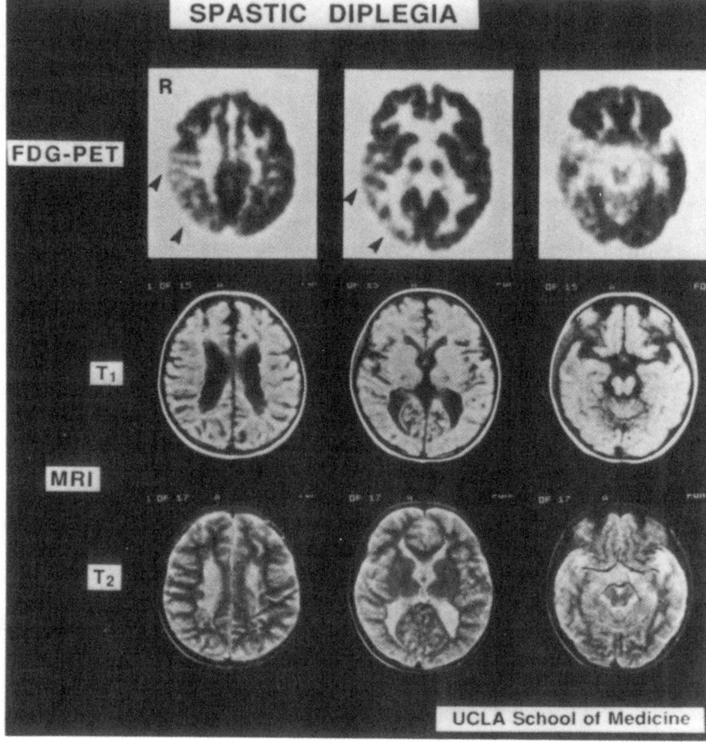

Figure 6–3. Magnetic resonance image and FDG-PET images of a child with spastic diplegic cerebral palsy. The MRI shows irregular contour to the walls of the lateral ventricles and high signal intensity in the periventricular white matter. The PET images reveal moderate hypometabolism in the right parieto-occipito-temporal cortex (arrows), which appears normal on MRI. In addition, there may be mild thalamic hypometabolism bilaterally (from Chugani, 1992).

Interview with the Parent

A family history of previous psychiatric disturbance and of developmental disorder in other family members must be elicited. Among the psychological issues that affect the parents' adjustment to the child, denial of the disability, self-blame, depression, projection, and dependency are most commonly encountered. To determine the degree of the parents' adaptation to the disabling condition, the following areas should be specifically covered in the parental interview (MacKeith, 1976; Richmond, 1972): First, it is important to clarify the extent of denial; do the parents have a realistic appreciation of the nature of the disability and its seriousness? Denial of the extent of the illness may place the child at risk. Secondly, whom do the parents talk to when they become concerned about their child; is there a close confiding relationship, or are the parents psychologically isolated? The third area deals with excessive guilt. Do the parents feel someone is to blame for the child's condition, e.g., the hospital staff, themselves? Self-blame and the frequently accompanying guilt is important to gauge because it may herald a depressive disorder. The parent may feel a sense of self-blame regarding his or her knowledge about child rearing or shame for producing a disabled child. A fourth area focuses on the parents' sense of adequacy in parenting. Do the parents feel adequate to take care of the child, or have they become excessively dependent on others? Do the parents anxiously and automatically follow directions from others? When excessive dependency occurs in caregivers, the physician may find the parents view themselves as helpless. Common behavior of the overwhelmed parents includes frequent telephone calls about minor illnesses and requests for the physician to make decisions for family members unrelated to treatment of cerebral palsy.

The parents' perception of the child's care must also be evaluated. Do the parents feel the care staff can be trusted to carry out procedures they do themselves at home? Not uncommonly, parents criticize caregivers as an expression of their projected fears and anxiety and may benefit from the opportunity to ventilate those feelings.

A final question relates to the parents' future plans for their child. In reviewing their future plans, it is particularly important to clarify if there is a genetic basis for the condition or if the parents believe there are genetic implications to the diagnosis. A test of the parents' coping ability is their capacity to invest energy in the care of each other as well as other family members and to make appropriate future plans for their child.

Interview with the Child (Special Considerations)

In the interview with the child, one must take into account both the child's developmental level and his means of most effective communication. Particular patience may be needed to understand the child's speech. In some instances, a letter board, speech synthesizer, or a facilitated communication procedure may be required for an effective interview. Initially, assistance from a speech pathologist may be helpful, but as familiarity with the communication equipment develops, assistance may be discontinued. Once communication is established using a communication device, the interview may proceed as it would with another child of equivalent mental age.

ADAPTATION TO THE DISABILITY

Family Adaptation

Because the parents are active participants in the child's care and often function as co-therapists, the parents must be confident and fully informed about treatment requirements. The parents' adaptation plays a major role in the child's development. Cerebral palsy varies in its expression from one individual to the next and this variability affects the parents' adjustment to the disability. Difficulty recognizing motoric disability in the early months of life can be quite stressful for family members. Although the parents may be concerned about a floppy infant, the physician frequently will recommend waiting several months or more to clarify the diagnosis. During this period, concerned parents often shop, going from one physician to another for consultation. Often parents will misinterpret the developing child's behavior.

Since the developmental disability becomes apparent before the age of 3, the life course of the child and the family is affected. For the best developmental outcome, it is essential that the parents make an early adjustment to the child's disability. A comprehensive service system of care is needed to aid in the adjustment process. Associated brain damage, cognitive impairment, social stigma, and nonverbal learning disabilities all increase vulnerability to a psychiatric disorder.

Adjustment Problems in the Child and Adolescent

With appropriate physical and psychological supports, the child with cerebral palsy may have an active school and family life. (Handicapped access to school and community facilities is particularly important.) Still, the following potential adjustment problems must be taken into account in management (Hurley and Sovner, 1987):

Dependency and Passivity

The child with cerebral palsy may become dependent on others and show a lack of assertion and assertiveness. Because of his dependency on others for physical care over long periods of time, the child may develop a lack of initiative in self-care. Moreover, an attitude of dependency may be fostered by the parents' difficulty in adapting to their child's disability. Parental guilt may lead to overprotection and an unwillingness to allow the child to have appropriate independence. Without appropriate psychological support, the child may have difficulty following through on individual objectives.

Hopelessness and Frustration

The inability to carry out tasks easily and with fluidity of movement may lead to considerable frustration, particularly for the athetoid individual. In addition, the sense of being different from others becomes more apparent with age. There may also be the sense of being a victim of an incurable condition.

Lack of Social Competence

This sense of hopelessness may be accompanied by doubts about social competence, which may take several forms. Among them are physical problems that are difficult to control, e.g., dribbling food or drooling saliva, incontinence of urine, and physical problems that socially isolate the child from others. Moreover, social competence may be influenced by social-emotional learning disability, leading to difficulty in attending to and understanding interpersonal social cues. Learning disabilities may lead to further incompetence in school, resulting in school failure.

Being stigmatized is an ongoing concern and may influence the child's care. Physical appearance, problems with activities of daily living (ADLs), and lack of social awareness may combine to produce social stigma. Moreover, higher functioning children with athetosis may be misdiagnosed as mentally retarded. The perception of being considered mentally retarded leads to more difficulty and may further compound the social adaptational problems. Social rejection becomes a concern following the onset of adolescence when peer group relationships assume additional importance. In adulthood, social rejection and discrimination also may occur in the workplace.

Guilt and Shame

The child, like the parents, may develop a sense of guilt or shame about the disability. With emerging self-awareness, the child may become increasingly aware of the burdens, both physical and financial, that he may cause other family members. The parental attitude toward the disability is crucial to help the child work through these feelings. With advancing age, the need for community services increases and the requirement for social support is greater for both child and parents.

PSYCHIATRIC DISORDERS OCCURRING IN INDIVIDUALS WITH CEREBRAL PALSY

Psychiatric disorders related to cerebral palsy fall into several general categories. Among these are psychiatric conditions secondary to the physical disability, i.e., adjustment disorder, personality trait disturbance, and difficulties in temperament. In addition, major psychiatric diagnoses may co-occur in a person with cerebral palsy.

Brain damage is a vulnerability factor in the establishment of psychiatric disorder. Brain dysfunction may lead to difficulty in inhibiting irrelevant environmental stimuli. In the Isle of Wight study that addressed this issue, Rutter, Graham, and Yule (1970) demonstrated that those children whose behavior was most affected were those who had a physical condition involving the brain. Yet the mechanism of how brain dysfunction results in behavioral abnormality remains unclear. Does brain dysfunction lead directly to behavioral disturbance, or does it increase the child's vulnerability to environmental stressors (Breslau, 1990)?

Persons with cerebral palsy may show increased rates of emotional lability, irritability, attention deficits, impulsiveness, and limited skills in social problem solving. Breslau (1990) interviewed 157 children with cerebral palsy, myelodysplasia, or multiple disabilities, along with 339 randomly selected controls and their parents. Increases in depressive symptoms and inattention were significantly associated with physical disabilities. Family environment was particularly important for depression in both groups, but this was not the case for inattention. Difficult temperament was found to be a vulnerability factor. This study demonstrates that parental–child problems, alone or in combination with a difficult temperament in the child, may lead to psychiatric disorder.

Those disabled children who have been overly protected may be at risk for separation anxiety disorder. Other children whose parents have difficulty setting appropriate limits on their behavior may develop oppositional defiant disorder. Attention deficits are common in children with cerebral palsy and must be carefully assessed. Stress-related brief psychotic reactions may occur and should be distinguished from schizophrenia and mood disorder. Major mental illness, both mood disorder and schizophrenia, may present for the first time in adolescence or in early adult life in persons with cerebral palsy; both conditions respond to psychotropic drug treatment. Mood disorder is a particular concern because major depression may go unrecognized or be misdiagnosed as an adjustment disorder. Furthermore, what appear to be accidents must be carefully monitored because they may result from an undetected mood disorder.

COMPREHENSIVE THERAPY

A comprehensive treatment approach (Kohn, 1990) includes general pediatric supervision, psychoeducational assessment and intervention, orthopedic management (Bleck, 1987), appropriate neurosurgical treatment of spasticity, physical and occupational therapy, and psychological support. Therapy has benefited from advances in rehabilitation technology. This includes the use of orthotics (braces), robotics, mobility and seating devices, and computer interfaces for the control of devices. Assistive and augmentative communication devices allow children early in life to make choices and come to understand cause-effect relationships. Parent education about treatment is essential and educational materials are widely available for parents (Blasco, Baumgartner, and Mathes, 1983).

Activities of Daily Living

The routine tasks of toileting, feeding, dressing, and transferring the child from one place to another must all be attended to for the child's comfort and to facilitate family adjustment. Feeding may be a particular problem for the parent of a child with cerebral palsy, and prolonged feeding sessions of an hour or more are not uncommon. Tongue thrust (i.e., forceful tongue protrusion on stimulation) may interfere with nipple insertion and the initiation of feeding. Tonic biting may occur when the gums are stimulated. The parent must be taught feeding techniques that position the infant to optimize muscle tone (inhibit excessive extensor tone), including methods of introducing the nipple and supporting the jaw.

The management of incontinence is an ongoing concern. The etiology of incontinence may be complex so psychological, cognitive, neurological, and neuromuscular factors must be considered. Toileting can be a difficult issue for family members, and the child or adolescent may be reluctant to participate in such programming. Family members and caregivers may not understand the child's reluctance to participate and may become angry over these incidents. Incontinence may occur sporadically and be related to spasticity of the bladder, leading to intermittent incontinence. The intermittently incontinent patient may not be believed by others; the behavior may be interpreted as showing a lack of motivation directed toward toilet training. With a lack of understanding from others, children may characterize themselves as lazy or feel hopeless about their lack of control of continence.

Psychotherapy

Psychotherapy with individuals who have cerebral palsy requires several adaptations. In particular, psychotherapy must be tailored to the associated features of the disabled person's disorder. Of most importance is the use of communication devices, e.g., communication boards and other special devices to facilitate communication. Considerable patience is required by the therapist for effective therapeutic interventions in the disabled person more so than in the nondisabled. Therapeutic intervention involves the child and family; for example, parents may need to be engaged in interpreting the disabled person's speech for the interviewer.

Initial therapeutic goals for the child focus on establishing an understanding of the presenting problem, an understanding of the nature of the disability, and an understanding of the child's feelings about it. Subsequent psychotherapeutic goals include improving self-control, learning to attribute responsibility for behavior to the self, utilization of problem-solving techniques to understand consequences, developing a vocabulary of emotional states, acknowledging another person's point of view as different from one's own, and an appreciation of the effect of one's behavior on others.

With parents, crisis intervention techniques are important and include anticipatory guidance and preventive interventions. Anticipatory guidance is especially important at times of predictable crisis. These include the time of diagnosis, early adaptation to the specific physical needs for child care, the time of school entry, entry into adolescence, and the time of completion of schooling. Preventive interventions are essential during the crisis itself. For example, school entry can be particularly difficult because previously unrecognized mental retardation may become evident at that time. If preventive interventions are unsuccessful and adaptive failure is demonstrated during the parental interview, then short-term therapy goals include dealing with denial, guilt and self-blame, projection, and excessive dependency.

Pharmacotherapy

Pharmacotherapy may be effective for treatment of behavior and mental disorders in the affected child. The parent and the child should be actively involved in deciding on the treatment procedure and, if medication is used for the child, it should be reviewed with him. Moreover, a careful baseline neurological examination is essential before initiating neuroleptic drug treatment. The child's cognitive level is a major consideration in monitoring drug side effects.

SUMMARY

Despite recent advances in medical care, more than 100,000 American children and adolescents are estimated to have neurological disability linked to cerebral palsy and the conditions associated with it, particularly mental retardation. The increased survival of preterm infants at risk for the disease has resulted in a focus on developmental changes *in utero* and efforts to prevent periventricular leukomalacia in the third trimester of pregnancy. Future efforts at prevention of cerebral palsy must emphasize factors and events occurring during pregnancy as well as those events that may predispose to preterm delivery.

Interventions for children with cerebral palsy require an understanding of the types of cerebral palsy, the associated disabilities, and the child's and family's adaptation to the disability. Times when family crises may be expected are at the time of initial diagnosis, during the preschool years, when entering school, during adolescence, and at the completion of schooling. With maturation, changes in function and the extent of impairment may occur. Newly recognized associated impairments may become more apparent with age, especially in regard to mental retardation and seizure disorders. Younger children who were ambulatory on crutches may become nonambulatory as they gain weight during adolescence. Parents may misinterpret the child's physically based difficulty with feeding, continence, or ambulation and attribute it to a lack of motivation.

The parents' role is vital in dealing with the problems associated with the disability. This is most poignantly demonstrated by Christy Brown, a talented poet with athetoid cerebral palsy whose autobiography *My Left Foot* was made into an Academy Award winning film. His poems demonstrate how internal working models may develop and the possibility of a creative life despite this disability.

In his poem "For My Mother," (Brown, 1971), Christy Brown writes:

You were a song inside my skin
a sudden sunburst of defiant laughter
spilling over the night-gloom of my half awakenings
a firefly of far splendid light
dancing in the dim catacombs of my brain.

In "Inheritance," he says:

Deafmute tongues of tongue-tied thoughts
flare across the oceanic wastes of a room
loud as an afternoon landscape
sharp as a knife in the ribs
blade-toothed serpentine whispers
lipping the crumbling ledges of my mind . . .
A hand lightly on my sleeve
and the loneliness of being on earth.

These poems highlight the importance of the parent and the joyfulness of a loving presence to a disabled person, the frustration of not being able to communicate, and the sense of loneliness that is experienced. Yet they also affirm the possibility for creativity and the aliveness of the person with cerebral palsy behind a motoric mask that externally hides individual expressivity.

REFERENCES

Accardo, P. J. (1982). Freud on diplegia: Commentary and translation. *American Journal of Diseases of Children,* 136:452–456.

______. (1989). William John Little (1810–1894) and cerebral palsy in the nineteenth century. *Journal of the History of Medicine and Allied Sciences,* 44:56–71.

Bax, M.C.O. (1964). Terminology and classification of cerebral palsy. *Developmental Medicine and Child Neurology,* 6:295–297.

Blair, E., and Stanley, F. (1985). Interobserver agreement in the classification of cerebral palsy. *Developmental Medicine and Child Neurology,* 27:615–622.

Blasco, P., Baumgartner, M., and Mathes, B. (1983). Literature for parents of children with cerebral palsy. *Developmental Medicine and Child Neurology,* 25:642–647.

Bleck, E. (1987). Orthopedic management of cerebral palsy. *Clinics in Developmental Medicine,* no. 99/100. Blackwell Scientific Publications, Oxford.

Breslau, N. (1990). Does brain dysfunction increase children's vulnerability to environmental stress? *Archives of General Psychiatry,* 47:15–20 .

Brown, C. (1971). *Come softly to my wake.* Secker and Warburg, London.

Capute, A.J., and Accardo, P.J. (1991). *Developmental disabilities in infancy and childhood.* Brookes, Baltimore, MD.

______, Palmer, F. B., Shapiro, B.K., Wachtel, R.C., Ross, A., and Accardo, P.J. (1984). Primitive reflex profile. *Monographs in developmental pediatrics,* Vol. 1. University Park Press, Baltimore.

Chugani, H.T. (1992). Functional brain imaging in pediatrics. *Pediatric Clinics of North America,* 39:777–796.

Cohen, P., and Mustacchi, P. (1966). Survival in cerebral palsy. *Journal of the American Medical Association,* 195:462.

Cox, A.O., and Lambrenos, K. (1992). Childhood physical disability and attachment. *Developmental Medicine and Child Neurology,* 34:1037–1046.

Crothers, B.S., and Paine, R.S. (1959). *The natural history of cerebral palsy.* Harvard University Press, Cambridge.

Espinoza, M.I., and Parer, J.T. (1991). Mechanisms of asphyxial brain damage, and possible pharmacologic interventions, in the fetus. *American Journal of Obstetrics and Gynecology,* 164:1582–1591.

Evans, P.M., Evans, S.J.W., and Alberman, E. (1990). Cerebral palsy: Why we must plan for survival. *Archives of Diseases of Childhood,* 65:1329–1333.

Ford, L.M. (1990). Results of N-methyl-D-aspartate antagonists in perinatal cerebral asphyxia therapy. *Pediatric Neurology,* 6:363–366.

Freud, S. (1968). *Infantile cerebral paralysis.* University of Miami Press, Coral Gables, FL.

Grether, J.K., Cummins, S.K., and Nelson, K.B. (1992). The California Cerebral Palsy Project. *Pediatric and Perinatal Epidemiology,* 6:339–351.

Hughes, I., and Newton, R. (1992). Genetic aspects

of cerebral palsy. *Developmental Medicine and Child Neurology,* 34:80–86.

Hurley, A., and Sovner, R. (1987). Psychiatric aspects of cerebral palsy. *Psychiatric Aspects of Mental Retardation Reviews,* 6:1–6.

Kohn, Jean G. (1990). Issues in the management of children with spastic cerebral palsy. *Pediatrician,* 17: 230–236.

Kuban, K.C.K., and Leviton, A. (1994). Cerebral palsy. *New England Journal of Medicine,* 330:188–194.

Little, W.J. (1861–1862). On the influence of abnormal parturition, difficult labor, premature birth, and asphyxia neonatorum, on the mental and physical condition of the child, especially in relation to deformities. *Transactions of the Obstetrical Society of London,* 3:293–344.

MacKeith, R. (1976). The restoration of parents as the keystone of the therapeutic arch. *Developmental Medicine and Child Neurology,* 18:285–86.

Menkes, J.H., and Curran, J. (1994). Clinical and MR correlates in children with extrapyramidal cerebral palsy. *American Journal of Neuroradiology* 15:451–457.

Minear, W. (1956). A classification of cerebral palsy. *Pediatrics,* 18:841.

Mutch, L., Alberman, E., Hagberg, B., Kodama, K., and Perat, M.V. (1992). Cerebral palsy epidemiology: Where are we now and where are we going? *Developmental Medicine and Child Neurology,* 34:547–551.

Naeye, R.L., Peters, E.C., Bartholomew, M., and Landis, R. (1989). Origins of cerebral palsy. *American Journal of Diseases of Children,* 143:1154–1161.

Nelson, K.B. (1988). What proportion of cerebral palsy is related to birth anoxia? *Journal of Pediatrics,* 112:572–574.

Nelson, K., and Ellenberg, J. (1978). Epidemiology of cerebral palsy. *Advances in Neurology,* 19:421.

______, and ______. (1986). Antecedents of cerebral palsy. *New England Journal of Medicine,* 315:81–86.

Osler, W. (1889). *The cerebral palsies of children.* P. Blakiston and Son, Philadelphia.

Powell, T.G., Pharoah, P.O.D., Cooke, R.W.I., and Rosenbloom, L. (1988a). Cerebral palsy in low-birthweight infants: I. Spastic hemiplegia: Associations with intrapartum stress. *Developmental Medicine and Child Neurology,* 30:11–18.

______, ______, ______, and ______. (1988b). Cerebral palsy in low-birthweight infants: II. Spastic diplegia: Associations with fetal immaturity. *Developmental Medicine and Child Neurology,* 30:19–25.

Richmond, J.B. (1972). The family and the handicapped child. *Clinical Proceedings of the Children's Hospital National Medical Center,* 8:156–164.

Riikonen, R.S., Kero, P.O., and Simell, O.G. (1992). Excitatory amino acids in cerebrospinal fluid in neonatal asphyxia. *Pediatric Neurology,* 8:37–40.

Rumeau-Rouquette., C., du Mazaubrun, C., Mlika, A., and Dequae, L. (1992). Motor disability in children in three birth cohorts. *International Journal of Epidemiology,* 21:359–366.

Rutter, M., Graham, P., and Yule, W.A. (1970). A neuropsychiatric study in childhood. *Clinics in Developmental Medicine,* no. 35/36. Spastics International Medical Publications in association with William Heinemann Books, Ltd., London.

Stanley, F. (1987). The changing face of cerebral palsy? *Developmental Medicine and Child Neurology,* 29:263–265.

______, and Alberman, E. (1984). The epidemiology of cerebral palsy. *Clinics in Developmental Medicine,* no. 87. Blackwell Scientific Publications, Oxford.

Torfs, C.P., van den Berg, B., Oechsli, F.W., and Cummins, S. (1990). Prenatal and perinatal factors in the etiology of cerebral palsy. *Journal of Pediatrics,* 116:615–619.

Vannucci, R.C. (1990). Current and potentially new management strategies for perinatal hypoxic-ischemic encephalopathy. *Pediatrics,* 85:961–968.

Volpe, J.J. (1992). Value of MR in definition of the neuropathology of cerebral palsy *in vivo. American Journal of Neuroradiology,* 13:79–83.

CHAPTER 7

LEARNING DISORDERS

Learning problems associated with emotional and behavior disorders are common in children referred to clinics and in general population epidemiologic surveys. Up to 15% of the school-age population may have academic difficulty during their school careers, (Gaddes, 1976). The exact prevalence of learning disorders in the academic skills areas is unknown because various studies have used different criteria to define cases. However, the U.S. Centers for Disease Control (1987) concluded that based on the available data, 5% to 10% was a reasonable estimate of persons with learning disabilities. Males outnumber females; however, the magnitude of the difference between males and females may, to some extent, reflect referral bias (Finucci and Childs, 1981). For some, difficulty in learning and achieving in academic settings is associated with mental retardation; for others, it may be secondary to emotional and behavioral difficulties. There is a third group, perhaps 3% to 6% of school-age children, whose learning problems may stem from domain-specific processing difficulties, such as specific reading disorder, and whose behavioral and emotional problems may be secondary to their specific deficits.

Learning deficits may be identified in children who are normally intelligent and in children who have a variety of disabling conditions, including children who have specific syndrome presentations. The passage of U.S. Public Law 94–142 was a major step forward in developing services and programs for these learning-disabled children in the United States. In the law, children with learning disorders are defined as follows:

> Those children who have a disorder in one or more of the basic psychological processes involved in understanding or in using language, spoken or written, which disorder may manifest itself in an imperfect ability to listen, think, speak, read, write, spell, or do math calculations. The term includes such conditions as perceptual handicaps, brain injury, minimal brain dysfunction, dyslexia, and developmental aphasia. The term does not include children having learning problems which are primarily the result of visual, hearing, or motor handicaps, of mental retardation, of emotional disturbances, or of environmental, cultural, or economic disadvantage. (U.S. Congress: Public Law 94–142, 1975)

The general terms "learning disabilities" and "learning disorders" have been applied to include academic skills impairments; however, it is essential to designate clearly the particular skill that is impaired. Academic impairments may involve reading, mathematics and expressive writing. The Public Law 94–142 definition is contrasted with the DSM-IV (APA, 1994) definitions of reading disorder, mathematics disorder, and disorder of written expression in the description that follows.

The Public Law includes only children with normal intelligence, whereas the DSM-IV definition allows for mentally retarded children with uneven cognitive profiles. Moreover, the

DSM-IV definition excludes children whose learning problems are due to known neurological disorders; Public Law 94–142 includes brain injury and dysfunction. The use of specific neuropsychological testing to identify the underlying cognitive abnormalities or impairments is leading to a more specific characterization of the DSM-IV disorders. Reading, expressive writing, and mathematics disorders involve different processing deficits, such as visuospatial or linguistic processes in different brain regions. Social-emotional learning disorders or nonverbal learning disabilities may be associated with mathematics disorder.

Early descriptions of learning disorders focused on presumed brain dysfunction as related to the various academic skills areas, so reading disorders have been referred to as dyslexia, writing disorders as dysgraphia, and arithmetic disorders as dyscalculia. These terms suggest groups with pure disorders of genetic or constitutional origin with a common etiology and the need for a particular form of treatment (Rutter and Yule, 1975; Yule and Rutter, 1985). However, there may be multiple factors involved that include environmental influences as well as specific brain dysfunction. Consequently, the terms "reading disorder," "mathematics disorder," and "disorder of written expression" are preferred.

This chapter reviews the history, definition and classification, epidemiology, etiology and pathogenesis, developmental perspective, natural history, diagnosis, clinical presentation, and treatment of reading disorder, spelling disorder, mathematics disorder, disorder of written expression, and social-emotional learning disorder. Specific evaluation instruments are reviewed in Part I, Chapter 3.

7.1 Reading Disorder

Proficiency in reading is often considered the key to success in other academic areas. Reading achievement is highly correlated with mastery in spelling and mathematics (Yule and Rutter, 1985) and lack of mastery in reading may prevent mastery in other basic skills areas. The greatest amount of research in learning disability is on reading disorders; however, in recent years an increasing amount of research has been focused on the other academic skills disorders. It has been found that poor readers are almost invariably poor spellers, but the converse is not necessarily true.

HISTORY

Reading disorders have been reported since the end of the last century when Hinshelwood (1895) and Morgan (1896) described reading retardation as cases of congenital word blindness. These early cases were conceptualized based on what was understood of alexia, or reading loss, with acquired brain damage. Subsequently, theoretical explanations for learning disabilities, particularly in reading, were offered, such as those by Orton (1928), who proposed incomplete or mixed cerebral dominance and suggested that delayed development of specialization in the left hemisphere might occur. Despite these early reports, before the 1940s, children in the United States who had reading problems were generally considered mentally retarded, emotionally disturbed, or socially disadvantaged.

During the 1940s, learning disorders were recognized in children with neurological dysfunction. One group of studies that focused on whether children with learning difficulties invariably had demonstrable brain damage concluded brain disorder was minimal and introduced the term "minimal brain damage" (Strauss and Lehtinen, 1947). Others raised the possibility that learning difficulties reflected a brain that functioned differently, rather than being damaged, and suggested "minimal brain dysfunction" (MBD), which became the accepted designation (Clements, 1966). The minimal brain dysfunction syndrome included learning deficits, perceptual-motor problems, poor coordination, overactivity, impulsivity, and subtle neurological signs.

Later, the term "specific learning disability" was introduced and, in general, described the same group of children (Farnham-Diggory, 1978). Although these formulations emphasized brain dysfunction, traditional sensorimotor-based neurological examinations did not demonstrate specific abnormalities. Treatment with medication was recommended, but it was found that although stimulant medication improved the hyperactivity and attentional problems frequently associated with learning disability, the specific learning problems themselves were not improved (Gittelman, 1983). Higher cortical functions were apparently involved in the learning-disabled rather than motor and/or sensory neurological abnormality. Therefore, neuropsychological and linguistic tests began to be used to supplement traditional psychological examinations to identify children with these disorders.

In 1968 a subcommittee of the World Federation of Neurology defined the term "specific developmental dyslexia" (Critchley, 1970) as "a disorder manifested by difficulty in learning to read despite conventional instruction, adequate intelligence, and socio-cultural opportunity." It was attributed to "fundamental cognitive disabilities which are frequently of constitutional origin." Developmental dyslexia is often considered to be synonymous with the DSM-IV category of reading disorder. The World Federation diagnosis of developmental dyslexia is based on general criteria lacking in etiologic specificity, an assumption of a constitutional basis, and considers that the mechanisms may be similar to acquired alexia or dyslexia in adults. Others have emphasized that there may be multiple subtypes involving several areas of higher cortical function. However, the term "reading disorder" is currently preferred because there may be several forms of dyslexia in childhood.

DEFINITION AND CLASSIFICATION

One way of categorizing reading problems is in terms of reading retardation and reading backwardness (Yule and Rutter, 1985). Reading retardation refers to a substantial discrepancy, e.g., 2 years, between mental age and reading age. In research studies, reading retardation may be operationalized using criteria such as 2 standard deviations below the average expected score. In addition, regression equations that incorporate both IQ and age have been used in epidemiologic research to deal with the problem of regression to the mean. Regression to the mean is necessary because children with very high or very low IQs do not read as well or as poorly as might be expected based on IQ scores. Reading backwardness refers to a substantial difference between chronological age and reading age so that a number of children with subaverage intelligence would be included who have general problems in learning. In the normally intelligent child, these terms frequently overlap.

An alternative approach is based on determining absolute reading deficiency, regardless of IQ; this approach is consistent with there being neurobiological differences among children who have reading disorders. Pennington et al. (1992) have reviewed the use of age versus IQ discrepancy-based definitions of reading disability.

Reading disorders are most commonly diagnosed on educational grounds based on detection in school and results from psychoeducational test batteries that are administered to children who have been identified as reading delayed. The DSM-IV diagnostic criteria for reading disorder are outlined in Table 7.1–1. In addition to the requirement of substandard reading achievement (criteria A), an impairment in adaptive functioning is also required (criteria B).

Children with severe reading disorder most likely constitute several subtypes, such as the cognitively based linguistic and visual subtypes originally suggested by Boder (1973) or the reading disorder syndromes summarized by Rapin (1982): (1) language disorder syndrome; (2) visual-spatial perceptual syndrome; (3) articulation and graphomotor discoordination syndrome; and (4) sequencing syndrome.

Another approach is to consider the distinct reading systems abnormalities identified in adults with brain damage. This approach emphasizes the recognition that there are several routes involved in reading words aloud. A better understanding of these distinct reading systems may be profitably studied in development. Marshall and Newcombe (1973) provided the first formal description of subtypes of dyslexia as an acquired reading disorder. In their information processing model, they wrote of visual registration being coded as visual address, then passing to phonological and semantic address boxes. They included visual dyslexia where there is confusion of orthographically similar letters (e.g., *b, d, p, q*) whether or not they appear in context. Other

Table 7.1–1. DSM-IV Diagnostic Criteria for Reading Disorder

315.00 Reading Disorder

A. Reading achievement, as measured by individually administered standardized tests of reading accuracy or comprehension, is substantially below that expected given the person's chronological age, measured intelligence, and age-appropriate education.

B. The disturbance in Criterion A significantly interferes with academic achievement or activities of daily living that require reading skills.

C. If a sensory deficit is present, the reading difficulties are in excess of those usually associated with it.

Coding note: If a general medical (e.g., neurological) condition or sensory deficit is present, code the condition on Axis III.

From APA, 1994.

categories that are currently used include grapheme-phoneme (surface) dyslexia, phonological dyslexia, and semantic (deep) dyslexia. Temple (1992) suggests that when the developmental forms are comparable to the acquired forms of surface dyslexia and phonological dyslexia, it is difficult to distinguish the child from the adult case.

Surface dyslexics show an overreliance on a phonological reading system and have poorly developed lexical reading systems (Coltheart et al., 1983). The problem is characterized by difficulty with letter (orthography) to sound (phonology) translation. The child may recognize letters but mispronounce them, especially when multiple sounds are associated with a particular letter (e.g., *disease* read as *decrease*). The child does best when reading aloud words with regular spelling to sound patterns (e.g., *habit*) than irregular words (e.g., *knoll*). They make regularization errors, confuse the meaning of homophonic words (e.g., *gate/gait*) but are accurate in reading regular words and matched nonwords. Temple (1985) suggests that prior to being translated into words, the word is segmented into chunks and that parsing into chunks which are too small may result in surface dyslexia. Errors occur when these chunks are blended into words.

Surface dyslexia is less common than phonological dyslexia, which occurs where reading of nonwords is significantly poorer than reading words; there are no regularization errors and no confusion with homophones (Temple, 1992). This may come about because the phonological route to reading is inaccessible in contrast to surface dyslexia where it is relied on excessively. In this syndrome, parsing may occur into word chunks that are too large. The spelling pattern is deviant at an earlier age.

An uncommon form has been referred to as semantic, or deep, dyslexia (Coltheart, 1980). These children are unable to read nonwords and do not master any phonological reading route; they make major semantic errors. The semantic interpretation of the word is incorrect so that, for example, *hen* is read as *egg* or *chicken*. It is rare because the multiple impairments that are needed to produce it may completely prevent the development of reading.

ASSOCIATED NEUROPSYCHIATRIC DISORDERS

The most frequently associated diagnosis with reading disorder is attention deficit disorder (Silver, 1981), which is estimated to occur in between 20% and 25% of children with reading disorder. Halperin et al. (1984) have identified a reading-disabled subgroup of attention deficit disorder with hyperactivity. Psychiatric disorder and delinquency are frequently associated with severe reading disorder. The relationship is strongest with antisocial disorders. Attention deficit disorder may be a predisposing factor for conduct disorder (Yule and Rutter, 1985). Moreover, children and adolescents with reading disorder may have other secondary emotional, social, and family problems. There are certain developmental disorders where specific academic skills may be deficient. Children with Tourette's disorder, neurofibromatosis, and seizure disorders are also at risk for reading disorder.

CLASSIFICATION OF READING DISORDER: A DEVELOPMENTAL APPROACH

A developmental approach to classification links underlying processing deficits with patterns of reading and spelling performance.

Although the details continue to be debated, the acquisition of reading seems to involve two systems: the lexical system (sight-reading) to process printed familiar words and a secondary phonological system to decipher unfamiliar words. Awareness of phonological structure requires knowledge of letter–sound correspondences. A developmental analysis may facilitate better understanding of how reading-disabled children compensate for their problems and lead to a more informal intervention strategy.

A developmental classification of reading and spelling difficulties emphasizes the stage where these academic skills are arrested (Frith, 1985). Reading-disordered children have difficulty when advancing from the early phase of acquisition, where reading is visually based (logographic) and proceeds through the use of partial cues, to the alphabetic phase where letter–sound associations are used for both reading and spelling. In the logographic stage, the child lacks strategies to decipher unknown words other than by visual approximation to known words; spelling is limited to a few rote words (Snowling, 1991). The logographic stage involves instant recognition of familiar words, that is, whole-word sight-reading based mainly on memorization through repetition. Errors are made because words are remembered by features like first word or length of the word. These children read words by sight recognition and have difficulty with nonwords; their spelling tends to be dysphonetic. The child reads some sight words but has difficulty with any unfamiliar words and makes semantic errors on familiar words (e.g., *truck* for *car*). During the alphabetic phase, the child uses phoneme-grapheme to sound out words, begins to decode, starting with left to right decoding, which depends on consistency between letters and sounds ($g + u + m$) and then using more complex rules. In this phase, letter–sound correspondences are utilized. When development breaks down at this initial stage, the problem resembles a phonological reading disorder. Developmental problems in this stage may lead to a failure to move from the alphabetic letter–sound phase to another phase where reading and spelling are automatic and independent of sound. Arrest at the alphabetic stage shows better spelling than reading. This third phase is referred to as orthographic and features both automaticity and flexibility. This involves instant analysis into orthographic units, e.g., morphemes without initial phonological conversion. There is difficulty in reading irregular words where the child must rely on sound; spelling errors are phonetic. This latter group resembles "surface dyslexia." Finally, some children may read well, but fail to make the final step to develop spelling competence (Frith, 1985; Snowling, 1991).

That children fail to make progress because of phonological difficulties, leading to an "arrest" at the visual, or logographic, stage is supported by a study by Snowling, Stackhouse, and Rack (1986). These authors identified children with developmental disorders in reading whose attainment was at two ability levels, 7 years' and 10 years' reading age. In both groups, nonwords were read significantly below age-level expectations after considering their word recognition levels and making comparisons with reading-age-matched normal controls. These children had significantly more difficulty than control children on phonological processing tasks. These cases offer support for failure in reading due to phonological difficulties with poor progression beyond the visual, or logographic, stage.

Evidence for an arrest at a later stage of reading development when reading and spelling are based on letter–sound association is found in individual case reports by Goulandris and Snowling (1991). They found that children with reading disorder may have severe phonetic spelling problems along with difficulty in reading irregular words and in distinguishing between written homophones (e.g., *leek/leak*). One of these case reports deals with J.A.S., an adult student, who demonstrated success on most phonological processing tasks, but had great difficulty with visual memory. Memory for sequences of abstract visual shapes was poor, and there was major difficulty in producing sequences of Greek letters, which were unfamiliar to her. On memory tests, performance was as low as a 6-year level. The authors suggest that this data is consistent with visual memory problems, leading to reading difficulty. A developmental approach may be particularly useful in linking the underlying deficits in processing with reading performance.

EPIDEMIOLOGY AND PREVALENCE

The Isle of Wight study by Rutter, Tizard, and Whitmore (1970), using statistical regression procedures, identified a prevalence of 3.5% of 10-year-olds and 4.5% of 14-year-olds who were 30 months retarded in reading. Others (Hynd and Cohen, 1983) have found slightly higher rates and estimate the prevalence at 3% to 6%. Because these prevalences are significantly higher than the 2.3% expected on statistical groups, creating a "hump" in the distribution, a neurobiological basis should continue to be pursued. Prevalence has been thought to be higher in males than females, with a sex ratio of 2.5 males to 1 female (Critchley, 1970).

More recent estimates (Shaywitz et al., 1990) showed little sex difference in a group of boys and girls selected from an epidemiologic sample. They identified 8.8% of boys and 6.5% of girls in second and third grade whose achievement scores were 1.5 standard deviations below expectations based on achievement tests. Yet, overall, affected males are identified more frequently than females by a ratio of at least from 1.8–2 to 1 in other studies (Finucci and Childs, 1981), so there is an increased risk for males.

ETIOLOGY

The etiology of reading disorder has been studied from both neurobiological and cognitive perspectives. Studies of etiology address biological causes and morphological markers that may prove useful in classification, early identification, and clarification of theoretical issues. Findings from autopsy studies, neuroimaging, and neurophysiologic investigations suggest that reading retardation may be associated with fundamental changes in brain anatomy and brain physiology; subgroups may show neurocortical deficits that lead to disruption of cognitive processing. Many of these studies relate to abnormality in perinatal brain development. A disorder of language in childhood, the most commonly replicated finding in reading retardation, may be influenced by early perceptual abnormalities that interfere with the establishment of normal cognitive and linguistic structures (Galaburda, 1993). In the past, abnormal eye movements, dysfunction of the vestibular system, difficulty with learning rules, differential sensitivity to light, and various visual problems have been suggested as the primary etiologies.

Anatomical abnormalities in cell migration have been identified in postmortem studies; a marker on chromosome 15 has been identified in some families (Smith et al., 1983), and EEG abnormality has been reported in some cases (Duffy et al., 1980). Cognitive impairment in phonemic segmentation of spoken and written words has been reported (Shankweiler and Crain, 1986). MRI studies of brain anatomy, animal models, PET scan studies of brain functions, event-related potentials, and cognitive testing have all been carried out in learning-disabled children. Neuroanatomical correlates of reading disorder may be useful in clarifying questions about subtyping.

Genetics

Specific reading disorder has been reported in family case studies for almost a century. The familial risk for reading disorder was studied by Vogler, DeFries, and Decker (1985) who estimated the risk to be 40% to a son whose father is affected, and 35% if his mother is affected, which represents a 5- to 7-fold risk over those without affected parents. For daughters, the risk of having an affected parent of either sex is around 17% to 18%, which is 10- to 12-fold greater than for daughters without affected parents. Similar familial risks in the 36% to 45% range have been reported by others; this risk is sufficiently significant that family history may be used to help screen for children at risk (Pennington, 1990). Concordance rates of reading disorder have also been studied in monozygotic and dizygotic twins to evaluate heritability. In the Colorado Family Reading Study (Vogler, DeFries, and Decker, 1985), differential regression to the mean in the co-twin was used to estimate heritability. Regression to the mean is a necessary part of the methodology in twin studies because there should be greater regression to the mean for co-twins who are dizygotic (because their relationship is 0.5; the relationship is 1.0 in monozygotic co-twins) than for monozygotic co-twins. When examining twins, one of whom was reading disordered, significant heritability for reading recognition and spelling was demonstrated, but not for reading comprehension (DeFries, Fulker, and LaBuda, 1987). Moreover, digit span, a reading-related skill that is a measure of verbal short-term memory, was also found to be heritable. Measures of perception and motor speed on the Colorado Perceptual Speed Test were not genetically influenced; however, more refined measures of perception should be included in future studies. The authors' findings suggest that about 30% of the cognitive phenotype can be attributed to heritable factors other than IQ. Stevenson et al. (1987) studied 13-year-old twins, some of whom were reading disordered. They found that although genetic factors were important in individual differences for reading ability and reading disability, general intelligence was of greater importance. These authors found significant heritability for spelling and spelling disability. They considered that a significant part of the variance for reading ability is related to genetic effects, but a substantial amount of the variance is also related to environmental factors. Their reading heritability results are at variance with all other twin studies, which may be due to the older age of their sample. However, their results are of interest regarding findings in older subjects.

Overall, these twin study results are consistent with findings that deficits in single-word recognition, rather than comprehension, are the more important deficit and that the precursor of this deficit is in phonological processing skills. That phonological coding deficits in reading-retarded children are highly heritable is demonstrated in additional studies of the performance of monozygotic and dizygotic twins with reading disability (Olson et al., 1989). However, orthographic coding was not found to be heritable. These findings suggest that phonological awareness, which is critical to reading acquisition, is impaired in reading disorder and that it is this deficit which is inherited. Although there are heterogeneous etiologies of reading disorder, but these may not affect reading directly, but rather alter the establishment of spoken language skills that are essential for later reading development (Pennington, 1990).

Several models of genetic transmission for reading disorders have been proposed. Existing studies support genetic heterogeneity, but do not identify a specific model. However, Pennington and colleagues (1991) provide epidemiologic data that supports major gene transmission for severe developmental reading disorder in some families. They reviewed four independently ascertained samples, which include 1,698 persons from 204 families. In three of these samples, a major gene locus transmission was thought to be the most probable mechanism and polygenetic transmission was suggested in the fourth sample. Although the authors concluded that gender differences occur, reading retardation remains etiologically heterogeneous even in those families where there is apparent dominant transmission.

Smith et al. (1983) have reported linkage of the reading disorder trait to chromosome 15; however, this finding has not yet been replicated by other groups. Different genes could be acting in different families; however, a single major gene locus may be an adequate explanation for genetic transmission in some pedigrees. Genetic influences on reading disorder might influence the development of the temporal lobe planum temporale region, leading to altered planum symmetry. Such alterations in structure and, most likely, connectivity could result in phonological processing problems for both spoken and written language.

Neuroanatomical Findings

Asymmetry of the brain normally occurs and is evaluated with magnetic resonance imaging (MRI), using the planum temporale (superior surface of the temporal lobe) as a marker (Rumsey et al., 1986). The planum temporale is larger in the left than in the right hemisphere as early as 29 weeks' gestation (Witelson and Pallie, 1973). Symmetry of the planum temporale has been reported significantly more commonly in severely reading-disordered children when compared with normal controls and children with attention deficit/hyperactivity disorder (Hynd et al., 1990). Moreover, the symmetry of the planum temporale has been associated with difficulties in phonological awareness. Larsen and colleagues (1990) measured the planum temporale in 19 eighth-grade students with severe reading disorder and controls and found that 70% of those with reading difficulties showed symmetry of the planum compared to 30% of the controls. Furthermore, among the reading-disordered subgroup with phonological deficits, 100% showed symmetry of the planum. This suggests that asymmetry of the planum is associated with normal phonological awareness. In other studies, congenital abnormalities in the corpus callosum have been related to reading disorder, particularly in the phonological aspects of reading (Temple et al., 1990). Positron emission tomography (PET) scan evaluations have demonstrated anomalies in cerebral blood flow in the left temporoparietal region, a brain region involved in language, in males with severe reading disorder (Rumsey et al., 1992). Hagman et al. (1992) have used PET to evaluate performance during an auditory processing task. Shaywitz et al (1995) used functional MRI to demonstrate that performance on a phonological matching task is lateralized to the left hemisphere in males, but occurs bilaterally in females. This sex difference may need to be considered in the evaluation of reading disorder.

Alterations in the pattern of brain asymmetry in language areas and the presence of minor cortical malformations have been described by Galaburda and colleagues in a neuroanatomical study involving four male and three female subjects with a diagnosis of severe reading disorder (Galaburda et al., 1985; Humphreys, Kaufmann, and Galaburda, 1990). These authors reported an absence of the usual pattern of left-sided asymmetry of the planum temporale. In addition, areas with ectopic neurons were found in the molecular layer of the perisylvian cortex in the frontal region involving the areas whose blood supply comes from the anterior and middle cerebral arteries. In three of the brains, multiple foci of glial scarring involving the same perisylvian region were interspersed between the ectopic area, suggesting that injury to these regions may have led to minor cortical malformations. They speculated that the malformations may have occurred in the second trimester, but that scars may occur somewhat later, perhaps in the second and third trimesters and in the early postnatal period.

An autoimmune etiology for similar brain changes has been proposed in humans and in an animal model (Galaburda, 1993). It is possible that ischemic injury to the developing cortex produced by autoimmune damage to the wall of the arterial blood vessels supplying the involved brain regions might result in scars and malformations. Family studies of the prevalence of reading retardation suggest the possibility that the trait for reading retardation may be related to factors which influence cerebral dominance and possibly the development of the immune system.

Animal models with immune disease and learning disorders show anatomical changes, with patterns of neocortical ectopic neurons and cortical scars comparable to those found in human studies. To investigate how minor malformations may result in apparent and clinically persistent cognitive dysfunction, strains of New Zealand black mice that spontaneously develop autoimmune disease have been studied. In these animals, regions with neocortical ectopic neurons and cortical scars associated with specific cortical neuronal subtypes, alterations in cortico-cortico connectivity, and modifications of behavior have been reported (Denenberg et al., 1991; Sherman, Galaburda and Geschwind, 1985; Sherman et al., 1987; Sherman et al., 1990). Additionally, these mice also show alterations in the usual pattern of brain asymmetry, which is consistent with an interaction of early developmental events and the development of cortical asymmetry (Rosen et al., 1989). These studies indicate that insults to the developing brain during the period of neuronal migration to the neocortex may also lead to abnormalities in these brain regions. However, immunopathology is only one of several possible hypotheses. Whatever the mechanism of the injury, it is congenital. Yet, despite the abnormality in the brain, the associated behaviors in the mouse model can be modified by early life experience in an enriched and complex environment (Schrott et al., 1992).

Neurophysiological Findings

Event-related brain potentials (ERPs) are one of the few approaches that allow the study of neural events associated with information processing (Regan, 1989). ERPs may provide information about sequence, timing, and, in some instances, the location of neural activity that is elicited by a particular stimuli prior to the production of a specific response. Consequently, severe reading disorders have been investigated using event-related potential measures. These studies indicate that physiological differences do exist between normal readers and those with reading disorder in regard to cognitive processing, especially that involving linguistic categories. Furthermore, linguistic stimuli may be treated, in part, as nonlinguistic stimuli by the reading disordered, and significant differences may exist in expectancy, attention, and brain signal processing (Landwehrmeyer, Gerling, and Wallesch, 1990). Moreover, disabled readers may fail to engage long-term semantic memory in their responses to visually presented primed and unprimed words (Stelmack and Miles, 1990).

Perceptual anomalies have been suggested in reading-retarded individuals, using visual-evoked potential studies. The visual system may be involved in reading disorder in that there may be a failure of the brain's visual circuits to keep proper timing. In some cases, there may be an abnormality which leads to slowing of one of the two major visual pathways so that two basic kinds of visual information are not processed in the right sequence in the lateral geniculate nucleus, the relay station through which visual information passes en route to the primary visual cortex. The ventral layers of this nucleus, the magnocellular system, has large cells that carry out fast processes for seeing motion, stereoscopic vision, depth perception, low contrast, and locating objects in space. The dorsal layers, the parvocellular system, has smaller cells that carry out slower processes for perceiving stationary images, color, detailed forms, and high contrast. It is thought that the magnocellular pathway is segregated from the parvocellular system in the retina and remains segregated through the lateral geniculate nucleus, the primary visual cortex, and the higher order visual cortices (Livingstone et al., 1991; Livingstone and Hubel, 1988) (Figure 7.1–1).

These visual systems were tested because it had been found that there was some slowness in the visual system response in children with reading disorder; when two visual stimuli were presented in rapid succession, the child would report one rather than two images. But, like normal children, both images were seen by the learning-disordered child if presented at a slower rate.

The visual systems have been studied through the investigation of the "flicker fusion rate," the fastest rate at which a contrast reversal of the perceived stimulus may be demonstrated. The flicker fusion rate is abnormally slow in children with severe reading disorders when contrast is low and spatial frequency is

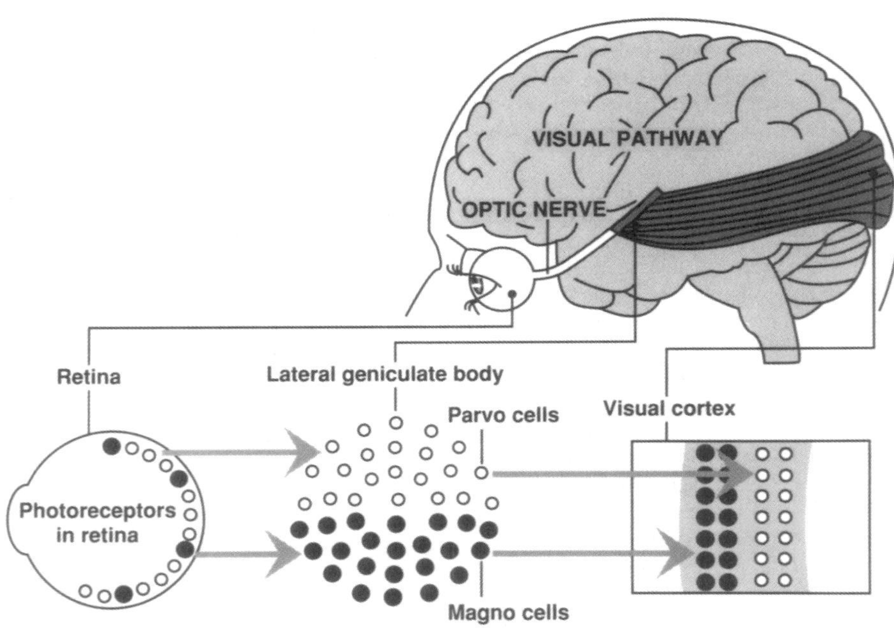

Figure 7.1–1. *Visual Pathways in the Brain.* In reading, light strikes photoreceptors in the retina; the information is then processed by magno cells and parvo cells in the lateral geniculate bodies. The signal then travels to the visual cortex for further processing. In a study of children with dyslexia, the magno cells were found to be smaller than normal, and low-contrast information processing was found to be slower than normal (from *New York Times,* 1991).

low (Lovegrove, Garzia, and Nicholson, 1990). In the flicker fusion rate test, dysfunctional readers and normal readers were shown a 36-rectangle flickering checkerboard pattern; the squares were reversed at different rates under high and low contrast (brightness) conditions and the transient and sustained visual-evoked potentials were recorded (Galaburda and Livingstone, 1993; Livingstone et al., 1991). At the high contrast, both visual systems should be operational, but at low contrast, only the fast magnocellular system should be responsive. The parvocellular pathway, which is known to be slow and relatively insensitive to contrast and color selective, functioned normally in their reading-disordered group, but the disordered group showed abnormalities when fast low-contrast stimuli were presented, indicating involvement of the magnocellular system. The presence of this physiologic abnormality in reading-retarded persons suggests a magnocellular deficit that occurs early in development. The magnocellular system involves the retina, the lateral geniculate nucleus, and the primary visual cortex; none of these regions are thought to be involved in coordinating cognitive functions.

Subsequently, the same investigators studied the magno- and parvocellular layers of the lateral geniculate nucleus in the brains of 5 reading-retarded and 5 control subjects and found that only the magnocellular cells were smaller in the reading-retarded group. This result is consistent with the physiologic finding of slower processing in the magnocellular system. The parvocellular cells did not show changes in size, although in some specimens, both the magno and the parvo layers showed structural disorganization. Overall, the magnocellular layers were more disorganized and the cell bodies appeared smaller in the dysfunctional readers; the magnocellular system was 27% smaller in the reading-disordered than the normal controls. In these two studies, the authors have provided the first neurophysiologic demonstration of a magnocellular defect in the visual system in severe reading retardation that could be matched to anatomical findings.

To read, information from the fast magnocellular system must precede the slower parvocellular system. Appropriate recognition of patterns may be necessary for the patterns to be interpreted at higher levels. Some retinal cells linked to the magnocellular system are specified for low-contrast fast stimuli and must be coordinated at higher levels. In the reading-retarded groups, high-contrast functioning seems to be intact, but significant differences are seen in low-contrast fast processing situations. If the magnocellular system is operating slowly, words might seem to blur, fuse, or jump off the page. In fact, deliberate image blurring, which reduces the contrast of high spatial frequencies, is capable of reestablishing normal temporal processing of words in some cases of reading disorders (Williams and Lecluyse, 1990). Colored light lenses are also being used in an attempt to alter the timing of these two systems and improve reading; findings are controversial.

Lehmkuhle et al. (1993) measured visual-evoked responses to evaluate visual information processing in the magnocellular and parvocellular visual systems in 8- to 11-year-old normal and reading-disordered children. Potentials were measured for targets with low and high spatial frequency in a normal or flickering field. The latencies of the early components of the visual-evoked potentials were longer in reading-disabled children than in normal readers when the low spatial frequency target was used, but no differences were seen with the high spatial frequency target. The authors conclude that the magnocellular responses are slowed in reading-disabled children, but there is no general slowing of the visual response. Additional studies are needed with larger samples to investigate a possible cause-effect relationship with reading disability, possibly resulting from a cognitive dysfunction secondary to a sensory-perceptual problem.

Tallal and Piercy (1973) have reported a defect in fast auditory processing in language/reading disorder, raising the possibility that fast processing is abnormal in both visual and auditory modalities. If so, these processing abnormalities might interfere with the acquisition of auditory and visual language and affect efficient language processing in those brain areas where fast processing is necessary to extract meaning from words. Tallal's group found that the fast components of the auditory system were impaired in young children with language learning problems, approximately 85%

of whom had trouble learning to read. Children were presented combinations of the same high and low tones and asked to repeat what they had heard. Normal children are able to discriminate tones presented to them at .08 seconds apart, but language-impaired children required 300 milliseconds between tones to discriminate them properly. When consonant sounds were artificially lengthened, using computer synthesis, the sounds were discriminated by the language-disordered children. Moreover, practicing with lengthened sounds led to better discrimination and improved speech. In keeping with these results, Galaburda (1993) presents preliminary data that the kinds of anatomical abnormality similar to those found in the visual thalamus may also be found in the auditory thalamus. He found that cell bodies in the medial geniculate nuclei of the thalamus, the relay station to the primary auditory cortex, tend to be smaller in size, especially those affecting the left hemisphere. This shift in size might represent a disruption of a large cell system that could produce difficulties in processing rapidly changing auditory information. In addition to visual and auditory processing problems, deficiencies in tactile discrimination may also occur in children with reading disorders; for example, if two fingers are touched in rapid succession, the child may sense that only one was touched.

Overall, these neurophysiologic studies are consistent with difficulties in processing rapidly changing information in several sensory channels. Children with these various sensory disabilities must make sense of the world without perceiving large amounts of fast-moving visual, auditory, and tactile information and apparently must rely on context, repetition, facial expression, and other strategies to do so.

Concurrent Investigation of Sensory-Cognitive and Linguistic Abnormality

Formulations of the underlying deficits in reading-disabled children emphasize both linguistic and sensory-cognitive mechanisms that are thought to be involved in normal language development. The proposed deficits include an inability to integrate rapidly presented nonlanguage auditory stimuli, limiting functioning of the transient visual system, deficits in syntactic processing, and deficits in verbal short-term memory (Shankweiler and Crain, 1986). These different aspects of processing have not been studied in the same sample of children. Most electrophysiologic studies have focused on aspects of processing within a single sensory modality. Consequently, there is little evidence to clarify whether the several deficits in reading disability that are reported arise from a similar underlying impairment or whether they co-occur in the same children. Neville et al. (1993) studied both behavioral and neurobiological aspects of language and nonlanguage processing in the same subjects. These authors investigated timing and organization of neurophysiologic processes within and between the hemispheres while children with reading disability and normal children processed sensory, cognitive, and language information.

Children who had early language impairments were initially identified at age 4 and displayed both expressive and receptive language problems. When retested at age 9, they were found to be reading disabled (Tallal, 1987). At least 85% of language-disordered children develop reading disability, and many reading-disabled children have early language development problems. The age of assessment distinguishes whether the language or the reading will receive primary emphasis in the study. These authors found that no single factor accounts for deficits of language impairment and reading disability. Many aspects of processing are affected but not homogeneously across children, suggesting a multiple factor and multiple subtypes framework. Some aspects of sensory and language processing were abnormal in the group as a whole; other aspects were abnormal only in subsets of the language-impaired, reading-disabled group. Evoked-response potentials during auditory sequencing processing were abnormal only in children who had difficulty on the Tallal repetition task, which is associated with language impairment. Early responses of visual event-related potentials to both language and nonlanguage stimuli were severely reduced in amplitude in the group as a whole. However, organization of event-related potentials that are linked to grammatical processing were found in only a subset, which was not the subset that had the abnormal auditory processing. The group as a whole also displayed abnormally large evoked-response potentials to sentence medial open class words and to sentence final words.

In regard to auditory-sensory processing, Tallal has shown that language-impaired children are impaired in their ability to discriminate and sequence rapidly presented nonverbal stimuli. She has suggested that a significant percentage of developmental language disorders arise in the inability to perceive the changing acoustic spectra that are characteristic of speech perceptions. This was demonstrated in the event-related potential study (Neville et al., 1993), which showed that the early auditory ERP component was delayed in latency and reduced in amplitude in those cases who scored most poorly on the repetition task. The reduction in amplitude of the ERP components occurred over the anterior regions of the right hemisphere. MRI studies in the same children showed reduced subcortical volumes in the right diencephalon and caudate compared to controls. These regions require further study of processing during focused auditory attention.

In the Neville et al. study, visual-sensory processing was also disturbed; nonlanguage visual processing was reduced, using the ERP tests. These effects were equivalent for both peripheral and central stimulation and for the various rates at which stimuli were presented, in contrast to Lovegrove, Garzia, and Nicholson (1990) who found abnormalities in the transient visual subsystem. (This system arises on the periphery of the retina and is most sensitive to low spatial frequencies and the high temporal ones.) Attention focused to central and peripheral visual space is thought to be mediated by separate neural systems. The visual system that processes central visual information and is most sensitive to high spatial and low temporal frequencies was normal in the reading-disabled subjects.

Studies in animals and in deaf adults suggest that the peripheral or transient visual system develops later and, therefore, may be more vulnerable to developmental insult. Lovegrove, Garzia, and Nicholson (1990) suggest that the transient system, or peripheral system, is important in reading because it permits the integration of information from successive fixations and produces better temporal resolution. A deficit in this system could diminish the integration of information across visual fixations, and within a fixation, may diminish the integration of foveal information. Yet the ERP studies, although they need to be replicated, show reduced visual ERPs to both peripheral and central foveal stimulation.

Overall, early sensory processing deficits are an important component of the reading disorder profile. Still, some affected children display aberrant processing of grammatical information that does not appear to be correlated with sensory deficits. As a group, these subjects placed more reliance on and/or must expend more effort to integrate words into the context of a sentence. This increased effort may be necessary to compensate for deficits in the earlier stages of language processing. Therefore, multiple factors are involved in the emergence of language processing deficits, and these deficits are heterogeneous across groups with reading disorders.

NEUROPSYCHOLOGICAL PHENOTYPE

The cognitive psychology of reading has been extensively reviewed by Pennington (1991). Neuropsychological testing procedures are utilized to establish the underlying deficits in reading disorder. Specifically, testing has established the components in reading that are impaired. Procedures for neuropsychological testing are described in Chapter 3.

Difficulty in word recognition is generally thought to be the central problem in reading disorder. Yet other components of information processing systems may also be involved because reading involves: (1) visual perception in order to recognize letters, (2) word recognition, and (3) comprehension. Despite considerable interest in these components, the greatest empirical support is for a language abnormality, although speed of information processing in each modality may be problematic. Word recognition is ordinarily accomplished through direct access or by phonological coding. For most children with reading disorder, interference in phonological coding is the major factor, although the direct access hypothesis to word recognition may be important for subgroups, and there may be associated visual or spatial processing problems. Difficulties with word recognition are commonly caused by a deficiency in the use of phonological coding to recognize words. In order to translate printed letters into words, the phonemes of the alphabet (individual speech sounds) and rapid coding ability are needed.

The major difficulty is in phonics, the ability to sound out words, which makes reading slower and less automatic which, in turn, distracts from comprehension. Furthermore, poor phonics ability makes spelling less accurate and less automatic. In reading, one moves from letters to phonological representation, and in spelling, from phonological representation to letters. That reading-disordered children have higher rates of spoken language problems, including articulation problems, name-finding problems, and difficulties remembering sequences, such as phone numbers and addresses, is consistent with this interpretation.

Evaluation of the phonological coding problems with written language reveals a primary deficit in phoneme segmentation skills and phonological coding. Phoneme segmentation is closely tied to later reading skill where breaking a word into phonemic segments utilizes awareness of the subsyllabic structure of individual phonemes and the ability to manipulate those phonemes. Moreover, the development of phoneme segmentation is influenced by sociocultural experiences so that lack of educational stimulation may lead to an apparent reading disorder.

Problems with phoneme segmentation may be tied to biological variation, lack of early language stimulation, and perhaps lack of practice in reading.

DEVELOPMENTAL COURSE

Reading disorders have been viewed as a specific problem of school-age children; however, reading difficulties are not simply related to maturational lags, but are developmental problems that must be considered throughout the life span. Although reading disorder is not diagnosable until beginning school, ordinarily at the end of the first or beginning of the second grade, precursors to reading disorder may be present before beginning school. These may include speech delay, articulation difficulties, difficulty learning the names of letters and colors, problems in word finding, difficulty in sequencing syllables and difficulties in remembering addresses, phone numbers, and other verbal sequences, including directions that involve several steps.

Longitudinal studies of the development of reading, based on testing at age 4 or 5, show that subsequent reading ability is predicted by phonological processing skills even when effects of IQ, sex, and age are parceled out (Pennington, 1991). Phoneme awareness and segmentation skills are most predictive of later reading ability. This suggests that children who have future reading problems have preexisting phonological processing difficulties during their preschool years. Before the age of 4, phoneme awareness has been demonstrated to be related to later reading problems but not to mathematics disorder (Maclean, Bryant, and Bradley, 1987). Furthermore, early knowledge of nursery rhymes predicts better phoneme awareness later in childhood.

Although differences in individuals in phoneme awareness may involve both genetic and environmental factors, the genetic aspects are being pursued to identify children at risk at age 4 and below. Scarborough (1990), in a longitudinal study of children at high familial risk for reading disorder, found that at age 2½ at-risk subjects were worse than siblings and normal controls in a test of natural language production but not on formal language tasks. These findings are consistent with an interpretation that reading disorder is related to developmental language disorder.

Outcome studies suggest that the reading gap remains relatively constant over time. Therefore, during the school years, it is not a question of a developmental lag and catching up, at least for most children, but rather developing means to compensate for the reading impairment. Children with reading disorder continue to have reading difficulties as adults; this is especially true in males. Pennington (1991) suggests that females with early reading problems may compensate more fully than males and may not be diagnosable on standard tests, although, when asked, they report continued reading difficulty. The developmental course may be variable so there can be considerable compensation by adulthood. Yet the deficit may continue to be problematic and, for some, presents a greater disability in adult life than in childhood. Still, most of those affected fall in the middle and show a basically constant lag on reading tests throughout life. It is not clear what the protective factors are that facilitate this compensation; however, being of female sex and the quality of intervention are recognized as important.

Most identified reading-disordered children finish high school and many go to college, yet overall, affected children finish fewer years of education and are less likely to enter the professions. There also may be an increased risk of emotional disorder in adulthood, but this is not yet confirmed. Adult outcome depends on overall cognitive and social abilities that may help to compensate for the consequences of a reading disorder and lead to success in adult life.

ASSOCIATED SPEECH AND LANGUAGE DISORDERS

Reading disorder may be part of a broader developmental language disorder or may be very specific with few or no language symptoms. Associated developmental speech disorders may be divided into three subtypes, i.e., problems in articulation, voice, and fluency. In an articulation disorder, speech sounds are mispronounced when individual sounds are substituted, omitted, distorted, or added. Ordinarily, competence in articulation occurs by age 8, although there may be variation in the age of mastery of certain sounds, such as the *s* and *z*. By age 5, 15% of children still show some problems in articulation, but the majority of these do not have enduring problems. The age of acquisition of words is also variable, ranging from approximately 6 to 30 months, and acquisition of phrases ranges from 10 to 44 months.

Articulation problems may be associated with problems in hearing, structural defects in the oropharynx, and neurological dysfunction that leads to poor coordination of the speech mechanism (dysarthria and/or dyspraxia). Articulation disorders involve those speech parts involved in word articulation, that is, tongue, lips, and teeth. Such neurological dysfunctions may be genetic or acquired. Moreover, articulation disorders may run in families that show a higher rate of reading and spelling difficulties among family members. Children with reading disorder do have a higher rate of articulation problems (Owen et al., 1971), and children with severe articulation problems have higher rates of reading disorder. The extent of the overlap between these groups requires further study.

Other general categories of developmental speech difficulty include voice and fluency disorders; however, these are not clearly associated with either learning disorders or developmental language problems. Voice disorders involve problems in volume, pitch, rate, or quality of speech related to the functioning of the vocal cords and pharynx in speech production. Although it is generally true that voice disorders are not associated with language problems, voice problems may be important in speech pragmatics. Because pitch, volume, intonation, contour, and other aspects of speech prosody are important in social communicative function, these aspects of voice need to be evaluated.

In a disorder of speech fluency (stammering, stuttering, and cluttering), the rhythm of speech is disrupted. Sounds, syllables, or words are repeated, prolonged, or not produced at all. The etiology of speech dysfluency is unclear but, in some instances, there may be a genetic mode of transmission, either polygenetic transmission or single-gene inheritance with environmental modification (Kidd and Records, 1979). The specific mechanisms involved in producing articulation disorders and dysfluency, such as stuttering, have not been identified.

HYPERLEXIA

Hyperlexia is a reading disorder where children demonstrate pervasive semantic processing difficulties. In hyperlexia, single-word reading precocity occurs in the absence of intensive instruction in children who have general cognitive and language deficiencies (Metsala and Siegel, 1992). An examination of hyperlexia, a disorder that is not infrequent in high-functioning children with autistic disorder (Whitehouse and Harris, 1984) and other children with developmental disorders, may further our understanding of processes and the organization of knowledge involved in reading.

In early stages in reading acquisition, the semantic system is apparently more developed than decoding skills; however, in hyperlexia the opposite seems to be the case. Knowledge of orthographic representations and sound–letter correspondences appear before semantic and syntactic processing in hyperlexia. Reading appears to be mechanical and based on bottom-up processing without comprehension.

Definition

Several definitions have been proposed for hyperlexia. Silberberg and Silberberg (1967, 1968) used the term to refer to children who recognized written words that would not be expected to be known at their intellectual level. Richman and Kitchell (1981) identified children as hyperlexic whose word recognition on the Wide Range Achievement Test (WRAT) was 2 years above that expected for their full-scale cognitive ability. The most interest in hyperlexia has focused on children who test in the moderate to severe range of mental retardation. A more appropriate definition may be to focus on single-word reading precocity, in the absence of instruction, in children with cognitive and language deficiencies because this focus is on an ability that is not learned.

Clinical Features

In hyperlexia, advanced word reading skills are observed in children with language and cognitive delays. Speech development is generally severely delayed, and there may be no conversational speech. Precocious word recognition skills are observed early in development during the first 2 to 3 years of life prior to formal reading instruction. Abnormalities in expressive language, such as dysarthria, echolalia, and perseveration, are common. Rote memory skills may be well developed.

Hyperlexia is generally viewed as a decoding skill with no, or limited, comprehension of the words that are sounded out; there may be a total absence of comprehension, recognition of single words, and sometimes simple sentence comprehension. Typically, children score in the moderate to severe range of mental retardation on standardized tests. Yet some studies have included children who tested in the normal range of intelligence (Goldberg and Rothermel, 1984; Richman and Kitchell, 1981; Welch, Pennington, and Rogers, 1987).

Hyperlexia and Reading Disorder

Hyperlexia has led to considerable interest in understanding the mechanisms of word recognition skills in children with pervasive deficits in cognition. Central nervous system involvement is suggested by reports of dysarthria, perseveration, echolalia, poor motor functioning, and attention deficits. It may be that processes governing word recognition are modular and may function independently of the general cognitive deficits in children with hyperlexia.

There are two opposing views regarding the relationship between their word decoding skills and the comprehension deficits. One view suggests that the same linguistic mechanism underlies both advanced word reading and deficient reading comprehension, and the other that the two processes are independent. In the unitary view, advanced word recognition is the result of bias in information processing, leading to an acute awareness of the physical features of stimuli and intense processing of physical attributes due to an inability to allocate processing capacity to higher level analysis (Rimland, 1964). In this model, language consists of mechanical associations rather than semantic and syntactic processing. Children, then, would decode words but bypass the semantic analysis system. Comprehension is minimal because of the lack of interaction between top-down semantic information processing and bottom-up decoding.

The second position suggests that deficient comprehension skills occur independently of special word recognition abilities (Pennington, Johnson, and Welsh, 1987; Welsh et al., 1987). In this model, word recognition skills are intact and do interact with semantic knowledge, if present. Poor comprehension, then, is the result of poor language and cognitive ability separate from intact word recognition abilities. The underlying mechanism of isolated word reading may not be atypical, using this model. However, processes that govern word recognition may function independently of general cognitive deficits in children with hyperlexia.

These two approaches have been considered in regard to the dual route theory of reading where children may show exceptional decoding by one route but impairment in semantic performance in the other. If hyperlexia is compared to surface dyslexia, comprehension in surface dyslexics may not be as impaired as in hyperlexics. In surface dyslexia, there is difficulty with irregular words and semantic confusion of homophones. However, hyperlexia has been compared to direct dyslexia where fewer errors were reported on exceptional words than regular words, but the words that were read were not understood. The direct dyslexics would read words through the lexical, whole-word route, but not have access to lexical semantic knowledge. The ability of hyperlexic children to recognize exceptional words, in addition to making some visual errors, suggests that one or more levels of units higher than the grapheme–phoneme correspondence are functional. In hyperlexics, regular consistent words were recognized more accurately than inconsistent regular words. From these comparisons, it does not appear that hyperlexics represent either an extreme form of reading impairment, that is, reading only by grapheme–phoneme correspondence or reading only by whole-word recognition, because they are able to recognize exceptional words that are not derived by grapheme–phoneme correspondences (Cobrinik, 1982). They are also able to read nonwords that are unfamiliar and not stored as whole-word units. It is suggested that hyperlexic children's isolated word recognition is deviant from normal only insofar as that normal readers use other forms of word knowledge, such as semantic knowledge and spoken word knowledge. Cognitive and language deficits may impede the development of other sources of lexical knowledge.

Overall, there is not a unitary underlying style or mechanism, such as excessive attention to detail, which causes both lowered comprehension and advanced word recognition. Instead, hyperlexics may be differentiated from other developmentally disordered children by their unimpaired ability to acquire orthographic to phonological correspondences. Their oral language comprehension seems to be comparable to that of children with similar cognitive abilities. Essentially, these children appear to read as skilled word decoders. The phenomenon of hyperlexia supports a relatively modular model of word recognition skills. Decoding skills appear to develop independently of other types of lexical knowledge.

When compared to children with developmental reading disorder, hyperlexic children are able to read nonwords, but are not able to perform on some phonemic awareness tasks. However, developmental reading-disordered children have difficulty reading non-words and perform poorly on these tasks. These differences may relate to the child's accessibility to cognitive consciousness, which perhaps could be measured by phonemic awareness tasks that are thought to be an important aspect of normal reading acquisition and a predictor of reading success but may not be necessary for hyperlexic children.

For the normal reader, both conceptual ability to understand a task and the stability of phonological representations allow intact sound-to-symbol structures to develop. Hyperlexic children may have difficulty understanding the task even though the phonological representations are well developed. Although both groups perform poorly on tasks of phonemic awareness, it appears that children with developmental reading disorders have an impairment in the development of specific phonological processes or a phonological processing module that has been spared in children with hyperlexic disorder.

TREATMENT

A variety of treatment approaches have been advocated for reading disorder (Gittelman, 1983). However, two basic approaches to treatment have been used. The first approach, which is process oriented, attempts to remediate nonreading deficits or deficits that are presumed to lead to reading dysfunction. The second approach, which is task oriented, focuses on the remediation of the deficient reading behavior, which is the primary symptom.

Perceptual Training

Treatment of nonreading deficits has emphasized perceptual training approaches. Perceptual training programs were introduced because they were compatible with early views that disabled readers show primary perceptual deficits, either in visual or auditory modalities. A visual perceptual training program that included exercises in form discrimination, spatial orientation, and visual coordination was introduced by Frostig (1969). With the popularization of intersensory integration models of reading dysfunction, intersensory perceptual training methods, such as the Fernald (1943) method which utilizes auditory, visual, and tactile kinesthetic modalities, were introduced. Other theories considered that poor reading was a result of delayed or deficient development of those neurophysiologic mechanisms that are involved in perceptual and motor development. These functions were thought by some to be necessary for the development of higher level cognitive function. This framework led to sensorimotor treatment, including the controversial Delacato (1966) approach, which involves creeping and crawling exercises to retrain the brain by influencing hemispheric specialization for necessary functions. This approach has been demonstrated to be completely ineffective.

These various approaches have been evaluated in terms of their long-term effectiveness in the remediation of reading disorder. Much of the assessment that has been done does not meet scientific research standards, generally because of inappropriate comparison or control groups. The evidence from control studies that is available does not support positive claims for these approaches to remediate reading disability or their utility in teaching normal or disadvantaged readers (Robinson, 1972). The recent research on visual pathways to the lateral geniculate ganglion, which suggest difficulties in speed of processing visual information and other data on speed of processing auditory and tactile information, is being evaluated in regard to treatment. The issue under consideration has to do with finding ways to facilitate processing speed to complement language-based approaches rather than to develop new elaborate, nonfocused perceptual training programs.

Remediation of the Reading Deficit

Academic therapies for treatment of reading disorder are varied and, in some instances, are poorly defined. There may be at least 45 different approaches to teach reading (Lovett, 1992). The structural techniques vary regarding the symbol systems utilized to introduce letter–sound correspondences, the extent that instruction is structured, and the level that printed language is segmented for instructional use. Although phonological coding is a skill that is deficient, it is so central to reading it must be approached directly. A frequently used remedial reading program is the Orton-Gillingham approach, which is a multisensory, synthetic, alphabetic method (Johnson, 1978). The child is instructed on individual letter–sound correspondences and then taught to establish associations that involve auditory, visual, and motor aspects of speech and of written language. Single words that have clearly recognizable phonetic structures are introduced, and longer words are learned through syllabication. Instruction begins with reading and writing simple words and then combining them into sentences.

Others have advocated different remedial approaches for different subgroups of reading disorders (Johnson and Myklebust, 1967). Recommendations were made for using synthetic phonics methods for reading-disordered children whose problems involve orientation of letters, visual perception, and memory, and whole-word or story methods for children whose difficulties involve phonics, auditory processing, and the generalization of letter–sound information. Others may have difficulties with word retrieval and phonological problems related to abilities to rhyme and sequence sounds and thus require a focus in this area.

A general orientation to instruction has also been recommended in the intervention. This includes focusing on deficient cognitive components of reading, including all components to the reading process, providing intensive interaction between the instructor and the child, maximizing the amount of instruction time on task, and moving slowly after demonstrating task mastery from one task to the next.

Despite these efforts, there continues to be a lack of evidence in regard to whether one method is better than another or whether certain children benefit more from one teaching method than from others (Gittelman, 1983). However, it is not that the approaches to teaching are ineffective, but rather the outcome studies have been difficult to interpret because of the lack of clear sample definition, the experimental design, and the rationalization for the treatment approach.

Recent approaches have included microcomputer programs to improve word recognition and decoding skills. Other computer programs are directed toward segmentation training. In these various training programs, transfer of treatment effects to learning situations is essential. Lovett et al. (1990) emphasize targeting phoneme segmentation deficits because these deficits interfere with the acquisition of word recognition skills. They found that their reading-disabled students did not segment spoken syllables spontaneously into smaller units and, therefore, had great difficulty breaking up the corresponding spelling units and then extracting rules. Problems in parsing a syllable into subunits was suggested as a factor in transfer failures, rather than a more global problem in understanding pattern similarities or acquiring rule knowledge (Lovett, 1991). Positive transfer of effects may be better achieved on spelling, perhaps because spelling training forces a reading-disabled child to deal with individual letters and to segment the subword units in writing and orally. Spelling involves visual and auditory rehearsal as well as motor copying practice, providing an additional code to retrieve letter sequences. Consequently, it may be that learning to spell a set of words may be used to facilitate their introduction as reading vocabulary. Results from continued control treatment trials may further increase our understanding of the nature of developmental reading disorder and provide new opportunities as the reading acquisition process is better understood.

In summary, treatment of reading disability is based on helping the child compensate for both reading disorder and the frequent accompanying language disorder. The first step is to develop an individualized tutoring program that utilizes a phonics-based approach to reading. For younger children, training in segmental language skills may also be needed. If a phonics program is not successful, then tutoring in basic phoneme awareness skills may be needed.

The school setting may allow the child to compensate by providing extra time on written tests; spelling errors should be noted but not lead to reduced grades; foreign languages should not be required; and oral examinations are preferred over written. It is particularly important that all of the child's teachers be aware of the child's problem areas to avoid the child's being labeled as lazy or incompetent. Parents must function as advocates for their child's treatment and help facilitate appropriate interventions as well as provide emotional support. The major adjustment difficulties related to reading disorder are reduced self-esteem, self-blame, and mood disorder. Both parents and teachers need to provide for successes in the child's areas of strength and monitor the child for associated psychological symptoms (Silver, 1989). However, parents should not become their child's primary tutor, not only because of their lack of training in reading but also because of inherent conflicts between the role of parent and the role of teacher, which may lead to emotionally charged disagreements (Pennington, 1991).

Pharmacological Treatment

Pharmacological approaches have also been utilized to treat reading disorders. Because attention is important for the development of fluent reading, attentional deficits have been treated pharmacologically. Psychostimulant medication, which is used to treat attention deficit disorder, has been considered to be potentially valuable for use in children with reading disorders. Gittelman, Klein, and Feingold (1983) combined remedial reading instruction with either placebo or methylphenidate drug treatment. Their results suggested some benefit in academic task performance, such as those involving math computation. However, children with pure reading disorder did not show any clear benefit in reading performance. In this study, two measures of reading showed nonsignificant differences, and the one test that showed some advantage did not lead to significant improvement in performance. Some studies have shown short-term improvement on laboratory tests of learning, but long-lasting improvement in academic achievement has not been demonstrated. The conclusion is that there is no justification for the use of stimulant medication alone, without academic treatment, and that the combined use of academic remediation with drug treatment may produce some improvement but, over a period of months, this advantage is neither "broad nor dramatic" (Gittelman, Klein, and Feingold, 1983). Children with attention deficit disorder, then, should be appropriately treated for the attention deficit disorder with drug treatment; however, expectations are limited in terms of educational improvement because the drug treatment is not targeted to the basic mechanism of the reading disorder.

More recently, pharmacological treatment of reading disorder has involved the use of piracetam, a drug structurally similar to the neurotransmitter gamma aminobutyric acid (GABA). It has been suggested that this medication may enhance performance on left hemispheric-dependent tasks (Tallal et al., 1986). Piracetam has been used for treatment of reading disorder because of suspected deficits involving left hemispheric function in some cases. A multisite double blind evaluation study with piracetam was conducted that involved 257 reading-disabled boys who were assessed during a 12-week placebo control study. Improved reading speed was observed in the treated subjects, but no significant effects were obtained for either reading accuracy or reading comprehension. A longer, 36-week multisite evaluation with 225 reading-disabled children showed small, but apparently reliable, improvement in oral passage reading (Wilsher et al., 1987). However, this subsequent study did not replicate the improvement in reading speed seen in the original study. Additional measures of information processing, language, and memory did not show improvement with piracetam treatment. There is some evidence of improved digit span (Tallal et al., 1986). Because learning-disabled children may show increased anxiety, anxiolytic medications have been prescribed. None of these studies have shown improvements in academic achievement related to drug use (Aman and Schroeder, 1990).

Overall, the results with piracetam have been interpreted to suggest that continued research on its role in improving reading rate may be of interest. Specifically, the effect of piracetam on word and syllable identification speed requires more study rather than a return to earlier measures of passage reading rate. The drug studies did not show improvement of the nonreading deficits that are associated with reading disorder. Piracetam medication, in isolation, cannot be recommended as a treatment for developmental reading disorder. Whether piracetam might be used in combination with other forms of treatment, for example, remedial reading instruction and/or training in phonological awareness, has not been assessed. Drug treatments might also be combined with recent neurophysiologic studies that suggest problems in visual and auditory processing speed.

The evidence seems to indicate that pharmacotherapy is not indicated to treat specific learning disorders but may be useful for coexisting behavioral problems.

REFERENCES

Aman, M.G., and Schroeder, S.R. (1990). Specific learning disorders and mental retardation. In B.J. Tonge, G.D. Burrows, and J.S. Werry (eds.), *Handbook of studies in child psychiatry*, pp. 209–224. Elsevier Science Publishers, Amsterdam.

American Psychiatric Association, Committee on Nomenclature and Statistics (1994). *Diagnostic and statistical manual of mental disorders*, 4th ed. Author, Washington, DC.

Boder, E. (1973). Developmental dyslexia: A diagnostic approach based on three atypical reading-spelling patterns. *Developmental Medicine and Child Neurology*, 15:663–687.

Centers for Disease Control. (1987). Assessment of the number and characteristics of persons affected by learning disabilities. In Interagency Committee on Learning Disabilities: *Learning Disabilities. A Report to the U.S. Congress*, p. 107. U.S. Department of Health and Human Services, Washington, DC.

Clements, S. (1966). *Minimal brain dysfunction in children* (National Institute of Neurological Diseases and Blindness, Monograph no. 3). U.S. Department of Health, Education, and Welfare, Washington, DC.

Cobrinik, L. (1982). The performance of hyperlexic children on an "incomplete words" task. *Neuropsychologia*, 20:569–577.

Coltheart, M. (1980). Deep dyslexia: A right hemispheric hypothesis. In M. Coltheart, K. Patterson, and J. Marshall (eds.), *Deep dyslexia*. Routledge and Kegan Paul, London.

______, Masterson, J., Byng, S., Prior, M., and Riddoch, J. (1983). Surface dyslexia. *Quarterly Journal of Experimental Psychology*, 35:469–496.

Critchley, M. (1970). *The dyslexic child*. Heinemann, London.

DeFries, J.C., Fulker, D.W., and LaBuda, M.C. (1987). Reading disability in twins: Evidence for a genetic etiology. *Nature*, 329:537–539.

Delacato, C.H. (1966). *Neurological organization and reading*. Charles C. Thomas, Springfield, IL.

Denenberg, V.H., Sherman, G.F., Schrott, L.M., Rosen, G.D., and Galaburda, A.M. (1991). Spatial learning, discrimination learning, paw preference, and neocortical ectopias in two autoimmune strains of mice. *Brain Research*, 562:98–104.

Duffy, F.H., Denckla, M.B., Bartels, P.H., and Sandini, G. (1980). Dyslexia: Regional differences in brain electrical activity by topographic mapping. *Annals of Neurology*, 7:412–420.

Farnham-Diggory, S. (1978). *Learning disabilities: A psychological perspective*. Harvard University Press, Cambridge.

Fernald, G.M. (1943). *Remedial techniques in basic school subjects*. McGraw-Hill, New York.

Finucci, J.M., and Childs, B. (1981). Are there really more dyslexic boys than girls? In A. Ansara, N. Geschwind, A. Galaburda, M. Albert, and N. Gartrell (eds.), *Sex differences in dyslexia,* pp. 1–9. Orton Dyslexia Society, Towson, MD.

Frith, U. (1985). Beneath the surface of developmental dyslexia. In K.E. Patterson, J.C. Marshall, and M. Coltheart (eds.), *Surface dyslexia,* pp. 301–330. Routledge and Kegan-Paul, London.

Frostig, M. (1969). *Move, grow, learn.* Follet, Chicago.

Gaddes, W. (1976). Learning disabilities: Prevalence estimates and the need for definition. In R. Knights and D.J. Bakker (eds.), *The neuropsychology of learning disorders.* University Park Press, Baltimore, MD.

Galaburda, A.M. (1993). Neurology of developmental dyslexia. *Current Opinion in Neurobiology,* 3:237–242.

Galaburda, A., and Livingstone, M. (1993). Evidence for a magnocellular defect in developmental dyslexia. *Annals of the New York Academy of Science,* 682:70–82.

______, Sherman, G.F., Rosen, G.D., Aboitiz, F., and Geschwind, N. (1985). Developmental dyslexia: Four consecutive patients with cortical abnormalities. *Annals of Neurology,* 18:222–233.

Gittelman, R. (1983). Treatment of reading disorders. In M. Rutter (ed.), *Developmental neuropsychiatry,* pp. 520–541. The Guilford Press, New York.

______, Klein, D.F., and Feingold, I. (1983). Children with reading disorders: II. Effects of methylphenidate in combination with reading remediation. *Journal of Child Psychology and Psychiatry,* 24:193–212.

Goldberg, T.E., and Rothermel, R.D. (1984). Hyperlexic children reading. *Brain,* 107:759–785.

Goulandris, N., and Snowling, M. (1991). Visual memory deficits: A possible cause of developmental dyslexia? Evidence from a single case study. *Cognitive Neuropsychology,* 8:127–154.

Hagman, J.O., Wood, F., Buschbaum, M.S., Tallal, P., Flowers, I., and Katz, W. (1992). Cerebral metabolism in adult dyslexic subjects assessed with positron emission tomography during performance of an auditory task. *Archives of Neurology,* 49:734–739.

Halperin, J.M., Gittelman, R., Klein, D.F., and Rudel, R.G. (1984). Reading-disabled hyperactive children: A distinct subgroup of attention deficit disorder with hyperactivity. *Journal of Abnormal Child Psychology,* 12:1–14.

Hinshelwood, J. (1895). Word blindness and visual memories. *Lancet,* 2:1566–1570.

Humphreys, P., Kaufmann, W.E., and Galaburda, A.M. (1990). Developmental dyslexia in women: Neuropathological findings in three cases. *Annals of Neurology,* 28:727–738.

Hynd, G.W., and Cohen, M. (1983). *Dyslexia: Neuropsychological theory, research, and clinical differentiation.* Grune & Stratton, New York.

Hynd, G.G., Semrud-Clikeman, M., Lorys, A.R., Novey, E.S., and Eliopulos, D. (1990). Brain morphology in developmental dyslexia and attention deficit disorder/hyperactivity. *Archives of Neurology,* 47:919–926.

Johnson, D.L. (1978). Remedial approaches to dyslexia. In A.L. Benton and D. Pearl (eds.), *Dyslexia: An appraisal of current knowledge.* Oxford University Press, New York.

______, and Myklebust, H.R. (1967). *Learning disabilities.* Grune & Stratton, New York.

Kidd, K.K., and Records, M.A. (1979). Genetic methodologies for the study of speech. In X.O. Breakfield (ed.), *Neurogenetics: Genetic approaches to the nervous system,* pp. 311–344. Elsevier-North Holland, New York.

Larsen, J.P., Hien, T., Lundberg, I., and Odegaard, H. (1990). MRI evaluation of the size and symmetry of the planum temporale in adolescents with developmental dyslexia. *Brain and Language,* 39:289–301.

Landwehrmeyer, B., Gerling, J., and Wallesch, C.W. (1990). Patterns of task-related slow brain potential in dyslexia. *Archives of Neurology,* 47:791–797.

Lehmkuhle, S., Garzia, R.P., Turner, L., Hash, T., and Baro, J.A. (1993). A defective visual pathway in children with reading disability. *New England Journal of Medicine,* 328:989–996.

Livingstone, M., and Hubel, D. (1988). Segregation of form, color, movement, and depth: Anatomy, physiology, and perception. *Science,* 240:740–749.

Livingstone, M.S., Rosen, G.D., Drislane, F.W., and Galaburda, A.M. (1991). Physiological and anatomical evidence for a magnocellular defect in developmental dyslexia. *Proceedings of the National Academy of Science, USA,* 88:7943–7947.

Lovegrove, W.J., Garzia, R.P., and Nicholson, S.B. (1990). Experimental evidence for a transient system deficit in specific reading disability. *Journal of the American Optometric Association,* 61:137–146.

Lovett, M.W. (1991). Reading writing, and remediation: Perspectives on the dyslexic learning disability from remedial outcome data. *Learning Individual Differences,* 3:295–305.

______, M.W. (1992). Developmental dyslexia. In S.J. Segalowitz and I. Rapin (vol. eds.) and F. Boller and J. Grofman (series eds.), *Handbook of neuropsychology: Vol. 7. Child neuropsychol-*

ogy, pp. 163–185. Elsevier Science Publishers, Amsterdam.

______, Warren-Chaplin, P.M., Ransby, M.J., and Borden, S.L. (1990). Training the word recognition skills of reading disabled children: Treatment and transfer effects. *Journal of Educational Psychology,* 82:769–780.

Maclean, M., Bryant, P., and Bradley, L. (1987). Rhymes, nursery rhymes, and reading in early childhood. *Merrill-Palmer Quarterly,* 33:255–282.

Marshall, J.C., and Newcombe, F. (1973). Patterns of paralexia. *Journal of Psycholinguistic Research,* 2:175–199.

Metsala, J. L., and Siegel, L.S. (1992). Patterns of atypical reading development: Attributes and underlying reading processes. In S.J. Segalowitz and I. Rapin (vol. eds.) and F. Boller and J. Grofman (series eds.), *Handbook of neuropsychology: Vol. 7. Child neuropsychology,* pp. 187–210. Elsevier Science Publishers, Amsterdam.

Morgan, W.P. (1896). A case of congenital word-blindness. *British Medical Journal,* 2:1378.

Neville, H.J., Coffey, S.A., Holcomb, P.J., and Tallal, P. (1993). The neurobiology of sensory and language processing in language-impaired children. *Journal of Cognitive Neuroscience,* 5:235–253.

Olson, R., Wise, B., Conners, F., Rack, J. and Fulker, D. (1989). Specific deficits in component reading and language skills: Genetic and environmental influences. *Journal of Learning Disabilities,* 22:339–348.

Orton, S.T. (1928). Word blindness in school children. *Archives of Neurology and Psychiatry,* 14:581–615.

Owen, F.W., Adams, P.A., Forrest, T., Stolz, L.M., and Fisher, S. (1971). Learning disorders in children: Sibling studies. *Monographs of the Society for Research for Child Development,* 36, serial no. 144.

Pennington, B.F. (1990). The genetics of dyslexia. *Journal of Child Psychology and Psychiatry,* 31:193–201.

______. (1991). *Diagnosing learning disabilities,* pp. 45–81. The Guilford Press, New York.

______, Gilger, J.W., Olson, R.K., and DeFries, J.C. (1992). The external validity of age- versus IQ-discrepancy definitions of reading disability: Lessons from a twin study. *Journal of Learning Disabilities,* 25:562–573.

______, ______, Pauls, D., Smith, S.A., Smith, S.D., and DeFries, J.C. (1991). Evidence for major gene transmission of developmental dyslexia. *Journal of the American Medical Association,* 266:1527–1534.

______, Johnson, C., and Welsh, M.C. (1987). Unexpected reading precocity in a normal preschooler: Implications for hyperlexia. *Brain and Language,* 30:165–180.

Rapin, I. (1982). *Children with brain dysfunction: Neurology, cognition, language, and behavior.* Raven Press, New York.

Regan, D. (1989). *Human brain electrophysiology: Evoked potentials and evoked magnetic fields in science and medicine.* Elsevier, New York.

Richman, L.C., and Kitchell, M.M. (1981). Hyperlexia as a variant of developmental language disorder. *Brain and Language,* 12:203–212.

Rimland, B. (1964). *Infantile autism: The syndrome and its implications for a neural theory of behaviour.* Appleton-Century-Crofts, Chicago.

Robinson, H.M. (1972). Visual and auditory modalities related to methods for beginning readers. *Reading Research Quarterly,* 8:7–39.

Rosen, G.D., Sherman, G.F., Mehler, C., Emsbo, K., and Galaburda, A.M. (1989). The effect of developmental neuropathology on neocortical asymmetry in New Zealand black mice. *International Journal of Neuroscience,* 45:247–254.

Rumsey, J.M., Andreason, P., Zametkin, A.J., Aquino, T., King, A.C., Hamburger, S.D., Pikus, A., Rapaport, J.I., and Cohen, R.M. (1992). Failure to activate the left temporoparietal cortex in dyslexia. An oxygen 15 positron emission tomographic study. *Archives of Neurology,* 49:527–534.

______, Dorwart, R., Vermess, M., Denckla, M.B., Kruesi, M.J., and Rapaport, J.L. (1986). Magnetic resonance imaging of brain anatomy in severe developmental dyslexia. *Archives of Neurology,* 43:1045–1046.

Rutter, M., Tizard, J., and Whitmore, K. (1970). *Education in health and behavior.* Longman, London.

______, and Yule, W. (1975). The concept of specific reading retardation. *Journal of Child Psychology and Psychiatry,* 16:181–197.

Scarborough, H. (1990). Very early language deficits in dyslexic children. *Child Development,* 61:1728–1743.

Schrott, L.M., Denenberg, V.H., Sherman, G.F., Waters, N.S., Rosen, G.D., and Galaburda, A.M. (1992). Environmental enrichment, neocortical ectopias, and behavior in the autoimmune NZB mouse. *Developmental Brain Research,* 67:85–93.

Shankweiler, D., and Crain, S. (1986). Language mechanisms and reading disorders: A modular approach. *Cognition,* 24:139–168.

Shaywitz, B.A., Shaywitz, S.E., Pugh, K.R., Constable, R.T., Skudlarski, P., Fulbright, R.K., Bronen, R.A., Fletcher, J.M., Shankweiler, D.P., Katz, L., and Gore, J.C. (1995) Sex differences in the functional organization of the brain for language. *Nature* 373:607–609.

Shaywitz, S.E., Shaywitz, B.A., Fletcher, J.M., and Escobar, M.D. (1990). Prevalence of reading disability in boys and girls: Results of the Connecticut Longitudinal Study. *Journal of the American Medical Association,* 264:998–1002.

Sherman, G.F., Galaburda, A.M., Behan, P.O., and Rosen, G.D. (1987). Neuroanatomical anomalies in autoimmune mice. *Acta Neuropathologica,* 74:239–242.

______, Galaburda, A.M., and Geschwind, N. (1985). Cortical anomalies in brains of New Zealand mice: A neuropathologic model of dyslexia? *Proceedings of the National Academy of Science, USA,* 82:8072–8074.

______, Stone, J.S., Press, D.M., Rosen, G.D., and Galaburda, A.M. (1990). Abnormal architecture and connections disclosed by neurofilament staining in the cerebral cortex of autoimmune mice. *Brain Research,* 529:202–207.

Silver, L.B. (1981). The relationship between learning disabilities, hyperactivity, distractibility, and behavioral problems. *Journal of the American Academy of Child and Adolescent Psychiatry,* 28:385–397.

______. (1989). Psychological and family problems associated with learning disabilities: Assessment and intervention. *Journal of the Academy of Child and Adolescent Psychiatry,* 28:319–325.

Silberberg, N.E., and Silberberg, M.C. (1967). Hyperlexia: Specific word recognition skills in young children. *Exceptional Children,* 34:41–42.

______, and ______. (1968). Case histories in hyperlexia. *Journal of School Psychology,* 7:3–7.

Smith, S.D., Kimberling, W.J., Pennington, B.F., and Lubs, H.A. (1983). Specific reading disability: Identification of an inherited form through linkage analysis. *Science,* 219:1345–1347.

Snowling, M.J. (1991). Developmental reading disorders. *Journal of Child Psychology and Psychiatry,* 32:49–77.

______, and Frith, U. (1986). Comprehension in "hyperlexic" readers. *Journal of Experimental Child Psychology,* 42:392–415.

______, Stackhouse, J., and Rack, J.P. (1986). Phonological dyslexia and dysgraphia: A developmental analysis. *Cognitive Neuropsychology,* 3:309–339.

Stelmack, R.M., and Miles, J. (1990). The effect of picture priming on event-related potentials of normal and disabled readers during a word recognition memory task. *Journal of Clinical and Experimental Neuropsychology,* 12:887–903.

Stevenson, J., Fredman, G., McLoughlin, V. and Graham, A. (1987). A twin study of genetic influences on reading and spelling ability and disability. *Journal of Child Psychology and Psychiatry,* 28:229–247.

Strauss, A.A., and Lehtinen, L.E. (1947). *Psychopathology and education of the brain-injured child.* Grune & Stratton, New York.

Tallal, P. (1987). Developmental language disorders. Interagency Committee on Learning Disabilities – Report to the U.S. Congress.

______, Chase, C., Russell, G., and Schmitt, L.R. (1986). Evaluation of the efficacy of piracetam in treating information processing, reading and writing disorders in dyslexic children. *International Journal of Psychophysiology,* 4:41–52.

______, and Piercy, M. (1973). Defects of non-verbal auditory perception in children with developmental aphasia. *Nature,* 16:468–469.

Temple, C.M. (1985). Surface dyslexia: Variation within a syndrome. In K. Patterson, J.C. Marshall, and M. Coltheart (eds.), *Surface dyslexia.* Routledge and Kegan-Paul, London.

______. (1992). Developmental and acquired disorders of childhood. In I. Rapin and S.J. Segalowitz (eds.), *Handbook of Neuropsychology: Vol 6. Child Neuropsychology,* pp. 93–114. Elsevier Science Publishers, Amsterdam.

______, Jeeves, M.A., and Vilarroya, O.O. (1990). Reading in callosal agenesis. *Brain and Language,* 39:289–301.

U.S. Congress. (1975) Public Law 94–142, *Education for All Handicapped Children Act of 1975.* U.S. Government Printing Office, Washington, DC.

Vogler, G.P., DeFries, J.C., and Decker, S.N. (1985). Family history as an indicator of risk for reading disability. *Journal of Learning Disabilities,* 18:419–421.

Welsh, M.C., Pennington, B.F., and Rogers, S. (1987). Word recognition and comprehension skills in hyperlexic children. *Brain and Language,* 32:76–96.

Whitehouse, D., and Harris, J. (1984). Hyperlexia in infantile autism. *Journal of Autism and Developmental Disorders,* 14:281–289.

Williams, M.C., and Lecluyse, K. (1990). Perceptual consequences of a temporal processing deficit in reading disabled children. *Journal of the American Optometric Association,* 61:111–121.

Wilsher, C.R., Bennett, D., Chase, C.H., Conners, C.K., Di Ianni, M., Feagans, L., Hanvik, L.J., Helfgott, E., Koplewicz, H., Overby, P., Reader, M.J., Rudel, R.G., and Tallal, P. (1987). Piracetam and dyslexia: Effects on reading tests. *Journal of Clinical Psychopharmacology,* 7:230–237.

Witelson, A., and Pallie, W. (1973). Left hemisphere specialization for language in the newborn: Neuroanatomical evidence of asymmetry. *Brain,* 96:641–647.

Yule, W., and Rutter, M. (1985). Reading and other learning difficulties. In M. Rutter and L. Hersov (eds.), *Child and adolescent psychiatry: Modern approaches,* pp. 444–464. Blackwell Scientific Publications, Boston.

7.2 Spelling Disorder

There is considerable overlap between reading and spelling difficulties; however, the processes involved in reading and spelling may be different. Frith (1978) suggested that there is no simple 1 to 1 sound–symbol correlation because sounds do not have natural segments and pronunciations change frequently. Mastery of spelling requires a considerable degree of linguistic competence, and an understanding of "meaning in context" may be as important as knowledge of sound–symbol correspondences. Spelling problems tend to last longer than reading problems. Phonological rather than visual skills are more important in the development of spelling, although visual memory for spelling patterns may play a major role in spelling proficiency.

INTERFACE OF SPELLING AND READING

It is sometimes thought that if a child has learned to read, then spelling will naturally follow; however, this is not necessarily true. Children may read words they cannot spell and may spell other words without being able to read them, which suggests reading and spelling skills have some independence from one another. Children who make spelling errors most commonly are poor readers rather than normal readers because reference to phonological cues is more common in spelling than in reading. The examination of spelling errors identifies dysphonetic and/or phonetic misspelling. Children may be able to spell phonetically regular words they are not able to read. Although a phonological analysis is essential in learning to spell, visual analysis is also required. In order to spell irregular words, word-specific knowledge is also needed. In spelling as in reading, there is more than one approach. One code is based on the sound elements of the word and the other on the meaning and structure of the whole word (Temple, 1993).

Children with both reading and spelling difficulties tend to have a more generalized language disorder, whereas those with specific problems in spelling, but little problem in reading, more often have phonetically accurate spelling errors. Frith (1983) referred to children who had both reading and spelling difficulties as dyslexic and those who only had spelling errors as dysgraphic. In the dysgraphic group, phonetic spelling errors occurred twice as often as nonphonetic errors; in the reading-disordered group, the two types of errors were equally frequent. Consequently, in the dysgraphics, the phonological route seemed intact because they were able to analyze speech sounds into phonemes. Although they did not show problems in reading, an increased difficulty in rhyming was noted. Phonological problems in spelling were associated with reading problems.

DEVELOPMENTAL ASPECTS

Children can spell words they are unable to read (Bryant and Bradley, 1980). This suggests an association between the strategies that are initially used in reading and in spelling, i.e., reading (visual) and spelling (phonological). The importance of phonological awareness in spelling is demonstrated by children's early attempts to invent the correct spelling of words and later when phonological skills are essential for spelling progress. Training in sound categorization may have a greater effect on spelling than on reading, indicating that phonological awareness may be particularly important for spelling progress (Goswami and Bryant, 1990).

Several models have been introduced supporting the view that spelling is initially phonological and the integration of different strategies used in reading and spelling is the eventual outcome in successful spelling. Frith (1985) suggests three stages in spelling: (1) logographic, where spelling is symbolic and not connected to phonology; (2) alphabetic, where children spell words out by working out all the phonemes in the words and representing them with letters; and (3) orthographic, where children begin operating on larger segments, using analogies in spelling and also morphemic units. Although these sequences are reasonable, the first stage may be brief and the methods used in the last two stages may overlap. As children approach these stages, the irregularity in the English writing system and its use of "th" and "sh" sounds, in addition to consonant clusters, make reading difficult because the irregularities are difficult to teach.

Children may utilize a phonological strategy in spelling in different ways. The constituent sounds, or phonemes, may be worked out alphabetically so each is represented by one letter, or the child may make analogies to similar sounding words and see the similarity in spelling between the two words. The analogies are based on segments, rather than phonemes. Rhymes are the most frequent phonological segments used for analogies in spelling. Beginning spellers may make use of rhymes and words, but then attempt to represent the segment by a single letter, which leads to errors, such as "cr" for "car." When children learn to spell, they may categorize words at the phonemic or the rhyme level.

But when does visual memory for the appearance of words, which is gained through reading, become linked to spelling? There seems to be a normal developmental integration so that although younger children may be able to spell words they cannot read, by age 10 this difference has essentially disappeared. For younger children, spelling is a more important contributor to this process of integration than reading. This may be because reflection on phonemic content that is necessary for spelling affects reading development by improving phonological awareness. As children grow older, they begin to use knowledge gained through reading as they approach spelling. Reading knowledge does result in the visual representation of particular letters and words. Consequently, these two skills seem to influence each other at different times and early spelling may help early reading, but when reading is well developed, children use their stored memories for spelling patterns and this knowledge improves spelling.

SPELLING DISORDERS

Studies of children with phonological difficulties show they also have difficulties in spelling (Goswami, 1992). However, children who become poor spellers may fail to integrate strategies they use in visual reading and spelling. Good readers who were poor spellers at age 14 were worse at manipulating sounds than good readers who were good spellers. Poor spellers who are also poor readers have the most difficulty in remediation (Frith, 1980). These children tend to have difficulties working out the relationship between letters and sounds in both reading and in spelling.

SPELLING REMEDIATION

The direct approach to spelling difficulties is to train for phonological awareness. Specific training in phonological awareness does improve spelling, but multisensory approaches are the most successful (Bradley and Bryant, 1983). In one method, the simultaneous oral spelling method (Bradley, 1981), the child is showed the word to be learned on a small card. The word is read aloud by the teacher and the child repeats the word and then copies it letter by letter, saying the name of each letter as it is written. Once the word has been written, the child repeats it once more and checks to see if the spelling is correct. This process is again repeated twice. In this approach, a visual component, seeing the word, an auditory component, spelling out the letters, and a motor component, writing them, are all utilized. Poor spellers do best when taught using all components simultaneously. For example, Bradley found that by using the complete approach, the children remembered 58% of words taught versus 30% to 35% taught when only one of the three components was included. This author suggests that simultaneous oral spelling is important in learning because it connects reading and spelling. Although visual inspection alone may help normal children learn to spell, children with spelling disorder require integration of each of these components.

REFERENCES

Bradley, L. (1981). The organisation of motor patterns for spelling: An effective remedial strategy for backward readers. *Developmental Medicine and Child Neurology,* 15:663–687.

______, and Bryant, P.E. (1983). Categorising sounds and learning to read: A causal connection. *Nature,* 310:419–421.

Bryant, P.E., and Bradley, L. (1980). Why children sometimes write words which they do not read. In U. Frith (ed.), *Cognitive processes in spelling,* pp. 355–370. Academic Press, London.

Frith, U. (1978). Spelling difficulties. *Journal of Child Psychology and Psychiatry,* 19:279–285.

______. (1980). Unexpected spelling problems. In U. Frith (ed.), *Cognitive processes in spelling,* pp. 495–515. Academic Press, London.

______. (1983). The similarities and differences between reading and spelling problems. In M. Rutter (ed.), *Developmental neuropsychiatry,* pp. 453–472. The Guilford Press, New York.

______. (1985). Beneath the surface of developmental dyslexia. In K. Patterson, M. Coltheart, and J. Marshall (eds.), *Surface dyslexia,* pp. 301–330. Routledge and Kegan-Paul, London.

Goswami, U. (1992). Phonological factors in spelling development. *Journal of Child Psychology and Psychiatry,* 33:967–975.

______, and Bryant, P.E. (1990). *Phonological skills and learning to read.* Erlbaum, Hillsdale, NJ.

Temple, C. (1993). *The brain: An introduction to the psychology of the human brain and behavior,* pp. 178–180. Penguin Books, London, England.

7.3 Mathematics Disorder

Mathematics disorder is a disorder of numerical competence and arithmetic skill that is manifest in children with normal intelligence and without neurological injuries (Temple, 1992). It may occur along with reading disorder, but is separable from this condition.

Four basic factors may be involved in math achievement: language, conceptualization, visual-spatial ability, and memory (Johnson, 1988). Proficiency in mathematics involves more than computational skills. It also includes a systematic plan toward problem solving and adequate working memory to complete the task. Good working memory of basic number facts is essential.

Mathematics disorder is a heterogeneous condition. There may be both intrinsic and extrinsic influences on the acquisition of academic skills in mathematics. The extrinsic factors relate to the complexity of mathematics, poor skill instruction, and lack of mastery of prerequisite math skills. Intrinsic skills relate to general intelligence, quantitative reasoning ability, and visual-spatial ability. Other factors are more attitudinal, such as attitude toward the subject, interest, and sociocultural background.

HISTORY

Hinshelwood (1917) suggested there are distinctive processes involved in number calculation. His belief in separate centers for processing numbers was initially based on the study of a patient with brain damage who, despite being alexic, retained the ability to read figures rapidly and fluently. He pointed out that differential abilities in mental arithmetic among normals who are not brain damaged is demonstrated by their different abilities. Hinshelwood claimed that the reverse is true in boys who excel in reading and other subjects, but have difficulty in arithmetic. In the same paper, Hinshelwood notes that others have recognized children who have difficulty in reading figures without corresponding difficulties in reading letters and words. Although Hinshelwood's primary interest was in disorders of word reading, he found that among 12 children with congenital word blindness, only 3 had difficulties which extended to the recognition of figures. In fact, 2 of his subjects were above average in arithmetic. He writes, "The visual memories of words and figures are deposited in distinct cerebral areas . . . probably close together and possibly contiguous . . . when defective development was more extensive and thus involved the figure area, then the inability to read included both words and figure" (Hinshelwood quoted by Temple, 1992).

In the 1930s and 1940s, children with mathematics disorders were found to have associated minimal brain damage or dysfunction. The recognition of minimal brain dysfunction with mathematical problems led to the concept of developmental mathematics disorder. The initial research on mathematics disorder addressed the relationship of visual-spatial skills to problems in numerical computation. Because of its involvement in visual-spatial skills, the right hemisphere was thought to be involved. However, the evidence supports the involvement of both hemispheres in computation and problem-solving tasks. Although children with math disorder, or dyscalculia (described later), generally show the same symptoms as adults with acalculia, there may be some differences in developing basic math concepts, in retrieval of number words and facts, and in forming numerals and sequencing them appropriately. Moreover, there may be differences in the application of computational skills to problem solving.

DEFINITION

The DSM-IV (APA, 1994) criteria for mathematics disorder are shown in Table 7.3–1. DSM-IV defines mathematics disorder as substantially substandard ability in mathematics, as shown in the table.

The essential feature of mathematics disorder is marked impairment in the development of mathematic skills that cannot be explained as an associated feature of reading disorder. The diagnosis is made if the impairment interferes with academic achievement or with activities of daily living that require mathematical skills. Mathematics disorder and disorder of written expression commonly occur in combination with reading disorder. When diagnostic criteria are met for more than one learning disorder, all should be diagnosed.

CLASSIFICATION

Rourke (1978) suggests there may be distinct types of math disorder. Some children with linguistic difficulties have particular difficulty in learning arithmetic tables. He suggests these difficulties may result from problems in verbal memory and left hemispheric impairment. Others have shown that calculation disturbances are most commonly associated with left posterior hemisphere lesions (Temple, 1992). Kosc (1974, 1979) proposed a classification based on the possible anatomical and physiological systems involved in the maturation of mathematics ability. Kosc goes on to suggest six different types of developmental math disorder including verbal dyscalculia, where there is difficulty with the verbal designation of particular mathematical terms, and practognostic dyscalculia, which results from difficulty manipulating objects mathematically. Difficulty in reading mathematical symbols is referred to as "lexical dyscalculia"; difficulty in writing these symbols is called "graphic dyscalculia." The other types are ideognostic dyscalculia, where there is difficulty in understanding mathematical ideas and working out the mental solutions to problems, and operational dyscalculia, which affects the execution of the operations themselves. It is suggested these forms may or may not occur in isolation, but are distinct.

Table 7.3–1. DSM-IV Diagnostic Criteria for Mathematics Disorder

315.1 Mathematics Disorder

A. Mathematical ability, as measured by individually administered standardized tests, is substantially below that expected given the person's chronological age, measured intelligence, and age-appropriate education.
B. The disturbance in Criterion A significantly interferes with academic achievement or activities of daily living that require mathematical ability.
C. If a sensory deficit is present, the difficulties in mathematical ability are in excess of those usually associated with it.

Coding note: If a general medical (e.g., neurological) condition or sensory deficit is present, code the condition on Axis III.

From APA, 1994.

Temple (1992) proposed an alternative classification based on the functional structure of the mature calculation system. She includes number processing dyscalculia (difficulty in processing numerical symbols or words; may impair reading, writing, repeating, or transcoding numbers or numbered words); number fact dyscalculia (impaired mastery of arithmetic facts, most commonly tables); and procedural dyscalculia (difficulty in planning and conducting the ordered sequence of operations that form an arithmetical calculation) (Temple, 1991). The number processing dyscalculia is analogous to verbal and practognostic dyscalculia, number fact dyscalculia to lexical and graphic dyscalculia, and procedural dyscalculia to ideognostic and operational dyscalculia.

The DSM-IV (APA, 1994) classification suggests that a number of specific skills may be impaired in mathematics disorder. These include: (1) linguistic skills involving mathematical terms and concepts as well as decoding written problems; (2) perceptual skills in recognizing numerical symbols; (3) attentional skills in copying correctly and following procedures; and (4) the mathematical skills described earlier.

ASSOCIATED DEFICITS

Math disorder may be associated with right hemispheric dysfunction involving the parietal lobe. Because right hemispheric dysfunction is commonly associated with social-cognitive difficulties, one may see deficits in social skills in addition to mathematics disorder. Moreover, demoralization and poor self-esteem may accompany school failure in mathematics.

EPIDEMIOLOGY

Math disorder occurs in approximately 6% of children. This estimate derives from school-aged children of normal intelligence who do not show adequate attainment in mathematics. It is not known within this group what percentage have a subtype of dyscalculia involving certain processing domains in the central nervous system. Epidemiologic assessment is complicated because achievement in mathematics may depend more on the quality and amount of instruction than is the case for reading. Math achievement is correlated with intelligence, reading achievement, and emotional state. It is uncommon for referrals to be made to special education for isolated math learning problems without another learning disability. A greater societal emphasis is also placed on skills in reading and writing than on math. It is unclear whether or not the prevalence is more common in males than females.

ETIOLOGY

The concept of developmental math disorder is based on studies of adults with acquired acalculia. The term "acalculia" has been used to designate an acquired disorder in calculation ability since the early years of this century. Symptoms of acalculia include difficulty in recalling number words, in forming numerals, and in doing mathematical calculations. The brain areas involved in acquired acalculia include the frontal, temporal, parietal, and occipital lobes. Consequently, the integrity of several cortical areas is needed for comprehensive calculation abilities. Although isolated acalculia is rare, it may be one symptom associated with others involving central nervous system dysfunction. Mathematics ability depends on a complex set of skills that involve both linguistic and spatial abilities. The search for etiology has focused on the neuropsychological basis of developmental math disorder. Initial studies suggested it was rooted in visual-spatial processing deficits that resulted from right hemispheric damage. Although acquired acalculia or dyscalculia in adults has not been shown to be specifically related to damage in the right hemisphere, assessment of these brain systems has been, and continues to be, the focus for developmental mathematics disorder.

In children, there has been considerable interest in determining an underlying cognitive deficit that might be characteristic of developmental math disorder. Rourke (1978) suggested that right hemisphere based visual-spatial skills are essential to the development of normal arithmetic ability. He reports that children with poor mathematics skills but who have adequate reading skills show defective visual perception, tactile perception, and psychomotor ability. He postulates that a resulting absence of understanding of arithmetic operations leads to failure in carrying out arithmetic tasks. The deficits he reports in the children with math disorder cover both spatial and perceptual elements. Rourke's model suggests that children who have normal mathematics skills should not have spatial and perceptual difficulties.

In students with relatively pure math disorder, which is not associated with reading and spelling problems, one subgroup shows impairment in perception, analysis, organization, and synthesis of nonverbal information (Pennington, 1991). This subgroup also shows deficits in psychomotor performance and nonverbal problem solving. Such studies lend support to the view that the right hemisphere may be impaired in children with developmental math disorder.

An etiologic hypothesis proposed by Geschwind and Behan (1983) is that excessively high levels of testosterone during intrauterine life may play an etiologic role. If testosterone levels are excessively high, or if the fetus is sensitive to testosterone, then differences might occur in cerebral hemispheric development. One proposal is that right hemispheric development may be enhanced by testosterone levels and the left hemispheric development slowed. It is hypothesized that this may lead to an imbalance between visual-spatial and language ability. This hypothesis has been used to explain differences in mathematics abilities between the two sexes. Although males generally have more difficulties with developmental problems, in adolescence more males may show extremely high achievement in mathematics.

Another hypothesis is based on the development of informational processing abilities (Fleischner and Garnett, 1987). It is proposed that proficiency in mathematics depends on certain abilities that develop with age. Ordinarily, a sequence of strategic behaviors associated with arithmetic learning take place. When children who are achieving normally and children with math learning problems are compared, differences have been reported in problem-solving strategies. In normal development, when children learn basic number facts, they use a series of strategies in succession, beginning with counting to find the answer; later, they reproduce the answer they have memorized. The reproduction of the answer most likely involves visual-spatial skills, sequencing ability, and memory. Students with math disorder may use less developed strategies than their normally achieving classmates. This developmental lag may be related to neurobiological dysfunction.

Math disorder is also associated with genetic syndromes, such as Turner syndrome. Girls with Turner syndrome have difficulty with math and with handwriting but do not necessarily have reading problems (Pennington, 1991). The brain dysfunction in Turner syndrome involves nonverbal rather than focal right hemispheric dysfunction and is not limited to the right hemisphere (Pennington, 1991). Individuals with Turner syndrome have a particular cognitive phenotype associated with problems in visual-spatial tasks (Alexander and Money, 1966; Garron, 1977).

THE INTERFACE OF READING AND MATH DISORDERS

Math disorder has also been associated with disorder of written expression in the developmental Gerstmann syndrome. This syndrome is made up of four symptoms: dyscalculia, dysgraphia, difficulty in left-right orientation, and finger agnosia. When acquired in neurological patients, it suggests involvement of the parietal lobe. Yet it is not accurate to consider these four characteristics as a parietal lobe syndrome because other parietal lobe signs may also occur with the Gerstmann signs with a similar frequency. The four symptoms selected by Gerstmann are not specific. Kinsbourne and Warrington (1963) identified seven children with developmental Gerstmann syndrome who had finger agnosia and at least two other characteristics of the syndrome, but none had difficulty with number concepts themselves. However, they did have difficulty using place values to represent and manipulate numbers. Children with Gerstmann syndrome do not exhibit abnormal reading. Studies of Gerstmann syndrome have not meaningfully identified underlying procedures that are impaired in developmental mathematics disorder.

Arithmetic, reading, and spelling all require the acquisition of a formal symbol code, which is conveyed through education. The nature and meaning of these symbols differ, however. Written nouns and adjectives address items and attributes that are seen in everyday life; numbers refer to groupings and qualities which may have an existence and be manipulated independently of concrete materials. For example, the planning and the strategies involved in carrying out long division does not have a clear parallel in literacy skills (Temple, 1992). Yet the implementation of both of these codes requires the acquisition of certain facts. In reading and spelling, grapheme-phoneme pairs must be understood. For arithmetic, facts, such as multiplication tables, must be learned. Difficulties may occur in carrying out either of these types of tasks. However, attempts to find clustering of reading and math problems have met with mixed results. There has not been a consistent co-occurrence of the two kinds of disorders.

CLINICAL PRESENTATION

The basic clinical feature in math disorder is a discrepancy between expected and actual achievement of math computation and problem solving. The discrepancy must take into account accurate assessment of cognitive ability and past educational experience.

The diagnosis of math disorder is generally not made until several years after beginning school. Although younger children have learned to count, it is ordinarily not until formal math instruction is begun that the diagnosis is made. Often the diagnosis is not made until the third grade, a time when problem solving becomes more complex and simple counting strategies are no longer successful. However, developmental math problems may be recognized in preschool or kindergarten for children who have difficulty in learning number names, problems counting by rote, problems committing number facts to memory, failure to develop means to solve common problems that involve understanding quantity and quality relationships, difficulties learning to print numbers, maintaining number alignment during computation, and slowness at computation. In addition, children with mixed difficulties will have particular difficulty with word problems and the graphic representation of number information.

The most common of these difficulties are a focus on processes of ordering or sequencing and those involving memory processes. If order is the primary issue, then misplacement of vertical and horizontal number sequences and transposition of numbers may be evident. With impaired memory, difficulties might include carrying numbers over, failure to follow the designated operational sign, and difficulty in remembering basic number facts.

Solving word problems is a particular issue in itself. Proficiency in doing them requires more than computational skills. Difficulty in solving word problems may go beyond problems in computation or reading deficits because the child may not develop a systematic plan to find a solution, but rather act immediately on the numbers found in the problem instead of analyzing to establish what data is needed to solve it. Solving word problems involves language ability, reading skill, background knowledge to understand the situation presented, and computational skills. Each case requires a careful analysis of the types of errors the child makes.

DIAGNOSIS

Both educational testing and psychometric testing are needed to establish the diagnosis of a math disorder. Individually administered intelligence tests are administered to clarify verbal and performance ability and overall cognitive capacity. They are followed by standardized achievement tests where mathematics ability is evaluated along with reading and spelling ability to identify discrepancies between ability and achievement. The extent of the discrepancy should be based on comparisons of standard scores and related to the IQ.

DIFFERENTIAL DIAGNOSIS

The differential diagnosis of a developmental math disorder includes other reasons for poor school achievement. Among these are mental retardation, borderline intelligence, poor educational experience, and frequent absences from school. It is essential to complete the educational history to establish whether or not inadequate instruction is a factor, rather than an intrinsic math disorder. Moreover, children with reading disorder and/or language disorder should also be assessed for math disorder.

TREATMENT

Special education and remedial education programs focus on the specific presenting problem. The educational program must emphasize the development of math skills in either small group or individual tutorial sessions. Debate continues about whether self-contained special education classrooms or resource room programs are the best means to provide supplementary teaching.

The treatment program focuses on enhancement of mathematical skills. A developmental treatment model is used that includes illustrations and specific, concrete exercises. Interactive computer programs have recently been introduced to teach mathematical reasoning to children.

When math materials are presented, it is important they be presented using concrete materials. A variety of such materials, such as blocks and counting devices, may be utilized.

Once basic concepts have been understood, the next step is to encourage students to automate number facts. This is necessary because complex computations require speed and accuracy in using basic number facts. Students with math disorder may be accurate but very slow in conducting basic computations. The slow speed at computations may affect their accuracy as they move on to more complex problems and begin to lose their focus as they move from one step to another. Computer-based interactive video programs have the advantage of being paced by the child. In this way, a problem that is difficult for particular students can be individualized. Computer software may be used to provide drill and practice in number facts, which may be helpful. By using graphics and, in some instances, animation, the computer may maintain motivation and interest when basic paper and pencil tests do not maintain attention. Finally, frequent follow-up and reevaluation is necessary to maintain progress.

REFERENCES

American Psychiatric Association, Committee on Nomenclature and Statistics. (1994). *Diagnostic and statistical manual of mental disorders,* 4th ed. Author, Washington, DC.

Alexander, D., and Money, J. (1966). Turner's syndrome and Gerstmann's syndrome: Neuropsychologic comparisons. *Neuropsychologia,* 4:265–273.

Fleischner, J.E., and Garnett, K. (1987). Arithmetic difficulties. In K. Kavale, S. Forness, and M. Bender (eds.), *Handbook of learning disabilities,* Vol. 1. College Hill, San Diego, CA.

Garron, D. (1977). Intelligence among persons with Turner's syndrome. *Behavioral Genetics,* 7:105–127.

Geschwind, N., and Behan, P. (1983). Laterality, hormones, and immunity. In N. Geschwind and A. Galaburda (eds.), *Cerebral dominance: The biological foundations,* p. ll. Harvard University Press, Cambridge.

Hinshelwood, J. (1917). *Letter, word and mind-blindness.* H. K. Lewis, London.

Johnson, D. (1988). Review of research on specific reading, writing, and mathematics disorders. In J.F. Kavanagh and T.J. Truss (eds.), *Learning disabilities: Proceedings of the National Conference,* pp. 79–177. York Press, Parkton, MD.

Kinsbourne, M., and Warrington, E.K. (1963). The developmental Gerstmann syndrome. *Archives of Neurology,* 8:490.

Kosc, L. (1974). Developmental dyscalculia. *Journal of Learning Disabilities,* 7:164–177.

______. (1979). To the problems of diagnosing disorders of mathematical functions in children. *Studies in Psychology,* 21:62–67.

Pennington, B.F. (1991). *Diagnosing learning disabilities,* pp. 111–134. The Guilford Press, New York.

______, Van Doorninck, W.J., McCabe, L.L., and McCabe, E.R.B. (1985). Neuropsychological deficits in early treated phenylketonurics. *American Journal of Mental Deficiency,* 89:467–474.

Rourke, B. (1978). Reading, spelling and arithmetic disabilities: A neuropsychological analysis. In H. Myklebust (ed.), *Progress in learning disabilities,* Vol. 4. Grune & Stratton, New York.

Temple, C.M. (1991). Procedural dyscalculia and number fact dyscalculia: Double dissociation in developmental dyscalculia. *Cognitive Neuropsychology,* 8:155–176.

______. (1992). Developmental dyscalculia. In S.J. Segalowitz and I. Rapin (vol. eds.) and F. Boller and J. Grafman (series eds.), *Handbook of neuropsychology: Vol. 7. Child neuropsychology,* pp. 211–222. Elsevier Science Publishers, Amsterdam.

7.4 Disorder of Written Expression

Impairment in the development of written expression occurs when there is significant interference with academic achievement or with those activities of daily living that require expressive writing skills. Difficulty in the expression of thoughts through written language may be the common communicative disability. Disorders of written expression (writing disorder) basically involve an impairment in the ability to compose written text (Critchley, 1968). Writing disorder is frequently associated with spelling errors, grammatical and punctuation errors within sentences, and poor paragraph organization. It is commonly associated with developmental reading disorder, developmental expressive and receptive language disorder, developmental math disorder, and developmental motor coordination disorders.

Children with this disorder are particularly at risk because reading disabilities tend to be given more credence by teachers than writing disorders. Those children who have both writing disorders and reading problems are among the most severely learning disabled. Their difficulties are often not considered as "legitimate" as reading or math disability. Moreover, the standardized tests of academic achievement may not identify a writing disorder so individualized instruction and remediation are not provided. It is not uncommon for writing problems to be ascribed to laziness, noncompliance, or poor motivation. Consequently, children with writing disorder are particularly vulnerable to frustration.

HISTORY

Writing is speech made visible and is thought to have been introduced by the Sumerians in Lower Mesopotamia about 5,000 years ago. The earliest known writing systems were based on pictograms that showed a specific image of the object being represented in the real world. Thus the pronunciation of the word in language may have been clear. Later, the pictogram evolved into the ideogram, which depicted not only the object but also ideas or concepts associated with it. For example, the ancient Egyptian hieroglyphics (sacred carvings) were originally thought to serve this function. Pictograms were stylized and became increasing abstract as they evolved into linguistic symbols. The Sumerian language is said to be logographic; a logogram is a written sign that stands for a single morpheme (a word form that is the minimal unit needed to convey meaning) or sometimes for a full word. Now the relationship between the symbol and its meaning required explicit instructions for its interpretation. Linguistic symbols assumed a semantic function and came to represent sounds (Temple, 1993).

The Greeks, in the 9th century B.C., borrowed the earlier symbols systems but found them to be inefficient in representing their language. They introduced symbols taken from the Phoenician system of consonants to represent individual sounds and added vowels to create an alphabetic system (Coe, 1992). Our own writing system owes its origins to the Greeks but is ultimately derived from the Roman alphabet. In alphabetic scripts language is broken down into phonemes, i.e., the individual consonants and vowels that make up the sounds of language. In phonetic writing, signs lose all resemblance to the original images of objects and denote only sounds. The Roman alphabet came to England in the 6th century, and stable spelling of words became standardized in the 16th century and was uniformly stabilized in the 17th century.

DEFINITION

In DSM-IV (APA, 1994), disorder of written expression replaces the previous designation of developmental expressive writing disorder. As shown in Table 7.4–1, writing skills are substantially below that expected based on chronological age, measured intelligence, and age-appropriate education.

In addition, the disorder leads to difficulty in academic achievement at school or in activities of daily living that require expressive writing skills. There may be an inability to compose written text, spelling errors, grammatical or punctuation errors within sentences, and poor paragraph organization. If there are only spelling errors or poor handwriting in the absence of other evidence of impaired written expression, the diagnosis is not given.

EPIDEMIOLOGY

No specific data is available on the frequency of disorder of written expression. It is estimated to be as common as reading disorder. Developmental language disorders and other academic skills disorders may be seen in first-degree relatives.

DIFFERENTIAL DIAGNOSIS

Difficulty in composition of written text generally is linked to the level of intellectual functioning. Still, some mildly retarded individuals may show expressive writing skills that are below their expected grade level despite available schooling. In these instances, a diagnosis of disorder of written expression should also be made along with mild mental retardation. Moreover, impaired vision and hearing may affect expressive writing and should be evaluated using appropriate screening tests. Inadequate schooling may lead to poor written expression, but in these instances, there is generally a history of school absence. Impaired motor coordination

Table 7.4–1. DSM-IV Diagnostic Criteria for Disorder of Written Expression

315.2 Disorder of Written Expression

A. Writing skills, as measured by individually administered standardized tests (or functional assessments of writing skills), are substantially below those expected given the person's chronological age, measured intelligence, and age-appropriate education.

B. The disturbance in Criterion A significantly interferes with academic achievement or activities of daily living that require the composition of written texts (e.g., writing grammatically correct sentences and organized paragraphs).

C. If a sensory deficit is present, the difficulties in writing skills are in excess of those usually associated with it.

Coding note: If a general medical (e.g., neurological) condition or sensory deficit is present, code the condition on Axis III.

From APA, 1994.

may influence handwriting but does not lead to a specific disorder of written expression. However, if poor handwriting is secondary to impaired motor coordination, a diagnosis of developmental coordination disorder should be considered.

ETIOLOGY

Children with writing disorders are a heterogeneous group. Many affected children have other difficulties, such as inattention and delayed math achievement (Johnson, 1988). The heterogeneity of the disorder is an important consideration because the approach to remediation will vary depending on the child's particular presentation. In identifying cases, the most important developmental tests are those which involve retrieval memory, that is, tasks which involve rapid naming, oral sentence formulation, digit span, and visual retrieval. These tests help identify children who are in need of services, but such tests also serve to identify children's strengths. The etiology of a disorder of written expression may be related to right hemispheric dysfunction and may coexist with a math disorder (Pennington, 1991).

In adults, Gerstmann syndrome occurs with acquired lesions in the dominant parietal lobe. There may be an analogous developmental disorder that involves poor handwriting and spelling, spelling errors being characterized by altered letter sequences, omissions, and substitutions. As stated earlier, developmental Gerstmann syndrome includes dysgraphia, right-left disorientation, finger agnosia, and dyscalculia (Kinsbourne and Warrington, 1963). Math skills are delayed but reading is at or above grade level. On psychometric testing, a higher verbal than performance IQ is reported, with particularly poor performance on coding subtests. The underlying deficit for Gerstmann syndrome is thought to be a deficit in sequential processing, but in developmental Gerstmann syndrome, involvement of both parietal lobes has been suggested.

DEVELOPMENTAL ASPECTS

Among the language skills, writing is the last to develop. Writing disorders frequently persist into secondary school for children with developmental language and/or reading disorder. A writing sample may reflect the child's difficulty in linguistic, motor, and cognitive development. Writing involves the complex integration of several skills, and a variety of developmental dysfunctions may present through the child's written output. The study of writing disorders and the writing process may contribute substantially to understanding how a particular child processes information.

Written language includes handwriting, spelling, and syntax. Many aspects of writing dysfunction may exist alone or in combination: illegibility, irregular letter formation, inconsistency in letter formation, mechanical problems in writing including punctuation and capitalization, poor grammar and sentence structure, misspellings of words, and slow rates of writing to dictation.

CLASSIFICATION OF DISORDER OF WRITTEN EXPRESSION

Denckla and Roeltgen (1992) have proposed a model that takes into account those cognitive systems involved in informational flow beginning after word and letter choices (i.e., linguistic spelling operations) have been completed and encoded with functional handwriting. The model proposes that at least six cognitive systems are involved in poor handwriting. These include the grapheme buffer, the graphemic system, the allographic store, praxis, motor planning, and finally, visual motor integration. This model is in the process of development and is not yet available to use in planning remediation.

Sandler et al. (1992) investigated the correlates of disorder of written expression in middle childhood through comparisons of children with disorder of written expression with learning-disabled children referred for other school problems. Based on an assessment of 190 children who functioned in the normal range of intelligence and were aged 9 through 15, they proposed a method of subtyping disorder of written expression.

Writing Disorder with Fine Motor and Linguistic Deficits

Children in this group showed delays in reading, involving both decoding and comprehension. Their writing was characterized by poor spelling with frequent dysphonetic spelling errors, suggesting poor phonetic skills. There were problems with punctuation and capitalization, and written language lacked sophistication. Written output was slow and problems in fine motor and in linguistic functions were identified on developmental examination. Finger agnosia and mirror movements were commonly reported. Some children had difficulty imitating finger apposition sequences. They performed poorly on subtests of written language, for example, tests of oral sentence formulation, picture naming, and rapid naming. They also showed difficulties on digit span tests.

Writing Disorder with Visual-Spatial Deficits

This group of children demonstrated normal reading skills, but their writing characteristically showed poor legibility and was not neat. Letter formations were inconsistent and poor spatial organization on the page was characteristic as were poorly defined margins, sloping lines, and inadequate or excessive spacing. Despite the fact that written output was slow, spelling and written language were not notably impaired. On neurodevelopmental testing, poor performance was noted on visual-spatial tasks, including form copying and visual vigilance tasks.

Writing Disorder with Attention and Memory Deficits

These children had difficulty decoding written words. They demonstrated poor spelling with errors that showed phonetic approximations, omissions, insertions, and a lack of consistency. Legibility of written words, mechanics, and writing rate, however, were not abnormal. Teachers reported attentional deficits.

On neurodevelopmental examination, there were particular difficulties in visual retrieval memory. Performance on visual vigilance tasks was poor, and although language skills were age appropriate, those linguistic tasks that place heavy demands on retrieving information from memory, such as picture naming and sentence formulation, were particularly deficient. Digit span performance was poor, and impulsivity and inattention were noted when demands were placed during the test situation.

Writing Disorder with Sequencing Deficits

This group of children showed strong reading skills both in decoding and comprehension, but had problems with math computation and showed significant discrepancies between their math and reading abilities. Their writing reflected poor spelling, illegibility, and poor mechanics. The formation of letters was not well automatized and there were characteristic spelling errors with omissions, insertions, and transpositions of letters. On neurodevelopmental testing, language skills were strong, but there was difficulty in some fine motor and visual sequencing tasks, even though auditory sequencing was less affected. Finger agnosia was common, as was poor performance on a finger sequencing task. Discrepancies were noted on the Wechsler Intelligence Scale for Children between verbal and performance subtests.

TREATMENT

Children with disorder of written expression are often not recognized in the school program. If they are able to read adequately, they may be overlooked or thought to be poorly motivated in writing. Early diagnosis with explanations to the child's parents and teachers are critical. Disorder of written expression must be taken quite seriously, because the stress of output difficulties may be considerable. Appropriate tests should be used to diagnose writing disorders, and the child's deficit should be made known to his current teachers and to teachers in subsequent years of schooling.

Once identified, a writing disorder becomes a challenge throughout a child's school career. Generally, these problems do not spontaneously remit with maturation, but may, in fact, intensify in secondary school where demands for written output continue to increase. Disorder of written expression in adolescents is frequently accompanied by a secondary loss of self-esteem because teachers may not fully appreciate the extent of the problem. The child's writing is constant visual evidence of deficiencies. Because normally intelligent children with writing problems may not have other academic weaknesses, their learning disorder may pass unnoticed.

The treatment involves sequential handwriting instruction in school and often tutoring. Specific therapeutic interventions include tasks involving teaching sequencing, e.g., the appropriate use of syllables, and the use of oral tests and other means to bypass the disability. Compensatory approaches involve the use of notetakers for the child, increased time for written tests, provision of copies of long written assignments from the blackboard, and the use of typewriter and computers.

REFERENCES

American Psychiatric Association, Committee on Nomenclature and Statistics. (1994). *Diagnostic and statistical manual of mental disorders.* 4th ed. Author, Washington, DC.

Coe, M.D. (1992). *Breaking the Maya code,* pp. 24–32. Thames and Hudson, Inc., New York.

Critchley, MN. (1968). Dysgraphia and other anomalies of written speech. *Pediatric Clinics of North America,* 15:639–650.

Denckla, M. B., and Roeltgen, D. P. (1992). Disorders of motor control and function. In S.J. Segalowitz and I. Rapin (vol. eds.) and F. Boller and J. Grafman (series eds.), *Handbook of neuropsychology: Vol. 7. Child neuropsychology,* pp. 455–476. Elsevier Science Publishers, Amsterdam.

Johnson, D. (1988). Review of research on specific reading, writing, and mathematics disorders. In J.F. Kavanagh and T.J. Truss (eds.), *Learning disabilities: Proceedings of the National Conference,* pp. 79–177. York Press, Parkton, MD.

Kinsbourne, M., and Warrington, E.K. (1963). The developmental Gerstmann syndrome. *Annals of Neurology,* 8:490–501.

Levine, M.D. (1987). *Developmental variation and learning disorders,* pp. 308–345. Educators Publishing Service, Cambridge, MA.

Pennington, B. P. (1991). *Diagnosing learning disabilities,* pp. 111–134. The Guilford Press, New York.

Sandler, A.D., Footo, M., Levine, M.D., Coleman, W.L., and Hooper, S.R. (1992). Neurodevelopmental study of writing disorders in middle childhood. *Developmental and Behavioral Pediatrics,* 13:17–23.

Temple, C. (1993). *The Brain: An introduction to the psychology of the human brain and behavior,* pp. 153–154. Penguin, London.

7.5 Social-Emotional Learning Disabilities

Learning-disabled children have both social and academic problems. Their social disabilities were initially attributed to persistent school failure, isolation from other children in special classes, and the high prevalence among them of behavioral patterns associated with attention deficit disorder that provoked disapproval from peers and teachers (Denckla, 1989). Subsequently, it became apparent that, in addition to poor academic skills, there were serious problems with social skills acquisition. Moreover, social skills were found to involve certain cognitive functions that were needed to discriminate social cues. As a result, the learning-disabled child often had difficulty in social understanding that led to chronic difficulties in interpersonal relationships with others. Children with these types of learning disorders neither appropriately interpreted emotional responses of others nor made correct inferences about others' emotional behavior. Consequently, they were often isolated, not actively engaged with their peer group, and were frequently rejected by peers. These learning disorders have been referred to as "nonverbal learning disability," "right hemispheric learning disability," or "social-emotional learning disabilities."

In this section, social-emotional learning disabilities will be reviewed, including historical background, assessment, clinical features, developmental perspective, subtypes, associated deficits, family history, differential diagnoses, and intervention.

HISTORY

In the 1970s Johnson and Myklebust (1971) identified children who performed poorly in mathematics and had difficulty interpreting social signals, in pretending, and in abstract thinking. Bryan (1977) and Bruininks (1978) evaluated learning-disordered children with poor social status in the classroom and reported that, as a group, they showed poor performance on a test of nonverbal affective signal detection. Children with this clustering of problems were referred to as having "nonverbal learning disabilities." This categorization was in keeping with a growing awareness by special educators that children with learning disabilities have psychosocial as well as academic problems.

With the identification of the category of nonverbal learning disabilities, the relationship between these children's nonverbal behavior and their social abilities and dysfunction received particular emphasis (Semrud-Clikeman and Hynd, 1990). When compared to their nondisabled peers, the learning-disabled child was found to be not as well liked and more likely to show anxiety, withdrawal, and mood disturbance. Brumbach, Staton, and Wilson (1980) reported the co-occurrence of depression, learning disability, attentional deficits, and left-sided neurological signs and suggested possible right hemispheric pathology. Weintraub and Mesulam (1983) described emotional, interpersonal, and cognitive components of "developmental learning disabilities of the right hemisphere." Subsequently, Voeller (1986) used the term "right hemispheric deficit syndrome." In Voeller's group, some children had radiologically documented right hemispheric lesions and the majority showed impaired social abilities, problems in attention, visuospatial deficits, and math disability.

With the recognition of right hemispheric involvement in the processing of social-emotional signals in addition to its role in spatial processing, comparisons were made with previous diagnostic categories and the term "social-emotional learning disability" (SELD) was introduced (Denckla, 1983). The presentation of social-emotional learning disability is distinguishable from other disorders. These patients do not meet the diagnostic criteria for autistic disorder or Asperger's syndrome, nor do the diagnoses of schizotypal or schizoid describe them fully (Wolff and Barlow, 1979). The more general term "social-emotional learning disability" (SELD) emphasizes the character of their disabling condition and could be applied to children whose presentation is not as severe as the more pervasively disabling conditions described by the DSM-IV (APA, 1994) pervasive developmental disorder (PDD) diagnostic categories. Although each of these conditions must be considered for children with deficits in social awareness, all are conditions with a relatively low prevalence, whereas children with social-emotional learning disorder may represent a larger group and overlap more with children who are routinely seen in psychiatric clinics for mood and disruptive behavior disorders. Recognition of social-emotional learning disorders has highlighted the need for better assessment instruments to recognize social dysfunction. Gillberg (1992) has suggested that these problems in social signal recognition be considered disorders of empathy.

Social signals involve specific patterns and sequences of facial, body, and limb movement, referred to as "body language," along with associated vocal intonation patterns, or prosody. These nonverbal patterns suggest information about the emotions and intentions of others. These patterns of behavior have been referred to in ethology as "social displays" (MacLean, 1970). Moreover, the right hemisphere has been shown to be specialized for processing these social-emotional signals; it has an advantage in processing facial affect (Ley and Bryden, 1979) and vocal affective prosody (Carmon and Nachshon, 1973; Heilman et al., 1984). Studies in adults who have right hemispheric damage show poor performance in tasks of facial affect recognition and in the interpretation of utterances from others that are emotionally intoned. Such right hemispheric disordered patients also have difficulty interpreting social context cues and understanding jokes, metaphors, and the implied meanings of others' behavior. This right hemispheric specialization is also seen in children with right hemispheric involvement who perform more poorly than peers with left hemispheric dysfunction and control subjects on facial recognition tasks (Voeller, Hanson, and Wendt, 1988).

ASSESSMENT

Clinical evaluation based on the assessment of right hemispheric dysfunction is designed to recognize perceptual processing problems, difficulty responding to social-emotional signals, and difficulty in producing social-emotional signals on demand. In addition, these children may have difficulty interpreting cartoons, metaphors, and proverbs.

Neuropsychological testing and educational tests for right hemispheric dysfunction focus on the child's ability to discriminate, name and match facial expression and prosodic affect expression, and to perform cross-modal matching of faces to intoned prosody, and prosody to face. Although these tests are experimental, they are in the process of being standardized.

CLINICAL CHARACTERISTICS

Clinically, children with social-emotional learning disabilities are generally referred for problems other than social dysfunction. A common complaint is an inability to make friends, but a desire to have friends. A referred child may be described as odd by other children so they make little attempt to relate to him. Furthermore, the child may not be invited to parties or to go out with other children; others may turn down invitations from the affected child. In school, the child may not join in and play with others during break time, and although he may join others at lunch time, the child is not considered part of the group. In addition, although children with SELD may be intelligent and have good general academic knowledge, they may be unaware that others are not interested in their particular preoccupations. In this sense, these children seem to be insensitive to the wishes and desires of others.

DEVELOPMENTAL PERSPECTIVE

The presentation of social-emotional learning disabilities may vary with age. Younger children may seem different to an observer but still enjoy physical contact, such as being held and picked up. As toddlers, they may play on the periphery of the group and, developmentally, not move beyond parallel play into imaginative play. They may be intrusive with other children, grab toys from others, and disrupt games without being aware of the effect of their behavior on their peers.

In school, the child may be isolated from his peer group and, if the child engages in play, may spend time with younger children. By adolescence, efforts to make social contact with others have often been abandoned so considerable time is spent alone playing with a computer or engaged in other isolated activities. The affected adolescent may have learned enough about social behavior to cope with, and perform adequately on, standardized tests of social-emotional ability, but may continue to have difficulty in everyday social interactions with others because more complex and transient feedback is required. Moreover, these adolescents may dress differently than their peers and be unaware they are singled out by their appearance. When observed in groups with other adolescents, those with this syndrome tend to be involved with their own interests rather than those of their peers.

POTENTIAL SUBTYPES OF SOCIAL-EMOTIONAL LEARNING DISABILITIES

The classification of social-emotional learning disorder has been based on consideration of domains or modules for processing social signals. Visual/facial, vocal/prosodic channels, and expressive/receptive systems may make up distinct neural systems that have neuroanatomic correlates (Voeller, 1991). In some instances, children with social-emotional learning disabilities may be impaired expressively but not receptively. Children with the expressive type of deficit often have a flattened range of facial affective expressions and/or robotic speech, yet they may be able to interpret expressions of others without major difficulty. However, those who have intact affective expression but receptive impairments in comprehension may express emotions but lack social understanding of others.

Some children may be able to comprehend and demonstrate affect through visual/facial channels better than through vocal/prosodic channels, or vice versa. Others, however, may have global involvement of both channels in receptive and expressive systems and present a mixed picture. The mixed group may appear remote, distant, and lacking in social warmth. In addition, some may lack a sense of social distance, moving inappropriately and uncomfortably close to others. Despite this variability in presentation, the core symptoms relate to difficulty in processing social-emotional information.

ASSOCIATED DEFICITS

As indicated earlier in the section on mathematics and written communication disorder (Chapters 7.3 and 7.4), these academic skills problems may be associated, and other visuospatial and attentional deficits may also be apparent. Some children will show motor skills difficulties. On neurological examination, left-sided findings may be demonstrated on a standard sensorimotor examination.

FAMILY HISTORY

The association of social deficits in other family members has been reported, but family history studies have, for the most part, addressed specific disorders, such as Asperger's syndrome and autistic disorder.

DIFFERENTIAL DIAGNOSIS

Social-emotional learning disabilities may occur in a variety of neuropsychiatric diagnoses. The most important consideration for the future is to develop neuropsychological tests related to measurement of social-emotional learning problems in children that can be used to clarify the co-occurrence of social-emotional learning disabilities with other diagnoses. These conditions should be distinguished from autistic disorder, Asperger's syndrome, and schizotypal personality by using specific diagnostic criteria, natural history, and the associated features. Other diagnoses that co-occur must be taken into account, such as the anxiety disorders, avoidant disorder, and overanxious disorder. Depression may co-occur as a specific disorder or as an adjustment disorder. In diagnosing depression, it is necessary to discriminate between a problem in affective expression, which may be an aspect of a nonverbal or social-emotional learning disorder, and depressive symptoms that relate to internal state changes.

Other co-occurring disorders are attention deficit disorder with or without hyperactivity (Landau and Milich, 1988) and mathematics disorder. The diagnosis of a mathematics disorder requires that social-emotional learning disabilities must also be considered. However, conduct disorder is usually not associated with social-emotional learning disabilities. The child with social-emotional learning disabilities may violate the rights of others because of his lack of awareness of others' rights, whereas the child with a typical conduct disorder is fully aware of social cues and uses that awareness to deliberately manipulate others. Yet some children with social-emotional learning disorder may fail to regulate their aggressive impulsiveness toward others, not take others' interests into account, and act in an inappropriate manner, leading to a co-occurring diagnosis of conduct disorder.

Impulsive and compulsive behavior may be associated with SELD as well. Some genetic disorders, such as the fragile X syndrome, have associated social deficits. In fragile X syndrome, gaze avoidance is a characteristic feature (see Chapter 10.3), yet children with fragile X syndrome may show social responses when the social context is appropriately established.

INTERVENTION

Social skills have been defined as cognitive functions and discrete behaviors that are performed in interactions with others (Schumaker and Hazel, 1984a; 1984b). Social skills, then, are discrete behaviors that are learned and performed in interactive situations. Among them are verbal responses, such as making a statement; nonverbal responses, such as eye contact and nodding "yes" or "no," and more covert nonverbal responses that involve the discrimination of social cues. Children with social-emotional learning disabilities have difficulty with their social skills and appear to lack social competence. Social competence is usually taken to mean a person has performed a social task adequately so that social skills are performed in a socially acceptable manner. Hazel et al. (1985) suggest that a socially competent person can discriminate appropriate social behavior, utilize appropriate skills in social context, carry out those skills fluently in appropriate combinations, accurately perceive another person's verbal and nonverbal cues, and flexibly respond to them.

Overall, social skills are learned responses, and social competence is the ability to perform social skills in a flexible sequence in a variety of situations. Children with social-emotional learning disabilities have both social skills deficits, in that the needed skills are lacking in their repertoire of behaviors, and also have a problem in social competence with accompanying social performance deficits. The treatment of their social-emotional learning disability must take each of these factors into account. A social-cognitive behavioral approach focuses on their difficulties in social perception, self-regulation, and rule-governed behavior. The social-emotional learning difficulty must be treated in the context of other co-occurring psychiatric diagnoses. Michelson et al. (1983) provide recommendations for social skills assessment and training. An effective social cognitive assessment provides elements to address social problem solving, self-control, affective understanding, and enhancement of self-esteem. The following are drawn from the PATHS (Providing Alternative Thinking Strategies) curriculum (Greenberg et al., 1992; Kusche et al., 1992):

1. Increased self-control, i.e., the ability to stop and think before acting when upset or confronted with a conflict situation. Lessons in this area also teach identification of problem situations through recognition of "upset" feelings.
2. Attributional processes that lead to an appropriate sense of self-responsibility.
3. Increased understanding and use of the vocabulary of logical reasoning and problem solving, e.g., "if . . . then" and "why . . . because."
4. Increased understanding and use of the vocabulary of emotions and emotional states; e.g., excited, disappointed, confused, guilty. Increased use of verbal mediation.
5. Increased ability to recognize and interpret similarities and differences in the feelings, reactions, and points of view of self and others.
6. Increased recognition and understanding of how one's behavior affects others.
7. Increased knowledge of, and skill in, the steps of social problem solving: stopping and thinking; identifying problems and feelings; setting goals; generating alternative solutions; anticipating and evaluating consequences; planning, executing, and evaluating a course of action; trying again if the first solution fails.
8. Increased ability to apply social problem-solving skills to prevent and/or resolve problems and conflicts in social interactions.

In summary, children with social-emotional learning disabilities may be of normal or above normal intelligence, have associated visuospatial deficits, attentional problems, and mathematics learning disorder, but their core deficit is in the social communicative disorder spectrum (Tanguay, 1990). Their symptoms may be based on underlying right hemispheric dysfunction in processing information of a social-emotional nature along with other cognitive deficits. Neurological signs involving the left side of the body may be present.

REFERENCES

American Psychiatric Association, Committee on Nomenclature and Statistics. (1994). *Diagnostic and statistical manual of mental disorders,* 4th ed. Author, Washington, DC.

Bruininks, V.L. (1978). Peer status and personality characteristics of learning disabled students. *Journal of Learning Disabilities,* 11:484–489.

Brumbach, R.A., Staton, R.D., and Wilson, H. (1980). Neuropsychological study of children during and after remission of endogenous depressive episodes. *Perceptual Motor Skills,* 550:1163–1167.

Bryan, T.M. (1977). Learning disabled children's comprehension of nonverbal communication. *Journal of Learning Disabilities,* 10:501–506.

Carmon, A., and Nachshon, I. (1973). Ear asymmetry in the perception of emotional non-verbal stimuli. *Acta Psychologia,* 37:351–357.

Denckla, M.B. (1983). The neuropsychology of social-emotional learning disability. *Archives of Neurology,* 40:461–462.

______. (1989). Social learning disabilities. *International Pediatrics,* 4:133–136.

Gillberg, C. (1992). The Emanuel Miller Memorial Lecture, 1991. Autism and autistic-like conditions: Subclasses among disorders of empathy. *Journal of Child Psychology and Psychiatry and Allied Disciplines,* 33:813–842.

Greenberg, M.T., Kusche, C.A., Calderon, R., Gustafson, R.N., and Coady, E.A. (1992). *The PATHS curriculum: Providing alternative thinking strategies (Special Needs Version): Vol. 2. Facilitating interpersonal understanding and problem solving skills.* University of Washington Press, Seattle.

Hazel, J.S., Sherman, J.A., Schumaker, J.B., and Sheldon, J. (1985). Group social skills training with adolescents: A critical review. In D. Upper and S. Ross (eds.), *Handbook of behavioral group therapy,* pp. 203–246. Plenum Press, New York.

Heilman, K.H., Bowers, D., Speedie, L., and Coslett, H.B. (1984). Comprehension of affective and nonaffective prosody. *Neurology,* 34:917–921.

Johnson, D.J., and Myklebust, H.R. (1971). *Learning disabilities.* Grune & Stratton, New York.

Kusche, C.A. Greenberg, M.T., Gustafson, R.N., Calderon, R., and Coady, E.A. (1992). *The PATHS curriculum: Providing alternative thinking strategies (Special Needs Version): Vol. 1. Facilitating and reinforcing emotional understanding and development.* University of Washington Press, Seattle.

Landau, S., and Milich, R. (1988). Social communication patterns of attention-deficit-disordered boys. *Journal of Abnormal Child Psychology,* 16:69–81.

Ley, R.G., and Bryden, M. (1979). Hemispheric differences in processing emotions and faces. *Brain and Language,* 7:127–138.

MacLean, P.D. (1970). *The triune brain in evolution: Role in paleocerebral functions.* Plenum Press, New York.

Michelson, L., Sugai, D.P., Wood, R.P., and Kazdin, A.E. (1983). *Social skill assessment and training with children.* Plenum Press, New York.

Schumaker, J.B., and Hazel, J.S. (1984a). Social skills assessment and training for the learning disabled: Who's on first and what's on second? Part I. *Journal of Learning Disabilities,* 17:422–431.

______, and ______. (1984b). Social skills assessment and training for the learning disabled: Who's on first and what's on second? Part II. *Journal of Learning Disabilities,* 17:492–499.

Semrud-Clikeman, M., and Hynd, G.W. (1990). Right hemispheric dysfunction in nonverbal learning disabilities: Social, academic and adaptive functioning in adults and children. *Psychological Bulletin,* 107:196–209.

Tanguay, P.E. (1990). Infantile autism and social communication spectrum disorders. *Journal of the American Academy of Child and Adolescent Psychiatry,* 29:854.

Voeller, K.K.S. (1986). Right-hemisphere deficit syndrome in children. *American Journal of Psychiatry,* 143:1004–1009.

______. (1991). Social-emotional learning disabilities. *Psychiatric Annals,* 21:735–741.

______, Hanson, J.A., and Wendt, R.N. (1988). Facial affect recognition in children: Comparison of the performance of children with right and left hemisphere lesions. *Neurology,* 38:1744–1748.

Weintraub, S., and Mesulam, M.M. (1983). Developmental learning disabilities of the right hemisphere: Emotional, interpersonal, and cognitive components. *Archives of Neurology,* 40:463–468.

Wolff, S., and Barlow, A. (1979). Schizoid personality in childhood: A comparative study of schizoid, autistic, and normal children. *Journal of Child Psychology and Psychiatry,* 20:29–46.

CHAPTER 8

TRAUMATIC BRAIN INJURY

Traumatic brain injury is a major cause of death and of disability among children, adolescents, and young adults and one of the most common causes of chronic brain syndromes in childhood. This chapter provides an overview of the epidemiology, types of trauma, recovery process, and long-term sequelae. The references provided offer more detailed information about these topics.

EPIDEMIOLOGY

It is estimated that 185 per 100,000 children from infancy to age 14 and 295 per 100,000 adolescents and young adults ages 15 to 24 are hospitalized each year for traumatic brain injury (Kraus and Nourjah, 1988). The risk is highest among the 15- to 19-year-olds where the rate is 550 per 100,000 (Jennett and Teasdale, 1981). The causes of traumatic brain injury are different depending on the age of the child. The younger children are more involved in falls and other forms of accidental injury; adolescents and young adults tend to be involved in motor vehicle accidents and violent assaults. The incidence is twice as high in males as in females, and children who live in poor psychosocial circumstances are at greater risk.

TYPES OF TRAUMATIC BRAIN INJURY

Neurological damage associated with head trauma can be produced in several ways. Closed head injuries typically involve acceleration and deceleration of the brain within the hard skull that leads to contusion of the brain and may result in subarachnoid hemorrhage. Different parts of the brain have different densities and, therefore, shearing stresses that develop during rapid brain movement cause injury. Furthermore, compression of blood vessels against the falx cerebri or tentorium may result in infarction of the areas these blood vessels supply. Open head injuries typically involve penetrating traumatic brain injury that causes specific and direct loss of neural tissue.

A common complication of traumatic brain injury is cerebral edema, but other complications include infection and hematoma formation both inside and outside the brain. Each of these complications results in neurological deficits, and the effects may be widespread. Furthermore, compensatory mechanisms that are involved in recovery from head trauma may themselves alter brain function. A child who has suffered traumatic brain injury is, therefore, likely to have both neurological and psychiatric difficulties depending on the brain regions involved. Multiple mechanisms lead to psychological symptom formation; both psychosocial and physiologic factors are involved.

RECOVERY FROM TRAUMATIC BRAIN INJURY

Children who experience severe traumatic brain injury usually follow a predictable postoperative course (Levin, Benton, and Grossman, 1982; Rosen and Gerring, 1986). The most important landmarks for recovery are related to the time of emergence from coma and the time of emergence from posttraumatic amnesia. Commonly, the Ranchos Los Amigos Scale is used to evaluate recovery following traumatic brain injury. The emergence from coma is generally defined as the point at which the patient is able to follow simple verbal commands. Concurrently, visual tracking of objects in the environment may be noted.

Immediately following emergence from coma, the child will not be able to form new memories. This time, from the accident to the time when new memories emerge, is referred to as posttraumatic amnesia (PTA). Another form of memory loss, retrograde amnesia for events before the accident, typically becomes shorter and shorter during the recovery process. PTA ends when the child is able to form new memories. The frequency of PTA is most likely related to concurrent injury to the temporal lobes that are associated with head trauma. However, older memories may be recalled that do not involve the temporal lobes. It is important to remember that children with severe head trauma rarely have specific memories of the accident itself. In summary, the milestones of recovery that are most important for future outcome are the length of coma and PTA.

COGNITIVE AND BEHAVIORAL SEQUELAE

Children and adolescents tend to have a better outcome after severe traumatic brain injury than those over age 21 (Filey et al., 1987; Knights et al., 1991; Kraus, Fife, and Conroy, 1987; Levin et al., 1987; Slater and Bassett, 1988). Despite this general rule, children who are younger than 7 may have a worse outcome (Kriel, Krach, and Panser, 1989) because they may be at increased risk of child abuse, which may be particularly traumatic and may involve multiple injuries. Furthermore, younger children may have a worse outcome based on the global effects of trauma on the developing brain (Johnston and Gerring, 1992). The duration of recovery of significant neuropsychological, behavioral, and emotional deficits may last several years following injury. Cognitive deficits are the major disability in traumatic brain injury (Cope et al., 1991).

The most common long-term sequelae of traumatic brain injury are cognitive and behavioral. The length of coma and the duration of posttraumatic amnesia are particularly important in regard to complete cognitive recovery. There is a strong inverse relationship between subsequent IQ and duration of coma according to Brink, Garrett, and Hale (1970). Others, such as Chadwick, Rutter, and Brown (1981), have correlated the persistence of cognitive deficits with the duration of PTA. These authors suggest that the more persistent deficits were found following more than 3 weeks of PTA. Furthermore, performance IQ was noted to be more affected than the verbal intelligence score in these children. Persistent verbal memory impairment has been reported for as long as 10 years and up after injury in a quarter of those studied (Gaidolfi and Vignolo, 1980). Rutter (1981) found that children showed behavioral disinhibition after severe closed traumatic brain injury with overtalkativeness, ignoring social conventions, impulsiveness, and poor personal hygiene.

PSYCHIATRIC SEQUELAE

Psychiatric sequelae may be divided into those that occur in the early phases of recovery and those that occur in later phases of recovery. The earliest sequelae are noted before the termination of PTA. During this time, behavioral and affective symptoms are related to the neurological presentation. The most common psychiatric diagnosis noted is that of delirium. Symptoms commonly noted include short attention span, agitation, hallucinations, and disturbances in the sleep/wake cycle.

Subsequently, posttraumatic psychiatric symptoms may be noted (Hill, 1989). Their occurrence relates to the severity of the injury, its location, the child's behavioral and emotional symptomatology prior to the accident, and the psychosocial interactions of the family during the phases of recovery (Rutter, 1981; Parker, 1994). Furthermore, the more severe the traumatic brain injury, the more likely it is that there will be psychiatric sequelae (Lehmkuhl and Thoma, 1990). All children in one prospective study of severely injured children who had premorbid psychiatric conditions showed posttraumatic psychiatric disorders (Brown et al., 1981). Furthermore, more than half of the children in this group who had no premorbid symptoms prior to the accident had developed psychiatric symptoms during a 28-month follow-up period. The greatest premorbid risks relate to previous difficulties with impulse control and disruptive behavior. A previous history of family dysfunction also increases the risk for subsequent symptomatology. Of particular importance are posttraumatic mood disorders, which include both depressive and manic symptoms.

TREATMENT

Advances in treatment focus on pharmacologic therapies that address post-traumatic neurochemical changes (McIntosh, 1993) and endogenous neuroprotective factors, interventions for post-traumatic seizures (Willmore, 1993), cognitive remediation (Ben-Yishay and Diller, 1993), and early intervention for psychiatric disorders.

REFERENCES

Ben-Yishay, Y., and Diller, L. (1993). Cognitive remediation in traumatic brain injury: Update and issues. *Archives of Physical Medicine and Rehabilitation* 74:204–213.

Brink, J.D., Garrett, A.L., and Hale, W.R. (1970). Recovery of motor and intellectual function in children sustaining severe head injuries. *Developmental Medicine and Child Neurology,* 12:565–571.

Brown, G., Chadwick, O., Shaffer, D., Rutter, M., and Traub, M. (1981). A prospective study of children with head injuries; III. Psychiatric sequelae. *Psychological Medicine,* 11:63–78.

Chadwick, O., Rutter, M., and Brown, G. (1981). A prospective study of children with head injuries; II. Cognitive sequelae. *Psychological Medicine,* 11:49–61.

Cope, D.N., Cole, J.R., Hall, K.M., and Barkans, H. (1991). Brain injury: Analysis of outcome in a post acute rehabilitation system; I. General analysis. *Brain Injury,* 5:111–125.

Filey, C.M., Cranberg, L.D., Alexander, M.P., and Hart, E.J. (1987). Neurobehavioral outcome after closed head injury in childhood and adolescence. *Archives of Neurology,* 44:194–198.

Gaidolfi, E., and Vignolo, L.A. (1980). Closed head injuries of school aged children: Neuropsychological sequelae in early adulthood. *Italian Journal of Neurological Science,* 2:65–73.

Hill, P. (1989). Psychiatric aspects of children's head injury. In D.A. Johnson, D. Uttley, and M. Wyke. *Children's Head Injury: Who Cares?* pp. 134–146. Taylor and Francis, London.

Jennett, B., and Teasdale, G. (1981). *Management of head injuries.* F.A. Davis Company, Philadelphia.

Johnston, M.V., and Gerring, J.P. (1992). Head trauma and its sequelae. *Pediatric Annals* 21:362–368.

Knights, R.M., Ivan, L.P., Ventureyra, E.C.G., Bentivoglio, C., Stoddart, C., Winogron, W., and Bowden, H.N. (1991). The effects of head injury in children on neuropsychological and behavioral functioning. *Brain Injury,* 5:339–351.

Krause, J.F., Fife, D., and Conroy, C. (1987). Pediatric brain injuries: The nature, clinical course, and early outcomes in a defined United States population. *Pediatrics,* 79:501–507.

______, and Nourjah, P. (1988). The epidemiology of uncomplicated brain injury. *Journal of Trauma,* 28:1637–1643.

Kriel, R.L., Krach, L.E., and Panser, L.A. (1989). Closed head injury: Comparison of children younger and older than 6 years of age. *Pediatric Neurology,* 5:296–300.

Lehmkuhl, M., and Thomas, W. (1990). Development in children after severe head injury. In A. Rothenberger (ed), *Brain and Behavior in Child Psychiatry.* pp. 267–282. Springer-Verlag, Berlin.

Levin, H.S., Amparo, E., Eisenberg, H.M., Williams, D.H., High, W.M.,Jr., McArdle, C.B., and Weiner, R.L. (1987). Magnetic resonance imaging and computerized tomography in relation to the neurobehavioral sequelae of mild and moderate head injuries. *Journal of Neurosurgery,* 66:706–710.

______, Benton, A.L., and Grossman, R.G. (1982). *Neurobehavioral consequences of closed head injury.* Oxford University Press, New York.

McIntosh, T.K. (1993). Novel pharmacologic factors in the treatment of experimental brain injury: A review. *Journal of Neurotrauma* 10:215–261.

Parker, R.S. (1994). Neurobehavioral outcome of children's mild traumatic brain injury. *Seminars in Neurology* 14:67–73.

Rosen, C.D., and Gerring, J.P. (1986). *Head injury: Educational reintegration.* College-Hill Press, Boston.

Rutter, M. (1981). Psychological sequelae of brain damage in children. *American Journal of Psychiatry,* 138:1533–1544.

Slater, E.J., and Bassett, S.S. (1988). Adolescents with closed head injuries. *American Journal of Diseases of Children,* 142:1048–1051.

Willmore, L.J. (1993). Post-traumatic seizures. *Neurology Clinics* 11:823–834.

CHAPTER 9

PERVASIVE DEVELOPMENTAL DISORDERS

The term "pervasive developmental disorder" (PDD) was introduced in DSM-III (APA, 1980) as a new designation. Childhood autism was placed in this category among the developmental disorders because it has more in common with other disturbances of development than with emotional disorders and is distinct from schizophrenia. In DSM-III-R (APA, 1987), this definition was broadened to include "a group of disorders characterized by qualitative impairments in the development of reciprocal social interaction, in the development of nonverbal and verbal communication skills, and in imaginative activity." This designation, PDD, to a considerable extent, includes children with Wing's and Gould's triad of impairments along an autistic continuum (Wing, 1988; Wing and Gould, 1979).

Basic categories and a residual category were introduced for pervasive developmental disorder in DSM-III. These were "infantile autism," "childhood onset pervasive developmental disorder," "residual autism," and an atypical category. "Infantile autism" had previously been included under the "childhood psychosis" or "childhood schizophrenia" designation and was now separated out as a discrete entity for the first time since its initial description in 1943. The category "childhood onset pervasive developmental disorder" focused on later symptom onset and included some cases previously diagnosed as childhood schizophrenia and possibly some cases of "Heller's syndrome." The categories included in pervasive developmental disorder were modified in DSM-III-R where "infantile autism" and "childhood onset pervasive developmental disorder" were merged into a general category "autistic disorder" with no specific age of onset required for the diagnosis, although age of onset was to be specified. "PDD not otherwise specified (NOS)" was added to include all other disorders that did not meet the criteria for "autistic disorder." The residual autism category was discontinued in DSM-III-R to allow the diagnosis to be made at any developmental level or age. With the introduction of ICD-10 (WHO, 1992) and DSM-IV (APA, 1994), the designation "pervasive developmental disorder" has been retained.

The retention of the "pervasive developmental disorder" (PDD) terminology is controversial (Happe and Frith, 1991). Originally, the term "pervasive developmental disorder" was chosen to encompass autism as well as a heterogeneous group of conditions that share similarities with autism (Volkmar and Cohen, 1991). However, in ICD-10, PDD includes nonautistic disorders as well. PDD is taken to mean that the disturbance in development is pervasive and involves more than one developmental line or domain. Moreover, the designation "pervasive" is contrasted to the more specific developmental disorders involving cognition or academic skills. The advantage of the term "PDD" is that it is a descriptive term which does not suggest a particular theoretical orientation about etiology, nor does it suggest a particular form of treatment. It is a generic term for a group of conditions, but it is controversial whether it should be considered a diagnosis in itself (Rutter and Schopler, 1992). Much of the debate about its use stems from the DSM-III-R category "PDD-NOS" being treated as though it were a diagnosis rather than a residual category for children with severe social communicative deficits.

Because some autistic individuals are higher functioning and test within the normal range in some cognitive domains, the use of the term "pervasive" for them has been questioned. The term "pervasive" is not specific enough and may be misleading because it might imply all functions are equally affected. Yet despite the sparing of some abilities and the presence of certain strengths, they may show autistic behavior that may be sufficiently severe to have a pervasive effect on their long-term outcome. In this sense, "pervasive" does not imply there are no areas of normal functioning. Consequently, children with problems in many domains of development, including social, language, communicative, and cognitive skills, are recognized by the "pervasive" category as in need of multiple services and intervention strategies.

Several alternatives have been offered for the term "pervasive," largely based on the past application of the term "PDD" exclusively to autistic and autistic-like conditions. Baird et al. (1991) view deficits in the social/cognitive domain as the specific-defining characteristic of these disorders just as reading disorder may be defined as linked to phonological processing deficits. Tanguay (1990) suggested the term "social communicative disorders" for disorders of social awareness and social contact. This designation addresses the basic disabilities of social and affective communicative dysfunction, including disorders in pragmatic language usage. Another alternative is "autistic spectrum disorder," or "autism and autistic-like conditions." These categories suggest deviation that may be inherent in the social and communicative lines of development as they relate to brain function. An even more global alternative designation is "disorder of social interaction, communication, and imagination." The choice is between focusing on the extent of disability (a pervasive disorder) or on the type of behavior disorder that results from the disruption of cognitive, communicative, social, and perceptual development. The ICD-10 approach of using "PDD" as a generic term has not been strictly followed in DSM-IV where the emphasis continues to be on the presence of autistic-like behavior.

Yet the term "pervasive" in ICD-10 and DSM-IV has been extended to include conditions that are basically nonautistic forms of pervasive developmental disorder. In both classifications, these include other disorders of infantile onset, such as Rett's disorder, and other childhood disintegrative disorders. In ICD-10, overactive disorder with mental retardation and stereotyped movements is also included. Syndromes associated with severe and profound mental retardation may be the most pervasive developmental disorders because they involve several developmental lines; these disorders require the most intensive interventions.

The strongest objection to the term "pervasive" in DSM-IV is that it does not describe the nature of the impairments it covers. Moreover, the "PDD" label does not indicate the severity of the impairment, although it recognizes the nature of the impairments primarily involve communication, socialization, and imagination. Furthermore, despite autism being included in the "PDD" designation, autistic disorder, in itself, is recognized as a disorder that has wide general recognition through parent groups and national organizations; increasingly refined techniques are being applied in its investigation. If one considers basic levels of organization at the biological level, there is an ongoing effort to find consistent abnormalities in the brains of autistic individuals, which requires well-defined cases. At the cognitive level, some functions, such as rote memory, may be preserved, and at the behavioral level, daily living skills may or may not be impaired. However, at the level of social adaptation, autism is pervasively disabling in the context of the world being a socially oriented one. Pervasive developmental disorder is best considered a general designation and not a diagnosis. This allows the focus to remain on the criteria for the specific categories included under this term. In the future, disorders in the social-cognitive domain may be better delineated. Neuropsychological testing procedures are being applied to clarify both executive function and social communicative deficits in autistic disorder (McEvoy, Rogers, and Pennington, 1993).

The next descriptor in pervasive developmental disorder is the term "developmental." The use of this term introduces a developmental perspective and places emphasis on the age of recognition or the age of onset of various disorders that occur in children. It implies disturbances and, in many instances, deviation from the normal developmental lines, particularly those that involve social and language communicative development. An early onset impacts later phases of development throughout the life span. Gillberg (1991) has noted that the designation "developmental" is appropriate for almost all cases, emphasizing the biological basis for autism is generally linked to developmental processes. Yet linking "pervasive" to development lacks specificity because the diagnosis covers both low- and high-functioning cases of varying degrees of severity. In regard to severity, pervasive developmental disorder has been described on a mild to severe spectrum. Such an approach has limitations because one must consider the natural history of autism and the fact that children may emerge from its socially withdrawn phase.

The term "pervasive developmental disorder" has been expanded to include both autistic-like and nonautistic disorders. In the following sections, the categories listed in DSM-IV and ICD-10 will be reviewed. These include autistic disorder, Asperger's syndrome, Rett's disorder, childhood disintegrative disorder, atypical autism, and overactive disorder associated with mental retardation and stereotyped movements. The last two of these categories are ICD-10 rather than DSM-IV categories; however, they are included here in the spirit of utilizing the term "pervasive developmental disorder" comprehensively until the specific deficits in the social communicative grouping can be better defined. Perhaps in a future classification the category of "social communicative disorder" or a similar designation will be used for those conditions rather than "pervasive developmental disorder." The descriptions used here include the clinical course and natural history because these features are essential in establishing the validity of a particular disorder.

REFERENCES

American Psychiatric Association, Committee on Nomenclature and Statistics. (1980). *Diagnostic and statistical manual of mental disorders,* 3rd ed. Author, Washington, DC.

American Psychiatric Association, Committee on Nomenclature and Statistics. (1987). *Diagnostic and statistical manual of mental disorders,* 3rd ed, revised. Author, Washington, DC.

American Psychiatric Association, Committee on Nomenclature and Statistics. (1994). *Diagnostic and statistical manual of mental disorders,* 4th ed. Author, Washington, DC.

Baird, G., Baron-Cohen, S., Bohman, M., Coleman, M., Frith, U., Gillberg, I.C., Gillberg, C., Howlin, P., Mesibov, G., Peeters, T., Ritvo, E., Steffenburg, S., Taylor, D., Waterhouse, L., Wing, L., and Zapella, M. (1991). Letter. Autism is not necessarily a developmental disorder. *Developmental Medicine and Child Neurology,* 33:363–364.

Gillberg, C. (1991). Debate and argument: Is autism a pervasive developmental disorder? *Journal of Child Psychology and Psychiatry,* 32:1169–1170.

Happe, F., and Frith, U. (1991). Is autism a pervasive developmental disorder? Debate and argument: How useful is the PDD label? *Journal of Child Psychology and Psychiatry,* 7:1167–1172.

McEvoy, R.E., Rogers, S.J., and Pennington, B.F. (1993). Executive function and social communication deficits in young autistic children. *Journal of Psychology and Psychiatry,* 34:563–578.

Rutter, M., and Schopler, E. (1992). Classification of pervasive developmental disorders: Some concepts and considerations. *Journal of Autism and Developmental Disorders,* 22:459–479.

Tanguay, P.E. (1990). Infantile autism and social communication spectrum disorder. *Journal of the American Academy of Child and Adolescent Psychiatry,* 29:854.

Volkmar, F.R., and Cohen, D.J. (1991). Debate and argument: The utility of the term pervasive developmental disorder. *Journal of Child Psychology and Psychiatry,* 32:1171–1172.

Wing, L. (1988). The continuum of autistic characteristics. In E. Schopler and G.M. Mesibov (eds.), *Diagnosis and assessment in autism.* Plenum Press, New York.

______, and Gould, J. (1979). Severe impairments in social interaction and associated abnormalities in children: Epidemiology and classification. *Journal of Autism and Developmental Disorders,* 9:11–29.

World Health Organization (1992). *International statistical classification of diseases and health related problems,* 10th Revision, Vol. l. Author, Geneva.

9.1 Autistic Disorder

Although initially described by Kanner in 1943, autistic disorder was not included in the diagnostic classification as a separate category until 1980 with the publication of DSM-III (APA, 1980). The diagnosis has stood the test of time and the DSM-IV (APA, 1994) clinical features are essentially those described by Kanner in his original description. Kanner generally excluded cases with known brain dysfunction and severe mental retardation. The eponym "Kanner's syndrome" was used for many years and has been retained by some authors when they describe idiopathic cases with a classical clinical course. In DSM-IV, the classic case is designated "autistic disorder" and the eponym is not used; however, other eponyms, such as Asperger's syndrome, are used. When considering cases, it is helpful to review Kanner's original description of cases that are drawn from his observations and those of the children's parents.

From its beginnings, "autism" was a term that focused on impairment in the development of social relations and social understanding. Recent developmental research has returned to the original theme of abnormality in social understanding so that affective development, social cognition, and interpersonal reciprocity are guiding themes in research. Autistic disorder may provide cues to a better understanding of how social cognition emerges and whether there is a social cognitive network in the brain.

This chapter reviews the history, definition and classification, epidemiology, clinical features, etiologies, models of autism, assessment, neuropsychological testing, developmental issues and perspectives, natural history, theoretical approaches, and treatment. It focuses on the spectrum of social communicative or autistic spectrum disorders in an attempt to understand the basic deficit in autistic disorder. The discussion includes the language disorder and the associated compulsive and stereotypic behaviors; however, the major emphasis is on social understanding and the development of social awareness from a neurobiological and a social interactional perspective.

HISTORY

> Since 1938, there have come to our attention a number of children whose condition differs so markedly and uniquely from anything reported so far, that each case merits—and, I hope, will eventually receive—a detailed consideration of its fascinating peculiarities. (Kanner, 1943)

In this first paragraph of his classic 1943 paper, *Autistic Disturbances of Affective Contact,* Leo Kanner initiated clinical and research interest into autistic disorder. The following year, he introduced the term "early infantile autism." How affective contact develops in children with autistic disorder remains a major theme in autism research more than a half century later. The designation "autism" was initially chosen to describe the sense of aloneness that seemed apparent to those who observed children with this developmental disorder. It does not refer to a retreat into fantasy, but rather an absence of social awareness of themselves as they relate to others. Yet aloneness does not necessarily mean lonely, which is a developmental acquisition that follows the emergence of a sense of self. Kanner felt this syndrome represented an innate inability, present from the becoming of life, to develop social relationships with others. He pointed out that these children failed to initiate socially meaningful anticipatory gestures; autistic children did not reach to be picked up, apparently did not respond to animate persons in the environment, and seemed to be "in a world of their own." Because social communicative interactions are among our most basic species-typical characteristics, the lack of affective contact remains an intriguing topic for research. It is both perplexing and demoralizing to family members who attempt in vain to make meaningful contact with these children. Resistance to social contact and other characteristics that now define the syndrome, such as delayed and deviant language development, restricted interest in activities, and stereotypical patterns of behavior, were described in the first case report.

At one time it was debated whether autism was related to an innate dysfunction within the individual or was the consequence of psychosocial deprivation. Neurobiological research has since demonstrated that it is an innate developmental disorder. With the recognition that autistic disorder is a neurobiologically based developmental disorder, child development research has begun to consider whether or not development in autistic individuals is essentially deviant and follows an autistic developmental line, or if, in general, development follows a sequence in these children similar to that of the nondisabled child. Because it is a developmental disorder, the role of the family is crucial, and teaching family members to understand the deficit allows them to respond to their children more effectively. Parental motivation in helping their children emerge from the autistic phase has led to the establishment of national organizations throughout the world, and in the United States to parental organizations in each state to help understand this perplexing condition.

DEFINITION AND CLASSIFICATION

Prior to 1980, when DSM-III was published, there was no specific category of "autistic disorder." Instead, the term "childhood schizophrenia" or "childhood psychosis" was broadly applied to children with severe psychiatric disturbances beginning in early life. In 1972 Rutter highlighted these differences in his paper, *Childhood Schizophrenia Reconsidered.* Gradually, autism was more clearly differentiated from schizophrenia in childhood, based on the age of onset, symptom presentation, and clinical course (Rutter, 1978). These autism criteria were based on distortions in the development of multiple basic psychological functions that are involved in the development of social skills and language, such as attention, perception, reality testing, and motor movement.

In DSM-III, 37 years after the original description, the basic criteria proposed by Kanner were incorporated in the Diagnostic and Statistical Manual III under the designation "pervasive developmental disorders—infantile autism." Over the years, several definitions had preceded the DSM-III definition. In 1978, at an international conference on autism in St. Gallen, Switzerland, Rutter had emphasized onset before 30 months, deviant social development, deviant language development, and stereotypical behavior, which were integral features of the diagnosis. The National Society for Autistic Children definition (1978) focused on the early onset of social and communicative abnormalities, including disturbances in the rates and/or sequences of development and unusual responses to sensory stimuli. Taking into account past definitions, the DSM-III definition for infantile autism specified an age of onset before 30 months of age, pervasive lack of responsiveness to others, deviant language development, unusual responses to the environment, and the absence of hallucinations and delusions found in schizophrenia. Further revisions were made in the revision of DSM-III, DSM-III-R (APA, 1987), because the original criteria were found to apply best to younger and more severely impaired individuals and were thought to be too restrictive. A residual category was included in DSM-III but was not commonly used (it was subsequently abandoned in DSM-III-R) because even the highest functioning autistic adults continue to have difficulties with social adaptation and communication. Although characteristic symptoms are less apparent, especially for those individuals who emerge from the severe, socially autistic phase, autistic children and adolescents continue to remain sufficiently symptomatic as they grew older so that the category "residual state" was not felt to describe them satisfactorily.

The DSM-III-R recognized the importance of changes in syndrome expression during development and included more developmentally focused criteria, leading to a change in the name of the category from "infantile autism" to "autistic disorder." Accordingly, the diagnostic criteria were broadened to take into account the entire age range and spectrum of functioning. Three broad categories were included: abnormal reciprocal social relations, disturbances in communication and imaginative play, and restricted range of activities and interests. To receive a diagnosis of autistic disorder in DSM-III-R, a child or adult needed to demonstrate at least 8 of 16 criteria, with a specified distribution over the three categories. An age of onset before age 30 months was no longer required as a criterion, but the time of onset or time of recognition of symptoms needed to be recorded. Furthermore, its differentiation from schizophrenia was further clarified so that an individual with an autistic disorder might have both diagnoses if the additional diagnostic criteria for schizophrenia, such as the presence of hallucinations and delusions, were present. Essentially, the diagnosis of the schizophreniform disorder or of schizophrenia was recognized as potentially co-occurring in a vulnerable autistic person. Moreover, the diagnosis of autistic disorder could be made in DSM-III-R, based on a current examination of the child without knowledge of early history. The major change in DSM-III-R was the introduction of the developmentally focused criteria. Yet DSM-III-R broadened the concept of autistic disorder substantially so that a greater number of false positive cases were reported (Volkmar et al., 1992a).

Volkmar et al. (1992b) compared the DSM-III, DSM-III-R, and ICD-10 (WHO, 1992) definitions of autism. In their sample, they found the ICD-10 approach identified cases similar to those identified by clinicians and, to a lesser degree, cases identified by the DSM-III, which tended to underdiagnose autism. The underdiagnosis in DSM-III seemed to be based on the description of the social deficit as a "pervasive lack of responsiveness to others." However, they found that the DSM-III-R overdiagnosed autism relative to the clinician's and the DSM-III and ICD-10 systems. Most of the additional cases that were diagnosed using DSM-III-R were felt to be atypical forms of pervasive developmental disorder rather than more clear-cut examples of autistic disorder. These authors concluded that the DSM-III-R system may have expanded the diagnosis to include atypical cases. Because DSM-III-R identified more cases that are atypical, this complicated its use for both clinical and research purposes; for that reason, additional modifications were proposed for DSM-IV.

Additional changes were made in DSM-IV to bring the diagnosis closer to that contained in the International Classification of Diseases (ICD-10) and to improve the diagnostic algorithm for DSM-III-R that was criticized as difficult to apply. The operationalization of the criteria and the developmental orientation introduced in DSM-III-R were maintained. The changes in DSM-IV were developed to provide greater simplicity in their application while maintaining compatibility with ICD-10 and clinical judgment. In developing the DSM-IV criteria, the historical issues that relate to too narrow a definition and too broad a definition were balanced along with the importance of considering symptoms that occurred at various ages during development. Thus criteria such as pervasiveness unrelatedness were not reintroduced because they apply primarily to the most severely autistic and generally to the younger child. The age of onset or recognition criterion was reintroduced, typical examples of behavior that were previously included along with the diagnostic criteria in DSM-III-R were removed, and efforts were made for better operationalization of criteria. In regard to the diagnostic algorithm, rather than 8 of 16 items, a total of 6 of 12 items are now required for the diagnosis. A requirement for qualitative impairments in social interaction and in communication and restricted interests and activities is maintained. The word "stereotyped" is now added to the latter category. Delays or abnormal functioning is required prior to age 3 in at least one of the following areas: social interaction, social communicative language, and symbolic or imaginative play. Moreover, with the inclusion of additional categories under the "pervasive developmental disorder" terminology, exclusionary criteria now include Rett's disorder and childhood disintegrative disorder. The diagnostic criteria for DSM-IV are shown in Table 9.1–1.

The diagnosis requires at least two items related to qualitative impairment in social interaction, one from the category of qualitative impairment in communication and one from the category of restricted repetitive and stereotyped patterns of behavior. Because examples are not given in DSM-IV, it is important to consult the descriptive text for specific examples that fit under each of the categories outlined.

Atypical Autism

Atypical autism is a specific category in ICD-10 but is not a specific category in DSM-IV, where it is included under "Pervasive Developmental Disorder Not Otherwise Specified." Atypical autism differs from classical autism in regard to either age of onset or the failure to meet all three sets of diagnostic criteria. Abnor-

Table 9.1–1. DSM-IV Diagnostic Criteria for Autistic Disorder

299.00 Autistic Disorder

A. A total of six (or more) items from (1), (2), and (3), with at least two from (1), and one each from (2) and (3):
  (1) qualitative impairment in social interaction, as manifested by at least two of the following:
    (a) marked impairment in the use of multiple nonverbal behaviors such as eye-to-eye gaze, facial expression, body postures, and gestures to regulate social interaction
    (b) failure to develop peer relationships appropriate to developmental level
    (c) a lack of spontaneous seeking to share enjoyment, interests, or achievements with other people (e.g., by a lack of showing, bringing, or pointing out objects of interest)
    (d) lack of social or emotional reciprocity
  (2) qualitative impairments in communication as manifested by at least one of the following:
    (a) delay in, or total lack of, the development of spoken language (not accompanied by an attempt to compensate through alternative modes of communication such as gesture or mime)
    (b) in individuals with adequate speech, marked impairment in the ability to initiate or sustain a conversation with others
    (c) stereotyped and repetitive use of language or idiosyncratic language
    (d) lack of varied, spontaneous make-believe play or social imitative play appropriate to developmental level
  (3) restricted repetitive and stereotyped patterns of behavior, interests, and activities, as manifested by at least one of the following:
    (a) encompassing preoccupation with one or more stereotyped and restricted patterns of interest that is abnormal either in intensity or focus
    (b) apparently inflexible adherence to specific, nonfunctional routines or rituals
    (c) stereotyped and repetitive motor mannerisms (e.g., hand or finger flapping or twisting, or complex whole-body movements)
    (d) persistent preoccupation with parts of objects

B. Delays or abnormal functioning in at least one of the following areas, with onset prior to age 3 years: (1) social interaction, (2) language as used in social communication, or (3) symbolic or imaginative play.

C. The disturbance is not better accounted for by Rett's Disorder or Childhood Disintegrative Disorder.

From APA, 1994.

mal and/or impaired development becomes apparent to others after 3 years of age when abnormalities are present in one or two of the following areas: reciprocal social interaction, communication, or stereotyped repetitive behavior, but not in all three areas. The DSM-IV definition suggests that atypical autism is most often seen in profoundly retarded individuals who, perhaps because of their low level of functioning, may not exhibit the specific behaviors needed for the diagnosis of autism. It may also include children with severe forms of specific developmental disorder of receptive language, atypical childhood psychosis, and other levels of mental retardation with autistic features. In DSM-IV, atypical autism refers to cases that do not meet the criteria for autistic disorder because of "late age of onset, atypical symptomatology, subthreshold symptomatology, or all of these." Moreover, criteria are not met for a specific pervasive developmental disorder, schizophrenia, schizotypal personality, or avoidant personality disorder. Although specific operational criteria are not given, it is suggested that the diagnosis of atypical autism be placed in parentheses when used, i.e., "PDD-NOS (Atypical Autism)."

Yet the use of the designation "atypical autism" for children with severe and profound mental retardation remains problematic. The idiopathic syndrome described by Kanner (1943) may be a genetic disorder and the use of the term "atypical autism" may suggest a link to a genetic condition when there is none. It is more parsimonious to describe the specific deficits that are observed. Perhaps in the next classification there will be a new designation for this group, such as "social communicative disorder associated with mental retardation, with or without stereotypies."

Moreover, social deficits are commonly found in severely and profoundly retarded individuals. Wing and Gould (1979) assessed social deficits in a large sample of disabled children and identified both autistic children and other groups of children with disabilities based on their social skills. Their categories include (1) the aloof child who pays little attention to social exchange; (2) the passive child who is more responsive but tends to avoid social interactions unless passively engaged; and (3) the active, but odd child, who may initiate interactions but does so in an inappropriate and stilted manner.

Differential Diagnosis

In the other pervasive developmental disorders, such as Asperger's syndrome, detection may occur somewhat later because these children have a higher intellectual level and less difficulty with communication skills (Asperger, 1944). However, children with childhood disintegrative disorder develop behavior changes after 2 or more years of clearly normal development. Children with Rett's disorder appear normal in the first months of life, but toward the end of the first year begin to show difficulty, although the diagnosis may not be made until somewhat later.

In addition to other forms of pervasive developmental disorder, the following diagnoses should be considered in the differential diagnosis: mixed receptive/expressive language disorder, with secondary socioemotional problems; reactive attachment disorder or disinhibited attachment disorder; mental retardation with associated emotional/behavior disorder; and schizophrenia of unusually early onset.

EPIDEMIOLOGY

There is general agreement, using a narrow definition of autistic disorder, that when strictly defined, prevalence rates are approximately 2 in 10,000. With less stringent criteria, the prevalence rates increase to 4 to 5 cases per 10,000 (Wing, 1993). This rate is somewhat higher using the DSM-III-R criteria (Volkmar et al., 1988). When prevalence rates of pervasive developmental disorder (children with autistic-like symptoms) are included, the general rate increases to 12 to 15 in 10,000 (Wing, 1993). The other categories of pervasive developmental disorder are less common than autism.

Epidemiologic investigations show that the rate is higher for boys than girls, with rates of 4 or 5 to 1 (Wing, 1993). When girls are involved, there is a tendency for them to be more severely affected (Lord, Schopler, and Revicki, 1982). The majority of autistic individuals, 75% to 80%, test within the mentally retarded range. Although autism was initially associated with higher social class, it is now evident that it is observed in families at all levels of education (Schopler et al., 1980). The age of onset in the majority of cases is within the first year or the second year of life. It is often difficult to determine the exact age of onset, so more commonly, the age of recognition is used. The most common age of recognition is in the first 2½ years of life. The diagnosis has been observed after a few months to a few years of normal development (Volkmar, Stier, and Cohen, 1985). Although family factors and higher cognitive functioning may delay case recognition, when careful histories are taken, the early symptoms ordinarily are recognized. Early detection of autistic symptoms in toddlers, by 18 months, is being investigated. Baron-Cohen, Allen, and Gillberg (1992) reviewed developmental screening of 41 18-month-old toddlers who were at high genetic risk and 50 randomly selected 18-month-olds using the CHAT (Checklist for Autism in Toddlers).

CLINICAL FEATURES

Social Deficits

The most essential feature of an autistic disorder is a qualitative abnormality in social interaction. The severity and nature of the social deficit varies with the child's age and developmental level.

In infancy, children with autistic disorder may resist cuddling and not mold to the parent, and they may not utilize anticipatory gestures when approached or when approaching others. When engaged with others, they may lack joint attention, which is demonstrated through an absence of pointing and utilizing eye contact to engage others' interest (or in failure to show pride of accomplishment in bringing items to show to others). As toddlers and during the preschool years, they may ignore others, or bump into them as if they were unaware of their existence. They may not turn when called or look at a person who is trying to engage them in conversation. This gaze avoidance may continue into school age and even into adulthood in a less striking form. Yet gaze avoidance is responsive to improvement by appropriate training.

As the higher functioning child emerges from the autistic phase, rather than being socially distant, he may become socially intrusive. The child may seem unaware of others' feelings and lack understanding of a negative impact of his behavior on others. There may be limited ability to interpret the tone of voice or facial expression so the usual exchanges between child and parent that are used to convey wishes or show pleasure or displeasure may have little long-term effect on the child's behavior. The higher functioning child will have difficulty making friends and engaging other children in play although, at a younger age, the child seemingly is not distressed by social isolation and may seek solitude. But in those who do seek to find friends, ostracism may be the result of their inadequate attempts to socialize. Moreover, autistic children are rigid in their social responses and must be taught simple social forms, such as greeting another person. The verbal autistic child may learn the social forms but may not apply them in context and have difficulty in this way.

Deficits in Communication and Imaginative Activity

The failure to acquire language at an expected age is the most frequent presenting concern by parents of preschool autistic children. All preschool children with this disorder have some form of developmental language difficulty. The difficulties are not simply expressive but involve impaired comprehension of language. Some may be mute, and others may understand very little of conversation directed toward them. Others develop language later but may speak unintelligibly and not use appropriate sentence structure. Those who speak late may have unintelligible jargon, which does not show communicative intent. This jargon may include bits and pieces of memorized information from cartoons, television commercials, or phrases they have heard. Their speech fluency may be misleading because they have comprehension problems, especially for questions that are addressed to them about their personal experiences and for connected speech. Others may speak more appropriately but become preoccupied with a narrow range of favorite topics and show little regard for the interest of the person with whom they are speaking. They may perseverate and ask the same question over and over, although they know the answer. In other instances, they may recite phrases they have heard, imitating exactly the tone of voice and rhythm of the speaker from whom the phrase was learned. Early in life, verbal autistic children may be echolalic and repeat a question rather than responding to it (immediate echolalic). This echolalia may be associated with a reversal of pronouns as the child refers to himself as "you" or by name, rather than using the word "I" appropriately.

Pragmatic language use, a form of nonverbal communication, is also deficient. This is seen most clearly when the autistic child does not use gestures or pantomime in conversation.

Although children normally begin to point with one finger at about 10 months to things they like and begin shaking their head "no" by a year, many autistic children are limited in developing these nonverbal behaviors. Instead of pointing, they may get things themselves or take the hand of a parent and move it toward the preferred object. Being unable to gesture their communicative intent, they may become distressed and cry or tantrum until an adult has guessed, by trial and error, what the child needs.

Verbal autistic children may speak in a monotone, either loudly or softly, and sometimes in a singsong manner. They usually have a deficiency in using rhythm and intonation (prosody) to clarify the meaning of another's speech. They must be taught how to participate in conversation, to maintain the topic, to take turns, to look at the conversational partner, to interpret tone of voice, facial expression, and body language.

Imaginative activities are limited and often consist of the repetition of parts of commercials or cartoons the child has observed. The abnormality in inner language development is also a characteristic feature and is most often demonstrated in observations of play routines.

Restricted Activities

Children with autistic disorder routinely show repetitive patterns of movement (stereotypies and mannerisms) that include hand flapping (especially when excited), twirling, rocking, head banging, finger posturing, and sensory preoccupations. Commonly, they may resist changes in routines in the environment and become quite distressed when a small object is moved to another location. Stereotypies with objects are common, such as flicking a string, turning light switches on and off, tearing paper into shreds, or turning a toy car over and spinning the wheels rather than rolling it appropriately. Children who are higher functioning may become preoccupied with letters or numbers, for example, the yellow pages in the telephone book. Other children use verbal stereotypies and may repeat the same statements over and over again. When efforts are made to change their routines, the child may resist and tantrum. A lack of the use of imagination in creative play is apparent from the preschool years. Preference is for manipulating or stimulating with objects, lining them up, and utilizing the same play figures in repetitive ways. Recognition that figurines used in play represent people is delayed. When higher functioning autistic children do show some form of pretend play, such as feeding a stuffed animal or figurine and putting it to sleep, the pretending is repetitious and lacks flexibility.

The higher functioning verbal autistic child may become preoccupied and become an expert on very limited topics, such as mapmaking or timetables. Once this topic is mastered, they may perseverate on a theme ideationally and want to speak about it continually. They become particularly preoccupied with classification and become collectors of small items like stones.

Intelligence

Initially autistic children were thought to show a broad range of intelligence and were frequently considered untestable, but potentially of normal intelligence. With better testing procedures, it became apparent that the autistic person was limited cognitively and, rather than normally intelligent, autistic children were considered to represent a group who were primarily mentally retarded. Currently, it is generally agreed that autistic children show the full range of intellectual competencies from profound mental retardation to superior intelligence. The modal IQ is in the moderately retarded range and approximately 20% have an IQ of 70 or above.

Intelligence testing is complicated because the full-scale IQ measures the activities of several brain systems. The subtests that are utilized test different cognitive skills, and the profile for an autistic person may be uneven. Therefore, a full-scale IQ may provide information that is of limited use and may be misleading in autistic persons with brain dysfunction. Most often autistic children have higher nonverbal or visual-spatial skills than auditory-verbal skills. This difference is the most apparent for younger children, and as the child grows and advances in age, the abilities may show less discrepancy. Commonly, splinter skills for a narrow range of abilities, such as calculation, rote verbal memory, and puzzle completion, may be noted despite overall limited cognitive ability.

Even though it may be difficult to test autistic children because of their distractibility, negativism, and difficulty comprehending, it should not be assumed they are untestable. If tasks are provided at the child's general cognitive level, he ordinarily can cooperate with an experienced tester.

Mood and Affect

Because of their lack of responsiveness, autistic children are often described as having a flat affect. Yet preschool children, particularly, are generally described as happy as long as environmental demands are not excessive. When demands are placed, they may become irritable and tantrum and be difficult to console. Older autistic children may show more labile affect, particularly during the phase of emergence from the socially withdrawn phase. Others may become aggressive and may pinch or hit without apparent provocation. Fearfulness may be noted and phobias may develop, particularly if these children have been startled in a situation where they do not understand the social context. Their fearfulness and anxiety may be situation specific. Tantruming is common, particularly when their routines are disrupted, and may be so severe that the family becomes organized around the child's routines to try to reduce the frequency of tantruming.

Attention and Arousal

The majority of autistic children have attention deficits and may be highly distractible; some are hyperactive. The child may be observed to wander from one activity to the next and not become engaged in any activity. Yet other autistic children may show extremely long attention spans for activities they have become preoccupied with. In these instances, they may stay with a single activity for long periods of time without apparent boredom.

Sleep

Sleep disturbances are common in autistic infants and may persist to school age. DeMyer (1979) found that about one third of infants had sleep difficulties, but half reported a worsening of sleep between ages 2 and 3 years. Waking once or twice at night is not uncommon. Alternations in sleep pattern may also be observed, with excessive sleepiness alternating with reduced sleep. Sleep disturbances show a poor response to medication.

Sensorimotor Abilities

Some classically autistic children may show excellent coordination; others are clumsy. The child who is well coordinated may be able to balance in remarkable ways, for example, standing on the edge of a chair and rocking back and forth. Both toe walking and hypotonia are frequently seen without evidence of specific neurological deficit. The autistic child may be late in walking and have difficulty imitating movements and learning to use specific tools (Rapin, 1991).

Abnormal responses to sensory input is a common problem. It may be particularly evident when autistic children place their hands over their ears to avoid auditory stimulation. An autistic child may be intolerant of loud sounds, but at other times, be unresponsive to sound and thought to be deaf. Difficulties in auditory processing may influence discrimination of speech sounds and affect language learning.

Autistic children may be fascinated with visual stimuli, such as watching a record turn, the rotation of a fan, spinning wheels in order to watch the rotation, and moving lights. The visual modality may be better developed than the auditory one, as demonstrated through excellent visual-spatial skills.

There may also be somatosensory abnormalities, such as insensitivity to pain. Children may bang their heads until there is a lump or bite their hands, leading to severe injury. In other instances, self-stimulation may involve excessive rubbing or masturbating. With the emergence from the autistic phase, excessive sensitivity to pain may be noted and, in some instances, an apparently minor toothache may lead to major changes in behavior until it is recognized. Some children may be tactually defensive and arch their backs and withdraw when touched or stroked.

Other sensory modalities may also be

involved; children may lick or smell objects they pick up and, in other instances, show strong taste aversions, leading to eating a very narrow range of foods.

Seizure Disorder

The prevalence of seizures in autistic children is greater than in the population at large. The likelihood of seizures, however, is related to the presence of mental retardation and motor dysfunction, e.g., those that have more extensive brain damage (Tuchman, Rapin, and Shjinnar, 1989). The onset of seizures increases gradually from childhood and reaches a peak during adolescence. About one quarter of adult autistic persons have been reported to have seizures. Seizures are least common in the high-functioning autistic group. When seizures do occur, there is no specific seizure type that is characteristic. Generalized, partial complex, atypical absence, and other types have been reported, either singularly or in combination (Rapin, 1991).

Autistic-like behavior has been associated with infantile spasms and the Lennox-Gastaut syndrome (Taft and Cohen, 1971). These disorders are associated with diffuse slow spike-wave complexes on the electroencephalogram (EEG) (Aicardi, 1986). Both are correlated with mental retardation. Of interest is the fact that infantile spasms are related to abnormalities in the REM sleep mechanism, a finding that seems unique to this form of seizure disorder. In addition, acquired epileptic aphasia (Landau-Kleffner syndrome), which is associated with unilateral or bilateral temporoparietal spike-wave discharges that may be activated during slow wave sleep, also has been associated with autistic symptoms in a significant proportion of children (Landau and Kleffner, 1957).

ETIOLOGIES

Although the autistic spectrum of behavioral and developmental features may be associated with a variety of brain disorders (Coleman and Gillberg, 1985), it is the form Kanner emphasized that most likely has a genetic basis. He was reluctant to diagnose severely mentally retarded children and those with known brain disorders as having autistic disorder. The known syndromes associated with autistic and autistic-like behavior are shown in Table 9.1–2.

The natural history of symptom development and outcome in these disorders is not necessarily the same as in classical autism as described by Kanner. These disorders should be followed carefully to establish the course of autistic symptoms in each of them.

There may have been difficulty in pregnancy or in the perinatal period in some children who have a later diagnosis of autism. However, such problems are variable and because they are not consistently present and have not been shown to be causally related, there is no evidence they provide useful indicators for the prevention of autism (Nelson, 1991).

Genetic Aspects

There is now substantial evidence that idiopathic autism is a genetic disease (Folstein and Rutter, 1988) rather than a syndrome with diverse organic etiologies (Coleman and Gillberg, 1985). Three epidemiologic studies of identical twins found high concordance rates ranging from 36% to 91% in contrast to a zero concordance rate among nonidentical twin pairs (Folstein and Rutter, 1977, 1988; LeCouteur, Bailey, and Rutter, 1989b; Steffenberg et al., 1989). These combined British twin samples support inheritance of cognitive and social abnormalities related to and including autistic disorder. LeCouteur, Bailey, and Rutter (1989b) reported 92% of identical twins were concor-

Table 9.1–2. Disorders Associated with Autism and Autistic-like Behavior

Fragile X (q27) chromosome abnormality
Other sex chromosome abnormalities
Tuberous sclerosis
Neurofibromatosis
Infantile spasms
PKU
Intrauterine rubella infection
Postnatal herpes infection
Lactic acidosis
Purine disorder
Hydrocephalus
Möbius syndrome
Duchenne muscular dystrophia
Rett's disorder

dant for a broader cognitive and/or social deficit phenotype, whereas only 10% of nonidentical were concordant. The recurrence risk in a family for the birth of another child with an autistic disorder following the birth of an autistic child is approximately 3%, or 60 to 100 times the base rate in the general population (Smalley, Asarnow, and Spence, 1988). The rate of mental retardation is not elevated among the siblings of autistic children. This suggests the specificity of genetic influences on cognitive and social abnormality rather than there being a generalized influence on brain functioning. It seems most likely that siblings and parents have an increased risk for social and cognitive deficits which are mild to minimal in degree but similar in kind to those found in autistic disorder (Folstein and Piven, 1991). Piven et al. (1990b) studied 67 adult siblings of 37 autistic individuals. They found that 3% of the siblings were autistic, 4.4% had severe social dysfunction, 15% had cognitive disorders, and 15% had been treated for an autistic disorder. Landa et al. (1992) studied social language use (pragmatics) in the parents of autistic individuals. Although mild in degree, disinhibited social communication, awkward/inadequate expression, and odd verbal interaction were reported. Landa, Folstein, and Isaacs (1991) compared spontaneous discourse narratives of parents of autistic persons and controls. Although similar in length, the narratives of the autistic parents were less complex and coherent and, in some instances, rambling and difficult to comprehend. These narrative-discourse deficits may also be associated with genetic liability.

In contrast, little evidence indicates that autism is associated with the more common causes of brain damage or that genetic abnormalities are specifically associated with autistic disorder. Although autistic-like behavior has been reported in the fragile X syndrome, Steffenberg et al. (1989) found fragile X syndrome in only 9% of 22 twin pairs with autistic-like behavior, and medical disorders were identified in only 10% of the British twin pairs. Piven et al. (1991a) found the fragile X marker in 2 of 75 cases (2.7%). Future fragile X screening should use specific DNA markers. Moreover, obstetrical complications or neonatal injury do not account for concordance in identical twins. In twins who were discordant for autism in the combined British study, most of the autistic co-twins had a greater number of minor congenital anomalies than their nonautistic co-twin (Bailey, 1993). As is the case for other developmental anomalies, the time that the anomaly occurs is thought to be in the prenatal period.

If obstetrical complications do occur, they may have their major effects on fetuses with preexisting intrauterine developmental anomalies. These findings are consistent with the lack of evidence that autistic disorder is associated with brain damage caused by obstetrical complications or any evidence of postmortem findings in autistic disorder that suggest obstetrical injury (Nelson, 1991). Moreover, autism is rarely associated with the most common causes of mental retardation, such as trisomy 21 and cerebral palsy. In fragile X syndrome, social deficits are reported in a proportion of cases, as noted earlier, but these cases do not follow the same clinical course as classical autism.

These findings suggest autistic disorder has a genetic etiology. However, the specific mode of inheritance is unclear, and it is possible there may be more than one genetic form with variable expression. The mode of inheritance may remain unclear until the broader autistic phenotype is defined with greater sensitivity and specificity. About half of the parents of autistic persons have mild neuropsychiatric disorders characterized by social language deficits (Landa et al., 1992). Recent research on human mutation involving unstable regions in chromosomes with the expansion of trinucleotide repeats may be fruitful, particularly if anticipation can be demonstrated in family pedigrees. To progress, genetic studies require better descriptions of the types of cognitive deficits, associated features, and, eventually, the identification of biological markers.

Neurochemistry

Neurochemical investigations in autistic disorder have focused primarily on neurotransmitter levels (Cook, 1990). Serotonin, dopamine, norepinephrine, endogenous opiates, thyroid hormone, and cortisol production have been evaluated. Although specific endocrine abnormalities have not been found, dysregulation of both cortisol (Hoshino et al., 1984) and of melatonin rhythms have been suggested (Ritvo et al., 1993). The most consistent finding is that of hyperserotoninemia, which has been demonstrated in 30% to 50% of autistic subjects whose whole blood serotonin levels are in the upper 5% of the normal range (Anderson et al., 1987). Piven et al. (1991c) measured serotonin levels in autistic subjects whose siblings had diagnoses of PDD or autistic disorder and found that levels were significantly higher in autistic subjects with an affected sibling. Investigations of the neurochemistry of the brain using positron emission tomography (PET) and immunocytochemistry have not been reported. However, Harris, Frost, and Dannals (unpublished) have carried out D_2 dopamine receptor PET scans with ^{11}C N-Methylspiperone in two adult autistic patients and found some postsynaptic increase in receptor density when contrasted to age-matched control subjects.

PET scan studies utilizing glucose metabolism and cerebral blood flow studies have yielded conflicting results. The initial study of 12 adult autistic males showed an increase in 2-fluoro-2-deoxy-D-glucose (FDG) uptake and a suggested increase in the cerebral metabolic rate for glucose in the frontal, parietal, temporal, and occipital cortex and hippocampus, thalamus, and basal ganglia (Rumsey et al., 1985). However, there was a substantial overlap between autistic and control groups. Additional analysis of this information from 15 autistic men showed less interhemispheric functional correlation between appropriate regions of the frontal and parietal lobes. Moreover, there was decreased intrahemispheric correlation between the frontal and parietal lobes and the striatum and thalamus (Horwitz, Rumsey, and Grady, 1987). There were similar trends in a second FDG PET study of 16 autistic children that did not reach statistical significance (DeVolder et al., 1987). A third PET study with 6 autistic adults did not show differences in cerebral blood flow, glucose utilization, or oxygen consumption (Herald et al., 1988). The first two studies were done under presumed resting conditions and the third was done listening to music; the age range and functional ability among subjects was variable. The differences may relate to the fact that autistic subjects become more anxious during clinical procedures and have difficulty attaining a true basal metabolic resting condition. Moreover, higher functioning autistic subjects may show less abnormality in brain function. Future studies require cortical activation techniques and larger, more uniform samples.

Nuclear magnetic resonance spectroscopy with phosphorus 31 has also been used to study *in vivo* neurochemistry of the brain in autistic subjects. Minshew et al. (1991) investigated 11 adolescent and young adult autistic males whose full-scale verbal and performance IQs were greater than 80. They found decreased levels of phosphocreatine and ATP and a borderline significant increase ($p < 0.007$) in phosphodiesters in the dorsal prefrontal cortex. The levels of NMR metabolites were compared with performance on language and neuropsychological tests. A decline in cognitive performance was demonstrated to correlate with a decline in labile high energy molecules in the brain along with an increase in metabolic breakdown products of membrane phospholipids. Minshew and Rattan (1992) suggest these metabolic findings may indicate abnormal dendritic integrity in the frontal cortex that may be consistent with neurophysiologic and neuropsychological dysfunction reported in the temporal lobes.

When functional studies and neuroanatomical studies are considered together, there is the suggestion of immaturity of the neuronal dendritic tree. The limbic system findings may reflect a reduction in connectivity of these structures with other brain regions. The combined findings are consistent with the incomplete development of distributed neural networks in frontal and parietal association cortex that are involved in complex information processing (Minshew and Rattan, 1992). Such deficits may be associated with abnormalities in those executive systems and social cognitive systems involved as information is transferred between brain regions.

Neuroanatomical Studies

Neuroanatomical studies have demonstrated abnormalities in the emotional or limbic brain and cerebellum (Courchesne, 1991; Raymond, Bauman, and Kemper, 1989). MRI findings of hypoplasia of cerebellar lobules VI and VII, pons, and fourth ventricle have not been replicated in high-functioning autistic subjects when contrasted with IQ-matched control subjects (Piven et al., 1992b). The same authors did find 5 of 13 autistic subjects had polymicrogyria and one had macrogyria. These abnormalities may reflect abnormal migration of neurons to the cortex. However, patients with and without these migrational abnormalities had the full syndrome of autistic disorder (Piven et al., 1990a). Bauman (1991, Bauman and Kemper, 1994) reported autopsy findings on six cases who were clinically diagnosed and met clinical criteria for an autistic disorder. These children had deficits in social interaction, disordered language development, and compulsive and ritualistic behavior. The age range was 9 to 29; five males and one female were studied. On standardized tests, four of the six cases tested in the severe range of mental retardation, one was mildly retarded, but one had a nonverbal IQ of 105 on the Leiter test. Two of the children died in drowning accidents, two died of sepsis, one was found dead in bed without any specific etiology, and the sixth had Ewing sarcoma. On gross examination, the brains appeared normal but weighed 100 to 200 grams above average. The brains were well formed and, on examination, externally the cortex appeared normal, as did the cerebellar lobes.

When the cases were studied, using whole-brain serial sections, abnormalities were found in the amygdala, hippocampus, septum, anterior cingulate, and mammillary body—all parts of the limbic system. Moreover, the olivary nucleus and the cerebellum showed abnormalities. The abnormalities found in the hippocampus and amygdala were bilateral. Many cells were present in these areas that were very small and closely packed together. Similar cellular changes were found in the diagonal band of broca in the septum. Abnormalities were also found in the entorhinal cortex and a persistent lamina desicans was apparent in the oldest case (age 29); the lamina desicans usually disappears by 15 months of age. When Golgi cell stains were used to study morphology, the dendrites were found to have reduced branching, especially less tertiary branching. Cell bodies were reduced in size. Central, medial, and cortical involvement of the amygdala was noted. The lateral part of the amygdala was involved only in the highest functioning case (IQ of 105), a boy with the most substantial behavioral difficulties. The medial nucleus of the amygdala (which may be involved in learning from experience) and the mammillary bodies were also reduced in this same case. Bauman concludes that this pattern represents a developmental curtailment in the growth of the limbic brain circuits.

These brain regions are important in processing environmental information, particularly social information. Damage to the amygdala has been linked to impaired recognition of emotion in facial expression (Adolphs et al., 1994) and to deficits in the capacity to recognize the direction of gaze (Allman and Brothers, 1994). Autistic children are inattentive to facial expression of emotion and may not interpret gaze normally. The neuroanatomical studies raise questions about the persistence of fetal circuits into later stages of development, leading to a dysfunctional means of processing information from the environment. That the effects of prenatal anatomical development may not become apparent until the particular circuits are integrated into new systems later in development is consistent with recognition of autistic disorder during the first 3 years of life rather than at birth.

The anatomical findings may relate to brain mechanisms involved in memory formation; both types of memory, representational memory and habit memory, need to be considered in interpreting these regional abnormalities. Habit memory may involve the corpus striatum and related brain regions and develops very early in life. However, representational memory develops later in life, generally in the second year in humans, and its development could be disrupted by these abnormalities.

In the cerebellum, there was a 60% to 90% reduction in Purkinje cells in the neocerebellum. Furthermore, there were abnormalities in the olivary nucleus. In fetal development, the cells from the olivary nucleus migrate prior to 30 weeks' gestation to connect to Purkinje cells in the cortex. These circuits normally attach into a single circuit, but apparently this did not occur in these autistic cases, suggesting the developmental disorder must have occurred prior to 30 weeks' gestation. The anatomical findings are consistent with developmental difficulties in learning, behavior, and emotional development seen in autistic cases. These findings need to be replicated with comparisons made to age-matched and mental age-matched control subjects.

ANIMAL MODELS

Several animal models for autistic disorder have been proposed. The oldest model is the Kluver Bucy syndrome where hypoemotionality, fearlessness, hyperexploration, and hypersexual behavior are produced through lesioning the limbic brain. Another animal model (Mishkin, 1978) is developmentally based and involves combined lesions of the amygdala and hippocampus in neonatal rhesus monkeys. The effects on development are studied following placement of lesions to the brain regions that are involved in memory formation (hippocampus) and in social-emotional behavior (amygdala).

The areas lesioned are two of the regions that were shown to be abnormal in Bauman's autopsy study. The effects of neonatal damage to the monkey's hippocampus and amygdala on later social and emotional behavior was evaluated on three occasions during later development. Disturbances in behavior were evaluated at 2 months, 6 months, and 6 to 7 years. At 2 months, the monkeys are described as passive, showed less exploration of the environment, and demonstrated temper tantrums. No specific abnormal behaviors were demonstrated at 2 months of age. At 6 months, the monkeys were found to be less social than controls. They had begun to explore the environment, had motor stereotypies, and showed a lack of facial expression. When followed up at 6 to 7 years of age, the monkeys continued to show less social behavior. They continued to explore the environment, demonstrated self-directed behavior (stereotypy), and lacked facial expression. Thus it is evident that damage to the limbic system areas involving the amygdala and hippocampus in neonatal monkeys produces long-lasting disturbances in their social and emotional behavior. The effects of neonatal lesions on developmental outcome require careful monitoring.

The Delayed Non-Matching to Sample (DNMS) task was used to evaluate the lesioned monkey. This task involves individual trials where the subject must discriminate between food and nonfood objects to obtain food rewards. There are two phases in each trial, a sample phase and a choice phase. During the sample phase, an object is presented and after a delay the sample object plus another novel object are presented and the subject must choose between them. The choice of a novel object leads to reward, but no reward is given when the other object is chosen. The objects used in the test include items such as toy blocks and jar lids. Mishkin (1978) found there was mild impairment on visual DNMS when either the amygdala or the hippocampus was lesioned. The deficit became severe when both of these brain regions were lesioned. Lesions in those brain regions that link the hippocampus and amygdala to the thalamus involving the fornix and amygdala pathways also led to deficits. When conducting this task with monkeys, Murray and Mishkin (1985) and Bachevalier (1991) found that the combined lesion caused the most severe deficit, the amygdala-alone lesion produced a moderate deficit, and no impairment was noted on this task with only a hippocampal lesion. Similar results were demonstrated on a tactile DNMS task. Therefore, DNMS tasks do provide sensitive measures for damage to the amygdala that are separable from those resulting from damage to the hippocampus.

However, the hippocampus is more involved in environmental tasks relying on spatial cues. A task requiring the use of a place system is the water maze task where a platform is fixed under water in a 5- to 6-ft diameter tank that is filled with cloudy or opaque water. Rats are placed in water at various locations until they learn the location of the platform. Ordinarily, rats will quickly learn the location of the platform and swim toward it, but with hippocampal lesions, they never learn where the platform is located. By contrast, rats with lesions to the amygdala are not impaired on this task. Findings from combined lesions of the hippocampus and amygdala do not differ from lesions only involving the hippocampus in rats.

Linking Animal Studies with Developmental Disorders

Bachevalier and Merjanian (1994) and Merjanian et al. (in press) have used the visual, tactile, and cross-modal DNMS along with a spatial location task, based on the water maze, in children with autistic disorder and Down syndrome.

When autistic and Down syndrome groups were matched for age, sex, and nonverbal mental age, the tactile and cross-modal matching tasks were too difficult to solve. On the visual Delayed Non-Matching to Sample task, there was substantial difference between children with Down syndrome and autistic disorder. The autistic group were superior to the Down syndrome group in dealing with the spatial location task. The authors attributed the differences they found to be related to the genuine abilities of the two groups rather than to attentional, motivational, and general cognitive abilities.

These animal lesion studies demonstrate that behavioral dysfunction may result from lesions to specific brain structures. Lesions of several different structures might lead to the same pathological behavior, and other dysfunctions may cause behaviors similar to those that could result from the lesions in animals. Moreover, the behaviors may be the result of damage to particular structures, but dysfunction results from disruption of functional connections to a neighboring brain area, or dysfunction in a brain system that is disrupted. Behavioral observations might implicate the involvement of particular brain structures in autistic individuals but are not sufficient to identify those structures precisely.

The components in the Delayed Non-Matching to Sample task that may be pertinent to autistic disorder include: (1) recognition memory; and (2) recent memory or sensitivity to novelty. Recent memory is a major component of the visual DNMS task and may be mediated by the amygdala but not the hippocampus. The implication is that a disruption of limbic memory systems in autism may be selective. Many autistic persons show excellent rote memory, possibly related to nonlimbic memory systems, or perhaps due to involvement of only one of the major limbic memory systems. Other forms of memory, such as skill learning or procedural learning, are intact in both the autistic and Down syndrome groups. However, that aspect of autobiographical memory that deals with memory of emotional experiences is not intact.

In summary, animal studies are important in understanding links between autistic behavior and neuroanatomy and provide a way to increase our understanding of lesions that are placed at different times during the developmental period.

MODELS OF AUTISM

Ethological Theory

Tinbergen and Tinbergen (1972) presented an ethological theory of the etiology of autism, based on their work on courting patterns of gulls and observations of young normal children in community settings and in their own homes. The emphasis was on the pattern of behavior related to conflicting emotions produced when a child approaches an adult. The autistic child was considered by them to be overly fearful and to experience conflict based on fear to approach despite a desire for contact. Tinbergen and Tinbergen suggested that social bonding may not occur because this motivational conflict is not resolved and the child remains fearful and overaroused. This overarousal results in stereotyped behavior and the failure of social bond development. Moreover, if the child is not approached in a sensitive manner, the disability may become more permanent. This model has been criticized since the autistic child does not have a normal nervous system, so observations from nonautistic children may not be applicable (Wing and Ricks, 1976).

Also inconsistent with the Tinbergens' approach is the finding that in children with a normal nervous system, studies of social bonding show that environmental deprivation leads to children's becoming indiscriminately and superficially friendly and attention seeking, resulting in a superficial quality to their interpersonal relationships. In addition, the impairment of social bond formation may lead to antisocial behavior. A child whose nervous system is apparently normal shows a different response to that seen in autism, where the child's social awareness is deviant. Moreover, the overarousal hypothesized by Tinbergen and Tinbergen has been difficult to measure or demonstrate.

Social avoidance and anxiety may be secondary consequences of an autistic disorder. Tinbergens' model is perhaps most useful in emphasizing the importance of a sensitive approach for children with developmental disorders who find it difficult to cope with new environmental settings and new people. Their orientation to the person does consider the high-functioning autistic child's social perplexity and, if adapted, could lead to a gentle, but firm, approach to the child rather than one based on strong direction and intimidation. However, their model is not an etiologic one because it does not take into account the neurobiological basis of autistic disorder.

Stereotypical behaviors may be seen in the earliest stages of normal development. At around 4 months of age, children will inspect their hands and fingers, and toddlers and younger children may demonstrate hand and limb flapping and jumping when they become excited, yet these patterns do not persist as occurs in autism. The normal child may also rock before falling asleep, cling to a special toy, produce echolalic speech, be shy and withdraw from strangers, and may even demonstrate some reversal of pronouns. But, in contrast to the autistic child, the normal child demonstrates these patterns of behavior rarely and then only briefly. Moreover, a normal child, unlike an autistic child, has a wide repertoire of other behaviors.

Children with autistic disorder show delays as well as deviance in their development. They may respond to only one component of a complex stimulus and show abnormalities of motor organization that affect their ability to imitate movements and communicative gestures. They show an inability to extract rules from experiences and severe deviance in their language development that affects all modalities of language. The autistic child shows severe impairment in the ability to classify and label experiences and to store ideas in symbolic form. This storage of metaphoric or symbolic information is important because these representations can be drawn into memory to interpret the present situation and plan for the future. Because of these learning difficulties, acquiring rules, developing language, and understanding the context of social relationships occurs by rote rather than through social understanding. New facts may not be associated to past experiences, particularly interpersonal ones.

Neurological Model

Damasio and Maurer (1978) proposed a model of autistic disorder involving the mesolimbic cortex, an area of cortex in the mesial aspect of the frontal and temporal lobe that is neurochemically distinct from adjacent brain regions. This area includes the cingulate gyrus, entorhinal area, perirhinal area, parahippocampal gyrus, and subicular and presubicular regions of the hippocampus. They postulated that impaired motility, communication, goal-directed behavior, attention, and perception could be explained due to dysfunction of this system and closely related areas of the frontal lobe and basal ganglia. These authors proposed that autistic persons and adults with frontal lesions show similarities in goal-directed behavior abnormality. This model stimulated interest among neuropsychologists. Recent studies using neuropsychological tests in autistic individuals do point to executive dysfunction so that the idea of frontal lobe dysfunction and limbic dysfunction should continue to be pursued (Bishop, 1993).

ASSESSMENT

The confirmation of the diagnosis of autistic disorder is generally based on the clinical history and neuropsychiatric interview and observational assessment. A variety of psychometric instruments are available for the assessment of autistic children (Parks, 1988). Among these are the Childhood Autism Rating Scale (CARS), which is made up of 15 scales that include different features of autism (Schopler et al., 1980; Schopler, Reichler, and Renner, 1988). The CARS distinguishes mildly to moderately autistic and severely autistic children. It is based on direct observation of the child. The CARS is useful for research and administrative classification of and for deriving a descriptive summary of the autistic behavior. It should be used in conjunction with diagnostic information from the child's history, and information from home, school, and community. For research purposes, the most comprehensive interview and observation scales are the Autistic Diagnostic Interview (ADI) (LeCouteur et al., 1989a) and the Autism Diagnostic Observation Schedule (ADOS) (Lord, 1988).

Frequently, parents will ask about electrophysiologic studies, neuroimaging, and blood and urine tests to establish a diagnosis. Only a minority of autistic children require extensive testing. The tests are most often done to reassure the family that the condition is not progressive and a known metabolic disorder or neurological condition is not present.

The history focuses on behaviors typically found in autistic children. The themes mentioned include the development of sociability, language, play, the presence of stereotypies, and abnormal responses to sensory stimuli. Although autistic symptoms ordinarily are not related to perinatal difficulties, birth history and history of infections and accidents that may involve the brain must be included in the history. Because of the potential genetic disorder, questions are asked about other family members with autism and other developmental disorders as well as specific psychiatric disorders, such as mood disorders, which have, in some instances, been related to autistic disorder in family studies (Piven et al., 1991b, 1992a).

The physical examination addresses signs of specific disorders that have been associated with autistic-like behavior, such as tuberous sclerosis, congenital rubella, and the fragile X syndrome. The mental status examination is primarily observational for younger children. It begins with attempting to engage the child in meaningful interactions and, for verbal children, in conversation. Assessment for imaginative play with representational toys is important. Although the diagnosis may be apparent in those who are severely affected, for those who are less severely affected, attention must focus on more subtle difficulties in the child's relatedness and play. Gaze avoidance, difficulty in initiating social communication, problems with joint attention, and stereotypies must be evaluated.

Testing should be carried out by an interdisciplinary team to establish the needed interventions. This includes psychological tests and speech and language tests that are done to establish baseline information about the child and to clarify the nature of the deficits. In some instances, a hearing test is necessary because of the complaint of language and speech delays. If the child cannot cooperate in standard behavioral audiometry, then brainstem auditory evoked response measures are carried out.

NEUROPSYCHOLOGICAL TESTING

Kanner (1943) suggested that autistic disorder is inborn, and this judgment is being confirmed by genetic research. The cognitive impairment is thought to be the result of the neurodevelopmental disorder. Pennington (1991) has reviewed the neuropsychological phenotype, including attention/arousal (Dawson and Lewy, 1989a, 1989b), long-term episodic memory (Bachevalier, 1991), executive function, and social cognitive deficits. Some early social cognitive processes are not specifically impaired in autism when compared to mental age controls. These include attachment behavior, self-recognition, person recognition, and differential responses in social situations (Pennington, 1991).

Specific patterns of cognitive and affective development are recognizable in autistic persons. They have uneven profiles on subtests of versions of the WISC and WAIS in contrast to IQ-matched controls. The major differences are on subtests dealing with verbal abstraction, sequencing, visual-spatial skills, and rote memory (Lockyer and Rutter, 1970). These deficits are thought to impair normal language acquisition and social functioning. In contrast to children with specific language delay, social functioning in adulthood is correlated with verbal IQ (Rutter, Mawhood, and Goode, 1991).

Social cognitive functioning has been studied in autistic persons, using the "theory of mind" paradigm (Astington, Harris, and Olson, 1988; Baron-Cohen, Leslie, and Frith, 1985; Leslie, 1987) where metarepresentational deficits are thought to impair an autistic person's comprehension of the mental states of others. Theory of mind refers to the ability of normal children to attribute mental states, i.e., beliefs, desires, and intentions, to themselves and to other people as a way of predicting and making sense of behavior. Autistic individuals may show significantly poorer performance on tests of their understanding of others' beliefs and knowledge. Yet their deficits may not be specific to social cognition; autistic persons also perform poorly on executive function tasks (Chapter 3), such as the Wisconsin Card Sort Test (WCST) and the Tower of Hanoi Test (Ozonoff, Pennington, and Rogers, 1991). These tests are designed to identify an inability or reduced ability to anticipate others' intentions, to systematically plan actions or respond spontaneously to novel events—the types of cognitive deficits that may underlie the disorder. McEvoy, Rogers, and Pennington (1993) suggest frontally mediated executive function abilities are the basis for performance on cognitive tasks, such as joint attention and theory of mind tasks that are unique to an autistic disorder. In nonverbal joint attention, the child uses gestures and eye contact to coordinate attention with another person to share his interest with them—for example, making eye contact and then pointing to a picture in a book. Mundy, Sigman, and Kasari (1994) found that deficits in joint attention were the most pronounced of the deficits in nonverbal communication and were consistently present across developmental levels. Although necessary for performance, executive dysfunction is not necessarily the core neuropsychological deficit in autistic disorder, which may involve affective and social cognitive domains as well.

Kanner's emphasis on disturbances in affective contact has been challenged by this focus on cognitive deficits. In keeping with Kanner, Hobson (1989, 1991) maintains that many problems of autistic children are related to a lack of capacity to form affective contact with others and a lack of ability to develop intimate friendships as they grow older despite their motivation to do so. In addition, they lack creative symbolic play and "flexible, context-sensitive" thinking and language. An autistic person's social problems are not fully accounted for by conceptual impairment in interpersonal understanding, although this may be an essential aspect of autism. Their lack of understanding of others' beliefs and desires may not be an adequate explanation for the quality of their nonverbal communication disorder and relationship difficulties. Severely mentally retarded children with mental ages of less than 3 may be socially responsive despite the absence of metarepresentational ability that becomes established by the mental age of 3 to 4 years.

The underlying neurobiological abnormality may involve both higher level cognitive processes and responses to affective stimuli. The lack of social relatedness in autism may be the result of an inborn incapacity to recognize and respond to emotional state expression in others. This is a difficult hypothesis to evaluate using neuropsychological tests because standard emotional recognition tasks are quite sensitive to cognitive influences. An alternative approach is to assess affective responsivity because individuals who do not understand a social or emotional event may show a decreased affective response.

Most autistic children are impaired in attending to and recognizing simple basic emotions and their expression and show abnormal emotional expression themselves. This may lead to a disturbance of affective contact, that is, a severe disruption in the experience of "interpersonal relations as interpersonal" (Hobson, 1989, 1991). Here, affective refers to the domain where bodily inner coordination and mental inner coordination are linked, and intraindividual forms of expressed bodily feeling are understood between persons as social experience. Stern (1985) has used the term "attunement" to describe these experiences of contact, and Trevarthen (1979) refers to them as "intersubjectivity."

DEVELOPMENTAL ISSUES

The establishment of interactional synchrony between parent and child is a critical component of early development. From 2 months of age onward, nonverbal interchanges between parent and child are stimulated by temporal patterns of spoken conversation. This early affective attunement is thought to be essential to facilitate language development. Interactional synchrony is beginning to be studied systematically in autistic children, based on studies of attunement and intersubjectivity.

DEVELOPMENTAL PERSPECTIVE

Bartak and Rutter (1976) described differences in function between mentally retarded and normally intelligent autistic children. They found that stereotypies occurred more frequently and that the extent of social deficit was greater in the mentally retarded group. Burack and Volkmar (1992) have followed up on these earlier observations and evaluated the development of low- and high-functioning autistic children. Autistic children in this study with an IQ below 50 were described as low functioning and those with an IQ of 50 or more as high functioning. These authors utilize a developmental perspective and discuss the similar sequence hypothesis and the similar structure hypothesis as they apply to autistic disorder. The similar sequence hypothesis addresses developmental sequences within specific developmental domains; the similar structure hypothesis focuses on the relationship among domains of functioning. In autistic disorder, this analysis is complicated by the occurrence of periodic marked developmental regressions with the loss of skills that sometimes may not return. These authors found that for receptive and expressive language communication, there is a similar sequence in their developmental progression. The autistic group did not differ in sequence of development from nonautistic, developmentally disabled peers within the domain of communicative function. Regressions occurred most commonly among the low-functioning autistic cases and may reflect fundamental etiologic differences between the groups. Because of these regressions, continued evaluation of the similar sequence hypothesis is necessary in the low-functioning autistic group of children.

However, the similar structure hypothesis does not apply to autistic individuals. Profiles of adaptive development in autism, when compared to nonautistic developmentally disabled children, show significantly greater scatter among a variety of adaptive behaviors. This was true for both the high- and low-functioning autistic groups. It was hypothesized that the extent of unevenness in development may relate to the degree of organicity (more evident in the lower functioning group). Future studies utilizing the developmental perspective in autism will need to take into account etiology, organic impairment, language skills, and the extent of intellectual functioning. Additional investigation is also needed to study the transition from one developmental stage to the next and to evaluate the extent that developmental milestones have been fully mastered by an autistic individual.

In reviewing the developmental perspective, Burack (1992) raises questions about how to interpret the "theory of mind" hypothesis in autistic disorder. The sequence of the development of skills that are involved in belief attribution or the relationship between belief attribution and general functioning are not discussed in detail in the traditional "theory of mind" hypothesis. However, Baron-Cohen (1992) indicates that there is evidence for both specific developmental delay and developmental deviance in acquisition of theory of mind in autistic disorder and suggests a mixture of deviance and delay, although he notes that longitudinal studies are necessary to clarify these issues. Moreover, Baron-Cohen suggests that "theory of mind" might be modular in that it may be biologically based, be vulnerable to specific damage while other processes remain intact, have distinct information processing characteristics, be domain-specific, and have its own evolutionary history. From a developmental perspective, he suggests the development of "theory of mind" has been hypothesized to begin in the early months of life with the origins of affective understanding, or at 9 to 12 months in the understanding of the relationship between attention and goal, or at 12 to 18 months with the onset of pretend play. A modular description may be compatible with a developmental delay model in which it fails to be "switched on" at the normal time in development but rather is switched on later. A modular model is also compatible with developmental deviance where two different components within a module, which are normally switched on together, but are not, resulting in abnormal modular function. The third alternative is a mixed delay/deviance model that may be most pertinent to the low-functioning autistic group which is most delayed in development.

NATURAL HISTORY

The classically autistic child may have a period of apparently normal early development. However, all elements of the behavioral syndrome have been recognized in the early months of life. Problems with feeding, lack of responsiveness to others, absent anticipatory gestures, and excessive quietness and cooperativeness during infancy have been reported, as have excessive irritability and screaming.

The impairment in autism involves all aspects of language and not only speech. In most autistic children, language development is deviant, with difficulties in both the comprehension of speech as well as the expression of ideas in speech. Autistic persons may be markedly impaired in their vocal and their nonvocal symbolic processes. Yet they may be good at nonsymbolic matching and assembly tasks.

The prognosis of autistic children is based

on intelligence scores and the level of functional language development (Cantwell, Baker, and Rutter, 1978; DeMyer et al., 1973). Language development at 5 years is a useful marker. Verbal and full-scale IQ scores are generally taken as an index of severity of the disorder; however, nonverbal IQ is essential to monitor because there may be discrepancies of 60 or more points between nonverbal and verbal scores in the preschool years. During the school years, academic achievement for the higher functioning group may be benefited by their memory skills. However, the presence of hyperlexia may lead to an overestimate of ability (Whitehouse and Harris, 1984).

Academic achievement and social adaptability may have improved over the past 20 years with the improvement in special education. Venter, Lord, and Schopler (1992) studied 58 high-functioning autistic children over an 8-year period. Verbal skills were the best predictor of social adaptive functioning. Academic achievement was related to intellectual functioning. Early nonverbal IQ showed a positive relationship to outcome. Academic performance was stronger than in previous reports on this study. Academic achievement declines when task demands for abstract reasoning exceed rote memory skills. Despite their academic achievement, high-functioning children may be placed in special education classes for social and emotional disturbances because of their deficits in interpersonal skills. In some instances, high-functioning autistic children who have been mainstreamed in grade school will return to special education during the high school years. Mild and moderately mentally retarded persons benefit from special education with teachers who have special training to understand the functioning of the autistic nervous system.

Approximately 15% to 20% of children who show some autistic behavior in their early years gradually emerge from the autistic phase; some make a relatively good social adjustment, although they may continue to have unusual and eccentric behaviors as adults (DeMyer, 1979; Kanner, 1971; Kanner, Rodriguez, and Ashenden, 1972; Rutter, 1970). Adult adjustment is judged based on independent living and employability. Moderately impaired individuals may work successfully in areas where their careful attention to detail and preoccupations can be channeled into jobs requiring completion of repetitive tasks. In job settings that require the least interaction with others they may be most successful. Other employees who are aware of an obvious disability may help and support them. Achievement by the group who are most successful academically may be limited by their social deficits, particularly by difficulty in language comprehension and poor judgment in social situations. Employers may not appreciate the extent of their limitations in problem solving and social adjustment. Social adjustment requires self-awareness of difference from others by the autistic person and special education programs specifically focused on social, language, and cognitive impairment.

Affective Responses in Autistic Individuals

It is essential to monitor affective development in autistic children (Gillberg, 1992). Aggression toward others, sadness in the context of frustration, and apparent joy is frequently reported. Although fear of specific objects, such as animals, may be expressed, a more general awareness of danger and understanding of dangerous situations is lacking. In general, an enhanced expression of affect precedes the emergence of social awareness of others. On emergence from the autistic phase, social perplexity and social intrusiveness are common. The transition from lack of social awareness and inattention to others is often heralded by exaggerated emotions and behavioral difficulty.

Studies of affect in autistic individuals evaluate their ability to comprehend affect in context (Fein et al., 1992). Autistic persons generally do not attend to faces or utilize information from faces in the same way as others do and may simply respond to faces as perceptual patterns. They may perform better than matched control subjects when faces are shown to them upside down. This suggests the lower portion of the face is used to recognize peers in contrast to normal children who use the upper portion (Langdell, 1978). Moreover, the autistic person's performance declines on these tasks when the mouth and forehead are covered, suggesting they may focus more on the mouth than on the eyes to identify facial expressions. They have more difficulty than IQ-matched mentally retarded persons in matching videotaped segments or pictures of gestures, vocalizations, and understanding the situational context of photographed or drawn pictures of facial expressions (Hobson, 1986a, 1986b). Yet autistic individuals who are matched on receptive language ability with mentally retarded control subjects are able to match photographs based on affect when the whole face is shown to them.

Older subjects who are nonretarded and have emerged from the autistic phase may show little difficulty comprehending emotional content in pictures of faces. Moreover, if given a choice on which cue to use to identify others, autistic children may use items of dress, such as hats, rather than facial expression to do so. Autistic children are less able to imitate an affect when asked to do so, or to imitate an affect demonstrated by another person (Langdell, 1981). Although autistic persons do not process affective and facial stimuli in the same way as others, this could be a comprehension problem. If, for example, an autistic person does not see another person as having feelings or thoughts, then facial expressions may not be meaningful indicators for them.

The autistic child's affective response must be observed in a variety of situations to clarify whether or not these children show a full range of emotions. Langdell (1981) surveyed familiar teachers and caretakers and found that the autistic children observed showed all affects except surprise. However, their affective responses were generally reported to be flat and not contingent on the particular situation observed. In addition, parents have reported that their autistic children's vocalizations were idiosyncratic and can only be understood by those who knew the child. When autistic children's own spontaneous facial expressions are observed—for example, how they respond to their image in a mirror—it was found that less positive affect and less self-consciousness was shown than in control children. Autistic children in the preschool years (age 2 to 4) showed fewer observed intervals of affective response, positive or negative, when interacting with familiar adults than mentally retarded controls (Shapiro and Hertzig, 1991; Snow, Hertzig, and Shapiro, 1987). Observations of how they respond to affective signals when interacting with others in an ambiguous situation is an essential aspect of their assessment. Learning to respond to another's affect may be a major developmental milestone.

THEORETICAL APPROACHES

Despite apparent normal development for the first few months of life, language and social development is deviant in autistic individuals. Yet there are advantages to evaluating the deficits in autism within the framework of normal development. These include deficits in imitation, emotional perception, metarepresentation, intersubjectivity, pragmatics, and symbolic play. The following three general models have been proposed: (1) the metarepresentational deficit hypothesis (Baron-Cohen, Leslie, and Frith, 1985); (2) the emotion theory (Hobson, 1989, 1991); and (3) the intersubjectivity model (Rogers and Pennington, 1991; Sigman, 1989; Stern, 1985; Trevarthen, 1979) (see Figure 9.1–1).

In Figure 9.1–1, the three models, metarepresentational theory, emotion (affective deficit) theory, and intersubjectivity theory, are outlined. In each instance, the relationship between deficits is hypothesized but not yet demonstrated.

Metarepresentational Model

The metarepresentational model is a cognitive model of autism based on a variety of measures of theory of mind. Metarepresentation refers to the ability to decouple primary accurate representations from their objective referents so they may be utilized to pretend or for pretense. These include false belief tasks, appearance reality tests, and storage sequencing tasks. The theory of development of mind (mentalizing) model refers to the ability to predict and explain the behavior of others in terms of the other's mental state, being aware of another's intentions, desires, and beliefs. From the child's point of view, knowing with another person, having wishes in regard to another person, and pretending are aspects of theory of mind.

The ability to understand others' intentions is not manifest at birth and apparently is not explained by learning. At the age of 1 year, infants attend to behavior and internally represent physical states of the world. For example, they can remember what they perceive in the external environment. These are referred to as

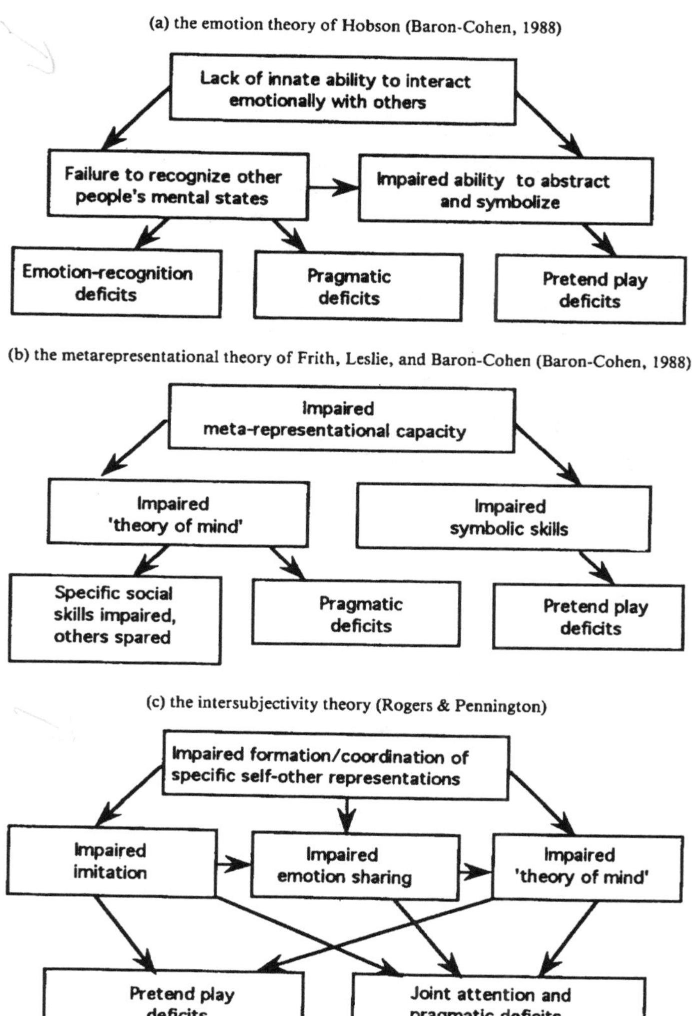

Figure 9.1–1. *Theoretical models of the primary deficits in autism.* These are (a) the emotion theory; (b) the metarepresentational theory; and (c) the intersubjectivity theory (from Rogers and Pennington, 1991).

first-order representations. In the second year of life, a second-order representational ability develops that allows children to represent mental states as well as physical states. This is known as the establishment of representational thought. Children not only attend to the behavior of others, but have the capacity to make sense of others' behavior by anticipating and deducing the other person's underlying mental states. By age 4, children normally acquire an understanding and concept of belief as they come to understand that people have different beliefs, including false beliefs.

About 80% of autistic subjects fail these tasks; about 80% of age-matched mentally retarded controls and mental age-matched or below nonretarded controls succeed. On metarepresentational tasks, autistic children show their difficulty in developing a "theory of others' minds." Such a theory is proposed as necessary to attribute mental states, i.e., thoughts and beliefs, to other people. A deficit in the theory of others' minds may result from a basic cognitive deficit in the ability to form metarepresentations. Metarepresentation refers to second-order representations that are abstractions, i.e., representations of others' mental representations. This theoretical approach assumes an autistic child is capable of developing a primary representation of another person's physical self, or their own physical self, just as a representation of a chair or a desk would be formed. Yet at a higher cognitive level, the autistic child is not able to move to the next step, that of comprehending another's mental state due to a deficit in this secondary representational ability. Consequently, the autistic child may be unable to represent another's mental state in his own mind.

The metarepresentational theory predicts that autistic children will be able to recognize themselves and to recognize others, but are impaired in understanding and making assumptions about another person's internal mental state. One example of the establishment of metarepresentation during development is in the capacity to substitute symbolically one object for another in play (Baron-Cohen, Leslie, and Frith, 1985) as play emerges in the second year of life. The metarepresentation hypothesis has been used to explain deficits in symbolic play, in communication pragmatics, in joint attention, and in theory of mind in autistic subjects.

Rogers and Pennington (1991) raise several questions in a critique of the metarepresentational theory of autistic disorder. First, the metarepresentational theory does not provide an adequate account of deficits in imitation, a capacity that develops earlier than joint attention and symbolic play in infants. Second, they suggest a specific link between metarepresentational ability and symbolic ability has not been proven. Third, metarepresentational theory implies a specific discontinuity in the establishment of a theory of others' minds whereas other developmental theories (Stern, 1985) indicate that development of intersubjectivity is a continuous process. Finally, although metarepresentation has been linked to joint attention by some authors, joint attention is not necessarily related to the establishment of metarepresentation. Therefore, the metarepresentational approach also does not fully account for the presence of sensorimotor imitation, affective deficits, or the possible continuous development of intersubjectivity during development.

Even though metarepresentation does not account for all the developmental abnormalities, a theory of mind deficit may account for certain symptoms of autistic disorder; the majority of young autistic children apparently do have this deficiency. That awareness of others' minds is a special human interpersonal ability is a position that has been taken by ethologists, attachment theorists, philosophers, and object relations theorists.

Emotion (Affective Deficit) Theory

Like Kanner, Hobson and many others suggest that an impairment in affectively patterned, intersubjective personal relations is basic to autism. Hobson (1989) suggests that the autistic child's deficits in symbolic play, cognition, and language result primarily from a problem in affective development that involves constitutionally based emotional reactivity. This includes deficits in emotional expression and perception and an inability to develop reciprocal affectively based relationships with others. Because of these deficits, the autistic child does not develop intersubjective awareness of self and others, which results in the child's failure to recognize other people as people with their own feelings, thoughts, wishes, and intentions. In addition, it leads to a severe impairment in the capacity to think abstractly and symbolically. Others have demonstrated deficits in an autistic person's perception and understanding of affect (Hertzig, Snow, and Sherman, 1989; MacDonald et al., 1989). Specific deficits in expression of the sharing of affect in autistic children, when compared to control groups, include reduced positive affect, increased negative affect, difficulty in recognizing emotional expression, reduced affective response toward a social partner, less use of gaze to communicate affect, and less mirroring of social signals from others, such as smiles. All of these studies have investigated the dynamics of interpersonal interactions. Studies that have found no differences in emotional perception between autistic and control groups have studied emotional perception statically, using verbally matched and

IQ-matched control groups. However, emotional perception deficits have been found in mentally retarded subjects. Consequently, questions have been raised about the primacy of an affective deficit in autism but not about the presence of this deficit in autistic persons.

A critique of the affective deficit hypothesis shows it has difficulty explaining imitation deficits; it should follow that they would be secondary to affective deficits. The research on imitation in infants indicates that their capacity for simple motor imitation occurs before affective development and self–other concepts develop. Moreover, some authors suggest that neonatal imitation precedes the development of self–other awareness. However, these early forms may not be true imitation but rather isopraxis (MacLean, 1990). Affective deficit theory emphasizes the need to incorporate affective deficiency into a theoretical formulation even though there may be disagreements about whether or not it is the primary deficit. Any theory must consider a connection between the development of affective mutuality and the development of awareness of others' minds.

Intersubjectivity Model

Intersubjectivity refers to reciprocal sharing of one's internal subjective experiences, whether or not they are affective or cognitive, with another person through imitative, affective, and communicative modes. In autistic disorder, an intersubjective deficit may be combined with other developmental deficits, such as mental retardation. The intersubjective model posits that the autistic child does not choose to withdraw from the social world or to avoid it, but rather has difficulty in accessing the social world through "physically mirroring affective mutuality," shared meanings and understanding of the interior life of others.

This model further posits that the basis for autism is in the deficient capacity to form or to manipulate particular internal representations of the self and others. These representations are basic to infant body imitation, affective mirroring, and sharing with others as well as awareness of others' subjective states. Rogers and Pennington (1991) suggest that, in normal development, imitation, emotion sharing, and theory of mind develop sequentially. Therefore, in autistic disorder, a deficit in one of these capacities will influence the development of the next. Figure 9.1–1 highlights the hypothetical relationship between primary and secondary deficits. Both imitation and theory of mind abilities are thought to have important roles in the establishment of symbolic play. Moreover, imitation, affect sharing, and theory of mind are all thought to be necessary for the development of joint attention, pragmatic language, and pretend play.

When autistic children are judged in the context of the interpersonal model proposed by Stern (1985), autistic individuals have an impairment in the development of the verbal self; disorders of language are common to all of them. Sigman (1989) suggests the young autistic child apparently does not develop an intersubjective self and has only a partial realization that inner subjective experiences may be shared with others. It is possible that inner subjective experiences may not be shared with others because autistic children do not recognize others have separate minds. This may be related to the autistic child's being unable to experience affective attunement.

In Stern's model, in the earliest phase of life an infant has only subjective experiences of the various internal organizations that are forming. Gradually, through internal and external perceptions, an infant distills and begins to organize the general qualities of experience. This emergent organization is active as the various domains of the self are formed. From 2 to 7 months, the infant develops a sense of a core self and a core other. Basic experiences that lead to the integration of the core self include (1) an impression of coherence among the infant's own experiences and behaviors; (2) a sense of affect as belonging to the infant; (3) memory of the self over a brief period of time; and (4) an initial view of the self as an agent of action. These experiences take place as a consequence of intense social interactions between the infant and others. A sense of a core other develops concurrently through experiences of being with another person who helps to regulate the infant's affect, attention, somatic state, or degree of cognitive engagement. The adult's role as a self-regulating other may allow the infant to construct the sense of an "evoked companion" or to internalize a working model of interpersonal relationships.

The sense of a subjective self begins to emerge between 7 to 9 months of age; the autistic child may show distortions in the sense of self stemming from this developmental period. Stern (1985) states, "The next . . . leap in the sense of self occurs when the infant discovers that he or she has a mind and other people have minds as well . . . infants gradually come upon the momentous realization that inner subjective experiences, subject matter of mind, are potentially sharable with someone else." Therefore, intersubjective relatedness involves not only the sharing of intentions and motives but also an activation of experiences, which includes changes in internal states of arousal and affect. The sharing of interpersonal activation experiences, which has been called "affective attunement" by Stern, results in the infant's sensing forms of feelings based on reference to the subjective state of another person (Sigman, 1989). The behaviors of others can then be recognized as signifying an interior state. The next stage in self-development takes place around 15 to 18 months. Now the child's ability to coordinate sensorimotor schemas with external actions or words allows the child's self to be an object of reflection, to engage in symbolic actions and to acquire language. The infant now is able to establish shared meaning with another about personal knowledge (Sigman, 1989).

For the autistic child, the emergent self appears to have developed, but it is uncertain whether the autistic child forms a core self and a core other in early life. Autistic individuals are able to differentiate between themselves and others and may show some coherence in their sense of themselves and are able to use themselves and others as agents of action as well as demonstrate they have memories of themselves in action; consequently, limited working models of internalized relationships may be developed. Therefore, development of the core self and core other may continue normally in early development until a major developmental distortion occurs related to the intersubjective self.

Failure to form an intersubjective self may be based on cognitive and/or affective deficits. This might involve a modal perception that Stern describes as an innate general capacity to take information from one sensory modality and translate it into another. What may be translated is an encoded amodal representation that might be recognized by the various sensory modalities. In Stern's theory, this amodal information processing is needed to establish the self. It is possible that autistic individuals are limited in their ability for amodal information processing or their lack of affective attunement could be central to an inherent affective unresponsiveness. Although the mechanism of early self-development remains hypothetical, a core 7- to 9-month-old child developmental task apparently is not fully mastered by an autistic child.

The intersubjectivity model acknowledges the importance of sharing of emotions in development and the incorporation of early and later self–other experiences. It incorporates areas not accounted for by the affective and metarepresentational models (Rogers and Pennington, 1991). For example, the affective deficit model does not fully account for the timing and role of the imitation impairment and the development of social processes, such as attachment, and the metarepresentational model does not account for deficits in imitation and in the sharing of emotions. Intersubjectivity theory also differs from the metarepresentational model because these metarepresentational deficits are considered to be primary and discontinuous. Still, intersubjectivity theory recognizes, as does the metarepresentational approach, the importance of having a theory of others' minds as a landmark in social development.

Overall, the intersubjectivity model integrates the major impairments in autistic disorder into a developmental framework. It includes both intact and deficient social skills and integrates other competing theories of autism and thereby accounts for similarities and differences between autistic people and comparison groups throughout development. In addition, it offers an alternative interpretation of the pragmatic and symbolic play deficits in autistic disorder. Each of the theoretical approaches recognizes that social deficits in autistic disorder are primary, long lasting, and reflect dysfunction in the neurobiological mechanisms that underlie human sociability. It is hypothesized that these deficits are linked to proposed dysfunction in the limbic and orbitofrontal brain regions.

TREATMENT

A misunderstanding of the application of psychological treatments has often led to a lack of emphasis on a comprehensive approach to treatment of autistic disorder. It is not the psychogenesis of autism that is the issue, but rather an understanding of the development of the autistic child and the functioning of the autistic nervous system that must be considered in establishing treatment. Programs that are developmentally based, affectively oriented, and tailored to specific known deficits in individual children with autistic disorder and other pervasive developmental disorders may lead to broad and positive changes in development, compensation for areas of deficit, and reduction of autistic symptomatology.

The goals of treatment are then based on the types of disabilities seen in autistic disorder (Howlin and Rutter, 1987). Treatment programs must be sensitive to the needs and perceptions of the autistic child (Simons and Sabine, 1987) and provide guidance to parents (Wing, 1985). The primary goal is to foster normal development and, in doing so, one must take into account what is known about the normal developmental process and also what is known about abnormal development in autistic disorder that interferes with the normal developmental process. The general goal is to focus on mechanisms that underlie normal growth and maturation to facilitate them but concurrently recognize that autistic features interfere. Even though the neurobiological basis of autistic disorder is well recognized and anatomic features are becoming increasingly apparent, intervention still may be effective in helping children compensate for their developmental deficits. Rutter (1983) suggests four general aims in the treatment of the autistic person: to promote cognitive development, to promote language development, to promote social development, and to promote overall learning. In addition to these, behavior reduction and behavior enhancement strategies are necessary, as is appropriate use of pharmacological interventions.

Cognitive development is promoted through the facilitation of active, meaningful experiences. Problems that are identified are self-isolation, which may be approached through planned periods of interaction; impaired understanding, which requires simplified communication and individualized treatment approaches; lack of initiative for social interaction, which requires structured direct learning experiences; and specific cognitive deficits, which must be targeted by the choice of appropriate learning tasks. Reduced cognitive capacity is also an issue and requires intervention that focuses on direct teaching at the appropriate developmental level.

Language development is enhanced through social/conversational exchanges to deal with social isolation and the lack of social reciprocity. Planned periods of interaction should be scheduled to promote social development. The problem with social reciprocity is addressed by emphasizing exercises that involve joint attention which structure reciprocal language exchange. The deficit in social communication or in pragmatic language difficulty leads to the problem of failure to use language socially. Direct teaching is necessary to teach the social use of language along with differential reinforcement and a focus on communication rather than simply focusing on speech. Pragmatic language involves teaching turn taking and other aspects of social communication. Language development may be limited and, consequently, direct teaching must emphasize the child's level of language comprehension. Moreover, the use of alternative modes is necessary, such as the use of signing. Treatment interventions will increase the use of language.

Promotion of social development requires intense personal interaction that is positive, comforting, and pleasurable to the child. The lack of social approach and lack of social reciprocity in social interaction require structured settings with intrusiveness on the part of the examiner to help the child remain focused on the social exchange. Here again, joint attentional exercises are necessary where the adult gets the child's attention and then requires the child to gesture or point to items that are needed and is encouraged to show things to the examiner. Personal caretaking may be problematic, particularly if the child is outside of the home and has not been instructed in personal hygiene and other aspects of personal care. A systematic program in social skills as they relate to personal care is required. The lack of social awareness characteristic of autistic disorder is addressed through direct teaching of skills that lead to social competence as well as early interpersonal programs, such as that described by Rogers and Pennington (1991).

A general approach to learning is necessary. First, the attention to environmental cues is essential. Because autistic children lack self-direction, structured learning is needed with an effort to break down learning tasks into small steps. There may be interference in remaining on task in the environment because of deviant behaviors that may require concomitant behavior reduction strategies. Moreover, autistic children often are overselective in their choice of activities, and considerable effort may be necessary to keep them on task after becoming aware of their specific interests. Generalization of learning to new situations is particularly important and requires that context specificity be considered. The focus is on natural environments at home and at school, limited use of residential treatment, and structure to facilitate generalization from one situation to another. A central problem in promoting learning is the autistic child's difficulty in understanding the meaningfulness of events. Their comprehension deficit requires that the teaching staff monitor learning carefully and focus on meaningfulness of events. Finally, lack of persistence to cope with challenges and the adversive response the child shows to failure require that, as much as possible, the environment provide error-free learning.

The basic principles of behavior modification are utilized in the treatment of autism. However, behavioral techniques must be developed based on a clear understanding of the deficits and the types of abnormal behavior associated with autistic disorder because these will determine what can be changed and the best approach to the patient. Attempts to use behavior management techniques without taking into account the specific characteristics of the autistic nervous system may lead to difficulty and potentially might result in failure or worsening of the autistic person's behavior. Moreover, the environment must often be adapted to the autistic person rather than expecting the autistic individual to adapt to it. The nature of the autistic deficit makes adaptability and generalization of targeted behaviors across settings difficult. A stable environmental context is necessary for treatment, and once this environment is established, it should not be changed without careful consideration of the contingencies that led to improvement.

When behavioral difficulties develop, the first step is to determine whether they are the result of environmental factors, which might include excessive social contact, excessive demand for change, or difficulty with staff who do not appreciate the individual characteristics of the autistic person. Stereotypies, which are characteristic in autistic disorder, may themselves be used as reinforcers as part of the behavioral program. It is often helpful to find a context for these behavioral patterns.

Behavior management strategies are utilized to eliminate nonspecific maladaptive behaviors. The behavioral approach is based on a functional analysis of behavior and application of learning theory. A careful functional analysis takes into account the possible role of medication, intercurrent illnesses, and seizure disorder. It involves a careful evaluation of preceding circumstances that increase or decrease the likelihood of the occurrence of a maladaptive behavior together with an analysis of succeeding circumstances that seem to be associated with either diminution or prolongation of the behavior. To employ a behavioral technique, it is essential to determine which environmental features influence a behavior, not in children in general but in this particular child.

For the most severely involved autistic persons, behavioral approaches are based on operant conditioning procedures rather than on cognitive understanding of rewards. For individuals who are less impaired, consequences are better understood and token economies may be established. Still, generalization may be limited so it is extremely important to address the individual's understanding regardless of level of intelligence.

The types of behavior most commonly targeted in behavior management programs are aggression and self-injurious behavior. For these and other disruptive behaviors, avoidance of precipitants, provision of help to establish coping skills, and differential reinforcement may be used as interventions. Differential reinforcement involves feedback to the child, rewards for positive behaviors, and behavior reduction procedures for negative behaviors. Fears may be addressed through controlled exposure, with desensitization, modeling, and the teaching of coping skills to deal with them.

The role of the parent is crucial for intervention with the autistic child. The parent has often been described as co-therapist and has an integral role in treatment. Parent counseling begins with clarification of the diagnosis and an explanation of the characteristics of an autistic disorder. A detailed history is appreciated because it may be reassuring to the parent to know that perplexing behaviors they have observed in their child are part of a known disorder. Schopler et al. (1984) have provided recommendations for working with parents derived from their experience in their TEACCH (*T*reatment and *E*ducation of *A*utistic and related *C*ommunication handicapped *CH*ildren) program.

Interpersonal Approaches to Treatment

The treatment approach to autistic disorder, based on the intersubjectivity model, must take into account the child's age and developmental level. The treatment model for preschool autistic children must incorporate the development of interpersonal relationships, pragmatic language development, the establishment of symbolic thought, and the use of play techniques.

Rogers and Lewis (1989) have developed a day treatment model for autistic children ages 2 through 6 based on the intersubjectivity model. Their emphasis is on providing positive affective experiences to aid in the development of interpersonal relationships, the use of pragmatic language therapy offered in a structured and predictable school setting, and the provision of these services through the medium of play. Play is emphasized as providing a means to facilitate assimilation and generalization of social-emotional, cognitive, and communicative skills just as it does for nonimpaired children. Adult–child social relationships are promoted through a specific adult working with an individual child on activities. The 1 to 1 adult–child contact, involving social games and reciprocal interactions, is essential to maintain attention and engagement. Other social relationships that must be encouraged focus on peer awareness and close proximity during play between children. The adult's role is to direct the autistic child's attention to their peers' activities. If conflicts between children emerge, the adult provides verbal and behavioral "scripts" to facilitate negotiation and problem solving. Moreover, the effect of one child's behavior on another is explicitly stated to highlight what has occurred. In adult–child interactions, positive affect is essential to enhance the child's attention to specific experiences and particularly to motivate them to continue activities. Close proximity facilitates imitation, is more likely to provide meaning to learning experiences, and may result in relationships that are pleasing to both adult and child.

Because communication difficulties are part of the diagnostic profile, adults working with autistic children must utilize reactive language strategies (Weiss, 1981). Using this approach, the adults interpret the child's potential verbal communicative and nonverbal gestural behaviors at the child's developmental level. This includes clarification and explanation about children's feelings, actions, apparent desires, and responses, which are then reflected back to them, taking into account the child's developmental language level. Those children lacking in speech are taught simple signs from the American Sign Language System, and preverbal gestures are used or prompted. Consistency is essential and repetition critical in teaching communication.

Because the transition from sensorimotor intelligence to representational, or symbolic, intelligence is essential for language development and is particularly impaired in these children, educationally oriented activities that demand mental representation are incorporated into the program. This includes activities organized around the establishment of symbolic play and preoperational grouping activities.

Play, adult–child social relationships, stimulation of positive affective experiences, communicative training, and an emphasis on representational thinking is carried out in a structured classroom with a well-developed daily routine. The social structure and the physical arrangements and the rhythm of the day's activities are used to provide an external structure to facilitate self-regulation and to help the child mediate, select, focus, and organize sensory stimulation. Distractors are identified for each child by evaluating activities with respect to their primary goals. Sensory stimulation is reduced when it becomes apparent the child is sensitive to that sensory modality. The treatment programs are provided by child psychiatrists, speech and language therapists, occupational therapists, and clinical child psychologists, who work with teachers in the classroom and develop individualized treatment programs for each child.

This comprehensive approach is an alternative to a strict behavior management approach, which focuses on acquisition of specific skills. The behavioral approach is ordinarily not developmentally oriented and may fail to recognize and target the specific deficits of an individual autistic child or place those targeted skills in a clearly meaningful developmental framework. If development is not considered in the establishment of treatment goals, then isolated skills may be trained that do not generalize well to other situations or to other skills. The comprehensive preschool approach emphasizes the individual child's specific deficits and takes into account symbolic processes, social relationships, and communication, and provides a structured environment to help remediate and compensate for them. The goal is to establish and promote developmental change.

Rogers and Lewis (1989) have evaluated this treatment model and demonstrated change in cognitive, communicative, social-emotional, perceptual-motor, and motor domains, using the early intervention profile and preschool profile (Schafer and Moersch, 1981), the Play-Observation Scale (Rogers et al., 1986), and the Childhood Autism Rating Scale (CARS) (Schopler et al., 1980). Of particular importance was the finding that ratings of symbolic play were significantly improved, although the effects were relatively modest. These changes are important because symbolic activities of autistic children are related to their cognitive and communicative abilities as they grow older. In addition, the symbolic play occurs in the context of environmental exploration of both the physical and social world. The enhancement of these skills over time is expected to facilitate long-term outcome.

Moreover, social relatedness improved using this approach. In the evaluation, the elements that were most essential were sensitivity by the adult to the child's verbal and nonverbal communications, structured social reciprocal interactions with the child, an emphasis on positive affective experiences, and the use of play in interaction with the child. This approach needs to be carried out in autistic children who are randomly assigned to other treatment modalities for comparison. Long-term follow-up is needed to evaluate the impact of treatment.

For the older verbal child who has emerged from the autistic phase and is socially perplexed, a social cognitive approach based on the intersubjectivity and metarepresentational deficits may be helpful. Intersubjectivity may be conceptualized as an appreciation of self–other representations and the ability to put oneself in the place of another person and empathetically respond. Issues that relate to understanding others' minds may be interpreted for the higher functioning child in the context of affective awareness. It is not uncommon for older and higher functioning autistic individuals to complain they are not able to read other people's thoughts and have difficulty anticipating the response of others to their overtures. The autistic person may find it difficult to gauge the depth of another's feeling about something, yet they may recognize the feeling state itself in the other person.

If mental state concepts can be taught, then specific instruction might be given to the autistic person on how to cope socially, i.e., social survival skills. Treatment based on the theory of mind approach might focus on compensating for, and remediation of, possible insensitivity to others' feelings, inability to take into account what other people know during a conversation, inability to read others' intentions, inability to appreciate the listener's level of interest in one's own conversation directed toward them, and inability to anticipate what others might think of one's actions.

Difficulties in reading others' intentions may make the autistic person the brunt of jokes by others; the autistic person may not appreciate when he or she is being teased or deceived after complying without question to an inappropriate request. Difficulty with reading the listener's level of interest in one's speech may lead to boring monologues about the limited special interests of the autistic person. Often autistic individuals are unaware that others do not share their enthusiasm for topics that interest them. An inability to anticipate others' responses to one's actions is seen frequently in the social interactions of autistic people.

Baron-Cohen and Howlin (1993) provide examples of some communicative errors; they list unwanted and inappropriate comments about personal appearance that may be interpreted by others as personal insensitivity (rather than curiosity based on simple observation), a lack of sense of the personal space of others, and requesting information that might be viewed as intimate by others. An inability to consider what other people know in conversation is demonstrated by a lack of understanding that another individual's experience is different from their own. The autistic person must be taught that when referring to events, the provision of background information for the other person is essential in order to establish a context.

An approach to teaching is to break down mental state understanding into simple principles to be taught through intensive training. For the nonautistic child, these principles do not need to be explicitly taught. Baron-Cohen and Howlin (1993) suggest the following fundamental basic principles be taught to autistic persons about mental states through the use of stories and discussion about their life experiences:

1. *Perception causes knowledge.* An individual will know that something happened only if it was seen or heard. This approach can be applied by introducing stories where the central character does not know that something has happened unless he actually saw that it occurred.
2. *Desires are satisfied by actions or objects.* If a person wants something, he will look to obtain it, but if he does not want it, he will refuse or avoid it. In children's stories, for example, if the children want their parents they will look for them, and when unpleasant problems occur, as when someone is chasing them, they will move away.
3. *Pretense involves object substitution or outcome suspension.* If a person pretends something will happen, he may do so to solve a problem or for fun. An example is when someone pretends an object is another thing, e.g., when a child pretends a block is a car.
4. *Deception involves making someone think something is false.* For example, if someone needs something, they may not try to obtain it directly, but use indirect means.
5. *Understanding emotion involves an awareness* that someone carries out a particular behavior based on how they are feeling at the time. For example, if someone is grieving, their crying means they are sad.

Teaching of mental state concepts requires that the autistic person has attained the mental age when these concepts are normally acquired, the mental age of at least 3½ to 4 years. Teaching how beliefs, desires, new knowledge, pretense, deception, and emotion are experienced by another person may involve a variety of techniques, including imaginative play with figurines, drama, explanation, pictures, the use of computer graphics, and the use of television.

Pharmacotherapy

There is no specific pharmacological treatment for the core deficits of autistic disorder. However, particular behavior syndromes and symptoms are targeted for medication use. These include attention deficits, hyperactivity, aggression, affective lability, compulsive behavior, self-injurious behavior, depression, psychotic symptoms, and depression. Before instituting pharmacotherapy, it is essential that the underlying basis for the target behavior be identified.

Attention deficit disorder may be diagnosed in some autistic children and teenagers. Although there has been confusion about the benefits of using stimulants (Aman and Singh, 1988), some autistic children do respond well to them, although side effects must be carefully monitored. Moreover, heterocyclic antidepressants may also be helpful for attention deficit symptoms. Clonidine has been successfully utilized for some characteristics of attention deficit disorder in autistic children (Fankhauser et al., 1992; Jaselskis et al., 1992).

Low doses of neuroleptics have been prescribed for severe overactivity, aggression, and for brief reactive and schizophreniform psychosis. Campbell et al. (1985) and Anderson et al. (1989) have demonstrated the effectiveness of low-dose neuroleptics and the absence of severe, long-term effects when low doses were utilized. Locascio et al. (1991) found that reduction in symptoms during short-term haloperidol treatment was not related to whether or not children developed dyskinesias in later long-term haloperidol administration. Malone et al. (1991) evaluated 14 autistic children who developed repeated haloperidol-related dyskinesias while participating in a long-term maintenance clinical trial. The dyskinesias tended to occur earlier and to last longer with subsequent introduction of medication. The dyskinesias were seen most commonly when haloperidol was withdrawn. Care is needed in the use of neuroleptics because autistic disorder is a lifelong condition and the risk of tardive dyskinesia must be considered, particularly when higher doses are used (Campbell et al., 1990a). The neuroleptics may be necessary to maintain a child with severe aggressive symptoms in his school program but should be used on a short-term basis.

Two other medications that have been used in the treatment of autistic disorder are buspirone (Realmuto, August, and Garfinkel, 1989) and propranolol (Ratey et al., 1987). Both medications have been used to deal with aggression and anxiety in autistic children; however, controlled studies are needed to clarify their efficacy.

Clomipramine (Gordon et al., 1993) has been shown to be superior to placebo and desipramine in reducing anger and compulsive and ritualistic behavior. Clomipramine was equal to desipramine and both drugs were superior to placebo in reducing hyperactivity. These results suggest controlled trials of other serotonin reuptake inhibitors, such as fluoxetine and sertraline, in the treatment of compulsive and ritualistic behavior because the latter medications have fewer side effects.

Mood stabilizers, such as lithium (Gadow, 1992) and carbamazepine, have been used to treat mood disorders and aggressive behavior that is related to mood lability. Smith and Perry (1992) emphasize that the primary indication for carbamazepine is for seizure disorders. Finally, naltrexone, an opium antagonist, has been successfully used as an adjunctive treatment for autistic children (Campbell et al., 1989; Campbell et al., 1990b). However, it is less effective than low doses of neuroleptics for target symptoms of aggression and impulsivity. In choosing the use of an opiate antagonist, it is important to consider sensory abnormalities in the autistic child. Because the opiate receptors are sensory neurotransmitters, some children will have an enhancement of their sensitivity to sound as a side effect of the use of naltrexone. Although naltrexone has been used for treatment of self-injurious behavior in autistic persons, to date results regarding its effectiveness are inconclusive.

FUTURE DIRECTIONS

Substantial progress has been made since autistic disorder was first described over fifty years ago by Leo Kanner; however, much remains to be done. Future research may emphasize genetic aspects, refinements in classification, identification of better diagnostic techniques, and new treatments. Better characterization of cases is essential to conduct genetic studies that will be benefited by a better understanding of underlying pathophysiological mechanisms involved in social cognition. Advances in neuroimaging, particularly in MRI, fMRI, and PET scanning, may be helpful in the characterization of subtypes.

REFERENCES

Adophs, R., Tranel, D., Damasio, H., and Damasio, A. (1994). Impaired recognition of emotion in facial expressions following bilateral damage to the human amygdala. *Nature,* 372:669–672.

Aicardi, J. (1986). *Epilepsy in children.* Raven Press, New York.

Allman, J., and Brothers, L. (1994). Faces, fear and the amygdala. *Nature,* 372:613–614.

Aman, M.G., and Singh, N.N. (eds.). (1988). *Psychopharmacology of the developmental disabilities.* Springer-Verlag, New York.

American Psychiatric Association, Committee on Nomenclature and Statistics. (1980). *Diagnostic and statistical manual of mental disorders,* 3rd ed. Author, Washington, DC.

American Psychiatric Association, Committee on Nomenclature and Statistics. (1987). *Diagnostic and statistical manual of mental disorders,* 3rd ed, revised. Author, Washington, DC.

American Psychiatric Association, Committee on Nomenclature and Statistics. (1994). *Diagnostic and statistical manual of mental disorders,* 4th ed. Author, Washington, DC.

Anderson, G.M., Volkmar, F.R., Hoder, E.L., McPhedran, P., Minderaa, R.B., Young, J.G., Hansen, C.R., and Cohen, D.J. (1987). Whole blood serotonin in autistic and normal subjects. *Journal of Child Psychiatry and Psychology,* 28:885–900.

Anderson, L.T., Campbell, M., Adams, P., Small, A.M., Perry, R., and Shell, J. (1989). The effects of haloperidol on discrimination learning and behavioral symptoms in autistic children. *Journal of Autism and Developmental Disorders,* 19: 227–239.

Asperger, H. (1944). 'Autistic psychopathy' in childhood. In U. Frith (ed.), *Autism and Asperger syndrome.* Cambridge University Press, New York.

Astington, J.W., Harris, P.L., and Olson, D.R. (eds.). (1988). *Developing theories of mind.* Cambridge University Press, New York.

Bachevalier, J. (1991). An animal model for childhood autism: Memory loss and socio-emotional disturbances following neonatal damage to the limbic system in monkeys. In C.A. Tamminga and S.C. Schulz (eds.), *Advances in neuropsychiatry and psychopharmacology,* Vol. 1, pp. 129–140. Raven Press, New York.

Bachevalier, J., and Merjanian, P. (1994). The contribution of medial temporal lobe structures in infantile autism: A neurobehavioral study in primates. In M.L. Bauman and T.L. Kemper (eds.). *The Neurobiology of Autism,* pp. 146–169, Johns Hopkins University Press, Baltimore, MD.

Bailey, A.J. (1993). The biology of autism. (Editorial). *Psychological Medicine,* 23:7–11.

Baron-Cohen, S. (1992). Debate and argument: On modularity and development in autism: A reply to Burack. *Journal of Child Psychology and Psychiatry,* 33: 623–629.

______, Allen, J., and Gillberg, C. (1992). Can autism be detected at 18 months? The needle, the haystack and the CHAT. *British Journal of Psychiatry,* 161:839–843.

______, and Howlin, P. (1993). The theory of mind deficit in autism: Some questions for teaching and diagnosis. In S. Baron-Cohen, H. Tager-Flusberg and D. Cohen (eds.), *Understanding other minds: Perspectives from autism.* Oxford University Press, New York.

______, Leslie, A., and Frith, U. (1985). Does the autistic child have a 'theory of mind'? *Cognition,* 21:37–46.

Bartak, L., and Rutter, M. (1976). Differences between mentally retarded and normally intelligent autistic children. *Journal of Autism and Childhood Schizophrenia,* 6:109–120.

Bauman, M.L. (1991). Microscopic neuroanatomic abnormalities in autism. *Pediatrics,* 87, Part 2 Supplement, pp. 791–796.

______, and Kemper, T.L. (1994). Neuroanatomic observations of the brain in autism. In M.L. Bauman and T.L. Kemper (eds.), *The Neurobiology of Autism,* pp. 119–145, Johns Hopkins University Press, Baltimore, MD.

Bishop, D.V.M. (1993). Autism, executive function, and theory of mind: A neuropsychological perspective. *Journal of Child Psychology and Psychiatry,* 34:279–293.

Burack, J.A. (1992). Debate and argument: Clarifying developmental issues in the study of autism. *Journal of Child Psychology and Psychiatry,* 33:617–621.

______, and Volkmar, F.R. (1992). Development of low- and high-functioning autistic children. *Journal of Child Psychology and Psychiatry,* 33:607–616.

Campbell, M., Anderson, L.T., Small, A.M., Locascio, J.J., Lynch, N.S., and Choroco, M.C. (1990b). Naltrexone in autistic children: A double-blind and placebo-controlled study. *Psychopharmacology Bulletin,* 26:130–135.

______, Locascio, J.J., Choroco, M.C., Spencer, E.K., Malone, R.P., Kafantaris, V., and Overall, J.E. (1990a). Stereotypies and tardive dyskinesia: Abnormal movements in autistic children. *Psychopharmacology Bulletin,* 26:260–266.

______, Overall, J.E., Small, A.M., Sokol, M.S., Spencer, E.K., Adams, P., Foltz, R.L., Monti, K.M., Perry, R., Nobler, M., and Roberts, E. (1989). Naltrexone in autistic children: An acute open dose range tolerance trial. *Journal of the American Academy of Child and Adolescent Psychiatry,* 28:200–206.

______, Small, A.M., Perry, R., and Green, W.H. (1985). Pharmacotherapy in infantile autism: Efficacy and safety. In C. Shagass, R.C. Josiassen, W.H. Bridger, K.J. Weiss, D. Stoff, and G.M. Simpson (eds.), *Biological psychiatry,* pp. 1489–1491. Elsevier, New York.

Cantwell, D.P., Baker, L., and Rutter, M. (1978). A comparative study of infantile autism and specific developmental receptive language disorder: IV. Analysis of syntax and language function. *Journal of Child Psychology and Psychiatry,* 19:351–363.

Coleman, M., and Gillberg, C. (1985). *The biology of the autistic syndromes.* Praeger, New York.

Cook, E. (1990). Autism: Review of neurochemical investigation. *Synapse,* 6:292–308.

Courchesne, E. (1991). Neuroanatomic imaging in autism. *Pediatrics,* 87, Part 2 Supplement, pp. 781–790.

Damasio, R., and Maurer, R. (1978). A neurological model for childhood autism. *Archives of Neurology,* 35:777–786.

Dawson, G., and Lewy, A. (1989a). Arousal, attention, and socioemotional impairments of individuals with autism. In G. Dawson (ed.), *Autism: Nature, diagnosis and treatment,* pp. 49–74. The Guilford Press, New York.

______, and ______. (1989b). Reciprocal subcortical-cortical influences in autism. In G. Dawson (ed.), *Autism: Nature, diagnosis and treatment,* pp. 144–173. The Guilford Press, New York.

DeMyer, M.K. (1979). *Parents and children in autism.* V.H. Winston and Sons, Washington, DC.

______, Barton, S., DeMyer, W.E., Norton, J.A., Allen, J., and Steel, R. (1973). Prognosis in autism: A follow-up study. *Journal of Autism and Childhood Schizophrenia,* 3:199–245.

DeVolder, A., Bol, A., Michel, C., Congneau, M., and Goffinet, A.M. (1987). Brain glucose metabolism in children with the autistic syndrome: Positron tomography analysis. *Brain Development,* 9:581–587.

Fankhauser, M.P., Karumanchi, V.C., German, M. L., Yates. A., and Karumanchi, S.D. (1992). A double-blind, placebo-controlled study of the efficacy of transdermal clonidine in autism. *Journal of Clinical Psychiatry,* 53:77–82.

Fein, D., Lucci, D., Braverman, M., and Waterhouse, L. (1992). Comprehension of affect in context in children with pervasive developmental disorders. *Journal of Child Psychology and Psychiatry,* 33:1157–1167.

Folstein, S.E., and Piven, J. (1991). The etiology of autism: Genetic influences. *Pediatrics,* 87, Part 2 Supplement, pp. 767–773.

______, and Rutter, M. (1977). Infantile autism: A genetic study of 21 twin pairs. *Journal of Psychology and Psychiatry,* 18:297–321.

______, and ______. (1988). Autism: Familial aggregation and genetic implications. *Journal of Autism and Developmental Disorders,* 18:3–30.

Gadow, K.D. (1992). Pediatric psychopharmacotherapy: A review of recent research. *Journal of Child Psychology and Psychiatry,* 33:153–195.

Gillberg, C.L. (1992). Autism and autistic-like conditions: Subclasses among disorders of empathy. The Emanuel Miller Memorial Lecture 1991. *Journal of Child Psychology and Psychiatry,* 33:813–842.

Gordon, C.T., State, R.C., Nelson, J.E., Hamburger, S.D., and Rapoport. J.L. (1993). A double-blind comparison of clomipramine, desipramine, and placebo in the treatment of autistic disorder. *Archives of General Psychiatry,* 50:441–447.

Herald, S., Frackowiak, R.S.J., LeCouteur, A., Rutter, M., and Howlin, P. (1988). Cerebral blood flow and metabolism of oxygen and glucose in young autistic adults. *Psychological Medicine,* 16:823–831.

Hertzig, M.E., Snow, M.E., and Sherman, M. (1989). Affect and cognition in autism. *Journal of the American Academy of Child and Adolescent Psychiatry,* 28:195–199.

Hobson, P. (1986a). The autistic child's appraisal of emotion. *Journal of Child Psychology and Psychiatry,* 27:321–342.

______. (1986b). The autistic child's appraisal of expressions of emotion. *Journal of Child Psychology and Psychiatry,* 27:671–680.

______. (1989). Beyond cognition: A theory of autism. In G. Dawson (ed.), *Autism: Nature, diagnosis and treatment,* pp. 22–48. The Guilford Press, New York.

Hobson, R.P. (1991). What is autism? *Psychiatric Clinics of North America,* 14:1–18.

Horwitz, B., Rumsey, J.M., and Grady, C. (1987). Interregional correlations of glucose utilization among brain regions in autistic adults. *Annals of Neurology,* 22:118.

Hoshino, Y., Ohno, Y., Yamamoto, T., Tachibana, R., Murata, S., Yokoyama, F., Kaneko, M., and Kamashiro, H. (1984). Dexamethasone suppression test in autistic children. *Japanese Journal of Clinical Psychiatry,* 26:100–102.

Howlin, P., and Rutter, M. (1987). *Treatment of autistic children.* John Wiley and Sons, New York.

Jaselskis, C.A., Cook, E.H., Jr., Fletcher, K.E., and Leventhal, B.L. (1992). Clonidine treatment of hyperactive and impulsive children with autistic disorder. *Journal of Clinical Pharmacology,* 12:322–327.

Kanner, L. (1943). Autistic disturbances of affective contact. *The Nervous Child,* 2:217–250.

______. (1971). Follow-up study of eleven autistic children originally reported in 1943. *Journal of Autism and Childhood Schizophrenia,* 1:119–145.

______, Rodriguez, A., and Ashenden, B. (1972). How far can autistic children go in matters of social adaptation? *Journal of Autism and Developmental Disorders,* 2:9–33.

Landa, R., Folstein, S.E., and Isaacs, C. (1991). Spontaneous narrative discourse performance of parents of autistic individuals. *Journal of Speech and Hearing Research,* 34:1339–1345.

______, Piven, J., Wzorek, M.M., Gayle, J.O., Chase, G.A., and Folstein, S.E. (1992). Social language use in parents of autistic individuals. *Psychological Medicine,* 22:245–254.

Landau, W.M., and Kleffner, F.R. (1957). Syndrome of acquired aphasia with convulsive disorder in children. *Neurology,* 7:523–530.

Langdell, T. (1978). Recognition of faces: An approach to the study of autism. *Journal of Child Psychology and Psychiatry,* 19:255–268.

______. (1981). *Face perception: An approach to the study of autism.* Unpublished doctoral dissertation, University of London.

LeCouteur, A., Bailey, A., and Rutter, M. (1989b). *Epidemiologically based twin study of autism.* Paper presented at the First World Congress on Psychiatric Genetics, Cambridge, England.

______, Rutter, M., Lord, C., Rios, P., Robertson, S., Holdgrafter, M., and MacLellan, J. (1989a). Autism Diagnostic Interview: A standardized investigator-based instrument. *Journal of Autism and Developmental Disorders,* 19:363–387.

Leslie, A.M. (1987). Pretense and representation:

The origins of 'Theory of Mind.' *Psychological Review*, 94:412–426.

Locascio, J.J., Malone, R.P., Small, A.M, Kafantaris, V., Ernst, M., Lynch, N.S., Overall, J.E., and Campbell, M. (1991). Factors related to haloperidol response and dyskinesias in autistic children. *Psychopharmacology Bulletin*, 27:119–126.

Lockyer, L., and Rutter, M. (1970). A five to fifteen year follow-up study of infantile psychosis: IV. Patterns of cognitive ability. *British Journal of Social and Clinical Psychology*, 9:152–163.

Lord, C. (1988). Autism Diagnostic Observation Schedule. *Journal of Autism and Developmental Disorders*, 19:185–212.

______, Schopler, E., and Revicki, D. (1982). Sex differences in autism. *Journal of Autism and Developmental Disorders*, 12:317–330.

MacDonald, H., Rutter, M., Howlin, P., Rios, P., LeCouteur, A., Evered, C., and Folstein, S. (1989). Recognition and expression of emotional cues by autistic and normal adults. *Journal of Child Psychology and Psychiatry*, 30:865–877.

MacLean, P.D. (1990). *The triune brain in evolution.* Plenum Press, New York.

Malone, R.P., Ernst, M., Godfrey, K.A., Locascio, J.J., and Campbell., M. (1991). Repeated episodes of neuroleptic-related dyskinesias in autistic children. *Psychopharmacology Bulletin*, 27:113–117.

McEvoy, R.E., Rogers, S.J., and Pennington, B.F. (1993). Executive function and social communication deficits in young autistic children. *Journal of Child Psychology and Psychiatry*, 34:563–578.

Merjanian, P.M., Nadel, L., Jans, D.S., and Granger, D.A. (in press). Involvement of the amygdala and hippocampus in autism: Review and empirical test.

Minshew, N., Pettegrew, J.W., Goldstein, G., Phillips, N.E., and Weldy, S.R. (1991). Correlations between in vivo brain phospholipid and high energy phosphate metabolism and cognitive functioning in autism. *Biological Psychiatry*, 29, 48A.

______, and Rattan, A.I. (1992). The clinical syndrome of autism. Developmental and acquired disorders of childhood. In I. Rapin and S.J. Segalowitz (eds.), *Handbook of neuropsychology: Vol 6. Child neuropsychology*, pp. 401–441. Elsevier Science Publishers, Amsterdam.

Mishkin, M. (1978). Memory in monkeys severely impaired by combined but not by separate removal of amygdala and hippocampus. *Nature*, 273:297–298.

Mundy, P., Sigman, M., and Kasari, C. (1994). Joint attention, developmental level, and symptom presentation in autism. *Development and Psychopathology*, 6:389–401.

Murray, E.A., and Mishkin, M. (1985). Amygdalectomy impairs crossmodal association in monkeys. *Science*, 228:604–606.

National Society for Autistic Children. (1978). National Society for Autistic Children definition of the syndrome of autism. *Journal of Autism and Developmental Disorders*, 8:162–167.

Nelson, K.B. (1991). Prenatal and perinatal factors in the etiology of autism. *Pediatrics*, Part 2 Supplement, 87:761–766.

Ozonoff, S., Pennington, B.F., and Rogers, S.J. (1991). Executive function deficits in high functioning autistic individuals: Relationship to theory of mind. *Journal of Child Psychology and Psychiatry*, 32:1081–1105.

Parks, S. L. (1988). Psychometric instruments available for the diagnosis and assessment of autistic children. In E. Schopler and G. Mesibov (eds.), *Diagnostic and assessment in autism.* Plenum Press, New York.

Pennington, B.F. (1991). Autism spectrum disorder. In B.F. Pennington, *Diagnosing learning disorders: A neuropsychological framework*, pp. 135–166. The Guilford Press, New York.

Piven, J., Berthier, M., Startstein, S., Nehme, E., Pearlson, G., and Folstein, S. (1990a). Magnetic resonance imaging evidence for a defect of cerebral cortical development in autism. *American Journal of Psychiatry*, 147:734–739.

______, Gayle, J., Chase, G.A., Fink, B., Landa, R., Wzorek, M.M., and Folstein, S.E. (1990b). A family history study of neuropsychiatric disorders in the adult siblings of autistic individuals [see comments]. Comments in *Journal of the American Academy of Child and Adolescent Psychiatry*, 31(2):370–371; *Journal of the American of Child and Adolescent Psychiatry*, 29:177–183.

______, Landa, R., Wzorek, M., and Folstein, S. (1991a). The prevalence of fragile X in a sample of autistic individuals diagnosed using a standardized interview. *Journal of the American Academy of Child and Adolescent Psychiatry*, 30:825–830.

______, Chase, G. A., Landa, R., Wzorek, M., Gayle, J., Cloud, D., and Folstein, S. (1992a). Psychiatric disorders in the parents of autistic individuals. See comments in *Journal of the American Academy of Child and Adolescent Psychiatry*, 31:370–371. *Journal of the American Academy of Child and Adolescent Psychiatry* (1991) 30:471–478.

______, Chase, G.A., Landa, R., Wzorek, M., Gayle, J., Cloud, D., and Folstein, S. (1991b). Psychiatric disorders in the parents of autistic individuals. *Journal of the American Academy of Child and Adolescent Psychiatry*, 30:471–478.

______, Nehme, E., Simon, J., Barta, P., Pearlson, G., and Folstein, S.E. (1992b). Magnetic resonance imaging in autism: Measurement of the cerebellum, pons, and fourth ventricle. *Biological Psychiatry,* 31:491–504.

______, Tsai, G.C., Nehme, E., Coyle, J.T., Chase, G.A., and Folstein, S.E. (1991c). Platelet serotonin, a possible marker for familial autism. *Journal of Autism and Child Development,* 21:51–9.

Rapin, I. (1991). Autistic children: Diagnosis and clinical features. *Pediatrics,* 87, Part 2 Supplement, pp. 651–760.

Ratey, J.J., Bemporad, J., Sorgi, P., Bick, P., Polakoff, S., O'Driscoll, G., and Mikkelsen, E. (1987). Open trial effects of beta-blockers on speech and social behaviors in 8 autistic adults. *Journal of Autism and Developmental Disorders,* 17:439–446.

Raymond, G., Bauman, M., and Kemper, T. (1989). The hippocampus in autism: Golgi analysis. *Annals of Neurology,* 26:483–484.

Realmuto, G.M., August, G.J., and Garfinkel, B.D. (1989). Clinical effect of buspirone in autistic children. *Psychopharmacology,* 9:122–125.

Ritvo, E.R., Ritvo, R., Yuwiler, A., Brothers, A., Freeman, B.J., and Plotkin, S. (1993). Elevated daytime melatonin concentrations in autism: A pilot study. *European Child and Adolescent Psychiatry,* 2:75–78.

Rogers, S.J., and Lewis, H. (1989). An effective day treatment model for young children with pervasive developmental disorder. *Journal of the American Academy of Child and Adolescent Psychiatry,* 28:207–214.

______, Herbison, J., Lewis, H., Pantone, J., and Reis, K. (1986). An approach for enhancing the symbolic, communicative, and interpersonal functioning of young children with autism and severe emotional handicaps. *Journal of the Division of Early Childhood,* 10:135–148.

______, and Pennington, B.F. (1991). A theoretical approach to the deficits in infantile autism. *Development and Psychopathology,* 3:137–162.

Rumsey, J., Duara, K., Grady, C., Rapoport, J.L., Margolin, R.A., Rapoport, S.I., and Cutler, N.R. (1985). Brain metabolism in autism: Resting cerebral glucose utilization as measured with positron emission tomography (PET). *Archives of General Psychiatry,* 42:448–455.

Rutter, M. (1970). Autistic children: Infancy to adulthood. *Seminars in Psychiatry,* 2:435–450.

______. (1972). Childhood schizophrenia reconsidered. *Journal of Autism and Childhood Schizophrenia,* 2:315–338.

______. (1978). Autism: Diagnosis and definition. In M. Rutter and E. Schopler (eds.), *Autism: A reappraisal of concepts and treatment,* pp. 1–25. Plenum Press, New York.

______. (1983). The treatment of autistic children. *Journal of Child Psychology and Psychiatry,* 26:193–214.

______, M., Mawhood, L., and Goode, S. (1991, April). *Adult follow-up of boys with autism or with a specific developmental disorder of receptive language (SDLD).* Paper presented at SRCD symposium on "Understanding the nature of autism from considering the course of development," Seattle.

Schafer, D.S., and Moersch, M.S. (eds.). (1981). *Developmental programming for infants and young children.* University of Michigan Press, Ann Arbor.

Schopler, E., Mesibov, G.B., Shigley, R.H., and Bashford, A. (1984). Helping autistic children through their parents: The TEACCH model. In E. Schopler and G.B. Mesibov (eds.), *The effects of autism on the family.* Plenum Press, New York.

______, Reichler, R., DeVillis, R., and Daly, K. (1980). Toward objective classification of childhood autism: Childhood Autism Rating Scale (CARS). *Journal of Autism and Developmental Disorders,* 10:91–103.

______, and Renner, B.R. (1988). *The Childhood Autism Rating Scale (CARS).* Western Psychological, Los Angeles.

Shapiro, T., and Hertzig, M.E. (1991). Social deviance in autism: A central integrative failure as a model for social nonengagement. In M.M. Konstantareas and J.H. Beitchman (eds.), *Pervasive developmental disorders,* pp. 19–33. W. B. Saunders Company, Philadelphia.

Sigman, M. (1989). The application of developmental knowledge to a clinical problem: The study of childhood autism. In D. Cicchetti (ed.), *The emergence of a discipline: Rochester Symposium on Developmental Psychopathology,* Vol. 1. Erlbaum, Hillsdale, NJ.

Simons, J., and Sabine, O. (1987). *The hidden child: The Linwood method for reaching the autistic child.* Woodbine House, Baltimore.

Smalley, S., Asarnow, R., and Spence, M. (1988). Autism and genetics: A decade of research. *Archives of General Psychiatry,* 45:953–961.

Smith, D.A., and Perry, P.J. (1992). Nonneuroleptic treatment of disruptive behavior in organic mental syndromes. *Annals of Pharmacotherapy,* 26:1400–1408.

Snow, M.E., Hertzig, M.E., and Shapiro, T. (1987). Expressions of emotion in young autistic children. *Journal of the American Academy of Child and Adolescent Psychiatry,* 26:836–838.

Steffenburg, S., Gillberg, C., Hellgren, L., Andersson, L., Gillberg, I., Jakobsson, G., and Bohman, M. (1989). A twin study of autism in Denmark, Finland, Iceland, Norway and Sweden. *Journal of Child Psychology and Psychiatry,* 30:405–416.

Stern, D.N. (1985). *The interpersonal world of the*

infant: A view from psychoanalysis and developmental psychology. Basic Books, New York.

Taft, L.T., and Cohen, H.J. (1971). Hypsarrhythmia and infantile autism. *Journal of Autism and Childhood Schizophrenia,* 1:327–336.

Tinbergen, E.A., and Tinbergen, N. (1972). Early childhood autism: An ethological approach. *Beihefte zur Zeitshrift für Tierpsychologie,* no. 10.

Trevarthen, C. (1979). Communication and cooperation in early infancy. A description of primary intersubjectivity. In M. Bullowa (ed.), *Before speech: The beginnings of human communication,* pp. 321–346. Cambridge University Press, Cambridge.

Tuchman, R.F., Rapin, I., and Shjinnar, S. (1989). Epilepsy in children with developmental language and autistic spectrum disorders. *Epilepsia,* 30:732.

Venter, A., Lord, C., and Schopler, E. (1992). A follow-up study of high-functioning autistic children. *Journal of Child Psychology and Psychiatry,* 33:489–507.

Volkmar, F.R., Bregman, J., Cohen, D.J., and Cicchetti, D.V. (1988). DSM-III and DSM-III-R diagnoses of autism. *American Journal of Psychiatry,* 145:1404–1408.

______, Cicchetti, D.V., Cohen, D.J, and Bregman, J., (1992a). Brief Report: Developmental aspects of DSM-IIIR criteria for autism. *Journal of Autism and Developmental Disorders,* 22:657–662.

______, ______, Bregman, J., and Cohen, D.J. (1992b). Three diagnostic systems for autism: DSM-III, DSM-III-R, and ICD-10. *Journal of Autism and Developmental Disorders,* 22:483–492.

______, Stier, D.M., and Cohen, D.C. (1985). Age of recognition of pervasive developmental disorder. *American Journal of Psychiatry,* 142:1450–1452.

Weiss, R. (1981). INREAL intervention for language handicapped and bilingual children. *Journal of the Division of Early Childhood,* 4:40–51.

Whitehouse, D.W., and Harris, J. (1984). Hyperlexia in infantile autism. *Journal of Autism and Developmental Disorders,* 11:31–44.

Wing, L. (1985). *A guide for parents and professionals.* Brunner/Mazel, New York.

______. (1993). The definition and prevalence of autism: A review. *European Child and Adolescent Psychiatry,* 2:61–74.

______, and Gould, J. (1979). Severe impairments of social interaction and associated abnormalities in children: Epidemiology and classification. *Journal of Autism and Developmental Disorders,* 9:11–29.

______, and Ricks, D.M. (1976). The aetiology of childhood autism: A criticism of the Tinbergens' ethological theory. *Psychological Medicine,* 6:533–543.

World Health Organization. (1992). *The ICD-10 classification of mental and behavioural disorders: Clinical descriptions and diagnostic guidelines.* Author, Geneva.

9.2 Asperger's Disorder

In 1944, the year following Kanner's original description of autistic disturbance of affective contact, Asperger identified a syndrome of social isolation in combination with odd and eccentric behavior that he labeled "autistic psychopathy." Although "autistic psychopathy" was used to indicate an abnormality of personality, this usage has led to some misunderstanding because, in English, psychopathy is generally associated with sociopathic behavior. To avoid misunderstanding, the eponym "Asperger's disorder" has been retained and included in the DSM-IV (APA, 1994) and ICD-10 (WHO, 1992) classifications.

In this section, the history, definition, epidemiology, etiology, relationship to autistic disorder, natural history, and treatment of Asperger's disorder will be reviewed.

HISTORY

In Asperger's studies (1944) of how children form groups, he suggested the failure to form a group was not based on intelligence but on not having a relationship with others, in "lack of contact" in establishing interpersonal relations. In the syndrome he described, Asperger stressed the children's failure to understand others' emotional expression and lack of understanding of how their own emotional expressions were uninterpretable by peers.

In Asperger's original description, he stated, "The children I will present all have in common a fundamental disturbance which manifests itself in their physical appearance, expressive functioning, and in their whole behavior. This disturbance results in severe and characteristic difficulties of social integration. In many cases, the social problems are so profound, they overshadow everything else." Asperger went on to say that the problems are compensated, in some instances, by a high level of original thought that may lead to exceptional achievements in later life. He viewed this syndrome as a type of personality disorder and suggested these children are exceptional human beings who must be given an exceptional education that takes into account their special difficulties. He went on to say that, despite their abnormality, they can fulfill their social role in the community if they find appropriate understanding, love, and guidance.

Despite Asperger's early description, during intervening years most clinical and research interests have focused on autistic disorder, rather than Asperger's disorder. Wing's (1981) paper was instrumental in renewing an interest in Asperger's disorder. Others (Frith, 1991; Tantam, 1988), following her lead, began to emphasize diagnosis, natural history, and treatment. Until the publication of Frith's monograph in 1991, Asperger's landmark paper was only available to the German-speaking reader.

DEFINITION

The decision to include Asperger's disorder in the U.S. Diagnostic and Statistical Manual for Mental Disorders (DSM-IV) and the International Classification of Diseases (ICD-10) psychiatric classification took place over a decade after infantile autism was introduced into the classification in 1980. The DSM-IV recommended criteria for Asperger's disorder are listed in Table 9.2–1.

Schopler (1985) has objected to the introduction of criteria for a disorder involving what might be regarded as the "autistic continuum" and suggests it may lead to diagnostic confusion. Although Wing (1991) agrees there may be an autistic continuum, she suggests several reasons for including Asperger's disorder as a separate entity.

First, the diagnosis of autistic disorder, in the minds of many in the general population, seems synonymous with a most severe disorder involving lack of speech, social isolation, lack of eye contact, hyperactivity, and preoccupation with stereotypies. Moreover, autistic disorder may occur in children with various levels of developmental disability; at least 75% of children with autistic disorder test in the mentally retarded ranges whereas children with Asperger's disorder test in the normal range. Additionally, the basic impairments in autistic disorder have not been clarified. Families often overlook or reject the diagnosis of autistic disorder if their children have better developed language and social abilities. Therefore, the use of another term, "Asperger's disorder," is appropriate as a designation for higher functioning individuals with social deficits.

Secondly, including Asperger's disorder as a separate entity encourages the identification of the genetic aspects that may be specific to this disorder. Thirdly, psychiatrists who work with adults tend to have a narrow view of the clinical picture of the autistic spectrum. The recent recognition of Asperger's disorder in adults has led to increasingly detailed characterization of cases (Tantum, Holmes, and Cordess, 1993) and renewed interest in identifying better means of intervention. It has also led to the recognition that an "autistic-like" person with normal intelligence may be undiagnosed in childhood.

It would seem appropriate to find new diagnostic terms rather than using an eponym for this disorder. "Kanner's syndrome" was used as the diagnostic category for many years and has now been abandoned for the diagnostic term "autistic disorder." With further refinements in classification, perhaps a better descriptive designation will be developed to describe what is now referred to as "Asperger's disorder."

EPIDEMIOLOGY

The general population prevalence of Asperger's disorder is unknown because of the lack of availability of large-scale epidemiologic studies. The syndrome appears to be considerably more common in boys than in girls and does not seen to be associated with social class or level of education of the parents (Wing, 1981). With the inclusion of this category in the diagnostic classification, epidemiologic studies can now be planned to identify prevalence rates in the general population (Gillberg and Gillberg, 1989).

Wing and Gould (1979) studied all mentally and physically disabled children under age 15 in an area of London to identify early childhood

Table 9.2–1. DSM-IV Diagnostic Criteria for Asperger's Disorder

299.80 Asperger's Disorder

A. Qualitative impairment in social interaction, as manifested by at least two of the following:
   (1) marked impairment in the use of multiple nonverbal behaviors such as eye-to-eye gaze, facial expression, body postures, and gestures to regulate social interaction
   (2) failure to develop peer relationships appropriate to developmental level
   (3) a lack of spontaneous seeking to share enjoyment, interests, or achievements with other people (e.g., by a lack of showing, bring ing, or pointing out objects of interest to other people)
   (4) lack of social or emotional reciprocity

B. Restricted, repetitive and stereotyped patterns of behavior, interests, and activities, as manifested by at least one of the following:
   (1) encompassing preoccupation with one or more stereotyped and restricted patterns of interest that is abnormal either in intensity or focus
   (2) apparently inflexible adherence to specific, nonfunctional routines or rituals
   (3) stereotyped and repetitive motor mannerisms (e.g., hand or finger flapping or twisting, or complex whole- body movements)
   (4) persistent preoccupation with parts of objects

C. The disturbance causes clinically significant impairment in social, occupational, or other important areas of functioning.

D. There is no clinically significant general delay in language (e.g., single words used by age 2 years, communicative phrases used by age 3 years).

E. There is no clinically significant delay in cognitive development or in the development of age-appropriate self-help skills, adaptive behavior (other than in social interaction), and curiosity about the environment in childhood.

F. Criteria are not met for another specific Pervasive Developmental Disorder or Schizophrenia.

From APA, 1994.

psychosis and severe mental retardation. They found two cases (0.6 in 10,000) that showed most of the characteristics of Asperger's disorder and four other cases (1.1 in 10,000) who had autistic characteristics in early life and later resembled Asperger's disorder. The authors point out that this study probably provides an underestimate of cases.

Their study raises two issues that must be taken into account in future epidemiologic studies. First, the two patients who were indentified were in the mildly mentally retarded range on cognitive testing. Asperger's original description was of children with normal intelligence; this requirement for normal cognitive functioning is included in DSM-IV diagnostic criteria. Secondly, the four additional cases they described had an early history that was typical of autistic disorder, yet Asperger described a different natural history for his population. Moreover, social-class variables need to be considered. Finally, the age of recognition will need to be taken into account because less severe cases of Asperger's disorder may not be recognized until adolescence.

ETIOLOGY

Genetics

Asperger felt the syndrome he identified was genetically transmitted, further noting the characteristics tended to cluster in families, especially the fathers of those with the syndrome (Wing, 1981). In regard to familial patterns, Ghaziuddin et al. (1993) have reported the diagnosis of Asperger's disorder in three siblings, using the ICD-10 criteria. In this family study, the authors proposed that Asperger's disorder may occur as a distinct clinical entity without overlapping with autistic disorder. This family report along with neuropsychological data provide further support for Asperger's disorder being pursued as a separate entity. Future genetic studies require more detailed evaluation of other family members. Twin pairs have also been identified.

Cases of Asperger's disorder have been reported that are associated with Tourette's syndrome (Kerbeshian and Burd, 1986), aminoaciduria (Miles and Capelle, 1987), and ligamentous laxity (Tantam, Evered, and Hersov, 1990). Morever, Gillberg (1989) found a variety of neurological abnormalities in 60% of 23 patients with Asperger's disorder. However, Asperger's original focus seems to have been on an idiopathic form without other identifiable disorders.

Laboratory Studies and Neuropathology

Tantam (1991) reports abnormal CT scans and EEGs in approximately one third of cases he studied. These findings will have to be pursued in a larger number of subjects. Detailed neuropathological studies are not available.

COMPARISON OF AUTISTIC DISORDER AND ASPERGER'S DISORDER

Since Asperger's (1944) original description of "autistic psychopathy," similarities have been reported to cases with autistic disorder. Although Asperger's disorder shares features with other disorders, including social-emotional learning disability Klin (et al., in press) (Chapter 7.5) and schizoid personality disorder (Wolff and Barlow, 1979), it is ordinarily categorized on the autistic continuum, yet there has been disagreement whether Asperger's disorder has clinical features sufficiently different from high-functioning autistic disorder to require a different name (Szatmari et al., 1986, Klin, 1994), or whether it is the same phenomenologically as high-functioning autistic disorder. However, there are some characteristic differences between the two disorders.

Intelligence

Asperger's cases tested in the normal range of intelligence, frequently had special abilities, first showed symptoms in the third year of life, and developed grammatical speech. Does higher cognitive functioning account for the differences? Autistic persons with intelligence in the normal range have fewer unusual responses to the environment, more normalized play, and more extensive interests, yet there are apparent differences in the clinical course of the two conditions (Bartak and Rutter, 1976).

Severity of Symptoms

Asperger considered that the children he described were not as disturbed as those with autistic disorder. The outcome of Asperger's disorder is generally good in contrast to autistic disorder where a good prognosis is seen in only 5% to 19% of cases (DeMyer, Hingtgen, and Jackson, 1981). The issue of severity raises the question: Which symptoms should be considered in comparing severity? Are there fundamental autistic symptoms found in both disorders, and are symptoms of equal severity in both conditions? Social impairments in both disorders do persist into adulthood even when language and interests have changed.

Interpersonal and Language Development

Gillberg (1991), in reviewing family studies of Asperger's disorder, finds a reduced capacity for an empathetic understanding of other people and odd, all-absorbing interests. In Asperger's disorder, the early development of attachment may not be quite normal, and there may be some abnormalities in language development. These abnormalities may be different in degree and distinct from the striking distortions in social and language development that are observed in an autistic disorder.

Motor Disorder

Unlike most persons with autistic disorder, those with Asperger's disorder tend to be clumsy, lack coordination of movement, and may have an awkward gait. Although individuals with autistic disorder may have motor skill difficulties, those with Asperger's disorder tend to show more striking motoric involvement (Ghaziuddin, Tsai, and Ghaziuddin, 1992).

Natural History

When the early history and outcome of children with Asperger's disorder were contrasted with those of high-functioning children with autistic disorder (Szatmari, Bartolucci, and Bremner, 1989), the high-functioning autistic individuals' histories showed more impairment in social responsiveness, communication, and restricted range of activities than those of the individuals with Asperger's disorder. There were also other differences between groups in that despite having the same IQ as the high-functioning individuals with autistic disorder, those with Asperger's disorder spent fewer years in special education. When cognitive profiles of children with Asperger's disorder and high-functioning autistic disorder were matched on verbal performance and full-scale IQ (Szatmari et al., 1990), there were few differences on standard intelligence achievement and neuropsychological tests. The Asperger's disorder group had higher WISC-R similarity scores than the high-functioning autistic disorder group, whereas the performance of the high-functioning autistic disorder group was greater than that of the Asperger's group on a test of motor speed and coordination. This study was complicated by the fact that the authors did not match the groups on mental age. Because the mental age of the high-functioning subjects with autistic disorder was significantly greater than that of the Asperger's cases, the lack of group difference might be accounted for by these differences in IQ score.

Neuropsychological Testing

A neuropsychological distinction has been suggested between autistic disorder and Asperger's disorder based on finding "theory of mind deficits" in an autistic disorder group (Ozonoff, Pennington, and Rogers, 1991) but not in a comparison group with Asperger's disorder. In this study, which must be replicated, the Asperger 's syndrome cases did show abnormality on an emotional perception task. These findings along with reports of multiple cases of Asperger's in one family (Ghaziuddin et al., 1993), and a different natural history, suggest a distinction between Asperger's disorder and autistic disorder.

Few empirical studies of neuropsychological test profiles in Asperger's disorder have been conducted and these have been confounded because of the confusion about the diagnostic categorization in case selection. Various studies have used different criteria to diagnose cases and assign them to groups, making it difficult to compare and interpret the results of these studies. Bowler (1989) found no group differences between adults with Asperger's disorder and adults with schizophrenia who were matched by IQ and nondisabled controls, using theory of mind tests. Deficits of metarepresentation, or theory of mind, have been found in autistic disorder.

Ozonoff, Rogers, and Pennington (1991) expanded the battery of tests of high-functioning autistic and Asperger's disorder individuals to include intellectual, neuropsychological, and social cognitive tests in patients who were matched on age, sex, and verbal IQ. The authors asked whether or not the neuropsychological profiles of Asperger's disorder and high-functioning autistic disorder were different, what deficits appear primary to Asperger's and high-functioning autistic disorder, and if the group shares a common primary deficit.

In making these comparisons, the Asperger's disorder group showed fewer autistic symptoms on the CARS than the high-functioning autistic disorder group and also had a significantly higher verbal intelligence score. There was a large discrepancy between verbal and performance IQ in the high-functioning autistic disorder group, which was not demonstrated in the Asperger's disorder group.

Analyses of the neuropsychological variables provided evidence for a subtype distinction. Each group was compared to a matched control group, direct comparisons were made between the two groups on neuropsychological tests, and a discriminate function analysis was carried out of the groups. A multivariate comparison was made of the neuropsychological profiles which showed that relative to matched controls, the high-functioning autistic disorder group performed poorly on executive function, verbal memory, and theory of mind tests. However, the Asperger's group differed from controls only on tests involving executive function and emotional perception, but did not show difficulties in theory of mind or in verbal memory. When the high-functioning autistic disorder and Asperger's groups were compared, the Asperger's disorder group performed better than the high-functioning autistic disorder group on theory of mind composite tests and verbal memory. An overall comparison of the two groups suggested that the better developed abilities in each group were among the least developed for the other group.

The discriminate function analysis results also suggested an empirical distinction between the high-functioning autistic disorder and the Asperger's disorder groups. The authors report that 80% of the high-functioning autistic disorder group and 70% of the Asperger's subjects were correctly classified. The best discrimination was in the theory of mind domain. These results confirm that the two syndromes can be distinguished with reasonable accuracy, but require additional validation by other investigators.

In regard to the primary deficit for the two groups, in the high-functioning autistic disorder group, deficits were widespread and involved executive function, second order theory of mind, and, particularly, verbal memory. For the Asperger's group executive function and emotional-perceptual deficits were found across subjects. No one particular deficit was found to be primary to each group. The only composite neuropsychological test scores wherein both groups were deficient was in executive function. Therefore, executive function measures rather than theory of mind measures are most similar for the two groups. The major difference between the Ozonoff, Rogers, and Pennington (1991) study and that of Szatmari et al. (1990) is that the first authors' cases had a higher mental age, and the domain which may be the most important to differentiate between the groups, theory of mind, was not tested in the Szatmari et al. study.

In summary, individuals with Asperger's disorder, unlike those with autistic disorder, can perform well on theory of mind tests and do not demonstrate verbal memory deficits that are found in high-functioning autistic subjects. In the future, additional research is needed that focuses on whether subjects with autistic disorder and those with Asperger's disorder respond differently to treatment and have a different prognosis. The distinction of Asperger's disorder from high-functioning autistic disorder is important in identifying homogeneous subgroups of patients for research studies. Autistic disorder is recognized as a heterogeneous condition with a variety of subtypes. The designation of Asperger's disorder as distinct is important for future epidemiologic and outcome studies. One question that remains from the Ozonoff et al. study is the clarification of early history in designating future cases. In their study, several cases had been identified with a diagnosis of autistic disorder or pervasive developmental disorder (PDD) and showed language deficits characteristic of those groups in early childhood. Therefore, half of their subjects showed progressive developmental progression from autistic symptomatology to Asperger's disorder. However, Szatmari et al. did not find any Asperger's disorder cases with a previous diagnosis of autistic disorder or PDD early in childhood. These investigations emphasize the importance of taking the early history into account in evaluating pervasive developmental disorder presentations.

MECHANISM OF SOCIAL DYSFUNCTION

The absence of theory of mind deficits in individuals with Asperger's disorder raises questions about the mechanism for their social dysfunction. Their peculiar preoccupations, lack of reciprocity in social interactions, and pragmatic language deficits have, in the past, been considered to be secondary to abnormalities related to theory of mind. An alternative explanation for their social deficit is that the combination of emotional perception and executive function problems could have led to a pragmatic and prosodic abnormality, possibly related to right hemispheric dysfunction. The narrow focus of interests may be tied to their executive function impairments, which might result in preoccupations and social communicative deficits. However, subjects with Asperger's disorder might be deficient in making inferences about others' mental states, but use strategies other than those based on the theory of mind strategies to make mental state attribution.

A final possibility is that theory of mind tests

are not sufficiently sensitive to detect deficits in high-functioning individuals. Other strategies may be helpful in identifying social deficits, which include role-taking measures that require a more naturalistic setting to evaluate social deficits in individuals with Asperger's disorder. Continued investigations of the mechanisms involved in Asperger's disorder may help to clarify the neuropsychological processing difficulties that underlie social communicative deficits.

TREATMENT

Individuals with social deficits have an increased vulnerability to psychiatric disorders; the lack of recognition of their developmental disorder may complicate their treatment by attributing a psychodynamic etiology to neurobiologically based symptoms.

The treatment of the social deficit in Asperger's disorder follows the same principles outlined for the social cognitive treatment of social-emotional learning disability (Chapter 7.5) and teaching mental state concepts (Chapter 9.1).

Tantam (1991) reported that 35% of 85 adult cases with Asperger's disorder had a major psychiatric diagnosis. The majority had mood disorders, but schizophrenia and obsessive compulsive disorder were also reported. Co-occurring mental illnesses should be treated, using appropriate drug therapy.

REFERENCES

American Psychiatric Association, Committee on Nomenclature and Statistics. (1994). *Diagnostic and statistical manual of mental Disorders,* 4th ed. Author, Washington, DC.

Asperger, H. (1944). Die "Autistischen psychopathen" im kindesalter. *Archiv für Psychiatrie und Nervenkrankheiten,* 117:76–136. Translated as `Autistic psychopathy' in childhood. In U. Frith (ed.), (1991), *Autism and Asperger syndrome,* pp. 37–92. Cambridge University Press, New York.

Bartak, L., and Rutter, M. (1976). Differences between mentally retarded and normally intelligent autistic children. *Journal of Autism and Childhood Schizophrenia,* 6:109–120.

Bowler, D.M. (1989, December). *Theory of mind in Asperger's disorder.* Paper presented at the London Conference of the British Psychological Society, London.

DeMyer, M.K., Hingtgen, J.N., and Jackson, R.K. (1981). Infantile autism reviewed: A decade of research. *Schizophrenia Bulletin,* 7:388–451.

Frith, U. (1991). *Autism and Asperger disorder.* Cambridge University Press, Cambridge.

Ghaziuddin, M., Metler, L., Ghaziuddin, N., Tsai, L., and Giordani, B. (1993). Three siblings with Asperger syndrome: A family case study. *European Child and Adolescent Psychiatry,* 2:44–49.

______, Tsai, L., and Ghaziuddin, N. (1992). A reappraisal of clumsiness as a diagnostic feature of Asperger syndrome. *Journal of Autism and Developmental Disorders,* 22:651–656.

Gillberg, C. (1989). Asperger syndrome in 23 Swedish children. *Developmental Medicine and Child Neurology,* 31:520–531.

______. (1991). Clinical and neurobiological aspects of Asperger syndrome in six family studies. In U. Frith (ed.), *Autism and Asperger syndrome,* pp. 122–146. Cambridge University Press, Cambridge.

______, and Gillberg, C. (1989). Asperger syndrome: Some epidemiological considerations: A research note. *Journal of Child Psychology and Psychiatry,* 30:631–638.

Kerbeshian, J., and Burd, L. (1986). Asperger's disorder and Tourette syndrome. *British Journal of Psychiatry,* 148:731–735.

Klin, A. (1994). Asperger syndrome. *Child and Adolescent Clinics of North America,* 3:131–148.

______, Volkmar, F.R., Sparrow, S.S., Cicchett, D.V., and Rourke, B.P. (in press). Validity and neurophysiological characterization of Asperger syndrome: Convergence with nonverbal learning disabilities syndrome. *Journal of Child Psychology and Psychiatry.*

Miles, S.W., and Capelle, P. (1987). Asperger's disorder and aminoaciduria: A case example. *British Journal of Psychiatry,* 147:397–399.

Ozonoff, S., Pennington, B.F., and Rogers, S.J. (1991). Executive function deficits in high-functioning autistic individuals: Relationship to theory of mind. *Journal of Child Psychology and Psychiatry,* 32:1081–1105.

______, Rogers, S.J., and Pennington, B.F. (1991). Asperger's disorder: Evidence of an empirical distinction from high-functioning autism. *Journal of Child Psychology and Psychiatry,* 132:1107–1122.

Schopler, E. (1985). Convergence of learning disability, higher-level autism, and Asperger's disorder. *Journal of Autism and Developmental Disorders,* 15:359.

Szatmari, P., Bartolucci, G., Finlayson, A., and Krames, L. (1986). A vote for Asperger's disorder. *Journal of Autism and Developmental Disorders,* 16:515–517.

_____, _____, and Bremner, R. (1989). Asperger's disorder and autism: Comparisons on early history and outcome. *Developmental Medicine and Child Neurology,* 31:709–720.

______, Brenner, R., and Nagy, J. (1989). Asperger's disorder: A review of clinical features. *Canadian Journal of Psychiatry,* 34:554–560.

______, Tuff, L., Finlayson, M.A.J., and Bartolucci, G. (1990). Asperger's disorder and autism: Neurocognitive aspects. *Journal of the American Academy of Child and Adolescent Psychiatry,* 29:130–136.

Tantam, D. (1988). Asperger's disorder. *Journal of Child Psychology and Psychiatry,* 29:245–255.

______. (1991). Asperger syndrome in adulthood. In U. Frith (ed.), *Autism and Asperger syndrome,* pp. 147–183. Cambridge University Press, Cambridge.

______, Evered, C., and Hersov, L. (1990). Asperger's disorder and ligamentous laxity. *Journal of the American Academy of Child and Adolescent Psychiatry,* 93:769–774.

______, Holmes, D., and Cordess, C. (1993). Nonverbal expression in autism of Asperger type. *Journal of Autism and Developmental Disorders,* 23:111–133.

Wing, L. (1981). Asperger's disorder: A clinical account. *Psychological Medicine,* 11:115–129.

______. (1991). The relationship between Asperger's disorder and Kanner's autism. In U. Frith (ed.), *Autism and Asperger syndrome,* pp. 93–121. Cambridge University Press, Cambridge.

______, and Gould, J. (1979). Severe impairments of social interaction and associated abnormalities in children: Epidemiology and classification. *Journal of Autism and Developmental Disorders,* 9:11–29.

Wolff, S., and Barlow, A. (1979). Schizoid personality in childhood: A comparative study of schizoid, autistic and normal children. *Journal of Child Psychology and Psychiatry,* 20:29–46.

World Health Organization. (1992). *The ICD-10 classification of mental and behavioural disorders: Clinical descriptions and diagnostic guidelines.* Author, Geneva.

9.3 Rett's Disorder

Rett's disorder is a category of pervasive developmental disorder in the current classification of mental disorders found in ICD-10 (WHO, 1992) and in DSM-IV (APA, 1994). In the past, the pervasive developmental disorder category focused on mental disorders that have associated qualitative impairments in social interaction, verbal and nonverbal communication skills, and imaginative activity as well as characteristic stereotypies. The period of social withdrawal is usually transient in Rett's disorder, so social deficits should not be the sole basis for its inclusion in this category. Moreover, the ICD-10 classification system has expanded the PDD category to include additional nonautistic conditions that involve multiple developmental lines. If the "PDD" category is used to designate pervasive disruption of developmental functions followed by a subsequent plateau after a period of normal development, then Rett's disorder and other childhood disintegrative diseases may be considered pervasive developmental disorders.

There has also been considerable debate regarding whether Rett's disorder is a degenerative disease, a neurodevelopmental disorder, or a mental disorder. Rett's disorder is considered to be a neurodevelopmental disorder rather than a degenerative disease because with age, there is no demonstrable progression in the neuropathology or neurophysiology as measured by EEG or evoked potential, nor is there regression demonstrated in developmental testing once the diagnosis is established. It is also not considered to be a dementia because there is no clearly demonstrated loss of skills. Although language use diminishes, there has been no unequivocal evidence of language loss. Even though Rett's disorder is associated with changes in head size (acquired microcephaly), ataxia, seizures, and pyramidal signs, these features are thought to be the consequence of a neurodevelopmentally based neurological or developmental neuropsychiatric disorder. Its most characteristic behavioral phenotypic feature is hand wringing, often associated with hand-to-mouth behavior, which is distinct from the hand biting stereotypies found in Lesch-Nyhan disease.

Rett's disorder is not unique among developmental conditions that are thought to be at the boundary between neurology and psychiatry. Both autistic disorder and Tourette's disorder have neurobiological bases, and seizures do occur in one third of low-functioning autistic children. Still, in Rett's disorder, the neurological features are more striking and seizure management may be particularly difficult. Even though Rett's disorder is included in the pervasive developmental disorder classification in DSM-IV, decisions about treatment of specific symptoms will determine which specialties are most actively involved. A better understanding of the neurobiological abnormality in Rett's disorder may lead to new possibilities for therapeutic intervention and perhaps provide insights into the normal processes in neural development that may lead to normal behavior or deviant behavior, if disrupted.

This section discusses the history, epidemiology, definition, natural history, etiology, neurochemistry, neuropathology, relationship to autistic disorder, natural history, assessment and treatment of Rett's disorder.

HISTORY

In a relatively inaccessible Austrian journal, Andreas Rett (1966) initially described his observations on 22 girls with what came to be known as Rett's disorder. Rett originally became aware of this syndrome when the nurse working with him in a mental retardation outpatient clinic pointed out the behavioral similarity between two girls who were waiting to be seen. Despite these early observations, it was not until 1983 when 35 cases from several countries (France, Portugal, Sweden) were reported by Hagberg et al. (1983) that the syndrome came to international attention. Subsequently, Rett's disorder has been investigated in many centers worldwide, an International Rett Syndrome Association (IRSA) has been established, and university centers in many countries are collaborating in research on this disorder. The Rett's disorder work group has published diagnostic criteria (Rett Syndrome Diagnostic Criteria Work Group, 1988) based on an international consensus.

EPIDEMIOLOGY

The prevalence of Rett's disorder is 1 in 10,000 to 12,000 girls, with no confirmed male cases (Hagberg, 1985; Kerr and Stephenson, 1985). It occurs in all ethnic groups. Survival into the fourth decade is common, although there have been some unexplained deaths in mid-childhood. For epidemiologic purposes, the diagnosis is clinical because no consistent biochemical or physiological markers have been identified. Although Rett's disorder occurs in girls, female sex is not indicated as a necessary criteria, based on the possibility of undiagnosed male cases. Deviant development is apparent by 15 months in 50%, by 18 months in 80%, and by age 2 in 100% of reported cases (Witt-Engerstrom, 1987).

DEFINITION

The inclusion of Rett's disorder in the ICD-10 and DSM-IV classifications of mental disorders has been controversial. The controversies have revolved around the diagnostic validity of Rett's disorder and the suitability of classifying Rett's disorder as a mental disorder rather than a neurological disorder, and more specifically, as a subtype of pervasive developmental disorder (Tsai, 1992).

Diagnostic criteria for Rett's disorder, developed by a group representing the Centers for Disease Control, the American Association of University Affiliated Programs, and the IRSA, are now being consistently applied worldwide (Rett Syndrome Diagnostic Work Group, 1988). The criteria are based on those adopted by a panel of international experts at the 1984 Rett Syndrome Conference (Hagberg et al., 1985), and are shown in Table 9.3–1.

The acceptance of these diagnostic criteria and their careful application to cases has confirmed the diagnostic validity of Rett's disorder. The diagnostic criteria have been used in more than 1,500 cases worldwide to establish the existence of this syndrome.

The DSM-IV diagnostic criteria for Rett's disorder are described in Table 9.3–2. The Work Group diagnostic criteria are broken down into necessary, supportive, and exclusion criteria (Table 9.3–1). Moreover, the diagnosis is considered to be tentative until 2 to 5 years of age. The necessary criteria include apparently normal prenatal and perinatal development and apparently normal psychomotor development through the first 6 months of life, normal head circumference at birth, but deceleration of head growth between 5 months and 4 years of age. There is a subsequent loss of acquired, purposeful hand skills and speech by 1 to 2 years of age (range 6 to 30 months). This is followed by the development of stereotypical hand movements, such as hand wringing/squeezing, clapping/tapping, mouthing, and washing/rubbing

Table 9.3–1. Rett Syndrome Diagnostic Criteria

Necessary Criteria

1. Apparently normal prenatal and perinatal period
2. Apparently normal psychomotor development through the first 6 months
3. Normal head circumference at birth
4. Deceleration of head growth between ages 5 months and 4 years
5. Loss of acquired purposeful hand skills between ages 6 and 30 months, temporally associated with communication dysfunction and social withdrawal
6. Development of severely impaired expressive and receptive language, and presence of apparent severe psychomotor retardation
7. Stereotypic hand movements such as handwringing/squeezing, clapping/tapping, mouthing, and "washing"/rubbing automatisms appearing after purposeful hand skills are lost
8. Appearance of gait apraxia and truncal apraxia/ataxia between ages 1 and 4 years

Supportive Criteria

1. Breathing dysfunction
   a. Periodic apnea during wakefulness
   b. Intermittent hyperventilation
   c. Breath-holding spells
   d. Forced expulsion of air or saliva
2. EEG abnormalities
   a. Slow waking background and intermittent rhythmic slowing (3–5 Hz)
   b. Epileptiform discharges, with or without clinical seizures
3. Seizures
4. Spasticity often with associated development of muscle wasting and dystonia
5. Peripheral vasomotor disturbances
6. Scoliosis
7. Growth retardation
8. Hypotrophic small feet

Exclusion Criteria

1. Evidence of intrauterine growth retardation
2. Organomegaly, or other signs of storage disease
3. Retinopathy or optic atrophy
4. Microcephaly at birth
5. Evidence of perinatally acquired brain damage
6. Existence of identifiable metabolic or other progressive neurologic disorder
7. Acquired neurologic disorders resulting from severe infections or head trauma

From The Rett Syndrome Diagnostic Criteria Work Group, 1988.

automatic movements. Between 1 and 4 years of age, severely impaired expressive and receptive language disorder, severe psychomotor retardation with gait apraxia, and truncal apraxia/ataxia become evident. During this phase, children may lose social interest and become socially withdrawn.

Supportive criteria for Rett's disorder are dysfunctional breathing, including periodic apnea during wakefulness, intermittent hyperventilation, breath-holding spells, and forced expulsion of air or saliva. EEG abnormalities include a slow waking background and intermit-

Table 9.3–2. DSM-IV Diagnostic Criteria for Rett's Disorder

299.80 Rett's Disorder

A. All of the following:
  (1) apparently normal prenatal and perinatal development
  (2) apparently normal psychomotor development through the first 5 months after birth
  (3) normal head circumference at birth

B. Onset of all of the following after the period of normal development:
  (1) deceleration of head growth between ages 5 and 48 months
  (2) loss of previously acquired purposeful hand skills between ages 5 and 30 months with the subsequent development of stereotyped hand movements (e.g., handwringing or handwashing)
  (3) loss of social engagement early in the course (although often social interaction develops later)
  (4) appearance of poorly coordinated gait or trunk movements
  (5) severely impaired expressive and receptive language development with severe psychomotor retardation

From APA, 1994.

tent rhythmic slowing associated with epileptiform discharges, with or without clinical seizures. Clinical seizures occur at some point in the course, as does spasticity (with some muscle wasting), dystonia, and peripheral basal motor disturbances. Scoliosis, growth retardation, and poorly developed small feet are reported. The diagnosis is possible, particularly in young children, without these supportive criteria.

The exclusion criteria for Rett's disorder include other conditions, such as intrauterine growth retardation, evidence of a metabolic storage disease, retinopathy at birth, evidence of perinatally acquired brain damage, identification of a known metabolic and progressive neurological disease, and acquired neurological disorders resulting from severe infections and head trauma. The presence of one or more of these conditions exclude the diagnosis of Rett's disorder.

NATURAL HISTORY

There is no specific diagnostic marker for Rett's disorder so the diagnosis must be made based on clinical criteria and the characteristic clinical presentation (Kerr, 1992). The clinical presentation is shown in Figure 9.3–1.

Rett's disorder variability in the clinical presentation depends on the patient's age and the stage of the illness. A diagnosis based on a single examination may lead to an inappropriate diagnosis if the full developmental profile and past history are not considered (Hagberg, 1989).

Both Naidu (Naidu et al. 1986; Naidu, 1992) and Kerr (1992) have provided comprehensive reviews of the natural history of Rett's disorder. Kerr (1992) has described the natural history of the Rett's disorder phenotype based on a review of over 520 cases who presented over a 10-year period. There are phases of apparently normal development, stagnation (6 to 18 months), regression and deterioration (age 1 to 3 years), and plateau (preschool to early school age). With advancing age, there may be further motor deterioration with spasticity and scoliosis.

From a developmental perspective, girls with Rett's disorder typically appear normal at birth and their head size is found to be in the normal range. There are ordinarily no problems in feeding or weaning. In early life, the child smiles, reaches out, examines objects, makes transfers, babbles, produces real words, and is described as sociable and cuddling. She may crawl and walk but will rarely run or climb.

When the early developmental history is carefully reviewed from family videotapes, some difficulties may be observed in the latter part of the first 6 months of life. In fact, a provisional diagnosis of Rett's disorder can be made as early as 6 months of age. The signs used to make an early diagnosis are early signs of hyp-

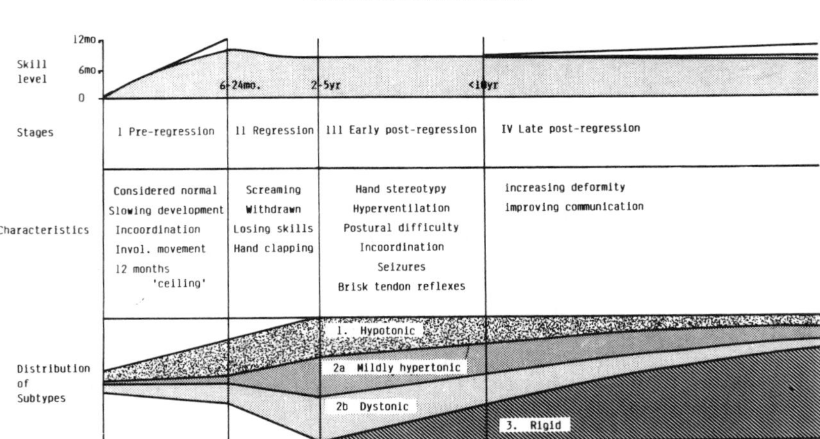

Figure 9.3–1. *Clinical presentation in Rett's Disorder.* This figure highlights skill level, stages of illness, characteristic features, and the various subtypes of Rett's disorder (with permision from Kerr).

tonia, reduced mobility, excessive repetitive activity, and failure to initiate play. There are distinct, although nonspecific, signs that suggest motor and cognitive dysfunction from birth and indicate the disorder may be clinically manifest before the characteristic regression begins.

Subsequently, there is an arrest or stagnation in development that starts near the end of the first year of life before the beginning of the regressive phase, which may take place as late as 2 years later. During this period, girls with Rett's disorder remain sociable and content, which may lead their caregivers to reassure themselves about these children's skills, yet their actual skill level remains at about the 1-year level. This phase of arrested development is followed by deceleration in growth of the occipitofrontal circumference of the head, which may indicate defective late infant cortical development.

In the absence of other associated diseases, the regressive phase begins during the first 6 to 30 months. Regression may be sudden or gradual, but in each case, it is the manipulative movements, particularly skilled hand movements, and language skills that are first affected. Motor milestones affected include abnormal crawling and poor coordination. In regard to fine motor development, the pincer grasp is established and lost. Concurrently, the child may develop episodes of crying and screaming, may become emotionally withdrawn from others, and may stop self-feeding. Gradually, hand stereotypies develop that are accompanied by jerky movements which may affect the face, mouth, trunk, and limbs. It is during this regressive phase that the behavioral pattern may suggest an autistic-like disorder because of the loss of the child's social interest in others, withdrawal, and stereotyped movements. Despite this, autistic disorder has rarely been specifically diagnosed at this age, although it sometimes is listed as part of the differential diagnosis. The characteristic regression, particularly as it relates to fine movement control mechanisms, suggests a disorder that is being progressively expressed but plateaus over time.

The fully established Rett's disorder is characterized by identifying a cluster of behaviors, including expressive movement patterns that may occur in a normal child, but in Rett's disorder, become "fractured gestures" (Kerr, 1992) and lose their normal integration. It is thought these repetitive movement patterns are normally modulated by higher cortical centers, but are released from normal inhibition in Rett's disorder due to lack of higher cortical control. These movement patterns may interfere as the child attempts routine activities and often leads to agitation, which can be reduced if involuntary movements are restrained and the child is guided and assisted at a task. With increasing age, breathing problems occur and a hyperventilation/apnea cycle is activated whenever the child is suddenly alerted by others or by environmental events. Even when awakened at night in a darkened room, a breathing dysrhythmia may be initiated that is linked to increased rates of repetitive movements of the hands, limbs, trunk, mouth, and face. Control of breathing appears normal during sleep, which suggests this is not simply a problem with the brainstem respiratory centers (Glaze et al., 1987).

Breath-holding spells with cyanosis, tremulousness, rigidity, and dystonic posturing may be mistaken for seizures (Naidu, 1992). However, seizures do occur with an average age of onset around age 4. All cases of Rett's disorder have abnormal EEGs, and clinical seizures are identified in 50%. Grand mal, focal, or generalized seizures, myoclonus, and atonic spells have been reported. The natural history is for severe early seizures, with reduction in intensity with advancing age, and cessation of seizure activity in the second decade in some cases.

As they grow older, spasticity is noted in some girls with Rett's disorder, with a tendency to develop muscle wasting, scoliosis, and lower limb deformities. These motor findings led to investigation of possible upper and lower motor neuron neurological abnormalities; however, the maintenance of locomotor ability in some patients and the recognition of early improvement in some manipulative skills occurring as late as the fourth decade of life are not consistent with a progressive neurological disorder. Examinations of the corticospinal tracts suggest their intactness, so that the movement difficulty primarily involves the proximal control of movement.

Despite these severe disabilities, some functions are relatively preserved. For example, the sensory organs are largely intact and spontaneous motor and emotional responses may occur.

ETIOLOGY

Genetics

The similarity of clinical features and natural history among subjects with Rett's disorder suggests a common cause. Evidence pointing to Rett's disorder as a genetic disorder includes twin studies where there is concordance in monozygotic twins and discordance in dizygotic twins, expression in the female sex, and the occurrence of familial cases (Zoghbi, 1988). Although familial cases are rare (less than 1%), their occurrence is greater than chance (Naidu, 1992). Two pairs of concordant monozygotic female twins have been reported, both of whom have typical Rett's disorder, but one is more severely disabled than the other. Of two pairs of dizygotic twins, consisting of female:female and male:female, each pair had one affected girl. Severe major mental illnesses, both schizophrenia and depression, have been reported in first-degree relatives; however, no clear-cut association has been demonstrated.

The most likely genetic hypothesis is that Rett's disorder is an autosomal dominant mutation that is lethal in males (Comings, 1986). However, Zoghbi et al. (1990b) suggest the possibility of nonrandom X chromosome inactivation in putative carriers leading to an X-linked mutation that is lethal in males. A matrilineal pattern of inheritance has been suggested based on a family with affected half sisters with the same mother and an aunt-niece pair. Genetic research has focused on the identification and study of translocations in rare familial cases. However, the majority of Rett's disorder cases are considered to be sporadic. There is one instance of a young woman with Rett's disorder who was sexually assaulted and subsequently gave birth to a child with Rett's disorder. Two patients with chromosomal translocations have been reported. The first has a balanced translocation between the short arm of X chromosome (p22.11) and the long arm of chromosome 3, and the second has a translocation between Xp11.22 and Xp22.11, also present in a mother and a sister with atypical features (Zoghbi et al., 1990a).

It is thought that the gene product potentially responsible for Rett's disorder is an important factor in the development of neural networks for processing of sensory signals. Failure in development of these systems might lead to the severe cognitive and executive function disabilities that are seen in Rett's disorder.

NEUROCHEMISTRY

The role of biogenic amines in Rett's disorder has been studied with direct measurement of neurotransmitter metabolites in cerebral spinal fluid and in D_2 PET scan studies. Zoghbi et al. (1985) found reductions of both MHPG, a metabolite of norepinephrine, and HVA, a metabolite of dopamine, in cerebrospinal fluid. However, changes in these neurotransmitter metabolites are not consistent and may be nonspecific because similar alterations may be found in epileptic patients (Goldstein et al., 1988; Perry et al., 1988). Postmortem brain studies have identified reduced levels of choline acetyl-transferase (CHAT) in brain (Wenk, Naidu, and Moser, 1989) and biogenic amines and metabolites (Lekman et al., 1989). Norepinephrine, serotonin, and muscarinic receptors sites showed minimal reduction and NMDA (glutamate) benzodiazepine binding sites were unchanged (Wenk, Naidu, and Moser, 1989).

Riederer et al. (1986) reported a reduction in ^{3}H-spiroperidol binding sites in the putamen of a patient with Rett's disorder, which indicates a reduction in the density of D_2 dopamine receptors. Harris et al. (1986) used the same ligand for *in vivo* positron emission tomography scanning in a 25-year-old woman with Rett's disorder and found low normal levels ($p = .10$) of dopamine density in the striatum. There was no reduction in cerebrospinal fluid neurotransmitter levels. Subsequent D_2 PET studies of Rett's disorder, using better quantification methods for D_2 receptors, have shown similar results. Since these studies were carried out, it has been reported the caudate may be smaller in proportion to other brain structures in Rett's disorder (Casanova et al., 1991). Because, unlike Parkinson's disease, the receptor number is reduced, Rett's disorder may not result from isolated dopamine denervation (Naidu et al., 1992). Substantial presynaptic reductions in dopamine are needed for there to be postsynaptic changes; therefore, future investigations should emphasize the presynaptic dopamine transport uptake ligands.

NEUROPATHOLOGY

The neuropathological findings in Rett's disorder are substantially different than those found in other conditions involving the basal forebrain and the dopamine and cholinergic systems, such as Huntington's disease, and Parkinson disease. The early onset of a disorder during development leads to a strikingly different presentation. This has been demonstrated in an animal model by Breese et al. (1984) who have shown that the behavioral outcome of neonatal lesions of the dopamine system in the neonatal animal is substantially different from the adult.

The most consistent finding at autopsy in Rett's disorder is low brain weight without evidence of dysgenesis or of changes in white matter. Neuropathological studies involving full brain serial sections (Bauman, 1991) found small densely packed cells noted in certain brain regions that appear normal. Although this is most evident in the hippocampus and amygdala, unlike similar studies in autistic cases, it is a generalized finding that also involves cortical areas. Bauman suggests that these findings reflect immaturity rather than morphological changes and that although cellular migration has occurred, maturation has not continued normally. Findings were similar in younger and older subjects. Studies by Armstrong (1992) cited similar abnormalities in the cortex with small closely packed neurons that show limited dendritic branching. These neuropathological findings provide evidence of an arrest or a lack of normal developmental progression. This may be followed by some subsequent reestablishment of function or perhaps a toxic neuronal reorganization.

These findings are consistent with the reports by Diamond (1990) that primitive brain systems may account for early, apparently normal development, and it is the failure of the development of other systems that develop later that accounts for subsequent developmental difficulty. Rakic (personal communication, 1992) has suggested the extent of developmental brain dysfunction may not become evident until the period of rapid synaptic development comes to an end during the second year of life as synaptic pruning occurs and neuronal reorganization takes place.

RETT'S DISORDER AND AUTISTIC DISORDER

Before international diagnostic criteria for Rett's disorder were established (Rett Syndrome Diagnostic Criteria Work Group, 1988), some cases were initially considered to be autistic disorder. Yet several studies, using both behavioral observation and family history information, have demonstrated both qualitative and quantitative differences between Rett's disorder and autistic disorder (Gillberg, 1987; Olsson and Rett, 1987; Percy et al., 1990). This has led to the recognition that Rett's disorder is distinguishable from autistic disorder in early life and is a distinct diagnostic entity. The clinical features of the two disorders are contrasted in Table 9.3–3. It is essential that psychiatrists and other professionals working in developmental neuropsychiatry clinics be aware of the clinical features and natural history of both conditions for appropriate classification.

Confusion with autistic disorder in the past has been based on loss of interest in, and awareness of, the environment that develops primarily during the phase of rapid developmental regression in Rett's disorder. Social withdrawal is one aspect of this regressive phase. With the gradual loss of purposeful hand movements, midline hand stereotypies develop which have been interpreted as autistic-like symptoms; however, these simple, central hand wringing and hand-to-mouth stereotypies differ from the typical complex, peripheral hand stereotypies seen in autistic disorder. Involuntary movements and difficulty initiating voluntary hand movements along with the extent of mental retardation further distinguish the girl with Rett's disorder from a child with an autistic disorder.

Language may develop in Rett's disorder, and the majority of girls pass through development with babbling, jargoning, early social reciprocity, and the development of single words; however, any verbal skills are generally lost by 18 months. There is no recovery from language loss. In autistic disorder, up to one third may use words in the first year and subsequently stop using them but may later recover language usage.

Accompanying the regressive phase, there is a deceleration in head circumference with eventual microcephaly, which does not occur in autistic disorder. As the regressive phase subsides, children with Rett's disorder show a prominent gait

Table 9.3–3. Contrasting Features of Rett's Disorder and Autistic Disorder

Rett's Disorder	Autistic Disorder
1. Normal social development, 6 to 12 months. Early social reciprocity and cuddling. May show social disinterest during regressive phase.	Social deficits may be recognized in the first year (limited social communication). May show lack of anticipatory gestures. Diagnosis uncommon before 15 to 18 months.
2. Microcephaly and growth retardation.	Normal head growth and physical development.
3. Midline hand clasping and loss of pincer grasp. Limited object manipulation.	Hand stereotypies with hand flapping and complex hand movements. Complex object manipulation.
4. Gait abnormality with truncal ataxia and apraxia.	Gait is generally normal although toe walking may be present.
5. Language consists of babbling, jargoning, early social reciprocity, and occasional use of single words. Language is lost by 18 months without recovery.	Limited language development with single words that are lost in the second year but subsequently recovered, depending on cognitive level.
6. Profound mental retardation.	Variable mental age. Most commonly moderate mental retardation.
7. Seizures of various types in 70%, beginning in early childhood.	Seizures (usually temporal-limbic complex) in 25%, beginning in adolescence.
8. MRI shows diffuse cortical atrophy.	No cortical atrophy on MRI.
9. Neuropathological findings reveal diffuse involvement of limbic brain and cortex.	Neuropathological findings reveal changes in limbic brain but not in cortex.

disturbance and those who were previously hypotonic show an increase in muscle tone and may develop hypertonia with hyperreflexia and rigidity. They walk with a wide-based gait or may become nonambulatory as early as 4 years and show fluctuations in muscle tone, scoliosis, and a movement disorder. By the third decade, 80% may be nonambulatory. In autistic disorder, ambulation is generally normal although toe walking may be present in some cases. Sleep disturbances are common in autistic children and in Rett's disorder. Eighty-five percent of girls with Rett's disorder meet diagnostic criteria for a sleep disorder with delayed sleep onset, night waking, and early morning waking. Magnetic resonance imaging (MRI) abnormalities have been reported in autistic subjects involving the cerebellum and other brain regions whereas in Rett's disorder imaging studies show diffuse cortical atrophy.

When girls are referred to pervasive developmental clinics because of concerns about behavior problems, behavioral regression, or stereotypies, the developmental history generally suggests a diagnosis of Rett's disorder. Referral most often occurs in the second phase of the disease because of social withdrawal, disruptive behavior, screaming, and hand-to-mouth stereotypies. On clinical examination, hyperventilation may be noted along with a clumsy ataxic gait. The child may demonstrate midline hand-wringing stereotypies and will frequently bring her hands to the mouth but generally will not bite the fingers. When the girls are placed on the floor, they may demonstrate their lack of purposeful hand movements by rocking into a sitting or standing position without using their hands to push themselves up. Older girls who have passed through the regressive phase will make eye contact and may demonstrate a social smile.

TREATMENT

The optimal treatment of the behavioral manifestations of Rett's disorder should be based on the underlying processes and mechanisms that lead to the clinical features. Thus far, there is not a definitive understanding of these processes, so continued multidisciplinary research is needed. Treatment is symptomatic and supportive and includes psychosocial and educational treatment, i.e., physical therapy, occupational therapy, and music therapy (Wesecky, 1986) as well as pharmacological treatment, particularly for seizure disorder.

According to a parent survey by Sansom et al. (1993), apparent anxiety attacks marked by expressions of panic and agitation were noted in 75% of children, and low mood and crying for no reason in 70% and 62%, respectively. The episodes of anxiety may respond to hydrotherapy, massage, and music therapies. In the same survey, 38% were reported to have self-injury to the hands, which was generally mild. However, self-injury did extend to other topographies, such as head banging. Behavior treatments have been utilized for severe self-injury (Iwata et al., 1986). Functional analysis of behavior indicated different functions for two forms of self-injurious behavior in Rett's disorder: automatic reinforcement by sensory stimulation and escape from social interactions (Oliver et al., 1993). However, behavior reduction approaches have generally been ineffective in reducing episodes of distress, hyperventilation, and hand stereotypies. Distraction and reinforcement of alternative incompatible behaviors (DRO procedures) along with comforting have been the most successful interventions (Sansom et al., 1993). Because of the language disorder, physical complaints or illnesses that result in physical pain, such as otitis media and dental caries, must be sought out.

Physical and occupational therapists focus on problems such as ataxia, spasticity, spinal deformity, loss of ambulation, poor hand function, feeding, irritability, and poor social awareness. Although none of these treatments alter the course of the disease, they may reduce symptoms that interfere with function and are aimed at maintenance of skills.

Physical therapy for the ataxia has emphasized segmental rolling, stimulation of balance using a therapy ball, and repetition of activities that require weight shifting. Spasticity has been addressed in physical therapy, using activities that reduce muscle tone. As girls with Rett's disorder grow older, they may lose the ability to walk; some may never have walked. For those who do walk, physical therapy activities emphasize the maintenance of weight bearing and focus on the prevention and correction of foot deformities. Arm splints have occasionally been useful in maintaining hand skills, such as those involved in self-feeding. Music therapy may have a calming effect, particularly during the second stage of the disorder when crying and screaming episodes and sleep disturbances are the most troublesome. The child's receptivity to rhythm and melodies has been utilized in music therapy and, in some girls, has resulted in a temporary cessation of stereotyped movements (Wesecky, 1986). Motion, such as rocking and riding in a car, may also reduce agitation.

Seizure disorders require the use of anticonvulsant medication. Several drug trials may be necessary due to the complexity of the seizures. The breathing abnormality sometimes leads to apneic episodes mixed with hyperventilation. The breathing abnormality occurs during wakefulness, but does not occur during sleep. It may be associated with syncopal episodes. This breathing disorder is not responsive to anticonvulsant medication.

A variety of other medications have been utilized in Rett's disorder to address its various behavioral manifestations. Initially, naltrexone was used to treat nighttime sleep problems; however, this treatment has not been demonstrated to be effective. Other treatments have included the utilization of antiobsessional medications to reduce stereotypic behavior, but, so far, these have been unsuccessful.

A major aspect of intervention is the provision of supportive activities for parents to carry out with their children. The phases of parent adjustment that have been outlined for other disorders are applicable to Rett's disorder. Parental education is the first step and may be supplemented by educational sessions in parent groups. An increased risk of mood disorder in the family has been suggested; however, this, too, has not been confirmed. Yet mood disorder should be considered when developing treatment plans for the child and family. Working with parents in parent associations and using parents as support for families with a newly diagnosed condition is an essential aspect of management.

REFERENCES

American Psychiatric Association, Committee on Nomenclature and Statistics. (1994). *Diagnostic and statistical manual of mental disorders,* 4th ed. Author, Washington, DC.

Armstrong, D. (1992). Neuropathology of Rett's disorder. Report of Rett Syndrome Symposium, Tokyo, November 1990. *Brain and Development,* 14(suppl.):S89–98.

Bauman, M. (1991, June). *Neuropathology of Rett's syndrome.* Rett's syndrome Symposium. Kennedy Institute, Baltimore.

Breese, G.R., Baumeister, A.A., McCown, T.J., Emerick, S.G., Frye, G.D., Crotty, K., and Mueller, R.A. (1984). Behavioral differences between neonatal and adult-6-hydroxydopamine treated rats to dopamine agonists: Relevance to neurological symptoms in clinical syndromes with reduced brain dopamine. *Journal of Pharmacology and Experimental Therapeutics,* 231:343–354.

Casanova, M.F., Naidu, S., Goldberg, T.E., Moser, H., Khoromis, S., Kumar, A., Kleinman, J.E., and Weinberger, D.R. (1991). Quantitative magnetic resonance imaging in Rett's syndrome. *Journal of Neuropsychiatry,* 3(1):67–72.

Comings, D.E. (1986). The genetics of Rett's syndrome: The consequences of a disorder where every case is a mutation. *American Journal of Medical Genetics,* 24(suppl.):383–388.

Diamond, A. (1990). Developmental time course in human infants and infant monkeys and the neural bases of inhibitory control in reaching. In A. Diamond (ed.), *The development and neural bases of higher cognitive functions,* pp. 637–669. Annals of the New York Academy of Sciences, Vol. 608, New York.

Gillberg, C. (1987). Autistic symptoms in Rett syndrome: The first two years according to mothers' reports. *Brain Development,* 9:499–501.

Glaze, D.G., Frost, J.D.,Jr., Zoghbi, H.Y., and Percy, A.K. (1987). Rett's syndrome: Characterization of respiratory patterns and sleep. *Annals of Neurology,* 21:377–382.

Goldstein, D.S., Naidu, N.S., Stull, R., Wyler, A.R., and Porter, R.J. (1988). Levels of catechols in epileptogenic and non-epileptogenic regions of the human brain. *Journal of Neurochemistry,* 50:225–229.

Hagberg, B. (1985). Rett's syndrome: Prevalence and impact on progressive severe mental retardation in girls. *Acta Pediatrica Scandanavica,* 74:405–408.

______. (1989). Rett syndrome: Clinical peculiarities, diagnostic approach, and possible cause. *Pediatric Neurology,* 5:75–83.

______, Aicardi, J., Dias, K., and Ramos, O. (1983). A progressive syndrome of autism, dementia, ataxia, and loss of purposeful hand use in girls: Rett's syndrome: Report of 35 cases. *Annals of Neurology,* 14:471–479.

______, Goutieres, F., Hanefeld, F., Rett, A., and

Wilson, J. (1985). Rett syndrome: Criteria for inclusion and exclusion. *Brain Development,* 7:372–373.

Harris, J.C, Wong, D.F., Wagner, H.N., Jr., Rett, A., Naidu S., Dannals, R.F., Links, J.M., Batshaw, M.L., and Moser H.W. (1986). Positron emission tomographic study of D-2 dopamine receptor binding and CSF biogenic amine metabolites in Rett syndrome. *American Journal of Medical Genetics,* 24(suppl.):S201–210.

Iwata, B.A., Pace, G.M., Willis, K.D., Gamache, T.B., and Hyman, S.L. (1986). Operant studies of self-injurious hand biting in the Rett syndrome. *American Journal of Medical Genetics,* 24(suppl.):S157–166.

Kerr, A.M. (1992). *The significance of the Rett syndrome phenotype.* In "From Genes to Behaviour," Society for the Study of Behavioural Phenotypes, 2nd International Symposium, Welshpool, UK, November 19–21. Paper no. 1.

______, and Stephenson, J.B.P. (1985). Rett's syndrome in the west of Scotland. *British Medical Journal,* 291:579–582.

Lekman, A., Witt-Engerstrom, I., Gottfries, J., Hagberg, B.A., Percy, A.K., and Svennerholm, L. (1989). Rett syndrome: Biogenic amines and metabolites in postmortem brain. *Pediatrica Neurologia,* 5:357–362.

Naidu, S. (1992). Rett Syndrome: An update. In Y. Fukuyama, Y. Suzuki, S. Kamoshita, and P. Casaer (eds.), *Fetal and perinatal neurology,* pp. 79–92. Karger, Basel, Switzerland.

______, Murphy, M., Moser, H.W., and Rett, A. (1986). Rett syndrome–natural history of 70 cases. *American Journal of Medical Genetics,* 24(suppl.):S61–72.

______, Wong, D.F., Kitt, C., Wenk, G., and Moser, H.W. (1992). Positron emission tomography in the Rett syndrome: Clinical, biochemical and pathological correlates. *Brain Development,* 14(suppl.):S75–79.

Oliver, C., Murphy, G., Crayton, L., and Corbett, J. (1993). Self-injurious behavior in Rett syndrome: Interactions between features of Rett syndrome and operant conditioning. *Journal of Autism and Developmental Disorders,* 23:91–109.

Olsson, B., and Rett, A. (1987). Autism and Rett syndrome: Behavioral investigations and differential diagnosis. *Developmental Medicine and Child Neurology,* 29:429–441.

Percy, A., Gillberg, C., Hagberg, B., and Witt-Engerstrom, I. (1990). Rett syndrome and the autistic disorders. *Neurology Clinics,* 8: 659–676.

Perry, T.L., Dunn, H.G., Ho, H.H., and Crichton, J.U. (1988). Cerebrospinal fluid values for monoamine metabolites, τ-aminobutyric acid, and other amino compounds in Rett syndrome. *Journal of Pediatrics,* 112:234–238.

Rett, A. (1966). Uber ein eigenartiges hirnatrophisches Syndrom bei Hyperammoniamie im Kindesalter. *Wiener Medizinische Wochenschrift,* 116:723–738.

Rett Syndrome Diagnostic Criteria Work Group. (1988). Diagnostic criteria for Rett syndrome. *Annals of Neurology,* 23:425–428.

Riederer, P., Weiser, M., Wichart, I., Schmidt, B., Killian, W., and Rett, A. (1986). Preliminary brain autopsy findings in progredient Rett syndrome. *American Journal of Medical Genetics,* 24(suppl.):S305–315.

Sansom, D., Krishnan, V.H.R., Corbett, J., and Kerr, A. (1993). Emotional and behavioural aspects of Rett syndrome. *Developmental Medicine and Child Neurology,* 35:340–345.

Tsai, L.K. (1992). Is Rett syndrome a subtype of pervasive developmental disorders? *Journal of Autism and Developmental Disorders,* 22:551–561.

Wenk, G.L., Naidu, S., and Moser, H. (1989). Altered neurochemical markers in Rett syndrome. *Annals of Neurology,* 26:A466.

Wesecky, A. (1986). Music therapy for children with Rett syndrome. *American Journal of Medical Genetics,* 24 (suppl.):S253–257.

Witt-Engerstrom, I. (1987). Rett syndrome: A retrospective pilot study on potential early predictive symptomatology. *Brain and Development,* 9:481–486.

World Health Organization. (1992). *The ICD-10 classification of mental and behavioural disorders: Clinical descriptions and diagnostic guidelines.* Author, Geneva.

Zoghbi, H.Y. (1988). Genetic aspects of Rett syndrome. *Journal of Child Neurology,* 3:S76–78.

______, Ledbetter, D.H., Schultz, R., Percy, A.K., and Glaze, D.G. (1990a). A *de novo* X;3 translocation in Rett syndrome. *American Journal of Medical Genetics,* 35:148–151.

______, Milstien, S., Butler, I.J., Smith, E.O., Kaufman, S., Glaze, D.G., and Percy, A.K. (1989). Cerebrospinal fluid biogenic amines and biopterin in Rett syndrome. *Annals of Neurology,* 25:56–60.

______, Percy, A.K., Glaze, D.G., Butler, I.J., and Riccardi, V.M. (1985). Reduction of biogenic amine levels in the Rett syndrome. *New England Journal of Medicine,* 313:921–924.

______, Percy, A.K., Schultz, R.J., and Fill, C. (1990b). Patterns of X chromosome inactivation in the Rett syndrome. *Brain and Development,* 12:131–135.

9.4 Childhood Disintegrative Disorder

Childhood disintegrative disorder is the most recent designation for a syndrome long known by the acronym "Heller's syndrome," or "disintegrative psychosis." It is a rare condition, but it has distinctive clinical features and a worse prognosis than autistic disorder. In some instances, this condition may show autistic-like features at its onset, although an important difference is apparent normal development for at least the first 2 years of life. In some cases, there may be an associated encephalopathy; despite this, the diagnosis is made based on a behavioral presentation. Loss of language and social skills generally occurs over a several-month period, which is followed by a plateau and possible limited improvement with maturation. In some instances, loss of skills is progressive, but this ordinarily is associated with a diagnosable neurological disorder.

In this section, the history, definition and diagnostic criteria, epidemiology, etiology, natural history, diagnostic assessment, and prognosis of childhood disintegrative disorder are discussed.

HISTORY

In 1908 Heller, a Viennese educator, suggested the designation "dementia infantilis" in a report on six children, drawn from a large number of mentally retarded children he had evaluated in 1905 and 1906, who showed a severe regression in development following 3 to 4 years of apparently normal development (Heller, 1908). He was impressed by the number of cases with similar past histories, which suggested to him a close connection among them. The children came from different countries and from different social backgrounds. Yet in each instance, without prior illness, early symptoms of character change, particularly changes in mood, were noted during the third to fourth year of life. Previously "placid or lively children. . . . became moody, negativistic, disobedient, often raging without reason, and whining; not rarely, they started to destroy their toys, of which they had made reasonable use before." He went on to describe anxiety states and suspected occasional hallucinations, which were followed by a regression that led within a few months to a loss of speech and moderate to severe mental retardation.

Language loss occurred gradually as words became distorted and sentences were no longer meaningfully produced until speech stopped altogether; receptive language was also lost. During this regressive process, motoric changes were also noted, which included tic-like movements, stereotypies, and motor restlessness. Each of the parents indicated their children had been normally intelligent before the onset of the disorder and, in some instances, gifted. Throughout their disorder, the children maintained "an intelligent facial expression." According to Heller, the "clear look in their eyes and the apparent attention which these children frequently seemed to pay to whatever went on around them" led to families' continually seeking additional advice regarding treatment. Although with therapeutic nursing they could be trained to feed themselves and to maintain hygiene, there was no recovery of lost functions. On neurological examination, there was a lack of focal neurological signs but motor functioning was maintained. By 1930 Heller had collected 28 cases, and in each instance, medical examinations had not been able to identify an underlying brain disorder (Heller, 1969). These cases were carefully distinguished from encephalitis lethargica and from early onset schizophrenia and found to differ from these disorders in their presentation.

Since these early descriptions, additional cases of Heller's syndrome have continued to be reported. Corbett (1987) has emphasized the appropriateness of the term "disintegrative" because the characteristic feature of the condition is a period of normal development, followed by disintegration with loss of previously acquired skills, and ultimately by a dementia of unknown etiology. Although the earlier terminology of "childhood psychosis" had included autism, schizophrenia, and Heller's syndrome (disintegrative psychosis), the DSM-III classification (APA, 1980) did not include it. In DSM-III, those conditions previously referred to as "early childhood psychosis" were grouped under the term "pervasive developmental disorders." DSM-III included two general categories: The first was "autism" and the second "childhood onset pervasive developmental disorder (COPDD)." This latter term was sometimes utilized for what previously had been called "childhood schizophrenia." DSM-III did not include the diagnosis of disintegrative disorder, most probably because previously reported cases were thought to be associated with unrecognized progressive neurological instances of "childhood onset pervasive developmental disorder" or dementia.

Yet disintegrative psychosis was included in ICD-9 (WHO, 1977). In that classification, it was defined as "normal or near-normal development in the first few years of life, followed by loss of social skills and of speech, together with a severe disorder of emotions, behavior, and relationships." In agreement with Heller's observations, loss of both speech and social competence took place over several months or more and was accompanied by the appearance of overactivity and stereotypies. The condition was noted to occur in the absence of known brain disease or damage (Rutter, 1985). The diagnoses of schizophrenia of childhood onset or autistic disorder were exclusionary criteria. In ICD-10 (WHO, 1992), a similar description is used.

Childhood disintegrative disorder was not included in the PDD classification largely because such children were thought to have an undiagnosed disorder of the central nervous system. Another consideration was the DSM-III-R (APA, 1987) position that the diagnosis of pervasive developmental disorder should be made on the basis of a current examination regardless of the past history. Most of the children with childhood disintegrative disorder were thought to exhibit an autistic-like clinical picture but with a different age of onset, and, therefore, might meet the broader DSM-III-R criteria of autistic disorder.

DEFINITION AND DIAGNOSTIC CRITERIA

In ICD-10, the diagnostic category used for Heller's Syndrome is "other childhood disintegrative disorder" to distinguish it from Rett's disorder, which also is designated as a specific pervasive developmental disorder. The diagnostic criteria closely follow Heller's original description and are based on apparent normal development up to the age of at least 2 years, which is followed by a definable loss of previously acquired skills. The loss of skills is accompanied by qualitatively abnormal social functioning with profound regression or loss in the use of language, and regression in the level of play, social skills, and adaptive behavior. There may also be a loss of bladder and bowel control, and sometimes difficulties in motoric behavior are found. Commonly, there is an associated loss of interest in the environment with stereotyped, repetitive motor mannerisms and an autistic-like impairment of social interaction and communication.

The disorder resembles the diagnosis of dementia in adult life, but differs in at least three ways: (1) no evidence of any known neurological disease or acquired brain damage (although brain dysfunction is usually inferred); (2) loss of skills may be followed by some degree of recovery; and (3) the early impairment in socialization and communication has deviant qualities that may have some similarity to autistic disorder and are not simply the consequences of a clear-cut intellectual decline.

In DSM-IV (APA, 1994), the diagnostic criteria are similar to ICD-10 but attempt greater operationalization. They specify the presence of age-appropriate verbal and nonverbal communication, social relationships, play, and adaptive behavior for at least the first 2 years of life. This normal developmental period is followed by a clinically significant loss of previously acquired skills in at least two areas, as shown in Table 9.4–1.

In addition, the same qualitative impairments noted in autistic disorder are included, which include qualitative impairment in social interaction and communication, and restricted, repetitive, and stereotyped patterns of behavior, interest, and activities (including motor stereotypies and mannerisms). Pervasive developmental disorder and childhood onset schizophrenia are exclusionary criteria. The inclusion in DSM-IV of the criteria for autistic disorder in this definition requires further study.

These descriptions do not emphasize the affective symptomatology and anxiety mentioned by Heller, nor do they emphasize deterioration in self-help skills that has been reported

Table 9.4–1. DSM-IV Diagnostic Criteria for Childhood Disintegrative Disorder

299.10 Childhood Disintegrative Disorder

A. Apparently normal development for at least the first 2 years after birth as manifested by the presence of age-appropriate verbal and nonverbal communication, social relationships, play, and adaptive behavior.
B. Clinically significant loss of previously acquired skills (before age 10 years) in at least two of the following areas:
   (1) expressive or receptive language
   (2) social skills or adaptive behavior
   (3) bowel or bladder control
   (4) play
   (5) motor skills
C. Abnormalities of functioning in at least two of the following areas:
   (1) qualitative impairment in social interaction (e.g., impairment in nonverbal behaviors, failure to develop peer relationships, lack of social or emotional reciprocity)
   (2) qualitative impairments in communication (e.g., delay or lack of spoken language, inability to initiate or sustain a conversation, stereotyped and repetitive use of language, lack of varied make-believe play)
   (3) restricted, repetitive, and stereotyped patterns of behavior, interests, and activities, including motor stereotypies and mannerisms
D. The disturbance is not better accounted for by another specific Pervasive Developmental Disorder or by Schizophrenia.

From APA, 1994.

previously and summarized by Volkmar (1992, 1994). As is the case in Rett's disorder, a loss of interest in the environment during the acute, early phases of the disorder should not be confused with the classic lack of social awareness characteristic of classical autistic disorder.

ASSOCIATED FEATURES

Cognitive skills are substantially reduced, and children, following the onset of the disorder, function in the mentally retarded range, most commonly in the severe to profound range of mental retardation. Stereotypic behaviors and unusual responses to the environment are commonly noted.

EPIDEMIOLOGY

Specific data on prevalence is not available, although the condition is noted to be rare. Childhood disintegrative disorder has been reported to be one tenth as common as autistic disorder (Burd, Fisher, and Kerbeshian, 1987; Volkmar and Cohen, 1989). Among case reports, the overall male to female ratio is approximately 4 to 1, which is similar to the ratio observed in autistic disorder. Onset is most commonly reported in the third year of life, although cases are reported in an age range from 1 to 9 years. The mean age of onset in a series of 76 cases summarized by Volkmar (1992) is 3.4 years. The average age of onset is later than the typical age of onset of autistic disorder, although there may be some overlap. Although an age of onset of less than 2 would not meet ICD-10 criteria, the clinical course must be taken into account in establishing the diagnosis.

ETIOLOGY

Although an apparent association with neurological disorders has been noted (Evans-Jones and Rosenbloom, 1978), the etiologic significance of association with another medical condition is not clear. Despite the fact that in a number of instances life change events, such as the birth of a sibling and various family crises, have been reported, these psychosocial stressors would not account for the severity and type of deterioration noted. In those instances where there is a known medical condition, such as measles encephalitis, or another viral condition, the behavioral diagnosis should be listed as accompanying this condition. However, the original description by Heller excluded any known condition. Whether there is a genetic etiology requires further investigation. Like autistic disorder, symptomatic changes in behavior may be related to associated neurological conditions; however, there is a genetic form of autistic disorder.

NATURAL HISTORY AND COURSE

In some instances, cases are described with an insidious onset over a period of weeks to months, and in other instances, with an abrupt onset of days to weeks. As originally described by Heller, there may be an early phase during which the child is more active, anxious, negativistic, and restless. The overall course is uniformly one of deterioration, resulting in a lower plateau of development (Hill and Rosenbloom, 1986; Kurita, 1988). The extent of recovery that is possible is unclear, but self-care skills have been taught in some cases (Kanner, 1973; Volkmar, 1992). The child must continue to be observed carefully for evidence of a diagnosable, although not yet recognized, progressive neurological disease. The disorder is lifelong and requires continuing care throughout life because impairment persists throughout lifetime. Additional information is needed to clarify the degree of recovery that is attainable. The major neurological complication is the onset of a seizure disorder.

SPECIAL CONSIDERATIONS IN ASSESSMENT

The assessment requires an extensive and detailed family history, with documented evidence of prior developmental milestones. The use of photographs and videotapes can be quite helpful to clarify the establishment of early developmental milestones. Examination of the child may be difficult because of behavioral deterioration, but should be as extensive as possible. In the early phases of the disorder, some communication may be possible with the child, but with continuing regression, language skills may be entirely lost. During an evaluation of the child, the phase of the illness is important to consider. The extent of the social interactive disturbance may be less severe and pervasive than that seen in classical autistic disorder. Autistic-like behavior may relate more to the child's general lack of awareness of the environment than to the specific deficits in social reciprocity observed in autistic disorder.

The neurological examination focuses on demonstrating a dementia of childhood onset. In Heller's original report, disintegrative disorder was observed in the absence of apparent neurological disease. However, because it is a diagnosis of exclusion, specific neurological diseases must be ruled out in making the diagnosis. In Volkmar's review of 77 cases (1992), the EEG was normal in 20 of 45 cases and abnormal in 21 cases. Seizures were reported in over 20%. The pattern of EEG abnormality and prevalence of seizure disorder is similar to that observed in lower functioning autistic children. Neurological diseases that should be ruled out include tuberous sclerosis (Creak, 1963), metachromatic leukodystrophy (Corbett, et al., 1977), neurolipidoses (Malamud, 1959), and subacute sclerosing panencephalitis (Rivinus, Jamison, and Graham, 1975).

Although some authors have used the diagnosis of childhood disintegrative disorder for children with known neurological disorders if the child had social and language deficits that fit into the pervasive developmental disorder diagnostic category, this practice is best avoided. The greater the child's age at the time of diagnosis, the more suspicious one should be of a diagnosable neurological disorder. The diagnosis of neurodegenerative diseases in childhood can be difficult, and often the failure to make the diagnosis is related to ignorance of the brain mechanisms that may be involved. Similar issues regarding diagnosis have been raised for autistic disorder, which may be associated with a variety of medical conditions when it presents as a symptomatic autistic disorder. The practical consideration in recognizing the behavioral presentation is finding a program that guarantees that social deficits are taken into account in treatment planning.

DIFFERENTIAL DIAGNOSIS

This is a diagnosis of exclusion, and autistic disorder is frequently the first consideration, even though the age of onset is later and the extent of deterioration in function after onset is substantially greater than that observed in autistic children. Elective mutism may be considered, but with that diagnosis, the child does not show deterioration in speech and language behavior but demonstrates communication skills only in certain contexts.

PROGNOSIS

In his review of 76 published cases with follow-up ranging from 1.2 to 22 years, Volkmar (1992) found that the course was static for about three quarters of the patients, with some minimal improvement noted in a minority. For example, when four of the published studies were combined for the purpose of follow-up statistics, 42% of the children were mute, 38% used single words or phrases, and 19% showed some capacity to speak in sentences. All children required special education services, and placement in residential settings was common. Overall function was in the moderate to severe range of mental retardation at follow-up.

REFERENCES

American Psychiatric Association, Committee on Nomenclature and Statistics. (1980). *Diagnostic and statistical manual of mental disorders,* 3rd ed. Author, Washington, DC.

American Psychiatric Association, Committee on Nomenclature and Statistics. (1987). *Diagnostic and statistical manual of mental disorders,* 3rd ed., revised. Author, Washington, DC.

American Psychiatric Association, Committee on Nomenclature and Statistics. (1994). *Diagnostic and statistical manual of mental disorders,* 4th ed. Author, Washington, DC.

Burd, L., Fisher, W., and Kerbeshian, J. (1987). A prevalence study of pervasive developmental disorders in North Dakota. *Journal of the American Academy of Child Psychiatry,* 26:700–703.

Corbett, J. (1987). Development, disintegration, and dementia. *Journal of Mental Deficiency Research,* 31:349–356.

______, Harris, R., Taylor, E., and Trimble, M. (1977). Progressive disintegrative psychosis of childhood. *Journal of Child Psychology and Psychiatry,* 18:211–219.

Creak, E. M. (1963). Childhood psychosis: A review of 100 cases. *British Journal of Psychiatry,* 109:84–89.

Evans-Jones, L.G., and Rosenbloom, L. (1978). Disintegrative psychosis in childhood. *Developmental Medicine and Child Neurology,* 20:462–470.

Heller, T. (1908). Dementia infantilis. *Zeitschrift für die Erforschung und Behandlung des Jugenlichen Schwachsinns [Journal for Research and Treatment of Juvenile Feeblemindedness],* 2:141–165.

______. (1969). Uber dementia infantilis. In J.G. Howells (ed.), *Modern perspective in international child psychiatry.* Oliver and Boyd, Edinburgh. (Translation of original work published 1930)

Hill, A.E., and Rosenbloom, L. (1986). Disintegrative psychosis of childhood: Teenage follow-up. *Developmental Medicine and Child Neurology,* 28:34–40.

Kanner, L. (1973). Dementia infantilis. In L. Kanner (ed.), *Childhood psychosis,* pp. 279–281. V. Winston, Washington, DC.

Kurita, H. (1988). The concept and nosology of Heller's syndrome: Review of articles and report of two cases. *Japanese Journal of Psychiatry and Neurology,* 42:785–793.

Malamud, N. (1959). Heller's disease and childhood schizophrenia. *American Journal of Psychiatry,* 116:215–218.

Rivinus, T.M., Jamison, D.L., and Graham, P.J. (1975). Childhood organic neurological disease presenting as a psychiatric disorder. *Archives of Disease in Childhood,* 50:115–119.

Rutter, M. (1985). Infantile autism and other pervasive developmental disorders. In M. Rutter and L. Hersov (eds.), *Child and adolescent psychiatry: Modern approaches,* pp. 545–566. Blackwell, London.

Volkmar, F.R. (1992). Childhood disintegrative disorder: Issues for DSM-IV. *Journal of Autism and Developmental Disorders,* 22:625–642.

______. (1994). Childhood disintegrative disorder. *Child and Adolescent Psychiatric Clinics of North America,* 3:119–129.

______, and Cohen, D.J. (1989). Disintegrative disorder or "late onset" autism? *Journal of Child Psychology and Psychiatry,* 30:717–724.

World Health Organization. (1977). *International classification of diseases,* 9th ed. Author, Geneva.

World Health Organization. (1992). *The ICD-10 classification of mental and behavioural disorders: Clinical descriptions and diagnostic guidelines.* Author, Geneva.

PART III

BEHAVIORAL PHENOTYPES

A growing body of evidence indicates that specific developmental disorders may be associated with particular patterns of behavior, temperament, and psychopathology. This has been studied most extensively in Down, fragile X, Williams, Lesch-Nyhan, and Prader-Willi syndromes. The term "behavioral phenotype" was introduced by Nyhan in 1972 to describe outwardly observable behavior that was so characteristic of children with genetic disorders that its presence suggests the underlying genetic condition. In speaking of compulsive self-mutilation in the syndrome he initially described, Lesch-Nyhan disease, Nyhan noted,

> We feel that these children have a pattern of unusual behavior that is unique to them. Stereotypical patterns of behavior occurring in syndromic fashion in sizable numbers of individuals provide the possibility that there is a concrete explanation that is discoverable. In these children, there are so many anatomical abnormalities, from changes in hair and bones to dermatoglyphics, that it is a reasonable hypothesis that their behaviors are determined by an abnormal neuroanatomy that would be discoverable, possibly neurophysiologically, ultimately anatomically . . . these children all seem self-programmed. These stereotypical patterns of unusual behavior could reflect the presence of structural deficits in the central nervous system (Nyhan, 1976, p. 235)

A behavioral phenotype, then, is a pattern of behavior that is reliably identified in groups of children with known genetic disorders and is not learned. With increasing attention to genetic disorders that are frequently associated with mental retardation, the number of identifiable behavioral phenotypes is continually increasing. Careful observations of behavior are becoming more and more important as the medical community focuses attention on intervention for genetic disorders. Rating scales are being developed to measure behavioral phenotypes and personality profiles (O'Brien, 1991, 1992). In addition to these behavioral phenotypes, isolated special abilities have been reported to occur in genetically based syndromes. These include special abilities in calculation and in music (Hill, 1978) that may potentially be related to the proposed modular organization of the central nervous system. A highly specialized "neuromodule" might switch on when the specific stimulus (e.g., music, visual material) reaches it at the right time. Finally, both physical and behavioral phenotypes have been described in syndromes caused by environmental events. Among these are developmental neurotoxic conditions, such as fetal alcohol syndrome. Although this condition is not a genetic disorder, there may be genetic vulnerability.

A review of early descriptions of behavior of children and adults with genetic syndromes reveals that the medical and psychological literature is replete with suggestions about specific personality, temperament, and behavioral attributes. An appreciation of behavioral characteristics that were associated with genetic disorders was present from the first reports. In the first description of a specific mental retardation syndrome by Langdon Down (1887), he commented on behavior that was characteristic of the syndrome subsequently named for him. He observed of children with Down syndrome, "They have considerable powers of imitation, even bordering on being mimics. Their humorousness and a lively sense of the ridiculous often colors their mimicry." Later he added, "Several patients who have been under my care have been wont to convert their pillow cases into surplices (vestments) and to imitate, in tone and gesture, the clergymen or chaplain which they have recently heard." He also commented on personality traits, saying, "Another feature is their great obstinancy—they can only be guided by consummate tact." Down's description of liveliness and pleasant temperament, fondness for music, and a love of mimicry entered the psychological literature, but more often problem behaviors were identified as characteristic of mental retardation syndromes rather than the prosocial ones he had suggested. In the first large-scale study on tuberous sclerosis (Critchley and Earl, 1932), peculiar and severe behavioral problems were identified in children and adults with that condition. Despite the early recognition of behavioral phenotypes, syndrome-specific behavioral and psychiatric features received little or no emphasis for many years.

Recent developments in the neurosciences are leading to a new interest in the biological bases of behavioral phenotypes. Applying this technology to study the brain and behavior requires the identification of well-defined syndromes for investigation. Moreover, the recognition of behavioral phenotypes has led to closer scrutiny of known conditions. Following Nyhan's paper, which addressed behaviors typical of the Lesch-Nyhan syndrome, Gath and Gumley (1986) carried out a comprehensive evaluation of Down syndrome subjects and found that behavioral problems were just as characteristic in Down syndrome as in other persons with mental retardation.

In addition to particular behavioral phenotypes, there is an interest in typical personality traits. A bibliography of publications from the American Psychological Association identifies an extensive list of personality attributes associated with mental retardation. Among these are personality traits of assertiveness, creativity, curiosity, dependency, egotism, emotional security, introversion, extroversion, negativeness, passiveness, persistence, suggestibility, and sociability.

Besides reports of unique personality characteristics, there are also studies of particular temperament features. Personality and temperament are viewed differently; personality is defined as a characteristic configuration of behavioral response patterns that a person evolves as a reflection of his individual adjustment to life, the totality of an individual's characteristics, whereas temperament is defined as an inherent constitutional disposition to react in a certain way to stimuli. Thomas and colleagues (Thomas et al., 1963; Thomas, Chess, and Birch, 1968) conducted a longitudinal study of temperament and identified the following temperament categories: activity level, rhythmicity, approach/withdrawal, adaptability, threshold to responsiveness, intensity of reaction, quality of mood, distractibility, attention span, and persistence. When these temperament characteristics were studied in 52 subjects with mental retardation syndromes who were matched with mental-age controls, Chess and Korn (1970) found that those with mental retardation were more intensively responsive, more distractible, less persistent, and had a shorter attention span. Moreover, Thomas et al. (1963) and Thomas, Chess, and Birch (1968) distinguished three temperament clusters that occurred in 65% of their longitudinal sample: easy (40%), difficult (10%), and slow to warm up temperaments (15%). When a particular mental retardation syndrome, Down syndrome, was studied looking at these temperament clusters, Baron (1972) and Gunn, Berry, and Andrews (1981) demonstrated both easy and difficult temperament in Down syndrome children; a typical temperament pattern was not demonstrated.

The temperament categories and personality traits are broad descriptors of individuals. Investigation into the biological basis of behavior in mental retardation syndromes requires greater specificity of behavior than these personality and temperamental variables.

In Nyhan's (1972) description of the behavioral phenotype, he suggested that a more specific biological focus might be identified for those stereotyped behaviors and compulsive behaviors that are consistently found in a few genetically based mental retardation syndromes. However, most available descriptions of genetically based syndromes restrict their attention to (1) physical features, including dysmorphology, motor problems, sensory disabilities, and other associated medical problems; and (2) an indication of developmental delays and developmental attainments that may be listed in the gross motor, intellectual, and linguistic domains. Following Down's description, there was interest in the behavioral phenotype in early publications, but interest declined in the intervening years.

Two main reasons may explain this lack of interest following the early reports by Down and others. First, there was a general negative reaction against eugenics and claims for genetic bases of personality (Bax, 1990). This negative reaction established a climate where it was not considered appropriate for academic investigators to emphasize the genetics of behavior. Secondly, there has been a major emphasis on learning theory and its applications to the field of mental retardation, where the majority of genetic disorders are found. There have been enormous strides in the education of even the most severely mentally retarded individuals. Advances in academic and social adaptive education, in conjunction with motor treatment, has placed greatest emphasis on how severely and multiply-disabled persons could attain greater degrees of independence and social integration. With the emphasis on normalization, severe disorders in learning tended to be deemphasized. Moreover, the occurrence of associated psychiatric and behavioral problems has been interpreted more often in terms of learning theory rather than their being unlearned behaviors associated with behavioral phenotypes. The focus has been on addressing the potential of individuals and their developmental possibilities. Yet this emphasis could not continue to ignore reports from families and clinical observations of characteristic patterns of behavior and stereotypies.

With the establishment of active and refined learning-based approaches and a better understanding of the interpretation of genetic findings, a reappraisal and revision of attitudes toward research with behavioral phenotypes has begun. O'Brien (1992) suggests three reasons for this. First, research findings have been reliably reported with various syndromes. Second, there are continued reports from family members as large family organizations have developed in the United States and other countries that describe characteristic behavioral patterns and interpersonal responses. Parent groups frequently report similar behavior problems and difficulties in management across syndromes when they meet. The interest of parent group members in improving the life of their children has led to additional hypotheses and more refined observations on behavioral characteristics. Third, new techniques in genetics provide new insights into the extent and mechanisms of the human genome as the basis of behavior, and advances in other aspects of neuroscience, including neurophysiology and neuroanatomy, provide additional means of designating brain mechanisms that may be involved. With the establishment of these new methods of evaluation and the identification of rating scales to measure behavioral phenotypes, there is now an increased focus on behavioral phenotypes in developmental neuropsychiatry. However, Flint and Yule (1994) counsel caution in deciding what to include in a behavioral phenotype, particularly in determining whether a behavior is characteristic of a syndrome. Finally, comprehensive study of children with different developmental disabilities may increase our appreciation for the relative contribution of genetic variables in the pathogenesis of specific affective and behavioral disorders.

The chapters that follow address a variety of syndromes where behavioral phenotypes have been recognized. They include cytogenetic disorders such as Down syndrome, metabolic disorders that are genetically based, such as phenylketonuria and Williams syndrome, and environmentally caused disorders with particular behavioral patterns, i.e., fetal alcohol syndrome and gestational use of cocaine. Some conditions with behavioral phenotypes have not been included, i.e., Lowe syndrome, Noonan syndrome, Smith-Magenis syndrome, neurofibromatosis, and Klinefelter syndrome. Others, such as Rett's disorder, where hand stereotypies are characteristic features, are described in Part II, "Developmental Disorders."

In these chapters cytogenetic disorders and other genetic disorders associated with behavioral phenotypes are clustered in Chapter 10, and genetic metabolic disorders associated with behavioral phenotypes are clustered in Chapter 11. In these chapters characteristic behaviors will be highlighted, findings on etiology discussed, potential neurochemical and neuroanatomical abnormalities considered, and interventions briefly reviewed. Behavior and pharmacological therapies have frequently had limited success in many of these conditions, so better characterization of the individual condition is essential to establish treatment. New methods in nuclear imaging and continuing investigations of neurotransmitter systems, endocrine rhythms, and sleep studies may provide information that will be helpful in the future in treatment.

REFERENCES

Baron, J. (1972). Temperamental profile of children with Down's syndrome. *Developmental Medicine and Child Neurology,* 14:640–643.

Bax, M. (1990). *Behaviours seen in children with mucopolysaccharidosis in behavioural phenotypes.* Abstracts and Syndrome Information Publications, Society for the Study of Behavioural Phenotype, Welshpool, U.K.

Chess, S., and Korn, S. (1970). Temperament and behavior disorders in mentally retarded children. *Archives of General Psychiatry,* 23:122–130.

Critchley, M., and Earl, C.J.C. (1932). Tuberous sclerosis and allied conditions. *Brain,* 55:311–346.

Down, J.L. (1887). *Mental affectations of childhood and youth.* J.A. Churchill, London.

Flint, J., and Yule, W. (1994). Behavioural phenotypes. In Rutter, M., Taylor, E., and Hersov, L. (eds.). *Child and adolesent psychiatry: Modern approaches,* p. 667. Blackwell Scientific Publications, Oxford.

Gath, A., and Gumley, D. (1986). Behavior problems in retarded children with special reference to Down's syndrome. *British Journal of Psychiatry,* 149:156–161.

Gunn, P., Berry, P., and Andrews, R.J. (1981). The temperament of Down's syndrome in infants: A research note. *Journal of Child Psychology and Psychiatry,* 22:189–194.

Hill, A.L. (1978). Savants: Mentally retarded individuals with special skills. *International Review of Research in Mental Retardation,* 9:277–298.

Nyhan, W. (1972). Behavioral phenotypes in organic genetic disease. Presidential address to the Society for Pediatric Research, May 1, 1971. *Pediatric Research,* 6:1–9.

______. (1976). Behavior in Lesch-Nyhan syndrome. *Journal of Autism and Childhood Schizophrenia,* 6:235–252.

O'Brien, G. (1991). *Behavioural measurement in mental handicap: A guide to existing schedules.* Society for the Study of Behavioural Phenotypes, Oxford, England.

______. (1992). Behavioural phenotypy in developmental psychiatry. *European Journal of Child and Adolescent Psychiatry,* 1(suppl.):1–61.

Thomas, A., Chess, S., and Birch, H.G. (1968). *Temperament and behavior disorders in children.* New York University Press, New York.

______, ______, ______, Hertzig, M.E., and Korn, S. (1963). *Behavioral individuality in early childhood.* New York University Press, New York.

CHAPTER 10

CYTOGENETIC AND OTHER GENETIC DISORDERS ASSOCIATED WITH BEHAVIORAL PHENOTYPES

10.1 Prader-Willi Syndrome

The Prader-Willi syndrome is of particular interest as a neuropsychiatric disorder because of the associated behavioral phenotype that involves compulsive hyperphagia and aggressive behavior. It is one of the five most common syndromes seen in birth defects clinics and is the most common dysmorphic form of obesity.

This chapter reviews the history, epidemiology, clinical features, behavioral phenotype, natural history, etiology, and treatment of Prader-Willi syndrome.

HISTORY

The first description of what is now known as the Prader-Willi syndrome was most probably that of Langdon Down (1887), who outlined the characteristic features in a woman who was 4 feet 4 inches tall, weighed 210 pounds, and had a voracious appetite, small hands and feet, and had not begun to menstruate by age 25. The eponymic Prader-Willi syndrome was initially described in 1956 as a new disorder involving obesity, short stature, cryptorchidism, and mental retardation (Prader, Labhart, and Willi, 1956).

EPIDEMIOLOGY

The incidence of Prader-Willi syndrome is estimated to fall between 1 in 10,000 and 1 in 30,000 live births. Over 90% of cases occur sporadically. The prevalence has been studied in Sweden in a large-scale epidemiologic study and found to be 12 in 100,000 in the survey population that ranged in age from infancy to age 25 years (Akefeldt, Gillberg, and Larsson, 1991). Life span is related to management of weight; with successful weight control, survival has been reported through the fifth decade (Clarke, Waters, and Corbett, 1989; Greenswag, 1987).

CLINICAL FEATURES

In addition to the obesity, short stature, cryptorchidism, and mental retardation that were originally described, additional characteristics now include hypogonadism, hypotonia, small hands and feet, and dysmorphic facies. Excessive daytime sleepiness is an associated feature. Moreover, there is an increased prevalence of scoliosis and other orthopedic abnormalities. Because of the obesity, heart failure and diabetes may occur as complications. The diagnostic characteristics are shown in Table 10.1–1.

BEHAVIORAL PHENOTYPE

The extent of cognitive impairment is variable, with some individuals testing in the normal

Table 10.1–1. Characteristics of Prader-Willi Syndrome

Infantile hypotonia
Failure to thrive
Small stature
Dysmorphic facial appearance
Small hands and feet
Atrophic scrotum, small testes and penis
Variable mental retardation (IQ 30 to 85)
Compulsive hyperphagia with obesity
Emotional lability and tantruming (particularly in adolescence)

range of intelligence, most in the mild to moderate range of mental retardation, and others testing in the severe range.

Children with Prader-Willi syndrome have been reported to manifest a behavioral phenotype that includes unusual food-related behavior (compulsive food seeking, hoarding, gorging), irritability, anger, a low frustration tolerance, and stubbornness. Studies employing standardized methods of assessment have substantiated these impressions and suggest that anxiety and compulsive behaviors are particularly common. As many as 50% of children and adults with Prader-Willi syndrome meet criteria for a behavior disorder.

The most disabling of these behavioral manifestations is compulsive eating, leading to obesity and the complications of severe obesity, such as respiratory impairment and diabetes. The hyperphagia, which has been consistently found, has received the most systematic behavioral evaluation. When not carefully supervised, patients may steal food and, in some instances, eat unpalatable food, although this can be avoided with appropriate supervision. Bray et al. (1983) found that one half of the patients in their sample got up at night to seek food. The management of their indiscriminate food taking and apparent difficulty with satiety is the major issue in clinical management.

Holm and Pipes (1976) and Holm, Sulzbacher, and Pipes (1981) evaluated food-related behavior in the Prader-Willi syndrome and also found that behavioral problems were most commonly related to food and included food stealing, foraging for food, gorging, and indiscriminate eating with little food selectivity. No special circumstances that resulted in food stealing or gorging were identified; it was noted that older children were preoccupied with food and eating and sometimes reported concerns about there not being enough food and often asked where the next meal would come from.

In addition to food-related compulsions, emotional lability with temper tantrums, stubbornness, negativism, skin picking, and scratching also have been identified as problems. A recent questionnaire survey involving 369 cases identified compulsive and impulsive aggressive behavior (Stein, Keating, and Zar, 1993). These authors used the Overt Aggression Scale, the Yale-Brown Obsessive-Compulsive Disorder Scale, a clinical global rating, and DSM-III-R (APA, 1987) criteria to diagnose self-stimulation and self-injury, compulsive behavior, and obsessive behaviors. They found that skin picking was the most common form of self-injury being observed in 19.6% of this sample. Other types of self-injury with lower frequency were nose picking, nail biting, lip biting, and hair pulling. The second behavioral problem area was compulsive behavior where food hoarding was the most severe manifestation and occurred in 17.7%. Other compulsive behaviors included counting, symmetrical arrangement of objects, checking, and hand washing, which were less common. Obsessive thinking was far less characteristic with only 1.4% being in the severe range on an item dealing with concerns about contamination.

Although the main concern is for food, worries about other situations and things have also been reported (Akefeldt, 1992). Interpersonal difficulties are common, especially for older children with Prader-Willi syndrome. Behavior may change with increasing age so children over age 7 become more irritable and more demanding and show more ritualistic behavior. Sulzbacher, Crinic and Snow (1981) found that behavioral problems identified in the preschool years persist through the school years and continue into adolescence and adulthood.

Personality

Although generally described as friendly and engaging when food needs are met, personality problems have been consistently reported in Prader-Willi syndrome (Hall and Smith, 1972). Dunn (1968) found that 8 of 17 patients over age 10 had emotional difficulties that ranged from temper tantrums to intermittent rage episodes and psychotic behavior. Barringer et al. (1991) identified temper tantrums, aggression, theft, and self-abuse. Older cases responded to real or imagined slights and frustrations that seemed insignificant to others with extreme "bellicosity." Turner and Ruvalcaba (1981) contrasted 10 institutionalized subjects during their adolescence and adult years with 10 non-Prader-Willi institutionalized, age-matched, mentally retarded subjects. The Prader-Willi group were found to be more verbally aggressive and self-assaultive (less than .001). They differed from other mentally retarded groups in having less sexual acting out behavior.

NATURAL HISTORY

Prader-Willi syndrome may present in infancy with severe hypotonia, poor cry and suck, and absent or reduced deep tendon reflexes. The feeding difficulties may lead to failure to thrive and may be associated with delayed locomotor milestones. During the second year of life, the hypotonia and weakness gradually improve, but commonly between ages 2 and 3, eating increases dramatically with rapid weight gain, resulting in obesity by school age. Learning disorders and mental retardation (usual IQ range is 40 to 50 extending up to the normal range) may not be recognized for the first time until school age.

ETIOLOGY

Genetic

A genetic abnormality involving a chromosome 15/15 translocation associated with typical Prader-Willi phenotype was described by Hawkey and Smithies (1976). This was followed by other reports of translocations of chromosome 15 suggesting an unbalanced translocation involving the proximal part of chromosome 15. The few familial cases appear to result from an unbalanced translocation. High-resolution chromosome banding and advanced molecular genetic techniques, using DNA probes, have been used to identify a small interstitial deletion in chromosome 15, with break points at the 15q11 and the 15q13 regions that is inherited from the patient's father. This pattern has been found in more than 80% of cases thus far studied. Maternal heterodisomy for chromosome 15 has also been described (Nicholls et al., 1989; Robinson et al., 1991) wherein the child inherits both members of the maternal chromosome pair but neither member of the paternal pair. Additional chromosome 15 anomalies have been described by these same authors. In the remainder of Prader-Willi syndrome cases, no chromosomal abnormalities have been identified; however, it is suspected that as technical progress continues, all cases will be shown to result either from a microdeletion involving 15q11-15q13 or from uniparental disomy. Those individuals with chromosome 15 deletion are more likely to show hypopigmentation than those without deletions, but other differences have not been consistently observed (Butler, 1990). Finally, there are animal models in genetically obese mice that are potentially relevant to the Prader-Willi syndrome. Mouse chromosome 7 has been evaluated for potential models for imprinted and nonimprinted components of human chromosome 15q11–15q13 (Nicholls et al., 1993).

Neuroanatomical Aspects

The presence of a developmental hypothalamic abnormality has been considered as potentially involved in the etiology. Hypothalamic dysfunction might account for the appetite control problems, disorders in gonadal development, the short stature, and possibly the emotional lability and unpredictable tantrums. Evans (1964) suggests the early symptoms of hypotonia and poor feeding might be related to abnormalities of the lateral nuclei in the hypothalamus and that subsequent problems with overeating might involve the ventromedial hypothalamic nuclei. Others have suggested (Clarren and Smith, 1977) that there might be a disturbance of the development of midline structures of the brain, which include the hypothalamus and the thalamus. Although midline abnormalities in the central nervous system have been reported and functional abnormalities in specific hypothalamic brain regions hypothesized, routine examination of the brain has not demonstrated specific abnormalities in the hypothalamus or other brain regions (Bray et al., 1983). Lesions in the ventromedial hypothalamus and in the temporal lobe, frontal lobe, septum amygdala, and dorsal tegmentum have been associated with hyperphagia and must also be considered. Despite these possibilities, ingestive behavior does not seem to be localized to a specific part of the brain. Selective destruction of serotonin pathways by the injection of neurotoxins into ventricles may also produce hyperphagia.

An abnormality in the central nervous system may lead to problems in circadian rhythms and bodily homeostasis. It has been suggested that there are two circadian pacemakers, a strong one (X), and a weaker one (Y) (Moore-Ede, Sulzman, and Fuller, 1982). The strong oscillator is approximately four times more effective in coupling brain systems than the weaker one. The X oscillator is thought to be involved in REM sleep, core body temperature regulation, plasma cortisol rhythms, and urinary potassium secretion. The Y oscillator is thought to be involved in driving slow wave sleep, skin temperature regulation, plasma growth hormone, and urinary calcium excretion. Inouye (1983) reports that the suprachiasmatic nucleus (SCN) pacemaker is linked to rhythmic activity in the ventromedial hypothalamus. Bray et al. (1983) demonstrated difficulties in the maintenance of core body temperature in Prader-Willi syndrome and noted that rectal temperature declined in 3 of 5 patients during exposure at 4° C, but in none of 4 obese controls. Besides temperature and REM sleep abnormalities, which may be independent of disturbed breathing, nocturnal oxygen desaturation, and probably excessive daytime sleepiness (Harris and Allen, 1985; Hertz et al., 1993), and abnormalities in respiratory rhythm have also been reported (Orenstein et al., 1977, 1980). Each of these circadian abnormalities might be related to hypothalamic dysfunction. In gastric loading experiments in 6 Prader-Willi cases (Robinson and McHugh, personal communication), eating abnormalities were noted when contrasted to obese controls. The Prader-Willi patients did not report a reduction in hunger with eating, but would suddenly stop eating, possibly related to the volume of food intake. Other evidence of compulsions related to food was noted by Bray et al. (1983) who found that salivation was not increased when the patients viewed food.

Abnormalities in biological rhythms have been studied by Tamarkin et al. (1982), who found that both melatonin and cortisol rhythms were abnormal in 3 of 16 cases of Prader-Willi syndrome when compared to obese controls. The cases with abnormal rhythms were those that were closest to ideal body weight for height. That circadian disturbances in hormonal rhythms were present in the group whose weight was closest to normal weight for height may be consistent with hyperphagia masking circadian disturbances in the more obese cases.

Sleep Cycle Disturbance

Excessive daytime sleepiness (EDS), daytime hypoventilation, and sleep apnea have been documented in Prader-Willi syndrome. Akefeldt (personal communication) matched obese males on body mass index (BMI), age, and intelligence with Prader-Willi patients and found PWS patients had significantly more excessive daytime sleepiness. Einfeld (1994) compared 60 children, adolescents, and young adults with PWS with an epidemiologic sample of 454 children, adolescents, and young adults and found significant increased prevalence of EDS ($p<000$). Children with Prader-Willi may have better sleep (i.e., increased slow wave sleep and decreased awakenings) when compared to sleep in adults (Hertz et al., 1993). In some cases, cataplexy and sleep onset REM periods without narcolepsy have been found (Vela-Bueno et al., 1984). Abnormal sleep architecture has been identified with unusual sleep stage transition from stage REM to stage 2 sleep. Sleep apnea and REM-related oxygen desaturation are present in mild forms in most subjects and are significantly correlated with increased obesity. Hertz et al. (1993) found abnormal REM sleep cycles with variable REM latency (often shortened) and fragmented REM sleep with multiple brief REM periods in both children (age 2 to 12) and adults (age 18 to 47). The REM abnormalities appeared to be independent of sleep-disordered breathing, nocturnal oxygen desaturation, and daytime sleepiness. The REM findings suggest a specific disruption in the timing of REM/non-REM cycles. These abnormalities are consistent with an underlying hypothalamic dysfunction. Uncontrolled appetite and hypogonadism also implicate the hypothalamus. Multiple sleep latency tests demonstrate the presence of daytime sleepiness (Harris and Allen, 1985; Hertz et al., 1993) with variable sleep apnea, which is often mild. Weight loss leads to improvement in the sleep apnea, but REM abnormality may persist despite weight loss (Harris and Allen, 1985). The sleep disorder in Prader-Willi syndrome is not narcolepsy (Harris and Allen, in press; Vela-Bueno et al., 1984) because the ancillary symptoms are not present and there is no HLA-DR15-DQ6 association with the Prader-Willi syndrome. The only symptoms of narcolepsy reported are excessive daytime sleepiness.

The mechanism of the REM sleep abnormality may be related to dysfunction in the posterior hypothalamus. Sakai et al. (1989) have described the role of the posterior hypothalamus in the regulation of wakefulness and paradoxical sleep. Brain transection experiments and single-unit recordings suggest that cholinergic afferents originating in the brainstem provide excitatory inputs to the posterior hypothalamic region. Such excitatory inputs occur during both REM sleep and wakefulness and appear to play a role in generalized cortical desynchronization during these sleep stages. Hertz et al. (1993) suggest that dysfunction in these systems may provide a basis for the REM cycle abnormality.

TREATMENT

Approaches to treatment include behavior management, family interventions, and pharmacological interventions. Behavioral approaches have focused primarily on the hyperphagia and food stealing and have utilized food restriction and behavior management techniques. Behavior analysis identifies social reinforcement and praise as most important in management. Indiscriminate eating makes it difficult to substitute low-calorie foods for higher-calorie foods because food preference is lacking. However, recognition of the lack of normal satiety has led to therapeutic diets that offer the greatest volume of food possible within caloric limitations.

Approaches to the family initially focus on the education of family members regarding the nature of the disorder and emphasize the importance of food restriction and behavior management. Total family involvement is essential because access to food in the environment must be controlled. Teachers, peers, and family members must be engaged in frequent monitoring of caloric intake, growth, and compliance with the behavior management program. Teaching appropriate behavior may be complicated because of learning difficulties and short-term memory problems in the Prader-Willi syndrome (Warren and Hunt, 1981). The learning disability profile must be considered in regard to treatment planning.

Despite the success of behavior treatments, the need for constant surveillance to monitor behavior is often resented by the patient and is difficult to generalize to home settings. For this reason, drug treatment for control of appetite might simplify management and could be helpful in the older patient who has tantrums and anxiety symptoms, particularly revolving around food. Psychopharmacological management and special diets, such as a ketogenic diet, have been tested with varying amounts of success.

A variety of medications have been introduced for the management of weight gain; however, medications have generally been reported to be of limited effectiveness. Agents with anorexic properties, such as dexedrine and methylphenidate, are most commonly used. These medications may produce temporary reduction in hyperphagia. In one case, the frequent alternation of methylphenidate and dexedrine led to better control of appetite (Harris et al., personal communication) than either drug alone. Other cases have been treated with fenfluramine, a drug that affects brain serotonin and brain glucose metabolism.

More recently, serotonin reuptake inhibitors, such as fluoxetine, have been investigated (Dech and Budow, 1991; Jerome, 1989). Jerome (1993) combined fluoxetine with lithium in a Prader-Willi patient with bipolar disorder. In the family survey of drug prescription in 369 Prader-Willi cases, approximately 17.5% were receiving serotonin reuptake inhibitors; 20.8%, neuroleptics; and 25%, stimulants. Naloxone has also been used for excessive eating (Kyriakides et al., 1980; Sullivan, 1980), and decreased food intake with naloxone was reported in 2 out of 3 cases in one open drug trial. Zlotkin, Fettes, and Stallings (1986) have reported similar findings with naltrexone. The rationale for the use of naloxone/naltrexone was suggested by an improvement in hyperphagia in genetically obese mice where this drug was thought to affect hypothalamic β-endorphin activity (Margules et al., 1978). Others have suggested that if naloxone has any effect on appetite, it could be related to delaying gastric emptying time through its effects on enkephalin receptors in the gastrointestinal tract. Naltrexone and fluoxetine have been successfully combined in one case report. This combination of medication led to substantial improvement in weight control, skin picking, and behavior (Benjamin and Buot-Smith, 1993). Still, none of these drug treatments for compulsive eating have been consistently effective and the positive effects are generally short lived.

Other pharmacological targets for intervention are the tantrums, aggressive behavior, and skin picking where serotonin reuptake inhibitors, neuroleptics, and stimulants have also been utilized. In addition, anticonvulsants have been used to regulate behavior for temper tantrums, mood disorder, and severe skin picking (Tu, Hartridge, and Izawa, 1992). Current treatment recommendations are for a combined treatment program that involves dietary management, behavior modification, family intervention and supportive family therapy, and drug treatment for targeted behavioral symptoms.

In the future, the type of circadian rhythm disturbance needs to be better delineated. Differences in behavior should be studied, taking into account the type of genetic abnormality—either a chromosomal deletion or maternal heterodisomy for chromosome 15. Future studies of hypothalamic function, using PET scanning, and more systematic neuroanatomical studies of the brain regions that are potentially involved are also needed.

REFERENCES

Akefeldt, A. (1992, November). *Behavior in Prader Willi syndrome—variations in the phenotype with age.* Paper presented at "From Genes to Behaviour," 2nd International Symposium, Society for the Study of Behavioural Phenotypes, Welshpool, UK.

______, Gillberg, C., and Larsson, C. (1991). Prader-Willi syndrome in a Swedish rural county: Epidemiological aspects. *Developmental Medicine and Child Neurology,* 33:715–721.

American Psychiatric Association, Committee on Nomenclature and Statistics. (1987). *Diagnostic and statistical manual of mental disorders,* 3rd ed., revised. Author, Washington, DC.

Barringer, D.M., Wallace, C.J., Elder, J., Burke, K., Oliver, T., and Blackmon, R. (1991). A behavioral approach to treatment of Prader Willi Syndrome. In V.A. Holm, S. Sulzbacher, and P.L. Pipes (eds.), *The Prader-Willi syndrome.* University Park Press, Baltimore.

Benjamin, E., and Buot-Smith, T. (1993). Naltrexone and fluoxetine in Prader-Willi syndrome. *Journal of the American Academy of Child and Adolescent Psychiatry,* 32:870–873.

Bray, G.A., Dahms, W.T., Swerdloff, R.S., Fiser, R.H., Atkinson, R.L., and Carrell, R.E. (1983). The Prader-Willi syndrome. A study of 40 patients and a review of the literature. *Medicine,* 62:77–80.

Butler, M.G. (1990). Prader-Willi syndrome: Current understanding of cause and diagnosis. *American Journal of Medical Genetics,* 35:319–332.

Clarke, D.J., Waters, J., and Corbett, J.A. (1989). Adults with Prader-Willi syndrome: Abnormalities of sleep and behavior. *Journal of the Royal Society of Medicine,* 82:21–24.

Clarren, S.K., and Smith, D.W. (1977). Prader-Willi syndrome: Variable severity and recurrence risk. *American Journal of Diseases of Children,* 131:798–800.

Dech, B., and Budow, L. (1991). The use of fluoxetine in an adolescent with Prader-Willi syndrome. *Journal of the American Academy of Child and Adolescent Psychiatry,* 30:298–302.

Down, J. L. (1887). *Mental affectations of childhood and youth.* J.A. Churchill, London.

Dunn, H.G. (1968). The Prader-Labhart-Willi Syndrome: Review of the literature and report of nine cases. *Acta Paediatrica Scandinavica,* 186(suppl.):1–38.

Einfeld S., Smith, A., Tonge B.J., Durvasula S., Florio T. (November 1994). Behavioural and emotional disturbance in Prader-Willi syndrome. Poster presentation, 3rd International Symposium, *Society for the Study of Behavioural Phenotypes,* Maastricht, Netherlands.

Evans, P.R. (1964). Hypogenital dystrophy with diabetic tendency. *Guys Hospital Reports,* 113:207–222.

Greenswag, L.R. (1987). Adults with Prader-Willi syndrome. *Developmental Medicine and Child Neurology,* 29:145–152.

Hall, B.D., and Smith, D.W. (1972). Prader-Willi Syndrome: A resume of 32 cases, including an instance of affected first cousins, one of whom is of normal stature and intelligence. *Pediatrics,* 81:286–293.

Harris, J.C., and Allen, R.P. (1985). Excessive daytime sleepiness in the Prader-Willi syndrome: Sleep apnea or idiopathic hypersomnolence. *Proceedings of the American Academy of Child Psychiatry,* 1:27.

Hawkey, C.J., and Smithies, A. (1976). The Prader-Willi syndrome with 15/15 translocation. *Journal of Medical Genetics,* 13:152–163.

Hertz, G., Cataletto, M., Feinsilver, S.H., and Angulo, M. (1993). Sleep and breathing patterns in patients with Prader Willi syndrome (PWS): Effects of age and gender. *Sleep,* 16:366–371.

Holm, V.A., and Pipes, P.L. (1976). Food and children with the Prader-Willi syndrome. *American Journal of Diseases of Children,* 130:1063–1067.

______, Sulzbacher, S., and Pipes, P.L. (1981). *The Prader-Willi syndrome.* University Park Press, Baltimore.

Inouye, S.T. (1983). Does the ventromedial hypothalamic nucleus contain a self- sustained circadian oscillator associated with periodic feedings? *Brain Research,* 279:53–63.

Jerome, L. (1989). Pharmacological therapeutic approaches for Prader-Willi syndrome. *Canadian Journal of Psychiatry,* 34:845–846.

______. (1993). Prader-Willi and bipolar illness. *Journal of the American Academy of Child and Adolescent Psychiatry,* 34:872–873.

Kyriakides, M., Silverstone, T., Jeffcoate, W., and Laurance, B. (1980). Effects of naloxone on hyperphagia in Prader-Willi syndrome. *Lancet,* i:876–877.

Margules, D.L., Moisset, B., Lewis, M.J., Shibuya, H., and Pert, C. (1978). β-endorphin is associated with overeating in genetically obese mice (ob/ob) and rats (fa/fa). *Science,* 202:988–991.

Moore-Ede, M.C., Sulzman, F.M., and Fuller, C.A. (1982). *The clocks that time us: Physiology of the circadian timing system.* Harvard University Press, Cambridge, MA.

Nicholls, R.D., Gottlieb, W., Russell, L.B., Davda, M., Horsthemke, B., and Rinchik, E.M. (1993). Evaluation of potential models for imprinted and nonimprinted components of human chromosome 15q11-q13 syndromes by fine-structure homology mapping in the mouse. *Proceedings of the National Academy of Sciences USA,* 90(5):2050–2054.

______, Knoll, J.H., Butler, M.G., Karam, S., and Lalande, M. (1989). Genetic imprinting suggested by maternal heterodisomy in non-deletion Prader-Willi syndrome. *Nature,* 342:281–185.

Orenstein, D.M., Boat, T.F., Owens, R.P., Horowitz, J.G., Primiano, F.P., Germann, K., and Doershuk, C.F. (1980). The obesity hypoventilation syndrome in children with the Prader-Willi syndrome: A possible role for familial decreased response to carbon dioxide. *Journal of Pediatrics,* 95:765–767.

______, ______, Stern, R.C., Doershuk, C.F., and Light, M.S. (1977). Progesterone treatment of the obesity hypoventilation syndrome in a child. *Journal of Pediatrics,* 90:477–479.

Prader, A., Labhart, A., and Willi, H. (1956). Ein syndrom von adipositas, kleinwuchs, kryptorchismus und oligophrenie nach myatonieartigem zustand in neugeborenenalter. *Schineizerische Medizinische Wochenschrift,* 86:1260–1261.

Robinson, W.P., Botttani, A., Xie, Y.G., Balakrishman, J., Binkert, F., Machler, M., Prader, A. and Schinzel, A., (1991). Molecular, cytogenetic and clinical investigations of Prader-Willi syndrome patients. *American Journal of Human Genetics,* 49:1219–1234.

Sakai, K., Mansari, E.L., Lin, J.S., Zhang, J.G., and Vanni-Mercier, G. (1989). The posterior hypothalamus in the regulation of wakefulness and paradoxical sleep. In M. Mancia and G. Marini (eds.), *The diencephalon and sleep,* pp. 171–198. Raven, New York.

Stein, D.J., Keating, J., and Zar, H. (1993, May). Compulsive and impulsive symptoms in Prader-Willi syndrome. *Abstracts in New Research (NR33).* Annual meeting of the American Psychiatric Association, San Francisco.

Sullivan, S.N. (1980). Naloxone and Prader-Willi syndrome [letter]. *Lancet* i (8178):1140.

Sulzbacher, S., Crinic, K.A., and Snow, J. (1981). Behavioral and cognitive disabilities in Prader Willi syndrome. In V.A. Holm, S. Sulzbacher, and P.L. Pipes (eds.), *The Prader-Willi syndrome.* University Park Press, Baltimore.

Tamarkin, L., Abastillas, P., Chen, H., McNemar, A., and Sidbury, J.B. (1982). The daily profile of plasma melatonin in obese and Prader-Willi syndrome children. *Journal of Clinical Endocrinology and Metabolism,* 55:491–495.

Tu, J-B, Hartridge, C., and Izawa, J. (1992). Psychopharmacogenetic aspects of Prader-Willi syndrome. *Journal of the American Academy of Child and Adolescent Psychiatry,* 31:1137–1140.

Turner, R., and Ruvalcaba, R.H.A. (1981). A retrospective study of the behavior of Prader-Willi syndrome versus other institutionalized retarded persons. In V.A. Holm, S. Sulzbacher, and P.L. Pipes (eds.), *The Prader-Willi syndrome.* University Park Press, Baltimore.

Vela-Bueno, A., Kales, A., Soldatas, C., Dobladez-Blanco, B., Campos-Castello, J., Espino-Hurtado, P., and Olivan-Palacias, J. (1984). Sleep in the Prader-Willi syndrome: Clinical and polygraphic findings. *Archives of Neurology,* 41:294–296.

Warren, J.L., and Hunt, E. (1981). Cognitive processing in children with Prader-Willi syndrome. In V.A. Holm, S. Sulzbacher, and P.L. Pipes (eds.), *The Prader-Willi syndrome.* University Park Press, Baltimore.

Zlotkin, S., Fettes, I., and Stallings, V. (1986). The effects of naltrexone, and oral β-endorphin antagonist, in children with Prader-Willi syndrome. *Journal of Endocrinology and Metabolism,* 63:1229–1232.

10.2 Angelman Syndrome

Angelman syndrome is a rare mental retardation syndrome associated with a characteristic physical and behavioral phenotype. Interest in Angelman syndrome has grown with the recognition that it involves a deficiency in the same region on chromosome 15 as the Prader-Willi syndrome—an example of genomic imprinting (Hall, 1990). Angelman syndrome demonstrates that the parental origin of genetic material may have a major effect on the clinical expression of a defect.

This chapter reviews the history, epidemiology, clinical presentation and phenotype, etiology, and treatment of Angelman syndrome.

HISTORY

Angelman syndrome was initially described in 1965 by Harry Angelman. It was reported only infrequently until 1987 when a small deletion of the long arm of chromosome 15 was recognized at 15q11–13 (Kaplan et al., 1987; Magenis et al., 1987). Following the recognition of its origins, additional research is under way to specify the genetic abnormality in Angelman syndrome.

EPIDEMIOLOGY

Angelman syndrome is a rare condition whose overall prevalence rate is unknown.

CLINICAL PRESENTATION AND PHENOTYPE

Pregnancy and delivery are generally described as normal, although birth weight is less than that of normal siblings. Feeding problems are common in the neonatal period, with difficulty in breast feeding, poor weight gain, and gastroesophageal reflux. Parents frequently describe tremulousness and jerky movements with handling during the first several months of life. Motor milestones are delayed and truncal hypotonia may be apparent. Independent walking generally is not achieved until 3 to 4 years of age, although some children may walk during their second year. A minority do not ambulate and may have associated scoliosis or cerebral palsy. The gait of a child with Angelman syndrome is ataxic, with a wide base and stiff legs. Because they maintain a characteristic posture with arms upheld and flexed and laugh frequently, the designation "happy puppet syndrome" has been used (Bower and Jeavons, 1967; Clayton-Smith, 1992; Robb et al., 1989). However, the appropriate characterization is "Angelman syndrome."

Seizure disorder occurs in approximately 80% of cases, with an onset between 18 and 24 months. Commonly, the first convulsion is a febrile one. A variety of seizure types are noted; myoclonic jerks and drop attack are most frequent. Seizures may be difficult to control and may occur episodically. Speech development is significantly delayed, generally with the acquisition of single words or rote phrases. Because of the speech disturbance, sign language may be needed for communication.

Physical Phenotype

Dysmorphic facial features are characteristic and become apparent during the second year of life (Clayton-Smith, 1992). The mouth is typically wide and smiling, with a thin upper lip, pointed chin, and prominent tongue with wide-spaced teeth. The head circumference is usually below the 50th percentile; however, approximately a quarter of cases are microcephalic. Approximately half of those affected have fair hair and skin, and most have blue eyes. About two thirds demonstrate alternating strabismus.

Behavioral Phenotype

Overall cognitive level is generally in the severe to profound range of mental retardation; however, it may be difficult to obtain accurate psychological testing because of the child's difficulties in speech and in coordination. Comprehension abilities are significantly better than expressive speech.

Children with Angelman syndrome appear happy and sociable. They laugh frequently and often inappropriately. Although the laughter is not uncontrollable, it occurs unexpectedly and with minimal stimulation. In addition to laughter, hand flapping may occur with excitement. There is no associated EEG change with the laughter. The happy, sociable appearance in a young severely retarded child provides clues to a diagnosis of Angelman syndrome before dysmorphic facial features are apparent. Sleep disturbances are also characteristic, with frequent nighttime waking.

ETIOLOGY

Angelman syndrome is a genetic disorder and may arise from several genetic mechanisms. Most reported cases are sporadic, but familial inheritance has been reported (Baraitser et al., 1987; Fisher et al., 1987; Kuroki et al., 1980). Approximately 60% of patients have a deletion of chromosome 15q11–13, which is demonstrable cytogenetically (Pembrey et al., 1989). In those cases where there is no apparent cytogenetic deletion, DNA analysis is necessary to demonstrate the deletion (Knoll et al., 1990). The deletion occurs at the same site on chromosome 15 as is seen in Prader-Willi syndrome. Despite deletions of the same chromosome region, these are distinct clinical phenotypes. Minor similarities occur in both syndromes, such as fair hair and blue eyes, but the major clinical features do not overlap. The chromosomes of the parents are reported to be normal. In Angelman syndrome, the deletion always arises on the chromosome 15 inherited from the mother, whereas in Prader-Willi syndrome the deletion is inherited on chromosome 15 from the father (Knoll et al., 1989; Ledbetter et al., 1981). The two disorders, Angelman syndrome and Prader-Willi syndrome, provide a human model for genomic imprinting, a phenomenon where genetic information is expressed differently depending on the parental chromosome inherited.

In 2% or 3% of Angelman syndrome cases, both chromosome 15s are inherited from a single parent; this form of inheritance is referred to as "uniparental disomy" (Malcolm et al., 1991). In this instance, there are no deletions, but both chromosome 15s are inherited from the father. It is possible that the fetus may have been trisomic for chromosome 15 and a maternal chromosome 15 was lost during early cell divisions in these cases so that the embryo survived. Parental chromosomes are ordinarily normal with uniparental disomy. However, in approximately 5% of families, there may be chromosomal rearrangements in the mother, such as translocations, which may give rise to Angelman syndrome and be passed on to a child due to predisposition of the 15q11–13 site. In this instance, there is a risk to subsequent children. Therefore, assessment of the parental chromosomes is necessary in all cases of Angelman syndrome so a chromosomal rearrangement can be ruled out.

Finally, in about 15% of families, the 15q11–13 deletion is not detected and uniparental disomy is not demonstrated. It is this group of families that has the highest risk of recurrence. It is speculated that siblings who are affected in these families inherit a small mutation from one of the maternal chromosome 15s. In these cases of familial Angelman syndrome, the mode of inheritance appears to be autosomal dominant with a 50% recurrence risk. Angelman syndrome will occur in this instance if the mutation is maternally transmitted due to genomic imprinting (Hamabe et al., 1991).

There are several genes in the 15q11–13 region. Further investigation of this region requires molecular studies to identify the gene sequences. One gene located in the 15q11–13 region is the gene for the GABA receptor β3 subunit (Wagstaff et al., 1991). Dysfunction of the GABA system may be relevant to the seizure disorder and the increased motor activity seen in these patients.

TREATMENT

Treatment begins with the recognition of the syndrome. Family counseling is initiated to assist with the associated clinical symptoms. Parental chromosome study is essential to rule out one of the rare familial forms. Adaptation to the child's mental retardation and clarification of the expected behavior disorder is crucial. Management of seizure disorder may be difficult and require multiple anticonvulsant drug trials. Sleep disturbances are common and may respond to a combination of pharmacotherapy and behavior management (Summers et al., 1992).

REFERENCES

Baraitser, M., Patton, M., Lam, S.T.S., Brett, E.M., and Wilson, J. (1987). The Angelman (happy puppet) syndrome: Is it autosomal recessive? *Clinical Genetics,* 31:323–330.

Bower, B.D., and Jeavons, P.M. (1967). The 'happy puppet' syndrome. *Archives of Diseases of Childhood,* 42:298–302.

Clayton-Smith, J. (1992). Angelman syndrome. *Archives of Disease in Childhood,* 67:889–891.

Fisher, J.A., Burn, J., Alexander, F.W., and Gardner-Medwin, D. (1987). Angelman (happy puppet) syndrome in a girl and her brother. *Journal of Medical Genetics,* 24:294–298.

Hall, J.G. (1990). Genomic imprinting: Review and relevance to human diseases. *American Journal of Human Genetics,* 46:103–123.

Hamabe, J., Kuroki, Y., Imaizumi, K., Sugimoto, T., Fukishima, Y., Yamaguchi, A., Izumikawa, Y., and Niikawa, N. (1991). DNA deletion and its parental origin in Angelman syndrome patients. *American Journal of Medical Genetics,* 41:64–68.

Kaplan, L.C., Wharton, R., Elias, E., Mandell, F., Donlon, T., and Latt, S.A. (1987). Clinical heterogeneity associated with deletions in the long arm of chromosome 15: Report of 3 new cases and their possible genetic significance. *American Journal of Medical Genetics,* 28:45–53.

Knoll, J.H.M, Nicholls, R.D., Magenis, R.E., Graham, J.M., Jr., Kaplan, L., and Lalande, M.(1990). Angelman syndrome—three molecular classes identified with chromosome 15q11–13 specific DNA markers. *American Journal of Human Genetics,* 47:149–154.

______, ______, ______, ______, Lalande, M., and Latt, S.A. (1989). Angelman and Prader-Willi syndromes share a common chromosome 15 deletion but differ in parental origin of the deletion. *American Journal of Medical Genetics,* 32:285–290.

Kuroki, Y., Matsui, I., Yamamoto, Y., and Ieshima, A. (1980). Happy puppet syndrome in two siblings. *Human Genetics,* 56:227–229.

Ledbetter, D.H., Riccardi, V.M., Airhart, S.D., Strobel, R.J., Keenan, B.S., and Crawford, J.D. (1981). Deletions of chromosome 15 as a cause of the Prader-Willi syndrome. *New England Journal of Medicine,* 304:325–328.

Magenis, R.E., Brown, M.G., Lacy, D.A., Budden, S., and LaFranchi, S. (1987). Is Angelman syndrome an alternate result of del(15) (q11q13)? *American Journal of Medical Genetics,* 28:829–838.

Malcolm, S., Clayton-Smith, J., Nichols, M., Robb, S., Webb, T., Armour, J.A., Jeffreys, A.J., and Pembrey, M.E. (1991). Uniparental paternal disomy in Angelman syndrome. *Lancet,* 337:694–697.

Pembrey, M.E., Fennell, S.J., Van den Berghe, J., Fitchett, M., Summers, D., Butler, L., Clarke, C., Griffiths, M., Thompson, E., Super, M., and Baraitser, M. (1989). The association of Angelman syndrome with deletions within 15q11–13. *Journal of Medical Genetics,* 26:73–77.

Robb, S.A., Pohl, K.R.E., Baraitser, M., Wilson, J., and Brett, E.M. (1989). The 'happy puppet' syndrome of Angelman: Review of the clinical features. *Archives of Diseases of Childhood,* 64:83–86.

Summers, J.S., Lynch, P.S., Harris, J.C., Burke, J.C., Allison, D.B., and Sandler, L. (1992). A combined behavioral/pharmacological treatment of sleep-wake schedule disorder in Angelman syndrome. *Journal of Developmental and Behavioral Pediatrics,* 13:284–287.

Wagstaff, J., Knoll, J.H., Fleming, J., Kirkness, E.F., Martin-Gallardo, A., Greenberg, F., Graham, J.M., Jr., Menninger, J., Ward, D., Venter, J.C. and Lalande, M. (1991). Localization of the gene encoding the GABA receptor beta3 subunit to the Angelman/Prader-Willi region of human chromosome 15. *American Journal of Human Genetics,* 49:330–337.

10.3 Fragile X Syndrome

The increased prevalence of mental retardation in males when compared to females has been recognized for over 50 years (Penrose, 1938). With the advent of chromosomal studies, a number of genetic conditions have been identified that are associated with the X chromosome. Among these, the fragile X syndrome is the most common form of inherited mental retardation and second only to Down syndrome as a known chromosomal cause of mental retardation; it is responsible for 30% of all X-linked mental retardation (Hagerman, 1992). Moreover, it is the most common heritable form because Down syndrome is rarely transmitted as a genetic disease from a Down syndrome parent to a Down syndrome child. Fragile X syndrome provides an example of a new mechanism of dynamic mutation involving heritable unstable DNA elements and is of interest to neuropsychiatry because of its behavioral phenotype, other associated behavioral features, and its potential association to other developmental neuropsychiatric disorders.

This chapter reviews the history, epidemiology, clinical features, behavioral phenotype, etiology, psychological and neuropsychological testing, developmental perspective, psychiatric aspects, and treatment of fragile X syndrome.

HISTORY

Familial X-linked mental retardation was first reported by Martin and Bell (1943). This report is now also known to be the first identified case of the fragile X syndrome. Additional families were described with X-linked mental retardation over the ensuing years. In 1969 a fragile cytogenetic marker site (Lubs, 1969), a constriction in the distal long arm of the X chromosome, was identified in a family with mentally retarded males in each of three generations. Although the fragile site served as a marker for the disorder, it could not be reliably demonstrated by cytogenetic techniques until 1977 when Sutherland found that special culture conditions, which involved deprivation of folate and thymidine from the culture medium, were needed to produce it. Thompson, McInnes, and Willard (1991) indicate that the fragile site becomes visible when chromatin does not condense during mitosis on the X chromosome at the Xq27.3 locus. This finding of the new culture media led to standardized chromosomal analysis as the method for fragile X testing.

Although it could be more reliably identified, fragile X syndrome remained a puzzle for geneticists because the combination of a single mutant gene and a specific cytogenetic abnormality was unique in genetics. In addition, the mode of inheritance was not clear; it could not be specifically assigned to either the dominant or recessive category. Those who inherited the fragile X mutation may or may not be mentally retarded, and risk for mental retardation in the fragile X carrier's offspring showed considerable variation (Sherman et al., 1985). Nonretarded transmitting males have no abnormality and a high percentage of carrier females also are cytogenetically normal. Moreover, not all cells in affected males showed the fragile site. These findings led to renewed and successful attempts at gene delineation, using positional cloning methods.

In 1991 Verkerk et al. used molecular cloning of DNA to identify the candidate FMR-1 (*f*ragile X *m*ental *r*etardation) gene for fragile X syndrome. Their group and several others (Oberle et al., 1991; Yu et al., 1991) found that a heritable unstable DNA sequence was characteristic of the FMR-1 gene. This sequence contained a CGG repeat sequence that was amplified and of varying lengths. The fragile X syndrome results from the amplification of the CGG repeat found in the FMR-1 gene. Amplification of the CGG repeat blocks transcription of the FMR-1 gene, leading to the absence of the FMR protein that results in mental retardation. Recognition of this DNA sequence facilitates the diagnosis and provides a rapid method of carrier detection and prenatal diagnosis (Sutherland et al., 1991). The FMR-1 protein (FMRP) is not synthesized in fragile X patients and its function is not known. Future studies on this protein are needed to understand the variable phenotype of this disease. Verheij et al. (1993) have reported on a methodology to isolate FMRPs, characterize them, and study their possible functioning.

EPIDEMIOLOGY

The prevalence of fragile X syndrome has been estimated to be 1 in 1,250 males and 1 in 2,500 females (Sherman, 1991; Webb et al., 1986). However, these figures are based on cytogenetic rather than molecular genetic procedures and, therefore, may represent an underestimation of the true prevalence. Among males, 20% to 50% of all cases of X-linked mental retardation is caused by the fragile X syndrome. Because of the X-linked characteristic, unlike Down syndrome, it is carried from one generation to the next. It has been found in all races, including blacks, whites, Orientals, and Australian aborigines.

Multiple studies of mentally retarded individuals in institutions have been carried out to identify the fragile X syndrome. If all individuals in an institution for mentally retarded persons are screened, the percentage with fragile X syndrome varies from 1.6% to 6.2%. However, if only those individuals at high risk with clinical features, such as macro-orchidism, are studied, then up to one third of males in institutional settings have been identified as having the fragile X syndrome. Using the other physical features, including long ears and hand changes, the yield may go up to 50%. Early screening studies of autistic individuals indicated that up to 25% of cases were associated with fragile X syndrome. However, more extensive experience with this disorder leads to the conclusion that the usual behavioral phenotype of fragile X syndrome is distinct from that of classical autistic disorder. Bailey et al. (1993) evaluated the prevalence of the fragile X anomaly in autistic twins and singletons and detected the anomaly in 1.6% of cases in males and in 5% of females. Because the number of females available for study was substantially less than the number of males, the authors suggest the prevalence in both sexes is most likely equal.

CLINICAL FEATURES

The presentation of the fragile X syndrome varies in relationship to puberty. Prepubertal males may have normal growth but have large heads (above the 50th percentile); as they grow older, other physical features become more apparent. Carrier females are not dysmorphic, but approximately one third test in the mildly mentally retarded range (Table 10.3–1).

The classical clinical features are macro-orchidism, large and prominent ears, and a narrow face (Hagerman, 1991a). Approximately 80% of adult males have one or more of these features. However, the individual features are not pathognomonic for fragile X syndrome and may be seen in other conditions and in normal individuals. Among these features, macro-orchidism is seen in 70% to 90% of adult males. Sutherland (1985), in reviewing 22 reports, found this characteristic in 87% of postpubertal males, but in only 21% of prepubertal males. Large prominent ears are a useful but nonspecific sign. Approximately 50% of males have an ear length that is 2 standard deviations or more above the mean of the general population. Another 30% will have normal-sized but prominent ears, protruding more than 30% out from the side of the head. The ear itself is well formed but the antihelical fold may be poorly developed. In the prepubertal patient, the ears may be the only prominent physical feature; ears are only occasionally low set. The third feature, a long and narrow face, is seen more commonly in the postpubertal group. Approximately one fourth of subjects have a face length that is more than 2 standard deviations above the mean.

Table 10.3–1. Clinical Features of the Fragile X Syndrome in Males*

Prepubertal
Delayed developmental milestones
Abnormal temperament (inattentive, hyperactive, impulsive)
Social deficits (gaze aversion)

Postpubertal
Mental retardation
Abnormal craniofacies (long jaw, prominent forehead, large ears, prominent jaw)
Macro-orchidism

Additional features
Strabismus
Joint hyperextensibility, pes planus
Mitral valve prolaspe
Soft, smooth skin

*Carrier females are not dysmorphic but about one third are mildly mentally retarded.

From Tarleton and Saul, 1993.

To account for these physical findings, it has been suggested that a connective tissue abnormality may be involved. This would be consistent with reports of hyperextensibility of finger joints and double-jointed thumbs. Furthermore, biopsies of the testicles have shown an increased interstitial volume with excessive connective tissue; however, fertility is normal. Other physical features are seen in less than 60% of the males with this condition, but are also probably related to connective tissue problems. The height of adult males tends to be reduced; 26% of 87 men were below the 5th percentile. Other associated features include seizure disorder in 20%, a diffusely abnormal EEG in 50%, strabismus, mitral valve prolapse, and soft, smooth skin.

The behavioral features and the cognitive profile are useful in identifying higher functioning individuals. Behavioral features are helpful in diagnosis, especially for prepubertal males who may not show the classical physical characteristics.

BEHAVIORAL PHENOTYPE

There is a substantial degree of genetic and phenotypic heterogeneity in the physical, cognitive, and behavioral phenotype. The behavioral phenotype has been the subject of considerable study and includes mental retardation and learning disabilities, language impairment, and neuropsychiatric disturbance, principally attention deficit/hyperactivity disorder and pervasive developmental disorder-like symptoms. Attentional difficulty and concentration problems are commonly associated, and hyperactivity may be a presenting symptom in nonretarded boys with fragile X syndrome. Self-injury, most commonly hand biting and scratching, may be elicited by excitement and by frustration. Hand flapping is a common stereotyped behavior. Fragile X females may be unaffected, although abnormalities in social interaction, thought process, and affect regulation have been reported in carriers (Reiss and Freund, 1990; Reiss et al., 1988). Both schizotypal features and depression have also been found in carriers.

Gaze Aversion

Gaze aversion is a striking feature of affected males. When greeting another person, there is remarkable consistency in gaze aversion over repeated trials in the same individual; nearly all fragile X males over the age of 8 or 9 avert gaze when greeting another person. Their idiosyncratic greeting is characterized by both head and gaze aversion combined with an appropriate recognition of the social partner (Wolff et al., 1989). Their greeting response is qualitatively different from the gaze aversion described in autistic individuals. Detailed analyses of the behavior ratings show a higher frequency of gaze avoidance in fragile X patients when compared to mentally retarded controls. Those with Down syndrome and nonspecific mental retardation do not show this behavioral pattern on greeting. The idiosyncratic gaze behavior in fragile X syndrome may potentially disrupt social interactions and interpersonal dialogues. Despite their apparent social anxiety and aversion to eye contact, males with fragile X syndrome are otherwise socially responsive and may be affectionate.

Speech and Language

Speech and language in fragile X syndrome is generally delayed even in those cases where the IQ is in the normal range. Deficits are present in both receptive and expressive language and include dysfluency, production of incomplete sentences, echolalia, palilalia (self-repetitions, e.g., reiteration of the speaker's own words and phrases in a perseverative manner in conversation), verbal perseveration, and poor fluency in conversation (Newell, Sanborn, and Hagerman, 1983). Compulsive utterances and shifts in speech pitch are common, and auditory processing and memory deficits are present. Cluttering, which refers to fast and fluctuating rates of talking with repetitions and disorganized speech, poor topic maintenance, and tangential comments are also characteristic (Hanson, Jackson, and Hagerman, 1986).

ETIOLOGY

Genetics

The genetics of fragile X syndrome reflect the major advances in human genetics that have taken place during the past two decades. Interestingly, the fragile site (located at Xq27.3) is expressed in only a minority of cells, and may be absent entirely, especially among asymptomatic male and female carriers. The proportion of positive cells in affected individuals ranges from less than 5% to greater than 40%, but is generally in the 10% to 40% range. Cytotoxic agents, such as methotrexate, may be added to the medium to increase fragile X expressivity.

DNA analysis allows more valid and reliable diagnosis in both males and females. DNA studies, using new probes that detect CGG repeat sequences, should be carried out to clarify the relationship between genetic findings and symptom presentation. Initial characterization of the mutation has begun; affected individuals exhibit a repetitive DNA base sequence (CGG) of considerable length within the FMR-1 gene. The number of CGG repeats appears to be related to phenotypic expression. It appears that approximately 230 repeats are required to produce the full clinical syndrome and between 52 and 230 repeats to produce the asymptomatic premutation carrier state; the normal range varies between 6 and 54 repeats (Tarleton and Saul, 1993). The intermediate premutation repeat length appears to be unstable and to predispose to a subsequent expansion and amplification of the abnormal region, which may grow in size. Excessive numbers of CGG repeats may induce methylation, which leads to subsequent reduction in expression of the gene.

There are at least two distinct mutation types, the premutation and the full mutation. Individuals with the premutation do not show the clinical syndrome but, in the full mutation, both males and females are at greater risk for severe neuropsychiatric disability related to inactivation of the adjacent candidate FMR-1 gene. In males, the extent of clinical involvement appears to correlate with the length of abnormal CGG repetitive sequence. When the premutation is passed from father to daughter, the premutation remains essentially unchanged in size. However, when it is passed from the mother, who is a carrier, the premutation may increase in size and potentially convert to the full mutation in both sons and daughters. Those children who inherit an X chromosome with the full mutation from their mother will also have the full mutation, and it often is even further increased in size. The premutation increases in size and potentially converts to a full mutation only when it is passed through the mother. It has been hypothesized that this amplification occurs during female gametogenesis and that sex-specific imprinting is involved. In addition to the mechanism described earlier, the fragile X syndrome phenotype has now also been reported in patients with a deletion of the FMR-1 gene (Gedeon et al., 1992; Wiegers, 1992; Wohrle et al., 1992).

The region of the X chromosome that is involved in the fragile X syndrome is in relatively close proximity to two other genes that may have importance to the neurobiology of the cerebellum. These are the GABAa-3 gene, which encodes a receptor subunit of gamma-aminobutyric acid (Bell et al., 1989), and the CDRP gene (cerebellar degeneration related protein). In the first instance, GABA is the primary neurotransmitter in the human cerebellum; it functions primarily as an inhibitory system. The second gene codes for a neuronal antigen that is a target for auto-antibodies in degeneration of the paraneoplastic cerebellum. Reiss et al. (1991) indicate that the proximity of these genes to the fragile X site suggests that other genes related to the development and possibly the maintenance of cerebellar structure might be located in this region. In addition, the L-1 neural adhesion gene, which is involved in neuron-neuron and axon-axon adhesion in cerebellar granular cell migration, an outgrowth of neurites to other neurites in Swann cells, is tightly linked to the Xq28 region. This adhesion gene plays an important role in brain development and could also potentially be influenced by the fragile X mutation. Continued investigations are needed to clarify the effects of the fragile X abnormality on brain development and will be benefited substantially by the identification of the protein product (Verheij et al., 1993).

Neuroimaging Studies

Reiss et al. (1991) examined a group of 14 males with fragile X syndrome, a comparison group of 17 males with other causes of developmental disability, and 18 males with normal IQ. The size of the posterior cerebellar vermis was found to be decreased, and the fourth ventricle increased in the males with fragile X syndrome when compared with males in either of the other two groups. No other brain areas or brain volumes differed significantly among any of these three groups of patients. These neuroanatomical findings are thought to be secondary to hypoplasia rather than atrophy. The patients with fragile X syndrome ranged in age from 2 to 43 years, with a mean age of 15.7 years; the broad range of males with fragile X syndrome was necessary to ascertain whether the decreased size was secondary to hypoplasia or due to atrophy. The magnetic resonance imaging (MRI) information showed the lack of a significant correlation between age and vermal size, making hypoplasia the more likely explanation.

Overall, it is the connections between the posterior vermis and other brain regions that may be most pertinent for the fragile X syndrome. As such, this region of the cerebellum is a component of the systems that are involved in the integration and modulation of both internal and external stimuli. Abnormalities in this brain region may be linked to deficits in processing and modulating sensory input, motor behavior, and language function.

PSYCHOLOGICAL AND NEUROPSYCHOLOGICAL TESTING

Psychological tests have been carried out to identify the extent of intellectual impairment and have identified the full range of mental retardation from borderline to profound. Intellectual impairment generally is in the mild to moderate range of mental retardation; the majority test in the moderate range, with IQs of 35 to 40. Verbal IQ frequently exceeds performance IQ in affected males and in nonretarded female carriers. Fragile X males perform poorly on certain subtests of the Wechsler Intelligence Scale for Children (WISC-R), including information, digit span, and arithmetic subtests, and higher on other subtests, such as picture completion and similarities (Chudley et al., 1983). With the introduction of the Kaufman Assessment Battery for Children (K-ABC) (Kaufman and Kaufman, 1983), sequential processing, or solving problems in serial or temporal order, and simultaneous processing, integrating stimuli into a Gestalt, have been evaluated in patients with fragile X syndrome. Consistent difficulties are reported with sequential processing tasks (Dykens, Hodapp, and Leckman, 1987). These difficulties in sequential processing may relate to weaknesses in auditory, visual, and motoric short-term memory. Weakness in math achievement is consistent with poor sequential processing skills and difficulties in retaining math facts.

Dykens and Leckman (1990) suggest that sequential processing deficits pervade cognitive, linguistic, and adaptive functioning. However, strengths in simultaneous processing may be helpful in adaptation in facilitating an understanding of the global meaning of stories or events. Relative strengths in simultaneous processing may relate to the ability to make perceptual inferences and to complete tasks that require perceptual closure.

Higher functioning fragile X males who test in the borderline to normal IQ range have been found to have learning disabilities that involve mathematics, visual-motor coordination, abstract reasoning, pragmatics, and attentional skills. Strengths include single-word vocabulary visual matching task, reading, and spelling skills (Pennington, O'Connor, and Sudhalter, 1991). These affected males with learning disability ordinarily express the fragile X chromosome in cytogenetic studies and may be distinguished from nonpenetrant carrier males who do not show these characteristics.

Psychological and neuropsychological testing has also been carried out in females who are heterozygous for fragile X syndrome. Approximately 40% to 50% of these heterozygous females are fragile X negative and have normal IQs. Of those who do express the fragile X chromosome, about 50% are cognitively impaired with an IQ in the borderline range or lower. These patients have been evaluated to clarify the extent of learning disability and emotional disability. Many heterozygous females will be unaffected, but despite normal intelligence, others have reported problems with mathematics, attention deficits, impulsivity, abstract reasoning, and staying on task in school (Hagerman, 1987; Wolff et al., 1988). When fragile X positive girls were evaluated, over 70% were receiving special education services; none of their sisters who were fragile X negative were in special education (Hagerman et al., 1992). Two thirds of the girls in special education had IQs below 85, and one third had IQs in the normal range. In those positive for fragile X, attentional problems, with and without hyperactivity, were identified. Overall, the problems in females appeared to be a milder version of the deficits that led to mental retardation in affected males.

Deficits in attention, short-term memory, and arithmetic seem most characteristic of the neuropsychological phenotype (Pennington, O'Connor, and Sudhalter, 1991). The profile of deficits suggests underlying problems in executive function and/or social cognition—domains that require further study. Moreover, initial neuropsychological studies of nonretarded fragile X positive heterozygotes have suggested significant frontal lobe deficits. These are demonstrated in problems with perseveration, distractibility, difficulty with maintaining mental set, and shifting topics (Mazzocco et al., 1992). Although left hemispheric functioning was not different when this group was compared to IQ-matched controls, mild deficits on right hemispheric tasks were noted in heterozygotes.

DEVELOPMENTAL PERSPECTIVE

The trajectory of intelligence may differ so that intellectual functioning of younger boys with fragile X syndrome may lie in the borderline to mildly mentally retarded range, whereas in adulthood, males may be diagnosed as severely retarded. This change over time has raised a question about there being a deceleration of IQ in fragile X males. A decline in IQ with a mental age plateau has been reported to begin in late childhood, lasting through the early adolescent years, i.e., through the age range of 10 to 15 years (Dykens et al., 1989). Others have suggested that the greatest drop takes place between 8 and 12 years.

There is general agreement that IQ test scores decline in many patients with fragile X syndrome. It has been postulated that the premature decline in intelligence may be related to factors responsible for the initiation of puberty and that the plateau in intelligence coincides with the beginning of pubertal development. It has also been hypothesized that the drop in IQ occurs primarily because abstract reasoning and symbolic language skills, which are stressed in intellectual assessment in tests for children, in later childhood may be specifically deficient in many fragile X males. These considerations raise the question whether IQ changes are due to changes in the developmental task facing the child or to changes in the maturation and development of the central nervous system.

A comprehensive study of the natural history of IQ change in the general population was completed through the New Zealand Multidisciplinary Health and Development Study. Children were evaluated longitudinally at ages 7, 9, 11, and 13, using the WISC-R. Very little measurable naturalistic change in IQ across middle childhood and early adolescence was identified. The reliable change that did take place appeared to be idiosyncratic and was not systematically associated with environmental changes (Moffitt et al., 1993). The question of change in task complexity versus maturational changes has also been considered for Down syndrome and in the development of normal children. In Down syndrome, decelerating rates of intellectual development have been reported from infancy through adolescence. In children with cerebral palsy, however, IQ has been reported to be relatively stable with some slight increases over time.

The IQ findings in fragile X syndrome suggest there may be a plateau in cognitive achievement that is reached earlier than that seen in the general population. Rather than overall IQ, an assessment of the neuropsychological profile of individuals with fragile X syndrome may be useful to clarify particular strengths and weaknesses, as outlined in Chapter 3 on neuropsychological testing. Despite the lack of progression in overall intelligence, adaptive behavior may continue to improve. Besides cognitive level, adaptive behavior has been evaluated in fragile X syndrome utilizing the Vineland Adaptive Behavior Scales, which assesses communication, daily living, and socialization skills. Using this approach, Dykens, Hodapp, and Leckman (1987) compared older fragile X subjects to other residents in a large institution and found that the fragile X males demonstrated significantly higher domestic daily living skills than their nonspecific mentally retarded and autistic peers. Their adaptive skills, in some instances, exceeded mental-age expectations. Improvements in adaptive ability must also be considered in the context of fragile X patients having a different natural history than those with other disorders.

Developmental Considerations in the Family

Fragile X syndrome provides an opportunity to examine the family environment and particularly the mother–child interaction in a way that may be unique among mental retardation syndromes. Because about one third to one half of the female carriers may have learning problems or mild to moderate mental retardation, boys with fragile X syndrome will frequently live in homes where their mothers and possibly their female siblings may have disabilities similar to, but less severe than, their own. In other families, no other member may have fragile X syndrome. Because of these variations in family constellation, the mother–child interaction and sibling–sibling interactions may be investigated to establish the environmental effect on an affected child who lives in a home either with or without other affected family members. Such research may provide additional information on the relationship of environmental factors to the degree of mental retardation.

In addition to the learning disabilities and mental retardation, carrier females may demonstrate anxiety symptoms, mood disorders, and schizotypal personality patterns (Reiss et al.,

1988). Research on mother–child interactions where the parent is depressed or schizophrenic has demonstrated important effects on development. Although not specifically investigated, the offspring of carrier females with cognitive and psychiatric difficulties may place boys with fragile X syndrome at greater risk for psychiatric disorder. Because of the variability in family constellation, intervention strategies need to be tailored to the particular problems for each individual family.

PSYCHIATRIC ASPECTS

There has been substantial interest in the identification of specific profiles of social, affective, and behavioral functioning among individuals with fragile X syndrome. Although initial reports described fragile X males as manifesting relatively normal patterns of emotional and behavioral functioning, more recent studies have highlighted the presence of neuropsychiatric symptomatology. Fragile X syndrome is associated with behavioral problems ranging from difficulties in social communication with strangers to pervasive developmental disorder, autistic disorder, and periodic violent outbursts of behavior. Other frequently described symptoms include gaze aversion, stereotypic behavior, attention deficits, and hyperactivity, as well as aggression and self-injury. Moreover, problems in visuomotor integration, as demonstrated in poor handwriting, motor delays, delays in sitting and walking, and hypotonicity have been noted. The difficulties in sensory integration may have been evident in early infancy and may be associated with histories of irritability, tantrums, problems with molding (arching or pulling away), and evidence of tactile defensiveness.

Autistic Disorder and Fragile X Syndrome

Males with fragile X syndrome can be sociable and friendly. Consequently, there has been controversy regarding the reported association between autistic disorder and fragile X syndrome. Although Brown et al. (1982) had suggested an association of autistic disorder with fragile X syndrome in five fragile X males who met the DSM-III (APA, 1980) diagnostic criteria, early screenings of individuals with autistic disorder did not identify fragile X positive patients. Subsequent screenings involving larger number of cases have identified an overall prevalence of approximately 7% fragile X positive cases with autistic disorder (Hagerman, 1990). Piven et al. (1991) found a prevalence of 2.7% (2 in 75) in a research study, using the Autism Diagnostic Interview (ADI) to elicit DSM-III-R (APA, 1987) criteria for autistic disorder.

Largo and Schinzel (1985) found one or more of the following features in 12 of 13 boys studied: poor eye contact, movement stereotypies, or social isolation. Repetitive hand mannerisms may occur and increase when the child is upset, angry, or frightened. These abnormalities along with language dysfunction and other behaviors, such as hand biting, tactile defensiveness, and perseveration, are recognized problems in fragile X syndrome and, in some instances, may have resulted in a diagnosis of autistic disorder.

Cohen et al. (1989) suggest that the mechanism involved in poor eye contact in fragile X males differs from that in non–fragile X males with autistic disorder in that poor eye contact in fragile X males is most likely related to aversion of mutual gaze. Up to 90% of males with fragile X show gaze avoidance and may turn their whole body away in greeting others (Wolff et al., 1989). Their hand stereotypies, vocal perseveration, severe attentional difficulties, and impulsivity may also interfere with social relatedness; executive dysfunction in the fragile X patient may be an important factor in their difficulties in social relatedness. Most verbal fragile X males express interest in social interactions, yet their neurophysiologic impairments may lead to apparent autistic-like behavior. Fragile X patients also appear to be overly sensitive to many stimuli and to become overwhelmed by them, which in their frustration may lead to social withdrawal, tantruming, and aggressive behavior. Their autistic-like behaviors may stem from problems in sensory integration, a factor that may also be present in subjects with autistic disorder. Overall, severe impairment in reciprocal social interaction is found in a significant minority of patients with the fragile X syndrome.

Ferrier et al. (1991) studied conversational skills in 18 individuals with fragile X syndrome and compared them to matched groups with autistic disorder and Down syndrome. The fragile X group used more eliciting forms in conversation than the other groups. Those with fragile X syndrome used partial self-repetition of their own statements to maintain the flow of conversation. Other authors have used the term "palilalia" to describe these partial repetitions, as noted earlier. Such repetition may be related to impaired auditory short-term memory and difficulty in formulating novel utterances to maintain one's "place" in the flow of conversation (Ferrier et al., 1991). Moreover, males with fragile X may have more difficulty pronouncing polysyllabic words and show dyspraxia. This tactic demonstrates an awareness of the interpersonal requirements of conversation and may allow the individual to maintain a conversation despite an expressive language disorder.

In this way, partial repetition is an aspect of functional communication. In contrast to the individuals with fragile X syndrome, those with autistic disorder use echolalia more often. Although there were no statistical differences between the groups in echolalia, the authors suggest that the fragile X individual is more likely to use echolalia with communicative intent, whereas this is less likely for the person with autistic disorder.

The autistic disorder group made many more multiply-inappropriate responses than either the fragile X or Down group. They showed failure to make appropriate verbal responses and failed to identify the referent. This response in persons with autistic disorder suggests an inability to maintain the focus of a conversational topic or to appreciate the speaker's needs. These findings emphasize the importance of studying the pragmatics of language in these conditions, particularly the analysis of verbal strategies in conversation.

Understanding the nature of the autistic disorder in fragile X syndrome has been complicated by the use of the DSM-III-R (APA, 1987) criteria that identified a higher percentage of individuals as autistic disorder than did DSM-III (1980). Future studies, using the DSM-IV (APA, 1994) criteria, which may be more specific than those in DSM-III-R, are needed to clarify the prevalence of the disorder in fragile X syndrome. In considering the diagnosis of autistic disorder, it is important that the natural history of the condition be taken into account as well as the symptom profile.

Einfeld, Molony, and Hall (1989) compared 44 fragile X positive males and 45 mentally retarded males who were matched for IQ and were fragile X negative. Using DSM-III-R criteria, 4 patients in each group were identified as having an autistic disorder. These authors concluded that autistic disorder was not associated with fragile X syndrome because the incidence was the same in the comparison group with mental retardation. Alternative explanations for the "autistic-like" symptoms include excessive social anxiety rather than autistic aloneness. Although fragile X syndrome has been proposed as a common cause of autistic disorder, the frequency of fragile X syndrome among previously diagnosed subjects with autistic disorder is not substantially different from that noted in the general mental retardation population.

Rather than focusing on a more global and composite diagnosis, such as autistic disorder, the behavioral characteristics of the fragile X behavioral phenotype itself should be emphasized in future investigations. Such studies might be limited to the behavioral phenotype of fragile X syndrome.

Because cerebellar abnormalities have been reported in MRI studies and in neuroanatomical studies in autistic disorder, Reiss et al. (1991) evaluated the MRI findings in individuals with fragile X syndrome who showed or did not show autistic-like behavior. They did not find an association between the diagnosis of autistic disorder in fragile X syndrome and the posterior vermis size or size of the fourth ventricle in the fragile X cases. This suggests that although posterior vermis hypoplasia may be an associated finding in both fragile X syndrome and autistic disorder, it may not be a specific marker for the development of autistic disorder or autistic-like behavior because fragile X patients with similar reductions in volume of the cerebellar lobules did not meet diagnostic criteria for autistic disorder. The role of cerebellar maldevelopment in autistic disorder remains to be clarified; Courchesne et al., (1994) have documented both hypoplastic and hyperplastic abnormalities of the cerebellar vermis in affected individuals. The language dysfunction that is characteristic of the fragile X syndrome, including palilalia, echolalia, perseveration, and cluttering, might be related to a cerebellar abnormality. The cerebellar vermis is also involved in auditory processing related to reception, modulation, and integration of speech and in the voluntary shift of selective attention between sensory modalities.

Attention Deficit Disorder

Attention deficit/hyperactivity disorder (AD/HD) has been reported in approximately 75% of boys with fragile X syndrome. However, the specificity of AD/HD for fragile X syndrome has been questioned. Reports of attention deficits and hyperactivity are commonly seen in younger subjects with fragile X syndrome; Fryns et al. (1984) found attentional problems in 21 study patients; however, these authors noted that the hyperactivity was no longer present after puberty. Hagerman et al. (1986), using the Connors Rating Scales in 37 males age 4 to 11, found that 73% of boys had a score of more than 2 standard deviations from the mean for hyperactivity; all of their subjects had concentration difficulties.

The findings of an abnormality in the cerebellar vermis on MRI are consistent with the findings of unusual responses to sensory stimuli and attentional dysfunction in fragile X syndrome (Reiss et al., 1991). The cerebellar vermis receives both direct and indirect sensory information from other brain regions, and the posterior vermis has been shown to receive tactile, auditory, and visual information. Moreover, connections with the brainstem reticular nuclei may link the cerebellar vermis to the modulation of attention. A role in hyperactivity might also be linked to cerebellar abnormalities because the cerebellar vermis has a role in the modulation and the execution of motor behaviors (Ghez, 1991).

TREATMENT

Although there is no cure, a variety of interventions are available that may make a difference in the developmental course and the behavior of the child with fragile X syndrome. The core professionals involved in treatment are the treating physician, psychologist, special education teacher, speech and language pathologist, and occupational therapist. Special education goals focus on relative strengths in memory, imitation, and reading and provide remediation for problem areas, such as mathematic and cognitive difficulties in reasoning. Speech and language therapists utilize both traditional language therapy and specific approaches to remediate pragmatic language deficits. Behavioral and emotional problems may be approached through cognitively based behavioral interventions and individual and family psychotherapy (Brown, Braden, and Sobesky, 1991).

Pharmacotherapy may be useful for inattentiveness, impulsivity, and overactivity (attention deficit disorder) in children with fragile X syndrome (Hagerman, 1991b). Hagerman, Murphy, and Wittenberg (1988) demonstrated improvement in two thirds of treated cases in a double-blind placebo controlled study with stimulant medication. Hilton et al. (1991) reported symptomatic improvement with imipramine in a case study of a boy with attention deficit disorder, enuresis, and initial insomnia. Behavioral problems, including attention deficit disorder, have been treated with folic acid in the past with mixed results; some children showed no change and others showed some improvement (Hagerman, 1991b). A specific subgroup of responders to folic acid supplementation has not been identified. Other behavioral symptoms, such as aggression and the psychiatric symptoms of depression and anxiety, may respond to pharmacotherapy. Further pharmacological trials are needed to determine if there are other characteristic behavioral profiles found in the fragile X syndrome that are drug responsive.

REFERENCES

General References

Davies, K.E. (1989). *The fragile X syndrome.* Oxford University Press, Oxford.

Hagerman, R.J., and Silverman, A.C. (1991). *Fragile X syndrome: Diagnosis, treatment, and research.* Johns Hopkins University Press, Baltimore.

Specific References

American Psychiatric Association, Committee on Nomenclature and Statistics. (1980). *Diagnostic and statistical manual of mental disorders,* 3rd ed. Author, Washington, DC.

American Psychiatric Association, Committee on Nomenclature and Statistics. (1987). *Diagnostic and statistical manual of mental disorders,* 3rd ed., revised. Author, Washington, DC.

American Psychiatric Association, Committee on Nomenclature and Statistics. (1994). *Diagnostic and statistical manual of mental disorders,* 4th ed. Author, Washington, DC.

Bailey, A., Bolton, P., Butler, L., LeCouteur, A., Murphy, M., Scott, S., Webb, T., and Rutter, M. (1993). Prevalence of the fragile X anomaly amongst autistic twins and singletons. *Journal of Child Psychology and Psychiatry,* 5:673–688.

Bell, M.V., Bloomfield, J., McKinley, M., Patterson, M.N., Darlison, M.G., Barnard, E.A., and Davies, K.E. (1989). Physical linkage of a GABA sub A receptor subunit gene to the DXS 374 locus in human Xq28. *American Journal of Human Genetics,* 45:883–888.

Brown, J., Braden M., and Sobesky, W. (1991). The treatment of behavioral and emotional problems. In R. J. Hagerman and A. C. Silverman (eds.), *The fragile X syndrome: Diagnosis, treatment, and research,* pp. 311–326. Johns Hopkins University Press, Baltimore.

Brown, W.T., Jenkins, E.C., Friedman, E., Brooks, J., Wisniewski, K., Raguthu, S., and French, J. (1982). Autism is associated with the fragile X-syndrome. *Journal of Autism and Developmental Disorders,* 12:303–308.

Chudley, A.E., Knoll, J., Gerrard, J.W., Shepel, L., McGahey, E., and Anderson, J. (1983). Fragile (X) X-linked mental retardation: I. Relationship between age and intelligence and the frequency of expression of fragile (X) (q28). *American Journal of Mental Retardation,* 92:436–446.

Cohen, I.L., Vietze, P. M., Sudhalter, V., Jenkins, E. C., and Brown, T. (1989). Parent-child gaze aversion patterns in fragile X males with autistic disorder. *Journal of Child Psychology and Psychiatry,* 30:845–856.

Courchesne, E., Saitoh, O., Yeung-Courchesne, R., Press, G.A., Lincoln, A.J., Haas, R.H., and Schreibman, L. (1994). Abnormality of cerebellar vermian lobules VI and VII in patients with infantile autism: Identification of hypoplastic and hyperplastic subgroups with MR imaging. *American Journal of Roentgenology,* 162:123–130.

Dykens, E., and Leckman, J. (1990). Developmental issues in fragile X syndrome. In R.M. Hodapp, J.A. Burack, and E. Zigler (eds.), *Issues in the developmental approach to mental retardation,* pp. 226–242. Cambridge University Press, New York.

______, Hodapp, R.M., and Leckman, J.F. (1987). Strengths and weaknesses in the intellectual functioning of males with fragile X syndrome. *American Journal of Mental Deficiency.* 92:234–236.

______, ______, and ______ (1989). Adaptive and maladaptive functioning of institutionalized and noninstitutionalized fragile X males. *Journal of the American Academy of Child and Adolescent Psychiatry,* 28(3):427–430.

Einfeld, S., Molony, H., and Hall, W. (1989). Autism is not associated with fragile X syndrome. *American Journal of Medical Genetics,* 34:187–193.

Ferrier, L.J., Bashir, A.S., Meryash, D.L., Johnston, J., and Wolff, P. (1991). Conversational skills of individuals with fragile-X syndrome: A comparison with autism and Down syndrome. *Developmental Medicine and Child Neurology,* 33:776–788.

Fryns, J.P., Jacobs, J., Kleczkowska, A., and Van Den Berghe, H. (1984). The psychological profile of fragile X syndrome. *Clinical Genetics,* 25:131–134.

Gedeon, A.K., Baker, E., Robinson, H., Partington, M.W., Gross, B., Manca, A., Korn, B., Poustka, A., Yu, S., Sutherland, G.R., and Mulley, J.C. (1992). Fragile X syndrome without CGG amplification has an FMR-1 deletion. *Nature Genetics,* 1:341–344.

Ghez, C. (1991). The cerebellum. In E.R. Kandel, J.H. Schwartz, and T.M. Jessell (eds.), *Principles of neural science,* 3rd. ed., pp. 634–637. Elsevier, New York.

Hagerman, R.J. (1987). Fragile X syndrome. *Current Problems in Pediatrics,* 17:621–674.

______. (1990). The association between autism and the fragile X syndrome. *Brain Dysfunction,* 3:218–227.

______. (1991a). Physical and behavioral phenotype. In R.J. Hagerman and A.C. Silverman (eds.), *The fragile X syndrome: Diagnosis, treatment, and research,* pp. 3–68. Johns Hopkins University Press, Baltimore.

______. (1991b). Medical followup and pharmacology. In R.J. Hagerman and A.C. Silverman (eds), *The fragile X syndrome: Diagnosis, treatment, and research,* pp. 282–310. Johns Hopkins University Press, Baltimore, MD.

______ (1992). Fragile X syndrome: Advances and controversy. *Journal of Child Psychology and Psychiatry,* 7:1127–1139.

______, Murphy, M., and Wittenberg, M. (1988). A controlled trial of stimulant medication in children with fragile X syndrome. *American Journal of Medical Genetics,* 33:513–518.

______, Jackson, A.W., Levitas, A., Rimland, B., and Braden, M. (1986). An analysis of autism in fifty males with fragile X syndrome. *American Journal of Medical Genetics,* 23:359–374.

______, ______, Amiri, K., Silverman, A.C., O'Connor, R., and Sobesky, W. (1992). Fragile X girls:

Physical and neurocognitive status and outcome. *Pediatrics,* 89:395–400.

Hanson, D.M., Jackson, A.W., and Hagerman, R.J. (1986). Speech disturbances (cluttering) in mildly impaired males with the Martin-Bell/Fragile X syndrome. *American Journal of Medical Genetics,* 23:195–206.

Hilton, D.K., Martin, C.A., Heffron, W.M., Hall, B.D., and Gregory, G.L. (1991). Imipramine treatment of ADHD in a fragile X child. *Journal of the American Academy of Child and Adolescent Psychiatry,* 30:831–832.

Kaufman, A., and Kaufman, N. (1983). *Kaufman assessment battery for children.* American Guidance Service, Circle Pines, MN.

Largo, R.H., and Schinzel, A. (1985). Developmental and behavioral disturbances in 13 boys with fragile X syndrome. *European Journal of Pediatrics,* 143:269–275.

Lubs, H.A. (1969). A marker X chromosome. *American Journal of Human Genetics,* 21:231–244.

Martin, J.P., and Bell, J. (1943). A pedigree of mental defect showing sex-linkage. *Journal of Neurology and Psychiatry,* 6:151-154.

Mazzocco, M.M., Hagerman, R.J., Silverman, A.C., and Pennington, B.F. (1992). Specific frontal lobe deficits among women with the fragile X gene. *Journal of the American Academy of Child and Adolescent Psychiatry,* 31:1141–1148.

Moffitt, T.E., Caspi, A., Harkness, A.R., and Silva, P.A. (1993). The natural history of change in intellectual performance: Who changes? How much? Is it meaningful? *Journal of Child Psychology and Psychiatry,* 34(4):455–506.

Newell, K., Sanborn, B., and Hagerman, R.J. (1983). Speech and language dysfunction in fragile X syndrome. In R.J. Hagerman and P.M. McBogg (eds.), *The fragile X syndrome: Diagnosis, biochemistry and intervention,* pp. 175–200. Spectra Publishing, Dillon, CO.

Oberle, I., Rousseau, F., Heitz, D., Kretz, C., Devys, D., Hanauer, A., Boue, J., Bertheas, M.F., and Mandel, J.L. (1991). Instability of a 550-base pair DNA segment and abnormal methylation in fragile X syndrome. *Science,* 252:1097–1102.

Pennington, B., O'Connor, R., and Sudhalter, V. (1991). Toward a neuropsychological understanding of fragile X syndrome. In R.J. Hagerman and A.C. Silverman (eds.), *The fragile X syndrome: Diagnosis, treatment and research,* pp. 173–201. Johns Hopkins University Press, Baltimore.

Penrose, L.S. (1938). A clinical and genetic study of 1280 cases of mental defect. *Medical Research Council Special Report Series,* No. 229. Medical Research Council, London.

Piven, J., Gayle, J., Landa, R., Wzorek, M., and Folstein, S. (1991). The prevalence of fragile X in a sample of autistic individuals diagnosed using a standardized interview. *Journal of the American Academy of Child and Adolescent Psychiatry,* 30:825–830.

Reiss, A.L., and Freund, L. (1990). Neuropsychiatric aspects of the Fragile-X syndrome. *Brain Dysfunction,* 3:9–22 .

______, Hagerman, R.J., Vinogradov, S., Abrams, M., and King, R.J. (1988). Psychiatric disability in female carriers of the fragile X syndrome. *Archives of General Psychiatry,* 45: 25–30.

______, Aylward, E., Freund, L.S., Joshi, P.K., and Bryan, R.N. (1991). Neuroanatomy of fragile X syndrome: The posterior fossa. *Annals of Neurology,* 29:26–32.

Sherman, S. (1991). Epidemiology. In R.J. Hagerman and A.C. Silverman (eds.), *The fragile X syndrome: Diagnosis, treatment, and research,* pp. 69–97. Johns Hopkins University Press, Baltimore.

Sherman, S.J., Jacobs, P.A., Morton, N.E., Froster-Iskenius, U., Howard-Pebbles, P.N., Nielson, K.B., Partington, M.W., Sutherland, G. R., Turner, G., and Watson, M. (1985). Further segregation analysis of the fragile X syndrome with special reference to transmitting males. *Human Genetics,* 69: 289–299.

Sutherland, G.R. (1977). Fragile sites on human chromosomes: Demonstration of their dependence on the type of tissue culture medium. *Science,* 197:265–266.

______. (1985). Heritable fragile sites on human chromosomes: XII. Population cytogenetics. *Annals of Human Genetics,* 49:153–161.

______, Gedeon, A., Kornman, L., Donnelly, A., Byard, R.W., Mulley, J.C., Kremer, E., Lynch, M., Pritchard, M., Yu, S., and Richards, R.I. (1991). Prenatal diagnosis of fragile X syndrome by direct detection of the unstable DNA sequence. *New England Journal of Medicine,* 325(24):1736–1738 (comment: 1720–1722).

Tarleton, J.C., and Saul, R.A. (1993). Molecular genetic advances in fragile X syndrome. *Journal of Pediatrics,* 122:169–185.

Thompson, M.W., McInnes, R.R., and Willard, H.F. (1991). *Genetics in medicine,* 5th ed., pp. 81–82. W.B. Saunders, Philadelphia.

Verheij, C., Bakker, C.E., de Graaff, E., Kuelemans, J., Willmesen, R., Verkerk, A.J.M.H, Galjaard, H., Reuser, A.J.J., Hoogeveen, A.T., and Oostra, B.A. (1993). Characterization and localization of the FMR-1 gene product associated with fragile X syndrome. *Nature,* 363:722–724.

Verkerk, A.J.M.H., Pieretti, M., Sutcliffe, J.S., Fu, Y.H., Kuhl, D.P., Pizzuti, A., Reiner, O., Richards, S., Victoria, M.F., Zhangi, F.P., Eussen, B., van Ommen, G., Blonden, L., Riggins, G., Chastain, J., Kunst, C., Galjaard, H., Caskey, C., Nelson, D., Oostra, B., and Warren, S. (1991). Identification of a gene (FMR-1) containing a CGG repeat coincident with a breakpoint cluster region exhibiting length variation in fragile X syndrome. *Cell,* 65:905–914.

Webb, T., Bundey, S.E., Thake, A.I., and Todd, J. (1986). Population incidence and segregation ratios in the Martin-Bell syndrome. *American Journal of Medical Genetics,* 23:573–580.

Wiegers, A. (1992, November). *Identical psychological profile and behavior pattern in different types of mutation in the FMR-1 region.* Paper presented at "From Genes to Behaviour," 2nd International Symposium, Society for the Study of Behavioural Phenotypes, Welshpool, UK.

Wohrle, D., Kotzot, D., Hirst, M.C., Manca, A., Korn, B., Schmidt, A., Barbi, G., Rott, H.D., Poustka, A., Davies, K.E., and Steinbach, P. (1992). A microdeletion of less than 250 kb, including the proximal part of the FMR-1 gene and the fragile X site, in a male with the clinical phenotype of fragile X syndrome. *American Journal of Human Genetics,* 51:299–306.

Wolff, P.H., Gardner, J., Lappen, J., Paccia, J., and Meryash, D. (1988). Variable expression of the fragile X syndrome in heterozygous females of normal intelligence. *American Journal of Medical Genetics,* 23:403–408.

______, ______, Paccia, J., and Lappen, J. (1989). The greeting behavior of fragile X males. *American Journal of Mental Retardation,* 93:406–411.

Yu, S., Pritchard, M., Kremer, E.J., Lynch, M., Nancarrow, J., Baker, E., Holman, K., Mulley, J.C., Warren, S.T., Schlessinger, D., Sutherland, G., and Richards, R. (1991). Fragile X genotype characterized by an unstable region of DNA. *Science,* 252:1179–1181.

10.4 DOWN SYNDROME

Down syndrome was the first mental retardation syndrome described and is the most common form of mental retardation. Approximately 7,000 infants are born in the United States each year with Down syndrome. Because of its frequency, the general population is most aware of Down syndrome and, in many minds, it is the prototypical form of mental retardation. It accounts for approximately one third of children in special education. The genotype, phenotype, and pathogenesis of Down syndrome continue to be rich areas of research.

This chapter reviews the history, epidemiology, etiology, clinical features, developmental perspective, personality development/behavioral phenotype, psychological adaptation, psychiatric disorders, and treatment of Down syndrome.

HISTORY

The first description of the child with Down syndrome is found in the writings of Esquirol (1838). Earlier physical descriptions of Down syndrome are rare when contrasted to other well-known pediatric conditions; this may be related to the life expectancy of adult women being low in medieval times—about 35 to 40 years—so that fewer women would have been giving birth in the ages when there is the highest risk.

J. Langdon Hayden Down (1826–1896) provided the first major classification and comprehensive description for what would later be called "Down syndrome." Down was medical superintendent of the asylum for idiots at Earlswood, England, from 1858 to 1868, and subsequently opened a private home for mentally retarded youth. From the beginning, he emphasized the need for early education of mentally retarded persons. In 1866 he proposed an ethnic classification of mental retardation in which he classified idiocy, a term he disliked, into three categories: congenital, congenital-accidental, and developmental (Down, 1866). He suggested Caucasian, Ethiopian, Malay, Aztec, and Mongolian forms of mental retardation. Although Down classified the congenital group according to ethnic similarities, he did not intend a negative view of any race. Rather, he hoped his classification system would confirm that mental retardation originates at birth, thereby avoiding parental guilt for the condition. Among these groupings, the Mongolian classification was retained and Down syndrome was known as "Mongolism" for many years afterward. Long before Down's description, facial stigmata characteristic of Down syndrome can be recognized in early paintings of children. In some instances, they appear as part of a crowd and, in others, as fairy characters or figures in the role of jester and even as a special child. There is also a legend of the changeling with strange-shaped eyes and ears who was placed in the cradle by the fairies, who stole the original baby and replaced it with one of their own. This legend may have been based on the unexpected birth of a child with Down syndrome who looked different from other members of the same family (Gath, 1985). Prior to Down's observations, Down syndrome more probably had been observed by physicians who may have considered it to be a variety of cretinism. For example, Séguin (1866) might have included Down syndrome under the category of "furfuraceous cretinism."

When Down syndrome was recognized and separated from cretinism, the degree of differentiation was often unclear. Wilbur, who rejected the ethnic classification, referred to Down syndrome as "that modified form of cretinism quite common in this country and in Great Britain" (Scheerenberger, 1983). Wilmarth (1889) suggested that those with Down syndrome were of "similar causative influence, and of prenatal origin, which was active during the formative stages of fetal existence." From the end of the last century until the 1950s, the etiology of Down syndrome was a common topic of medical discussion (Penrose and Smith, 1966; Rynders and Pueschel, 1982). Suspected causes were numerous, including parental alcoholism, syphilis, and smallness of the amnionic sac. Because Down syndrome occurred commonly in older mothers, it was hypothesized to be the result of maternal endocrine imbalance.

Advances in cytogenetics, resulting in improved techniques for the examination of human chromosomes, eventually led to the recognition of the chromosomal basis of Down syndrome. The underlying cytogenetic abnormality (trisomy 21) was identified by Lejeune, Gautier, and Turpin in 1959. It was the first syndrome to have a chromosomal anomaly demonstrated as the pathological basis for the characteristic physical features.

EPIDEMIOLOGY

Down syndrome occurs in approximately 1 in 600 live births (Hook, 1982). The incidence of Down syndrome is affected by maternal age and the availability of prenatal diagnoses. With advancing age, the risk of chromosome 21 nondisjunction is increased. The incidence is 1 in 1,400 for maternal age 20 to 24, but rises to 1 in 900 at age 30, 1 in 100 at age 40, and 1 in 25 among women 45 and older (Thompson, McInnes, and Willard, 1991). Most likely, there is significant fetal loss, particularly among older parents. Prenatal diagnostic procedures, including amniocentesis and chorionic villus sampling, have made it possible to identify the Down syndrome chromosomal abnormality early in gestation so that elective termination of pregnancy is possible. A variety of other potential risk factors have been studied, including demographic variables (e.g., geographic location, race, ethnicity, season of birth); parental variables (e.g., socioeconomic status, maternal smoking or infection, paternal age); and environmental exposures (e.g., fluoride, ionizing radiation). None of these have been found to affect the incidence of Down syndrome in a predictable and consistent manner.

The life expectancy of adults with Down syndrome is variable, but some individuals live well into their 70s. Early deaths are correlated with associated congenital anomalies, particularly cardiac malformations, which lead to death in early life or, in other instances, in the late teens to late 20s. Life expectancy has been considerably enhanced by surgical procedures and the availability of antibiotic treatment.

ETIOLOGY

Genetic

Down syndrome arises from an abnormality on chromosome 21; the chromosome 21 pair is the smallest of the 23 human chromosome pairs and includes about 1.5% of the total genetic material. Gene mapping studies have demonstrated that only 10% to 20% of chromosome 21, the 21q22 band on the long arm, is involved in Down syndrome. Despite the size of the region, the presence of an additional copy of this chromosome leads to profound changes in the development of affected individuals.

Three main types of Down syndrome are recognized. Most cases are caused by meiotic nondisjunction of autosomal chromosome pair

21, which results in the triplication of the entire 21st chromosome (Lejeune, Gautier, and Turpin, 1959). This is a nonfamilial form of Down syndrome and makes up approximately 95% of all cases. The recurrence risk is approximately 1 in 200. Because of the frequency of this type, Down syndrome is often referred to as "trisomy 21." The second type, which makes up approximately 4% of Down syndrome, involves translocation of a portion of chromosome 21q to another chromosome. This usually involves an unbalanced Robertsonian translocation between chromosome 14 and 21q for example, 46, XX,-14,+t (14q21q). Although this ordinarily is a new mutation, one parent may carry a balanced translocation, leading to a recurrent risk of 1 in 4. There may also be a 21q21q translocation that usually originates as an isochromosome; 90% of these are new mutations, but if a parent is a carrier, the recurrence risk is 1 in 2 future progeny will have either Down syndrome or monosomy 21. The third type is the mosaic form, which is generally said to occur in 1% to 2% of cases, but most likely, the occurrence is higher than this because the mosaic form may go undiagnosed. For mosaicism, there are two cell lines, one is trisomic and one is normal; the proportions vary from one child to the next. The mosaic forms are usually associated with less severe impairment.

Genetic studies have localized the core clinical phenotype of Down syndrome (facial and hand anomalies, congenital heart disease, mental retardation) to 21q22 (particularly the 21q22.3 segment). However, it is probable that a larger segment of proximal 21q plays a role in the development of many associated features of the syndrome.

CLINICAL FEATURES

The physical phenotype is characteristic and most commonly includes the following: upturned, outward slanting eyes, epicanthus, wide nasal bridge, brush field spots, large posterior fontanelle, brachycephaly, low nuchal hair line, single transverse palmar crease, large cleft between first and second toe, and relatively short upper arms. Hypotonia in infancy is usually present, but becomes less apparent as the child matures. The majority show short stature; 15% are hypothyroid by the time they reach adolescence. Approximately 50% have structural congenital heart lesions of varying severity and about 15% have a full atrial ventricular septal defect. Approximately 7% have congenital upper intestinal obstruction; 1% have a diagnosis of leukemia.

Behavioral features are also characteristic. Cognitive abilities are very variable, with about 10% functioning in the low normal range; however, the majority function in the mentally retarded ranges of intelligence. The majority have specific speech and language delays regardless of the extent of their cognitive ability. Although thought to have a characteristic personality and frequently described as happy and fun loving, the majority react to demand situations in a negative way and are often described as stubborn. Approximately 25% have attention deficit disorder.

DEVELOPMENTAL PERSPECTIVE

A developmental perspective in Down syndrome addresses whether temperament, social-emotional, cognitive, and representational development follow the same stages, sequences, and structures as in nonimpaired children. In addition, qualitative and quantitative differences must be considered between those with Down syndrome and those who are developing normally. Moreover, the developmental perspective asks whether or not there is a pattern in the development of children with Down syndrome that is specific to this particular condition.

In the past, development in Down syndrome has sometimes been considered to be qualitatively different than that of nonimpaired children. In children who have been referred to as "cultural-familial" mentally retarded, the sequence and order of developmental stages has been shown to be similar to that of non-mentally retarded persons, although development proceeds at a slower rate. This is referred to as the similar sequence hypothesis. In addition, a similar structure hypothesis has been proposed which posits that children with cultural-familial mental retardation utilize the same structures as they master developmental tasks. Finally, there is a similar response hypothesis which states that children who are culturally-familially retarded may respond in a similar way to life events, e.g., response to failure (Zigler and Balla, 1977).

Children with a neurobiological cause of their mental retardation, a genetic disorder, or a metabolic disorder were previously thought to follow different developmental pathways and diverge from the typical developmental course. Cicchetti and Pogge-Hesse (1982) indicate this may not be the case and suggest the developmental perspective be utilized to assess progress in Down syndrome and other neurobiological etiologies of mental retardation. Consequently, Cicchetti and Ganiban (1990) utilized aspects of Werner's (1957) organismic model and Piaget's (1952) structural model to study development in Down syndrome. In these models, an individual plays an active role in his development. Patterns of behavior are evaluated in terms of the organization between the parts and the whole; that is, a dynamic relationship between the individual and the environment is suggested.

In both of these developmental theories, development involves differentiation and hierarchical integration and results in a series of qualitative reorganizations. Differentiation results in parts that are distinct and separate; hierarchical organization ensures the organization of disparate parts into a more complex organism. Developmental theory posits an active organism, one which is inherently and spontaneously active, rather than being activated by external forces. This view contrasts with the behavioral view that conceptualizes the child as a passive recipient of external stimuli.

Development is characterized by regular and invariant sequences, leading toward a well-defined end point. Development is orderly and sequential, with transitions from one phase of development to the next. It consists of changes in internal mental structures and not in behaviors alone. Behavioral change is viewed as reflecting changes in underlying mental structures. Moreover, development occurs in a context and involves not only language and cognitive development but also social, emotional, motivational, and personality development (Hodapp and Zigler, 1990). Considering these aspects of development, developmental tasks include the development of self-image and mastery motivation. Development involves interaction with the environment and a series of transactions between the environment and the developing child.

The developmental perspective has been applied to the child with Down syndrome and is an important consideration in working with Down syndrome individuals. Children with Down syndrome traverse the same sequences of development as nonretarded children (Hodapp and Zigler, 1990). However, children with Down syndrome do show a slowing trajectory of IQ as they develop. In sensorimotor development, they develop through the six Piagetian stages in the expected order and, in language development, proceed from prelinguistic communication, to holophrases, into complex grammatical speech.

Because of the similar sequence of development, intervention efforts may proceed with the expectation that children with Down syndrome will follow a normal sequence in a particular domain. Consequently, knowledge about normal development in that domain may be used in an intervention program. Research on normal development is applicable to children with Down syndrome.

Although children with Down syndrome follow a similar sequence of development, they do have particular difficulties in certain areas; consequently, they have a different structure to their intelligence than mental-age-matched nonretarded children. When matched on mental age to normally intelligent children, those with Down syndrome perform worse on certain tests and better on others. The most common deficit involves language functioning. When 18 mentally retarded children with Down syndrome and 18 nonretarded children were matched on the Bayley Scales of Infant Development (Mahoney, Glover, and Finger, 1981) on both expressive language and receptive language, Down syndrome children were behind normal children of equivalent mental age. This language deficit may be related to lower levels of vocal imitation skills in those with Down syndrome. Yet not all aspects of language are deficient in Down syndrome. When evaluated in terms of conversational skill, i.e., the ability to maintain a conversation, take turns and give answers to questions, mental-age-matched children with Down syndrome showed better conversational skills than normal children of the same mental age. This suggests that within language some areas, such as social aspects of language, may be less impaired in Down syndrome children, whereas others, the more grammatical and relational aspects, are specifically deficient. The finding that the social aspects of language are strengths is consistent with the finding that Down syndrome children show better performance than expected for their mental ages on tasks of social maturity. Overall, social adaptation, simple visuospatial skills, and babbling seem less delayed than overall levels of mental abilities. Still, difficulties in expressive language, abstract thinking, and dealing with complex stimuli place those with Down syndrome at a disadvantage when compared to mental-age-matched peers.

Besides sequence and structure, the trajectory of development must also be considered. In Down syndrome, developmental trajectory does not seem to have a constant or near-constant form, as is seen in normally developing children. Studies in the infancy period suggest a deceleration in the rate of intellectual growth over time in Down syndrome infants (see Figure 10.4–1).

In one study (Dicks-Mireaux, 1972), Down syndrome infants progressed approximately 12 weeks in the first 16 weeks of life, which gave them a developmental quotient of 75; 20 weeks in the first 28 weeks, resulting in a developmental quotient of 71; 30 weeks in the first 40 weeks, leading to a developmental quotient of 75; and 45 weeks in the first 78 weeks, leading to a developmental quotient of 58. Overall, the rate of development is apparently slowed toward the end of the first year and thereafter.

Using a developmental perspective, a decelerated rate of growth implies a difference between Down syndrome children and normal children. In normally developing children, there are no consistent progressive declines in the rate of development over the years. Several theories have been advanced to explain the deceleration of IQ in those with Down syndrome, although the specific etiology is not known. McCall, Eichorn, and Hogarty (1977) suggest that 2 months, 8 months, 13 months, and 21 months are transition points in development. At those times, a different factor structure of intelligence was shown to emerge among nonmentally retarded children in the Berkeley growth studies; new tasks were characterized by intelligent behavior at each of these points. It has been hypothesized that Down syndrome children and some other children with disabilities fall behind at these cognitive transition points.

Affect relates to the extent to which an individual may appropriately evaluate an experi-

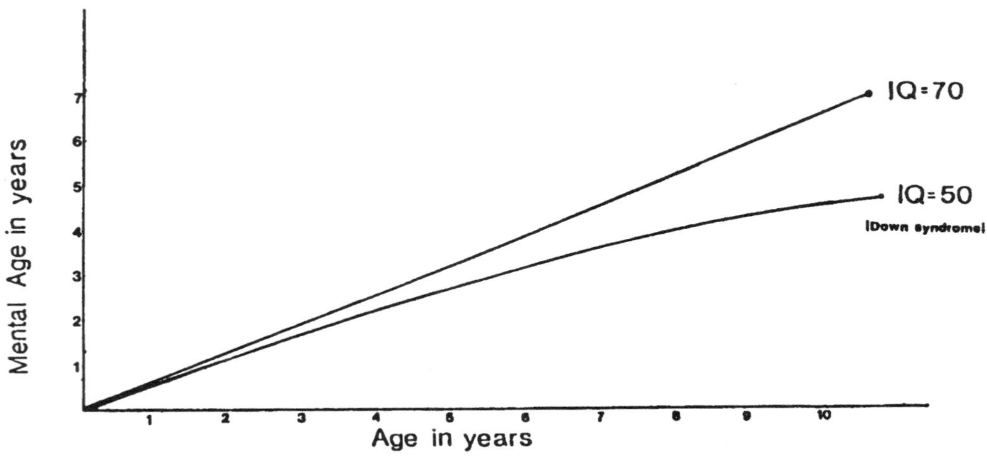

Figure 10.4–1. *Declining IQ in Down syndrome children.* This figure demonstrates the gradual decline in mental age (MA) relative to chronological age (CA) over time (from Hodapp and Zigler, 1990).

ence. Socioemotional development has been evaluated in Down syndrome, emphasizing the organization of affect, motivation, cognition, and play. Because children with Down syndrome develop at a slower rate, convergences and discontinuity in development may be magnified. Children with Down syndrome follow a developmental course similar to that of the nondisabled, as stated earlier. They move from being stimulus bound or reactive to the environment to becoming actively involved in shaping their experiences and pass through the same stages of development as normally developing children in an orderly fashion and gradually acquire more complex skills. Moreover, coherence in their development is demonstrated which parallels that of normally developing, nonimpaired children. Changes in the Down child's ability to evaluate and represent the world are seen in the development of affect, attachment, play, language, and self-systems (Beeghly, Weiss-Perry, and Cicchetti, 1990; Cicchetti and Ganiban, 1990).

Despite the similarities in development, certain differences are also apparent when comparisons are made to normally developing children. In general, the intensity of reactions to experience is weaker; differences are apparent in linguistic skills, pragmatics, and cognitive development. In language, syntactic and vocabulary skills are slower to develop than pragmatic and cognitive skills so that, when matched with nonimpaired children, syntax and vocabulary are less developed. The reason for linguistic differences is not clear, although one factor relates to less intense interactions with caregivers during the period of language development.

Overall, although infants with Down syndrome are not identical in their function to mental-aged-matched nondisabled children, a developmental approach shows organization and coherence in their early development. Additional investigation is necessary to establish developmental organization in older children and adults with Down syndrome.

PERSONALITY DEVELOPMENT/ BEHAVIORAL PHENOTYPE

Since Down's (1866) early report, children with Down syndrome have generally been assumed to have a pleasant manner, to be happy, amiable, and easygoing. Commonly, when an infant or older child deviates from this stereotype and shows negative reactions and irritability, the family may blame themselves. Yet studies of temperament in both infants and older individuals with Down syndrome do not confirm this personality stereotype. Gunn, Berry, and Andrews (1981) reported that a specific temperamental profile was not identifiable. On the Carey Scale, both easy and difficult temperaments were noted just as they are in children who do not have Down syndrome. Twenty percent (5 in 25) of infants with Down syndrome were rated as having difficult temperaments and showed irregular eating and sleeping habits, slow adaptation to change, and had negative reactions to new situations—all patterns that persisted into adolescence. This study recalls the negative personality traits Down commented on in his early paper, saying their great obstinacy requires that they "can only be guided by consummate tact."

In evaluating temperament in children with Down syndrome, they differ from normal youngsters along several dimensions. As the child with Down syndrome develops, the ability to respond to the environment is affected by the interaction of cognitive ability and reactivity, which is restricted by the genetic disorder. Changes in temperament, then, are affected by the developmental course of brain maturation. Although at certain developmental periods abilities may be organized in a similar way, for Down syndrome infants, the intensity of their expression may be specific to the disorder. When Down's patients are evaluated, using Rothbart and Derryberry's (1981) view of temperament as an organization of reactive capacities, emotionality, cognitive and self-regulatory abilities, differences are noted on parent reports. Individuals with Down syndrome may be less reactive to stimulation and possess higher threshold levels to respond. As a consequence of these patterns of reactivity, they may be more passive and less reactive. Moreover, the timing of shifts and changes in temperament may vary because of differences in neurological maturation.

Even though specific personality features have not been confirmed in studies of Down syndrome, there are features of a behavioral phenotype. Down originally had noted that his patients had considerable powers of imitation, "even bordering on being mimics. They are humorous and have a lively sense of the ridiculous which often colors their mimicry." The finding of increased imitational ability has been reported as a trait independent of intelligence in a German study (Huffner and Redlin, 1976). These authors compared individuals with Down syndrome with both mentally retarded and nonretarded persons matched for age.

PSYCHOLOGICAL ADAPTATION

Because Down syndrome can be diagnosed prenatally or at birth, the parents' adjustment to the disorder begins earlier than in many mental retardation syndromes. The integration of an affected child with Down syndrome into the family is enhanced by increasing knowledge about the life course of the person with Down syndrome. Parent support groups and special school programs are of considerable benefit in aiding in this understanding and in helping parents anticipate the needs of their child and make future plans. Placement outside the home is now uncommon and home rearing and management is the norm. Families make use of a variety of professionals to help them adapt to the diagnosis, yet adaptation is a continuing lifelong adjustment. Adolescents and adults with Down syndrome may have mothers who are in their 50s or 60s when they are completing special education.

The risk of occurrence of Down syndrome is greatest for mothers over 35 years of age; particular psychological problems in adjustment emerge when an older mother has an affected child. Still, Gath and Gumley (1984) found no specific evidence that older mothers had more difficulty in child rearing than younger parents. Some of the older mothers were happy for the companionship of a disabled child; however, a smaller percentage (4% in the Gath and Gumley study) had a child with Down syndrome as their first child and this was particularly stressful for them.

As children with Down syndrome reach adolescence and adulthood, they will often witness younger siblings moving beyond them in their cognitive development. The younger siblings may not understand the needs of their older brother or sister with Down syndrome and may not fully appreciate his or her feelings when the same responsibilities and privileges are not granted to them. The difficulties may be greatest in large sibships and in families with lower socioeconomic status. Because of sibling-related problems, sibling groups and sibling counseling and support are essential to alleviate or reduce interpersonal stress.

The presence of congenital abnormalities involving the cardiovascular system and gastrointestinal tract, leukemia, and infections are more common in children with Down syndrome. Psychological adjustment also may be complicated by hearing problems, secondary to recurrent ear infections or otosclerosis. Consequently, comprehensive medical care and counseling are important components in working with the family toward an optimum psychological adjustment. These congenital anomalies require intensive individual parent care and may lead to enhanced emotional bonding between the parent and child. Cytryn (1975) noted that the majority of infants with Down syndrome were delayed in demonstrating attachment behavior and initiated less direct social contact with their parents. However, those individuals with congenital heart disease who required more personal care were found to be closer to the normal expected age in displaying such attachment. These findings suggest that attachment may be enhanced by increased interpersonal involvement with the Down infant. But continued intense interpersonal involvement with the parent throughout the school years may lead to excessive dependency and difficulty with autonomy. Dependency may become most apparent when demands for more independent behavior are introduced in adolescence, upon entry into a special work group, in supportive employment activities, or in a group home.

In summary, the majority of children with Down syndrome survive school age, reach adulthood, enter into adult special day programming, and outlive their parents. Each phase in the life cycle of an individual with Down syndrome has its periods of predictable transitional adjustment. Birth, entry into school, emergence into adolescence, and transition from school to special work programs or supportive employment activities in the community each entail special psychological adjustment.

PSYCHIATRIC DISORDERS

A range of psychiatric diagnoses have been demonstrated in Down syndrome, including disruptive behavior disorders, such as conduct disorder and attention deficit disorder, emotional disorders, adjustment disorders, and major mental illness including psychoses with origins in childhood. Anorexia nervosa has been reported but occurs rarely in Down syndrome (Szymanski and Biederman, 1984).

Behavior and Emotional Disorders

Gath and Gumley (1986a, 1986b) compared children and adolescents with Down syndrome with a group of children without Down syndrome who attended the same school, who had comparable motor and verbal disabilities, and who were matched for age, sex, and intellectual functioning. Eighty-seven percent of children with Down syndrome lived at home with at least one natural parent, as did 89% of the control group. Using standardized parent ratings, supplemental ratings of specific behavioral concerns of parents whose children had Down syndrome, along with teacher ratings, these investigators demonstrated that both groups had behavioral and emotional abnormalities. Thirty-two percent of 98 adolescents with Down syndrome were thought to be behaviorally deviant versus 35% of a control group. The parents of children and adolescents with Down syndrome rated 15% of their children as having severe problems. Hyperkinetic and bizarre behavior counted for most of the differences between this group and the control group. Parents seem to consider that behavior management problems were expected in children with Down syndrome due to their low adaptive behavior. The family environment was an important factor in the type of behavioral symptoms expressed. Those adolescents from more dependent family settings had more emotional and mood disorders; those from homes where there was discord and conflict were at greater risk for antisocial behavior.

Mood Disorders

Mood disorders have been reported in approximately 10% of individuals with Down syndrome. Difficulty in the diagnosis of mood disorders may account for an earlier lack of recognition (Earl, 1934; Sovner and Hurley, 1983; Sovner, Hurley, and Labrie, 1985). In the assessment of affective disorders in Down syndrome, the more common depressive moods associated with unhappiness, bereavement (McLoughlin, 1986), or demoralization must be distinguished from a true major depressive disorder. In an individual with Down syndrome, the person's developmental level has an impact on the clinical presentation. The aspects of depression that involve self-blame and worthlessness may be difficult to elicit in individuals with Down syndrome due to their cognitive level. Thoughts of guilt, helplessness, and hopelessness about the future follow a developmental course, so criteria for depression must be modified to take developmental level into account (Harris, 1988). For example, at a mental age of 5 or 6 years, the ability to distinguish between accidental and intentional behavior becomes evident. At a mental age of 4 or 5 years, children are aware of others, being proud or ashamed of them. However, a mental age of about 8 years is required before children talk about being proud or ashamed of themselves.

In a severely and profoundly retarded person, behavioral change in eating, sleeping, or activity level, and loss of interest in usual interests, rather than the cognitive symptoms, provide the primary cues to diagnosis of a mood disorder (Reid, 1982). Moreover, presenting symptoms of aggression, withdrawal, or somatic complaints may be present and, when they are present, affective disorder should be considered. It is particularly important to determine that the mood disturbance is primary, not secondary, to another disorder.

Alzheimer's Disease

An association of Alzheimer's disease and Down syndrome has been suggested (Nadel, 1988; Solitare and Lamarche, 1966). Virtually all adults with Down syndrome who are older than 35 years of age will show brain tissue changes that are similar to those found in autopsy studies of individuals with Alzheimer's disease. An association of early senility with Down syndrome has been suggested since the original description of the syndrome (Fraser, 1876). Despite repeated evidence of neuropathological findings (Roper and Williams,

1980), which are identical to those seen in Alzheimer's disease patients and those with Down syndrome who are over 35 years of age, there does continue to be controversy in regard to the extent of the clinical correlation. The prevalence of symptoms of Alzheimer's disease in older institutionalized populations of persons with Down syndrome is estimated to be from 17% to 39% (Dalton and Cropper, 1977; Thase, 1988). When the clinical and neuropathological studies are reviewed (Cutler et al., 1985), the prevalence of clinical dementia in older adults with Down syndrome is variable. The onset of Alzheimer-like symptoms frequently occurs long after age 35, the age when definitive neuropathological findings are present. Moreover, although poor performance on neuropsychological tests may well be related to neuropathological findings, longitudinal study of individual persons is needed to clarify whether definite reductions in ability regularly occur over time and what the pattern of occurrence is.

Despite apparent decline in cognitive skills, which is based on cross-sectional studies, many older adults with Down syndrome do continue to function at premorbid levels despite suspected changes in brain function. In a study of 42 adults with Down syndrome (Berry et al., 1984), mental development continued well into the third and fourth decade of life. In a positron emission tomographic study (Schwartz et al., 1983), a higher rate of brain glucose metabolism was found when Down syndrome patients in their twenties were compared to age-matched control subjects. A lower rate, however, was noted in a 51-year-old man. Despite the metabolic rate being somewhat lower in the 51-year-old, his parents reported his performance had actually improved in recent years. Silverstein, Herbs, and Nasuta (1986) studied 413 individuals with Down syndrome in a control study, using the Cline Development Evaluation Report. These authors could not demonstrate age-related reduction in adaptive behavior in their sample. Overall, the prevalence of Alzheimer-like symptoms has been reported in about one third of older patients with Down syndrome.

TREATMENT

The treatment of the preschool and school-age child with Down syndrome requires interventions for mental retardation, the associated congenital anomalies that involve multiple organ systems, social developmental issues, language disorder, behavioral disorder, and the family's adjustment to the disability. In adolescence and young adulthood, new problems may arise that require ongoing medical treatment. Among these are hypothyroidism, hearing difficulty, and orthopedic problems.

Psychotherapy may be necessary for the parents or for the affected individual throughout childhood and into adolescence and adulthood to deal with developmental crises. Behavior treatment programs may need to be instituted for disruptive behavior. Pharmacotherapy may be indicated for attention deficit disorder, mood disorder, and behavior disorders.

REFERENCES

Berry, P., Groeneweg, G., Gibson, D., and Brown R.I. (1984). Mental development of adults with Down syndrome. *American Journal of Mental Deficiency,* 89(3):252–256.

Beeghly, M., Weiss-Perry, B., and Cicchetti, D. (1990). Beyond sensorimotor functioning: Early communicative and play development of children with Down syndrome. In D. Cicchetti and M. Beeghly (eds.), *Children with Down syndrome: A developmental perspective,* pp. 329–368. Cambridge University Press, New York.

Cicchetti, D., and Ganiban, J. (1990). The organization and coherence of developmental processes in infants and children with Down syndrome. In R.M. Hodapp, J.A. Burack, and E. Zigler (eds.), *Issues in the developmental approach to mental retardation.* Cambridge University Press, New York.

______, and Pogge-Hesse, P. (1982). Possible contributions of the study of organically retarded persons to developmental theory. In E. Zigler and D. Balla (eds.), *Mental retardation: The developmental-difference controversy.* Erlbaum, Hillsdale, NJ.

Cutler, N.R., Heston, L.L., Davies, P., Haxby, J.V., and Schapiro, M.B. (1985). Alzheimer's disease and Down's syndrome: New insights. *Annals of Internal Medicine,* 103:566–578.

Cytryn, L. (1975). Studies of behavior in children with Down's syndrome. In E.J. Anthony (ed.), *Explorations in child psychiatry.* Plenum, New York.

Dalton, A.J., and Cropper, D. (1977). Down's syndrome and aging of the brain. In P. Mittler (ed.), *Research to practice in mental retardation: Vol. 3. Biomedical aspects.* University Park Press, Baltimore.

Dicks-Mireaux, M. (1972). Mental development of infants with Down's syndrome. *American Journal of Mental Deficiency,* 77:26–32.

Down, J.L. (1866). Observations on an ethnic classification of idiots. *London Hospital, Clinical Lecture and Report,* 3:259–262.

Earl, C.J.C. (1934). Primitive catatonia of idiocy. *British Journal of Medical Psychology,* 14:230.

Esquirol, J. (1838). *Des maladies mentales considérées sous les rapports médical, hygiénique et médico-legal.* 2 vols. Ballière, Paris.

Fraser, J. (1876). Kalmuc idiocy: Report of a case with autopsy. With notes on sixty-two cases by A. Mitchell. *Journal of Mental Science,* 22:169–179.

Gath, A. (1985). Chromosomal anomalies. In M. Rutter and L. Hersov (eds.), *Child and adolescent psychiatry: Modern approaches,* pp. 123–124. Blackwell Scientific Publications, London.

______, and Gumley, D. (1984). Down's syndrome and the family: Follow-up of children first seen in infancy. *Developmental Medicine and Child Neurology,* 26:500–508.

______, and ______. (1986a). Behavior problems in retarded children with special reference to Down's syndrome. *British Journal of Psychiatry,* 149:156–161.

______, and ______. (1986b). Family background of children with Down's syndrome and of children with a similar degree of mental retardation. *British Journal of Psychiatry,* 149:161–171.

Gunn, P., Berry, P., and Andrews, R.J. (1981). Temperament of Down's syndrome infants: A research note. *Journal of Child Psychology and Psychiatry,* 22:189–194.

Harris, J. (1988). Psychological adaptation and psychiatric disorders in adolescents and young adults with Down syndrome. In S. Pueschel (ed.), *The young person with Down syndrome: Transition from adolescence to adulthood,* Paul H. Brookes, Baltimore, MD.

Hodapp, R.M., and Zigler, E. (1990). Applying the developmental perspective to individuals with Down syndrome. In D. Cicchetti and M. Beeghly (eds.), *Children with Down syndrome: A developmental perspective.* Cambridge University Press, New York.

Hook, E.B. (1982). Epidemiology of Down syndrome. In S.M. Pueschel and J.E. Rynders (eds.), *Down syndrome. Advances in biomedicine and the behavioral sciences,* pp. 11–18. Ware Press, Cambridge, MA.

Huffner, U.T.E., and Redlin, W. (1976). Imitation responses in mongoloid children. *Zeitschrift fur Klinische Psychologie. Forschung und Praxis,* 5(4), 277–286.

Lejeune, J., Gautier, M., and Turpin, R. (1959). Etudes des chromosomes somatiques de neuf enfants mongoliens. *C. R. Academy of Science,* 248:1721.

Mahoney, G., Glover, A., and Finger, I. (1981). The relationship between language and sensorimotor development among Down syndrome and developmentally normal children. *American Journal of Mental Deficiency,* 86:21–27.

McCall, R.B., Eichorn, D., and Hogarty, P. (1977). Transitions in early mental development. *Monographs of the Society for Research in Child Development,* 42.

McLoughlin, I.J. (1986). Bereavement in the mentally handicapped. *British Journal of Hospital Medicine,* 35:256–260.

Nadel, L. (ed.). (1988). *The psychobiology of Down syndrome.* MIT Press, Cambridge, MA.

Penrose, L., and Smith, G. (1966). *Down's anomaly.* Little, Brown, Boston.

Piaget, J. (1952). *The origins of intelligence in children.* International Universities Press, New York.

Reid, A.H. (1982). *The psychiatry of mental handicap.* Blackwell Scientific Publications, Boston.

Roper, A.H., and Williams, R.S. (1980). Relationship between plaques, tangles, and dementia in Down's syndrome. *Neurology,* 30:639–644.

Rothbart, M., and Derryberry, D. (1981). The development of individual differences in temperament. In M. Lamb and A.L. Brown (eds), *Advances in developmental psychology,* Vol. 1, pp. 37–86. Erlbaum, Hillsdale, NJ.

Rynders, J., and Pueschel, S. (1982). History of Down syndrome. In S. Pueschel and J. Rynders (eds.), *Down syndrome: Advances in biomedicine and the behavioral sciences.* Ware Press, Cambridge, MA.

Scheerenberger, R.C. (1983). *A history of mental retardation.* Paul H. Brookes, Baltimore.

Schwartz, M., Duara, R., Haxby, J., Grady, C., White, B.J., Kessler, R.M., Day, A.D., Cutler, N.R., and Rapoport, S.I. (1983). Down's syndrome in adults: Brain metabolism. *Science,* 221:781–783.

Séguin, E. (1866). *Idiocy and its treatment by the physiological method.* William Wood, New York.

Silverstein, A.B., Herbs, D., and Nasuta, R. (1986). Effects of age on the adaptive behavior of institutional individuals with Down syndrome. *American Journal of Mental Deficiency,* 6:659–662.

Solitare, G.B., and Lamarche, J.B. (1966). Alzheimer's disease and senile dementia as seen in mongoloids: Neuropathological observations. *American Journal of Mental Deficiency,* 70:840–848.

Sovner, R., and Hurley, A. (1983). Do the mentally retarded suffer from affective illness? *Archives of General Psychiatry,* 40:61–67.

______, ______, and Labrie, R. (1985). Is mania incompatible with Down's syndrome? *British Journal of Psychiatry,* 146:319–320.

Szymanski, L., and Biederman, J. (1984). Depression and anorexia nervosa of persons with Down syndrome. *American Journal of Mental Deficiency,* 89:246–251.

Thase, M. (1988). The relationship between Down syndrome and Alzheimer's disease. In L. Nadel (ed.), *The psychobiology of Down syndrome.* MIT Press, Cambridge, MA.

Thompson, M.G., McInnes, R.R., and Willard, H.F. (1991). Genetics in medicine, 5th ed. Philadelphia, W.B. Saunders, p. 215.

Werner, H. (1957). The concept of development from a comparative and organismic point of view. In D. Harrid (ed.), *The concept of development.* University of Minnesota Press, Minneapolis.

Wilmarth, A. (1889). Mongolian idiocy. *Proceedings of the Association of Medical Officers of the American Institutions for Idiotic and Feeble-minded Persons,* pp. 57–61 (quoted in Scheerenberger, 1983).

Zigler, E., and Balla, D. (1977). Motivational and personality factors in the performance of the retarded. In E. Zigler and D. Balla (eds.), *Mental retardation: The developmental-difference controversy,* pp. 9–26. Erlbaum, Hillsdale, NJ.

10.5 Sotos Syndrome

Sotos syndrome, or cerebral gigantism, is a disorder characterized by rapid growth, with no evidence of an endocrine disorder. Those with this disorder may have behavioral difficulties in childhood and learning difficulties.

This chapter describes the history, epidemiology, clinical features and behavioral phenotype, etiology, and treatment of Sotos syndrome.

HISTORY

Sotos syndrome was described by Sotos et al. in 1964 as a syndrome of excessively rapid growth with acromegalic features and nonprogressive neurological disorder. Since the original description, at least 200 cases have been described. With increasing experience with this disorder, the behavioral phenotype as well as the physical phenotype have been investigated (Cole and Hughes, 1990; Finegan et al., 1994).

EPIDEMIOLOGY

Prevalence information is not available. Although rare, based on the number of published cases, this disorder may not be uncommon in children who present with large body size, learning and behavioral difficulties, and clumsiness (Dodge, Holmes, and Sotos, 1983).

CLINICAL FEATURES AND BEHAVIORAL PHENOTYPE

There is considerable variation in presentation of Sotos syndrome. Hughes and Cole (1991) suggested the following diagnostic criteria: (1) distinctive facial features; (2) period of accelerated growth in early childhood; (3) advanced bone age evidenced during development; and (4) early developmental delay. On reaching adolescence, the rate of growth may be within the normal range. The diagnosis may be complicated in that the facial features become less obvious as the child grows older and advanced bone age may not be found at the time of diagnosis. Evidence of accelerated growth may be absent in early infancy.

Birth weight and length are above the 90th percentile in most affected infants and a large head size may be noted. In a classical case, growth is rapid and by 1 year of age, the infants are over the 97th percentile in height. Accelerated growth generally continues for the first 4 to 5 years of age and then a normal rate is observed. Puberty ordinarily occurs at the normal time but may be slightly early. Hands and feet are large, with thickened subcutaneous skin tissue. The head is large and the jaw is prominent. The eyes show an antimongoloid slant and hypertelorism may be evident. There is a characteristic awkward gait and clumsiness so that children who are involved have difficulty in coordinated activities, such as riding a bicycle and participating in sports activities.

X-rays of the skull show a large skull size with a high orbital roof and increased interorbital distance. Growth hormone levels and results of other endocrine studies are usually normal, and there are no distinctive laboratory markers of the syndrome. Seizure disorder is frequent and occurs in about 50%; however, in many instances, seizures are expressed primarily as febrile convulsions. Abnormal electroencephalograms are common. Intelligence ranges from severe mental retardation to the average range (Finegan et al., 1994).

Behavioral Phenotype

Behavioral difficulties and learning disorders are prominent features. Common problems include aggressiveness and destructiveness, poor social relationships, and irritability (Rutter and Cole, 1991; Varley and Crnic, 1984). Behavioral difficulties reported in more than 50% of these children include a low frustration tolerance, sleep problems, ritualistic and compulsive patterns of behavior. ADHD was identified in 38% (10/27) on a parent rating scale (Finegan et al., 1994). Autistic disorder has been reported in Sotos syndrome (Morrow, Whitman, and Accardo, 1990).

ETIOLOGY

The cause of Sotos syndrome is unknown and it is not clear whether all patients have the same underlying defect. Most reported cases are sporadic. In those instances where familial inheritance is reported, autosomal dominance has been suggested (Winship, 1985). However, in some instances, the question of autosomal recessive inheritance has been raised. There may be an increased risk for tumor formation in that hepatic carcinoma, Wilm's tumor, ovarian and parotid tumors have been reported. Scores on intelligence tests are variable. Most children have severe learning difficulties and there is an increased risk for mental retardation. Not all children show global cognitive delay, but many have the uneven cognitive profile pattern of learning disorder (Bloom et al., 1983).

TREATMENT

Diagnosis is important to clarify for the family that the child has a known disorder. The diagnosis is generally made in younger children based on facial features, accelerated growth, and associated developmental delay. Behavior management and social skills training are important aspects of intervention.

REFERENCES

Bloom, A.S., Reese, A., Hersh, J.H., Podruch, P.E., Weisskopf, B. and Dinno, M. (1983). Cognition in cerebral gigantism: Are the estimates of mental retardation too high? *Journal of Developmental and Behavioural Pediatrics,* 4:250–252.

Cole, T.R.P., and Hughes, H.E. (1990). Sotos syndrome. *Journal of Medical Genetics,* 27:571–576.

Dodge, P.R., Holmes, S.J., and Sotos, J.F. (1983). Cerebral gigantism. *Developmental Medicine and Child Neurology,* 25:248–251.

Finegan, J.K., Cole, T.R.P., Kingwell, E., Smith, M.L., Smith, M., and Sitarenios, G. (1994). Language and behavior in children with Sotos syndrome. *Journal of the American Academy of Child and Adolescent Psychiatry,* 33:1307–1315.

Hughes, H.E., and Cole, T.R.P. (1991). Sotos syndrome: Diagnostic criteria and natural history. *Proceedings of the Greenwood Genetic Centre,* 10:73.

Morrow, J.D., Whitman, B.Y., and Accardo, P.J. (1990). Autistic disorder in Sotos syndrome: A case report. *European Journal of Pediatrics,* 149:567–569.

Rutter, S.C., and Cole, T.R.P. (1991). Psychological characteristics of Sotos syndrome. *Developmental Medicine and Child Neurology,* 33:898–902.

Sotos, J. F., Dodge, P.R., Muirhead, D., Crawford, J.D., and Talbot, N.B. (1964). Cerebral gigantism in childhood. A syndrome of excessively rapid growth with acromegalic features and non-progressive neurological disorder. *New England Journal of Medicine,* 271:109–116.

Varley, C.K., and Crnic, K. (1984). Emotional, behavioural and cognitive status of children with cerebral gigantism. *Journal of Developmental and Behavioral Pediatrics,* 5:132–134.

Winship, I.M. (1985). Sotos syndrome—autosomal dominant inheritance substantiated. *Clinical Genetics,* 28:243–246.

10.6 Turner Syndrome

Turner syndrome results from an X chromosomal abnormality associated with physical, neuropsychological, and behavioral phenotypes. It provides an opportunity to study the effects of having one rather than two copies of a gene or genes on the X chromosome that are required for normal physical development and cognition.

This chapter describes the history, epidemiology, clinical features and phenotype, natural history, etiology, diagnosis, and treatment of Turner syndrome.

HISTORY

In 1938 Henry Turner addressed the Association for the Study of Internal Secretions and described seven women who failed to develop secondary sexual characteristics (Turner, 1938). He presented a description of a syndrome consisting of sexual infantilism, short stature, webbed neck, and cubitus valgus, now known as Turner syndrome. Otto Ullrich (1930) had previously published a report of a girl with similar features; therefore, the syndrome is sometimes referred to as Ullrich-Turner syndrome. It was later found that affected women have elevated levels of urinary gonadotropins and that the gonads consist of rudimentary elongated streaks that contain no germinal elements.

Turner syndrome was recognized as a genetic disorder in 1959 when Charles Ford and his colleagues described a patient with 45 chromosomes who lacked one X chromosome (Ford et al., 1959). Therefore, her karyotype was designated as X0 (now known as 45,X). Since that time, cytogeneticists have demonstrated that Turner syndrome is almost uniformly associated with a sex chromosome abnormality; there is considerable reluctance to make the diagnosis if the karyotype is normal. Shaffer (1962) was the first to describe a specific cognitive profile associated with Turner syndrome.

EPIDEMIOLOGY

Turner syndrome is one of the most common chromosomal abnormalities with an estimated frequency of 3% among early fetuses, but with a live female birth frequency of only 1 in 2,500 to 5,000 (Connor and Loughlin, 1991). It occurs most commonly at conception; it is thought that 99% of affected fetuses are spontaneously aborted. Life expectancy for surviving infants is not affected; however, there is a risk of hypertension in adult life.

CLINICAL FEATURES AND PHENOTYPE

The essential features are short stature, premature ovarian failure *in utero,* with streak ovaries, and a characteristic profile on neuropsychological testing. The phenotype is outlined in Table 10.6-1.

Physical Phenotype

Most 45,X patients may be recognized at birth because of characteristic edema on the dorsum of their hands and feet and loose skin folds at the nape of the neck. Low birth weight and short stature are common. In childhood, clinical manifestations include webbing of the neck, a low posterior hairline, small mandible, prominent ears, epicanthic folds, high-arched palate, a broad chest with apparent wide-spaced nipples, cubitus valgus (increased carrying angle at the elbow), and hyperconvex fingernails. When height is measured, short stature is evident and below the 3rd percentile. Short stature may be detected in the early years of life, at school age, or at puberty when sexual maturation fails to occur. The mean adult height is 146 ± 5.3 cm. Associated defects are common and include coarctation of aorta in about one sixth, isolated nonstenotic bicuspid aortic valve in approximately a third, and hypertension. Renal anomalies and bilateral otitis media are not uncommon, nor are goiter and bowel disease.

Neurobehavioral, Psychological, and Neuropsychological Phenotype

Intelligence is generally within the normal range. Swillen et al. (1993) found average intelligence (IQ 90 to 109) in 25 of 50 (50%) of preschool, school-age, and adolescent girls (4 to 20 years) tested. Low normal/borderline intelligence was found in 16 of 50 (32%) and

Table 10.6–1. Phenotype of Turner Syndrome

Poor viability *in utero*
Short stature
Prepubertal ovarian failure
Anatomical abnormalities
Webbed neck
Increased carrying angle of the elbow (cubitus valgus)
Congenital swelling of the hands and feet (lymphedema)
Aortic narrowing (coarctation)
High arched palate
Low posterior hairline
Low-set ears
Kidney and urinary tract anomalies
Short fourth metacarpals
Multiple pigmented nevi (moles)
Fingernail and toenail deformities
Other features
Glucose intolerance
Hypothyroidism
Cognitive deficit in the ability to analyze visual-spatial relationships

mental retardation in 5 of 50 (10%); 1 mildly, 2 moderately, and 2 severely mentally retarded. Of these, 2 individuals with "classical" Turner syndrome were mentally retarded. Moreover, 3 of 10 (30%) of those with "rare" karyotypic anomalies (X/X or X/autosomal translocations; ring chromosome X) were mentally retarded. These findings of mental retardation are consistent with those in other studies (Fryns, Kleczkowska, and Van den Berghe, 1990; Kleczkowska et al., 1990; Van Dyke et al., 1991). Eight percent (4 of 50) were above average or gifted in contrast to the expected 30% in the general population. When the cognitive profile was evaluated in the Swillen et al. (1993) study, the average verbal IQ score (VIQ) was 98 and performance IQ (PIQ) was 87. The reduced performance score was attributed to poor performance on visuospatial tasks of the intelligence tests with lowest scores on the WISC-R subtests: picture completion, block design, and object assembly.

Although intelligence is usually in the normal to low normal range, a specific neuropsychological phenotype has been suggested. The neurocognitive profile shows an extensive spatial deficit (Shaffer, 1962). It involves disorders of space-form perception, spatial skill, left-right discrimination, visuomotor coordination, visual memory, drawing, arithmetic, motor learning, and difficulty in following a route. Generally, verbal skills are not impaired, although there may be difficulties with verbal fluency (Temple, 1992).

Another approach to IQ assessment involves the study of monozygotic (MZ) twins discordant for Turner syndrome, using standardized psychological tests. Weiss et al. (1982) reported an affected Turner twin's performance IQ was 18 points below that of her sister, whereas their verbal IQs differed only by 7 points. In another twin case, the twin with Turner syndrome showed a depressed performance IQ and a lower perceptual organization score relative to her twin. The neurobehavioral phenotype has been studied in another set of monozygotic twins discordant for Turner syndrome, using extensive neuropsychological testing (Reiss et al., 1993). Test results in this study suggest that psychological processes that are affected by X monosomy may involve multiple domains rather than being localized in a single domain, such as spatial cognition. When these monozygotic twins were compared, the twin with Turner syndrome (45,X) showed relative deficits when compared with her sister in those psychoeducational and neuropsychological domains that involve visual-perceptual and visual-motor skills, speed of response, and executive function. The twin with Turner syndrome scored within an average to above average range for her age group in IQ; her twin scored in the above average to superior range. On specific neuropsychological testing for the visual-perceptual subdomain, the Turner syndrome twin performed on a level 6 years or more below that of her sister on the Face Recognition Task. In the visual-motor domain, the Turner twin's scores were substantially reduced on block design (WISC-R), on object assembly (WISC-R), and on completion of the Rey-Osterrieth complex figure. Reduced speed was a factor in the low performance on the first two of these tests. She performed normally on a Judgment of Line task, suggesting no difficulty in recognizing angular displacement and position of lines that vary in spatial orientation. However, she did have difficulty with discriminating faces where the arrangement of elements is more subtle. Poor performance on these tests is related to right posterior parietal lesions. (The twins showed similar responses on memory tasks that involved both visual and verbal information.) On attentional tasks, the Turner syndrome twin had a slower reaction time on the Test of Variables of Attention (TOVA). This result may be linked to speed of response that was also evident on other tasks. A slowness in preparedness to act or to anticipate action may be associated with prefrontal neural structures and their subcortical pathways.

In regard to nonverbal tasks, the Turner syndrome twin showed particularly poor performance on the street map test. Success on this test requires a combination of visuospatial and executive function. Deficits are associated with right parietal and left frontal lobe lesions. The pattern of errors suggested an inability to reverse her right-left orientation in space and then to transfer this reversal to the map. Because of differences in age between the times the twins were tested, these results might relate to a difference in maturity between the twins; however, other investigators have found right-left confusion in Turner syndrome. The Turner syndrome twin scored below her sibling on the controlled word fluency test and on the Consistent Long-Term Retrieval (CLTR) task from the selective reminding task. Each of these tasks are associated with cognitive processes that involve organization, strategy use, and response monitoring.

On most verbally based neuropsychological tasks other than on the narrative story component, the Turner syndrome twin was comparable to her sister. This task requires skills in the use of pragmatic language in making inferences. Such tasks are linked with frontal lobe functioning and related to executive function ability. The narrative story task difficulty might relate to executive dysfunction in use of the basic elements of language.

Since Shaffer's (1962) first report of the Turner syndrome cognitive profile, impairment of spatial abilities has been consistently reported. Reports in the 1960s focused on impairment in space-form perception (Money, 1963), directional sense (Alexander, Walker, and Money, 1964), and constructional ability (Alexander, Ehrardt, and Money, 1966). In the 1970s the focus shifted to visual-motor integration and visual-spatial memory (Silbert, Wolff, and Lilienthal, 1977) and road map skills, right-left orientation, and visuomotor drawing (Waber, 1979). In the 1980s investigators maintained an interest in visuomotor memory (Pennington et al., 1985) and visuomotor integration (McCauley et al., 1987) but also turned to impairments in other areas, such as speed and accuracy of mental rotation (Rovet and Netley, 1982) and affect discrimination (McCauley, Ito, and Kay, 1985; McCauley et al., 1987).

These studies suggested that children with Turner syndrome have particular problems with tasks involving the right hemisphere which is thought to be involved in visuospatial tasks and affect discrimination. However, impairment of performance IQ and nonverbal function is not necessarily associated with right hemispheric impairment in women (Inglis and Lawson, 1981). Moreover, their cognitive deficits are not restricted to spatial abilities, because impairments in verbal fluency and performance on the Wisconsin Card Sort are also found that suggest frontal lobe, especially left frontal lobe, involvement (Waber, 1979). Reiss et al. (1993) also found disorders in executive function (frontal lobe), and visuospatial and visual-perceptual functioning (right posterior parietal lobe) in the X monosomic member of monozygotic twins discordant for Turner syndrome. Pennington et al. (1985) found general impairment of long-term memory. Pennington (1991) suggests that brain dysfunction in Turner syndrome is either diffuse or primarily nonverbal rather than specific to the right hemisphere.

NATURAL HISTORY

The incidence of prematurity is high for X monosomy, with over a quarter of affected children born 2 to 4 weeks and a third born more than 4 weeks before the expected birth date in one study (Swillen et al., 1993). Their average height at birth was reduced (45.7 cm). In this study, the mean age at diagnosis was 3 years, 7 months, but diagnosis was made at birth or before age 1 year in half of the sample. The diagnosis was not suspected until school age (6 to 12 years) in 20%.

To clarify the behavioral profile, children were evaluated on the parent Child Behavior Checklist (CBCL) (4 to 16 years) and the youth self-report (11 to 18). In the youngest age group (aged 4 to 6 years), hyperactivity was common and was expressed in easy distractibility and difficulty in completing tasks. The hyperactivity improved with age and, by puberty, some degree of hypoactivity was demonstrable. Overall, the majority of Turner girls, as they grow older, are quiet and show immaturity in their behavior and in their fantasy life.

In regard to social functioning, the younger girls (age 4 to 5) did not have behavioral difficulties and were integrated into peer groups. By elementary school age (6 to 11), interaction with peers was decreased. These girls tended to remain at home more and preferred to read and to draw. Academically, they were described by their parents as compliant and interested in schoolwork. By puberty, social interactions with peers were less evident (age 12 to 16 years) and there was less tendency to seek out contact with peers. With the teenage group, on the CBCL youth self-report, social withdrawal, feeling alone, being disliked by classmates and peers, and being unable to change their situation were described.

The cognitive profile, particularly the visuospatial and nonverbal learning deficit, may affect school integration and school results. Yet despite their deficits, the majority of Turner girls (90%) attended normal school although they required intervention for learning problems in mathematics and scientific drawing. Common interventions included growth hormone therapy (two thirds of the group) and identification and remediation of medical problems, such as mild hearing loss, myopia, and renal abnormalities.

With change in age and following hormonal treatment, the improvement in the visuospatial deficit has been evaluated. Waber (1979) and others have suggested that, with maturation, there is compensation for visuospatial task deficits. Nielson and Nyborg (1981) demonstrated a positive influence of estrogen therapy of short duration (less than 2 years) on the ability to problem-solve in girls with Turner syndrome. Swillen et al. (1993) found better results on visuospatial tasks in the 16- to 20-year age group, a group where hormonal substitution therapy was started between ages 15 and 16. The meaning of the improvement in visuospatial functioning will require longitudinal study because other psychological or physical factors may be influential.

ETIOLOGY

Genetic Aspects

Monosomy X is found in over 90% of aborted fetuses and mosaic 45,X, 46,XX in most of the rest. However, there are a wide variety of karyotypes observed in live born girls with Turner syndrome. The X chromosome is of maternal origin in 75% of cases. In approximately 50% of the live births, the karyotype is 45,X; (it is possible that a small number of undetected normal cells are present in these infants that prevent abortion). The next most frequent form is an isochromosome of the long arm of X [46,Xi(Xq)] or mosaic 46,Xi(Xq)/45,X (13% to 17%). This is followed by mosaic monosomy X with a normal female cell line (45,X/46,XX) (15%), ring X [(46Xr(X) or 45,X/46Xr(X)] (7%), and mosaic monosomy X with a normal male cell line (45,X/46,XY) (4%). Deletions of the short arm of the X and other abnormalities make up the remainder. Individuals who have 45,X/46,XY are at risk for both masculinization and gonadoblastoma.

In the mosaic form (45,X/46,XX), the abnormalities are milder and less frequent. An affected mosaic newborn usually has no recognizable physical features. However, short stature is frequent and may be the initial presenting manifestation. Abnormalities of the second X may be present in mosaicism. In all cells, there may be partial deletions of X and ring chromosomes. Sexual maturation fails to occur in the 45,X and the 45,X/46,XX patients. Yet despite the absence of the second X chromosome, fertility has been reported in children with the 45,X presentation. The physical phenotype of Turner syndrome is sometimes seen with an apparently normal karyotype (Zinn, Page, and Fisher, 1993).

Epstein (1990) has suggested that two copies of certain genes normally present on the homologous portion of the X and Y chromosomes are necessary to prevent the occurrence of short stature, thus the absence of one X chromosome or a segment of it leads to short stature. The genetic mechanism leading to short stature is not clear. Hall (1991) suggests three general approaches to understanding the relationship between karyotype and growth in Turner syndrome: (1) short stature may relate to the absence of bands on the short or long arm of the X chromosome; (2) short stature may relate to the ratio of normal to abnormal cells in mosaic cases; and (3) short stature may be linked to the placenta's karyotype and be related to placenta dysfunction.

In addition, imprinting could be a factor in short stature. It may make a difference whether it is a maternal or paternal X chromosome that is missing in the disorder. Brown and Willard (1990) found that at least four areas of the short arm of the X chromosome escape inactivation and these areas might be involved in growth. Hall (1991) suggests that a combination of these hypotheses may be involved in producing short stature.

Neuroanatomy and Neuroimaging

Abnormalities in learning and behavior in children with Turner syndrome may reflect differences in brain development and function. Although there have been a small number of autopsy studies, findings have been variable. These findings include abnormalities in cerebral cortical organization and developmental abnormalities in the posterior fossa, particularly in the midline cerebellum (Molland and Purcell, 1974). Brain-imaging studies also include reports of agenesis of the corpus callosum in mentally retarded adolescent females with the 45,X karyotype (Kimura, Nakajima, and Yoshino, 1990). One PET scan study was carried out in 5 individuals with Turner syndrome who had a variety of chromosomal abnormalities (Clark, Klonoff, and Hayden, 1990). The PET scan results were consistent with decreased glucose metabolism in the parietal and occipital cortex bilaterally.

One MRI study has been completed in monozygotic twins discordant for Turner syndrome. To clarify the nature of the chromosomal anomaly in these twins, a karyotype analysis was carried out that showed 50 of 50 cells in one twin to have the 45,X chromosome constitution and 50 of 50 cells in the other to have a normal 46,XX karyotype. Moreover, DNA fingerprinting showed the twins shared 42 bands and the X chromosome retained by the patient with Turner syndrome was of maternal origin. The Turner twin showed short stature (below the 1st percentile) and relatively mild physical stigmata of Turner syndrome. Total cerebrum, hemispheric, cerebellar, and basal ganglia volumes for both sisters were in the normal range. However, when the sisters were compared, total cerebral volume was slightly larger (3.6%) in the Turner syndrome sister and the cerebral spinal fluid volume was 25% greater in the Turner twin; it was relatively increased over her entire brain. This finding was accompanied by small, although proportional, decrease in gray matter volume (4.4%). These results suggest that X monosomy may result in a mild, generalized hypoplasia during neurodevelopment.

There was also an indication of differences between the twins in specific brain regions. The greatest differences were in the right prefrontal, right posterior parietal, occipital, and left parietal perisylvian cortical regions. Neuroanatomical differences were also noted in the posterior fossa. Impaired growth of midline structures in the posterior fossa in the X monosomy twin were suggested by enlargement of the fourth ventricle and cisterna magna coupled with decreased size of the cerebellar vermis, medulla, and pons. An abnormal growth of midline structure has also been reported in fragile X syndrome so the involvement of similar neuroanatomical regions in very different syndromes may indicate a vulnerability of midline regions in the posterior fossa to genetic insult. These regional anatomical findings might potentially be related to inefficiency in processing information and/or in the modulation of attention, sensory input, and motor outflow.

Additional imaging studies of children with X monosomy and appropriately matched controls are needed to confirm these differences and to further explore brain–behavioral associations in Turner syndrome.

Neurophysiology

Event-related potentials (ERPs) and reaction time (RT) were measured in untreated prepubertal and peripubertal (ages 9 to 14) and postpubertal (ages 15 to 20 years) individuals with Turner syndrome and contrasted with those from a normal matched controlled group (Johnson, Rohrbaugh, and Ross 1993). These studies allowed the assessment of the roles of both congenital and maturational brain changes as possibly etiologic for cognitive deficits in Turner syndrome. The clinical procedure involved presenting each individual subject with a series of auditory stimuli. The subject was asked to either count one of the two stimuli or rapidly press a button to discriminate between them. The ERPs in the 9- to 14-year group were essentially the same as those for age-matched controls, but in the 15- to 20-year-olds, the ERPs were more like those of the younger Turner group and the younger age-matched controls. A late frontal negative slow wave (Nc) in the older subjects with Turner syndrome did not show the normal maturational course where the amplitude and duration of this component decreases with age. The latencies, amplitudes, and scalp distributions of other ERP components, with the exception of slightly greater amounts of N1 amplitude in the younger Turner syndrome subjects, were the same at all ages for Turner syndrome subjects and their controls.

In regard to behavior, both Turner syndrome groups had longer reaction times than their matched controls. This was consistent with the ERP results. The event-related brain potential and reaction time results illustrate two types of abnormalities in Turner syndrome females. The ERP results indicate an age-dependent maturational defect; the reaction time results suggest an age-independent defect from the beginning of life, a congenital abnormality. These results suggest that the cognitive and motor abnormalities in Turner syndrome result from a combination of factors. Apparently both congenital and maturational abnormalities are involved to varying degrees and are related to the cognitive deficits in Turner syndrome. The event-related potential data suggest that, for auditory stimuli, both sensory and stimulus evaluation processes were intact and did not contribute to the pattern of deficits. When looking at all age groups, the largest deficits were in the response processing operations. Event-related potentials were particularly valuable in this study to clarify relative contributions of the different sources of sensory, cognitive, and motor deficits in Turner syndrome subjects and in clarifying the temporal characteristics of these deficits.

Psychiatric and Psychosocial Aspects

Preschool children with Turner syndrome are usually described as outgoing, but during the school-age years they become increasingly reserved and overadapted. The effect of short stature on development may be a major factor in their emotional development. Older girls surveyed tend to report feelings of inferiority and depression and develop anxiety about sexuality and male partnership. Difficulties in concentration, eating difficulties, including anorexia nervosa, abnormal peer relationships, and depression in adult life have been reported (Muhs and Lieberz, 1993).

An association of Turner syndrome and anorexia nervosa has been suggested based on case reports of anorexia nervosa in Turner syndrome and the relative rarity of both conditions. The first case reports of both diagnoses in the same individual were published in 1963. Since then, case reports have been reported from the United States, Europe, Australia, and Asia. Of 21 published case reports, 16 are 45,X and 5 are 45,X/46,XX mosaicism (Muhs and Lieberz, 1993). In 12 of these patients, anorexia nervosa occurred in association with hormonal treatment. In 5 of these, symptoms began shortly after the initiation of hormonal therapy, and in 7 patients, 1 to 6 years following the introduction of hormonal treatment. The beginning of anorexia nervosa in Turner syndrome is similar to the usual age of onset of the disorder; patients manifested anorexia nervosa between 13 and 23 years of age. However, in a third of cases, the anorexia nervosa occurred without pubertal onset. In 15 of the cases, psychological factors were ascertained that related to symptom onset, and in 6 cases, none were specifically described.

Muhs and Lieberz (1993) suggest that rather than a genetic connection between the two disorders, there is a confluence of hereditary factors and environmental factors. Psychological factors that may increase vulnerability to anorexia nervosa are social immaturity and overcompliance. Moreover, the initiation of hormonal therapy focuses the child's and family's attention on adolescent sexual development. The impact of hormonal treatment on self-awareness and behavior must receive careful consideration. Whether the anorexia nervosa is psychologically based and linked to parental overprotection and overcompliance as a personality factor in the child or whether there is a biological basis requires further exploration. If the girl with Turner syndrome is conflicted about sexual development as she enters into adolescence, the physical changes that accompany the institution of hormonal treatment may potentially trigger symptom formation. However, the majority of girls with Turner syndrome do not develop anorexia nervosa. They usually view hormonal therapy positively as providing an opportunity for improved self-esteem in peer groups and an opportunity to become more normalized. Rather than wanting to interrupt the process of maturation and stop the growth of secondary sexual features, the majority are eager to facilitate their development. When anorexia nervosa did develop in these accumulated cases reports, it was not a transient eating impairment but characteristically was a long-lasting illness. In 11 of the case reports where duration is included, the duration was up to 20 years.

Although rare, the occurrence of anorexia nervosa in Turner syndrome suggests careful attention to preparation for entry into puberty and encouragement of independence in the preadolescent years.

DIAGNOSIS

Chromosomal analysis should be carried out in those suspected of having Turner syndrome. Those girls who have partial Y chromosome material are managed differently because there is an increased risk of gonadoblastoma. Endocrine tests include measurements of gonadotropins, particularly follicle stimulating hormone (FSH); FSH is generally elevated even in infancy. In girls over 10 years of age, plasma levels are elevated and at the menopausal level. By adolescence, urinary gonadotropins are elevated. Growth hormone secretion in response to stimulation is normal.

TREATMENT

With appropriate medical intervention and psychological support in adapting to the ovarian dysfunction and short stature, psychiatric symptoms can be reduced. However, psychosocial interventions may be necessary to prepare the child to accept treatment. Replacement therapy with estrogen is essential, but there is disagreement about the optimal age to initiate it. The individual with Turner syndrome should be involved in this decision.

A detailed psychoeducational evaluation should be carried out early in the child's school career when the diagnosis is known. If the diagnosis becomes evident during the later school-age years, then psychoeducational assessment should become part of the treatment plan. If a learning disability is demonstrated, appropriate placement is necessary with proper remediation, especially in dealing with math skills. For those individuals with Turner syndrome who have attentional problems, the school environment should be one that limits distractions and provides structure to facilitate time on task. If attention deficit/hyperactivity disorder is present, then pharmacotherapy may be necessary to facilitate the child's participation in the classroom.

Because of the spatial deficits, when new material is introduced, the format of introduction should be one that relies on good verbal skills and less on visuospatial processing (Rovet, 1993). Teachers should limit the requirement to copy from the board and use graphs and maps in their instruction. When visual aids are used, explicit instruction is necessary in helping the child to use them. The sequence of teaching should be coordinated in a way that mastery occurs in learning, and modest gains should receive recognition and reward. In the school environment, opportunities for appropriate social development should be provided and peer relationships encouraged. Vocational planning is necessary to choose areas where visuospatial dysfunction will be less of a limitation. Educational evaluation should be coordinated with treatment of physical symptoms, such as the use of growth hormone therapies and replacement therapies. Because educators may be unaware of the nature of the learning problems in Turner syndrome, fact sheets and information on effective teaching may be needed. Finally, a teaching program is best carried out on a case-by-case basis because of the heterogeneity within the syndrome.

REFERENCES

Alexander, D., Ehrardt, A., and Money, J. (1966). Defective figure drawing, geometric and human in Turner syndrome. *Journal of Nervous and Mental Diseases,* 42:161–167.

______, Walker, H.R., and Money, J. (1964). Studies in direction sense in Turner syndrome. *Archives of General Psychiatry,* 10:337–339.

Brown, C.J., and Willard, H.F. (1990). Localization of a gene that escapes inactivation to the X chromosome proximal short arm: Implications for X inactivation. *American Journal of Human Genetics,* 46:273–279.

Clark, C., Klonoff, H., and Hayden, M. (1990). Regional cerebral glucose metabolism in Turner syndrome. *Canadian Journal of Neurological Science,* 17:140–144.

Connor, J.M., and Loughlin, S.A.R. (1991). Molecular genetic analysis in Turner syndrome. In M.B. Rande and R.G. Rosenfeld (eds), *Turner syndrome: Growth promoting therapies,* pp. 3–8. Elsevier, Amsterdam.

Epstein, C.J. (1990). In R.G. Rosenfeld and M.M. Grumbach (eds.), *Turner syndrome,* pp. 13–25. Marcel Decker, New York.

Ford, C.E., Jones, K.W., Polani, P.E., de Almeida, J.C., and Briggs, J.H. (1959). A sex-chromosome anomaly in a case of gonadal dysgenesis (Turner syndrome). *Lancet,* i:711–713.

Fryns, J.P., Kleczkowska, A., and Van den Berghe, H. (1990). High incidence of mental retardation in Turner syndrome patients with ring chromosome X formation. *Genetic Counseling,* 1:161–165.

Hall, J.G. (1991). The relationship between karyotype and growth in Turner syndrome. In M.B. Ranke and R.G. Rosenfeld (eds.), *Turner syndrome: Growth promoting therapies,* pp. 9–12.

Inglis, J., and Lawson, S. (1981). Sex differences in the effects of unilateral brain damage on intelligence. *Science,* 212:693–695.

Johnson, R., Jr., Rohrbaugh, J.W., and Ross, J. L. (1993). Altered brain development in Turner syndrome: An event-related potential study. *Neurology,* 43:801–808.

Kimura, M., Nakajima, M., and Yoshino, K. (1990). Ullrich-Turner syndrome with agenesis of the corpus callosum. *American Journal of Medical Genetics,* 37:227–228.

Kleczkowska, A., Dmoch, E., Kubien, E., Fryns, J.P., and Van den Berghe, H. (1990). Cytogenetic findings in a consecutive series of 478 patients with Turner syndrome. The Leuven experience 1965–1989. *Genetic Counseling,* 1:227–233.

McCauley, E., Ito, J., and Kay, T. (1985). Psychological functioning in girls with the Turner syndrome and short stature. *Journal of the American Academy of Child and Adolescent Psychiatry,* 25:105–112.

______, Kay, T., Ito, J., and Treder, R. (1987). The Turner syndrome: Cognitive deficits, affective discrimination and behavioral problems. *Child Development,* 58:464–473.

Molland, E.A., and Purcell, M. (1974). Biliary atresia and the Dandy-Walker anomaly in a neonate with 45,X Turner syndrome. *Cortex,* 115:227–230.

Money, J. (1963). Turner syndrome and parietal lobe functions. *Cortex,* 9:385–393.

Muhs, A., and Lieberz, K. (1993). Anorexia nervosa and Turner syndrome. *Psychopathology,* 6:29–40.

Nielsen, J., and Nyborg, H. (1981). Sex hormone treatment and spatial ability in women with Turner syndrome. In W. Schmid and J. Nielsen (eds.), *Human behavior and genetics,* pp. 167–181. Elsevier, Amsterdam.

Pennington, B.F. (1991). *Diagnosing learning disabilities,* p. 114. The Guilford Press, New York.

______, Heaton, R.K., Karzmark, P., Pendleton, M., Lehman, R., and Schucard, D. (1985). The neuropsychological phenotype in Turner syndrome. *Cortex,* 21:391–404.

Reiss A.L., Freund L., Plotnick L., Baumgardner T., Green K., Sozer A .C., Reader, M., Boehm C., and Denckla, M.B. (1993). The effects of X monosomy on brain development: Monozygotic twins discordant for Turner syndrome. *Annals of Neurology,* 34:95–107.

Rovet, J. F. (1993). The psychoeducational characteristics of children with Turner syndrome. *Journal of Learning Disability,* 26:333–341.

______, and Netley, C. (1982). Atypical hemispheric lateralization in Turner syndrome subjects. *Cortex,* 18:377–385.

Shaffer, J.W. (1962). A specific cognitive deficit observed in gonadal aplasia (Turner syndrome). *Journal of Clinical Psychology,* 18:403–406.

Silbert, A., Wolff, P.H., and Lilienthal, J. (1977). Spatial and temporal processing in patients with Turner syndrome. *Behavioral Genetics,* 7:11–21.

Swillen, A., Fryns, J.P., Kleczkowska, A., Massa, G., Vanderschueren-Lodeweyck, M., and Van den Berghe, H. (1993). Intelligence, behaviour and psychosocial development in Turner syndrome. A cross-sectional study of 50 preadolescent and adolescent girls (4–20 years). *Genetic Counseling,* 4:7–18.

Temple, C. (1992). Developmental and acquired disorders of childhood. In I. Rapin and S.J. Segalowitz (eds.), *Handbook of Neuropsychology: Vol 6. Child Neuropsychology*, pp. 93–114. Elsevier, Amsterdam.

Turner, H.H. (1938). A syndrome of infantilism, congenital webbed neck, and cubitus valgus. *Endocrinology*, 23:566–574.

Ullrich, O. (1930). *Über Typiche Kombinationsbilder Multipler Abartungen. Zeitschrift für Kinderheilkunde*, 49:271–276.

Van Dyke, D.L., Wiktor, A., Robinson, J.R., and Weiss, L. (1991). Mental retardation in Turner syndrome. *Journal of Pediatrics*, 118:415–417.

Waber, D.P. (1979). Neuropsychological aspects of Turner syndrome. *Developmental Medicine and Child Neurology*, 21:58–70.

Weiss, E., Loevy, H., Saunders, A., Pruzansky, S., and Rosenthal, I.M. (1982). Monozygotic twins discordant for Ullrich-Turner syndrome. *American Journal of Medical Genetics*, 13:389–399.

Zinn, A.R., Page, D.C., and Fisher, E.M.C. (1993). Turner syndrome: The case of the missing sex chromosome. *Trends in Genetics*, 9:90–93.

10.7 Tuberous Sclerosis Complex

Tuberous sclerosis is one of several neurocutaneous syndromes, which are also known as phakomatoses, or ectodermal dysplasias. These disorders present with lesions, both of the skin and central nervous system, and may also have associated ocular and visceral abnormalities. Among these disorders, tuberous sclerosis has most commonly been associated with behavioral manifestations, particularly overactivity and socially impaired behaviors. Tuberous sclerosis is now referred to as "tuberous sclerosis complex" because it involves all tissues; consequently, multiple organs are affected (Gomez, 1991). In addition to the brain and retina, the skin, kidneys, heart, and lungs are most frequently involved. It is a disorder that involves cellular migration, differentiation, and proliferation. An alternative name, epiloia (epilepsy and anoia, or mindlessness), is inappropriate and pejorative for a disorder where up to 30% may function in the normal range of intelligence (Hunt, 1993).

This chapter reviews the history, epidemiology, diagnostic criteria, clinical features and phenotype, etiology, neurodevelopmental aspects, genetic counseling, and treatment of tuberous sclerosis complex.

HISTORY

The first description of tuberous sclerosis complex is probably that of von Recklinghausen. In 1862 he described an infant with sclerotic areas in the brain and cardiac tumors to the Obstetrical Society of Berlin (von Recklinghausen, 1862). Subsequently, Bourneville (1880) introduced the term "tuberous sclerosis" in his description of the pathological findings in the brains of three severely mentally retarded individuals. In his third case, a 15-year-old girl with a history of seizures since infancy, severe mental retardation, and a facial rash he referred to as acne rosacee, he found that many cerebral convolutions had hard, raised, opaque, whitish areas of increased density on postmortem examination. According to Gomez (1988), Rayer had previously published a description of the facial skin lesions. In 1908 Heinrich Vogt established the association between the cerebral sclerosis of brain convolutions and the facial angiofibromas (Vogt, 1908). Vogt's work led to the designation of the classic triad of seizures, mental retardation, and adenoma sebaceum, a characteristic now recognized as facial angiomatosis. He also found that renal and cardiac tumors were aspects of the disease process. With the emergence of radiological examinations of the skull, brain calcifications were identified and the skull x-ray became a tool for diagnosis.

Subsequently, it has been recognized that additional organ systems are involved in tuberous sclerosis complex, mental retardation is not essential to the diagnosis, and the manifestations can be more subtle than initially thought. Critchley and Earl (1932) recognized hypomelanotic macules in the skin. Since their observations, these circumscribed areas have been identified as the earliest visible sign of tuberous sclerosis complex.

The familial occurrence of tuberous sclerosis complex was first reported in 1913 (Gomez, 1988). Later, Gunther and Penrose (1935), and after them Nevin and Pearce (1968), suggested the genetic mechanism involves dominant inheritance and a high mutation rate. Lagos and Gomez (1967) reappraised the characteristics of the tuberous sclerosis complex. In reviewing patients seen at the Mayo Clinic over a 30-year period, they found that 38% of 69 patients had average intelligence. All of the mentally retarded patients had seizures, but only 69% of those with average intelligence did. Current efforts to understand the etiology of this condition focus on establishing genetic markers, using the techniques of molecular neurobiology.

EPIDEMIOLOGY

Early studies estimated the prevalence of tuberous sclerosis complex to be approximately 1 in 30,000 (Gunther and Penrose, 1935). More recent studies (Hunt and Lindenbaum, 1984) found a prevalence of 1 in 29,000 in patients under 65 years of age. However, prevalence estimates were higher in the younger age groups, namely, 1 in 20,000 for those under 30 years and 1 in 15,000 in those below age 5.

Recent research based on population studies suggests the birth incidence of tuberous sclerosis complex may be as frequent as 1 in 8,000 to 12,000 (Nakauchi, 1990; Sampson et al., 1989) if one emphasizes the multisystem nature of the disorder. The prevalence is higher than previously expected, following recognition that affected individuals may be of normal intelligence, may not have seizures, and may have few skin lesions. The availability of magnetic resonance imaging (MRI) and CT scanning along with renal and cardiac ultrasound have increased awareness of the condition and led to better delineation of lesions. Less than half of those affected with tuberous sclerosis complex are believed to have learning disabilities, but a higher proportion than previously expected test in the severe range of mental retardation. Use of the classic triad of mental retardation, epilepsy, and adenoma sebaceum (facial angiofibromas) may have resulted in an underdiagnosis of tuberous sclerosis complex (Gomez, 1988); Gomez found the complete classic triad present in less than 30% of cases. Revised diagnostic criteria are now available for population studies to determine the prevalence of tuberous sclerosis complex in the general population.

DIAGNOSTIC CRITERIA

The diagnosis of tuberous sclerosis complex is straightforward in patients with classical clinical features; however, diagnosis is more difficult in patients with more subtle findings. For diagnosis of the latter, the National Tuberous Sclerosis Association has prepared the criteria shown on Table 10.7–1 (Roach et al., 1992).

As shown in the table, the criteria include primary, secondary, and tertiary features and based on these criteria, the diagnosis may be definite, probable, or suspect. Lesions that are not well characterized will lead to an initial presumptive diagnosis until confirmation is possible. As indicated in the table, one secondary feature and two tertiary features lead to a suspect or probable diagnosis.

CLINICAL FEATURES AND PHENOTYPE

There is considerable variability in the range and extent of physical and mental disorders in tuberous sclerosis complex. The characteristic cerebral lesions are sclerotic patches (tuberous) that are scattered throughout the cortical gray matter. The tumors are made up of collections of astrocytes, neurons, and unusual giant cells without the cellular organization normally seen in the cerebral cortex. In addition to these lesions, glial nodules occur in a periventricular distribution. The cerebral lesions are present at birth and gradually enlarge and become calcified with age. Growth of the periventricular tumors may lead to large masses, which may obstruct the foramen of Monro. Facial angiofibromas are the characteristic skin lesions and consist of small bright red or brownish nodules that occur in a butterfly distribution on the nose and cheeks. When examined histologically, these lesions consist of a mixture of fibrous tissue and blood vessels. They become apparent between 2 and 5 years of age and by late childhood may be seen in over 80% of patients. In addition, hypopigmented macules on the skin

Table 10.7–1. Diagnostic Criteria for Tuberous Sclerosis Complex (TSC)

I. Primary features
   1. Facial angiofibromas*
   2. Multiple ungual fibromas*
   3. Cortical tuber (histologically confirmed)
   4. Subependymal nodule or giant cell astrocytoma (histologically confirmed)
   5. Multiple calcified subependymal nodules protruding into the ventricle (radiographic evidence)
   6. Multiple retinal astrocytomas*

II. Secondary features
   1. Affected first-degree relative
   2. Cardiac rhabdomyoma (histologic or radiographic confirmation)
   3. Other retinal hamartoma or achromic patch*
   4. Cerebral tubers (radiographic confirmation)
   5. Noncalcified subependymal nodules (radiographic confirmation)
   6. Shagreen patch*
   7. Forehead plaque*
   8. Pulmonary lymphangiomyomatosis (histologic confirmation)
   9. Renal angiomyolipoma (radiographic or histologic confirmation)
   10. Renal cysts (histologic confirmation)

III. Tertiary features
   1. Hypomelanotic macules*
   2. "Confetti" skin lesions*
   3. Renal cysts (radiographic evidence)
   4. Randomly distributed enamel pits in deciduous and/or permanent teeth
   5. Hamartomatous rectal polyps (histologic confirmation)
   6. Bone cysts (radiographic evidence)
   7. Pulmonary lymphangiomyomatosis (radiographic evidence)
   8. Cerebral white matter "migration tracts" or heterotopias (radiographic evidence)
   9. Gingival fibromas*
   10. Hamartoma of other organs (histologic confirmation)
   11. Infantile spasms

Definite TSC: 1 primary feature, 2 secondary features, or 1 secondary plus 2 tertiary features.
Probable TSC: Either 1 secondary plus 1 tertiary feature, or 3 tertiary features.
Suspect TSC: Either 1 secondary feature or 2 tertiary features.

*Histologic confirmation is not required *if* the lesion is clinically obvious.
From Roach et al., 1992.

of the arms, trunk, and legs are ordinarily present at birth. These macules may be irregular or oval in outline and range in size from a few millimeters to several centimeters. When two or more of these skin lesions are found in an infant, the diagnosis of tuberous sclerosis complex is suggested. Other skin manifestations include thickened areas of skin generally over the back (Shagreen patches) and fibromas of the gingiva and in the periungual area.

Benign tumors are also found in many organs, especially the kidneys, heart, liver, spleen, and lungs. In about 80% of patients, renal tumors are present and may lead to renal failure due to compression of the ureters or renal pelvis. Rhabdomyomas of the heart may be asymptomatic but also may cause arrhythmia, cardiac failure, and sudden death in infancy. Cystic malformations and tumor nodules in the lungs may result in pneumothorax. Approximately 50% of patients have retinal lesions that are seen near the edge of the optic disk. These lesions generally do not impair vision.

Convulsions are the most common clinical sign related to brain involvement and are apparent in 80% of patients and occur in those with and without mental retardation. Infantile spasms may be seen during the first year of life in about a third of cases (Riikonen and Simell, 1990). Grand mal and psychomotor seizures characteristically occur later in childhood. There is also an increased incidence of strokes and brain hemorrhage.

Behavioral Phenotype

The behavioral phenotype includes mild to severe mental retardation in approximately 70% of patients, and behavioral disturbances. The syndrome is associated with a variety of behavior disorders, including autistic disorder (Smalley et al., 1992), Asperger's disorder, and socially impaired behaviors. Thirty-five percent show evidence of hyperactivity and/or attention deficit disorder. Thirty-five percent show evidence of obsessive and ritualistic behaviors, and sleep problems are noted in 60%. Over one third show aggressive or self-injurious behavior (self-biting, self-hitting, head banging) (Hunt, 1993; Hunt and Dennis, 1987). Developmental delay or learning difficulties were reported in 80% of 300 (240/300) cases surveyed in England (Hunt, 1993). Sleep-related problems may be associated with epileptic activity.

Jambaque et al. (1991) reviewed neuropsychological aspects in relation to epilepsy and MRI findings in 23 affected children: 7 with normal intelligence, 10 with mental retardation, and 6 with mental retardation and autistic disorder. There was a positive association between the number of lesions with IQ, behavioral problems, and severity of epilepsy. In children with autistic disorder both posterior lesions and frontal lobe dysfunction were observed.

Hunt (1992) followed up a group of patients with tuberous sclerosis to clarify the natural history of behavior problems between age 5 and young adulthood (age 18 and older). The most common problems identified were socially impaired behavior (pervasive developmental disorder), overactivity, rage outburst/physical aggression, self-mutilation, and pica. There was a decrease in socially aloof, noncommunicative, and obsessive behaviors that were associated with earlier pervasive developmental disorder diagnoses made between age 5 and early adulthood. Overactive behavior also showed a substantial reduction over time; however, rage outbursts and aggression remained constant.

Sleep disorders have been reported in approximately two thirds of cases and are one of the most common behavioral manifestations. Sleep disturbances include night waking, early morning waking, and seizure-related sleep problems. Hunt and Stores (1994) surveyed the parents of 40 children (age 2.5 to 15 years) with tuberous sclerosis complex, using standardized rating instruments, to establish the prevalence of sleep problems and their relationship to seizure disorders and pervasive developmental disorder. Comparisons were made with nondisabled children and a mixed group with learning disabilities. The authors asked if sleep problems were due to seizure activity or related to social maladaptation in developing appropriate patterns of acceptable sleep behavior due to pervasive developmental disorder. Children were grouped as having no seizures or controlled seizures (11%) and seizures with varying degrees of severity (29%) as well as pervasive developmental disorder (25%) and no pervasive developmental disorder (15%). Disrupted sleep was a severe problem in tuberous sclerosis complex in contrast to the age-matched control group. There was no difference in the prevalence of sleep disturbance in patients with tuberous sclerosis complex with and without pervasive developmental disorder. However, there was a significant difference in sleep problems in those with seizures in contrast to those without seizures. In the group with seizures, 72% had severe problems with night waking and 59% had difficulty settling to sleep. For those with controlled or no seizures, none had severe problems with nighttime waking and 18% had major problems in settling to sleep. The authors concluded that the sleep disturbance was significantly associated with seizures and daytime behavioral problems but not to pervasive developmental disorder and high levels of parental stress.

Nighttime polysomnograms indicate that severe and persistent sleep disorders are most commonly related to seizures or sleep-related epileptic events. Curatolo et al. (1992) studied

9 children, age 16 months to 14 years, using all-night polysomnography. All patients had a seizure disorder and were receiving anticonvulsant treatment. Sleep architecture was normal in 3 of 9 cases. In the other 6 cases, reduced REM sleep, or REM sleep fragmentation, increased number and duration of wakings after sleep onset, and reduced sleep efficiency were noted. Severe abnormalities of sleep architecture were most apparent in patients with uncontrolled, generalized, or partial seizures. The pattern of sleep disturbance varied among the types of epilepsy. Sleep was normal in 3 seizure-free patients.

Parent reports of the extent of sleep disturbance indicated that parents underestimated their children's sleep problems. These authors conclude that sleep abnormalities are a consistent feature and parallel the severity of seizure disorders. Sleep disturbance is related to daytime behavior problems and is disruptive to family life.

Autistic Disorder in Tuberous Sclerosis Complex

Among behavior disorders associated with tuberous sclerosis complex, pervasive developmental disorder is commonly reported (Critchley and Earl, 1932; Curatolo and Cusmai, 1987; Fisher et al., 1987; Hunt and Dennis, 1987; Lawlor and Maurer, 1987; Mansheim, 1979). Smalley et al. (1992) confirmed this in a review of the literature of case reports on problems other than mental retardation and seizures. In 50 cases, 36% had a diagnosis of autistic disorder or autistic-like behavior. Among published studies of behavior problems in tuberous sclerosis complex, the prevalence ranges from 17% to 58% compared to a prevalence of 0.05% in the general population. Hunt and Shepherd (1993) carried out a prevalence study of tuberous sclerosis in the west of Scotland and detected 9 out of 21 (43%) of these children to have characteristics of pervasive developmental disorder.

Because an association between autistic disorder and tuberous sclerosis complex would indicate an increased frequency of tuberous sclerosis complex among autistic subjects compared to the general population, Smalley et al. (1992) reviewed the prevalence of tuberous sclerosis complex in 5 epidemiologic and 2 clinically based studies of autistic disorder. The prevalence of tuberous sclerosis complex among autistic populations ranged from 0.4% to 3%. If only those autistic subjects with seizures were identified, the frequency was greater. These same authors systematically examined 13 tuberous sclerosis complex cases, using the Autism Diagnostic Interview (ADI) (Le Couteur et al., 1989). They identified 7 of 13 cases who were clinically referred as having autistic disorder and found that these cases were similar to nontuberous sclerosis complex probands on two domains of the ADI, the social and communicative domains. However, the tuberous sclerosis complex group showed fewer repetitive rituals. Moreover, there were more male tuberous sclerosis complex probands with autistic disorder than female, although the sex ratio is equal in tuberous sclerosis complex. Within the tuberous sclerosis complex group, those with autistic disorder had significantly more seizures and mental retardation than those without autistic disorder. It should be noted that although a structured interview with the parents was conducted, the children were not evaluated using the Autism Diagnostic Observation Scale (ADOS). Hunt and Dennis (1987) have suggested that the natural history of pervasive developmental disorder symptoms in tuberous sclerosis complex may be different than that of classical autistic disorder; in particular, there is a reduction in autistic symptomatology in adolescence.

Several mechanisms have been considered to understand the association between autistic disorder and tuberous sclerosis complex. These include similar brain abnormalities, such as cell migrational abnormality, the location of the tumors in specific brain regions that might relate to autistic-like behavior, and seizure foci in similar brain regions. A second possibility is that insults to the central nervous system might occur at a similar time in neurodevelopment as may occur in classical autistic disorder. In addition, the relationship of infantile spasms to the occurrence of autistic disorder must be considered. Smalley et al. (1992) also suggest that linkage dysequilibrium among closely linked genetic loci be considered as well.

Several studies suggest that the majority of reported cases of children with tuberous sclerosis complex and autistic disorder have a history of infantile spasms (Curatolo and Cusmai, 1987; Hunt and Dennis, 1987; Taft and Cohen, 1971). In the Hunt and Dennis study, 57% of children with tuberous sclerosis complex had infantile spasms and were autistic compared to 13% in a series of Finnish children whose infantile spasms had other etiologies (Riikonen and Amnell, 1981). The diagnosis of autistic disorder is complicated by the presence of severe mental retardation and infantile spasms. All cases in the Hunt and Dennis study with autistic behavior were severely mentally retarded.

Curatolo et al. (1991) hypothesized that there are two groups of patients with autistic behavior and tuberous sclerosis complex. In one group, the onset of the autistic behavior is before the age of 2, and in the second group, the onset is between ages 3 and 5. For the first group, those children with infantile spasms, they found parietotemporal cortical lesions on MRI. In the second group who presented with partial motor seizures or asymmetrical spasms and developmental delay, MRI demonstrated both frontal and posterior tubers. Moreover, they found severe autistic behavior in children with secondary generalized epilepsy whose cortical tubers involved both posterior and frontal regions. These authors suggest that some behaviors shown in children with tuberous sclerosis complex are neurobiologically based and that mental retardation, epilepsy, and autistic behavior may all be aspects of an underlying brain dysfunction. They suggest that the anatomic localization of the cortical tubers, the kind of epilepsy, and the age of onset of symptoms must be evaluated to better understand the mechanisms involved.

These findings suggest an early intervention program that emphasizes recognition of seizure disorder, an assessment of sleep disturbance, and possibly infant stimulation programs as means to try to minimize the extent of these disturbances in tuberous sclerosis complex. If, in fact, the symptomatology is related to the localization of the cortical tubers, their early detection with magnetic resonance imaging may be of prognostic value. Subsequent studies, using EEG, MRI, and PET scanning, are required to clarify associations that may be related to particular brain regions.

Smalley et al. (1992) found a strong association of seizures, mental retardation, and autistic disorder but did not find that all autistic-like tuberous sclerosis complex individuals were mentally retarded. Moreover, even though all autistic-like tuberous sclerosis complex subjects had seizures with onset in the first year of life, 75% of nonautistic tuberous sclerosis complex subjects had seizures as well. These authors suggest that if seizures and/or cortical tuber positioning is responsible for the presence of autistic disorder, then a sex difference would be predicted regarding seizure activity and localization of tumors. However, to date such differences have not been examined systematically. The mechanism requires further study, although Smalley et al. (1992) hypothesize that the association, at least in part, is independent of seizure onset at age 1 and mental retardation. Interpretation of the extent of the association of autistic disorder and tuberous sclerosis complex must be cautiously assessed. The role of the infantile spasms and cortical tubers requires further consideration. Because infantile spasms may interfere with REM sleep, Curatolo et al. (1992) studied REM sleep and found reduced REM sleep or an increased REM sleep fragmentation in 6 of 9 cases studied, as described earlier. The relationship between REM sleep fragmentation and behavior in this disorder requires further investigation.

ETIOLOGY

Genetics

Tuberous sclerosis complex is inherited as an autosomal dominant trait with variable penetrance and a high mutation rate. The clinical findings are quite variable even within the same family and discordance has been noted among homozygous twins (Gomez, Kuntz, and Westmoreland, 1982). Clinical diagnosis may be difficult in individuals with few clinical findings. There is no reliable molecular marker. Not only is phenotypic heterogeneity common, but genetic heterogeneity also occurs. Conneally (1991) suggests this is locus heterogeneity in which the same phenotype can result from genes at two or more loci.

Fryer et al. (1987) demonstrated linkage between tuberous sclerosis complex and the

ABO blood group locus and suggested assignment to the distal long arm of chromosome 9 at q34. Others (Northrup et al., 1992) have provided additional evidence for linkage to chromosome 9, but have also suggested linkage to a locus elsewhere. However, in about one third of families, tuberous sclerosis complex can be tied to chromosome 9. Linkage of tuberous sclerosis complex to the gene for adult kidney disease on chromosome 16 has received strong support, and this may account for the majority of patients. Therefore, at least two chromosomal locations may be involved in tuberous sclerosis complex. Nellist et al. (1993) have confirmed linkage to a locus on the long arm of chromosome 9. They suggest the gene is proximal to the dopamine β-hydroxylase area and distal to the gelsolin area.

The rate of spontaneous mutation varies from 56% to 86% depending, to some extent, on the completeness of assessment of the extended family (Fleury et al., 1980; Roach, 1993). Linkage to chromosome 9q34 in the region that includes the gene for dopamine β-hydroxylase and to chromosome 16p13 in an area known to include genes for adult polycystic kidneys has been reported (Kandt et al., 1992); however, there are families who do not show linkage to chromosome 9 or 16. A previous linkage to chromosome 11 is not proven.

NEURODEVELOPMENTAL ASPECTS

Tuberous sclerosis complex involves abnormal cellular differentiation, aberrant neuronal migration, and excessive cell proliferation. Each of these processes contributes to the formation of various brain lesions in this disorder. Neurons migrate from the germinal matrix to the developing cerebral cortex along radial glial fiber pathways. Similar processes are followed in other brain regions, such as the cerebellum. The neuron assumes a bipolar configuration and migrates toward the developing cortex. The glial cell bodies remain in the ventricular region as their processes arborize and as they move along the cerebral wall. Because several migrating neurons follow the same glial fiber in succession, those neurons that arise from a common proliferative region tend to reach the same cortical area. Therefore, the disruption of normal neuronal migration pathways may produce areas of poorly developed cortex that are similar to the focal cortical hypoplasia seen in tuberous sclerosis complex. Such lesions may lead to greater neurological impairment than the cortical tubers themselves.

Once a glial fiber is established, neuronal migration along that fiber is thought to be nonselective. As a result, neurons from one developing brain region may migrate along glial fibers from another brain region. Moreover, neurons may influence the growth and proliferation of glial cells in culture. Roach (1993) points out that when glial cells are grown without neurons, they proliferate rapidly but are poorly differentiated. Such changes are mediated via an interaction between the neuron and glial cell membrane (Crossin, 1991). Components of the membrane surface may modulate cell interactions and influence the extent of neuronal migration along glial pathways and also glial differentiation and glial proliferation. Roach (1993) points out that in this way a single molecular defect at the cell membrane might lead to the various types of brain lesions that are characteristic of tuberous sclerosis complex. There are several different constituents of cell surface that might result in similar morphological changes. Although neuronal cell adhesion molecule (NCAM) has been suggested as a candidate gene for tuberous sclerosis complex (Crossin, 1991), dysfunction or absence of other cell surface markers could also be involved in inhibiting neuronal migration, facilitating glial proliferation, and perhaps altering cellular differentiation. Roach (1993) suggests that there are many different cell surface modulators and any of these might produce similar morphological patterns so that individuals who are indistinguishable phenotypically might have different abnormal genes that could be on different chromosomes. Such a mechanism would be consistent with the finding of markers on both chromosome 9 and chromosome 16.

GENETIC COUNSELING

With the prospect of two or more gene sites, the likelihood of identifying a single product to use in carrier detection and antenatal diagnosis is reduced. Moreover, because the majority of cases are the results of new mutation, carrier detection is not an option for many families.

Genetic counseling is straightforward if one parent has evidence of tuberous sclerosis complex; however, counseling is less clear for a family with only a single affected child. The parent should be examined with ultraviolet light and also have a retinal examination. The use of radiological evaluation and ultrasound studies lead to a low yield for families who do not have any physical findings of tuberous sclerosis complex. If there is an affected child, however, then parents without signs should consider a CT or MRI scan or renal ultrasound. However, it is not possible to exclude the possibility of tuberous sclerosis complex and there is a 2% to 3% recurrent risk for apparently unaffected parents. This could be related to gonadal mosaicism or reduced penetrance.

Antenatal diagnosis may be feasible, using antenatal visualization of cardiac tumors by ultrasonography (Crawford, Garrett, and Tynan, 1983). However, even in the rare instance when changes are detected *in utero,* no specific treatment is available for the disorder. In well-studied families, Roach (1993) notes that linkage analysis of chorionic villus specimens has been used in families known to have tuberous sclerosis complex at a specific gene locus (Connor, Loughlin, and Whittle, 1987). This approach may be utilized in such families but presents ethical dilemmas in regard to assessment of the severity of the disorder if pregnancy termination is a consideration.

TREATMENT

The prognosis for tuberous sclerosis complex varies considerably. Those with mild involvement may have productive lives; however, those with severe mental deficiency and those with seizure disorder will require extensive medical and psychosocial intervention.

Epidemiologic studies are needed to establish the frequency of the disorder and provide additional information on signs, symptoms, and complications. This information is particularly important when normal parents who are affected seek genetic counseling. Genetic counseling is essential in working with families; both physical and behavioral phenotypes should be discussed in detail. Both parents should be examined for evidence of skin, retinal, or brain involvement related to the disorder. If one parent has a diagnosis of tuberous sclerosis complex, this suggests a 50% likelihood of occurrence of the disorder in subsequent children.

A comprehensive management program includes treatment of seizures, assessment of intellectual function, and appropriate diagnosis of associated neuropsychiatric disorders. Interventions are psychoeducational and behavior therapy focused on the learning problems and mental retardation, pharmacological to treat co-occurring diagnoses such as attention deficit disorder, and surgical to address the complications of enlarging tumors, particularly those near the foramen of Monro. The family needs considerable support to deal with stresses caused by unpredictable behavior, inappropriate social behavior in public, and sleep disturbance. In one third of Hunt's (1993) sample of 300 families, difficulties were present in all three of these areas.

REFERENCES

Bourneville, D.M. (1880). Sclerose tubereuse des circonvolutions cérébrales: Idiotie et épilepsie hémiplégique. *Archives of Neurology (Paris),* 1:81–91.

Conneally, P.M. (1991). Locating disease genes through linkage. In W.G. Johnson and M.P. Gomez (eds.), Tuberous sclerosis and allied disorders: Clinical, cellular, and molecular studies. *Annals of the New York Academy of Sciences,* 615:253.

Connor, J.M., Loughlin, S.A., and Whittle, M.J. (1987). First trimester exclusion of tuberous sclerosis. *Lancet,* i:1269.

Crawford, D.C., Garrett, C., and Tynan, M. (1983). Cardiac rhabdomyomata as a marker for the antenatal detection of tuberous sclerosis. *Journal of Medical Genetics,* 20:303–304.

Critchley, M., and Earl, C.J.C. (1932). Tuberous sclerosis and allied conditions. *Brain,* 55:311–346.

Crossin, K.L. (1991). Cell adhesion molecules in embryogenesis and disease. *Annals of the New York Academy of Sciences,* 615:172–186.

Curatolo, P., Bruni, O., Cortesi, F., and Giannoti, F. (1992, November). *Sleep disorders in tuberous sclerosis.* Paper presented at "From Genes to Behaviour," 2nd International Symposium, Society for the Study of Behavioural Phenotypes, Welshpool, UK.

______, and Cusmai, R. (1987). Autism and infantile spasms in children with tuberous sclerosis.

Developmental Medicine and Child Neurology, 29:550–551.

______, ______, Cortesi, F., Chiron, C., Jambaque, I., and Dulac, O. (1991). Neuropsychiatric aspects of tuberous sclerosis. *Annals of the New York Academy of Sciences,* 615:8–16.

Fisher, W., Kerbeshian, J., Burd, L. and Kolstoe, P. (1987). Tuberous sclerosis and autism. *Journal of the American Academy of Child and Adolescent Psychiatry,* 26:700–703.

Fleury, P., deGroot, W.P., Delleman, J.W., Verbeeten, B.,Jr., and Frankenmolen-Witkiezwicz, I.M. (1980). Tuberous sclerosis: The incidence of sporadic cases versus familial cases. *Brain Development,* 2:107–117.

Fryer, A.E.D., Chalmers, A., Connor, J.M., Fraser, I., Povey, S., Yates, A.D., Yates, J.R., and Osborne, J.P. (1987). Evidence that the gene for tuberous sclerosis is on chromosome 9. *Lancet,* i:659–661.

Gomez, M.R. (1988). *Tuberous sclerosis,* 2nd ed. Raven Press, New York.

______. (1991). Phenotypes of the tuberous sclerosis complex with a revision of diagnostic criteria. In W.G. Johnson and M.P. Gomez (eds.), Tuberous sclerosis and allied disorders: Clinical, cellular, and molecular studies. *Annals of the New York Academy of Sciences,* 615:1–7.

______, Kuntz, N.L., and Westmoreland, B.F. (1982). Tuberous sclerosis, early onset of seizures, and mental subnormality: Study of discordant monozygous twins. *Neurology,* 32:604–611.

Gunther, M., and Penrose, L.S. (1935). The genetics of epiloia. *Journal of Genetics,* 31:413–430.

Hunt, A. (1992, November). *A longitudinal study of the behavior of 23 people with tuberous sclerosis from age 5 to adulthood.* Paper presented at "From genes to behaviour," 2nd International Symposium, Society for the Study of Behavioural Phenotypes, Welshpool, UK.

______. (1993). Development, behavior, and seizures in 300 cases of tuberous sclerosis. *Journal of Intellectual Disability Research,* 37:41–51.

______, and Dennis, J. (1987). Psychiatric disorder among children with tuberous sclerosis. *Developmental Medicine and Child Neurology,* 29:190–198.

______, and Lindenbaum, R.H. (1984). Tuberous sclerosis: A new estimate of prevalence in the Oxford region. *Journal of Medical Genetics,* 21:272–277.

______, and Shepherd C. (1993). A prevalence study of autism in tuberous sclerosis. *Journal of Autism and Developmental Disorders,* 23:323–339.

______, and Stores, G. (1994). Sleep disorder and epilepsy in children with tuberous sclerosis: A questionnaire-based study. *Developmental medicine and child neurology,* 36:108–115.

Jambaque, I., Cusmai, R., Curatolo, P., Cortesi, F., Perrot, C., and Dulac, O. (1991). Neuropsychological apects of tuberous sclerosis in relation to epilepsy and MRI findings. *Developmental Medicine and Child Neurology,* 33:698–705.

Kandt, R.S., Haines, J.L., Smith, M. Northrup, H., and Gardner, R.J. (1992). Linkage of an important gene locus for tuberous sclerosis to a chromosome 16 marker for polycystic kidney disease. *Nature Genetics,* 2:37–41.

Lagos, J.C., and Gomez, M.R. (1967). Tuberous sclerosis: Reappraisal of a clinical entity. *Proceedings of the Mayo Clinic,* 42:26–49.

Lawlor, B.A., and Maurer, R.G. (1987). Tuberous sclerosis and the autistic syndrome. *British Journal of Psychiatry,* 150:396–397.

Le Couteur, A., Rutter, M., Lord, C., Rios, P., Robertson, S., Holdgrafer, M., and McLennan, J. (1989). Autism diagnostic interview: A standardized investigator-based instrument. *Journal of Autism and Developmental Disorders,* 19:363–386.

Mansheim, P. (1979). Tuberous sclerosis and autistic behavior. *Journal of Clinical Psychiatry,* 40:97–98.

Nakauchi, Y. (1990). Epidemiologic observation of tuberous sclerosis in Japan. In Y. Ishibashi and Y. Hori (eds.), *Tuberous sclerosis and neurofibromatosis: Epidemiology, pathophysiology, biology and management,* pp. 13–21. Elsevier, Amsterdam.

Nellist, M., Brook-Carter, P.T., Connor, J.M., Kwiatkowski, D.J., Johnson, P., and Sampson, J.R. (1993). Identification of markers flanking the tuberous sclerosis locus on chromosome 9 (TSC1). *Journal of Medical Genetics,* 30:224–227.

Nevin, N.C., and Pearce, W.G. (1968). Diagnostic and genetical aspects of tuberous sclerosis. *Journal of Medical Genetics,* 5:273–280.

Northrup, H., Kwiatkowski, D.J., Roach, E.S., Dobyns, W.B., Lewis, R.A., Herman, G.E., Rodriguez, E., Jr., Daiger, S.P., and Blanton, S.H. (1992). Evidence for genetic heterogeneity in tuberous sclerosis: One locus on chromosome 9 and at least one locus elsewhere. *American Journal of Human Genetics,* 51:709–720.

Riikonen, R., and Amnell, G. (1981). Psychiatric disorders in children with earlier infantile spasms. *Developmental Medicine and Child Neurology,* 23:747–760.

______, and Simell, O. (1990). Tuberous sclerosis and infantile spasms. *Developmental Medicine and Child Neurology,* 32:203–209.

Roach, E.S. (1993). Tuberous sclerosis. In R.N.

Rosenberg, S.B. Prusiner, S. DiMauro, R.L. Barchi, and L.M. Kunkel, (eds.), *The molecular and genetic basis of neurological disease*, pp. 791–800. Butterworth-Heinemann, Boston.

______, Smith, M., Huttenlocher, P., Bhat, M., Alcorn, D., and Hawley, L. (1992). Report of the Diagnostic Criteria Committee of the National Tuberous Sclerosis Association. *Journal of Child Neurology*, 7:221–224.

Sampson, J.R., Scahill, S.J., Stephenson, J.B.P., Mann, L., and Connor, J.M. (1989). Genetic aspects of tuberous sclerosis in the west of Scotland. *Journal of Medical Genetics*, 26:28–31.

Smalley, S.L., Tanguay, P.E., Smith, M., and Gutierrez, G. (1992). Autism and tuberous sclerosis. *Journal of Autism and Developmental Disorders*, 22:339–355.

Taft, L.T., and Cohen, H.J. (1971). Hypsarrhythmia and infantile autism: A clinical report. *Journal of Autism and Childhood Schizophrenia*, 1:127–336.

Vogt, H. (1908). Zur Diagnostik der tuberosen Sklerose. *Zeitsschrift für die Erforschung und Behandlung Des Jugenduchen Schwachsinns auf Wissenschaftlicher Grundlage*, 2:1–12.

von Recklinghausen, F. (1862). Ein Herz von einem Neugeborenen welches mehrere theils nach aussen, theils nach den Hohlen priminirende Tumoren (Myomen) trug. *Verhandlungen Der Gesellschaft Für Geburtschilfe*, 20:1–2.

10.8 Cornelia de Lange Syndrome (Brachmann-de Lange Syndrome)

The Cornelia de Lange syndrome is a mental retardation syndrome marked by a distinctive facial appearance, characteristic hands and feet, associated abnormalities in growth, and other minor physical abnormalities. Diagnosis is made on clinical grounds because there are no distinctive biochemical or chromosomal markers. It is associated with a behavioral phenotype that may include self-injurious behavior.

This chapter describes the history, epidemiology, etiology, clinical features and phenotype, and treatment of Cornelia de Lange syndrome.

HISTORY

The Dutch pediatrician Cornelia de Lange described two unrelated affected girls in 1933, using the designation "typus degenerativis Amstelodamensis," naming the syndrome after the city where her first case was evaluated (deLange, 1933). Subsequently, the name "Amsterdam dwarf" was used; however, because dwarfism is not an invariable characteristic of the disorder (Filippi, 1989), this term was not continued. Brachmann had previously reported a similar condition in 1916 (Brachmann, 1916). Brachmann's patient, unlike that of de Lange's, had webbing at the elbows, malformed forearms, and oligodactyly, but like de Lange's case, was similar in regard to failure to thrive, microbrachycephaly, and hirsutism. Because of this previous report, the syndrome is sometimes known as the Brachmann-de Lange syndrome. Meinecke and Hayek (1990) reported a case closely resembling the case described by Brachmann in 1916 and suggest that the similarity of this case is an additional factor in referring to the syndrome as the Brachmann-de Lange syndrome. Both names are used in the literature. However, de Lange's original report is more comprehensive and the U.S. national organization is referred to as the Cornelia de Lange Syndrome Foundation.

Following de Lange's reports on two unrelated girls, 21 cases were reported during the following three decades, all from European countries. In 1963 English and American publications began to appear. Three extensive reviews of cases were reported by Ptacek et al. (1963), Schlesinger et al. (1963), and Jervis and Stimson (1963). Since then, papers about the de Lange syndrome have appeared more frequently. With the increasing numbers of case reports, variability of expression of the disorder has been noted (Greenberg and Robinson, 1989).

EPIDEMIOLOGY

The prevalence of the Cornelia de Lange syndrome is about 1 in 40,000 to 100,000 live births. Boys and girls are equally affected. Most cases occur sporadically in otherwise normal families; however, the possibility of both autosomal recessive and autosomal dominant inheritance has been raised by several authors (Frijns et al., 1983; Kumar, Blank, and Griffiths, 1985; Robinson, Wolfsberg, and Jones, 1985).

ETIOLOGY

Genetics

Familial occurrence of the Cornelia de Lange syndrome has been described, including several cases that are consistent with autosomal dominant inheritance (Robinson, Wolfsberg, and Jones, 1985). There is one three-generation family, and at least four sets of sibling pairs have been reported. Autosomal dominant inheritance has been suggested, with germ line mosaicism as the explanation for recurrence in siblings. Because of the severity of the disorder, reproduction is rare but can occur. Mosher et al. (1985) reported pregnancy in a woman with de Lange syndrome who delivered a normal-appearing female infant; one would expect approximately 50% risk for having an affected offspring. De Die-Smulders et al. (1992) reported a mother and moderately mentally retarded son, both with typical facial features of the syndrome. These authors suggest that the most severe cases are due to fresh mutations of an autosomally dominant gene. De Die-Smulders et al. (1992) also suggest that there may be two forms of the disorder, a severe form and a mild form. The severe form is associated with severe growth and mental retardation, typical facies, and, frequently, upper arm malformations. The milder form lacks the ulnar upper limb reduction defect, and the other manifestations are milder. Because there is no definitive biochemical or other diagnostic test, clinical diagnosis of mildly affected individuals may be difficult. In their case report, there is genetic anticipation in that the child shows a more severe disorder than the mother. They suggest that in all convincing autosomal dominant cases, the transmitting parent is the mother, which might indicate genomic imprinting. Additional data is needed on the pattern of inheritance in light of the recently described genetic disorders that involve the inheritance of unstable trinucleotide repeat sequences, such as fragile X syndrome and Huntington's disease.

Several chromosomal anomalies have been suggested. Falek, Schmidt, and Jervis (1966) suggested a relationship between chromosome 3 and the de Lange syndrome. Others have suggested that chromosome 3 is not clearly associated. Several differences have been suggested between the de Lange syndrome and the duplication 3q syndrome, although there is overlap (Wilson, Dasouki, and Barr, 1985). Moreover, a ring chromosome abnormality involving chromosome 3 has been suggested (Lakshminarayana and Nallasivam, 1990). The question of chromosomal location requires further evaluation.

Although specific fetal markers are not available, Bruner and Hsia (1990) suggest suspicion when the triad of low maternal alphafetoprotein, early onset intrauterine growth retardation (IUGR), and characteristic ultrasound findings are present.

CLINICAL FEATURES AND PHENOTYPE

Infants with Cornelia de Lange syndrome demonstrate failure to thrive with feeding difficulties and gastroesophageal reflux that may be life threatening. Regurgitation, vomiting, and swallowing problems may lead to aspiration pneumonia in early life. Sexual development is normal, with reproduction being limited by the degree of social impairment seen in this disorder. The most common clinical findings are shown in Table 10.8–1.

The physical phenotype is characterized by growth failure, distinctive facial features, and limb abnormality. Specific facial features include characteristic eyebrows that are well defined, arched, and fan out laterally to join (synophrys). Eyelashes are frequently long and curled. The nose is small and upturned, with a long philtrum, and a mouth that is turned down with thin lips. Limb abnormalities range from small limbs (micromelia) to severe reductions in limb size (phocomelia) confined to the upper limbs. Other associated abnormalities include

Table 10.8–1. Characteristic Features of De Lange Syndrome

Birth weight below 5½ lb (2,500 g), often following full-term pregnancy
Retarded mental development, usually severe
Retarded physical growth, usually severe
Generalized hirsutism
Microbrachycephaly
Synophrys, usually associated with long eyelashes
Anteverted nostrils, usually associated with depressed nasal bridge
Prominent philtrum (i.e., elongated and/or protruding)
Thin lips, turned down at angles of mouth
Limitation of extension at elbows
Single transverse palmar crease
Proximally placed thumbs
Clinodactyly of fifth fingers
Severely malformed upper limbs, ranging from oligodactyly to phocomelia
Webbing of second and third toes

From Berg et al., 1970.

hearing loss and other physical abnormalities, including bowel duplication or malformation and congenital heart disease. In mild cases, typical facial features may not be evident until the second year of life (Greenberg and Robinson, 1989). Dermatoglyphics and radiological findings are important in confirming the diagnosis (Filippi, 1989).

Behavioral Phenotype

Mental retardation is characteristic and is usually severe. Speech is limited, ranging from an absence of speech to single words in those with severe mental retardation. However, language problems are also found in the higher functioning group and may require speech therapy (Cameron and Kelley, 1988). In the mild form, mental abilities may range up to the borderline or normal range. Behavior characteristics include avoidance of being held, stereotypical movements, and twirling, which some have referred to as autistic-like features. Although some children with the de Lange syndrome are "placid and good natured," others show irritability, destructiveness, self-mutilation (Bryson et al., 1971; Johnson et al., 1976; Nyhan, 1972; Shear et al., 1971), and bruxism (Berg et al., 1970).

Psychosocial Aspects

Beck (1987) assessed 36 de Lange patients, aged 5 to 47 years, with a median age of 16 years. Self-injury was found in 6 of 36 (17%) and consisted of finger biting. Limited social interaction was apparent in the younger cases. Forty-four percent had no language, which is consistent with other reports of language disorder in the severely involved group. Only 10 patients (27%) had useful language. The voice showed a characteristic hoarseness, and speech was dysphonic, which is consistent with previous findings by Fraser and Campbell (1978).

The subjects were evaluated using the Vineland Social Maturity Scale. Severe physical disabilities made scoring difficult in 6 patients. The social quotients from the other cases varied from 2.2 to 99.5. Of the patients scored, 81% had scores of less than 52. The abnormalities noted were specific retardation in verbal communication and other cognitive skills. Relatively high scores were shown for mental age in regard to self-help. Fifteen of the patients lived in large institutions for the mentally retarded, 3 lived in hostels or boarding school, and 1 lived in her own home. Two patients, both of whom were severely retarded, did not attend any regular daily activity. The authors indicate that patients with de Lange syndrome will not be able to live without support in the community and that they are particularly retarded in their verbal communication, although they may function relatively well given their mental age and self-care skills. They are relatively able to cope with everyday needs, although help in social skills and particularly with communication is needed.

TREATMENT

The initial aspects of treatment focus on family recognition of the disability and identification of this particular syndrome. Because of the potential overlap with other syndromes, such as duplication of 3q, a karyotype should be obtained to help clarify the diagnosis. There are national family associations for the Cornelia de Lange syndrome, and parent groups are important to provide support for newly diagnosed cases. Self-injurious behavior requires early intervention and behavior treatment. In evaluating self-injurious behavior, physical discomfort is important to identify. In some instances, physical discomfort associated with delayed dentition has been related to self-injury. Massage has been reported to reduce severe self-injury in one case study of a girl with the Cornelia de Lange syndrome (Dossetor, Couryer, and Nicol, 1991). When reflux vomiting is present and associated with behavior disorder, surgical treatment (Nissen fundoplication) may lead to improvement in temperament. Hearing loss is common (Marres, Cremers, and Jungbloet, 1989), as is impaired language development. Appropriate interventions are required for both of these conditions. A comprehensive approach that attends to educational, language, medical, and psychosocial needs is essential to facilitate long-term development.

REFERENCES

Beck, B. (1987). Psycho-social assessment of 36 de Lange patients. *Journal of Mental Deficiency Research*, 31:251–257.

Berg, J.M., McCreary, B.D., Ridler, M.A.C., and Smith, G.F. (1970). *The de Lange syndrome.* Pergamon Press, New York.

Brachmann, W. (1916). Ein Fall von symmetrischer Monodactylie durch Ulnadefekt, mit symmetrischer Flughautbildung in den Ellenbogen, sowie anderen Abnormalitaten. *Jahrbuch für Kinderheilknde ünd Physische Erziehung*, 84:225–235.

Bruner, J.P., and Hsia, Y.E. (1990). Prenatal findings in Brachmann-de Lange syndrome. *Obstetrics & Gynecology*, 76:966–968.

Bryson, Y., Sakati, N., Nyhan W.L., and Fish, C.H. (1971). Self-mutilative behavior in the Cornelia de Lange syndrome. *American Journal of Mental Deficiency*, 76:319–324.

Cameron, T.H., and Kelly, D.P. (1988). Normal language skills and normal intelligence in a child with de Lange syndrome. *Journal of Speech & Hearing Disorders*, 53(2):219–222.

de Die-Smulders, C., Theunissen, P., Schrander-Stumpel, C., and Frijns, J.P. (1992). On the variable expression of the Brachmann-de Lange syndrome. *Clinical Genetics*, 41(1):42–45.

de Lange, C. (1933). Sur un type nouveau dégénération (typus Amstelodamensis). *Archives de Médicine des Infants*, 36:713–719.

Dossetor, D.R., Couryer, S., and Nicol, A.R. (1991). Massage for very severe self-injurious behaviour in a girl with Cornelia de Lange syndrome. *Developmental Medicine and Child Neurology*, 33:636–644.

Falek, A., Schmidt, R., and Jervis, G.A. (1966). Familial de Lange syndrome with chromosome abnormalities. *Pediatrics*, 37:92–101.

Filippi, G. (1989). The de Lange syndrome: Report of 15 cases. *Clinical Genetics*, 35:343–363.

Fraser, W.I., and Campbell, B.M. (1978). A study of six cases of de Lange Amsterdam dwarf syndrome with special attention to voice, speech, and language characteristics. *Developmental Medicine and Child Neurology*, 20:189–198.

Frijns, J.P., Kleczkowska A., Verresen, H., and van den Berghe, H. (1983). Germinal mosaicism in achondroplasia: A family with 3 affected siblings of normal parents. *Clinical Genetics*, 24:156–158.

Greenberg, F., and Robinson, L.K. (1989). Mild Brachmann-de Lange syndrome: Changes of phenotype with age. *American Journal of Medical Genetics*, 32(1): 90–92.

Jervis, A.G., and Stimson, C.W. (1963). De Lange syndrome. The Amsterdam type of mental defect with congenital malformations. *Journal of Pediatrics*, 63:634–645.

Johnson, H.G., Ekman, P., Friesan, W., Nyhan, W.L., and Shear, C. (1976). A behavioral phenotype in the de Lange syndrome. *Pediatric Research*, 10:843–850.

Kumar, D., Blank, C.E., and Griffiths, B.L. (1985). Cornelia de Lange syndrome in several members of the same family. *Journal of Medical Genetics*, 22:296–300.

Lakshminarayana, P., and Nallasivam, P. (1990). Cornelia de Lange syndrome with ring chromosome 3. *Journal of Medical Genetics*, 27(6):405–406.

Marres, H.A., Cremers, C.W., and Jongbloet, P.H. (1989). Hearing levels in the Cornelia de Lange syndrome. A report of seven cases. *International Journal of Pediatric Otorhinolaryngology*, 18(1):31–37.

Meinecke, P. and Hayek, H. (1990). Brief historical note on the Brachmann-de Lange syndrome: A patient closely resembling the case described by Brachmann in 1916. *American Journal of Medical Genetics*, 35:449–450.

Mosher, G.A., Schulte, R.L., Kaplan, P.A., Buehlker, B.A., and Sanger, W.G. (1985). Pregnancy in a woman with the Brachmann-de Lange syndrome. *American Journal of Medical Genetics*, 22(1):103–107.

Nyhan, W.L. (1972). Behavioral phenotypes in organic genetic disease. *Pediatric Research*, 6:1–9.

Ptacek, L.J., Opitz, J.M., Smith, D.W., Gerritsen, T., and Waisman, H.A. (1963). The Cornelia de Lange syndrome. *Journal of Pediatrics,* 63:1000–1020.

Robinson, L.K., Wolfsberg, E., and Jones, K.L. (1985). Brachmann-de Lange syndrome: Evidence for autosomal dominant inheritance. *American Journal of Medical Genetics,* 22:109–115.

Schlesinger, B., Clayton, B., Bodian, M., and Vernon Jones, K. (1963). Typus degenerativus amstelodamensis. *Archives of Diseases of Childhood,* 38:349–357.

Shear, C., Nyhan, W., Kirman, B., and Stern, J. (1971). Self-mutilative behavior as a feature of de Lange syndrome. *Journal of Pediatrics,* 78:506–509.

Wilson, G.N., Dasouki, M., and Barr, M.,Jr. (1985). Further delineation of the dup(3q) syndrome. *American Journal of Medical Genetics,* 22(1):117–123.

CHAPTER 11

GENETIC METABOLIC DISORDERS ASSOCIATED WITH BEHAVIORAL PHENOTYPES

11.1 Lesch-Nyhan Disease

Lesch-Nyhan disease is a sex-linked recessive disease caused by an inborn error of purine nucleotide metabolism. It is caused by an almost complete deficiency of the enzyme hypoxanthine-guanine phosphoribosyltransferase (HPRT), which is involved in the purine salvage pathway. Self-injury is the major behavioral manifestation; this behavior was sufficiently characteristic that Nyhan (1972) introduced the term "behavioral phenotype" to describe it. Lesch-Nyhan disease is of psychosocial and psychiatric importance because of the suffering experienced by the involved child and his family, the unique behavioral phenotype, the resources required for lifelong patient supervision, and because an understanding of the neurobiological basis of this disease may contribute to a better comprehension of brain mechanisms involved in self-injurious and compulsive behaviors.

This chapter reviews the history, prevalence and epidemiology, definition and clinical features, developmental course, etiology, and treatment of the behavioral manifestations of Lesch-Nyhan.

HISTORY

Lesch-Nyhan disease was initially described in 1964 in two brothers, aged 4 and 8 years, by Michael Lesch, then a medical student, and William Nyhan, MD. The younger brother had been diagnosed with cerebral palsy and presented with hematuria. Both he and his brother were found to be mentally retarded and had choreoathetosis, renal stones, and self-biting. Subsequently, HPRT was identified as the missing enzyme involved in this metabolic disorder (Seegmiller, Rosenbloom, and Kelley, 1967). It was later determined that there is essentially a continuous spectrum of enzyme activity in mutant hemizygous subjects, ranging from nondetectable to about 50% of normal levels. The majority of patients with classical Lesch-Nyhan disease have low or undetectable levels of the HPRT enzyme, rarely more than 1%. In 1979 Becker et al. localized the gene to the long arm of the X chromosome (q26-q27). The complete amino acid sequence for HPRT was described by Wilson et al. in 1982 and the organization of the human HPRT gene (~44 kb; 9 exons) is described by Kim et al. (1986).

PREVALENCE AND EPIDEMIOLOGY

The prevalence of the classical syndrome is generally estimated at 1 in 100,000 to 1 in 380,000 (Crawhall, Henderson, and Kelley, 1972). However, based on the number of known cases in the United States, it may be as rare as 1 in 800,000 to 1 in 1.2 million. In addition, partial variants show considerable differences in the extent of residual HPRT activity (Page et al., 1981; Page and Nyhan, 1989). The incidence of partial variants is not known. Those with the classical syndrome rarely survive the third decade; however, life span is apparently normal for the partial variants.

DEFINITION AND CLINICAL FEATURES

Features of Lesch-Nyhan disease include hyperuricemia, mental retardation, cerebral palsy with early choreoathetosis and later spasticity and torsion dystonia, dysarthric speech, and compulsive self-injury, usually beginning with the eruption of teeth (Lesch and Nyhan, 1964). The extent of mental retardation is ordinarily in the mild to moderate range; however, test scores are influenced by difficulty in test administration due to the movement disorder and the dysarthria so that overall intelligence may be underestimated (Anderson, Ernst, and Davis, 1992) and sometimes extends into the normal range. The age of onset of self-injury may be as early as 1 year or rarely as late as the teens (Watts et al., 1982). Children demonstrate self-mutilation initially through self-biting, which is intense and causes tissue damage, often leading to amputation of fingers and loss of tissue around the lips. The biting often results in extraction of primary teeth. With increasing age, they also may self-mutilate by picking the skin with their fingers. Severe self-injurious behavior may lead to institutional placement. In type, the behavior is different from that seen in other mental retardation syndromes of self-injury where self-hitting and head banging are the most common initial presentations. The self-injury occurs although all sensory modalities, including the pain sense, are intact. Moreover, the intensity of the self-injurious behavior requires that the patient be restrained. Despite their movement disorder, when restraints are removed, the patient may appear terrified and quickly and accurately place a hand in the mouth. The child may ask for restraints to prevent elbow movement. When restraints are placed, the child may appear relaxed and more good humored (Nyhan, 1976). Patients' dysarthric speech may result in interpersonal communication problems; however, the higher functioning children can express themselves and participate in their treatment. Hemiballismic arm movements can also create difficulty because the raised arm is sometimes misinterpreted as a threatening gesture by others rather than an aspect of the movement disorder.

Behavioral Phenotype

The self-mutilation is conceptualized as a compulsive behavior that the child tries to control but generally is unable to resist. With increasing age, he becomes more adept at finding ways to control the self-injury, including enlisting the help of others to protect himself against these impulses. However, self-injury may progress to deliberate self-harm (Anderson and Ernst, 1994).

Self-injurious behavior usually is expressed as self-biting; however, other patterns of self-injurious behavior may emerge with time. Characteristically, the fingers, mouth, and buccal mucosa are mutilated. The biting pattern is often asymmetrical in that the patient mutilates the left or right side of the body and may become anxious if he perceives this side of the

Table 11.1–1. Forms and Frequency of Self-Injury Reported in 40 Subjects with Lesch-Nyhan Disease

Biting	Number	Nonbiting	Number
Lips	33	Arm, leg, or head out at doorway	35
Fingers	29	Arching and head snapping	34
Arms	16	Head banging	30
Tongue	14	Feet under wheelchair	23
Shoulders	8	Fingers in spokes	17
		Eye poking	13

From Anderson and Ernst, 1994.

body is threatened. Patterns of self-injury are shown in Table 11.1–1.

A characteristic language pattern may also become evident. This language pattern consists of repeated ambivalent statements that occur most commonly with anxiety, and coprolalia (vulgar speech). Other associated maladaptive behaviors include later-developing head or limb banging, eye poking, pulling fingernails, and psychogenic vomiting. Moreover, the patient may be compulsively aggressive and inflict injury to others through pinching, grabbing, or by using verbal forms of aggression. Frequently, the patient will apologize for this behavior immediately afterward and say the behavior was out of his control.

Cognitive Level

Children and adolescents with Lesch-Nyhan disease commonly test in the 40 to 60 IQ range, although some test higher than this into the low normal range of intelligence (Scherzer and Ilson, 1969). It is generally thought that these scores represent a low estimate of their overall abilities because of the difficulties in testing them and their limited life experiences (Anderson, Ernst, and Davis, 1992). Their behavioral difficulties and self-injury may interfere with learning.

DEVELOPMENTAL COURSE

At birth, infants with Lesch-Nyhan disease have no neurological dysfunction and may develop normally for 4 to 6 months before developmental retardation and neurological signs become apparent. However, before the age of 4 months, hypotonia, recurrent vomiting, and difficulty with secretions may be evident. At approximately 8 to 12 months of age, extrapyramidal signs appear, including athetosis, chorea, and dystonia. By around 12 months, pyramidal tract signs become evident with hyperreflexia, sustained ankle clonus, positive Babinski, and scissoring.

ETIOLOGY

Genetics/Metabolic

The gene involved in Lesch-Nyhan disease is on the X chromosome so the disorder occurs almost entirely in males. Occurrence in females is extremely rare (Ogasawara et al., 1989; van Bogaert et al., 1992). The metabolic abnormality is the result of an abnormal gene product—a deficiency in the enzyme hypoxanthine-guanine phosphoribosyltransferase (HPRT) (Sweetman and Nyhan, 1972). This enzyme is normally present in each cell in the body and is highest in the brain, especially in the basal ganglia. Its absence prevents the normal metabolism of hypoxanthine, resulting in excessive uric acid production and manifestations of gout without specific drug treatment (i.e., allopurinol). The full disease requires the virtual absence of the enzyme (Figure 11.1–1). Other syndromes with partial HPRT deficiency are associated with gout without the neurological and behavioral symptoms. Page and Nyhan (1989) have reported that HPRT levels are related to the extent of motor symptoms, presence or absence of self-injury, and possibly to the level of cognitive function.

Hypoxanthine accumulates in the cerebral spinal fluid, but uric acid does not because it is not produced in the brain and does not cross the blood-brain barrier from the blood. There are a variety of abnormalities in this disease not related to increased uric acid in body fluids.

The etiology of the neurological symptoms is not clearly established; however, abnormalities in neurotransmitter metabolism have been demonstrated (Baumeister and Frye, 1985; Lloyd et al., 1981) in three autopsied cases. The behavior is not caused by hyperuricemia or excess hypoxanthine because partial variants with hyperuricemia do not self-injure and infants treated for hyperuricemia alone from birth do develop self-injury. The hyperuricemia itself results from the absence of the HPRT enzyme in the purine salvage pathway. If the hyperuricemia is untreated, it may lead to renal failure and death at an early age.

Partial deficiency in HPRT is associated with hyperuricemia and variable neurological dysfunction; its severity is inversely correlated with the amount of residual HPRT activity. Most commonly, partial HPRT deficiency leads to a severe form of gout, with normal cerebral functioning.

Anatomical and Biochemical Studies

In investigating a biological basis for the behavior disorder in this disease, both anatomical and neurochemical studies have been undertaken (Harris, 1992a). No appreciable morphological abnormality in any part of the brain, including the basal ganglia where changes might be expected, given the motor symptoms, have been demonstrated. Watts and associates (1982) reported no abnormality with detailed histopathology and electron microscopy of 13 brain regions in one case studied.

Biochemical alterations also might be involved and underlie the abnormalities seen in the nervous system. This possibility might be assessed in three ways (Harris, 1987): (1) direct measurement of neurotransmitters in brain tissue; (2) measurement of neurotransmitters and their metabolites in cerebrospinal fluid; and (3) clinical response to neurotransmitter precursor treatment. Lloyd et al. (1981) have directly examined different brain regions postmortem from 3 patients (ages 13, 14, and 27) who died with Lesch-Nyhan disease for indices of dopamine, norepinephrine, serotonin, gamma-aminobutyric acid (GABA), and acetylcholine function in basal ganglia and other brain areas. Lloyd's group compared the pathological material from patients with age-matched control subjects without neurological disease. They found that all 3 patients with Lesch-Nyhan disease had very low HPRT levels (less than 1% in striatal tissue and 1% to 2% of control values in the thalamus and cortex). The finding that the phosphoribosyl transferase for adenine, another amino purine, was normal in these patients demonstrated there was no general deficit in purine metabolism.

A general reduction in the dopamine neurotransmitter system was found in those areas of the brain containing dopamine neurons. Low dopamine levels and decreased homovanillic acid (HVA), its main metabolite, as well as low levels of the synthesizing ezymes, dopamine decarboxylase, esterase, and hydroxylase, were noted in terminal-rich dopamine areas including the caudate nucleus, putamen, and nucleus accumbens. There was a functional loss of 65% to 90% of the nigrostriatal and mesolimbic

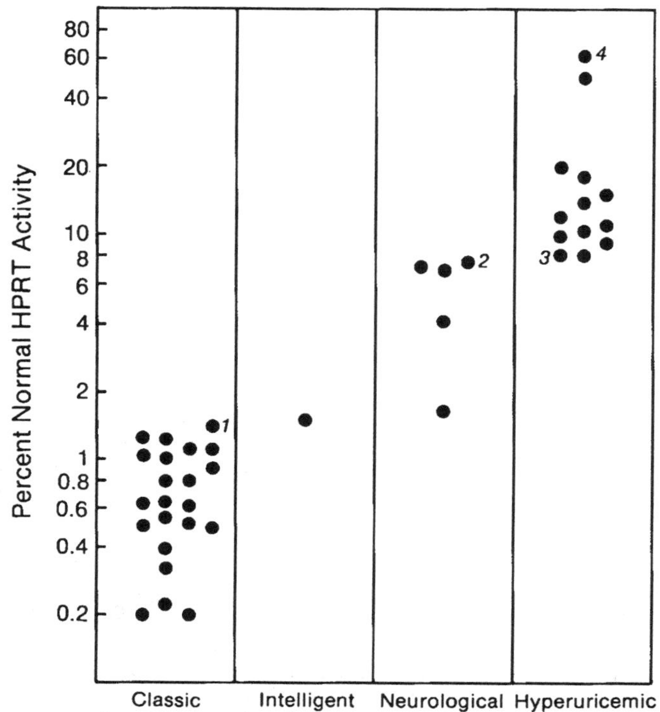

Figure 11.1–1. HPRT-deficient phenotypes and their corresponding enzyme activities. As the percentage of normal HPRT activity increases, there is a reduction in the severity of the clinical presentation (from Page and Nyhan, 1989).

dopamine terminals. The cell body region where these fibers originate, the substantia nigra, had normal dopamine levels. There was then a decrease in dopamine level in the terminal areas, but the cell bodies of origin were apparently preserved. Therefore, the neurochemical changes in this disorder may be related to functional abnormalities, perhaps resulting from a diminution of arborization or branching out of dopamine terminals and dendrites rather than cell loss. This would suggest a neurodevelopmental disorder rather than a degenerative disease. There was also a decrease in striatal cholinergic function, but norepinephrine and GABA from representative areas were normal, whereas serotonin was slightly elevated.

In regard to blood and cerebral spinal fluid measurements of neurotransmitters and their metabolites, several authors have found changes in Lesch-Nyhan disease (Silverstein et al., 1985). Serum dopamine β-hydroxylase has been reported to be altered in these patients, and low levels of HVA were observed in the cerebral spinal fluid (CSF) of one case of Lesch-Nyhan disease. The major serotonin metabolite, 5-hydroxy indoleacetic acid, has also been reported to be decreased.

A third approach to study neurotransmitters is the use of precursor treatment. There are reports in several patients that the administration of the serotonin precursor L-5-hydroxytryptophan, both with and without a peripheral decarboxylase inhibitor (carbidopa), leads to beneficial effects in Lesch-Nyhan disease. This response would be consistent with a variation in serotonin levels in brain regions despite the changes noted by Lloyd and co-workers (1981) in the brain areas they studied. Nyhan (1976) and Mizuno and Yugari (1975) suggest temporary improvement with the administration of a serotonin precursor. However, long-term improvement has not been demonstrated with a serotonin precursor. When the drug was given without interruption for several months, the self-injury reappeared during intervals of up to 3 months. Kopin (1981) suggests that a diazepam binding site may be involved in producing some of the behavioral manifestations of Lesch-Nyhan disease. He further suggests that future studies of interactions between neurotransmitters and neuromodulators that regulate brain function might have impact on developing a rational approach to chemotherapy.

Animal Models

A relationship between dopaminergic supersensitivity and self-injury has been demonstrated in experimental animals (Breese et al., 1984a; 1984b; 1990). These authors gave 6-hydroxydopamine (6-OHDA) to neonatal and adult rats and found that the age at which neural function is disrupted is an important factor in the type of motor and behavioral symptoms observed after a neural insult to basal ganglia structures. The rats treated with 6-OHDA in the neonatal period demonstrated self-mutilation when challenged as adults with L-dopa or a D_1 dopamine agonist. This self-injurious behavior was not noted in the adult rats treated with 6-OHDA. Based on these data, the neonatal 6-OHDA treated rat was suggested to be a model of the dopamine deficiency observed in Lesch-Nyhan disease. Rats who were not HPRT-deficient were given injections of 6-OHDA at 5 days of age to denervate basal ganglia regions. These brain regions developed supersensitive dopamine receptors. Self-biting was seen in the lesioned animals when they were challenged as adults with a dopamine agonist; however, untreated adult rats did not show this behavior. Goldstein et al. (1985) found dopamine-induced self-mutilative biting behavior in monkeys with unilateral ventral tegmental lesions lending further support to the dopamine hypothesis. Similar studies in monkeys were carried out by Goldstein et al. (1985), who found that the self-injury was elicited by specific dopamine agonists. The effect is thought to be predominantly on the D_1 dopamine receptor because these effects were blocked by a D_1 dopamine antagonist.

The HPRT-Deficient Mouse

Molecular genetic techniques combined with techniques to manipulate the developing mouse embryo make it feasible to produce genetic animal models of human neurological diseases. The HPRT-deficient mouse has been introduced as an animal model of Lesch-Nyhan disease (Figure 11.1–2).

As shown in the figure, embryonic stem (ES) cells are isolated from a pregnant mouse

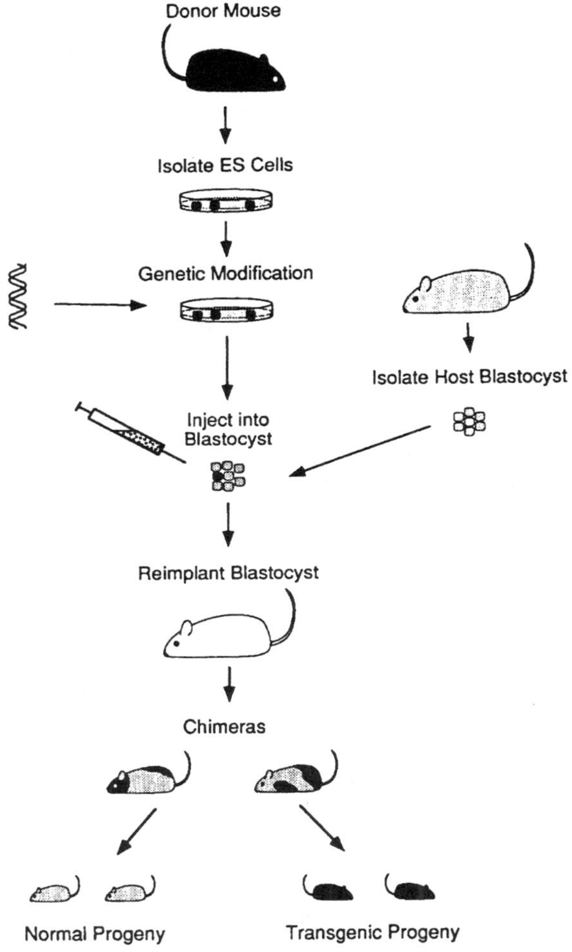

Figure 11.1–2. *Development of HPRT-deficient mice.* Embryonic stem cells are isolated from a donor mouse embryo (shown in black), genetically modified *in vitro,* and microinjected into a host blastocyst (shown in gray). The mixed blastocyst is then implanted into a pseudopregnant female (shown in white), and allowed to develop. Chimeric mice (black and gray) are bred further, producing either normal (gray) or transgenic (black) offspring (from Jinnah, Gage, and Friedmann, 1990).

with identifiable coat color that acts as a donor. The embryonic stem cells are grown in cell culture and then genetically modified with the insertion of genetic material or through mutation of endogenous genes. Modified embryonic stem cells are microinjected into a blastula that is isolated from another mouse who ordinarily has a different coat color. The blastula is then reimplanted into a female host mouse and develops *in utero.* The inserted stem cells then are incorporated into the developing fetuses, and progeny which contain genetically altered cells are chimeras that can be identified by their mosaic coat colors.

As adults, these chimeras, where genetically modified cells have been involved in the establishment of the germ cell line, may then transmit the altered gene to their own offspring. It takes several generations to produce an affected animal, using these embryonic stem cell techniques that depend on whether the needed phenotype can be produced in the heterozygous, homozygous, or hemizygous condition.

For Lesch-Nyhan disease, these techniques have been used to produce two HPRT-deficient strains of mice. One strain was produced by retroviral interruption of the human HPRT gene in the embryonic stem cells (Kuehn et al., 1987). Another model was produced through the selection of embryonic stem cells for spontaneous mutations in the HPRT gene (Hooper et al., 1987). In both instances, the mouse strains produced have nondetectable levels of HPRT. However, neither strain showed the spontaneous behavioral abnormalities or neurological presentation seen in patients with Lesch-Nyhan disease. Both tests of cognitive functions and motor functions are intact in these animals.

The absence of behavior changes in the mice was unexpected. Originally, it was thought that uricase, which is present in rodents but not in primates, may act in a protective manner to lessen behavioral manifestations because uric acid, which normally builds up in the blood in Lesch-Nyhan disease, would not do so in mice due to the presence of this enzyme. However, this explanation does not explain the inability of allopurinol, a xanthine oxidase inhibitor that prevents the accumulation of uric acid, to improve the behavior disorder in patients with Lesch-Nyhan disease.

In this HPRT-deficient transgenic mouse model of Lesch-Nyhan disease (Hooper et al., 1987), reduction in dopamine of 40% or more (Jinnah, Gage, and Friedmann, 1990) has been demonstrated in the caudate nucleus in the deficient strain of mice when compared to littermate controls. Reductions in the dopamine transporter of 35% to 40% also have been identified in the same species (Jinnah, personal communication). These results indicate an abnormality in the dopamine system despite apparently normal spontaneous behavior.

Pharmacological challenge studies were carried out in the HPRT mice. When amphetamine was administered in high doses to these mice (amphetamine stimulates release and inhibits uptake of monoamine neurotransmitters), significant increases in stereotypic and locomotor behavior were observed in contrast to control animals (Jinnah, Page, and Friedmann, 1991). Moreover, older mice (22 to 24 months) developed trauma to their ears and to their flanks from overgrooming, a type of mouse stereotypical behavior (Williamson, Hooper and Melton, 1992). Due to the response to amphetamine and the changes with aging, additional investigations have been carried out on the behavior of HPRT-deficient mice.

Because differences in purine metabolism between mice and humans could be responsible for the different manifestations between species, the purine pathway was evaluated in both species and comparisons were made (Jinnah, Page, and Friedmann, 1993) (Figure 11.1–3). The HPRT was completely absent in brain tissue homogenates, indicating the absence of HPRT-mediated purine salvage. Despite this, the animals had apparently normal brain purine content. It was concluded that *de novo* purine synthesis is accelerated four- to fivefold in the mutant animals.

An alternative explanation is that other pathways are involved in the synthesis of purines. Because it is possible that the regulation of the nucleotide pool differs between humans and mice, wild-type mice were studied. The study of wild-type mice revealed less dependency in mice than humans on HPRT to salvage purines. Wu and Melton (1993) found that although HPRT is the primary enzyme for purine salvage in humans, an alternative pathway, the APRT pathway, may also be important in mice. These investigators used purine analogs to inhibit APRT activity and were able to induce self-injurious behavior in young HPRT-deficient mice by using 9-ethyladenine to block APRT activity without producing general toxic effects. When 9-ethyladenine was given to 2 male and 3 female individually caged outbred 9- to 12-month-old mice with HPRT deficiency, all 5 animals developed self-inflicted injury between 48 and 130 days after the injections. Similar injuries did not occur in age-matched uninjected HPRT-deficient mice. The injury primarily involved the ears, neck, back, and flanks and was produced by excessive grooming. Severe self-biting, leading to skin damage,

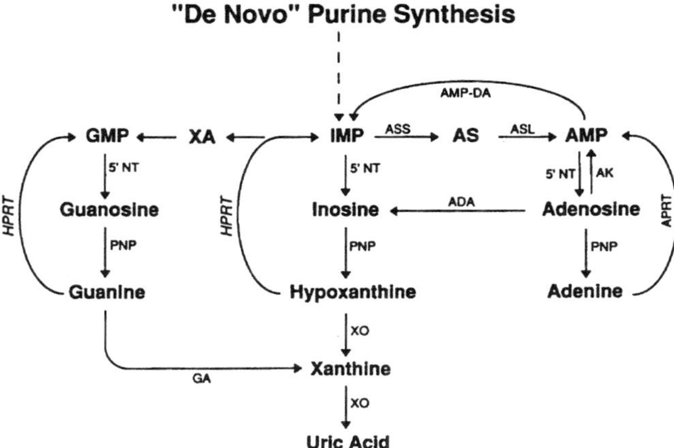

Figure 11.1–3. *Metabolic pathway for purine nucleotides.* Abbreviations: 5'NT, 5'-nucleotidase; ADA, adenosine deaminase; AMP, adenylic acid; AMP-DA, adenylic acid deaminase; APRT, adenine phosphoribosyltransferase; AS, adenylosuccinate; ASL, adenylosuccinate lyase; ASS, adenylosuccinate synthetase; GA, guanase; GMP, guanylic acid; HPRT, hypoxanthine-guanine phosphoribosyltransferase; IMP, inosinic acid; PNP, purine nucleoside phosphorylase; XA, xanthylic acid; XO, xanthine oxidase (from Jinnah, Gage, and Friedmann, 1990).

was also seen but was difficult to distinguish from biting or nibbling that did not cause physical injury. The grooming, nibbling, and biting are all characteristic stereotypic mouse behaviors. Subsequently, the experiment was repeated with 6- to 8-week-old mice, with similar findings, although the extent of self-injury was not as severe. These findings demonstrate the importance of understanding metabolic pathways in developing animal models. This mouse behavior suggests a model for compulsive patterns of behavior (i.e., compulsive grooming) but the self-biting in the mice is not identical to that seen in Lesch-Nyhan disease. A more specific mouse model of Lesch-Nyhan disease, combined HPRT/APRT-deficient mice, is being developed to clarify the impact of deficiency of combined enzyme loss on behavior (Melton, personal communication).

The self-injury that occurs in Lesch-Nyhan disease is a compulsive behavior; other forms of compulsive behavior are noted as well. Investigations of animal models involving APRT or combined APRT and HPRT lesions may lead to a better understanding of the basis of compulsive behaviors in general as well as those associated with Lesch-Nyhan disease. Furthermore, in the mouse model, the absence of the HPRT gene does lead to molecular abnormalities in the dopamine system, which seem to be expressed primarily in the caudoputamen rather than in other dopamine pathways (Jinnah, Langlais, and Friedmann, 1992; Jinnah et al., 1994). Because of this preferential involvement of the nigral-striatal system, greater elucidation of the mechanisms of compulsive behavior might be sought in investigations of animal models such as these.

TREATMENT

Understanding the molecular disorder has led to effective drug treatment for those aspects of the disease that are related to uric acid accumulation and subsequent arthritic tophi, renal stones, and neuropathy. However, reduction in uric acid has not influenced the neurological and behavioral aspects. In fact, some children have been treated from birth for the elevation in uric acid and have behavioral and neurological symptoms despite never having high levels of uric acid.

The focus on medical management emphasizes the prevention of renal failure by pharmacological treatment of hyperuricemia through administration of allopurinol and efforts to reduce self-mutilation through behavior management, the use of restraints, and/or removal of teeth. Pharmacological approaches to reduce anxiety and spasticity have met with mixed results. Of the psychopharmacological agents used, the drug reported by parents to be the most effective is diazepam.

Bone Marrow Transplantation and Gene Therapy

Based on the possibility that the central nervous system damage is produced by a circulating toxin, a bone marrow transplantation was carried out in the United States in a 22-year-old Lesch-Nyhan patient (Nyhan et al., 1986). The authors postulated that because specific gross neuropathology has not been demonstrated, an unknown neurotoxic substance of low molecular weight might cause central nervous system dysfunction. Restoration of HPRT activity in the hematopoetic system might protect the central nervous system from this possible toxin. Although the transplantation was successful and restored the HPRT activity in the patient's peripheral blood cells to near the normal range, there was no change in neurological symptoms or behavior. Positron emission tomography (PET) scanning was carried out before and after the bone marrow transplantation with 11_C NMSP, a D_2 dopamine receptor ligand, but no changes were demonstrated in receptor density following the transplantation (Harris, 1992b). Because it might be too late to reverse the cerebral symptoms in an adult, a second bone marrow transplantation was attempted in Germany (Endres et al., 1991) in a 16-month-old boy who had begun to show signs of psychomotor retardation. The patient did not survive the procedure and died on day 10 following the transplantation. The cause of death is unknown; however, there was no evidence of septicemia or graft-versus-host reaction.

Another approach to replace HPRT enzyme activity involved the use of partial exchange transfusion. Two patients received partial exchange transfusions every 2 months for 3 to 4 years (Edwards, Jeryc, and Fox, 1984). Although erythrocyte HPRT activity was 10% to 70% of normal during this period, no reduction of neurological or behavioral symptoms was evident.

Because of the lack of success with bone marrow transplantation and enzyme transfer using partial exchange transfusion, it has been suggested that the HPRT gene should be targeted to cells (Sege-Peterson, Nyhan, and Page, 1993) in the central nervous system to address the neurological and behavioral symptoms. This approach has been taken by infecting mice *in vivo* by direct intrathecal injection of a recombinant herpes simplex type 1 virus vector containing the human HPRT gene (Palella et al., 1989). In these animals, human HPRT was detected in the brains but not in tissues outside the central nervous system. It is not clear whether this viral vector led to the synthesis of human HPRT protein in these mice.

Behavior Treatment

The motivation for self-injury as well as the biological basis of self-injury must be considered in treatment programs. Behavioral techniques alone, using operant conditioning approaches, have not proved to be an adequate general treatment and have limited effectiveness in Lesch-Nyhan disease. Still, Nyhan (1976) notes that behavioral procedures do have some selective success in reducing self-injury. However, generalization outside the experimental setting may be problematic (Nyhan, 1976) and patients under stress may revert to their previous self-injurious behavior.

Behavioral approaches for Lesch-Nyhan disease must focus on reducing the self-injurious behavior and treating phobic anxiety associated with being unrestrained (Bull and LaVecchio, 1978; LaVecchio, 1990). A behavior treatment program utilizes several techniques, among which are systematic desensitization, extinction, and differential reinforcement of other (competing) behaviors (DRO). In addition to these behavioral approaches, stress management has been recommended to assist patients to develop more effective coping mechanisms.

Systematic desensitization is utilized to treat the anxiety the patient shows to being unrestrained. The procedure begins with the collection of baseline data to evaluate the child's response to the removal of each of the physical restraints; an individual with Lesch-Nyhan disease may react more forcefully when one restraint is removed in contrast to another. The restraints are then gradually removed through the systematic desensitization procedure, beginning with the least anxiety-provoking restraint and moving to the most anxiety-provoking restraint. A variety of procedures may be used, including elbow restraints with stays that can be removed one at a time, or the use of gloves whose thickness can be gradually reduced (Fisher et al., 1992). With restraint fading, there may be increased agitation and irritability.

Extinction procedures are utilized because any reinforcement, either positive or negative, may increase the frequency, duration, and intensity of self-injury rate; rates of self-injury may become sensitive to environmental social contingencies. The behavioral approach avoids the use of any procedure that directly attends to the child's behavior or is contingent on it. In the extinction procedure, any attempt made by the patient to injure himself or others is ignored by ceasing all physical contact and turning one's head away. In this procedure, no verbal comments are made, the staff member does not appear angry or disturbed, and eye contact is avoided. The individual with Lesch-Nyhan disease will periodically inflict injuries. These injuries will be anxiety provoking to the caregivers, so it is important the child receive minimal reinforcement while they occur. It is common that substantial positive reinforcement may take place if attention is paid to wounds. If any injury occurs, care must be taken not to pay excessive attention to the injury. Conversation about the injury should be avoided as much as possible even though the child or adolescent may attempt to engage the parent or caregiver in conversation to draw attention to it.

Patients with Lesch-Nyhan disease do not respond to contingent electric shock or other behavioral measures that ordinarily result in a suppression of self-injury. Instead, an increase in self-injury is observed when aversive methods, such as shock, are utilized (Anderson et al., 1977). Duker (1975) reported that behavior reduction strategies, such as contingent electric finger shock with response prevention, increased self-injury in 5 cases studied; however, time-out plus reinforcement of non–self-injurious behavior led to substantial reduction in a controlled setting. In some instances, the affected person will choose another means of self-injury when the targeted means is prevented.

Use of Restraints

In a survey conducted by Anderson and Ernst (1994), 18 (45%) of patients surveyed were restrained 100% of the time, 8 (20%) were restrained 75% of the time, and 5 (12%) were never in restraints. The time in restraints was associated with the age of onset of self-injury in that the older the patient was at the onset of self-injury, the less time was used for restraint. Twenty-nine (72%) were always restrained at night and 8 (20%) were never restrained at night. All cases who were never restrained at night had a significantly later onset of self-injury.

The individual with Lesch-Nyhan disease frequently participated in making decisions in regard to restraints and the type of restraints used. Of the group surveyed, 14 (35%) were always in control when restraints were used. Nineteen (47%) sometimes participated and 5 (12½%) never participated. Half of the group insisted on being restrained in a particular way and 17 (42%) insisted on restraint techniques that would be considered logically ineffective, like a lightweight glove, small bandage, or something else which could not physically prevent biting. When parents were surveyed about their family member's attitude toward restraints, 35 to 40 (87.5%) said he was at ease when restrained and liked to be restrained. Only 3 (0.7%) said they did not want to have restraints on. Two thirds of the parents felt the time of restraint was about right, although a quarter felt it was excessive. The time in restraints may potentially be reduced with systematic treatment programs.

Dental Management

Twenty-four out of 40 (60%) had had teeth extracted to prevent self-injury. In the families where this was done, the family members endorsed tooth extraction as a way to manage self-biting. Fifteen of 40 (37.5%) had tried a protective mouth guard designed by a dentist. Of this group, 75% said it never worked and 3 (20%) found the mouth guard was helpful.

Anxiety Management

Anxiety may present itself through posturing, facial grimacing, and increases in choreoathetoid and spastic movements. In working with the affected person in a medical setting, careful explanation should be given about what is to follow when initiating a medical or behavioral procedure. These explanations are given at a cognitive level the patient is able to understand. The patient should give permission to respond before proceeding with the behavior program. In addition to explanations, relaxation procedures may be taught, particularly those that encourage the patient to relax various body parts. Music may be used in conjunction with stress-reducing exercises.

Parental Intervention

When surveyed regarding the most effective methods of intervention for self-injury, most parents selected stress reduction and awareness of the patient's needs as the most effective (Anderson and Ernst, 1994). Those interventions characterized as awareness of needs and stress reduction were used more often than behavioral interventions and punitive interventions. Families reported that their most common method for dealing with self-injury was attending to physical comfort (66% rated this as very helpful). This was followed by adjusting restraints, talking to the child, finding something more interesting, and getting what the child needed. The least commonly used interventions were the strict behavioral approaches, such as stopping talking and turning away, or taking away something that is liked. However, positive behavioral techniques of reinforcing appropriate behavior by paying more attention to the child or adolescents when they were "being good" were rated effective by almost half of the families.

Pharmacotherapy

Drug treatments using diazepam, haloperidol, clomipramine, L-dopa, and pimozide (Watts et al., 1982) have not been successful in eliminating self-injury. Watts et al. noted that because self-injurious behavior in other conditions commonly responds to aversive techniques and Lesch-Nyhan cases proved insensitive to aversive methods, an abnormality in neurotransmitters such as serotonin, which may be involved in aggressive behavior and in punishment learning, requires consideration. He suggested an imbalance in dopamine/serotonin systems or dopamine in interaction with another neurotransmitter system as etiologic.

Another approach is to use dopamine agonist or antagonist treatment. Fluphenazine, which is a mixed D_1/D_2 dopamine antagonist, has been used to treat self-injury in 2 patients with Lesch-Nyhan disease (Goldstein et al., 1985), based on the Breese animal model mentioned earlier. Motor control was found to be improved and self-injurious behavior was decreased in one 20-month-old patient who demonstrated self-biting of the fingers at 18 months. However, after discontinuation of fluphenazine, there was definite worsening of the self-injury in contrast to before treatment. A second patient, aged 15 years, showed no improvement on fluphenazine, and when it was discontinued after a month, showed a worsening of symptoms with increased biting behavior. Although there is a report of improvement in self-injury in 1 of these 2 Lesch-Nyhan disease patients with this medication, 3 other patients seen by another investigator did not improve. When Harris et al. (1991) found no clinical response (i.e., reduction in the rate of self-injurious behavior) to a fixed dose of fluphenazine, they used PET scanning to evaluate this drug's effect on the D_1 receptor. A 7 mg single dose of fluphenazine (blood level 4.1 ng/ml) was administered and showed limited blocking of a D_1 dopamine antagonist (SCH 23390) that binds to this receptor. They concluded that fluphenazine is not an effective D_1 antagonist and that other more specific D_1 antagonists are needed to evaluate the D_1 dopamine model of self- injurious behavior.

In the Anderson and Ernst (1994) parent survey, 35 of 40 (87.5%) had used medication for self-injury or agitation. Approximately half of the group had tried medication specifically for self-injury and the same number had tried it for agitation. Most parents viewed these as related problems, and ratings for the effectiveness of self-injury were similar to those for agitation. Seven classes of medications were tried in the 40 patients surveyed (some used more than one of these): benzodiazepines in 21 patients, neuroleptics in 13, antidepressants in 4, opiate antagonists in 4, chlorohydrate in 1, beta blockers in 1, and Sinemet in 1. Of 35 patients who used medication, 20 were continuing to use medications at the time of the survey. The medications judged most effective on a short- and long-term basis were the benzodiazepines, particularly diazepam. Neuroleptics were used by 13 patients and 4 patients were using them long term. Naltrexone, which had been utilized by 4 patients, was not found to be effective. None of the families reported the use of medication specifically for compulsive behaviors.

FUTURE DIRECTIONS

Continuing genetic investigation using restriction enzyme analysis may further clarify the specific genetic abnormality in the classical Lesch-Nyhan disease. Identification of dopamine receptors in the caudate and putamen is now feasible. Dopamine findings suggested by Lloyd et al.'s (1981) study are being investigated *in vivo,* using positron emission tomography (PET) (Gjedde et al., 1986; Wong et al., 1988, 1991, 1994). Wong et al. (1994) have found a 29% reduction in dopamine transporter sites in the caudate and a 67% reduction in the putamen in 8 Lesch-Nyhan disease patients when contrasted to nomal control subjects. F-18 fluordeoxyglucose PET studies carried out by Palella et al., (1985) suggest reduced metabolic activity in the same brain regions.

Future treatment studies will need to take into account the existence of a variety of mutations in the HPRT gene structure. Why partial HPRT deficiency does not lead to behavioral symptoms remains unclear; perhaps neurotrophic factors are active to stimulate the dopamine system with minute amounts of the enzyme present. Finally, it is advisable to study combined drug and behavior treatment. An emphasis on parent training and stress reduction is of particular importance for drug compliance and generalization of treatment effects. As in other inborn errors, continuous family support is essential.

REFERENCES

Anderson, L.T., Dancis, J., Alpert, M., and Hermann, L. (1977). Punishment learning and self-mutilation in Lesch-Nyhan disease. *Nature,* 265:461–463.

______, and Ernst, M. (1994). Self-injury in Lesch-Nyhan disease. *Journal of Autism and Developmental Disorders,* 24:67–81.

______, ______, and Davis, S.V. (1992). Cognitive abilities of patients with Lesch-Nyhan disease. *Journal of Autism and Developmental Disorders,* 22(2):189–203.

Baumeister, L., and Frye, G.D. (1985). The biochemical basis of the behavior disorder in the Lesch Nyhan syndrome. *Neuroscience and Biobehavioral Reviews,* 9:169–178.

Becker, M.A., Yen, R.C., Itkin, P., Goss, S.J., Seegmiller, J.E., and Bakay, B. (1979). Regional localization of the gene for human phosphoribosylpyrophosphate synthetase on the X chromosome. *Science,* 203(4384):1016–1019.

Breese, G.R., Baumeister, A.A., McCown, T.J., Emerick, S.G., Frye, G.D., Crotty, K., and Mueller, R.A. (1984a). Behavioral differences between neonatal and adult-6-hydroxydopamine treated rats to dopamine agonists: Relevance to neurological symptoms in clinical syndromes with reduced brain dopamine. *Journal of Pharmacology and Experimental Therapeutics,* 231:343–354.

______, ______, ______, ______, ______, ______, and ______. (1984b). Neonatal-6-hydroxydopamine treatment: Model of susceptibility for self-mutilation in Lesch-Nyhan syndrome. *Pharmacology, Biochemistry and Behavior,* 21:459–461.

______, Criswell, H.E., Duncan, G.E., and Mueller, R.A. (1990). A dopamine deficiency model of Lesch-Nyhan disease—the neonatal-6-OHDA-lesioned rat. *Brain Research Bulletin,* 25(3):477–484.

Bull, M., and Lavecchio, F. (1978). Behavior therapy for a child with Lesch-Nyhan syndrome. *Developmental Medicine and Child Neurology,* 20:368–375.

Crawhall, J.C., Henderson, J.F., and Kelley, W.N. (1981). Diagnosis and treatment of the Lesch-Nyhan syndrome. *Pediatric Research,* 6:504.

Duker, P. (1975). Behavioral control of self-biting in a Lesch-Nyhan patient. *Journal of Mental Deficiency Research,* 19:11–19.

Edwards, N.L., Jeryc, W., and Fox, I.H. (1984). Enzyme replacement in the Lesch-Nyhan syndrome with long-term erythrocyte transfusions. *Advances in Experimental Medicine and Biology,* 165 (Pt. A):23–26.

Endres, W., Helmig, M., Shin, Y.S., Albert, E., Wank, R., Ibel, H., Weiss, M., Haborn, H.B., and Haas, R. (1991). Bone marrow transplantation in Lesch-Nyhan disease. *Journal of Inherited Metabolic Disease,* 14(2): 270–271.

Fisher, W., Piazza, C., Chinn, S., Bowman, L., Grace, N., and Taras, M. (1992, April). *Restraint fading in the treatment of self-injury among clients with Lesch-Nyhan syndrome and other conditions.* Presentation at the Developmental Neuropsychiatry Conference, Kennedy Krieger Institute. Baltimore, MD.

Gjedde, A., Wong, D.F., Harris, J., Dannals, R.F., Ravert, H.T., Wilson, A.A., Williams, J., Links, J., Scheffel, U., O'Tuama, C., Fanaras, G., Moser, H., Naidu, S., Nyhan, W., Wagner, H.N., and Braestrup, C. (1986). Quantification of D_1 and D_2 dopamine receptors in Lesch Nyhan syndrome as measured by positron tomography. *Society for Neuroscience Abstracts,* 12:486.

Goldstein, M., Anderson, L.T., Reuben, R., and Dancis, J. (1985) Self-mutilation in Lesch-Nyhan disease is caused by dopaminergic denervation. *Lancet,* i:338–339.

Harris, J.C. (1987). Behavioral phenotypes in mental retardation syndromes. In R. Barrett and J. Matson (eds.), *Advances in developmental disorders,* Vol. 1, pp. 77–106. Jai Publishing, New York.

______. (1992a). Neurobiological factors in self-injurious behavior. In J.K. Luiselli, J.L. Matson, and N.N. Singh (eds.), *Self-injurious behavior: Analysis, assessment, and treatment,* pp. 59–92. Springer-Verlag, New York.

______. (1992b November). Using PET scanning to investigate a behavioral phenotype: Imaging the dopamine system in the Lesch-Nyhan syndrome. Paper presented at "From Genes to Behaviour" 2nd International Symposium *Society for the Study of Behavioural Phenotypes,* Welshpool, UK, Paper 21.

______, Wong, D.F., Yaster, B., Dannals, R., Nyhan, W., Hyman, S., Naidu, S., Fisher, W., Piazza, C., Wilson, A.A., Ravert, H., and Wagner, H.N., Jr. (1991). Clinical investigation of the dopamine hypothesis of self-injurious behavior in the Lesch-Nyhan syndrome. *Society for Neuroscience,* 17:678 (abstract).

Hooper, M., Hardy, K., Handyside, A., Hunter, S., and Monk, M. (1987). HPRT-deficient (Lesch-Nyhan) mouse embryos derived from germ line colonization by cultured cells. *Nature,* 326:292–295.

Jinnah, H.A., Gage, F.H., and Friedmann, T. (1990). Animal models of Lesch-Nyhan syndrome. *Brain Research Bulletin,* 25(3):467–475.

______, Langlais, P.J., and Friedmann, T. (1992). Functional analysis of brain dopamine systems in a genetic mouse model of Lesch-Nyhan syndrome. *Journal of Pharmacology and Experimental Therapeutics,* 263:596–607.

______, Page, T., and Friedmann, T. (1991). Inherited impairment of purine recycling in the mouse: Consequences for brain purine and dopamine systems. *Society for Neuroscience,* 17:410 (abstract).

______, ______, and ______. (1993). Brain purines in a genetic mouse model of Lesch-Nyhan disease. *Journal of Neurochemistry,* 60(6):2036–2045.

______, Wojcik B.E., Hunt, M., Narang, N., Lee K.Y., Goldstein, M., Wamsley, J.K., Langlais, P.J., and Friedmann, T. (1994). Dopamine deficiency in a genetic mouse model of Lesch-Nyhan disease. *The Journal of Neuroscience,* 14:1164–1175.

Kim, S.H., Moores, J.C., David, D., Respess, J.G., Jolly, D.J., and Friedmann, T. (1986). The organization of the human HPRT gene. *Nucleic Acids Research,* 14(7): 3103–3118.

Kopin, I. (1981). Neurotransmitters and Lesch-Nyhan syndrome. *New England Journal of Medicine,* 305:1148–1149.

Kuehn, M.R., Bradley, A., Robertson, E.J., and Evans, M.J. (1987). A potential animal model for Lesch-Nyhan syndrome through introduction of HPRT mutations into mice. *Nature,* 326:295–298.

LaVecchio, F. (1990). *Behavioral management and Lesch-Nyhan syndrome.* Guidelines for parents and professionals (unpublished). Tufts University, Boston.

Lesch, M., and Nyhan, W.L. (1964). A familial disorder of uric and acid metabolism and central nervous system function. *American Journal of Medicine,* 36:561–570.

Lloyd, K.G., Hornykiewicz, O., Davidson, L., Shannak, K., Farley, I., Goldstein, M., Shibuya, M., Kelly, W.N., and Fox, I.H. (1981). Biochemical evidence of dysfunction of brain neurotransmitters in the Lesch-Nyhan syndrome. *New England Journal of Medicine,* 305:1106–1111.

Mizuno, T., and Yugari, Y. (1975). Prophylactic effect of L-5-hydroxytryptophan on self-mutilation in the Lesch-Nyhan syndrome. *Neuropaediatrie,* 6:13–23.

Nyhan, W. (1972). *Behavioral phenotypes in organic genetic disease.* Presidential address to the Society for Pediatric Research, May 1, 1971. *Pediatric Research,* 6:1–9.

______. (1976). Behavior in Lesch-Nyhan syndrome. *Journal of Autism and Childhood Schizophrenia,* 6:235–252.

______, Page, T., Gruber, H.E., and Parkman, R. (1986). Bone marrow transplantation in Lesch-Nyhan disease. *Birth Defects,* 22(1):113–117.

Ogasawara, N., Stout, J. T., Goto, H., Sonta, S., Matsumoto, T., and Caskey, C. T. (1989). Molecular analysis of a female Lesch-Nyhan patient. *Journal of Clinical Investigation,* 84(3):1024–1027.

Page, T., Bakay, B., Nissinen, E., and Nyhan, W.L. (1981). Hypoxanthine guanine phosphoribosyl transferase variants: Correlation of clinical phenotype with enzyme activity. *Journal of Inherited Metabolic Disease,* 4:203.

______, and Nyhan, W.L. (1989). The spectrum of

HPRT deficiency: An update. *Advances in Experimental Medicine and Biology,* 253A:129–132.

Palella, T.D., Hichwa, R.D., Ehrenkaufer, R.L., Rothley, J.M., Eider, W., McQuillan, M.A., Young, A.B., and Kelley, W.N. (1985). F-18 fluordeoxyglucose PET scanning in HPRT patients. *American Journal of Human Genetics,* 37(4) Suppl:A70.

______, Hidaka, Y., Silverman, L.J., Levine, M., Glorioso, J., and Kelley, W.N. (1989). Expression of human mRNA in brains of mice infected with a recombinant herpes simplex virus-1 vector. *Gene,* 80:137.

Scherzer, J.E., and Ilson, J.B. (1969). Normal intelligence in the Lesch-Nyhan syndrome, *Pediatrics* 41:71–90.

Sege-Peterson, K., Nyhan, W.L., and Page T. (1993). Lesch-Nyhan disease and HPRT deficiency. In R.N. Rosenberg, S.B. Prusiner, S. DiMauro, R.L. Barchi, and L.M. Kunkel (eds.), *The molecular and genetic basis of neurological disease,* pp. 241–258. Butterworth-Heinemann, Boston.

Seegmiller, J.E., Rosenbloom, F.M., and Kelley, W.N. (1967). Enzyme defect associated with a sex-linked human neurological disorder and excessive purine synthesis. *Science,* 155:1682.

Silverstein, F.S., Johnston, M.V., Hutchinson, R.J., and Edwards, N.L. (1985). Lesch-Nyhan syndrome: CSF neurotransmitter abnormalities. *Neurology,* 35:907–911.

Sweetman, L., and Nyhan, W.L. (1972). Further studies of the enzyme composition of mutant cells. *Archives of Internal Medicine,* 130:214–220.

van Bogaert, P., Ceballos, I., Desguerre, I., Telvi, L., Kamoun, P., and Ponsot, G. (1992). Lesch-Nyhan syndrome in a girl. *Journal of Inherited Metabolic Disease,* 15:790–791.

Watts, R.W.E., Spellacy, E., Gibbs, D.A., Allsop, J., McKeran, R.O., and Slavin, G.E. (1982). Clinical, post-mortem, biochemical and therapeutic observations on the Lesch-Nyhan syndrome with particular reference to the neurological manifestations. *Quarterly Journal of Medicine,* 201:43–78.

Williamson, D.J., Hooper, M.L., and Melton, D.W. (1992). Mouse models of hypoxanthine phosphoribosyltransferase deficiency. *Journal of Inherited Metabolic Disease,* 15:665–673.

Wilson, J.M., Tarr, G.E., Mahoney, W.C., and Kelley, W.N. (1982). Human hypoxanthine-guanine phosphoribosyltransferase. Complete amino acid sequence of the erthyrocytes enzyme. *Journal of Biological Chemistry,* 257:10978–10985.

Wong, D.F., Bropussolle, E.P., Ward, G., Villemagne, V., Dannals, R.F., Links, J.M., Zacur, H.A., Harris, J., Naidu, S., Braestrup, C., Wagner, H.N., Jr., and Gjedde, A. (1988). *In vivo* measurement of dopamine receptors in human brain by positron emission tomography: Age and sex differences. *Annals of the New York Academy of Science,* 515:203–214.

______, Harris J., Marenco S., Yokoi F., Alexandrescu C., Chan B., Dannals R.F., Mathews, W., Musachio, J., Ravert, H.T., and Breese, G. (1994). Dopamine reuptake sites measured by [^{11}C] WIN 35,428 are decreased *in vivo* in Lesch-Nyhan disease. *The Journal of Nuclear Medicine,* 35:130 (abstract 5).

______, ______, Naidu, S., Shaya, E., Yaster, M., Dannals, R.F., Wilson, A.A., Ravert, H., and Wagner, H.N.,Jr. (1991). *In vivo* human dopamine receptor quantification in self-injurious behavior syndromes. *Society for Neuroscience,* 17:1092 (abstract).

Wu, C.L., and Melton, D.W. (1993). Production of a model for Lesch-Nyhan syndrome in hypoxanthine phosphoribosyltransferase-deficient mice. *Nature Genetics,* 3(3):235–240.

11.2 Williams (Williams-Beuren) Syndrome

Williams syndrome is a specific neurodevelopmental disorder associated with a characteristic physical, linguistic, and behavioral phenotype that provides a unique opportunity to study personality development and linguistic functioning in a well-defined population of children with known cognitive deficits (Bellugi et al., 1992). The syndrome is characterized by congenital facial and cardiovascular anomalies (supervalvular aortic stenosis and peripheral pulmonary stenosis), failure to thrive, and mental retardation that are often accompanied by transient idiopathic infantile hypercalcemia.

Adolescents with Williams syndrome have expressive language abilities that are apparently better than expected for their mental age. Because of their relatively well-developed language abilities, the investigation of Williams syndrome allows the study of the dissociability of components of language and other cognitive brain systems. In mentally retarded patients with Williams syndrome, linguistic abilities may be selectively spared—which is the opposite of what occurs in normally intelligent children with language learning disability.

This chapter reviews the history, epidemiology, definition and clinical features, etiology, neuropsychological test profile, language processing, language and cognition, neuroanatomical and neurophysiological studies, developmental and behavior characteristics, and treatment of Williams syndrome.

HISTORY

Williams syndrome was initially identified in 1961 by the British cardiologist J.C.P. Williams and colleagues, who described a syndrome with supravalvular aortic stenosis, a specific heart defect, mental retardation, and unusual facial appearance (Williams, Barratt-Boyes, and Lowe, 1961). However, the earliest reports of Williams syndrome individuals most probably represent a subgroup of children with severe idiopathic infantile hypercalcemia (Fanconi et al., 1952; Lightwood, 1952). This severe group has been distinguished from the epidemic of mild idiopathic infantile hypercalcemia that occurred in Britain and Europe following the Second World War. These milder cases of hypercalcemia apparently resulted from hypervitaminosis D, which was caused by excessive supplementation of infant foods provided by the British and other European governments during the war. After World War II, it became increasingly apparent that the severe hypercalcemia subgroup had a constellation of physical and behavioral features that included idiopathic infantile hypercalcemia, mental deficiency, elfin face, failure to thrive, and congenital heart disease, especially supravalvular aortic stenosis.

The early reports of Williams syndrome emphasized that both physical and behavioral manifestations are characteristic. Jones and Smith (1975) were among the first to document the clinical aspects when they reported on 19 cases with characteristic facial features. These authors clarified that many of the children with the more severe forms of idiopathic hypercalcemia in infancy and others with supravalvular aortic stenosis had similar facial features. An earlier report (von Arnim and Engel, 1964) summarized four studies describing the psychological features. These include an unusual command of language combined with a loquacious and highly sociable interpersonal manner against a background of insecurity and anxiety; others confirmed that children with Williams syndrome are generally polite with an open and gentle manner. Subsequently, Preus (1984) suggested the "unusual friendly behavior" be considered a diagnostic feature. Still other investigators emphasized mental retardation, with test scores most commonly falling in the mild to moderate range (Bennett, LaVeck, and Sells, 1978).

As more cases were identified, the primary emphasis was placed on the facial features, mental retardation, and cardiac malformation, and less emphasis was placed on the supravalvular aortic stenosis and infantile hypercalcemia in case reports. Yet the early recognition of abnormal elevations in calcium levels and subsequent recognition of increased calcitonin secretion continue to be important aspects of research (Culler, Jones, and Deftos, 1985).

EPIDEMIOLOGY

The prevalence of Williams syndrome is unknown, but the incidence is estimated to be between 1 in 20,000 to 1 in 50,000 live births (Greenberg, 1990). Over 1,000 persons with Williams syndrome are known to the National Williams Syndrome Association in the United States; most are less than 20 years of age. There are thought to be other unreported or unrecognized adult cases in the United States. Life expectancy may be reduced if there is congenital heart disease, but this is not the rule.

DEFINITION AND CLINICAL FEATURES

The cluster of unusual facial features is one of the most characteristic aspects of Williams syndrome. The typical facial features include broad forehead, medial eyebrow flare, depressed nasal bridge, stellate pattern in the iris, widely spaced teeth, and full lips. Their full prominent cheeks, wide mouth, short turned-up nose, and flat nasal bridge have often been described as distinctive elfin-like faces. Although referred to as "elfin" face, the term "Williams syndrome face" is preferable (Burn, 1986; Greenberg, 1990). Other physical characteristics include growth retardation and low birth weight, digestive disorders in infancy, apparent auditory sensitivity, mild microcephaly, renal and cardiovascular (supravalvular aortic stenosis and peripheral pulmonary artery stenosis) abnormalities, and delays in development.

There is a phenotypically distinctive psychological profile with personality and behavior characteristics that are distinctive from other mental retardation syndromes. Approximately 95% of affected children have moderate to severe learning difficulties although, overall, their verbal abilities are superior relative to their visuospatial and motor skills. They present with an apparently good command of language although their language comprehension is ordinarily more limited than their expressive language abilities. Expressive language tends to be fluent and articulate at a superficial level and is pseudomature and sometimes described as verbose. There is characteristic social disinhibition and friendliness toward adults, including strangers. Dilts, Morris, and Leonard (1990) describe a characteristic behavioral phenotype beginning in infancy that consists of six factors, as shown in Table 11.2–1.

Children with Williams syndrome show increased rates of emotional and behavioral disturbances when compared to other children at similar levels of mental retardation. There is characteristic overactivity, poor concentration, sleep and eating difficulties, excessive anxiety, and poor peer relationships. Hyperacusis is found in over 90% of cases.

Williams syndrome typically presents in infancy, with difficulties in feeding, irritability, constipation, and failure to thrive. Over 60% of affected infants are found to have increased levels of blood calcium. Because of the hypercalcemia, treatment with a low calcium and vitamin D restricted diet may be instituted. With the implementation of the diet, serum calcium tends to drop to the normal level, although it may also decrease with the passage of time without major dietary changes. Despite the improvement in the hypercalcemia, the physical features and psychological profile persist.

ETIOLOGY (GENETIC)

Williams syndrome is associated with a hemizygous deletion that includes the elastin locus on chromosome 7q11-23, but the specific gene or genes that result in the full behavioral phenotype has not been identified (Ewart et al., 1993). This deletion has been found in 97% of 300 cases evaluated (Morris, personal communication). This deletion accounts for the associated congenital heart disease, particularly the supravalvular aortic stenosis (SVAS), since disruption of the elastin gene is also found in isolated SVAS, and may account for the associated connective tissue abnormalities. Because the

Table 11.2–1. A Behavioral Phenotype in Williams Syndrome

1. Multiple developmental motor disabilities affecting strength, balance, coordination, and motor planning
   a. Poor development in the use of tools for skills in play, self-care, school, domestic care, hobbies, and vocation
   b. Adaptive skill acquisition below that expected for cognitive level
2. Sensory integration dysfunction, i.e., hyperactivity
   a. Hypersensitivity to sound
   b. Hypersensitivity to vestibular input, or "gravitational insecurity"
3. Temperament
   a. Emotional insecurity and anxiety
      1. Tendency to worry perserveratively
      2. Interpersonal sensitivity
   b. Activity
      1. Attention deficit/hyperactivity disorder exemplified by
         (1) Distractibility to both internal and external events
         (2) Impulsivity
         (3) Poor rule-governed behavior
   c. Sociability
      1. Social attention seeking
      2. Personal, enthusiastic
      3. Loquacious; high frequency of engaging question asking
      4. Problems making and keeping friends
4. Delayed expressive and receptive language skills with simultaneous age-appropriate grammar and articulation
5. Better reading than mathematics ability
6. Cognitive dysfunction on a continuum, ranging from mental retardation to learning disabilities

Modified from Dilts, Morris, and Leonard, 1990.

deletion extends beyond the elastin locus, Ewart et al. propose that the neurobehavioral features may result from the loss or disruption of one or more contiguous genes, and the extent of mental retardation might be related to the size of the defect.

Most cases of Williams syndrome that have been identified have occurred sporadically; however, familial occurrence has been reported with affected parents or siblings. There are a few confirmed cases of parent to child transmission. Williams syndrome has also been formally reported in 4 sets of concordant monozygotic (MZ) twins (Murphy et al., 1990). There are no known cases of discordance in MZ twins and no documented reports of concordance in dizygotic twins. Hokama and Rogers (1991) reported discordance for Williams syndrome in a single dizygotic twin. This occurrence in one DZ twin is consistent with a mutational event as a cause of Williams syndrome.

Earlier cytogenetic and molecular studies of chromosome 15 have been reported in Williams syndrome. Kaplan et al. (1987) reported an interstitial deletion of 15q11-q12 and discussed two other reports of chromosome 15 involvement. In reviewing the evidence for chromosome 15 involvement, Greenberg (1990) notes that in qualitative and quantitative DNA studies with probes that map to 15q-q13, no molecular deletions were found. Subsequently, Colley et al. (1992) reported an unbalanced 13;18 translocation in Williams syndrome. Finally, Jones (1990) suggested a defect in the processing of the calcitonin gene might result in an underproduction of calcitonin and an abnormality in processing of the calcitonin gene-related peptide (CGRP). CGRP has biological effects on the central nervous system, cardiovascular system, and gastrointestinal system. It is also expressed in fibers in the nucleus of cranial nerve VIII. Each of these systems is prominently affected in Williams syndrome. However, Russo et al. (1991) investigated the possibility of mutation in the calcitonin/calcitonin gene related peptide (CGRP) but did not detect deletions or rearrangements in the gene locus as the cause of deficient expression of calcitonin in Williams syndrome. Thus, it is currently believed that contiguous gene deletions on chromosome 7 account for the clinical and neurobehavioral features of Williams syndrome.

NEUROPSYCHOLOGICAL TEST PROFILE

Standardized achievement tests and IQ measures were utilized in the initial studies of psychological functioning in Williams syndrome. However, standard tests did not identify the unusual neuropsychological profile that is seen in adolescent subjects with Williams syndrome. Earlier evaluations, based on standardized batteries of psychological tests, showed inconsistent findings. For example, verbal abilities were shown to surpass nonverbal abilities in some studies (Udwin, Yule, and Martin, 1987), whereas other investigators showed different findings (Crisco and Dobbs, 1988). It became apparent that in these studies verbal abilities were being assessed with psychological instruments which confound linguistic and other cognitive processing. Another factor in the initial studies was the age of the subjects, which varied from one study to the next. Bellugi et al. (1992) have dealt with both these issues by using neuropsychological test batteries that evaluate domain-specific functions and specifically focusing on the neuropsychological profile of younger versus older children. There may be marked differences in language and cognitive milestones in younger and older subjects where delays may be seen in each of these areas (Thal, Bates, and Bellugi, 1989).

Because tests of various domains make up general intelligence, IQ scores may not demonstrate differences between linguistic and cognitive domains. Specific tests are needed to evaluate relationships between and within domains of higher cortical functioning and to relate them to underlying neural structures.

A neuropsychological battery for Williams syndrome must probe linguistic processing at different structural levels in addition to assessing general problem solving and evaluating spatial cognition. Bellugi et al. (1992) evaluated over 50 Williams syndrome children and approximately the same number of a Down syndrome group. They provided data on 6 adolescents who were carefully matched in age and

IQ from the Down and Williams syndrome groups who ranged in age from 10 to 20 years. The mean age was 14.4 years for the Williams syndrome and 15.4 years for the Down syndrome group. The full-scale IQ was 50.8 for Williams syndrome adolescents and 48.8 for Down syndrome adolescents. Children with both syndromes attended similar classrooms for the educable mentally retarded. The adolescents with Williams and Down syndrome generally came from the same classrooms for mild to moderately retarded persons. There were differences in the neuropsychological profile with dissociations between linguistic and cognitive abilities being most characteristic for Williams syndrome.

Despite the similarities of both groups in cognitive ability, the children with Williams syndrome had remarkable linguistic abilities. For example, a 15-year-old studied by Bellugi et al. (1992) said, "You're looking at a professional book writer. My books will be filled with drama, action, and excitement. And everyone will want to read them. I'm going to write books, page after page, stack after stack . . . I'll start on Monday." She was able to spontaneously create original stories that involved imaginary events and could also compose lyrics for songs. However, her full-scale IQ is 49, and at age 15, she fails all Piagetian seriation and conservation tasks that are normally mastered by age 7. She attends a special school for the mentally retarded and has reading, writing, and math skills comparable to those of a child in first grade. Her visuospatial abilities are those of a 5-year-old child. This case vignette demonstrates an unusual dissociation of language from other cognitive functions that is found in a subgroup of children with Williams syndrome.

LANGUAGE PROCESSING IN WILLIAMS SYNDROME

Analysis of expressive language and neuropsychological tests of language processing and comprehension indicate that lexical and grammatical abilities are relatively well developed in contrast to other nonverbal abilities in Williams syndrome adolescents. Traditional IQ tests do not examine these linguistic functions. For example, on the vocabulary tests of the WISC-R, subjects are asked the meaning of words and the score is based on the ability to produce definitions, which is both a linguistic and cognitive skill. When persons with Williams syndrome and Down syndrome are compared on these tasks, those with Williams syndrome have a better understanding of the words and are able to provide more appropriate contexts for their use. Moreover, the Williams syndrome subjects were able to give associational responses to vocabulary words. Bellugi et al. (1992) give as an example the word "contagious" where the children with Williams syndrome were able to provide a list of symptoms, such as "hay fever, cough, and runny nose" but were not able to define the word as referring to a disease that is easily spread. Their associations were detailed and appropriate, whereas those with Down syndrome were not able to provide scorable responses at all. Moreover, when persons with Williams syndrome used unusual words in spontaneous conversation, they also demonstrated their understanding of the words' meanings.

Bellugi et al. (1992) found significant group differences in semantic abilities on tests of lexical knowledge, such as the Peabody Picture Vocabulary Test. On this test, when subjects hear a word they are asked to pick out the appropriate picture from an array of pictures. In contrast to those with Down syndrome, some with Williams syndrome performed at or above mental-age level. This suggests that in some individuals with Williams syndrome aspects of referential lexical knowledge may be better than expected for mental age. On another test of semantic fluency, subjects were asked to generate as many examples as they could of a particular semantic category, such as foods and animals, in 60 seconds. The Williams syndrome subjects produced more words over a series of trials than those with Down syndrome and had no difficulty accessing multiple words from a given general semantic category in the time provided to respond. In some instances, the number of words produced was comparable to norms for chronological age in the general population.

On a test of word fluency, adolescent subjects with Williams syndrome in this study produced not only words within a particular category but also produced low-frequency word choices. For example, in the animal category, *ibex, yak,* and *unicorn* were all listed. The ability to generate such words on a word fluency generation task is not typical for mentally retarded persons and may relate to good verbal memory (Finegan et al., 1995). For the most part, in mental retardation syndromes, the number of items is clearly linked to mental age, suggesting a delay rather than a deviance in their development. In Williams syndrome, because of the differences in their responses, their linguistic function is deviant rather than delayed.

In regard to expressive language, there was a clear difference between the adolescent Williams syndrome and Down syndrome groups, as shown in mean length of utterance, noun phrase complexity, verb phrase complexity, and embeddings (Bellugi et al., 1992). Despite delays in the onset and emergence of language milestones, older subjects with Williams syndrome expressive language is complex and ordinarily grammatically correct. This has been documented on a number of tests that evaluate linguistic structures, indicating syntactic function in Williams syndrome is appropriate for mental age in comparison to nonlinguistic cognitive abilities. Linguistic competence in both production and comprehension is substantially greater than that seen in matched mentally retarded subjects with Down syndrome, but is not necessarily greater than matched children with nonspecific developmental disabilities (Gosch, Stading, and Pankau, 1994).

Udwin and Yule (1990) studied expressive language in 43 school-age children with Williams syndrome and found a subgroup, representing 37% of the sample, who produced more speech, more complex utterances, more social phrases, and more complex communicative functions than the rest of the Williams syndrome group. They concluded that hyperverbal speech is present but is not a consistent manifestation of the syndrome in school-age children. When contrasted with mentally disabled control children, more of the Williams syndrome group had an overfamiliar manner and used more adult vocabulary and social phrases. These authors found that children with Williams syndrome performed better than control children on verbal subtests of the Rivermead Behavioral Memory Test. They indicate that it is possible superior verbal memory helps children with Williams syndrome recall phrases and vocabulary they have heard other people use and they then use in situations which are similar but perhaps "subtly inappropriate situations" (Udwin and Yule, 1990). These authors further indicate that in a more structured and circumscribed language sampling setting, other differences may be found between the speech of Williams syndrome children and control children. Bellugi et al. (1992) have carried out these special language tests, as indicated, and found differences. However, additional evaluation of expressive language is necessary because there is disagreement about whether all children with Williams syndrome have hyperverbal speech. Moreover, it is possible the language of children with Williams syndrome is stereotyped and repetitious and that this feature is not demonstrable without repeated testing. In addition, their verbal abilities, when contrasted to their impaired visuospatial abilities, may suggest a greater verbal ability than, in fact, they have.

LANGUAGE AND COGNITION

Bellugi et al. (1992) investigated cognitive abilities that have been thought to be prerequisites for the development of specific linguistic structures to clarify the relationship between linguistic and cognitive abilities in Williams syndrome. The authors ask, Are specific linguistic abilities dependent on the development of specific cognitive prerequisites or can the two domains be dissociated? It has generally been assumed that language and cognitive development are closely intertwined and that language is a major aspect of a general symbolic representation system whose development leads to, but also constrains, language acquisition (Bates et al., 1979). Another model argues that linguistic mental structures are unique and there are learning mechanisms specific for language (Fodor, 1983). In normal development, distinguishing linguistic and nonlinguistic functions is difficult so findings in Williams syndrome, where linguistic function is relatively intact, may provide new information about long-standing debates regarding the relationship between language and cognition. Williams syndrome individuals display surprisingly good performance when formal language tests are administered. In Williams syndrome, specific linguistic abilities do not depend on previous development of specific cognitive functions and the two domains seem to be dissociable. This was demonstrated when the authors used Piagetian tests of conservation skills that are typically mastered by normal children before age 8, as noted earlier. The skills tested included space, numbers, substance, continuous and discontinuous quantity, and weight. The mastery of these concepts has been considered a prerequisite for the acquisition of passive sentences (Sinclair, 1975). Subjects with Williams syndrome do produce full passive sentences and can comprehend semantically reversible sentences, e.g., "The dog is chased by the man." When adolescents with Williams syndrome were tested for reversible passive sentences, they had a perfect score although mental-age-matched adolescents with Down syndrome performed at a chance level.

Spatial Cognition

Although, in the linguistic domain, adolescents with Williams syndrome show higher function than expected based on their mental age, specific difficulties have been demonstrated in spatial cognition. Adolescents with Williams syndrome show specific spatial deficits in tasks involving spatial construction, spatial orientation, copying geometric shapes, and all aspects of drawing. This is shown in Figure 11.2–1.

In the figure, age- and IQ-matched subjects with Down syndrome and Williams syndrome were asked to draw a bicycle. The drawing by the child with Williams syndrome is disorganized and shows little resemblance to a bicycle, whereas that of the child with Down syndrome demonstrates a recognizable form of a bicycle. When asked to draw pictures, the child with Williams syndrome may give a fluid and coherent description of the task at hand despite the limitation in his drawing ability. Figure 11.2–2, the drawing of an elephant by an adolescent with Williams syndrome whose IQ is 49, is shown adjacent to her verbal description of an elephant (Bellugi et al., 1992).

The drawing of the elephant is unrecognizable and would not be identifiable without the labels provided by the adolescent. The verbal description, however, demonstrates spared linguistic abilities and imaginative abilities. Despite the comprehensive language description, the drawing shows severe visuospatial impairment. The verbal description and the drawing highlight the dissociation between language and visuospatial skills in Williams syndrome.

The psychological profile in Williams syndrome is uneven within spatial domains. When

Drawing of a Bicycle
Age and IQ Matched WS and DS Subjects

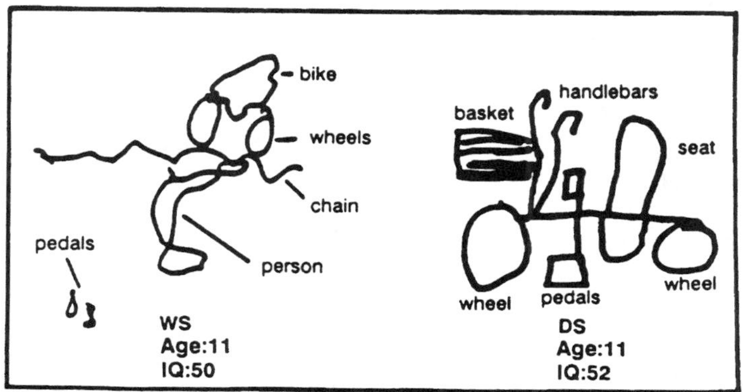

Figure 11.2–1. Contrasting visuospatial ability in selected persons with Williams syndrome and Down syndrome. The Williams syndrome drawing lacks spatial organization and integration of parts and could not be recognized without the verbal labels, whereas the Down syndrome drawing, although simplified, shows better spatial organization, closure, and integration of parts (from Bellugi et al., 1992).

Drawing of an Elephant

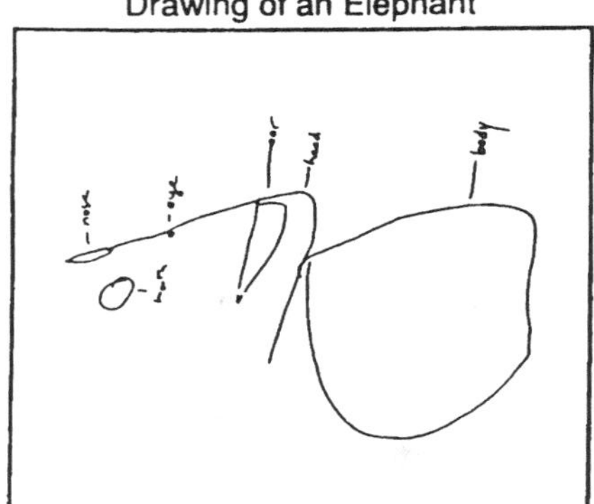

Verbal Description of Elephants

And what an elephant is, it is one of the animals. And what the elephant does, it lives in the jungle. It can also live in the zoo. And what it has, it has long gray ears, fan ears, ears that can blow in the wind. It has a long trunk that can pick up grass, or pick up hay....If they're in a bad mood it can be terrible...If the elephant gets mad it could stomp; it could charge. Sometimes elephants can charge, like a bull can charge. They have big long tusks. They can damage a car...It could be dangerous. When they're in a pinch, when they're in a bad mood it can be terrible. You don't want an elephant as a pet. You want a cat or a dog or a bird...

18 year old Williams Subject

Figure 11.2–2. The dissociation between visuopatial and language capacities in selected Williams syndrome individuals is dramatically illustrated in an 18-year-old with an IQ of 49. The drawing of the elephant is fractionated and impoverished and without the labels would be unrecognizable. This is juxtaposed with an elaborate verbal description of elephants (from Bellugi et al., 1992).

contrasted to age- and mental-age-matched subjects with Down syndrome, both groups perform poorly on a standardized visuoconstructive measure, the developmental test of motor integration (Beery and Buktenica, 1967). The adolescents with Williams syndrome performed at a mean age equivalent of 4 years, 8 months, and those with Down syndrome at a mean age of 5 years, 6 months. Moreover, the Williams syndrome subjects demonstrated difficulties in integrating component parts on visuoconstruction tasks; for example, they might draw a triangle made of circles. Subjects were asked to copy common objects on command from memory and through copying a model, for example, a flower, a bicycle, or a house. The drawing of a bicycle, as shown in Figure 11.2–1, is distinctly abnormal. The Down's drawing shows a better spatial organization, closure, and integration of parts than does the Williams syndrome drawing, which lacks both spatial organization and integration. Williams syndrome subjects performed similarly to patients with right hemisphere lesions in the parietal lobe who will depict parts of an object as scattered on the page without integrating them into a functional whole and do not show perspective, depth, or spatial orientation (Anderson, 1988).

The approach to spatial tasks can be demonstrated, using block design subtests of the WISC-R. Although adolescents with both Williams and Down syndrome perform poorly on this task, they fail in distinctly different ways. Children with Down syndrome maintain the overall configuration of the blocks but produce errors of internal detail similar to those seen in patients with left hemisphere dysfunction. Those with Williams syndrome fail to maintain the overall configuration of the blocks and exhibit a fragmented approach, which is more typical of right hemisphere damaged patients. Although equivalently impaired, when contrasted to a mental-age control group, the processing differences between the groups are easily demonstrated.

On the Delis hierarchical processing task, impaired visuospatial processing has also been documented by Bellugi et al. (1992). In this test a larger (global) form is created by spatial arrangement of repeated smaller (local) forms. In the test, for example, one stimulus is a large printed "D" formed out of 15 small x's. To study spatial abilities, this test has advantages over standard clinical measures because it clearly demarcates features perceived as parts and as wholes. The Williams and Down syndrome subjects were presented these hierarchical stimuli for 5 seconds and asked to reproduce the figure after a 5-second delay. Age-matched normal subjects produced both local and global forms; both Williams and Down syndrome subjects were impaired in this 50-item task. The Williams syndrome subjects were more impaired in accuracy for depicting the global form; the Down syndrome subjects were more impaired than the Williams subjects in accuracy for the local forms. Therefore, even though both groups were matched on overall cognitive ability and showed equal impairment on some spatial tasks, there are distinctions between them in the spatial construction of parts versus wholes. Patients with unilateral right hemisphere lesions perform like Williams syndrome subjects and tend to be impaired in local forms; left lesion patients show performances similar to those of Down syndrome subjects (Delis, Kiefner, and Fridlund, 1988). These findings are also important in regard to the perception that mentally retarded individuals show a nonspecific pervasive developmental disorder with generalized cognitive deficits. Comparisons between these two mental retardation syndromes demonstrate that without extrinsic brain injury or a space-occupying lesion, uneven spatial profiles with deficits in the visuospatial domain may be demonstrated.

Facial Recognition

Although adolescents with Williams syndrome show spatial cognitive dysfunctions, they may be unimpaired in other visuospatial abilities. Subjects with Williams syndrome showed a selective ability to discriminate unfamiliar faces when tested with the Benton Test of Facial Recognition (Benton et al., 1983). When contrasted to developmental norms in individuals with normal intelligence, those with Williams syndrome performed at the level of normal 13-year-olds, which is close to the level of normal adults. The matched Down syndrome subjects, however, showed severe deficits on this task. Adolescents with Williams syndrome respond quickly and show correct responses in this complex task, which involves recognition and discrimination of faces that have been spatially transformed. Performance on the facial discrimination tasks, despite generally impaired spatial cognition, may be a unique neuropsychological marker of Williams syndrome (Bellugi et al., 1992).

These findings on neuropsychological tests demonstrate an uneven profile of specific deficits and perseverations within and across domains of language and spatial cognitive functioning. The dissociations in Williams syndrome may provide clues to understand brain structure and function. Neuropsychological testing, then, may be linked to neuroanatomical studies with magnetic resonance imaging and studies of the functional organization of the brain, using event-related potentials.

NEUROANATOMICAL AND NEUROPHYSIOLOGIC STUDIES

Neuroanatomical Studies

Jernigan and Bellugi (1990) studied gross brain morphology in MRIs in adolescents with Williams syndrome. These authors looked specifically for right hemispheric abnormalities that might be consistent with the psychological test profiles suggesting spared language, but marked visuospatial deficits. However, no gross abnormalities were noted in the initial examination. Comparisons were then made with age- and IQ-matched cases of Down syndrome.

Because the two syndromes have different neurobehavioral profiles in regard to language and cognition, the authors asked whether or not there were quantitative differences between the two groups in cerebral and cerebellar volumes. They found that both Williams syndrome and Down syndrome subjects had reduced cerebral volumes; approximately 77% of equivalent volume of young normal controls for Down syndrome and 80% for Williams syndrome. Although there was a significant volume reduction for both groups, the proportion of cerebral gray matter was similar to that observed in normal controls.

When cerebellum and brainstem were compared, in Down syndrome these brain regions were more reduced in size than the cerebrum. In contrast, subjects with Williams syndrome showed no reduction in overall size of cerebellar structures and, in fact, cerebellar volumes were significantly larger than those in Down syndrome. The Down syndrome patients showed 69% reductions in cerebellar volume when contrasted to controls, but in Williams syndrome the findings were essentially identical to normal controls. Because of the overall reductions in brain size, there is an abnormal cerebellar to cerebral volume ratio in Williams syndrome. In a subsequent study, Jernigan et al. (1993) reconfirmed their findings of cerebral hypoplasia of equal degree in the two groups and reduction in cerebellar size in Down syndrome but not in Williams syndrome. Moreover, in Williams syndrome, whereas paleocerebellar vermal lobules make up a smaller area on midsaggital sections, the neocerebellar lobules are actually larger. The authors note that these findings suggest some frontal and temporal limbic structures are relatively preserved in Williams syndrome, whereas some basal ganglia and diencephalic structures are relatively preserved in Down syndrome.

Overall comparisons of the size of structures within the cerebrum in Down syndrome and Williams syndrome support brain differences in these two disorders. Although the cerebrum is small in Williams syndrome, the frontal cortex has an essentially normal volume in relationship to the posterior cortex. But in Down syndrome, the frontal cortex is disproportionately reduced in volume. In Williams syndrome, some limbic structures of the temporal lobe, i.e., amygdala and hippocampus, seem to be spared in relation to other cerebral structures; in Down syndrome these structures show substantial reduction in volume. Yet the volumes of several other subcortical structures, including the thalamus, putamen, and globus pallidus, are normal in Down syndrome despite reductions in overall brain size.

Galaburda et al. (1994) have documented changes in brain structure in an autopsied case of Williams syndrome. Features of cortical architectonic differentiation, including increased cell packing density, horizontal disposition of neurons, immature vascular development, and weak myelination, suggest developmental arrest between late fetal development (end of second trimester) and the second year of life. Dysplastic features and ectopic neurons suggest processes that go beyond developmental arrest. The horizontal disposition of neurons may reflect incomplete connectivity. There is also evidence of migrational abnormalities leading to anomalous layering of the cortex. These authors suggest links to the neurobehavioral profile based on several neuroanatomical findings. The finding of curtailment in the development of the dorsal parietal regions and the posterior temporal areas along with the thinning of relevant portions of the corpus callosum may, according to them, be linked to the visuospatial deficits. The relatively preserved size of the frontal lobes and most of the temporal lobes are consistent with MRI findings. Cytoarchitecturally, the exaggerated horizontal organization of neurons was most apparent in the visual cortex and consistent with the visuospatial deficits. However, increased cell packing density was found throughout the cortex.

Neurophysiologic Studies

The timing and organization of those neural systems that are active during sensory cognitive and language processing have been investigated in Williams syndrome, using the event-related potential (ERP) technique. This is a noninvasive technique that allows millisecond by millisecond monitoring of brain activity that precedes, accompanies, and/or follows certain kinds of cognitive processing (Bellugi et al., 1992). This procedure has been utilized to study the basis of these patients' increased sensitivity to sounds, or hyperacusis. The auditory recovery cycle was studied for evidence of hyperexcitability at any stage through information processing in the auditory pathway. In addition, auditory sentence processing was evaluated to clarify whether there are preserved language capabilities in otherwise mentally retarded adolescent subjects with Williams syndrome and to contrast them to control subjects.

In Williams syndrome, there is an unusual sensitivity to certain environmental sounds that becomes apparent when the patient is aware of sounds before others and also shows an aversion to sounds which are not usually aversive in the general population. Subjects with Williams syndrome were asked to listen to tones that were presented at different repetition rates to establish the rate of recovery or refractory period of the auditory sensory-evoked response. The overall morphology of the ERPs was similar in Williams and control subjects over both the left and right hemisphere. However, subjects with

Williams syndrome showed larger responses at higher repetition rates, which suggests their responses were less refractory and, therefore, more excitable than in normal subjects. The effect that was demonstrated was evident only over the temporal cortex and only occurred with auditory stimulation. The authors concluded that similar brain systems were activated in the Williams syndrome subjects and normal control subjects when they listened to tones, but subjects with Williams syndrome showed hyperexcitability. When an analogous study was conducted in the visual recovery cycle paradigm, there was no difference between subjects with Williams syndrome and normal controls, indicating this effect is specific to auditory processing. These neurophysiologic studies suggest that hyperacusis may be mediated by hyperexcitability that is specific to certain cortical areas which are utilized to process acoustic information.

ERPs were also recorded to auditory presented words that form sentences. In the analysis, responses to open and closed class words and sentence medial position were compared. Moreover, one half of the sentences were contextually constrained and ended with an expected word that was semantically appropriate; the other half ended with an anomalous unexpected word that was semantically inappropriate. Bellugi et al. (1992) give an example of the latter as "I take my coffee with cream and paper." Previous ERP studies have shown that semantically primed or expected events elicit a sustained positivity in normal subjects after an initial response but that semantically anomalous unexpected information produces a negative peak. On this test, in contrast to normal subjects, subjects with Williams syndrome displayed highly abnormal responses within the first 200 to 300 milliseconds following word onset. The Williams subjects showed a large positivity that was not apparent in control subjects at any age. This effect, which was demonstrated primarily over the temporal brain region, might be related to hyperacusis. Moreover, subjects with Williams syndrome did not display the expected asymmetry, with the left temporal region more negative than the right, which is normally seen by about age 7. This finding indicates there may be an unusual pattern of brain organization underlying their language disorder. The neural systems involved in processing certain aspects of language may then be different in Williams syndrome when contrasted to controls. There are similarities in responses to semantically anomalous sentence endings, but the negative peak predicted is larger in Williams syndrome. Overall, the neurophysiologic studies suggest that some brain systems which mediate the preserved language in mentally retarded Williams syndrome subjects do differ from those that mediate language in the general population.

DEVELOPMENTAL AND BEHAVIORAL CHARACTERISTICS

Cognitive skills range from severe mental retardation to average mental ability, although the mean cognitive level is within the mild range of mental retardation. Academic achievement is commensurate with cognitive level; most persons with Williams syndrome speak with mental age-appropriate grammatical and articulation skills. However, the onset of language is delayed (Mervis and Bertrand, in press). On a parent questionnaire (Dilts, Morris, and Leonard, 1990), 96% of parents reported hypersensitivity to sound and exaggerated startle responses in their children. Their increased sensitivity seems to contribute to behavioral and learning problems, perhaps related to their being highly distracted by background noise. In addition, parents reported ongoing anxiety in regard to their anticipation of experiencing disturbing sounds. The hypersensitivity to sound was apparent from infancy onward and may contribute to crying in the first months of life following loud door closing, hand clapping, and vacuuming.

Motor development was delayed and many parents reported their child to be cautious when walking downstairs or along uneven surfaces. Adaptive skill acquisition related to fine and gross motor ability was lower than expected for age and cognitive level. Adaptive skill acquisition was a problem because it was related to poor development in the use of tools. In one third of 56 patients school age to adulthood, the ability to spread or cut with a knife was not present. Among 17 adults, 2 were competitively employed. One had married but divorced due to genetic issues around the diagnosis.

On the Achenbach Child Behavior Checklist, 48 Williams syndrome children, ranging in age from 4 to 16, were assessed (Dilts, Morris, and Leonard, 1990). Two thirds were rated above the 98th percentile on the hyperactivity scale. Distractibility was also frequently described and almost half of the group, ranging in age from 5 to 16, were enuretic.

The problems in sensory integration, sensitivity to sound, adaptive skills, overactivity, distractibility, and emotional insecurity with excessive worrying placed the child at increased risk for a psychiatric diagnosis. The risk of psychiatric diagnosis is compounded by living in a family where frequent arguing and psychosocial stresses are evident.

TREATMENT

Treatment begins with the recognition of the disorder followed by a careful description to family members about its characteristic features. The first year of life is often stressful for parents due to feeding problems, vomiting, and constipation. For those infants with hypercalcemia, in some instances, hydrocortisone has been used, and in other instances, a low calcium diet recommended. There is some evidence of vitamin D sensitivity. The hypercalcemia usually abates between 9 and 18 months of age. Specific treatments are then directed toward specific manifestations of the syndrome, particularly for congenital heart disease. As the children grow older, they are responsive to their physical and social environments. Despite their sociability, physical problems associated with Williams syndrome may influence infant attachment behavior, especially their feeding and other gastrointestinal problems. Early motor development is delayed and these developmental problems, in conjunction with physical symptoms, may affect early mother–child attachment. Because more attention to the child is required due to illness, the attachment may be intense. Attachment may also be enhanced by the child's attractive smile and social interest in people. Parents may become protective of their children in the early months of life because of the child's failure to thrive and slow development and the parental efforts to protect the child from sounds in the environment that are distressing. Additional attention may be drawn to the child because of his or her problems in sensory integration in terms of oversensitivity to vestibular input. There may be anxiety based on difficulty in modulating sensations which arise when the vestibular system is stimulated through head movement or change of position.

During the toddler phase, children with Williams syndrome may be hesitant to walk and sit down, and crawl rather than step. Climbing a ladder or sliding on a playground slide may be frightening for the child who has difficulty with vestibular modulation. Insecurity in regard to balance may further enhance the child's tendency to cling physically to a parent or caregiver.

As the child with Williams syndrome seeks a sense of autonomy and to master his environment, difficulty in the mastery of basic skills may complicate this developmental phase. Problems may emerge in dressing and toileting skills and lead to increasing dependence on others. Confidence may come in the area of language development where, through imitation, the child may find success in verbal communication to compensate for difficulties in manual mastery. As the child grows older and begins to use language more effectively, language use may be particularly important in coping. Self-directed mastery may emerge from success or failure in utilizing approval and being successful in work tasks. However, given their multiple motor disabilities and skill deficits along with attentional problems and distractibility, as well as problems in the mastery of tool use, self-directed mastery may be thwarted.

The older child with Williams syndrome who is distractible and has poor manual skills may have adaptive problems. The child may seek to compensate for these deficits through social conversation and by showing interest in others. Older children may have physical difficulties related to joint limitation and hypertonia.

Treatment takes into account interpersonal, physical, and behavioral aspects of Williams syndrome. For those children with extreme attentional problems and hyperactivity, pharmacological management may be helpful. Parent training and parent education are crucial in preventing psychological and psychiatric complications of Williams syndrome. The parent functions as a co-therapist for the child in working with the physician.

REFERENCES

Anderson, R.A. (1988). The neurobiological basis of spatial cognition: Role of the parietal lobe. In J. Stiles-Davis, M. Kritchevsky, and U. Bellugi (eds.), *Spatial cognition: Brain basis and development,* pp. 57–80. Erlbaum, Hillsdale, NJ.

Bates, E., Benigni, L., Bretherton, I., Camaioni, L., and Volterra, V. (1979). *The emergence of symbols: Cognition and communication in infancy.* Academic Press, New York.

Beery, K.E., and Buktenica, N.A. (1967). *Developmental test of visual-motor integration.* Modern Curriculum Press, Cleveland, OH.

Bellugi, U., Bihrle, A., Neville, H., Doherty, S., and Jernigan, J. (1992). Language, cognition, and brain organization in a neurodevelopmental disorder. In M.R. Gunnar and C.A. Nelson (eds.), *Developmental behavioral neuroscience: The Minnesota Symposia on Child Psychology,* 24:201–232.

Bennett, F.C., LaVeck, B., and Sells, C.J. (1978). The Williams elfin faces syndrome: The psychological profile as an aid in syndrome identification. *Pediatrics,* 61:303–305.

Benton, A.L., Hamsher, K., Varney, N.R., and Spreen, O. (1983). *Test of facial recognition, Form SL.* Oxford University Press, New York.

Burn, J. (1986). Williams syndrome. *Journal of Medical Genetics,* 2:389–395.

Colley, A., Thakker, Y., Ward, H., and Donnai, D. (1992). Unbalanced 13/18 translocation and Williams syndrome. *Journal of Medical Genetics,* 29:63–65.

Crisco, J.J., and Dobbs, J.M. (1988). Cognitive processing of children with Williams syndrome. *Developmental Medicine and Child Neurology,* 4:650–656.

Culler, F.L., Jones, K.L., and Deftos, L.J. (1985). Impaired calcitonin secretion in patients with Williams syndrome. *Journal of Pediatrics,* 107:720–723.

Delis, D.C., Kiefner, M.G., and Fridlund, A.J. (1988). Visuospatial dysfunction following unilateral brain damage: Dissociations in hierarchical and hemispatial analysis. *Journal of Clinical and Experimental Neuropsychology,* 10:421–431.

Dilts, C.V., Morris, C.A., and Leonard, C.O. (1990). Hypothesis for development of a behavioral phenotype in Williams syndrome. *American Journal of Medical Genetics Supplement,* 6:126–131.

Ewart, A.K., Morris, C.A., Atkinson, D., Jin, W., Sternes, K., Spallone, P., Stock, D., Leppert, M., and Keating, M.T. (1993). Hemizygosity at the elastin locus in a developmental disorder, Williams syndrome. *Nature Genetics,* 5:11–16.

Fanconi, G., Girardett, P., Schlesinger, B., Butler, N., and Black. J. (1952). Chronische hypercalcamie, konbiniert mit osteoklerose, hypoazotamie, minderwuchs und kongenitalen missbildungen. *Helvetica Pediatrica Acta,* 4:314–349.

Finegan, J., Smith, M.L., Meschino, W., Bolan, P., and Sitarenios, G. (1995). Verbal memory in children with Williams syndrome. Abstracts. *Society for Research in Child Development,* 10:395.

Fodor, J.D. (1983). Phrase structure parsing and the island constraints. *Linguistics and Philosophy,* 6:163–223.

Galaburda, A.M., Wang, P.P., Bellugi, U., and Rossen, M. (1994). Cytoarchitectonic anomalies in a genetically based disorder: Williams syndrome. *Neuroreport,* 5:753–757.

Gosch, A., Stading, G., and Pankau, R. (1994). Linguistic abilities in children with Williams-Beuren syndrome. *American Journal of Medical Genetics,* 52:291–296.

Greenberg, F. (1990). Williams syndrome professional symposium. *American Journal of Medical Genetics Supplement.* 6:85–88.

Hokama, T., and Rogers, J.G. (1991). Williams syndrome in one dizygotic twin. *Acta Pediatrica Japonica,* 33:678–680.

Jernigan, T.L., and Bellugi, U. (1990). Anomalous brain morphology on magnetic resonance images in Williams syndrome and Down syndrome. *Archives of Neurology,* 47:529–533.

______, Bellugi, U., Sowell, E., Doherty, S., and Hesselink, J.R. (1993). Cerebral morphological distinctions between Williams and Down syndromes. *Archives of Neurology,* 50:186–191.

Jones, K.L. (1990). Williams syndrome: An historical perspective of its evolution, natural history, and etiology. *American Journal of Medical Genetics Supplement,* 6:89–96.

______, and Smith, D.W. (1975). The Williams elfin faces syndrome: A new perspective. *Journal of Pediatrics,* 86:718–723.

Kaplan, L.C., Wharton, R., Elias, E. Mandell, F., Doulon, T., and Lott, S.A. (1987). Clinical heterogeneity associated with deletions of the long-arm of chromosome 15: Report of three new cases and their possible genetic significance. *American Journal of Medical Genetics,* 28:45–53.

Lightwood, R. (1952). Idiopathic hypercalcemia with failure to thrive. *Archives of Diseases of Childhood,* 27:302.

Mervis, C.B., and Bertrand, J. (in press). Relations between cognition and language: A developmental perspective. In L.B. Adamson and M.A. Romski (eds.), *Research on communication and language disorders: Contributions to theories of language development.* Brookes, New York.

Murphy, M.B., Greenberg, F., Hughes, M., and DiLiberti, J. (1990). Williams syndrome in twins. *American Journal of Medical Genetics,* 6(suppl.):97–99.

Preus, M. (1984). The Williams syndrome: Objective definition and diagnosis. *Clinical Genetics* , 25:422–428.

Russo, A.F., Chamany, K., Klemish, S.W., Hall, T.M., and Murray, J.C. (1991). Characterization of the calcitonin/CGRP gene in Williams syndrome. *Americam Journal of Medical Genetics,* 39:28–33.

Sinclair, H. (1975). The role of cognitive structures

in language acquisition. In E. Lenneberg and E. Lenneberg (eds.), *Foundations of language development: A multidisciplinary approach*, pp. 223–238. Jossey-Bass, San Francisco.

Thal, D., Bates, E., and Bellugi, U. (1989). Language and cognition in two children with Williams syndrome. *Journal of Speech and Hearing Research*, 3:489–500.

Udwin, O., and Yule, W. (1990). Expressive language of children with Williams syndrome. *American Journal of Medical Genetics*, 6(suppl.):108–114.

______, ______, and Martin, N. (1987). Cognitive abilities and behavioral characteristics of children with idiopathic infantile hypercalcaemia. *Journal of Child Psychology and Psychiatry*, 28:297–309.

von Arnim, G., and Engel, P. (1964). Mental retardation related to hypercalcemia. *Developmental Medicine and Child Neurology*, 6:366–377.

Williams, J.C.P., Barratt-Boyes, B.G., and Lowe, J.B. (1961). Supravalvular aortic stenosis. *Circulation*, 24:1311–1318.

11.3 Phenylketonuria

Phenylketonuria (PKU) and hyperphenylalaninemia designate a group of inborn errors of metabolism of phenylalanine, an essential amino acid for protein synthesis in mammalian tissues. In both conditions, there is impairment of phenylalanine oxidation resulting in elevated tissue and serum phenylalanine. The primary enzymatic defect may involve phenylalanine hydroxylase or dihydropteridine reductase, or it may involve one of the sequential enzymatic steps in the synthesis of the cofactor biopterin.

PKU has become a model to study the consequences of inborn errors of metabolism related to mental retardation. Animal models (Lipton et al., 1967) have been developed and dietary modifications have been utilized to prevent the mental retardation that is almost certain for untreated individuals (Bickel, Gerrard, and Hickmans, 1953, 1954). This metabolic disorder may also serve as a model to understand the consequences of central norepinephrine and dopamine depletion on behavior in neuropsychiatry, particularly on executive function and attentional processes.

Because of the success of this nutritional intervention to prevent brain damage, PKU is a model for the interface of a genetic disorder with the environment. In this condition, the brain of the fetus apparently develops normally despite the lack of the fetal synthesizing enzyme in the liver. Because a critical period for human brain growth and development takes place over the first 6 months of the neonatal period and little cell division takes place in the brain after 5 months, the need for intervention in early life is critical.

This chapter reviews the history, epidemiology, clinical features and phenotype, etiology, animal studies, diagnosis, and intervention and treatment of phenylketonuria.

HISTORY

Folling (1934, 1971; Folling, 1994) first described PKU based on his finding of excessive phenylpyruvic in the urine of affected patients. He referred to this condition as "oligophrenia phenylpyrouvica" to emphasize the mental retardation that was associated with it. The condition was first referred to as "phenylketonuria" by Penrose (Penrose, 1935; Penrose and Quastel, 1937). In 1947 Jervis was able to identify the metabolic error by showing that feeding phenylalanine to patients with PKU did not result in the production of tyrosine, whereas a prompt rise in tyrosine was seen in normal subjects (Jervis, 1947). In 1953 Jervis found that a liver extract from a patient with PKU lacked the ability to convert phenylalanine to tyrosine, although the conversion readily occurred in normal subjects (Jervis, 1953). By 1954 a diet therapy based on phenylalanine restriction was identified by Bickel, Gerrard, and Hickmans. Subsequently, the development of a simple method for screening blood phenylalanine concentration led to mass screening of neonates for hyperphenylalaninemia (Guthrie, 1961; Guthrie and Susi, 1963). During the ensuing years, a spectrum of phenylalanine hydroxylase deficiency has been reported. As stated, defects have been identified in other aspects of the metabolic pathway, including defects in dihydropteridine reductase (Kaufman et al., 1975), the cofactor reducing enzyme, as well as defects in the synthesis of the cofactor biopterin (Kaufman et al., 1978).

Following the development of mass screening programs and the institution of dietary restriction, the long-term outcome of the dietary treatment on both mental retardation and behavior has assumed increasing importance.

EPIDEMIOLOGY

PKU is an autosomal recessive disorder that occurs about once in 10,000 to 15,000 live births in North America and was once a major cause of mental retardation (Nyhan and Haas, 1993; Partington and Laverty, 1978). Varying rates have been reported in different countries, e.g., 1 in 4,500 in Ireland and 1 in 60,000 in Japan (Tourian and Sidbury, 1983). With the initiation of early screening programs worldwide and treatment of the metabolic disorder, the epidemiologic focus has shifted to the study of the prevalence of learning and behavioral problems as they relate to the discontinuation of the low phenylalanine diet.

CLINICAL FEATURES AND PHENOTYPE

Untreated PKU

The clinical features of untreated PKU include the mental manifestations, neurological dysfunction, and systemic symptoms that vary from one patient to the next. In classical untreated PKU, the most consistent feature is mental retardation, which becomes apparent in mid-infancy. In later childhood, 98% of untreated individuals have an IQ less than 70, although in the majority it is less than 30 (Tourian and Sidbury, 1983). Severe behavior problems including hyperactivity, destructiveness, impulsiveness, uncontrolled rage attacks, and self-injury have been reported. Moreover, psychiatric diagnoses including autistic disorder (Chen and Hsiao, 1989; Friedman, 1969) and schizophrenia-like symptoms have been reported. Because of a disturbance in pigment formation, the affected child usually has fair, lightly pigmented skin, blond hair and blue eyes. Photosensitivity and sclerodermoid changes may be apparent. An eczematous rash is noted in 20% to 40% and a "mousy" (animal-like) odor is reported (Nyhan and Haas, 1993; Tourian and Sidbury, 1983). General physical development and nutritional state is usually normal, and there are no specific dysmorphic features, although mild microcephaly may be apparent. Approximately 25% of affected children have grand mal convulsions. Hyperreflexia has been reported in approximately 50%; spastic cerebral palsy may also occur.

Delayed Treatment of PKU

The effects of dietary treatment on patients who have been diagnosed late is unclear and largely confined to individual case reports (Hoskin, Sasithan, and Howard, 1992; Marholen et al., 1978; McKean, 1971). Dietary withdrawal at age 8 in 27 late-treated patients resulted in a mean drop of 6 points in IQ score (Smith et al., 1978). Follow-up of these patients suggests greater vulnerability to develop both behavioral and neurological changes than affected children who receive early treatment. Agitation, fidgetiness, tics, and intention tremor were noted on examination. Although the brain damage that results from untreated PKU cannot be reversed, dietary treatment may reduce the extent of the associated behavioral disturbance.

Early Treatment of PKU

The availability of national registers of children with PKU allows prospective studies of large groups of children to be carried out. Using 8-year-olds from the PKU registry (Smith et al., 1988) in England, schoolteachers assessed the frequency of abnormal behavior on the Rutter Behavior Questionnaire in 544 children diagnosed in infancy and maintained on the PKU diet. All children began dietary treatment before 4 months of age. Two matched control subjects were assessed for each patient. Compared with the controls, patients receiving a strict low phenylalanine diet (average phenylalanine concentration less than 600 μmol/L) were 1.5 and 1.7 times, respectively, more likely to have deviant behavior; those on the less well-controlled diet were 2.5 and 1.9 times, respectively, more likely to show deviant behavior. Patients more often had mannerisms, hyperactivity, and signs of anxiety. They were less responsive and more solitary than controls but they were not more aggressive, untruthful, or disobedient, nor did they have more school absences. In this study, there was a greater risk of behavior disturbance in the patients with the higher phenylalanine concentrations (after allowing for the effects of gender and social class); however, even children with what by present criteria would be regarded as well-controlled phenylalanine concentrations (less than 600 μmol/L) showed a greater frequency of abnormal behavior than did the control children.

ETIOLOGY

Metabolic Aspects

Phenylketonuria is a disorder of amino acid metabolism involving the liver enzymes responsible for converting dietary phenylalanine to tyrosine. Two enzymes, phenylalanine hydroxylase and dihydropteridine reductase, and two cofactors, tetrahydrobiopterin (BH_4) and reduced pyridine nucleotide, are required for the hydroxylation of phenylalanine to tyrosine. There is an excessive production of phenylpyruvic acid, phenylacetic acid, and phenylacetylamine. Phenylalanine hydroxylase deficiency is associated with an irreversible defect involving the developing brain (mental retardation) and toxic, but reversible, effects such as neuropsychological and behavioral dysfunction if the diet is discontinued. Well-documented neurochemical consequences of phenylalanine accumulation include the impairment of brain protein synthesis, myelin turnover, and neurotransmitter amine synthesis (Guttler and Lou, 1986). The impairment in lipid and protein synthesis may influence myelinization and lead to decreased dendritic proliferation. In addition, phenylethylamine, another metabolite, has been implicated in neuropsychiatric symptoms (Wolf and Mosnaim, 1983; Wyatt et al., 1977).

Neurotransmitter Effects

Following the introduction of early treatment of PKU with a special phenylalanine restricted diet, an inverse relationship has been found between phenylalanine levels and the urinary excretion of dopamine and serotonin. An inverse relationship between blood phenylalanine levels and cerebrospinal fluid (CSF) concentrations of HVA and 5-HIAA has been regularly reported (McKean, 1972). The effect of the discontinuation of diet in PKU on the synthesis of dopamine, norepinephrine, and serotonin has been evaluated and the possible relationship between low levels of these neurotransmitters and impaired performance (Guttler and Lou, 1986; Krause et al., 1985; Lou et al., 1987; Pennington et al., 1985; Schaefer et al., 1974) on neuropsychological tests has been suggested.

The synthesis of serotonin, dopamine, and norepinephrine then are impaired in untreated PKU with either a decreased concentration in the blood or a decreased excretion in the urine of these substances, or of their metabolites, 5- hyroxyinoleacetic acid (5-HIAA) and homovanillic acid (HVA). Evidence suggests that phenylalanine competes with tyrosine and tryptophan transport into the brain, which may be a factor in the decreased synthesis of dopamine and serotonin. Because they cannot convert phenylalanine to tyrosine, tyrosine levels are low in the brain. The conversion of tyrosine to L-dopa is the major rate-limiting step for the synthesis of dopamine and norepinephrine. High levels of phenylalanine lead to catecholamine depletion in the brain through reduction in brain tyrosine. In PKU, depression in the central levels of dopamine and norepinephrine is expected. Butler et al. (1981) have found reduced levels in untreated individuals with PKU. Moreover, in phenylalanine loading studies in which the blood levels of early-treated individuals with PKU are manipulated, reductions in dopamine precursors and metabolites are found (Krause et al., 1985; Lou et al., 1985). In addition, lowered serotonin levels have been identified and may be caused by the inhibition by phenylalanine of serotonin precursor uptake. As a result, serotonin metabolism apparently is more disturbed than dopamine metabolism (Nielsen, Lou, and Guttler, 1988). Studies in phenylalanine-deficient mouse mutants show reductions in neurotransmitter receptor density and connectivity (Hommes, 1994).

Genetic Aspects

The gene for human phenylalanine hydroxylase is localized on chromosome 12q and has been cloned (Di Lella et al., 1986). Restriction fragment length polymorphism haplotypes have been identified (Lou et al., 1987) that may provide genetic linkage information for prenatal diagnosis or for heterozygote detection in 75% of families (Woo et al., 1983).

EEG and Neuroimaging Studies

The EEG is frequently abnormal (Barashnev et al., 1982; Behbehani, 1985; De Giorgis et al., 1983) in untreated children with PKU. Nineteen of 37 patients in one study had paroxysms of staring, nystagmoid eye movements, and absence or generalized clonic seizures. That were more severe in those with IQs of 35 or less, but all cases had abnormal EEGs. Hypsarrhythmia is common in untreated younger individuals with PKU. In treated children with

PKU, the EEG tends to be normal. Changes that do occur are primarily slowing with occasional focal sharp waves.

In untreated PKU, cerebral atrophy with enlarged ventricles has been reported (Behbehani, 1985). A PET study (Yanai et al., 1987) showed decreased glucose utilization in the caudate and putamen. An MRI study was carried out on 15 known individuals with PKU (Pearsen et al., 1990). Varying degrees of symmetric high-signal intensity of the white matter was seen in the posterior cerebral hemispheres. Anterior hemisphere involvement was only seen in association with severe signal intensity changes. Involvement of the cerebral cortex, brainstem, and cerebellum was not demonstrated. No structural changes were detected. Eight of 15 subjects showed mild cortical atrophy. IQ scores were not correlated with the degree of signal change on magnetic resonance imaging. The authors suggest that although distinct abnormalities are seen, there is no clear association with the clinical severity of the disease. Future imaging studies require more careful neuropsychological testing of the subjects.

Neuropsychological Testing

Despite early treatment, children with PKU may have more subtle specific cognitive deficits that may not be identified using traditional cognitive testing procedures. Pennington et al. (1985) have suggested a prefrontal dysfunction hypothesis in early-treated PKU. This hypothesis proposes a relatively specific effect on neurochemistry in children with PKU. In the prefrontal dysfunction hypothesis, the main effects on cognition in PKU are thought to be specific to the dopamine depletion because this neurotransmitter system is more specifically involved through projections to the neurocortex. Dopamine depletion may impair prefrontal functioning and lead to reductions in executive functions. Executive function may be a behavioral marker for prefrontal functioning in the developing organism; it includes the ability to maintain an appropriate problem-solving set for the attainment of a future goal, as described in Chapter 3. This involves set maintenance for strategic planning, impulse control, organized search, and flexibility of thought. The executive function processes also involve self-monitoring.

Welsh and Pennington (1988) utilized four tasks: visual search, verbal fluency, motor planning, and the Tower of Hanoi test to evaluate executive function in 11 preschool early-treated children with PKU (mean age 4.6 years). These children were compared to age- and IQ-matched unaffected peers. The authors hypothesized that children with early-treated PKU may be selectively impaired on executive function measures even though they are still on the diet. Children were evaluated for executive functions, including set maintenance, planning, and organized search. The children with PKU were found to be significantly impaired on an executive function composite score. Moreover, the executive function composite score was negatively correlated with the concurrent and mean lifetime phenylalanine levels. These results suggest that the prefrontal dysfunction hypothesis of phenylketonuria is supported in these children.

These results further suggest that the use of standardized intelligence measures as the primary means of assessing early-treated PKU does not provide an adequate assessment. Executive function measures that evaluate planning and the ability to shift set may prove to be a more sensitive means to evaluate cognitive development in affected children. These test findings are similar to those found in children with attention deficits, suggesting that understanding the mechanism of the brain in PKU may be helpful in eliciting the abnormality seen in children with other forms of attention deficit disorder.

Moreover, these results provide evidence that executive functions may be dissociable from other cognitive skills, such as recognition memory, which was also tested in the Welsh et al. (1990) study. A broader implication of these findings on the neuropsychological phenotype in PKU in these children is that the mechanisms underlying executive functions may be important in validating theories of intelligence.

In addition to their deficits in executive functions, a specific deficiency in solving complex spatial problems has been reported (Brunner, Berch, and Berry, 1987). These authors presented a task that involved the assembly of various shapes and compared the performance of 16 patients with PKU to that of 11 sibling controls. Their results suggest that the choice of problem-solving strategy, attention span, and the correctness of mental representation may be affected despite efforts to maintain appropriate phenylalanine levels in the blood.

ANIMAL STUDIES

Behavioral changes associated with PKU have been documented in animal studies (Andersen and Guroff, 1972; Anderson, Rowe, and Guroff, 1974; Chamove, 1980; Fulton et al., 1980). Several authors have investigated phenylalanine dietary alterations in rhesus monkeys (Chamove, 1980; Fulton et al., 1980). Infant rhesus monkeys were fed a diet high in phenylalanine or p-chlorophenylalanine for the first 12 months of life, or their mothers were fed a diet high in phenylalanine during pregnancy. When tested during the first year of life with familiar peers and during the second year with unfamiliar stimulus animals, they showed less play and other positive social behavior and more withdrawal, aggression, and emotional reactivity than did the two control groups. Finally, Diamond et al. (1994) have documented impaired performance in a rat model of PKU. Rat pups were impaired on delayed alternation, a behavioral task that is linked to functions of the prefrontal cortex. Task performance was linked to reduced dopamine metabolism in the prefrontal cortex. Such behavioral changes require further confirmation in mutant PAH-deficient mice (McDonald, 1994).

DIAGNOSIS

Metabolic Disorder

The diagnosis is suspected from a positive screening test for phenylalanine but must be confirmed by a quantitative test for phenylalanine and tyrosine in the blood. In classical PKU, the phenylalanine level is more than 20 mg/dl and tyrosine is low. The normal level for each of these substances is 1 mg/dl. In addition to classical PKU, where there is less than 1% normal enzyme activity, there is a benign form of hyperphenylalaninemia where phenylalanine levels are below 10 mg/dl on a normal diet and enzyme activity is 5% of the normal enzyme activity. Mentally retarded untreated patients have been described whose serum concentrations are between 10 and 20 mg/dl.

Behavioral Disorder and Diet

Parent ratings may be used to identify problem behaviors in diet-treated children. Schor (1983) asked parents of children with PKU to complete behavior rating forms for their children who were ages 3 through 7 years old. Of the 16 children with PKU studied, 15 were on phenylalanine-restricted diets at the time of the study. When ratings were compared with children in a private pediatrics practice, children with PKU were significantly less persistent than their siblings and were more rhythmic and more intense. There was a significant correlation between blood phenylalanine levels and persistence ratings, with those children having higher blood levels tending to be rated as less persistent than children having lower blood levels.

The effects of terminating the diet on learning and behavior are of particular importance (Holtzman, Welcher, and Mellits, 1975; Seashore et al., 1985). Assessments (Holtzman et al., 1986; Koch et al., 1982; Matthews et al., 1986) before and after dietary discontinuation have also been conducted using parent ratings. Social quotients of 16 early-treated children with PKU (Matthews et al., 1986) were assessed before and after discontinuation of dietary therapy. The records of those whose low phenylalanine diets had been discontinued at an average age of 5.5 years were reviewed for evidence of deterioration in functioning. Serum phenylalanine levels and Vineland Social Quotients before and after diet discontinuation were investigated using a repeated measures analysis of variance. Social quotients decreased significantly following discontinuation and were inversely correlated with serum phenylalanine levels.

Comprehensive assessments of individual children with early and later treatment for PKU have been conducted. Behbehani (1985) studied dietary termination in 22 early- and late-treated patients with phenylketonuria. Diet termination occurred in the eighth year. For evaluation of possible functional CNS deficits, they applied psychometric tests, measured psychomotor behavior, and studied neurophysiological status and polysomnograms. EEG findings were studied visually and the rhythms of the different phases of sleep were quantified by computerized spectral analysis. EEG studies were carried out during diet therapy when phenylalanine levels in blood were low, after a period of 4 months of elevated phenylalanine blood levels, and at least 2 years after diet termination. Compared to the findings before diet termination in these patients, there were no significant changes in the sleep EEG seen after termination on visual inspection or on spectral analysis. However, minor EEG changes were present in early- treated children and overtly pathological EEG changes were seen in late-treated PKU patients with cerebral damage, both before and after diet termination. The authors suggest that central nervous system morphology changes may include altered synaptic maturation that may have occurred in an early phase of development before the diet therapy was implemented for the late-treated group. When children on the diet were assessed individually, disturbed attention on the continuous performance test, emotional lability, spatial disorders, poorly developed ability to develop an "internal plan of action," and reduced schoolwork capacity were reported (Anderson and Siegel, 1976). Realmuto et al. (1986), using a structured interview, found psychiatric disorder in 6 of 13 children who were currently being treated for PKU, 3 had attention deficit/hyperactivity disorder, and 6 of 13 had a past history consistent with the diagnosis of attention deficit disorder.

Several studies have been carried out in mentally retarded adults with PKU to evaluate the effects of diet on behavior (Harper and Reid, 1987; Marholin et al., 1978; Wyatt et al., 1977;). Harper and Reid used a restricted protein diet to successfully treat a 54-year-old profoundly retarded female patient with PKU for her behavior disorder. In another study, the effects of a low phenylalanine diet on 6 mentally retarded phenylketonuric adults were assessed (Wyatt et al., 1977) in a controlled manner. An ABA individual-subject design was used to assess the effects of a low phenylalanine diet on social and motor behavior. Following a baseline during which the subjects ingested a normal phenylalanine diet (phase A), a low phenylalanine diet (phase B) was administered in a double-blind fashion. Finally, the baseline condition (phase A) was reinstated (normal diet). The low phenylalanine diet resulted in few significant behavioral changes for those subjects in which proper methodologic controls were employed. However, for 2 of 6 subjects motor behavior, including stereotypy and tremor, seems to have been ameliorated.

Clarke et al. (1987) studied 7 adolescents with PKU who had been on unrestricted diets for 2 to 11 years. Serial neuropsychological testing was carried out over two consecutive 4- to 5-week periods while maintaining a low phenylalanine diet that was supplemented in a triple-blind fashion with either high phenylalanine or low phenylalanine. Six of the seven subjects with PKU showed slower baseline median choice reaction times when matched to a control group of similar age, gender, handedness, and full-scale IQ (WISC-R). The tests showed a highly significant improvement during the low phenylalanine phase of the study. Overall, the adolescents with PKU on unrestricted diets were found to have a neuropsychological deficit that was out of proportion to their overall mental ability. The neuropsychological deficit appeared to be partly reversible by returning to dietary phenylalanine restriction even though they had tolerated hyperphenylalaninemia for several years on unrestricted diets.

Clarke and Yapa (1991) reported a case of anorexia nervosa beginning at age 14.5 years in a mildly retarded girl (full-scale IQ of 60) with phenylketonuria. She was on a low phenylalanine diet from 4 months of age until 3 years of age when it was discontinued by the family. Subsequently, she was hyperphenylalaninemic. During hospitalization for anorexia nervosa at age 15.5 years, a low phenylalanine diet was started along with psychotherapy, leading to improvement of the anorexia nervosa. Clarke and Yapa speculate that there may be a worsening of complex spatial processing with high phenylalanine which may have contributed to the body image distortion characteristic of anorexia nervosa in this patient.

To evaluate the relationship of behavioral changes to dietary control, both blood and urinary levels of phenylalanine and its metabolites have been monitored. The metabolites of phenylalanine, i.e., phenylacetate, phenyllactate, phenylpyruvate, and phenylethylamine, were measured (Michals and Matalon, 1985) in the urine of PKU patients. In general, correlation was found between serum phenylalanine levels and excretion of these metabolites. However, there were individual variations in the quantities and type of metabolites excreted that could not be explained by the blood phenylalanine levels. Increase in the excretion of phenylalanine metabolites was found in patients who were considered to have good blood phenylalanine control. These preliminary studies indicate that the current practice of allowing a wide range of blood phenylalanine in the treatment of PKU may have to be reexamined. Because these metabolites are neurotoxic (Smith, Howells, and

Hyland, 1986), they may afford a new parameter for the study of PKU not only regarding the prevention of mental retardation but also with regard to behavior and learning disabilities.

These studies and others (Anderson and Siegel, 1976; Holtzman et al., 1986; Hudson, Mordaunt, and Leahy, 1970; Koch et al., 1982) in children and adults highlight the need for ongoing assessment of dietary management and the importance of considering behavioral and learning problems at follow-up. Behavioral disturbances are present in many patients with early-treated PKU and are more prevalent in those with higher phenylalanine concentrations. Behavioral problems may compound the intellectual problems that are often present; emotional stress and neurological dysfunction are their likely causal factors. The increased frequency of deviant behavior may be a result of an interaction of psychological stress and neurological impairment. There is a need for more precise identification of the mechanisms responsible for the behavioral findings to develop appropriate strategies for prevention. Behavioral disorders, including attention deficit disorder and pervasive developmental disorder, may be associated with PKU. The occurrence of these diagnoses suggests a possible contribution of inborn errors to the understanding of the mechanisms involved in producing these neuropsychiatric conditions.

The evidence linking disturbed behavior and impaired cognitive function to elevated phenylalanine concentrations justifies a policy of controlling phenylalanine intake as strictly as possible. If untreated, affected children are ordinarily developmentally delayed and develop moderate to severe mental retardation, although normal intelligence has rarely been reported in untreated cases.

INTERVENTION AND TREATMENT

The effective use of the Guthrie test on the fourth or fifth day of life, which is mandatory in newborn screening throughout the world, leads to case identification (Lemieux et al., 1988) and has made untreated PKU a rare condition. If diagnosed within the first few days of life, PKU is treatable by dietary management. Treatment involves a low phenylalanine diet, with close monitoring of blood phenylalanine levels throughout the first 7 or 8 years of life (levels must not exceed 7 to 10 times normal values during the first 8 years). Because phenylalanine is an essential amino acid, control of the dietary intake permits the patient to have only that amount of phenylalanine that is needed for normal protein synthesis. One of several phenylalanine-poor or phenylalanine-free commercial formulas are used. They are supplemented with standard formula and low-protein foods. For older children, special regular diets are prepared. Subsequently, a relaxed diet (e.g., plasma levels 15 to 18 times normal, or below 900 to 1,100 μmol/L) with some restriction of phenylalanine intake has been advised (Smith et al., 1978; Waisbren et al., 1987); however, dietary modifications are under continuing review. The strict diet (average phenylalanine concentration less than 600 μmol/L.) may interfere with the development of a normal social life and, for the younger child, is a consideration in choosing preschool programs (Waisbren et al., 1987). In older children, there may be parent–child conflict over the diet especially if family relationships are tense or if the child is temperamentally difficult. Many parents claim to be able to predict when phenylalanine concentrations are high by observing their child's behavior, and recent experimental studies have found that short-term phenylalanine excess alters behavior and cognitive function. The outcome of early-treated cases is usually good, and with treatment a normally independent life in adulthood is to be expected, although a mean IQ of 5 points less than that of siblings has been reported (Dobson et al., 1976).

The prediction of later intelligence is an area of ongoing investigation (Waisbren et al., 1987). Besides parental IQ and the age when treatment was started, the age at which phenylalanine levels are consistently greater than 15 mg/dl is an important factor in predicting subsequent IQ. However, it is now recognized that despite dietary treatment, cognitive, emotional, and behavioral problems may occur (Krause et al., 1985; Matthews et al., 1986; Pennington et al., 1985; Stevenson et al., 1979; Smith et al., 1988). Early studies focused on intelligence as an outcome measure, but more recent investigations have focused on problems in learning (Dobson et al., 1976; Dobson et al., 1977) and behavior (Brunner, Jordan, and Berry, 1983) that have psychosocial implications. There are also atypical forms of PKU and mild hyperphenylalaninemia that may affect intelligence and personality development (Waisbren, Schnell, and Levy, 1984).

In cases of PKU where phenylalanine levels are three to five times the normal level (6–10 mg/dl), levels generally considered "safe," cognitive deficits were found in tasks that involved the dorsolateral prefrontal cortex (Diamond, 1994).

The tasks involved holding information in mind while exercising inhibitory control over inclinations to act. The biological mechanism involved in this cognitive deficit may be linked to reduced dopamine metabolism in this brain region, perhaps the consequence of reduced tyrosine availability. In addition, another dopamine-related function, sensitivity to visual contrast, was also reduced thus providing additional data documenting dopaminergic involvement.

There is one case report of correction of PKU in a child who received a liver transplantation for cirrhosis of the liver whose etiology was unrelated to the PKU (Vajro et al., 1993). Such findings are consistent with somatic gene therapy as an alternative to dietary therapy. In this approach (Eisensmith and Woo, 1994), a functional hepatic phenylalanine hydroxylase (PAH) gene is implanted into the liver. These authors have corrected the phenylalanine deficit in a PAH-deficient mouse strain and demonstrated complete reconstitution of enzyme activity. Although the effect is transient, the development of new vectors suggests the possibility of corrective somatic gene therapy in the future.

Maternal Phenylketonuria

Affected women (Koch et al., 1986; Schalock and Copenhaver, 1973) are likely to give birth to children with congenital abnormalities and mental retardation as a result of the exposure of the fetus to high levels of maternal phenylalanine, unless they return to a diet before becoming pregnant. Phenylketonuric women planning pregnancy should begin a carefully monitored low phenylalanine diet, which should be monitored beginning before conception and continued until delivery. Guttler et al. (1990) reported on 26 maternal PKU pregnancies that were treated prior to conception. In two cases, a strict diet (phenylalanine concentrations less than 0.6 μmol/L) was introduced prior to planned pregnancy that occurred after being on the diet for several months. Serum phenylalanine was monitored weekly during the pregnancies so that phenylalanine levels remained in the range of 0.18 to 0.42 μmol/L. Healthy children were delivered with normal head circumference. At age 4 years and 10 years, their IQs were 119 and 105, respectively. Preconceptional dietary treatment in this study led to children with normal performance unlike their older siblings who were born following untreated pregnancies. These results highlight the importance of preconceptional treatment.

In a PKU pregnancy, phenylalanine metabolites require careful monitoring. One study (Smith, Howells, and Hyland, 1986) demonstrated large quantities of phenylalanine metabolites in urine despite a modest elevation of serum phenylalanine in a pregnant mother. Animal studies suggest a possible mechanism for these effects. When mice, *in utero,* were exposed to enzyme inhibition that has been shown to affect amino acid transport in adults, the young mice showed altered motor behavior at 40 days of age. The findings suggest that interference with blood-brain amino acid transport *in utero* has long-term consequences. Additional investigations are needed in relation to maternal phenylketonuria.

Robertson and Schulman (1987) addressed ethical issues in PKU pregnancies. In maternal PKU, the mother can prevent harm to her baby by returning to the unpleasant diet that prevents the infant from developing mental retardation. Informing, counseling, and access to medical care are essential for these mothers. Prenatal diagnosis (Scriver and Clow, 1988) is available that provides the choice of aborting an affected fetus. Because this is a treatable condition, most parents have the experience of raising a nonretarded affected child. However, Scriver (Scriver and Clow, 1988) suggests that some families may choose to be tested because they would not consider having additional children otherwise.

Family Treatment

Parents of children with PKU experience stresses that may disrupt family life. McBean (1971) surveyed 59 Scottish families who collectively had a total of 204 children, 79 with phenylketonuria. The families were divided into two groups. In the first, the diagnosis was made late so that a mentally retarded child was in the family. In the second, the index case was ascertained by screening in the newborn period. The families were then interviewed and asked the following specific questions: (1) their reaction to the PKU screening test; (2) their reaction to the diagnosis of phenylketonuria in the infant and their appreciation of what the diagnosis meant; (3) their understanding of the diet and the problems involved in following through with it; (4) their thoughts about the future for the infant; (5) the effect on the family and on their marriage of the child with PKU; (6) their attitude toward having additional children.

The initial Guthrie test for PKU was wanted; the parents were anxious that it be done. When the screening test was positive, the request for a second confirmatory test was stressful, particularly if relations with the medical staff were not secure. The hospital admission for the assessment of an apparently normal infant was remembered as a particularly unhappy time. When told of the diagnosis of phenylketonuria, all the parents acknowledged feelings of anxiety and disbelief and found it difficult to assimilate the facts about the disorder during the first interview. The mode of inheritance of the disease, which was discussed at the time when the diagnosis was given, was a difficult one for many parents to understand. Most parents appreciated that they both were involved in the transmission of the disorder; however, grandparents tended to blame one or the other side of the family. Frequently, the parents had not understood what was thought by the professional staff to have been an adequate and full explanation of the disorder.

All parents expressed considerable difficulty in understanding the administration of the diet as well as accepting the consequences of dietary neglect. When there was no previous experience of a retarded or phenylketonuric child, it was difficult for the parents to appreciate the form the mental retardation might take or how quickly it would occur. The fear of mental deterioration if the diet was not followed sometimes led to an increased involvement of the mother with the child with PKU. When some mothers found that dietary indiscretion does not lead to immediate mental retardation, they were inclined to question the diagnosis.

When asked about the future of the child with PKU, some parents feared that special schooling might be necessary. Others were more concerned with the supervision of the diet while the child was away from home. Very few parents mentioned long-term concerns, such as secondary school or future work plans. Fewer still looked ahead to the possibility of marriage for the child or childbearing. Although there was not significant evidence that the child with PKU specifically caused marital disharmony, if it already existed, the disorder increased it through providing an additional stress.

Many mothers wanted to have more children but feared the possibility of another affected child. The avoidance of pregnancy posed great problems for those mothers whose religious beliefs forbade artificial methods of contraception. Others, using natural methods of contraception or none at all, were often preoccupied with the possibility of conception and with the fear of having further children with PKU.

Based on this pilot study, McBean (1971) suggests that the parents be informed through simple and repeated explanations of the cause of phenylketonuria, the course of the disease, and the reasons underlying treatment. Although pamphlets may be helpful, alone they are inadequate. For all of the families, the moment of initial diagnosis is traumatic. Genetic counseling was particularly hard if a family already had two or more affected children or knew of other families where this situation had occurred. There is a need for constant emotional and practical support, which must be available for as long as the diet continues and may be necessary for even longer to help in dealing with the problems of the adolescent treated child with PKU.

In the years since McBean's study was carried out, there has been considerable experience in working with families. Pueschel, Yeatman, and Hum (1977) used questionnaires, informal group meetings, and individual interviews with parents and their children with phenylketonuria to understand their attitudes and experiences surrounding discontinuance of the phenylalanine-restricted diet. These authors stressed the importance of understanding changing social interactions as termination of the restricted diet progresses. Preparatory discussions with parents and children prior to the change in diet should be held to avoid undue stress and conflict in such families.

Reber, Kazak, and Himmelberg (1987) have provided another systematic study of family factors. They studied 41 young children with early-treated PKU and their families to determine relationships between dietary phenylalanine control and patient functioning and family functioning. Children received neuropsychological tests and parents completed behavior checklists on their child. Parents also completed four self-report measures to evaluate family adjustment, stress, and social interaction. Significant correlations were found between phenylalanine control subjects and affected patients' intelligence test scores and lifetime phenylalanine control. Children with PKU had lower social competence scores than the comparison control group. The parent-report measures of family psychological adjustment, stress, interaction, and socioeconomic status did not show significant association with children's dietary phenylalanine control. Family cohesion and adaptability correlated positively with the patients' cognitive performance. Mothers of children with PKU perceived their families to be significantly less cohesive (more separated) and less adaptable (more rigid) than control mothers of children without PKU. Fathers of children with PKU perceived their families to be less adaptable. The reduced cohesion and rigidity in families may have negative effects on test performance by children with PKU. These findings suggest that both metabolic and family factors should be considered in evaluating the outcome of early-treated PKU. Longitudinal study of families whose children have PKU is needed to clarify the effects of the illness on family cohesion and adaptability.

REFERENCES

Andersen, A.E., and Guroff, G. (1972). Enduring behavioral changes in rats with experimental phenylketonuria. *Proceeding of the National Academy of Science, USA,* 69(4):863–867.

______, Rowe, V., and Guroff, G. (1974). The enduring behavioral changes in rats with experimental phenylketonuria. *Proceeding of the National Academy of Science, USA,* 71(1):21–25.

Anderson, V.E., and Siegel, F.S. (1976). Behavioral and biochemical correlates of diet change in phenylketonuria. *Pediatric Research,* 10(1):10–17.

Barashnev, Y.I., Korneichuk, V.V., Klembovsky, A.I., and Klyushina, L.A. (1982). Role of the liver in the pathogenesis of cerebral disorders in phenylketonuria. *Journal of Inherited Metabolic Diseases,* 5:204–210.

Behbehani, A.W. (1985). Termination of strict diet therapy in phenylketonuria. A study on EEG sleep patterns and computer spectral analysis. *Neuropediatrics,* 16:92–97.

Bickel, H., Gerrard, J., and Hickmans, E.M. (1954). The influence of phenylalanine intake on the chemistry and behavior of a phenylketonuric child. *Acta Paediatrica Scandinavica,* 43:64–77.

______, ______, and ______. (1953). Influence of phenylalanine intake on phenylketonuria. *Lancet,* ii:812.

Brunner, R.L., Berch, D.B., and Berry, H. (1987). Phenylketonuria and complex spatial visualization: An analysis of information processing. *Developmental Medicine and Child Neurology,* 29:460–468.

______, Jordan, M.K., and Berry, H.K. (1983). Early treated phenylketonuria: Neuropsychologic consequences. *Journal of Pediatrics,* 102:831–835.

Butler, I.J., O'Flynn, M.E., Seifert, W.E., and Howell, R.R. (1981). Neurotransmitter defects and treatment of disorders of hyperphenylalaninemia. *Journal of Pediatrics,* 98:729–733.

Chamove, A.S. (1980). Dietary and metabolic effects on rhesus social behavior: Phenylalanine-related dietary alterations. *Developmental Psychobiology,* 13(3):299–307.

Chen, C.H., and Hsiao, K.J. (1989). A Chinese classic phenylketonuria manifested as autism. *British Journal of Psychiatry,* 155:251–253.

Clarke, D.J., and Yapa, P. (1991). Phenylketonuria and anorexia nervosa. *Journal of Mental Deficiency Research,* 35:165–170.

Clarke, J.T., Gates, R.D., Hogan, S.E., Barrett, M., and MacDonald, G.W. (1987). Neuropsychological studies on adolescents with phenylketonuria returned to phenylalanine-restricted diets. *American Journal of Mental Retardation,* 92:255–262.

De Giorgis, G.F., Antonozzi, I., Del Castello, P.G., Rosano, M., and Loizzo, A. (1983). EEG as a possible prognostic tool in phenylketonuria. *Electroencephalography and Clinical Neurophysiology,* 55:60–68.

Diamond, A. (1994). Phenylalanine levels of 6–10 mg/dl may not be as benign as once thought. *Acta Pediatrica (Suppl),* 407:89–91.

______, Ciaramitaro, V., Donner, E., Djali, S., Robinson, M. (1994). An animal model of early-treated PKU. *Journal of Neuroscience,* 14:3072–3082.

Di Lella, A.G., Kwok, S.C., Ledley, F.D., Marvit, J., and Woo, S.L. (1986). Molecular structure and polymorphic map of the human phenylalanine hydroxylase gene. *Biochemistry,* 25:743–749.

Dobson, J.C., Kushida, E., Williamson, M.L., and Freidman, E.G. (1976). Intellectual performance of 36 phenylketonuric patients and their nonaffected siblings. *Pediatrics,* 58:53–58.

______, Williamson, M.L., Azen, C., and Koch, R. (1977). Intellectual assessment of 111 four year old children with phenylketonuria. *Pediatrics,* 60:822–827.

Eisensmith, R.C., and Woo, S.L.C. (1994). Gene therapy for PKU. *Acta Pediatrica (Suppl),* 407: 124–129.

Folling, A. (1934). Über ausscheidung von Phenylbrenztraubensaure in den Harn als Stoffwechselanomalie in Verbindung mit Imbezillitat. *Zeitschrift Physiologische Chemie.,* 227:169–176.

______. (1971). The original detection of phenylketonuria. In H. Bickel, F. Hudson, and L. Woolf (eds.), *Phenylketonuria,* pp. 1–3. Georg Thieme Verlag, Stuttgart, Germany.

Folling, I. (1994). The discovery of phenylketonuria. *Acta Pediatrica (Suppl)*, 407:4–10.

Friedman, E. (1969). The autistic syndromes and phenylketonuria. *Schizophrenia*, 1:249–261.

Fulton, T.R., Triano, T., Rabe, A., and Loo, Y.H. (1980). Phenylacetate and the enduring behavioral deficit in experimental phenylketonuria. *Life Sciences*, 27(14):1271–1281.

Guthrie, R. (1961). Blood screening for phenylketonuria. *Journal of the American Medical Association*, 178:863.

______, and Susi, A. (1963). A simple phenylalanine method for detecting phenylketonuria in large populations of newborn infants. *Pediatrics*, 32:338–343.

Guttler, F., and Lou, H. (1986). Dietary problems of phenylketonuria: Effect on CNS transmitters and their possible role in behaviour and neuropsychological function. *Journal of Inherited Metabolic Diseases*, 9(suppl. 2):169–177.

______, ______, Andresen, J., Kok, K., Mikkelsen, I., Nielsen, K.B., and Nielsen, J.B. (1990). Cognitive development in offspring of untreated and preconceptionally treated maternal phenylketonuria. *Journal of Inherited Metabolic Diseases*, 13:665–671.

Harper, M., and Reid, A.H. (1987). Use of a restricted protein diet in the treatment of behaviour disorder in a severely mentally retarded adult female phenylketonuric patient. *Journal of Mental Deficiency Research*, 31:209–212.

Holtzman, N.A., Kronmal, R.A., van Doorninck, W., Azen, C., and Koch, R. (1986). Effect of age at loss of dietary control on intellectual performance and behaviour of children with phenylketonuria. *New England Journal of Medicine*, 314:593–598.

______, Welcher, D.W., and Mellits, E.D. (1975). Termination of restricted diet in children with phenylketonuria: A randomized controlled study. *New England Journal of Medicine*, 293:1121.

Hommes, F.A. (1994). Loss of neurotransmitter receptors by hyperphenylalaninemia in the HPH-5 mouse brain. *Acta Paediatrica (Suppl)*, 407:120–121.

Hoskin, R.G., Sasithan, T., and Howard, R. (1992). The use of a low phenylalanine diet with amino acid supplement in the treatment of behavioural problems in a severely mentally retarded adult female with phenylketonuria. *Journal of Intellectual Disability Research*, 36:183–191.

Hudson, F.P., Mordaunt, V.L., and Leahy, I. (1970). Evaluation of treatment begun in the first three months of life in 184 cases of phenylketonuria. *Archives of Diseases of Childhood*, 45:5–12.

Jervis, G.A. (1947). Studies on phenylpyruvic oligophrenia: The position of the metabolic error. *Journal of Biological Chemistry*, 169:651.

______. (1953). Phenylpyruvic oligphrenia deficiency of phenylalanine-oxidizing system. *Proceedings of the Society of Experimental and Biological Medicine*, 82:514–515.

Kaufman, S., Berlow, S., Summer, G.K., Milstien, S., Schulman, J.D., Orloff, S., Spielberg, S., and Pueschel, S. (1978). Hyperphenylalaninemia due to a deficiency of biopterin. *New England Journal of Medicine*, 299:673.

______, Holtzman, N.A., Milstien, S., Butler, I.J., and Krumholz, A. (1975). Phenylketonuria due to a deficiency of dihydropteridine reductase. *New England Journal of Medicine*, 293:785.

Koch, R., Azen, C.G., Friedman, E.G., and Williamson, M.L. (1982). Preliminary report on the effects of diet discontinuation in PKU. *Journal of Pediatrics*, 100:870–875.

______, Gross-Friedman, E., Wenz, E., Jew, K., Crowley, C., and Donnell, G. (1986). Maternal phenylketonuria. *Journal of Inherited Metabolic Diseases*, 9(2):159–168.

Krause, W., Halminski, M., McDonald, L., Dembure, P., Salvo, R., Freides, D., and Elsas, L. (1985). Biochemical and neuropsychological effects of elevated plasma phenylalanine in patients with treated phenylketonuria. *Journal of Clinical Investigation*, 75:40–48.

Lemieux, B., Auray-Blais, C., Giguere, R., Shapcott, D., and Scriver, C.R. (1988). Newborn urine screening experience with over one million infants in the Quebec Network of Genetic Medicine. *Journal of Inherited Metabolic Diseases*, 11(1):45–55.

Lipton, M.A., Gordon, R., Guroff, G., and Udenfriend, S. (1967). P-chlorophenylalanine-induced chemical manifestations of phenylketonuria in rats. *Science*, 156:248.

Lou, H.C., Guttler, G., Lykelund, C., Bruhn, P., and Niederwieser, A. (1985). Decreased vigilance and neurotransmitter synthesis after discontinuation of dietary treatment of phenylketonuria in adolescents. *European Journal of Pediatrics*, 144:17–20.

______, Lykkelund, C., Gerdes, A.M., Udesen, A.M., and Bruhn, P. (1987). Increased vigilance and dopamine synthesis by large doses of tyrosine or phenylalanine restriction in phenylketonuria. *Acta Pediatrica Scandanavia*, 76:560–565.

Marholin, D., 2nd, Pohl, R.E., 3rd, Stewart, R.M., Touchette, P.E., Townsend, N.M., and Kolodny, E.H. (1978). Effects of diet and behavior therapy on social and motor behavior of retarded phenylketonuric adults: An experimental analysis. *Pediatric Research*, 12(3):179–187.

Matthews, W.S., Baraba, G., Cusack, E., and Ferrari, M. (1986). Social quotients of children with phenylketonuria before and after discontinuation of dietary therapy. *American Journal of Mental Deficiency,* 91(1):92–94.

McBean, M.S. (1971). The problems of parents of children with phenylketonuria. In B. Bickel, F.P. Hudson, and L.I. Woolf (eds.), *Phenylketonuria,* pp. 280–282. Georg Thieme Verlag, Stuttgart, Germany.

McDonald, J.D. (1994). The PKU mouse project: Its history, potential and implications. *Acta Paediatrica (Suppl),* 407:22–23.

McKean, C.M. (1971). Effect of totally synthetic low phenylalanine diet on adolescent phenylketonuric patients. *Archives of Diseases in Childhood,* 46:606-615.

______. (1972). The effects of high phenylalanine concentrations on serotonin and catecholamine metabolism in the human brain. *Brain Research,* 47:469–476.

Michals, K., and Matalon, R. (1985). Phenylalanine metabolites, attention span and hyperactivity. *American Journal of Clinical Nutrition,* 42(2):361–365.

Nielsen, J.B., Lou, H.C., and Guttler, F. (1988). Effects of diet discontinuation and dietary tryptophan supplementation on neurotransmitter metabolism in PKU. *Brain Dysfunction,* 1:51–56.

Nyhan, W.L., and Haas, R. (1993). Inborn errors of amino acid metabolism and transport. In R.N. Rosenberg, S.B. Prusiner, S. DiMauro, R.L. Barchi, and L.M. Kunkel (eds.), *The molecular and genetic basis of neurological disease,* p. 151. Butterworth-Heinemann, Boston.

Partington, M.W., and Laverty, T. (1978). Long term studies of untreated phenylketonuria I: Intelligence or mental ability. *Neuropadiatrie,* 9(3):245–254.

Pearsen, K.D., Gean-Marton, A.D., Levy, H.L., and Davis, H.R. (1990). Phenylketonuria: MR imaging of the brain with clinical correlation. *Radiology,* 177:437–440.

Pennington, B., van Doorninck, W.J., McCabe, L.L., and McCabe, E.R.B. (1985). Neuropsychological deficits in early treated phenylketonuric children. *American Journal of Mental Deficiency,* 89:467–474.

Penrose, L.S. (1935). Inheritance of phenylpyruvic amentia (phenylketonuria). *Lancet,* ii:192–194.

______, and Quastel, J.H. (1937). Metabolic studies in phenylketonuria. *Biochemistry Journal,* 31:266.

Pueschel, S.M., Yeatman, S., and Hum, C. (1977). Discontinuing the phenylalanine-restricted diet in young children with PKU: Psychosocial aspects. *Journal of the American Diet Association,* 70(5):506–509.

Realmuto, G.M., Garfinkel, B.D., Tuchman, M., Tsai, M.Y., Chang, P., Fisch, R.O., and Shapiro, S. (1986). Psychiatric diagnosis and behavioral characteristics of phenylketonuric children. *Journal of Nervous and Mental Diseases,* 174(9):536–540.

Reber, M., Kazak, A.E., and Himmelberg, P. (1987). Phenylalanine control and family functioning in early treated phenylketonuria. *Journal of Developmental and Behavioral Pediatrics,* 8(6):311–317.

Robertson, J.A., and Schulman, J.D. (1987). Pregnancy and prenatal harm to offspring: The case of mothers with PKU. *Hastings Center Reports,* 17(4):23–33.

Schaefer, G.J., Barrett, R.J., Sanders-Bush, E., and Vorhees, C.V. (1974). Chloroamphetamine: Evidence against a serotonin mediated learning deficit in PKU. *Pharmacology, Biochemistry, and Behavior,* 2(6):783–789.

Schalock, R.L., and Copenhaver, J.H. (1973). Behavioral effects of experimental maternal hyperphenylalaninemia. *Developmental Psychobiology,* 6(6):511–520.

Schor, D.P. (1983). PKU and temperament: Rating children three through seven years old in PKU families. *Clinical Pediatrics (Philadelphia),* 22(12):807–811.

Scriver, C.R., and Clow, C.L. (1988). Avoiding phenylketonuria: Why parents seek prenatal diagnosis. *Journal of Pediatrics,* 113(3):495–497.

Seashore, M.R., Freidman, E., Novelly, R.A., and Bapat, V. (1985). Loss of intellectual function in children with phenylketonuria after relaxation of dietary phenylalanine restriction. *Pediatrics,* 75:226–232.

Smith, I., Beasley, M.G., Wolff, O.H., and Ades, A.E. (1988). Behavior disturbance in 8-year-old children with early treated phenylketonuria. Report from the MRC/DHSS Phenylketonuria Register. *Journal of Pediatrics,* 112(3):403–408.

______, Howells, D., and Hyland, K. (1986). Pteridines and monoamines: Relevance to neurological damage. *Postgraduate Medicine Journal,* 62:113–122.

______, Lobascher, M.E., Stevenson, J.E., Wolff, O.H., Schmidt, H., Grubel-Kaiser, S., and Bickel, H. (1978). Effect of stopping the low-phenylalanine diet on intellectual progress of children with phenylketonuria. *British Medical Journal,* 2:723–726.

Stevenson, J.E, Hawcroft, J., Lobascher, M., Smith, I., Wolff, O.H., and Graham, P.J. (1979). Behavioural deviance in children with early treated phenylketonuria. *Archives of Diseases in Childhood,* 54:14–18.

Tourian, A., and Sidbury, J.B. (1983). Phenylketonuria and hyperphenylalaninemia. In J.B. Stanbury, J.B. Syngaarden, D.S. Fredrickson,

J.L. Goldstein, and M.S. Brown (eds.), *The metabolic basis of inherited disease,* pp. 270–286. McGraw-Hill, New York.

Vajro, P., Strisciuglio, P., Houssin, D., Huault, G., Laurent, J., Alvarez, F., and Bernard, O. (1994). Correction of phenylketonuria after liver transplantation in a child with cirrhosis [letter]. *New England Journal of Medicine,* 329 (5):363.

Waisbren, S.E., Mahon, B.E., Schnell, R.R., and Levy, H.L. (1987). Predictors of intelligence quotient and intelligence quotient change in persons treated for phenylketonuria early in life. *Pediatrics,* 79(3):351–355.

______, Schnell, R., and Levy, H.L. (1984). Intelligence and personality characteristics with untreated atypical phenylketonuria and mild hyperphenylalaninemia. *Clinical and Laboratory Observations,* 105(6):955–958.

Welsh, M.C., and Pennington, B.F. (1988). Assessing frontal lobe function in children: Views from developmental psychology. *Developmental Neuropsychology,* 4:199–230.

______, ______, Ozonoff, S., Rouse, B., and McCabe, E.R.B. (1990). Neuropsychology of early-treated phenylketonuria: Specific executive function deficits. *Child Development,* 61:1697–1713.

Wolf, M.E., and Mosnaim, A.D. (1983). Phenylethylamine in neuropsychiatric disorders. *General Pharmacology,* 14(4):385–390.

Woo, S.C.L., Lidsky, A.S., Guttler, F., Chandra, T., and Robson, K.J.H. (1983). Cloned human phenylalanine hydroxylase gene allows parental diagnosis and carrier detection of classical phenylketonuria. *Nature,* 306:151–155.

Wyatt, R.J., Gillin, J.C., Stoff, D.M., Majo, E.A., and Tinklenberg, J.R. (1977). Betaphenylethylamine and the neuropsychiatric disturbances. In E. Usdin, D.A. Hamburg, and J.D. Barchas (eds.), *Neuroregulators and psychiatric disorders,* pp. 31–45. Oxford University Press, New York.

Yanai, K., Iinuma, K., Matsuzawa, T., Ito, M., Miyabayashi, S., Narisawa, K., Ido, T., Yamada, K., and Tada, K. (1987). Cerebral glucose utilization in pediatric neurological disorders determined by positron emission tomography. *European Journal of Nuclear Medicine,* 13:292–296.

11.4 Galactosemia

Galactosemia is a rare autosomal recessive disorder of carbohydrate metabolism where there is a deficiency of one of three enzymes involved in galactose metabolism; galactose-1-phosphate uridyl transferase (GALT) is the most common of these and its absence is referred to as classical galactosemia. Deficiency of these enzymes causes a failure in the metabolism of galactose to glucose, which is an essential source of calories for the newborn infant. Galactosemia refers to the presence of galactose in the blood; galactose and its metabolites, especially galactose-1-phosphate (gal-1-p), build up in tissue and adversely affect carbohydrate energy metabolism. Without treatment, infants with classical galactosemia characteristically are jaundiced, fail to thrive, develop hepatomegaly, and are vulnerable to hypoglycemia, sepsis, cataract formation, and brain damage. Those who survive may be left with residual cataracts and physical and mental retardation. The response to treatment has suggested a relatively benign disorder; however, despite the response of acute neonatal symptoms to treatment, long-term outcome remains problematic. Reduced intellectual functioning, speech problems, learning disability, and ovarian failure have been documented even though dietary treatment was closely followed (Lehotay, 1993). These characteristics suggest a recognizable cognitive and behavioral phenotype.

This chapter describes the history, epidemiology, clinical features and cognitive/behavioral phenotype, etiology, newborn screening, and treatment of galactosemia.

HISTORY

The first report of galactosemia was that of von Reuss (1908), "Sugar Excretion in Infancy," who reported on a breast-fed infant with failure to thrive, hepatosplenomegaly, and galactosemia. He noted that urinary galactose excretion stopped when milk products were removed from the diet. Classical galactosemia was observed by Goeppert in 1917 in an infant and siblings, pointing to a heritable basis for the disorder (Goeppert, 1917). It was further characterized in 1935 by Mason and Turner, who introduced the term "chronic galactemia" in describing a patient with failure to thrive, hepatomegaly, proteinuria, and galactosuria, who was successfully treated by removal of milk from the diet (Mason and Turner, 1935). Affected infants generally died in the first months of life unless started on a galactose-free diet early in life. Schwarz and co-workers (1956) first suggested the site of the metabolic block and demonstrated that gal-1-p accumulated in blood cells. That same year, Isselbacher et al. (1956) showed that GALT was missing from red blood cells in patients with galactosemia. Subsequently, abnormalities were found in the two other enzymes that are involved in galactose synthesis: galactokinase (GALK) and epimerase. Neither of the last two conditions is common, and neither causes the severe abnormalities seen with GALT deficiency.

EPIDEMIOLOGY

Galactosemia is a rare disorder of carbohydrate metabolism in which there is a deficiency of the enzymes galactose-1-phosphate uridyl transferase (GALT), galactokinase (GALK), or epimerase (Levy and Hammersen, 1978). Based on the screening of 19 million neonates by 1987 in the United States, the incidence is 1 in 62,000 births. Worldwide the highest incidence is 1 in 26,000 (Ireland) and the lowest is 1 in 667,000 in Japan; the range is from 35,000 to 89,000 in 10 other countries where data is available (Levy, 1993). Because GALT deficiency is the most common, the majority of case studies focus on this condition; GALK and epimerase deficiencies are extremely rare. Besides the GALT mutations that produce severe galactosemia, there are alleles that may confuse estimates of gene frequency for galactosemia. The most important of these is the Duarte variant. GALT activity expressed by the Duarte allele is approximately one half of that expressed by the normal allele (Beutler, 1993). Eleven percent of the Caucasian population are heterozygous for the Duarte allele.

CLINICAL FEATURES AND COGNITIVE/BEHAVIORAL PHENOTYPE

Clinical Features

Galactosemic infants usually appear normal at birth, but lose more weight than their normal peers when milk is introduced and fail to regain their birth weight. Symptoms ordinarily occur the second half of the first week of life after initiating milk feeding; if milk is withheld, the initial symptoms are milder. Early symptoms include food refusal, vomiting, jaundice, lethargy, hepatomegaly, edema, an increase in intracranial pressure, and ascites. Sepsis is common and may lead to death in the first weeks of life. The cause of increased susceptibility to infection is unknown but may relate to impaired white cell function secondary to the accumulation of galactose metabolites (Levy et al., 1977). Death may ensue within days from liver and kidney failure. In addition, nuclear cataracts of the eyes may appear within days or weeks and become irreversible. Aldose reductase, which is involved in an accessory metabolic pathway in the reduction of free galactose leading to the production of galactitol, has been implicated in both lenticular cataract development and cerebral edema.

Clinical expression can be variable; milder cases may show vague digestive problems, retarded physical and mental development, hepatic enlargement and cataracts, as well as milk intolerance. These patients, who make up about 15% of patients identified on newborn screening, appear to be variants of galactosemia and may follow a milder clinical course (Donnell, 1993).

Infants have been delivered with severe manifestations of galactosemia, suggesting prenatal onset of the disease *in utero*. Galactose-1-phosphate is present in cord blood of all affected infants, suggesting this compound may accumulate in fetal tissue and might affect development.

An association between galactosemia, infertility, and premature ovarian failure has been reported although a galactose-restricted diet was initiated early in infancy (Hoefnaegel, Wurster-Hili, and Child, 1979; Kaufman et al., 1986; Kaufman et al., 1981). The etiology of premature ovarian failure is unknown, although Kaufman et al. (1993) suggest it may be linked to a deficiency in ovarian uridine diphosphate galactose (UDPgal) which might lead to ovarian damage due to decreased synthesis of essential macromolecules containing galactose. Apparently, even minor variants of galactosemia are associated with infertility and premature menopause (Cramer et al., 1989). However, despite ovarian damage, a few women have achieved fertility and delivered; in at least one instance, after giving birth to a normal child, a 21-year-old galactosemic woman developed secondary amenorrhea. Another woman had three children. Other patients with GALK deficiency who have been examined had normal levels of erythrocyte UDPgal and have normal ovarian function (Kaufman et al., 1993).

Neurological complications may occur in galactosemia despite well-documented dietary control. Nelson et al. (1992) reported on magnetic resonance imaging studies in 67 transferase-deficient galactosemic patients (31 male, 36 female; median age 10 years). Among these, 22 patients had mild cerebral atrophy, 8 had cerebellar atrophy, and 11 showed multiple small hyperintense lesions in the cerebral white matter on T2-weighted images. Those patients over 1 year of age did not show the normal reduction in peripheral white matter signal intensity that is expected developmentally on T2-weighted images. The authors suggest this abnormal signal intensity may be due to altered myelin formation that is secondary to the inability to make adequate and/or normal galactocerebroside. Thus it appears that delay in myelination with a more generalized diminution in white matter may be characteristic of galactosemia. Koch et al. (1992) describe two siblings who are mentally retarded and have a progressive neurological disorder characterized by hypotonia, hyperreflexia, dysarthria, ataxia, and a postural and kinetic tremor. Magnetic resonance imaging showed moderate cortical atrophy, a lack of normal myelination, and multifocal areas of increased signal (T2-weighting) in the periventricular white matter.

Cognitive and Behavioral Phenotype

Intellectual development, with careful dietary management, is generally reported to be in the normal range. However, compared to their normal siblings, some affected children may have a slight reduction in intelligence; others test in the mild to moderate range of mental retardation (Fishler, 1993). Visuospatial deficits commonly occur (Komrower, 1982; Komrower and Lee, 1970). Waggoner, Buist, and Donnell (1990), in a survey of 350 cases, found developmental delay, speech abnormality, ovarian dysfunction, and growth retardation on follow-up that was independent of the time after birth when dietary restriction had begun.

Waisbren et al. (1983) studied 8 children and found that all of them had delayed speech or early speech problems, and all but one had later language disorders in at least one area. These deficits were most apparent in expressive language where immediate recall and word retrieval skills were most clearly affected. Receptive language skills were relatively intact. Speech production (articulation) problems were found in 5 of the 8 children and were linked to both motor planning and language deficits in word retrieval. Nelson (1993) also reports articulation problems in 62% (15 of 24) of the children with galactosemia he tested. He describes verbal dyspraxia, i.e., lack of ability to "plan and direct a series of coordinated movements" involving speech in 54% (13 of 24), and other forms of developmental or functional articulation problems in 8% (2 of 24). In addition, he notes the presence of both gross and fine motor problems, difficulty in sequencing, and difficulty performing rapid alternating movements.

Fishler et al. (1966, 1972) and Fishler (1993) reported on assessments of 71 treated patients with galactosemia—38 females and 33 males who have been followed for up to 35 years since initial diagnosis. Findings are reported in infants and preschool children (11 months to 5½ years), school-age children (6 to 16 years), and adults (17 to 40 years). Intelligence tests of siblings and parents were carried out for comparison. For the infant and preschool group (19 subjects), the mean development quotient (DQ)/IQ was 93 with a range of 44 to 122. Mental retardation was found in some cases despite good dietary control.

The IQ range was 50 to 112, with a mean of 85, for the children and adolescents (29 subjects). All attended school but only half (14 of 29) of secondary school students were in their appropriate grade placement. Five were held back but in regular classes; 5 were in classes for the mentally retarded (3 mild and 2 moderate), and 1 was in a class for aphasic children. Two thirds (20 of 29) demonstrated mild to moderate visual-perceptual problems that affected their school performance. Difficulties were noted in handwriting, reading, and arithmetic, requiring special class programs or tutoring. Almost half (13 in 29) had abnormal EEGs. Social and personal adjustment was poor, and both shyness and poor social skills were noted. Hyperactivity was not reported by teachers. Parents reported dependency in the younger children and problems in adolescents' maintaining the diet. The social restrictions related to the diet in conjunction with possible temperamental features and the increased risk of learning problems are risk factors for behavioral disorder.

The IQ varied from 58 to 111, with a mean of 89, in those between ages 17 to 40 years. Of the 6 youngest subjects who were in high school, 3 were in special education classes and 3 were in regular classes. Only 4 of the high school subjects pursued higher education in college or graduate school. Visual-perceptual problems were found in 50% of the older subjects but tended to be less severe than in younger subjects. Twenty-eight percent had abnormal EEGs. In the 20 oldest patients, when the IQs for 11 males and 9 females were compared using the WAIS, a statistically significant difference was found between males (IQ of 97) and females (IQ of 84). Both male verbal (97) and performance (101) scores were significantly higher than the female verbal (84) and performance (85) scores. The lowest subscale scores for both sexes were in arithmetic and block design. Significant group differences in intelligence were not found between patients and family members. In 33 parent pairs, the IQ range for fathers was 87 to 138 (mean 110) and for mothers 70 to 127 (mean 106). The IQ range of heterozygote siblings was 91 to 123 (mean 105) for boys and 86 to 125 (mean 105) for girls. Normal siblings tested essentially in the same IQ range as the heterozygote siblings.

Studies of emotional and behavioral development have demonstrated that children who are treated have increased rates of behavioral problems (Fishler et al., 1966). The younger children tend to be fearful and anxious. Older children were reported to be aggressive and to have interpersonal difficulties. The behavioral difficulties may arise as a result of residual brain dysfunction and as a response to psychosocial problems in the family and at school because of the need to follow a very specific dietary regimen.

ETIOLOGY

Genetics

Galactosemia is transmitted as an autosomal recessive condition. Enzyme methods are available to confirm the diagnosis and to identify carriers, i.e., heterozygous individuals (Beutler et al., 1966). The gene encoding the human GALT enzyme has been cloned and characterized by Reichardt and Berg (1988). The cDNA sequence was subsequently revised by Flach, Reichardt, and Elsas (1990). This genetic accomplishment provides the means to address fundamental questions that remain unresolved regarding the genetics and pathogenesis of galactosemia.

Several mutations have been identified (Reichardt et al., 1992). Reichardt (1992, 1993) completed molecular analyses of the DNA, mRNA, and protein in 15 galactosemic patients and found that galactosemia was predominantly associated with missense mutations (point mutations that change a codon specific for one amino acid and specify another amino acid instead). There were nine missense mutations, three splicing mutations, three GALT protein polymorphisms, and one silent nucleotide substitution. The most common mutation, Q188R, has a frequency of only one in four in the patient population examined. Three classes of disease-causing mutations have been reported: CRM+ missense mutations (the most common class), CRM- missense mutations, and splicing mutations. The finding that galactosemia is heterogeneous at the molecular level is consistent with the well-documented clinical variability observed in this disorder. Eight of the nine galactosemia missense mutations occur in evolutionarily well-conserved domains, indicating they may affect functionally and/or structurally important residues.

Metabolic Aspects and Proposed Pathochemistry

The metabolism of galactose requires that it be phosphorylated and isomerized to glucose. The three enzymes, GALK, GALT, and epimerase, are needed to convert galactose-1-phosphate to glucose-1-phosphate, which is subsequently metabolized to glucose or glycogen. In addition to its importance as a major source of calories in the newborn, galactose and its derivatives serve as important components of glycolipids and glycoprotein (Beutler, 1993).

Several hypotheses have been proposed to account for poor long-term outcome because the pathochemistry is only partially understood. The first by Gitzelmann and Steinmann (1984) suggests there is continuous self-intoxication resulting from the endogenous production of galactose-1-phosphate from UDPgal. Because UDP-gal 4′-epimerase allows galactose to be generated from glucose, transferase-deficient patients can form galactose-1-phosphate in the absence of exogenous galactose. This mechanism might lead to self-intoxication. In addition, the accumulation of other toxic intermediators from abnormal galactose metabolism may, in an unknown way, adversely affect other metabolic processes. For example, galactitol has been implicated in cataract formation (Gitzelmann and Steinmann, 1984), but this has not been fully substantiated. The second theory, proposed by Ng and colleagues (1989), based on findings that there is a depletion of cellular UDPgal in galactosemia (Holton, de la Cruz, and Levy, 1993), postulates an impairment of the synthesis of complex substances containing galactose. Because uridine sugar complexes act as galactose donors, a deficiency of UDPgal might influence the synthesis of gangliosides and other molecules involved in the functioning of the central nervous system (Beutler, 1993). Finally, the emergence of the disease may involve both of these metabolic mechanisms and others as well; no single abnormality may be responsible for toxicity when it occurs. Various factors may produce a synergistic toxicity that may be more important at one time in prenatal or postnatal development than another.

Animal Studies

When rats are fed high concentrations of galactose, they may develop cataracts and show changes in peripheral nerves; however, this approach only simulates the disorder in part because it does not offset the amount of product available for further metabolism (Beutler, 1993). Eliseeva, Soloveva, and Morozkova (1975) studied patterns of behavior and neural processes in rats with symptoms of galactosemia. Impairment of neural processes, particularly in "internal inhibition," in galactosemic rats was established. Galactosemic rats, in comparison with a galactose-resistant rat substrain, showed evidence of low conditioning rates and a lower level of responding in a two-way shuttle-box avoidance test. Significant changes in motor activity in repeated open-field testing were not found in galactosemic rats. In the active avoidance acquisition task analysis, the capacity for the retention of the acquired task was impaired, suggesting problems in memory storage in the galactosemic animals.

NEWBORN SCREENING

Neonatal screening for PKU began in 1962. The success of that screening program led to the introduction of neonatal screening for other disorders, and in 1963 an assay was developed that was subsequently used to screen newborns for galactosemia. The advantages of screening is that it lowers mortality, provides data that may be used for future prenatal diagnosis, reduces hospital costs related to sepsis and other disease-related complications, and allows the early introduction of improved treatments as they become available (Koch, 1993).

Several approaches have been used for galactosemia screening. These include the use of microorganisms to determine the amount of galactose in the blood sample, direct measurement of the activity of the GALT enzyme, and direct enzymatic techniques for measuring galactose and gal-1-phosphate. Levy (1993) suggests that as microplate technology, which can be automated, replaces other technology for newborn screening of galactosemia, direct techniques that measure gal-1-phosphate may become the method of choice. Following screening, secondary tests are necessary to establish which enzyme is deficient.

TREATMENT

Parents should be fully informed about the clinical features of the disease, its mode of inheritance, and treatment. Prenatal diagnosis is feasible to allow pregnancy options to families at risk (Ng et al., 1977). Because the lactose in milk is the primary source of galactose for the infant, milk and its products must be withheld from the infant's diet. The removal of galactose from the diet causes a rapid improvement of the acute toxicity syndrome in the first 24 hours. Brain damage can be largely prevented by the administration of a galactose-free or a low galactose diet beginning shortly after birth.

The diet is highly restrictive and is necessary throughout the individual's life. Therapy for galactosemia requires the total elimination of galactose from the diet. During the perinatal period, lactose-containing formula may be replaced with soy formula that contains very small amounts of galactose in unusable form or special formulas that are essentially free of galactose such as nutramigen. Dietary treatment is most effective for galactokinase deficiency. Strict dietary maintenance may lead to psychosocial problems; consequently, ongoing counseling is essential for the child and the parents. Both family therapy and behavior therapy interventions may be needed to address behavioral disorders. For school management (Gershen, 1975), regular developmental and speech/language testing is essential; speech therapy and special education are commonly required. Structured individual psychiatric interviews to ascertain potential DSM-IV diagnoses in patients with galactosemia or their parents have not been reported.

The response to dietary treatment has led to the belief that galactosemia is a relatively benign disorder which can be easily treated and that patients respond well to dietary maintenance. Neonatal symptoms do respond well, but long-term outcome continues to be problematic. Regardless of how early the treatment is begun, many affected persons develop complications, e.g., speech defects, reduced intelligence, neuropsychological deficits, learning disability, ovarian failure (in females), and, in some cases, late neurological syndromes (ataxia syndrome) despite early dietary restriction (Segal, 1992).

These long-term effects have been attributed to possible toxicity occurring both *in utero* and postnatally. Metabolic questions in regard to possible chronic toxicity due to accumulation of galactose from the breakdown of endogenous sources and depletion of essential metabolites of galactose will need to be resolved to improve outcome. Segal (1992) suggests that several new therapeutic strategies be considered. These include augmentation of residual transferase activity (folic acid, progesterone), interdiction of aldose alternative pathways (aldose reductase inhibition), replacement of depleted metabolites (inositol, nucleotide sugars, e.g., uridine), and gene therapy with replacement of the defective uridyl transferase gene (a prospect that currently is a long way off).

SUMMARY

Dietary galactose restriction had long been considered a satisfactory treatment for galactosemia because early and well-treated children with galactosemia show satisfactory general health and growth and, for the most part, test in the normal range on cognitive tests. However, despite early diagnosis and the institution of the galactose-free diet, there appears to be an inability to fully prevent mental retardation, ovarian failure, speech deficits, and visual-perception problems using the traditional dietary approach. In addition, there have been reports of neurologic ataxia syndromes in older patients despite adequate dietary maintenance, and problems in social adaptation have become apparent as larger numbers of patients are studied. These findings have led to renewed interest in the pathochemistry of the disorder, both prenatally and postnatally, the behavioral phenotype, and the long-term psychosocial outcome. New forms of treatment are being evaluated that may reduce these long-term complications.

REFERENCES

Beutler, E. (1993). Disorders of galactose metabolism. In R.N. Rosenberg, S.B. Prusiner, S. DiMauro, R.L. Barchi, and L.M. Kunkel (eds.), *The molecular and genetic basis of neurological disease,* p. 123. Butterworth- Heinemann, Boston.

______, Baluda, M.C., Sturgeon, P., and Day, P.W. (1966). The genetics of galactose-1-phosphate uridyl transferase deficiency. *Journal of Laboratory and Clinical Medicine,* 68:646–658.

Cramer, D.W., Harlow, B.L., Barbieri, R.L., and Ng, W.G. (1989). Galactose-1-phosphate uridyl transferase activity associated with age at menopause and reproductive history. *Fertility and Sterility,* 51:609–615.

Donnell, G. (1993). Clinical aspects and historical perspectives of galactosemia. In G.N. Donnell, F. de la Cruz, R. Koch, and H.L. Levy (eds.), *Galactosemia: New frontiers in research,* pp. 1–18. U.S. Department of Health and Human Services, Washington, DC. NIH Publication No. 93–3438.

Eliseeva, A.G., Soloveva, N.A., and Morozkova, T.S. (1975). [Higher nervous activity in rats with symptoms of hereditary galactosemia]. Issledovanie vysshei nervnoi deiatel'nosti krys, obladaiushchikh priznakami nasledstvennoi galaktozemii. *Genetika,* 11:72–79.

Fishler, K. (1993). Intellectual development in galactosemia. In G.N. Donnell, F. de la Cruz, R. Koch, and H.L. Levy (eds.), *Galactosemia: New frontiers in research,* pp. 53–64. U. S. Department of Health and Human Services, Washington, DC. NIH Publication No. 93–3438.

______, Donnell, G.N., Bergren, W.R., and Koch, R. (1972). Intellectual and personality development in children with galactosemia. *Pediatrics,* 50:412–419.

______, Koch, R., Donnell, G., and Graliker, B.V. (1966). Psychological correlates in galactosemia. *American Journal of Mental Deficiency,* 71:116–125.

Flach, J.E., Reichardt, J.K., and Elsas, L.J.,II. (1990). Sequence of a cDNA encoding human galactose-1-phosphate uridyl transferase. *Molecular and Biological Medicine,* 7:365–369.

Gershen, J.A. (1975). Galactosemia: A psychosocial perspective. *Mental Retardation,* 13:20–23.

Gitzelmann, R., and Steinmann, B. (1984). Galactosemia: How does long-term treatment change the outcome? *Enzyme,* 32:37–46.

Goeppert, F. (1917). Galaktosurie nach Milchzuckergabe bei angeborenem, familiarem, chronischem Leberleiden. *Klinische Wochenschrift,* 54:473–477.

Hoefnaegel, D., Worster-Hili, D., and Child, E.L. (1979). Ovarian failure in galactosemia. *Lancet,* ii:1197.

Holton, J. B., de la Cruz, F., and Levy, H.L. (1993). Galactosemia: the uridine diphosphate galactose deficiency-uridine treatment controversy. *Journal of Pediatrics,* 123: 1009–1014.

Isselbacher, K.J., Anderson, E.P., Kurahashi, E., and Kalckar, H.M. (1956). Congenital galactosemia, a single enzymatic block in galactose metabolism. *Science,* 123:635–636.

Kaufman, F.R., Donnell, G.N., Roe, T.F., and Kogut, M.D. (1986). Gonadal function in patients with galactosemia. *Journal of Inherited Metabolic Disease,* 9:140–146.

______, Kogut, M.D., Donnell, G.N., Goebelsmann, V., March, C., and Koch, R. (1981). Hypergonadotropic hypogonadism in female patients with galactosemia. *New England Journal of Medicine,* 304:994.

______, Ng, W.G., Xu, Y.K., and Donnell, G.N. (1993). Ovarian dysfunction and galactosemia. In G.N. Donnell, F. de la Cruz, R. Koch, and H.L. Levy (eds.), *Galactosemia: New frontiers in research,* pp. 99–107. U.S. Department of Health and Human Services, Washington, DC. NIH Publication No. 93–3438.

Koch, R. (1993). Panel discussion: Biochemical considerations. In G.N. Donnell, F. de la Cruz, R. Koch and H.L. Levy (eds.), *Galactosemia: New frontiers in research,* pp. 195–196. U. S. Department of Health and Human Services, Washington, DC. NIH Publication No. 93–3438.

Koch, T.K., Schmidt, K.A., Wagstaff, J.E., Won, G.N., and Packman, S. (1992). Neurologic complications in galactosemia. *Pediatric Neurology,* 8:3.

Komrower, G.M. (1982). Galactosemia–thirty years on. The experience of a generation. *Journal of Inherited Metabolic Disease,* 5:96–104.

______, and Lee, D.H. (1970). Long-term follow-up of galactosaemia. *Archives of Diseases in Childhood,* 45:367–373.

Lehotay, D.C. (1993). Current controversies about galactosemia. *Clinical Biochemistry,* 26:69–74.

Levy, H.L. (1993). Newborn screening for galactosemia. In G.N. Donnell, F. de la Cruz, R. Koch, and H.L. Levy (eds.), *Galactosemia: New frontiers in research,* p. 36. U.S. Department of Health and Human Services, Washington, DC. NIH Publication No. 93–3438.

______, and Hammersen, G. (1978). Newborn screening for galactosemia and other galactose metabolic defects. *Journal of Pediatrics,* 92:871–877.

______, Sepe, S.J., Shih, V.E., Vawter, G.F., and Klein, J.O. (1977). Sepsis due to Escherichia coli in neonates with galactosemia. *New England Journal of Medicine,* 297:823–825.

Mason, H.H., and Turner, M.E. (1935). Report of case with studies on carbohydrates. *American Journal of Diseases of Childhood,* 50:359–374.

Nelson, C.D. (1993). Speech disorders. In G.N. Donnell, F. de la Cruz, R. Koch, and H.L. Levy (eds.), *Galactosemia: New frontiers in research,* pp. 65–67. U.S. Department of Health and Human Services, Washington, DC. NIH Publication No. 93–3438.

Nelson, M.D., Jr., Wolff, J.A., Cross, C.A., Donnell, G.N., and Kaufman, F.R. (1992). Galactosemia: Evaluation with MR imaging. *Radiology,* 184:255–261.

Ng, W.G., Donnell, G.N., Bergren, W.R., Alfi, O., and Golbus, M.S. (1977). Prenatal diagnosis of galactosemia. *Clinica Chimica Acta,* 74:227–235.

______, Xu, Y.K., Kaufman, F.R., and Donnell, G.N. (1989). Deficit of uridine diphosphate galactose in galactosemia. *Journal of Inherited Metabolic Disease,* 12:257–266.

Reichardt, J.K. (1992). Genetic basis of galactosemia. *Human Mutation,* 1:190–196.

______. (1993). Galactosemia is caused by missense mutations: Molecular studies and implications for therapy. In G.N. Donnell, F. de la Cruz, R. Koch, and H.L. Levy (eds.), *Galactosemia: New frontiers in research,* pp. 199–213. U.S. Department of Health and Human Services, Washington DC. NIH Publication No. 93–3438.

______, Belmont, J.W., Levy H.L., and Woo, S.L.C. (1992). Characterization of two missense mutations in human galactose-1-phosphate uridyl transferase: Different molecular mechanisms for galactosemia. *Genomics,* 12:596–600.

______, and Berg, P. (1988). Cloning and characterization of a cDNA encoding human galactose-1-phosphate uridyl transferase. *Molecular and Biological Medicine,* 5:107–122.

Segal, S. (1992). The enigma of galactosemia. *International Pediatrics,* 7:75–82.

Schwarz, V., Goldberg, L., Komrower, G.M., and Holzel, A. (1956). Some disturbances of erythrocyte metabolism in galactosaemia. *Biochemistry Journal,* 62:34–40.

von Reuss, A. (1908). Sugar excretion in infancy. *Wiener Medicinische Wochenschrift,* 58:799–808.

Waggoner, D.D., Buist, N.R.M., and Donnell, G.N. (1990). Long-term prognosis in galactosemia: Results of a survey of 350 cases. *Journal of Inherited Metabolic Diseases,* 13:802–818.

Waisbren, S.E., Norman, T.R., Schnell, R.R., and Levy, H.L. (1983). Speech and language deficits in early-treated children with galactosemia. *Journal of Pediatrics,* 102:75–77.

11.5 Adrenoleukodystrophy

Adrenoleukodystrophy (ALD) is an inborn error of metabolism that results in the accumulation of saturated very long-chain fatty acids (VLCFA) in several target organs. It is the most common inherited peroxisomal disorder, affecting 1 in 15,000 to 20,000 Caucasian males. It is a progressive, nonselective condition involving the central and peripheral nervous systems and is characterized by progressive demyelination and adrenal insufficiency (Conner and Rosenberg, 1992). Early in the course of the illness, problems in learning and behavior may lead to psychiatric referral. Subsequently, changes in cognition and the manifestations of spinocerebellar degeneration, progressive limb and truncal ataxia, slurred speech, and spasticity, become evident.

This chapter describes the history, clinical features and behavioral phenotype, diagnosis, etiology, and treatment of adrenoleukodystrophy.

HISTORY

Adrenoleukodystrophy was originally reported in 1923 by Siemerling and Creutzfeldt. These authors emphasized the progressive leukodystrophy and skin pigmentation abnormalities. In 1970 Blaw introduced the term that is generally now used, "adrenoleukodystrophy." The characteristic cytoplasmic inclusions in the adrenal cortex in Schwann cells were described by Powers and Schaumberg (1974). These inclusions were demonstrated by Johnson, Schaumberg, and Powers (1976) to be saturated very long-chain (C24 or longer) cholesterol esters. Moser et al. (1984a) have provided an extensive description of the biochemistry, diagnosis, and treatment, based on a survey of over 300 cases.

CLINICAL FEATURES AND BEHAVIORAL PHENOTYPE

There are several characteristic phenotypes of adrenoleukodystrophy (ALD): X-linked childhood onset ALD, X-linked adult onset adrenomyeloneuropathy, neonatal ALD, and adrenal insufficiency (Addison's disease) without neurological disease (ADO) (Goto et al., 1986; Moser et al., 1984a). Heterozygote female carriers may exhibit some neurological symptoms (Moser et al., 1984a; O'Neill et al., 1984; Simpson, Rodda, and Reinecke, 1987). In addition, prolonged evoked response latencies and elevated very long-chain fatty acids have been demonstrated in some asymptomatic carriers.

The most common form is the X-linked childhood ALD whose age of onset is ordinarily between 4 and 8 years. The initial symptoms include difficulty with auditory and visual processing along with early changes in behavior. These progress to impaired vision, pseudobulbar affect, ataxia, dementia, and spastic quadriparesis. In 20% of involved males, Addison's disease is evident (Moser et al., 1984a). In the adult onset form, adrenomyeloneuropathy (AMN) symptoms appear in the second or third decade of life and progress more slowly. The neonatal form shows greater involvement of the gray matter and presents with seizures, severe mental retardation, retinopathy, and hepatomegaly.

Behavioral Phenotype

The child with ALD usually comes to medical attention during infancy or early childhood. In the X-linked childhood onset form, subtle changes in affect, behavior, and attention are among the early symptoms of the leukodystrophies (Brown et al., 1985). Frequently, nonmedical management is attempted by schools, parents, or counselors prior to the discovery of the specific diagnosis. In some instances, psychiatric disorders are diagnosed and children are placed in school programs for the emotionally disturbed, or in other instances, in programs for learning disabilities. Learning disabilities and attention deficit, with or without hyperactivity, may be early diagnoses. A common problem is an alteration of the sleep-wake cycle; the child may have difficulty getting to sleep and staying asleep. Muscle spasms may awaken the child at night as part of the disease.

DIAGNOSIS

In addition to the clinical features, both CT and MRI scans are important in case assessment. CT imaging shows reduced attenuation of the cerebral white matter, particularly involving the parietal and occipital lobes. On MRI, increased signal is found in the white matter on T2-weighted images. Motor and sensory nerve conduction velocities are reduced. Central and peripheral latencies are prolonged for visual-evoked potentials. Saturated very long-chain fatty acids are elevated in the sphingomyelin of plasma and cultured fibroblasts in each of the forms of ALD, including the carrier state (Moser et al., 1984a; Sakai et al., 1988).

ETIOLOGY

Genetics

The principal biochemical abnormality in ALD is the accumulation of very long-chain fatty acids (VLCFA) because of impaired β-oxidation in peroxisomes. The childhood onset ALD and adult onset AMN are inherited as X-linked recessive disorders, but the neonatal form is inherited as an autosomal recessive disorder. The possibility of clinical disease in female carriers is explained by the Lyon hypothesis of random inactivation. There is a close linkage between ALD and the genetic loci for glucose-6-phosphate-dehydrogenase. It maps close to the red/green color pigment gene cluster in Xq28. Sack and Morrell (1993) identified overlapping deletions in patients that specifically implicate this region as the likely site for the ALD gene. Mosser et al. (1993, 1994) concluded that the gene coding for the normal oxidation of VLCFA-CoA, VLCFA-CoA synthetase, could be the candidate gene for ALD. These authors used positional cloning to identify a gene partially deleted in 6 of 85 patients with ALD. The authors isolated complementary DNAs by exon connection and screening of DNA libraries. The deduced protein sequence (ALDP) shows considerable sequence identity to a peroxisomal membrane protein that is involved in peroxisome biogenesis. ALDP apparently encodes a putative peroxisomal transporter molecule that might be involved in the import of VLCFA-CoA synthetase. Braun et al. (1995) have identified mutations in a gene encoding peroxisomal membrane protein in patients with different clinical expressions of X-ALD, i.e., childhood ALD, AMN, and ADO.

Prenatal diagnosis of ALD is possible by testing for the C26:0 to C22:0 fatty acid ratio in cultured amniocytes. Saturated long-chain fatty acid levels have also been determined in cultured chorionic villi. These two techniques may allow almost 80% detection accuracy in heterozygotes and affected family members. About 15% to 20% of women have false negative tests. It is hoped that with genetic DNA testing, this false negative rate can be substantially improved.

TREATMENT

The alteration of the lipid content of cell constituents has been shown to alter the morphology, physiology, and enzyme function of cell membranes. Medical therapies for ALD are based on reducing dietary intake or in inhibiting synthesis of very long-chain fatty acids. Early dietary therapies, as well as treatment with immunosuppression, were not successful (Kishimoto et al., 1980). Bone marrow transplantation may produce a marked reduction in plasma in very long-chain fatty acids without clinical improvement (Moser et al., 1984b) and may arrest the progression of the disease in selected cases (Aubourg et al., 1990; Moser et al., 1992).

New approaches to dietary treatment have followed Rizzo et al.'s (1989) finding that the synthesis of saturated very long-chain fatty acids was reduced in cultured fibroblasts from ALD patients if they were grown with monounsaturated fatty acids. This procedure resulted in a decrease in cellular C26:0 concentration. As a result of these studies, ALD patients were placed on a diet enriched in oleic acid. A reduction in plasma C26:0 concentration was demonstrated in these cases, and some adult patients with AMN showed improved peripheral nerve conduction velocity on the diet; however, the course of clinical deterioration was not stopped. This regimen was subsequently supplemented by adding erucic acid (C22:1) to those patients who were taking long-term oleic acid. Further reductions were noted in C26:0 levels, and the C26:0 composition of plasma sphingomyelin and phosphatidylcholine could be normalized by 4 months. However, to date, the clinical course of the disease has not been clearly altered (Moser, 1993; Uziel et al., 1991; Wong, 1992), although trials are continuing using this combination of dietary treatments. Maeda et al. (1992) reported a 5-year-old boy with visual, mental, and motor disturbances that were progressive. He was treated with the oleic acid/erucic acid combination. Five months later, his ability to swallow was enhanced and T2-weighted magnetic imaging of the brain showed regression of a high intensity area of the parieto-occipital white matter. Despite single-case reports such as these showing slight clinical improvement, the oleic acid/erucic acid combination has shown limited benefits (Kaplan et al., 1993). Moser (1993), in studies of over 100 patients, found that while on the diet functional impairment may continue to progress slowly in those who have become symptomatic. In 7 cases, lesions progressed on MRI despite the diet. In asymptomatic cases who are still neurologically intact, the question of whether the disease can be postponed or prevented is unresolved. Moser (1993) found that in one patient who began the dietary treatment at age 3 and had excellent dietary control, the severe form of the illness developed. Fifty-three of 61 asymptomatic cases have remained well on a dietary regimen, but the follow-up time is limited. Follow-up studies are complicated by the fact that 50% of untreated patients will not develop the childhood onset form but may develop the adult onset form and would be expected to remain well in childhood regardless of therapy. Another test of the diet involved the use of pattern-reversal visual-evoked responses for the evaluation of visual pathways before and after treatment. Of 108 patients tested, none improved. Bone marrow transplantation may be a more promising avenue of treatment because cells with the gene are transfused. Moreover, now that the gene is identified (Mosser et al., 1993), gene therapy may be possible. Family members must be involved and informed about these advances. The anguish the family experiences has been characterized in the film *Lorenzo's Oil,* which graphically depicts the difficulties that families face with this illness.

Clinically, deterioration in function becomes evident as the leukodystrophy progresses so that a major therapeutic focus is to maintain muscle tone and support bulbar muscle functions. All patients have some altered muscle tone at some point in the illness; acute episodic changes in muscle tone present as periodic muscle spasms. Because bulbar muscle control is needed for normal respiratory, toilet, eating, and normal gastrointestinal activity, handling of oral secretions and nutritional support becomes essential. This requires changes in feeding patterns with the introduction of pureed and soft foods. In some instances, as the ability to handle liquids is lost, more invasive approaches, including the use of nasogastric tubes, nasoesophageal tubes, or a gastrostomy, may be required to administer medication, water, and food. As the child becomes more dependent, efforts are needed to help him maintain awareness of what is going on around him. This involves structuring his day and helping him use his remaining abilities to participate in his care.

In the United States, the Education Act for All Handicapped Children ensures that the children have the right to a free and appropriate education. Because children with leukodystrophies have problems in learning and attention and may have cognitive disorders as they grow older, the coordination of school services becomes particularly important. The purpose of the education program is to enhance the quality of life and provide as normal a life as possible. When the child can no longer attend school, home and hospital teaching services are needed and may focus on positioning, handling, and transporting techniques as well as relaxation procedures. Physical therapists and occupational therapists along with a teacher certified to work with the multiply disabled are needed and must coordinate their efforts.

Medication may be needed for a variety of associated problems, including the sleep disorder, the attention deficits, and the treatment of the muscle spasms. The management of these symptoms is often problematic for parents because the child frequently requires one-to-one supervision. As difficulties in understanding and in processing auditory and visual experience, and interpreting what is heard or seen occur, the child requires additional support. The family must fill in the missing information to help the child compensate for his loss of functioning.

From a family's perspective, grief, frustration, and anger about the lack of a specific therapy and the experience of dealing with progressive deterioration affects the patient, the family, the physician, and other professionals who are involved in care. With the introduction of experimental dietary treatments, one must work carefully with the family to minimize discomfort and help them to cope with the inconvenience of the diet and the additional time needed for care.

Work with the family involves symptomatic support in regard to ongoing difficulties in management as they emerge. Continuous supportive counseling is necessary to deal with issues surrounding any confusion or delay in the initial diagnosis, questions about screening of siblings, and day-to-day management. The severity of medical problems is compounded by the necessity of coping with a fatal illness that threatens family functioning. Parent organizations are available and families should be encouraged to contact them. The United Leukodystrophy Foundation publishes a newsletter for parents as well as mailings regarding current research, provides opportunities to talk to other parents about patient management, and offers an opportunity to share personal experiences in coping with the disorder. Through helping one another, the family can enhance its own ability to cope with the situation.

As family members begin to understand the severity of the condition and experience more stress, they may begin to withdraw investment in the child. The treating professions play a major role in helping the family maintain confidence and hope. To the degree that the final phase of the illness is adequately supported, the parents may develop a realistic and meaningful perspective on the individual child's life as part of the family and reintegrate.

REFERENCES

Aubourg, P., Blanche, S., Jambaque, I., Rocchiccioli, F., Kalifa, G., Naud-Saudreau, C., Rolland, M.O., Debre, M., Chaussain, J.L., Griscelli, C., Fischer, A., and Bougneres, P. (1990). Reversal of early neurologic and neuroradiologic manifestations of X-linked adrenoleukodystrophy by bone marrow transplantation. *New England Journal of Medicine* 322:1860–1866.

Blaw, M.E. (1970). Melanodermic type leukodystrophy (adrenoleukodystrophy). In P.J. Vinken and G.W. Bruyn (eds.), *Handbook of clinical neurology,* Vol. 10, pp. 128–133. American Elsevier, New York.

Braun, A., Ambach, H., Kammerer, S., Rolinski, B., Stöckler, S., Rabl, W., Gärtner, J., Zierz, S., and Roscher, A.A. (1995). Mutations in the gene for X-linked adrenoleukodystrophy in patients with different clinical phenotypes. *American Journal of Human Genetics,* 56:854–861.

Brown, F.R., III, Stowens, D.W., Harris, J.C., and Moser, H.G. (1985). Leukodystrophies. In R.T. Johnson (ed.), *Current therapy in neurologic disease,* pp. 313–317. B.C. Decker, Philadelphia.

Conner, K.E., and Rosenberg, R.N. (1992). The hereditary ataxias. In N. Rosenberg, S.B.

Prusiner, S. DiMauro, R.L. Barchi, and L.M. Kunkel (eds.), *The molecular and genetic basis of neurological disease*, pp. 705–708. Butterworth-Heinemann, Boston.

Goto, I., Kobayashi, T., Antoku, Y., Tobimatsu, S., and Kuroiwa, Y. (1986). Adrenoleukodystrophy and variants. Clinical neurophysiological and biochemical studies in patients and family members. *Journal of the Neurological Sciences*, 72:103–112.

Johnson, A.B., Schaumberg, H.H., and Powers, J.M. (1976). Histochemical characteristics of the striated inclusions of adrenoleukodystrophy. *Journal of Histochemistry and Cytochemistry*, 24:725–730.

Kaplan, P.W., Tusa, R.J., Shankroff, M.A.S., Heller, J., and Moser, H.W. (1993). Visual evoked potentials in adrenoleukodystrophy: A trial with glycerol trioleate and Lorenzo oil. *Annals of Neurology*, 34:169–174.

Kishimoto, Y., Moser, H.W., Kawamura, Y., Platt, M., Paliante, S.L., and Fenselau, C. (1980). Adrenoleukodystrophy: Evidence that abnormal very long chain fatty acids of brain cholesterol esters are of exogenous origin. *Biochemical and Biophysical Research Communications*, 96:69–76.

Maeda, K., Suzuki, Y., Yajima, S., Asano, J., Yamaguchi, S., Matsumoto, N., Borel, J., Moser, H.W., and Orii, T. (1992). Improvement of clinical and MRI findings in a boy with adrenoleukodystrophy by dietary erucic acid therapy. *Brain and Development*, 14:409–412.

Moser, H. (1993). Lorenzo's oil therapy for adrenoleukodystrophy: A prematurely amplified hope. *Annals of Neurology*, 34:121–122.

______, Moser, A.B., Singh, I., and O'Neill, B.P. (1984a). Adrenoleukodystrophy: Survey of 303 cases: Biochemistry, diagnosis, and therapy. *Annals of Neurology*, 16:628–641.

______, Tutschka, P.J., Brown, F.R., 3rd, Moser, A.E., Yeager, A.M., Singh, I., Mark S.A., Kumar, A.A., McDonnell, J.M., White, C.L., 3rd, Maumenee, I.H., Green, W.R., Powers, J.M., and Santos, G.W. (1984b). Bone marrow transplant in adrenoleukodystrophy. *Neurology*, 34:1410–1417.

______, Moser, A.B., Smith, K.D., Bergin, A., Borel, J., Shankroff, J., Stine, O.C., Merette, C., Ott, J., Krivit, W., and Shapiro, E. (1992). Adrenoleukodystrophy: Phenotypic variability and implications for therapy. *Journal of Inherited Metabolic Disease*, 15:645–664.

Mosser, J., Douar, A.M., Sarde, C.O., Kioschis, P., Feil, R., Moser, H. Poustka, A.M., Mandel, J.L., and Aubourg, P. (1993). Putative X-linked adrenoleukodystrophy gene shares unexpected homology with ABC transporters. *Nature*, 361:726–730.

______, Lutz, Y., Stoeckel, M.E., Sarde, O., Kretz, C., Douar, A.M., and Lopez, J. (1994). The gene responsible for adrenoleukodystrophy encodes a peroxisomal membrane protein. *Human Molecular Genetics*, 3:265–271.

O'Neill, B.P., Moser, H.W., Saxema, K.M., and Marmion, C.C. (1984). Adrenoleukodystrophy: Clinical and biochemical manifestations in carriers. *Neurology*, 34:798–801.

Powers, J.M., and Schaumberg, H.H. (1974). Adrenoleukodystrophy: Similar ultrastructural changes in adrenal cortical cells and Schwann cells. *Archives of Neurology*, 30:406–408.

Rizzo, W.B., Leshner, R.T., Odone, A., Dammann, A.L., Craft, D.A., Jensen, M.E., Jennings, S.S., Davis, S., Jaitly, R., and Sgro, J.A. (1989). Dietary erucic acid therapy for X-linked adrenoleukodystrophy. *Neurology*, 39:1415–1422.

Sack, G.H.,Jr., and Morrell, J.C. (1993). Adrenoleukodystrophy: Overlapping deletions point to a gene location in Xq28. *Biochemical & Biophysical Research Communications*, 191:955–960.

Sakai, T., Antoku, Y., Tsukamoto, K., Imanishi, K., Iwashita, H., and Goto, I. (1988). Carrier detection for adrenoleukodystrophy by high-performance liquid chromatography. *Experimental Neurology*, 100:556–562.

Siemerling, E., and Creutzfeldt, H.C. (1923). Bronzekrankheit and skleroriesende encephalomyelitis (diffuse sclerose). *Archives of Psychiatry*, 68:217–244.

Simpson, R.H.W., Rodda J., and Reinecke, D.J. (1987). Adrenoleukodystrophy in a mother and a son. *Journal of Neurology, Neurosurgery, and Psychiatry*, 50:1165–1172.

Uziel, G., Bertini, E., Bardelli, P., Rimoldi, M., and Gambetti, M. (1991). Experience on therapy of adrenoleukodystrophy and adrenomyeloneuropathy. *Developmental Neuroscience*, 13:274–279.

Wong, V. (1992). Adrenoleukodystrophy in a Chinese boy. *Brain and Development*, 14:276–277.

11.6 Mucopolysaccharidoses

The mucopolysaccharidoses (MPS) are a group of inherited disorders caused by specific enzyme defects leading to the incomplete degradation and storage of mucopolysaccharides (glycosaminogylcans). They are classified according to the precise type of acid hydrolase deficiency. The storage product is heparan sulfate, dermatan sulfate, keratan sulphate, or chondroitin 4/6 sulphates. The majority of these conditions are identifiable by their characteristic facial appearance along with skeletal deformities and physical features associated with involvement of other organ systems. The descriptive term "gargoylism," which was used in the past, graphically illustrates the altered physical appearance that can be of particular psychosocial importance. However, in Sanfilippo syndrome, the most common form, it is not physical appearance but developmental delay and a change in behavior that is most characteristic.

This chapter describes the history, epidemiology, clinical features and phenotype, etiology, and treatment of this group of diseases.

HISTORY

In 1917 Hunter described two brothers who showed the clinical features of the X-linked recessive form of the mucopolysaccharidoses and, in 1919, Hurler reported on two unrelated boys. Following these early reports, all the mucopolysaccharidoses were referred to as "Hurler disease." Other noneponymic names were suggested, such as "gargoylism," because of the characteristic coarse facial features (Ellis, Sheldon and Capon, 1936).

In 1952 Brante demonstrated the storage of mucopolysaccharide in the liver of patients with Hurler disease and coined the term "mucopolysaccharidoses" (Brante, 1952). Subsequently, the characterization of mucopolysaccharides in tissues and urine led to the delineation of the other mucopolysaccharidoses.

Van Hoof and Hers (1964) discovered that the liver from a patient with Hurler disease contained distended lysosomes, suggesting storage, and proposed that the mucopolysaccharidoses are caused by defects of lysosomal hydroxylases. Matalon and Dorfman (1972) identified the enzyme, α-L-iduronidase, in human and other mammalian tissue. They found that deficiency of this enzyme leads to Hurler disease. Following the discovery of this lysosomal defect, enzyme defects in other mucopolysaccharidoses were discovered.

The current classification includes the following syndromes: Hurler (MPS I H), Hurler-Scheie disease (MPS I H/S), Scheie (MPS I S; formerly MPS V), Hunter (MPS II, Types A and B), Sanfilippo (MPS III, Types A–D), Morquio (MPS IV), Maroteaux-Lamy (MPS VI, Types A and B), and Sly (MPS VII). Although ordinarily the presentation is severe, mild variants of several of these disorders have been described, most often in the Hunter and Sanfilippo syndromes.

EPIDEMIOLOGY

The prevalence of the mucopolysaccharidoses has not been fully established. Population studies have been carried out in the Netherlands showing that Sanfilippo A syndrome is the most common form of the mucopolysaccharidoses; the frequency is estimated to be approximately 1 in 24,000 (Van de Kamp et al., 1981). The incidence of Hunter syndrome has been assessed in British Colombia where the incidence is estimated at 1 in 78,000 live births (Lowry and Renwick, 1971), but in Israel, the prevalence was reported to be 1 in 36,000 (Schaap and Bach, 1980).

CLINICAL FEATURES AND PHENOTYPE

The clinical features depend on the specific enzyme deficiency, the end organ involved, and the accumulation of the storage product. If the brain is not involved, there is no mental retardation. Children who are affected with any of the mucopolysaccharidoses have common clinical findings that vary in severity. Affected babies appear normal at birth, with only slight developmental delays in their first 6 to 12 months of life, and early milestones, such as walking and single-word use, may be present. This is followed by developmental delay and physical changes that become apparent by the end of the first year in the severe forms but not until early childhood in the milder variants. Mental deterioration with mental retardation is also characteristic of the severe forms, but intelligence in childhood may be normal in the milder variants. Mental retardation is not found in some children with Hunter syndrome, Hurler-Scheie, Morquio, and Maroteaux-Lamy syndromes. This period of apparent early normality with a later decline in function is important to address with families. The severe form is a particular challenge to family adaptation. Behavioral problems related to central nervous system involvement may be present in the severe forms and may be complicated by poor interpersonal management. Death may occur in the school-age years and early teens in the most severe forms.

In the milder variants, survival into adulthood requires ongoing specific support for the young person who is affected. A specific metabolic diagnosis is particularly important in regard to prognosis and genetic counseling for this group (Epstein et al., 1976). Psychological adaptation to the disability is influenced by the extent of mental retardation and the type of associated physical features; those with milder forms commonly become aware of their differences from others and become distressed about them.

On physical examination, hepatosplenomegaly, chronic nasal discharge, and loud breathing are found. Following the first year of life, the coarse facial features become apparent. (An exception to this, however, is Sanfillipo syndrome wherein the facial appearance may be normal in the early years of life.) The head is ordinarily large, the nasal bridge depressed, the nose is broad, and the mouth is generally open revealing a large tongue. In some of the mucopolysaccharidoses, clouding of the corneas is apparent and ordinarily is detected by 1 year of age. Hearing difficulties are associated and are more pronounced in the Hunter syndrome. Children with most of the mucopolysaccharidoses are growth retarded, although in the Sanfilippo and Scheie syndromes linear growth is not affected.

Sanfilippo Syndrome

A behavioral phenotype of severe behavioral disturbances, particularly hyperactivity, aggression, and sleep disturbances, is characteristic of Sanfilippo syndrome. Based on a review of 62 cases, Cleary and Wraith (1993) describe three phases in the emergence of the neuropsychiatric disorder in the severe form of Sanfilippo syndrome. In the first phase, between ages 1 and 3 to 4 years, a mucopolysaccharidosis is generally not considered in the differential diagnosis because somatic abnormalities are lacking and the child's appearance is normal. However, during this phase, developmental delay becomes apparent, particularly in regard to language development and recurrent ear, nose, and throat disease and bowel disturbances require clinical attention; approximately 50% complete toilet training. Gross motor milestones are ordinarily not delayed.

Behavioral disturbances, heralded by frequent and severe temper tantrums, become apparent around the ages of 3 to 4 years. The child becomes hyperactive and shows a reduction in attention span; increased aggression and destructive behaviors follow. Panic attacks may also be noted when the child is introduced into an unfamiliar environment. Severe sleep disturbances become evident during this phase and are frequently associated with reversal of the day-night sleep pattern. At about 10 years of age, the child enters the third and final stage of the disease. The intensity of the aggressive behavior lessens, but falling is common as the sense of balance is lost. Due to impairment in swallowing, aspiration of food becomes a concern and may lead to the placement of a nasogastric tube. Seizure disorder may occur, commonly of the generalized or tonic clonic type. With increasing spasticity and joint stiffness, most children are wheelchair bound by their mid-teens.

Besides the severe presentation, a mild variant of Sanfilippo syndrome has been described most commonly in the B variant (van Schrojenstein-de Valk and van de Kamp, 1987; Wraith, Danks, and Rogers, 1987). Van Schrojenstein-de Valk and van de Kamp (1987) found that preschool development was apparently normal in 6 of 7 cases, but mental retardation became evident during the elementary school years. None of the mild group developed seizures or disturbances of hearing or vision in this study; however, all had episodes of severe sleep disturbance. In the mild form, behavioral disturbance and nonspecific mental retardation, which may be mild to profound, may be the only features apparent before adulthood; somatic findings are unremarkable. After age 20, dementia and behavioral disturbance emerge and may become severe by the 30s and 40s.

ETIOLOGY

With the exception of Hunter syndrome, the mucopolysaccharidoses are inherited as autosomal recessive diseases; Hunter syndrome is an X-linked recessive disorder. Carrier detection and prenatal diagnoses are available for each of the mucopolysaccharidoses.

TREATMENT

There is no generally agreed-upon effective treatment for the mucopolysaccharidoses. Symptomatic treatment is needed for associated systemic problems that vary among the syndromes. Ear, nose, and throat problems commonly require early intervention. Tonsils and adenoids removal is often necessary, as is the surgical correction of hernias and the provision of shunts for hydrocephalus (depending on the disorder). In those syndromes, such as Sanfilippo, where sleep is affected, the effects of hypnotic medications are variable; both choral hydrate and benzodiazepines have been used. In some instances, physical restraint at night is necessary; an elastic bed belt has been used with some success because it allows freedom of movement in bed while preventing the child from getting out of bed (Cleary and Wraith, 1993).

The hyperactivity and aggressiveness that accompany dementia, in those syndromes with central nervous system involvement, respond poorly to behavior management techniques. However, structured daily routines and the creation of a safe home environment to prevent injury are important. Although there are no reports of systemic drug trials, various pharmacotherapeutic agents, primarily neuroleptics, have been used to target the aggressive behavior. Intervention for associated behavioral problems requires a careful assessment of each individual patient to determine cognitive level and the patient's understanding of the nature of the illness.

Treatment must focus on helping the family adapt to living with a child with a mucopolysaccharidosis. The study described here for families dealing with Hunter syndrome is illustrative of the types of difficulties that are encountered. Psychosocial problems in Hunter syndrome (MPS II), an X-linked recessive condition, were investigated in a national study in the United Kingdom (Young and Harper, 1981). The sample consisted of families who volunteered for interview and cases chosen from hospital records; there was no control group and specific rating instruments were not used. Visits were made to 33 sets of parents with a total of 44 affected sons, 27 with the severe form and 17 with the mild form of the disease. Information about the behavioral pattern in a further 22 boys was obtained from hospital records. Serious behavioral disturbance was reported in 36 of the 38 severely affected boys. The mildly affected boys generally adapted to the condition but often suffered from stigma related to their physical appearance. Adaptation to adult life after leaving special schooling was problematic for the mildly involved, highlighting the need for long-term support for the families and the boys themselves.

In the early onset severe group, the initial behavioral complaint was overactivity, commonly beginning in the second year and continuing to age 8 or 9 years when the disease process progressed to the point that the boys were more inactive and lethargic. Overactivity was noted in 29 of 38 cases along with severe sleep disturbance in 4 and less severe sleep problems in the others. Eighteen were described as oppositional and noted to have tantrums when demands were made of them. Aggression toward others was reported in 16 out of 38 and, in some instances, related to rapid growth in the early years of life. However, 10 boys were described as particularly affectionate and playful. The prevalence of aggression and oppositional behavior in this group is comparable to the prevalence of behavior disorder in other reports of behavioral disturbance in severely mentally retarded persons. The rate of hyperactivity is quite high and reported to be unresponsive to pharmacotherapy.

In the mild form of Hunter syndrome (MPS II), overactivity, sleep disturbance, and violence were not reported. Of 28 mild cases, 3 were oppositional regarding school attendance and two had episodes of aggression during adolescence. In the mild form, the rate of disorder was similar to the rates in the general population. Special services introduced in early childhood may be responsible for the low rate in the mild form and were utilized to maintain the low rate. Although the boys themselves were not interviewed, adjustment to their physical appearance was reported by their parents to be an issue in their teen years.

In regard to family adjustment, Young and Harper found that most families indicated they had received considerable psychosocial support from professionals. Of 21 sets of parents whose children were severely involved, 16 were doing well at the time of interview, despite persistent parental guilt about the disorder. Two mothers had received psychiatric care and one marriage had terminated; however, premorbid parental adjustment before the child's birth is not provided by the authors. For the 12 families whose boys were mildly affected, mothers expressed more distress, perhaps related to the chronicity of the disorder, and three marriages had ended in divorce. Particular concern was expressed by the parents in regard to adult support services.

In another study, Crocker and Cullinane (1972) addressed clinical and educational issues for families and personality development in the children with Hurler syndrome (MPS I) and Hunter syndrome (MPS II). These authors emphasized specific problems faced by families including orthopedic, cardiac, and ENT management and describe the work of an interdisciplinary team involved in the management of three cases. They studied (1) response to the diagnosis; (2) the family's view of long-term needs; (3) reaction to genetic consequences; (4) continuing parental adjustment; (5) household emotional tone; and (6) response to guidance. The first family denied the disorder, did not plan for long-term care, avoided the mental retardation initially, then showed painful acknowledgment, and avoided the genetic issues. The mother became clinically depressed and the father left home, the emotional tone was one of chronic mourning, and the diagnosis was not accepted. The second family showed prolonged bereavement regarding the diagnosis, was cautious about the future, but showed partial acceptance of the mental retardation. Disappointment was evident and they avoided thinking about the hereditary aspect; however, this family did maintain a precarious marriage, and used some support services. The third family accepted the diagnosis, made plans for the future, accommodated to the diagnosis, although they had some difficulty regarding the siblings' anxieties, worked together to cope with problems, oriented their attention to the child, and effectively used medical and psychosocial guidance. The first family remained disorganized, the second was continuously reintegrating, and the third was maturely adapted to the diagnosis.

To facilitate mature adaptation, Crocker and Cullinane (1972) suggest (1) establishment of a relationship with the family early on, preferably before the diagnosis is reached; (2) identification of parental attitudes relevant to positive adaptation and initiation of contact with parent organization and community support groups; (3) formulation of the specifics of the patient care program and developing a clear outline of how they can be accomplished; (4) orientation of the program toward the family's rights and needs; (5) attention to the needs of siblings; (6) continuous regular support for parents; and (7) provision of genetic counseling along with information about new research related to the disorder.

Parent associations have been formed to provide group support to family members to cope with the difficulties associated with these disorders. In a multiethnic culture, transcultural understanding of the parents' belief systems is critical to gain their cooperation for treatment and their participation in parent groups (Handelman, Menahem, and Eisenbruch, 1989).

Bone Marrow Transplantation and Gene Therapy

Bone marrow transplantation has been suggested for this group of diseases, but success has been variable among the individual mucopolysaccharidoses (Hobbs et al., 1981; Krivit and Shapiro, 1991). Bone marrow transplantation is generally effective to reverse upper airway disease and organomegaly, but is generally not effective for brain involvement. Successful bone marrow transplantation may ameliorate coarse facial features and decrease the mucopolysacchariduria. Careful long-term follow-up studies are needed to clarify the optimal age for bone marrow transplantation and its efficacy to reverse the neurological features.

In the future, gene therapy with autologous transplantation may become possible. cDNA for the specific enzymes that are associated with the mucopolysaccharidoses, when available, may make it feasible to introduce normal genes into the hematopoietic system of patients with mucopolysaccharidoses (Desnick and Schuchman, 1991).

REFERENCES

Brante, G. (1952). Gargoylism: A mucopolysaccharidosis. *Scandinavian Journal of Clinical Laboratory Investigation,* 4:43–46.

Cleary, M.A., and Wraith, J.E. (1993). Management of mucopolysaccharidosis Type III. *Archives of Disease in Childhood,* 69:403–406.

Crocker, A.C., and Cullinane, M.M. (1972). Families under stress. The diagnosis of Hurler's syndrome. *Postgraduate Medicine,* 51(3):22–39.

Desnick, R.J., and Schuchman, E.H. (1991). Human gene therapy: Strategies and prospects for inborn errors of metabolism. In R.J. Desnick (ed.), *Treatment of genetic diseases,* pp. 239–259. Churchill-Livingstone, New York.

Ellis, R.W.B., Sheldon, W., and Capon, N.B. (1936). Gargoylism (chondro-osteo-dystrophy, corneal opacities, hepatosplenomegaly, and mental deficiency). *Quarterly Journal of Medicine,* 5:119–139.

Epstein, C.J., Yatziv, S., Neufeld, E., and Liebaers, I. (1976). Genetic counselling for Hunter syndrome [letter]. *Lancet,* ii(7988):73–78.

Handelman, L., Menahem, S., and Eisenbruch, I.M. (1989). Transcultural understanding of a hereditary disorder: Mucopolysaccharidosis VI in a Vietnamese family. *Clinical Pediatrics* 28:470–473.

Hobbs, J.R., Hugh-Jones, K., Barrett, A.J., Bryom, N., Chambers, D., Henry, K., James, D.C., Lucas, C.F., Rogers, T.R., Benson, P.F., Tansley, L.R., Patrick, A.D., Mossman, J., and Young, E.P. (1981). Reversal of clinical features of Hurler's disease and biochemical improvement after treatment by bone-marrow transplantation, *Lancet,* ii:709–712.

Hunter, C. (1917). A rare disease in two brothers. *Proceedings of the Royal Society of Medicine,* 10:104–116.

Hurler, G. (1919). Uber Einen Type multipler Abortunge, Vorwiegent am Skelet System. *Zeitschrift fur Kinderheilkunde,* 24:220–234.

Krivit, W., and Shapiro, E.G. (1991). Bone marrow transplantation for storage diseases. In R.J. Desnick (ed.), *Treatment of genetic diseases,* pp. 203–221. Churchill-Livingstone, New York.

Lowry, R.B., and Renwick, D.H.G. (1971). Relative frequency of Hurler and Hunter syndromes. *New England Journal of Medicine,* 284:221.

Matalon, R., and Dorfman, A. (1972). Hurler's syndrome: Alpha-L-iduronidase deficiency. *Biochemistry Biophysics Research Communications,* 47:959–964.

Schaap, T., and Bach, G. (1980). Incidence of mucopolysaccharidoses in Israel: Is Hunter disease a "Jewish disease"? *Human Genetics,* 56:221.

Van de Kamp, J.J.P., Niermeijer, M.F., VonFingura, K., and Giesberts, M.A.H. (1981). Genetic heterogeneity and clinical variability in the Sanfilippo syndrome (types A,B, and C). *Clinical Genetics,* 20:152.

Van Hoof, F., and Hers, H.G. (1964). The ultrastructure of hepatic cells in Hurler's disease (gargoylism). *Comptes Rendus Hebdomadaires Séances de L'Académie de Sciences,* 259:1281–1283.

van Schrojenstein-de Valk, H.M., and van de Kamp, J.J. (1987). Follow-up on seven adult patients with mild Sanfilippo B disease. *American Journal of Medical Genetics,* 28:125–129.

Wraith, J.E., Danks, D.M., and Rogers, J.G. (1987). Mild Sanfilippo syndrome: A further cause of hyperactivity and behavioural disturbance. *Medical Journal of Australia,* 147:450–451.

Young, I.D., and Harper, P.S. (1981). Psychosocial problems in Hunter's syndrome. *Child Care Health Development,* 7:201–209.

CHAPTER 12.1

BEHAVIORAL TOXICITY/GESTATIONAL SUBSTANCE ABUSE

12.1 Fetal Alcohol Syndrome

Fetal alcohol syndrome (FAS) is one of the most commonly recognized causes of mental retardation. Yet alcohol exposure during the prenatal period is preventable if recommended guidelines regarding alcohol use are followed by mothers. The economic cost of fetal alcohol syndrome has been estimated, taking into account growth deficiency, the need to surgically repair structural deficits, and the treatment of mental retardation and perceptual and learning problems, to be at least $320 million a year in the United States (Abel and Sokol, 1987). Mental retardation alone, related to fetal alcohol syndrome, may account for as much as 11% of the annual cost of all mentally retarded institutionalized residents in the United States and 5% of the cost of all congenital anomalies (Charness, Simon, and Greenberg, 1989). The psychosocial cost is substantial.

This chapter describes the history, epidemiology, clinical features, behavioral phenotype, natural history, etiology, and treatment of fetal alcohol syndrome.

HISTORY

In 1968 Lemoine et al. described anomalies observed in 127 children of alcoholic parents, thus emphasizing effects of alcohol on the developing fetus (Lemoine et al., 1968). Jones et al. (1973) outlined the pattern of malformation in the offspring of chronic alcoholic mothers and described the characteristics of the fetal alcohol syndrome. Subsequently, it has become apparent that prenatal alcohol exposure is associated with a more extensive range of abnormalities which include physical, cognitive, and behavioral dysfunction.

EPIDEMIOLOGY

Fetal alcohol syndrome is a common cause of mental retardation with a worldwide incidence of approximately 1.9 in 1,000 live births (Abel, 1990; Abel and Sokol, 1987). When those children who are less severely involved are included, the estimated incidence may reach 1 in 300 live births (Olegard et al., 1979). Despite its frequency, the syndrome may go unrecognized because physicians may not systematically inquire about alcohol use (Donovan, 1991) and may not recognize the extensive spectrum of the effects of prenatal exposure (Abel, 1990; Little et al., 1990).

CLINICAL FEATURES

Over 80% of children with fetal alcohol syndrome show prenatal and postnatal growth deficiency, microcephaly, infantile irritability, mild to moderate mental retardation, and a characteristic facial appearance (Clarren and Smith,

1978; Jones, 1986; Jones et al., 1973). Approximately half are poorly coordinated, hypotonic, and have attention deficits. An additional 20% to 50% have other birth defects including eye and ear anomalies and cardiac anomalies. Those children who are exposed to alcohol *in utero* who do not show growth retardation or congenital anomalies may demonstrate more subtle changes, such as increased risk for attention deficit disorder with hyperactivity, motor clumsiness, speech disorders, and fine motor impairment (Streissguth, 1986). These more subtle abnormalities are referred to as "fetal alcohol effects." Table 12.1–1 indicates the characteristics of fetal alcohol syndrome and also lists the fetal alcohol effects.

BEHAVIORAL PHENOTYPE

The behavioral phenotype is characterized by subnormal intellectual functioning, particularly in arithmetic, and difficulty understanding cause and effect and generalizing from one situation to another. Inattention, poor concentration, impaired judgment, memory deficits, and problems in abstract reasoning are also characteristic. Behavioral problems related to impulsivity and hyperactivity include oppositional and conduct disorders.

NATURAL HISTORY

Fetal alcohol syndrome is not only a childhood disorder; the cognitive and behavioral effects and psychosocial problems may persist through adolescence into adulthood. Streissguth et al. (1991) studied the manifestations of fetal alcohol syndrome in 61 adolescents and adults. After puberty, the faces of patients with fetal alcohol syndrome or those who had fetal alcohol effects were not as distinctive. The patients generally remained short and microcephalic but their weight was close to the mean for age. The average IQ was 68, although the range of IQ

Table 12.1–1. Features Observed in Fetal Alcohol Syndrome/Fetal Alcohol Effects

Growth
- Prenatal and postnatal growth deficiency†
- Decreased adipose tissue‡

Performance
- Mental retardation†
- Developmental delay
- Fine-motor dysfunction
- Infant irritability,† child hyperactivity,‡ and poor attention span
- Speech problems
- Poor coordination, hypotonia‡
- Cognitive, behavioral, and psychosocial problems

Craniofacial
- Microcephaly†
- Short palpebral fissures†
- Ptosis§
- Retrognathia in infancy†
- Maxillary hypoplasia‡
- Hypoplastic long or smooth philtrum†
- Thin vermillion of upper lip†
- Short upturned nose‡
- Micrognathia in adolescence‡

Skeletal
- Joint alterations including camptodactyly, flexion contractures at elbows, congenital hip dislocations
- Foot position defects
- Radioulnar synostosis
- Tapering terminal phalanges, hypoplastic finger and toe nails‖
- Cervical spine abnormalities
- Altered palm crease patterns§
- Pectus excavatum§

Cardiac
- Ventricular septal defect‖
- Atrial septal defect§
- Tetralogy of Fallot, great vessel anomalies‖

Other
- Cleft lip and/or cleft palate‖
- Myopia,‖ strabismus§
- Epicanthal folds§
- Dental malocclusion
- Hearing loss, protuberant ears
- Abnormal thoracic cage
- Strawberry hemangiomata§
- Hypoplastic labia majora§
- Microophthalmia, blepharophimosis
- Small teeth with faulty enamel‖
- Hypospadias, small rotated kidneys, hydronephrosis‖
- Hirsutism in infancy‖
- Hernias of diaphragm, umbilicus or groin, diastasis recti‖

From American Academy of Pediatrics Committee on Substance Abuse and Committee on Children with Disabilities, 1993.

Principal (†,‡) and associated (§,‖) features observed in 245 affected individuals. †>80%; ‡>50%; § 26% to 50%; ‖ 1% to 25% of patients.

scores widely varied. Average academic functioning was at the second- to fourth-grade levels, although arithmetic deficits were most characteristic. Maladaptive behaviors included poor judgment, distractibility, difficulty perceiving social cues, and problems in modulating mood. The family environment continued to be unstable. None of the subjects in the study were age appropriate regarding their socialization and communication skills.

ETIOLOGY

Genetics

Discordance in dizygotic twins affected by alcohol exposure *in utero* suggest that genetic factors may lead to susceptibility to fetal alcohol syndrome. Two male twins reported by Christoffel and Salafsky (1975) revealed one twin who was clearly affected; the other would not have been detected if the sibling had not been so severely involved. The twin who was more severely affected weighed approximately 500 grams less at birth than the sibling and had anomalies not present in the other twin, such as low-set, posteriorly rotated ears. At 5 years of age, the twins were less discordant in appearance and only one was described as hyperactive (Miller, Israel, and Cuttone, 1981). Santolaya et al. (1978) reported on dizygotic twins who were not apparently different at birth in weight, length, or head circumference, but differed at 11 months in psychomotor development and in physical features. Palmer et al. (1974) reported dizygotic twins who were slightly discordant in regard to physical features. Chasnoff (1985) reported on a pair of dizygotic girls who were discordant in regard to birth weight, length, and head circumference. At 18-month follow-up, they were different in physical appearance (facial stigmata) and in weight. Tsukahara, Eguchi, and Kajii (1986) studied mothers and their daughters with fetal alcohol syndrome. All of the mothers were positive for aldehyde dehydrogenase 2, the enzyme that metabolizes aldehyde to acetic acid, yet 4 of the 5 girls with fetal alcohol syndrome did not have this enzyme.

Neuropathology

Microcephaly is commonly reported in fetal alcohol syndrome and suggests an underdevelopment of the brain. The most common abnormalities reported are the underdevelopment or absence of the corpus callosum and enlarged lateral ventricles. Ferrer and Galofre (1987) observed decreased numbers of dendritic spines on the apical dendrites and abnormal morphology of the spines on the apical and basilar dendrites of cortical pyramidal cells in a 4-month-old with fetal alcohol syndrome. These neuropathological changes are of interest because dendritic spine abnormalities have been reported to be related to mental retardation (Purpura, 1974). Dendritic changes have also been observed in animal studies with prenatal exposure to alcohol; these changes were correlated with decreased learning ability (Abel, Jacobson, and Sherwin, 1983).

TREATMENT

Prevention

The first approach to treatment relates to prevention. There is no clearly established safe dose of alcohol for pregnant women. Those mothers of children with fetal alcohol syndrome drank more alcohol and drank excessively early in gestation when contrasted with those with less severe clinical features. Alcohol use in late pregnancy is primarily associated with prematurity and infants who are small for gestational age rather than with fetal alcohol syndrome (Jones et al., 1974). One prospective study of 31,604 pregnancies found that the consumption of 1 to 2 drinks a day was associated with an increased risk of giving birth to a baby who was growth retarded (Mills et al., 1984).

The Committee on Substance Abuse and the Committee on Children's Disabilities of the American Academy of Pediatrics (1993) recommends that because there is no known safe amount of alcohol consumption during pregnancy, abstinence from alcohol for women who are pregnant or who are planning a pregnancy is recommended. The committee recommends special efforts toward education about the harmful effects of alcohol, that identified children be referred for early educational services, and that federal legislation for print and broadcast alcohol advertisements read: "Drinking during pregnancy may cause mental retardation and other birth defects. Avoid alcohol during pregnancy."

Intervention

Both attention deficit disorder and autistic-like behavior have been described (Nanson, 1992). Nanson and Hiscock (1990) studied 20 children (aged 5 to 12) with fetal alcohol syndrome (FAS) or fetal alcohol effect (FAE) and compared them to 20 age-matched children with attention deficit disorder (ADD) and 20 age-matched normal control children on reaction time and vigilance tasks. Their parents completed questionnaires about their child's activity level and overall functioning. In addition each children completed the short form of an IQ test. The children with either FAS or FAE showed attentional deficits and behavioral problems. However, the FAS group was significantly more impaired intellectually than the FAE group or normal controls. Future studies will require IQ-matched controls. Still, these findings suggest that the treatments used to facilitate learning in children with attention deficit disorder may also benefit children with FAS or FAE. Moreover, psychotherapy may be indicated for their attention and behavioral problems.

Nanson (1992) also studied 6 children with a diagnosis of fetal alcohol syndrome who also fulfilled the criteria for diagnosis of autistic disorder. This group was compared with 8 other FAS children, of similar ages and functional levels, without autistic-like behaviors. The autistic-like FAS children tested in the moderately to severely retarded range. The autistic-like behavior described is consistent with the social deficits previously described in FAS; however, pervasive developmental disorder NOS may be a more appropriate designation for this group because autistic-like behavior has not been commonly associated with prenatal alcohol exposure. Appropriate educational and treatment resources are needed to address the social deficits, particularly in those cases where autistic-like behavior is described.

A comprehensive treatment program begins with parental acknowledgment of the etiology of fetal alcohol syndrome and treatment, as indicated, for alcohol misuse and abuse. Parental counseling should include discussion of the physical and behavioral phenotype. The family should be advised about the need for special educational programs and assisted in behavior management. Family therapy is often required to help family members cope with the developmental disorder. The impact of the disorder on the family has been poignantly described by Michael Dorris in *The Broken Cord,* his book about raising an adopted son with fetal alcohol syndrome (Dorris, 1989).

REFERENCES

Abel, E.L. (1990). *Fetal alcohol syndrome.* Medical Economics Books, Oradell, NJ.

______, and Sokol, R.J. (1987). Incidence of fetal alcohol syndrome and economic impact of FAS-related anomalies. *Drug and Alcohol Dependency,* 19:51–70.

______, Jacobson, S., and Sherwin, B.T. (1983). In-utero alcohol exposure: Functional and structural brain damage. *Neurobehavioral Toxicology and Teratology,* 5:363–366.

American Academy of Pediatrics Committee on Substance Abuse and Committee on Children with Disabilities. (1993). Fetal alcohol syndrome and fetal alcohol effects. *Pediatrics,* 91:1004–1006.

Charness, M.E., Simon, R.P., and Greenberg, D.A. (1989). Ethanol and the nervous system. *New England Journal of Medicine,* 321:442–454.

Chasnoff, I.J. (1985). Fetal alcohol syndrome in twin pregnancy. *Acta Geneticae et Gemellologiae,* 34:229–232.

Christoffel, K.K., and Salafsky, I. (1975). Fetal alcohol syndrome in dizygotic twins. *Journal of Pediatrics,* 87:963–967.

Clarren, S.K., and Smith D.W. (1978). The fetal alcohol syndrome. *New England Journal of Medicine,* 298:1063–1067.

Donovan, C.L. (1991). Factors predisposing, enabling, and reinforcing routine screening of patients for preventing fetal alcohol syndrome: A survey of New Jersey physicians. *Journal of Drug Education,* 21:35–42.

Dorris, M. (1989). *The Broken Cord.* Harper & Row, New York.

Ferrer, I., and Galofre, E. (1987). Dendritic spine anomalies in fetal alcohol syndrome. *Neuropediatrics,* 18:161–163.

Jones, K.L. (1986). Fetal alcohol syndrome. *Pediatrics in Review,* 8:122–126.

______, Smith, D.W., Ulleland, C.N., and Streissguth, A.P. (1973). Pattern of malformation in offspring of chronic alcoholic mothers. *Lancet,* i:1267–1271.

______, ______, Streissguth, A.P., and Myrianthopoulos, N.C. (1974). Outcome in offspring of chronic alcoholic women. *Lancet,* i:1076–1078.

Lemoine, P., Harrousseau, H., Borteryu, J.P., and Menuet, J.C. (1968). Les enfants de parents alcooliques: Anomalies observées à propos de 127 cas. [The children of alcoholic parents: Anomalies observed in 127 cases.] *Quest Médicale,* 21:476–482.

Little, B.B., Snell, L.M., Rosenfeld, C.R., Gilstrap, L.C., 3rd, and Gant, N.F. (1990). Failure to recognize fetal alcohol syndrome in newborn infants. *American Journal of Diseases of Childhood,* 144:1142–1146.

Miller, M., Israel, J., and Cuttone, J. (1981). Fetal alcohol syndrome. *Journal of Pediatric Ophthalmology and Strabismus,* 18:6–15.

Mills, J.L., Graubard, B.I., Harley, E.E., Rhoads, G.G., and Berends, H.W. (1984). Maternal alcohol consumption and birth weight: How much drinking in pregnancy is safe? *Journal of the American Medical Association,* 252:1875–1879.

Nanson, J. L. (1992). Autism in fetal alcohol syndrome: A report of six cases. *Alcoholism,* 16(3): 558–565.

______, and Hiscock, M. (1990). Attention deficits in children exposed to alcohol prenatally. *Alcoholism,* 14(5): 656–661.

Olegard, R., Sabel, K.G., Aronsson, M., Sandin, B., Johansson, P.R., Carlsson, C., Kyllerman, M., Iversen, K., and Hrbek, A. (1979). Effects on the child of alcohol abuse during pregnancy: Retrospective and prospective studies. *Acta Paediatrica Scandanavia Supplement,* 225:112–121.

Palmer, R.H., Ouellette, E.M., Warner, L., and Leichtman, S.R. (1974). Congenital malformations in offspring of a chronic alcoholic mother. *Pediatrics,* 53:490–494.

Purpura, D.P. (1974). Neuronal migration and dendritic differentiation: Normal and aberrant development of human cerebral cortex. In *Mead Johnson Perinatal Developmental Medicine,* 6. Marco Island, FL.

Santolaya, J.M., Martinez, G., Gorostiza, E., Aizpiri, J., and Hernandez, M. (1978). Alcoholismo fetal. *Drogalcohol,* 3:183–192.

Streissguth, A.P. (1986). The behavioral teratology of alcohol: Performance, behavioral, and intellectual deficits in prenatally exposed children. In J.R. West (ed.), *Alcohol and brain development,* pp. 3–44. Oxford University Press, New York.

______, Aase, J.M., Clarren, S.K., Randels, S.P., Ladue, R.A., and Smith, D.F. (1991). Fetal alcohol syndrome in adolescents and adults. *Journal of the American Medical Association,* 265:1961–1967.

Tsukahara, M., Eguchi, T., and Kajii, T. (1986). Fetal alcohol syndrome: Analysis of five families (School of Health Sciences University of Tokyo). *Japanese Journal of Human Genetics,* 31:170–171.

12.2 Behavioral Toxicity: Cocaine

The natural history of intrauterine drug exposure on social, cognitive, and emotional development is receiving increasing attention. Growing up in a substance-abusing family, following prenatal drug exposure, is an area of particular concern. Initial investigations that focused on the consequences of cocaine use in the newborn period and during early infancy have been extended to toddlers, preschoolers, and school-age children. When developmental toxicity occurs with a known therapeutic agent, such as diphenylhydantoin, or a physical agent, such as X-irradiation, standard testing procedures are established as part of a developmental neurotoxicity assessment. However, there is no standard testing for substances of abuse, such as cocaine. Therefore, problems only become apparent when difficulties are noted in children. The contribution of substances of abuse to the overall incidence of developmental toxicity is increasing.

Research into these drug effects is complicated by polysubstance abuse and adulteration of street drugs. Therefore, it is difficult to impose the same standards of control in research in human studies of prenatal drug effects in regard to dosage, time schedule, and purity of the substances used as is the case in animal studies. Furthermore, findings are difficult to interpret because, in addition to drug use, prenatal and perinatal factors, poverty, postnatal child rearing environment, and environmental factors all contribute to developmental outcome. All of these factors need to be taken into account in interpreting behavioral results. However, morphological changes associated with drug use have been identified with some consistency.

This chapter reviews the history, epidemiology, etiology, clinical features, intervention, and future directions of prenatal exposure to cocaine. It considers the evidence for a behavioral phenotype related to prenatal cocaine exposure.

HISTORY

In the 1930s there were epidemics of cocaine and alcohol abuse in the United States, which subsided. By the 1960s and 1970s heroin, alcohol, and marijuana again had become the more commonly abused drugs. During the 1960s, following the thalidomide tragedy, pregnant women became more aware of the effects that the substances they ingested had on the developing fetus. Although teratology and developmental toxicology had been developed in the earlier part of this century, the thalidomide tragedy led to general recognition of the role of chemical exposure in human developmental toxicity. It became clear that the exposure to chemicals during development may have long lasting, but often subtle, postnatal consequences in humans (Vorhees, 1986). In the 1970s the recognition of fetal alcohol syndrome led physicians to attend to recreational drugs that might be used during pregnancy. This was followed by descriptions of a neonatal abstinence syndrome found in newborns who underwent withdrawal from cocaine abused by their mothers during pregnancy. By the 1980s the use of cocaine as a drug of choice by women of childbearing age in large parts of the United States became an important new focus in perinatal medicine.

Cocaine is a drug that had been viewed as safe and nonaddictive and because it was not injected, it had become attractive to women as a recreational drug. Now it became apparent that cocaine could cause major problems for the developing fetus. Even though multiple drug use is the most common pattern for drug users, of all the current recreational drugs cocaine has some of the most substantial effects on pregnancy and neonatal outcome.

In 1985 Chasnoff et al. provided the first published report of the effects of cocaine on pregnancy and neonatal outcome. These authors recorded a high rate of spontaneous abortions, abruptio placentae, and neonatal neurobehavioral deficiencies. Subsequently, a high rate of premature labor and delivery (MacGregor et al., 1987), intrauterine growth retardation, sudden infant death (Chasnoff, Burns, and Burns, 1987a), malformation of the genitourinary tract (Chasnoff, Chisum, and Kaplan, 1988), and a risk for intrauterine cerebrovascular accidents (Chasnoff et al., 1986) were reported. Bingol et al. (1987) also reported an increased rate of malformations and intrauterine growth retardation.

EPIDEMIOLOGY

Establishing the incidence of intrauterine drug abuse is complicated because the majority of infants who are exposed to drugs may never be diagnosed. However, the advent of newborn urine toxicology testing has made a significant contribution to the study of prenatal drug use and allows better estimates of prevalence.

In 1989 the National Association of Perinatal Addiction, Research and Education (Chasnoff, 1989) surveyed 40 hospitals seeking an estimate of the number of women diagnosed as having used an illicit drug during pregnancy. In reports from 36 of these hospitals, 11% of infants were exposed to an illicit drug at some point during gestation. There was no difference between public and private hospitals. Based on this information, it was estimated that 375,000 infants born in 1989 had been exposed to an illicit substance at some point during pregnancy.

Another approach to data on drug exposure is to survey all women of childbearing age. In 1988 NIDA conducted a household survey of illicit drug use by women (National Institute on Drug Abuse, 1991). For women 18 to 25, 22% of white women, 21% of black women, and 16% of Hispanic women indicated they had used an illicit drug, usually cocaine or marijuana, in the month prior to questioning. For adolescent girls aged 12 to 17, 15% of white girls, 8% of black girls, and 11% of Hispanic girls had used an illicit substance, usually marijuana or cocaine, in the month before the survey. Based on these data, the Institute of Medicine (1990) estimated that between 350,000 and 625,000 individuals were born in the United States in 1988 who had been exposed to an illicit substance. Using this same methodology, Gomby and Shiono (1991) estimated that between 550,000 and 739,000 infants were exposed to an illicit substance. These studies were followed by population-based evaluations of community prevalence of drug use during pregnancy (Chasnoff, Landress, and Barrett, 1990). In one Florida county, every woman entering prenatal care was enrolled and had a urine test at the first prenatal visit. The overall prevalence rate for a positive finding for cocaine, marijuana, or heroin was approximately 14%. No difference was found between racial groups. Moreover, marijuana and cocaine were by far the two most important drugs found in the women's urine. Similar findings have been reported in other communities. Yet these rates may still be low because urine toxicology generally detects the use of drugs in the 48 hours prior to testing. Specifically, cocaine can be found in the urine for only 6 to 8 hours after use, whereas the primary metabolite of cocaine, benzoylecgonine, does persist for up to 48 hours.

Surveys of newborns for illicit substances utilize analysis of meconium (Ostrea et al., 1992). Because meconium is formed during the second and third trimesters of pregnancy, it provides a window on the last 20 weeks of gestation. Meconium sampling demonstrated the prevalence rate of exposure to be 44% among 3,010 newborn infants in a Detroit public hospital. Yet only 11% of the mothers admitted to drug use and only 6% of the newborns who were tested showed a positive finding on urine toxicology. Although further refinements are needed in meconium testing, this is a promising approach to newborn detection. Other approaches include hair analysis; however, this is a new methodology that requires further development. Information about fetal hair growth in the last parts of pregnancy might potentially give information on timing of exposure.

For epidemiologic studies, combining several approaches is necessary to establish previous exposure to illicit substances. Both a substance abuse history and urinary screening are necessary; mass meconium screening may become available in the future. Ostrea, Romero, and Yee (1993) have described a meconium drug test for mass screening. Assessing the substance abuse history without urinary screens would have led to a quarter of patients using cocaine being missed in one study (Zuckerman et al., 1989). Moreover, if the substance abuse history had not been taken and urinary screens were used alone, 50% would have been missed in this study. Therefore, a combination of both of these approaches is essential.

A majority of women who use cocaine during pregnancy are polydrug users (Singer, Garber, and Kleigman, 1991). Multiple drug use has been attributed to the withdrawal, or "crash," which follows cocaine's euphoric effects. Drug users typically use alcohol, marijuana, or heroin to reduce these withdrawal effects. Moreover, women who abuse cocaine may also have an increased likelihood of poor nutrition and be at increased risk for infectious diseases, particularly sexually transmitted diseases, including the human immunodeficiency virus (HIV). All of these factors must be considered in epidemiologic studies.

ETIOLOGY

Cocaine may lead to placental dysfunction (vasocontracture effects), structural changes (vascular compromise), and neurobehavioral abnormalities (postsynaptic junction neurotoxicity). When evaluating cocaine use in pregnancy, maternal factors, including timing and dose of cocaine, maternal and fetal factors, such as the metabolic rates of cocaine, and genetic characteristics of the mother and fetus must be considered.

Pharmacological Effects

An assessment of the pharmacological and physiological effects of cocaine in pregnancy must also take into account multiple drug use which may vary throughout the period of pregnancy. One pattern is binge use of cocaine along with continuous or intermittent use of other substances (Chasnoff, 1992). In addition, cocaine may be inhaled, smoked, or injected so the method of administration may affect outcome. Moreover, concentrations of cocaine dose may vary from one community to another and contaminants may be introduced with the cocaine prior to its being taken.

Cocaine is a central nervous system stimulant and inhibits nerve conduction in the peripheral nervous system. In adults, the principal pharmacological effects in the brain are due to an inhibition of active reuptake of dopamine, norepinephrine, and serotonin. Specific effects are reduced appetite and reduced need for sleep, cardiovascular changes including vasoconstriction and tachycardia, and occasional cardiac arrhythmias or acute myocardial infarcts, and the blocking of nerve conduction by prevention of transient inflow of sodium ions, leading to local anesthesia. Neurological complications in adults include seizures, headaches, elevations in body temperature, and brief loss of consciousness (Cregler and Mark, 1986).

Cocaine is metabolized primarily through the plasma cholinesterase system, with the primary metabolic product being benzoylecgonine. During pregnancy there may be a down regulation of the maternal cholinergic system, which results in a more prolonged exposure to the action of cocaine. Because the placenta plays a major role in drug elimination for the fetus, drug elimination time in the fetus is strongly related to the elimination characteristics of the mother. Moreover, differences in placental vascularity may mediate the effects of cocaine, as shown in studies of discordant abnormalities in monozygotic twins (Fogel, Nitkowsky, and Gruenwald, 1965).

Because cocaine rapidly crosses the placenta by simple diffusion, fetal peak blood levels are reached as quickly as 3 minutes (Mofenson and Corracio, 1987; Stewart, Inaba, and Lucassen, 1979). In the fetus, having crossed the placenta, cocaine has the same direct actions on the fetal cardiovascular system as seen in the maternal system. These cardiac changes may well relate to the direct effects of cocaine as well as indirectly from fetal hypoxia.

The mechanism for these changes may be cocaine's effects on blocking neurotransmitter reuptake, leading to increased catecholamine plasma levels that act at noradrenergic sites (Fischman et al., 1976) in the fetus. In animal studies using pregnant ewes (Moore et al., 1986), cocaine exposure leads to uterine artery blood flow changes, with a dose-dependent reduction in flow of about 40%, which is followed by fetal hypoxia. Similarly, direct effects on smooth muscle by catecholamines may increase uterine contractions.

Effects on CNS Development and Behavior

The fetus may be at special risk for central nervous system (CNS) abnormality because of cocaine's effects as a reuptake blocker of biogenic amines (Pitts and Marwah, 1987). An increased availability of these transmitters at neuroreceptor sites may increase neuronal excitability. Chronic exposure to cocaine might lead to down regulation of postsynaptic dopamine receptors in the brain (Spear, Kirstein, and Frambes, 1989). Because reduced dopamine activity in the frontal cortex may be related to attention deficits and hyperactivity, offspring of cocaine-using females might be at risk to develop attention deficit disorder. Wiggins et al. (1989) found that cocaine levels in the fetal brain were 109% to 151% of those in the maternal blood. Exposure to these increased levels of cocaine during early development, particularly in the first trimester, could result in an increased risk of abnormal differentiation of the major neurotransmitter systems and affect glial cell functioning and neuronal migration and growth as well (Lanier, Dunn, and van Hartesveldt, 1976).

Dow-Edwards (1989) found that cocaine exposure results in long-term alterations in animal behavior in rats and suggested the presence of changes in central pathways. In her study, females were more sensitive to cocaine than males; brain effects were noted at a dose where little general systemic toxicity was seen. If these rat experiments are a model for effects on the human nervous system, then cocaine exposure may place children at risk for neurochemical and neurobehavioral disorders.

Overall, fetal exposure to cocaine may lead to risk indirectly through pharmacological effects on both maternal and fetal blood vessels and directly through effects on neurotransmitter systems. These combined effects, along with hypoxia and malnutrition, can result in prematurity and abnormality of the developing central nervous system.

Teratogenic Effects

Whether cocaine is a teratogen continues to be controversial. Cocaine can affect the unborn infant not only during periods of embryonic differentiation in the first trimester of pregnancy but also throughout gestation (Jones, 1991). The primary support for cocaine's teratogenic effects comes from experimental animal studies that compare congenital defects found in drug-exposed animals to those seen in infants born to mothers who have used the drug during pregnancy. Animal studies suggest that cocaine exposure during pregnancy is a risk factor, leading to long-term alterations in brain functioning and perhaps in cognitive development. Overall, despite some reports of congenital neurological abnormalities, cocaine seems to be a relatively weak teratogen. Interpretation of the animal studies as applicable to human infants must still be considered with caution as they relate to human development. Moreover, animal studies have not taken into account multiple drug use and the interaction of a variety of postnatal environmental factors that may influence outcome during development. Lack of consideration of postnatal and perinatal factors may lead to an exaggeration of the negative impact of prenatal cocaine exposure.

CLINICAL FEATURES

Infant gestational age, birth weight, head circumference, and length have been found to be decreased and the rate of low birth weight increased in studies of the offspring of cocaine-using women. Although other factors may interact in producing small infants, cocaine use does seem to be independently associated with both decreased birth weight and decreased head circumference. Such impaired head growth may reflect reduced intrauterine brain growth (Bingol et al., 1987). Reduced head circumference at birth is a marker for poor developmental outcome. Although the combination of alcohol and heroin also lead to reduced head size, the impact of cocaine on head growth appears to be independent of the use of alcohol (Chasnoff et al., 1992; Frank et al., 1990).

In addition to abnormal growth patterns, congenital anomalies involving the genitourinary tract, heart, central nervous system, as well as limb reduction abnormalities, have been reported. A potential mechanism for all of these anomalies appears to be interruption of the intrauterine blood supply, with later disruption of embryonic development. Although relatively uncommon, these problems most likely relate to vascular accidents that might occur at any time during pregnancy, not only in the first trimester. Anomalies involving the gastrointestinal system could be secondary to disruption of blood flow through the mesenteric arteries.

Cerebral infarctions (Chasnoff et al., 1986) were one of the earliest complications reported from cocaine use. Dixon and Bejar (1988) reported a variety of difficulties, including intraventricular hemorrhage, subarachnoid hemorrhage, white matter cavitation, and cerebral infarction. Each of these defects may relate to vascular disruption.

Sudden infant death syndrome (SIDS) has been evaluated in infants exposed to cocaine because both heroin and tobacco used during pregnancy have been reported to increase its occurrence. However, Bauchner et al. (1988) could not document this increased rate of SIDS. These authors do suggest that SIDS might be associated with polydrug use and environmental factors in mothers who have used cocaine. Cocaine use does lead to changes in respiratory pattern, cardiac conduction, and abnormality of the autonomic nervous system. These potential effects, along with multiple drug use, must be taken into account when considering the reports of SIDS in cocaine-exposed infants.

Neurobehavioral Profiles

Although approximately 25% to 30% of infants exposed to cocaine *in utero* may have physical difficulties, neurobehavioral problems seem more common. Other drugs, such as alcohol, tobacco, and marijuana, may affect behavior in the neonate, but cocaine seems to account for the most clearly documented changes when formal assessments are used (Chasnoff et al., 1989; Chasnoff et al., 1992). These neurobehavioral changes do not specifically reflect neonatal withdrawal from the drug, as is the case with heroin, but rather neurotoxic effects (Chasnoff et al., 1989).

Infants exposed to cocaine have low thresholds for overstimulation and their caregivers may need to provide considerable assistance to deal with their overexcitable nervous systems. Studies, using the Neonatal Behavioral Assessment Scale (NBAS) (Brazelton, 1984), generally demonstrate variability in the severity of the response deficits and rate of recovery. Those areas most clearly affected are motor behavior (coordination of motor activities and reflexes), state control (variability in state of arousal in response to challenge), and orientation (ability to interact actively with the outside world by attending to and responding to auditory and visual stimuli) (Griffith, 1988; Lester et al., 1991; Mayes et al., 1993; Singer, Garber, and Kleigman, 1991).

Motor behaviors elicited by drug use include hypertonicity with rigid posturing and hyperextension, hyperactivity reflexes, and poor coordination of sucking and swallowing. Some infants may be hypotonic and lethargic at birth. State control may be poorly organized, with infants "shutting themselves off" from external stimulation and showing abrupt responses with changes in stimulation.

Some authors, such as Coles et al. (1992), found that NBAS scores for newborns were within a clinically normal range despite cocaine or alcohol exposure. Others, such as Mayes et al. (1993), have demonstrated impaired habituation performance on the NBAS in cocaine-exposed neonates in contrast to non-cocaine-exposed neonates. These authors point out that the habituation response demonstrates a reduction in attention to repetitive, familiar, or redundant stimuli and is closely related in function to the regulation of attention. Monoamine regulation involves basic modulation of arousal and attention and, therefore, is associated with these neurobehavioral capacities. Depressed habituation performance may indicate early evidence of impairment in basic attention and self-regulational processes. In the newborn, habituation may provide protection as the infant is exposed to multiple novel stimuli. Habituation is involved in some type of information processing and encoding for the infant and, later in infancy, predicts performance on the Bayley scales, language production, comprehension, and full-scale individual test performance at 4 years of age (Bornstein, 1989). In the Mayes paper, although the subjects did not use opiates, they did, in some instances, use alcohol and marijuana, so combined drug exposure cannot be completely ruled out. Long-term follow-up of the infants involved in the Mayes study who showed deficits in their habituation response is necessary to clarify long-term developmental outcome.

Eisen et al. (1990) also found significant differences in habituation performance on the NBAS. In the Eisen et al. study, the neonates were urine-screen positive only for cocaine, and their mothers denied opiate use.

These studies are of particular interest because habituation is involved with attention and information processing, and possibly learning (Bornstein, 1985). Because the dopaminergic system may be involved with attentional systems linked to the habituation process, Eisen et al.'s findings potentially link habituation performance to a neurochemical mechanism. Moreover, animal studies show a relationship between prenatal cocaine exposure and impaired early associative learning (Dow-Edwards, 1989; Spear, Kirstein, and Frambes, 1989). Cocaine's primary effects on the developing brain involve the ontogenesis of catecholamines, particularly dopamine, and associated effects on neurotransmitter-regulated patterns of synaptogenesis and axonal proliferation (Dow-Edwards, 1988; Lauder, 1991).

Cocaine effects have also been evaluated by Lester et al. (1991), using cry analysis. These authors analyzed cry patterns in cocaine-exposed infants and found that exposed infants in the study showed two neurobehavioral patterns. These two patterns, direct (excitable) and indirect (depressed), were ascribed then to direct neurotoxic effects for the excitable group and the indirect effects to intrauterine growth retardation for the depressed group. The excitable cry characteristics were considered to be direct effects. They were of higher fundamental frequency, higher and more variable first format frequency, and of longer duration. The indirect effects were considered secondary to low birth weight and were associated with longer latency, fewer utterances, lower amplitude, and more dysphonation. These findings are consistent with a pattern of underaroused neurobehavioral function (Corwin et al., 1992; Golub, 1991).

Long-term behavioral outcome studies of cocaine-exposed infants have been complicated by the chaotic lifestyle of many families where family members continue to abuse various substances. However, Howard et al. (1989) and Rodning, Beckwith, and Howard (1989) found that a group of 18-month-old children exposed to cocaine *in utero* showed significant lower developmental scores than nonexposed infants from similar backgrounds. They found that prenatal drug exposure had adverse effects on developmental processes, which extended into the second year of life. On standardized developmental tests, these children scored in the low average range; however, they showed deficits in self-initiation, self-organization, and follow-through without assistance from the examiner on tasks. In free play situations, they demonstrated less representational play and showed less sustained attention to play. Because representational play and language acquisition may be linked, these children are at risk for problems in language development. They tended to scatter toys, pick them up, and put them down, rather than engage in fantasy play and exploration with them. The disorganization in their play at 18 months may be related to their neurobehavioral dysregulation as newborns. Disorganization was evident in cognitive, social, and affective spheres.

Chasnoff et al. (1992) followed up a group of cocaine/polydrug-exposed infants for 2 years and contrasted them with a group exposed to marijuana and/or alcohol and another group with no drug exposure. During the first year of their life, the drug-exposed infants showed catch-up growth and their mean weight and length were similar to non-drug-exposed infants. Yet mean head circumference remained smaller during the first 2 years of life. The Bayley scales (1969) of infant development revealed mean developmental scores of the cocaine-exposed infants that were not significantly different from those in the control group. However, a larger number of the cocaine-exposed infants were greater than 2 standard deviations below the standardized mean on the Bayley scales, suggesting developmental delay. In this study, cocaine exposure was said to be the best predictor of head circumference. Small head size and developmental scores for infants between 12 and 24 months were significantly correlated so that those at greatest risk at age 2 were the infants who had a small head circumference at birth and did not catch up in head size during their first 2 years of life. These authors conclude that head growth may be an important clinical marker to predict 2-year development in children exposed to cocaine *in utero.*

By 3 years of age in this same group, no differences were found in overall performance of drug-free and cocaine-exposed children (Griffith, Azuma, and Chasnoff, 1994) on the Stanford-Binet Intelligence Scale (Thorndike, Hagen, and Sattler, 1986). However, the mean head circumference continued to be significantly smaller at 3 years for the cocaine-exposed infants. Moreover, approximately one third of the drug-exposed children demonstrated delays in normal language development and/or difficulties with attention and self-regulation. The 3-year follow-up study points out the importance of evaluating attention and executive functions in addition to standardized intelligence scales in follow-up studies. The identified speech and language difficulties of various types were responsive to speech therapy. Problems in self-regulation were linked to the low threshold for overstimulation and to low frustration tolerance. These children did best in one-to-one testing situations but showed difficulty in behavior regulation when placed in more complex situations. When environmentally challenged, some of the children with difficulties in self-regulation withdrew and others showed increased activity or impulsiveness, or a combination of these behaviors. Inconsistency and lack of predictability in the child's environment for this subgroup of drug-exposed children may lead to disruptive behavioral disorders.

Continued longitudinal follow-up is necessary during the school years for drug-exposed children. Not all children exposed to substances of abuse *in utero* have a poor prognosis; the early focus on there being severe learning and behavioral problems has been exaggerated. The overall developmental outcome from intrauterine cocaine exposure may be good if environmental risk factors are taken into account and early intervention programs are made available. Still, the interaction of environmental risk factors with difficulties in self-regulation does place them at risk for emotional, behavioral, and learning problems.

INTERVENTION

The most important aspect of intervention is prevention. There is no safe dose of cocaine to be used in pregnancy; therefore, abstinence is essential. A high level of suspicion for cocaine use is necessary among physicians caring for women of childbearing age because substance abuse is one of the most frequently missed diagnoses in obstetrics, and, probably, in pediatrics. Risk factors that suggest suspicion of substance abuse include lack of prenatal care, abruptio placentae, prematurity, evidence of intrauterine growth retardation, and vascular accidents (e.g., cerebral infarction, limb reduction anomaly). Neonatal apnea, seizures, or cardiac arrhythmias should also arouse suspicion. Chasnoff (1992) emphasizes the importance of eliciting a maternal substance abuse history and a urine or meconium (when available) screen when suspicions are aroused. If the history is positive and the child has a characteristic presentation, then therapy is multidimensional and should address the clinical presentation in the child (both physical and behavioral) and the parent. A mother using illicit drugs should not breast feed. Cocaine rapidly crosses into breast milk with levels measurable up to 48 hours after the last injection (Chasnoff, Lewis, and Squires, 1987b). Infant exposure to cocaine may continue through breast feeding. Because of the risk to the newborn for substance abuse, several states have passed laws mandating prenatal testing.

Child abuse is closely linked to substance abuse; it has been estimated that 50% of child abuse and neglect cases in New York City involve substance abuse (Marriott, 1987). These findings suggest that careful attention be paid to the postnatal rearing environment. Substance use in parents and parent–infant attachment should be carefully assessed. Rodning, Beckwith, and Howard (1991) evaluated the quality of attachment and home environments in children who were prenatally exposed to PCP and cocaine with a control group of infants from similar ethnic backgrounds. They found that the majority of drug-exposed infants were insecurely attached to their caregivers. Moreover, they did not differ in the quality of attachment in three caregiving environments, i.e., care by the biological mother, care by other family member, or foster care. These authors found that most of the drug-exposed children showed disorganized behavior, such as "dazed expression," aimless wandering about the room, excessive crying on reunion with the caregiver, confusing a stranger with the caregiver, and stereotypies. Overall, they were confused in communicating affect.

All children whose mothers continued to use drugs were insecurely attached, but half of the children whose mothers were abstinent were securely attached. When drug use was discontinued, parent–infant relationships could potentially improve.

Patterns of behavior associated with substance-using mothers included the infant being ignored, requests being rejected, insensitivity to communications, less physical response to distress, and poor quality of physical contact. Yet the authors found that difficulties in establishing an attachment also occur in good foster care settings, suggesting that temperamental factors in the children related to drug exposure may be factors in the establishment of attachment. More intensive therapeutic foster care may be needed.

Overall, the treatment program must take into account physical and psychological change secondary to intrauterine drug use and the postnatal nurturing environment (especially as it relates to substance use and mood disorder in the parents). Without early intervention, or despite it, for some children, special school programs that provide small groups, behavior management programs, and structure will be necessary. Ongoing parent training is also required.

FUTURE DIRECTIONS

Future programs must consider drug education for adolescents and young adults of childbearing age, multimodal treatment approaches for affected infants and children, and continued research in the mechanisms of the disorder. Multiple drug abuse will continue to be an issue in evaluating future studies. Advances in positron emission tomography (PET) scanning with ligands that bind to cocaine receptors, such as WIN 35,428, allow *in vivo* identification of the effect of cocaine on the brain (Scheffel, Boja, and Kuhar, 1989). This ligand has been used in Lesch-Nyhan disease and may potentially be used to evaluate cocaine effects.

REFERENCES

Bauchner, H., Zuckerman, B., McClain, M., Frank, D., Fried, L.E., and Kayne, H. (1988). Risk of sudden infant death syndrome among infants with in-utero exposure to cocaine. *Journal of Pediatrics,* 13:831–834.

Bayley, N. (1969). *Manual for the Bayley Scales of Infant Development.* Psychological Corporation, New York.

Bingol, N., Fuchs, M., Diaz, V., Stone, R.K., and

Gromish, D.S. (1987). Teratogenicity of cocaine in humans. *Journal of Pediatrics,* 110:93–96.

Bornstein, M. (1985). Habituation as a measure of visual information processing in human infants: Summary, systemization, and synthesis. In G. Gottlieb and N. Krasnegor (eds.), *Development of audition and vision during the first year of postnatal life: A methodological overview,* pp. 253–295. Ablex, Norwood, NJ.

______. (1989). Stability in early mental development: From attention and information processing in infancy and language and cognition in childhood. In M.H. Bornstein and N.A. Krasnegor (eds.), *Stability and continuity in mental development: Behavioral and biological perspectives,* pp. 147–170. Erlbaum, Hillsdale, NJ.

Brazelton, T.B. (1984). *Neonatal Behavioral Assessment Scale.* Spastics International, Philadelphia.

Chasnoff, I.J. (1989). Drug use and women: Establishing a standard of care. *Annals of the New York Academy of Science,* 562:208–210.

______. (1992). Cocaine, pregnancy, and the growing child. *Current Problems in Pediatrics,* 22:302–321.

______, Burns, W.J., Schnoll, S.H., and Burns, K.A. (1985). Cocaine use in pregnancy. *New England Journal of Medicine,* 313:666–669.

______, Bussey, M.E., Savich, R., and Stack, C.M. (1986). Perinatal cerebral infarction and maternal cocaine use. *Journal of Pediatrics,* 108:456–458.

______, Burns, K.A., and Burns, W.J. (1987a). Cocaine use in pregnancy: Perinatal morbidity and mortality. *Neurobehavior, Toxicology and Teratology,* 9:291–293.

______, Lewis, D.E., and Squires, L. (1987b). Cocaine intoxication in a breast-fed infant. *Pediatrics,* 80:836–838.

______, Chisum, G.M., and Kaplan, W.E. (1988). Maternal cocaine use and genitourinary tract malformations. *Teratology,* 37:201–204.

______, Griffith, D.R., Freier, C., and Murray, J. (1992). Cocaine/polydrug use in pregnancy: Two-year follow-up. *Pediatrics,* 89:284–289.

______, ______, MacGregor, S., Dirkes, K., and Burns, K. (1989). Temporal patterns of cocaine use in pregnancy. *Journal of the American Medical Association,* 261:1741–1744.

______, Landress, H.J., and Barrett, M.E. (1990). The prevalence of illicit-drug or alcohol use during pregnancy and discrepancies in mandatory reporting in Pinellas County, Florida. *New England Journal of Medicine,* 322:1202–1206.

Coles, C.D., Platzman, K.A., Smith, I., James, M.E., and Falek, A. (1992). Effects of cocaine and alcohol use in pregnancy on neonatal growth and neurobehavioral status. *Neurotoxicology and Teratology,* 14:23–33.

Corwin, M.J., Lester, B.M., Sepkoski, C., McLaughlin, S., Kayne, H., and Golub, H.L. (1992). Effects of in utero cocaine exposure on newborn acoustical cry characteristics. *Pediatrics,* 89:1199–1203.

Cregler, L.L., and Mark, H. (1986). Medical complications of cocaine abuse. *New England Journal of Medicine,* 315:1495–1500.

Dixon, S.D., and Bejar, R. (1988). Brain lesions in cocaine and methamphetamine exposed neonates. *Pediatric Research,* 23:405A.

Dow-Edwards, D.L. (1988). Developmental effects of cocaine. *NIDA Research Monograph,* 88:290–303.

______. (1989). Long-term neurochemical and neurobehavioral consequences of cocaine use during pregnancy. *Annals of the New York Academy of Science,* 562:280–289.

Eisen, L.N., Field, T.M., Bandstra, E.S., Roberts, J.I.P., Morrow, C., Larson, S.K., and Steele, B.M. (1990). Perinatal cocaine effects on neonatal stress behavior and performance on the Brazelton Scale. *Pediatrics,* 88:477–480.

Fischman, M.W., Schuster, C.R., Resnekov, L., Schick, J.F., Krasnegor, N.A., Fennell, W., and Freedman, D.X. (1976). Cardiovascular and subjective effects of intravenous cocaine administration in humans. *Archives of General Psychiatry,* 33:983–989.

Fogel, B.J., Nitkowsky, H.M., and Gruenwald, P. (1965). Discordant abnormalities in monozygotic twins. *Journal of Pediatrics,* 66:64–72.

Frank, D.A., Bauchner, H., Parker, S., Huber, A.M., Kyei-Aboagye, K., Cabral, H., and Zuckerman, B. (1990). Neonatal body proportionality and body composition after in-utero exposure to cocaine and marijuana. *Journal of Pediatrics,* 117:622–626.

Golub, H.L. (1991). Neurobehavioral syndromes in cocaine-exposed newborn infants. *Child Development,* 62:694–705.

Gomby, D.S., and Shiono, P.H. (1991). Estimating the number of substance-exposed infants. *The Future of Children: Drug Exposed Infants,* 1:17–25.

Griffith, D.R. (1988). The effects of perinatal cocaine exposure on infant neurobehavior and early maternal-infant interactions. In I.J. Chasnoff (ed), *Drug use in pregnancy: Mother and child,* pp. 105–113. MTP Press, Boston.

______, Azuma, S., and Chasnoff, I.J. (1994). Three-year outcome of children exposed prenatally to drugs. *Journal of Child and Adolescent Psychiatry,* 33:20–27.

Howard, J., Beckwith, L., Rodning, C., and Kropenske, V. (1989). The development of young children of substance-abusing parents: Insights from seven years of intervention and research. *Zero to*

Three/National Center for Clinical Infant Programs, 9:8–12.

Institute of Medicine. (1990) The need for treatment. In D.R. Gerstein and H.J. Harwood (eds.), *Treating drug problems,* pp. 80–87. National Academy Press, Washington, DC.

Jones, K.L. (1991). Developmental pathogenesis of defects associated with prenatal cocaine exposure: Fetal vascular disruption. *Clinical Perinatology,* 18:139–146.

Lanier, L.P., Dunn, A.J., and van Hartesveldt, C. (1976). Development of neurotransmitters and their function in brain. *Review of Neuroscience,* 2:195–256.

Lauder, J.M. (1991). Neuroteratology of cocaine: Relationship to developing monoamine systems. *NIDA Research Monograph,* 114:233–247.

Lester, B.M., Corwin, M.J., Sepkoski, C., Seifer, R., Pevcker, M., McLaughlin, S., and Golub, H.L. (1991). Neurobehavioral syndromes in cocaine-exposed newborn infants. *Child Development,* 62:694–705.

MacGregor, S.N., Keith, L.G., Chasnoff, I.J., Rosner, M.A., Chisum, G.M., Shaw, P., and Minogue, J.P. (1987). Cocaine use during pregnancy: Adverse perinatal outcome. *American Journal of Obstetrics and Gynecology,* 157:686–690.

Marriott, M. (1987, November 15). Child abuse cases swamping New York City's family court. *New York Times,* p. 17.

Mayes, L.C., Granger, R.H., Frank, M.A., Schottenfeld, R., and Bornstein, M.H. (1993). Neurobehavioral profiles of neonates exposed to cocaine prenatally. *Pediatrics,* 91:778–783.

Mofenson, H.C., and Corracio, T.R. (1987). Cocaine. *Pediatric Annals,* 16:864–874.

Moore, T.R., Sorg, J., Miller, L., Key, T.C., and Resnik, R. (1986). Hemodynamic effects of intravenous cocaine on the pregnant ewe and fetus. *American Journal of Obstetrics and Gynecology,* 155:883–888.

National Institute on Drug Abuse. (1991). *National household survey on drug abuse: Population estimates 1990.* U.S. Department of Health and Human Services, Washington, DC. Publication No. (ADM) 91–1732.

Ostrea, E.M., Romero, A., and Yee, H. (1993). Adaptation of the meconium drug test for mass screening. *Journal of Pediatrics,* 122:152–154.

______, Brady, M., Gause, S., Raymundo, A.L., and Stevens, M. (1992). Drug screening of newborns by meconium analysis: A large-scale, prospective, epidemiologic study. *Pediatrics,* 89:107–113.

Pitts, D.K., and Marwah, J. (1987). Cocaine modulation of central monoaminergic neurotransmission. *Pharmacology, Biochemistry, and Behavior,* 26:453–461.

Rodning, C., Beckwith, L., and Howard, J. (1989). Characteristics of attachment, organization and play organization in prenatally drug-exposed toddlers. *Development and Psychopathology,* 1:277–289.

______, ______, and ______. (1991). Quality of attachment and home environments in children prenatally exposed to PCP and cocaine. *Development and Psychopathology,* 3:351–366.

Scheffel, W., Boja, J.W., and Kuhar, M.J. (1989). Cocaine receptors: In vivo labeling with ^{3}H-(-) cocaine, ^{3}H WIN 35,065–2, and ^{3}H-WIN 35,428. *Synapse,* 4:390–392.

Singer, L.T., Garber, R., and Kleigman, R. (1991). Neurobehavioral sequelae of fetal cocaine exposure. *Journal of Pediatrics,* 119:667–672.

Spear, L.P., Kirstein, C.L., and Frambes, N.A. (1989). Cocaine effects on the developing central nervous system: Behavioral, psychopharmacological, and neurochemical studies. *Annals of the New York Academy of Science,* 562:290–307.

Stewart, D.J., Inaba, T., and Lucassen, M. (1979). Cocaine metabolism: Cocaine and norcocaine hydrolysis by liver and serum esterases. *Clinical Pharmacology and Therapeutics,* 25:464–468.

Thorndike, R.L., Hagen, E.P., and Sattler, J.M. (1986). *Stanford-Binet Intelligence Scale,* 4th ed. Riverside Publishing Company, Chicago.

Vorhees, C.V. (1986). Origins of teratology. In E.P. Riley and C.V. Vorhees (eds.), *Handbook of teratology,* pp. 3–22. Plenum Press, New York.

Wiggins, R.C., Rolsten, C., Ruiz, B.W., and Davis, C.M. (1989). Pharmacokinetics of cocaine: Basic studies of route, dosage, pregnancy and lactation. *Neurotoxicology,* 10:367–382.

Zuckerman, B., Frank, D.A., Hingson, R., Amaro, H., Levenson, S.M., Kayne, H., Parker, S., Vinci,. R., Aboagye, K., Fried, L.E., Cabral, H., Timperi, R., and Bauchner, H. (1989). Effects of maternal marijuana and cocaine use on fetal growth. *New England Journal of Medicine,* 320:762–768.

PART IV

DEVELOPMENTAL PSYCHOPATHOLOGY

Developmental psychopathology addresses child psychopathology, its relationship to nondisordered behavior, and the origins of maladaptive behavior that do not appear in clinical form until adulthood (Sroufe and Rutter, 1984). Developmental psychopathology investigates the origins and course of individual patterns of behavioral maladaptation. Among developmental disorders, the age of onset is variable, there are multiple causes, and there may be a variety of transformations in behavior that may lead to a complex course. In developmental psychopathology, the application of developmental principles are applied to high-risk and deviant populations. Knowledge of normal development is applied to children with atypical presentations to understand the natural history of their disorder and to recognize how studying deviant behavior may enhance our understanding of normal development. Its goal is to understand the mechanisms and processes through which risk factors lead to the emergence of disorder (Cicchetti, 1989; Rutter, 1988). Behavior and development are viewed within a social context, and the transactional nature of interactions is assessed. Disordered behavior is not viewed as a static condition, but is considered as part of a dynamic transaction. It is a comprehensive approach that seeks to integrate information derived from developmental psychology, clinical psychology, psychiatry, sociology, physiologic sciences, neurosciences, and epidemiology. It involves investigation of developmental continuities and discontinuities throughout the life span. This requires concern with etiology, developmental course, the predisposing factors, and the outcome of disordered behavior. In addition, developmental psychopathologists are concerned with both internal and external factors that may promote or inhibit the development of either competence or resiliency in children and adults. To understand these processes, development is studied from infancy through adulthood.

In Part IV, several disorders of childhood will be discussed from a developmental perspective. The most common of these is attention deficit/hyperactivity disorder (see Chapter 13); it is frequently linked to other disruptive behavior disorders. In this sense, attention deficit/hyperactivity disorder is a risk factor for other disruptive behavior disorders. The child's behavior itself affects the adult and the transactional interactions between them.

Schizophrenia is reviewed in Chapter 14. Schizophrenia has often been viewed as a disorder of late adolescence and adult life, yet its developmental origins are becoming more apparent with recent research. In this chapter, a developmental perspective will be assumed and evidence will be reviewed for a neurodevelopmental hypothesis of schizophrenia.

In Chapter 15, obsessive and compulsive symptoms that begin in childhood and are associated with developmental conditions, such as Tourette's disorder, are discussed. Compulsive behaviors may interfere with the conduct of normal routines and become particularly problematic for the family.

Chapter 16 focuses on sleep disorders, which are common in children with developmental disability and are often difficult to treat. This chapter will review some of the more common sleep difficulties as well as the sleep cycle itself as it relates to development.

The final chapter of Part IV, Chapter 17, discusses maladaptive behavior in severe developmental disability. Aggressive behavior, self-injurious behavior, and oppositional defiant behavior are common accompaniments of developmental disorders.

REFERENCES

Cicchetti, D. (1989). Developmental psychopathology: Some thoughts on its evolution. *Development and Psychopathology,* 1:1–4.

Rutter, M. (1988). Epidemiological approaches to developmental psychopathology. *Archives of General Psychiatry,* 45:486–495.

Sroufe, L.A., and Rutter, M.R. (1984). The domain of developmental psychopathology. *Child Development,* 55:17–29.

CHAPTER 13

ATTENTION DEFICIT/ HYPERACTIVITY DISORDER

Attention deficit/hyperactivity disorder (AD/HD) is the most common diagnosis for children who are seen in psychiatric clinics. It is estimated to involve 2% to 6% of children nationwide and is a factor in one third of referrals to psychiatric clinics. In addition to their attentional problems, difficulties with social perception and social awareness commonly occur, leading to psychosocial difficulties. Still, it is not pure attention deficits but rather impulsivity, overactivity, inappropriate social behavior, and problems in interpersonal relationships that lead to these clinic referrals. Oppositional defiant disorder, conduct problems, poor self-attitude, mood disorder, and anxiety symptoms are frequently associated.

This chapter will review attention deficit/hyperactivity disorder with an emphasis on the associated social cognitive and affect regulation problems that lead to dysfunctional relationships in the family and at school. It will review the history, classification, epidemiology, etiology, diagnostic criteria, developmental approach, and treatment for this disorder. The DSM-IV designation is AD/HD. This abbreviation is used throughout the chapter except when specific studies are referenced that used the DSM-III or DSM-III-R criteria, in which case the abbreviations ADD or ADHD are used.

HISTORY

Attentional difficulties and overactivity were recognized in disabled children during the second half of the last century. The first reports are in textbooks on mental retardation (Ireland, 1877; Tredgold, 1908). The nonretarded hyperactive child entered the folklore of the late 1800s with Reverend Dr. Heinrich Hoffman's popular poem "The Story of Fidgety Phillip" (1862). Yet the associated behavioral aspects in nonretarded children were not well described until the beginnings of this century when George Still, assistant physician to the Hospital for Sick Children in London, gave three lectures under the title "Some Abnormal Psychical Conditions in Children." In these Coulstonian Lectures (1902), Still described an "abnormal incapacity for sustained attention, restlessness, fidgetiness, violent outbursts, destructiveness, noncompliance, choreiform movements, and minor congenital anomalies." His focus, however, was on a defect in moral self-control in children, and he emphasized the psychosocial aspects of their attentional problems when he wrote, "Interesting as these disorders may be as an abstruse problem for the professed psychologist to puzzle over, they have a real practical—shall I say social—importance which I venture to think has been hardly sufficiently recognized." He goes on to describe their problems in self-control in social situations. It is in this area that the child's difficulty impacts on family functioning.

Still's stated intention was to describe a morbid defect in volition. He used the term "moral self-control" to refer to "the control of action for the good of all" and pointed out that moral control can exist only when there is a sufficient cognitive understanding of one's relationship to others. However, Still maintained that intellectual understanding is not enough; volitional control is also necessary. He went on to describe developmental aspects of these conditions and referred to the slow and gradual development of inhibitory volition as the child grows older. He suggested it is a lack in the inhibitory nature of volition to "overpower" a stimulus that leads to excessive activity. He also pointed out that inhibitory volition becomes directed toward those forms of activity that are the most instinctive, for example, the expression of emotions.

Still viewed moral control as multiply determined and acknowledged that later outcome depended on the cognitive interrelationship with the environment, with moral consciousness, and with volition. In his subsequent lectures, he provided examples to demonstrate that mental retardation, a purely cognitive defect, was not the cause of a self-control deficit because nonretarded individuals may show far more severe behavioral defects than those who are mentally retarded. He offered a series of case examples of defects in moral control and categorized them as congenital cases, those acquired following brain injury, those with permanent symptoms, those with temporary symptoms, and those where behavioral control was cyclical.

In subsequent years, different aspects of Still's original description have been emphasized (Taylor, 1986). Barkley (1990) describes several periods, noting an initial focus on the brain-damaged child (1900 to 1960), then a specific emphasis on hyperactivity (1960 to 1969), followed by the ascendance of attention deficits (1970 to 1979), and, finally, the establishment of diagnostic criteria and the waning of attention deficits (1980 to 1989). Barkley (1990) offers a renewed focus on volitional control and emphasizes the importance of rule-governed behavior along with problems associated with inhibitory control. These changing views are discussed next.

In the United States, attention deficits came to medical attention following the 1917–1918 encephalitis pandemic. Children who survived often had significant behavioral and cognitive difficulties (Bender, 1942; Bond and Appel, 1931; Ebaugh, 1923; Hohman, 1922; Kessler, 1980). The children who were affected in the encephalitis epidemic often developed overactivity, attention deficits, and impulse control problems, whereas affected adults were more likely to develop Parkinsonian symptoms as a sequelae. Such different presentations, depending on the age of the insult, highlighted the importance of the onset of the disorder during the developmental period. The fact that the occurrence of an infectious disease in infancy or in childhood could lead to a different behavioral presentation than the onset in adulthood was an early basis for a developmental perspective on brain–behavior relationships.

These early studies concluded that not only encephalitis but other cerebral lesions, such as measles infection, birth trauma, lead toxicity, head trauma, and seizures, can cause severe restlessness; less severe behavioral symptoms may result from interpersonal difficulties or stress. The term "organic drivenness" was used by Kahn and Cohen (1934) to describe the behavioral abnormality thought to be a consequence of brainstem involvement that led to behavioral disorganization. Levin (1938) suggested that severe restlessness in children resulted from pathological changes in forebrain structures. In regard to treatment, Bradley (1937) and Bradley and Bowen (1940) reported that benzedrine reduced hyperactivity and improved attention in children with behavioral difficulties.

By the 1940s the concept of hyperactivity and inattention had been broadened further, so that hyperactivity alone was often considered adequate evidence for a diagnosis of brain damage (Strauss and Werner, 1943). Strauss and Lehtinen (1947) attributed brain injury to children who presented with these behavioral characteristics although brain pathology was not clearly documented by history or on examination. Yet Strauss and Werner (1943) did see similarities between hyperactive children and adults who lost control after neurological injury or stroke. Strauss referred to this as the "brain-injured child syndrome," and Strauss and Lehtinen suggested approaches to education. In the 1950s it came to be known as the "Strauss syndrome."

By the late 1950s (Laufer and Denhoff, 1957; Laufer, Denhoff, and Solomons, 1957), the diagnostic term "hyperkinetic impulsive disorder" was used for children with emotional and conduct problems. Hyperkinetic impulse disorder was identified as a condition involving the brain in children who had no overt evidence of brain damage; its designation as a disorder was considered to be a corrective to the prevailing psychodynamic view that focused primarily on the parents' contribution to causing children's problems. The identification of positive drug treatment effects on behavior and findings of abnormalities on physiologic testing in identified children were followed by a dramatic increase in both biological and pharmacological research on this condition.

Critical reviews began to appear in the 1960s that questioned whether there was an identifiable brain syndrome in children, suggesting, instead, multiple syndromes. Such reviews (Birch, 1964; Rapin, 1964) acknowledged that behavioral symptoms may result from brain damage but questioned whether the term "brain damage" was appropriate for children with behavioral problems who had only equivocal evidence of dysfunction on neurological examination. The confusion about the appropriate label was highlighted by a task force that found 37 different labels were being used for the same type of clinical presentation (Clements, 1966). The task force found that neurological, psychiatric, and educational terms were all being applied to the same children and suggested the name of the disorder be changed. Recommendations included "minimal brain dysfunction" (MBD), "minimal cerebral dysfunction" (MCD), and "central nervous system dysfunction." In each instance, the word "damage" was removed from the diagnostic label. Of these, "minimal brain dysfunction" became the most commonly used term (Wender, 1971). Minimal was used to distinguish it from maximal cerebral dysfunction, such as that seen in cerebral palsy, some mental retardation syndromes, and other brain-related syndromes. The prevailing view on hyperactivity was that it was part of a brain dysfunction syndrome but of milder degree than previously considered. Despite the lack of agreement regarding etiology, the term "MBD" gained widespread use. Moreover, it was recognized that although brain damage could cause behavioral symptoms, genetic factors might also be important. Because many children do not have evidence of prenatal, perinatal, or postnatal involvement, a genetic and developmental basis was considered. Moreover, parents were noted to have similar problems to those of their children during their own childhood and, in some instances, into adulthood. In addition, the environment played a role in modifying the behavioral presentation.

Yet like brain damage before it, "minimal brain dysfunction" gradually was also recognized as too vague, overly inclusive, and not supported by symptoms of neurological dysfunction. With increasing scrutiny, MBD was gradually replaced by labels that focused on specific cognitive, learning, and behavior disorders, such as dyslexia, learning disability, and finally, hyperactivity. In this period, the emphasis increasingly shifted to hyperactivity as the most important symptom of MBD. Still, affected children continued to be recognized as at the mercy of background stimulation and as having difficulty in concentrating and in inhibiting stimuli. Chess (1960), in discussing activity as the defining feature, stressed the need for objective evidence of this, separated hyperactivity from brain damage, and concurred that the behavior was not the result of dysfunctional parenting. These distinctions prepared the way for the inclusion of hyperkinetic behavior into the American Psychiatric Association's 1968 Diagnostic and Classification System.

CLASSIFICATION

With the introduction of the second edition of the American Psychiatric Association's *Diagnostic and Statistical Manual* (APA, 1968), a new section was added on child and adolescent disorders and the syndrome of childhood hyperactivity formally entered the system of classification as "hyperkinetic reaction of childhood or adolescence." In DSM-I (APA, 1952), the term "reaction" accompanied many diagnostic categories, e.g., affective reaction, schizophrenic reaction, because of concerns about prematurely creating a rigid nosological concept of disease. With the publication of DSM-II, the term "reaction" was, for the most part, eliminated so that affective disorder and schizophrenia were introduced as specific categories. However, the term "reaction" continued to be applied to a newly created childhood category, hence the designation "hyperkinetic reaction" under the category of behavior disorders of childhood and adolescence. These disorders were considered to be more stable, internalized, and resistant to treatment than transient situation disturbance, that is, more pervasive. The hyperkinetic reaction was characterized by "overactivity, restlessness, distractibility, and short attention span, especially in young children; the behavior usually diminishes in adolescence."

In North America, with the introduction of DSM-II (APA, 1968), the "hyperkinetic reaction of childhood or adolescence" was seen as a behavioral syndrome with characteristic excessive activity. It was thought to be a common disturbance that was not necessarily associated with brain damage and, in fact, was possibly a normal variant of temperament in some instances. In Great Britain, however, hyperkinetic disorder continued to be seen as extremely uncommon. In the Isle of Wight survey, Rutter, Graham, and Yule (1970) found that hyperkinetic behavior was infrequent in the total population of 9-year-olds. In Great Britain, the brain-damaged model seems to have persisted, and the syndrome was thought to be highly uncommon and, when present, associated primarily with epilepsy, mental retardation, and hemiplegia (Taylor, 1988).

During the 1970s features other than the hyperactivity emphasized in DSM-II were increasingly addressed, especially distractibility and short attention span. The existence of a pure syndrome of hyperactivity was questioned (August and Stewart, 1982). The concept of MBD faded as critical reviews appeared, such as those of Rutter (1977, 1982) emphasizing that MBD symptoms were not well defined, the condition was heterogeneous, there was poor internal correlation among symptoms, and the symptoms lacked specific etiological significance and showed no common course or outcome. During the 1970s additional research (Douglas, 1972) highlighted the importance of sustained attention and impulse control in the diagnosis. Douglas found that these children had particular difficulty on vigilance tasks and tasks of sustained attention, using a continuous performance test. Variability in their task performance was the most significant feature. She emphasized deficits in investment, organization, and maintenance of attention and effort, inability to inhibit impulsive responding, inability to modulate arousal levels to meet specific situational demands, and a strong inclination to seek immediate environmental reinforcement. This and subsequent research on attention led to the renaming of the disorder "attention deficit disorder" (ADD) in 1980, with the publication of a third edition of the U.S. *Diagnostic and Statistical Manual* (APA, 1980). Deficits in sustained attention and impulse control were recognized as having greater clinical significance than hyperactivity. This new focus provided some increased specificity because research on hyperactivity had shown no clear delineation between normal and abnormal levels of activity, although Porrino and colleagues (1983) subsequently did demonstrate that activity was quantitatively greater in a group of affected children.

The DSM-III criteria provided greater emphasis on inattention and impulsivity as defining features and included a specific symptom list with numerical cut-off points for symptoms, guidelines for age of onset and duration of symptoms, and exclusionary criteria. DSM-III also created subtypes of attention deficit disorder with hyperactivity (ADDH) and without hyperactivity. Children with attention deficit disorder without hyperactivity were characteristically less active than those with ADDH, lethargic, learning disabled, and tended to daydream (Carlson, 1986).

During the 1980s research criteria also were developed (Barkley, 1982; Loney, 1983). Loney and others (Loney, Langhorne, and Paternite, 1978; Milich and Landau, 1989; Milich, Loney, and Landau, 1982) focused on differentiating the symptoms of hyperactivity from those of aggression or conduct disorder. She demonstrated that a short list of symptoms for hyperactivity could be empirically separated from a short list of aggressive symptoms. The demonstration of a separate aggression cluster established that negative outcomes of hyperactivity during adolescence and young adulthood most likely may be due to the concurrent presence and extent of aggression because both symptoms co-occur. Purely aggressive children did not show substantial problems with attention; purely hyperactive children did. In addition, greater psychopathology in the families of hyperactive children was found to be related to the extent of aggressiveness in the children. Aggression was more likely to be associated with environmental circumstances and family dysfunction; hyperactivity was linked to developmental immaturity. Efforts to subtype ADHD increasingly focused on associated language-based learning disabilities, pervasive versus situational hyperactivity, and co-occurring symptoms of anxiety, depression, and compulsive behavior. Co-occurring symptoms began to be studied in reference to response to pharmacological interventions.

An international symposium on research diagnostic criteria for attention deficit disorder was convened (Sergeant, 1988), and the following criteria were suggested for subjects enrolled in research study: (1) reports of problems with activity and attention from two independent sources, e.g., home, school, psychiatric clinic; (2) endorsement of at least three or four difficulties with activity and three or four with attention; (3) age of onset before 7; (4) duration of 2 years; (5) significantly elevated scores on parent-teacher ratings of attention deficit disorder symptoms; and (6) exclusion of autistic disorder and psychosis.

The diagnostic criteria in the DSM-III revision published in 1987 were changed. "Attention deficit disorder with hyperactivity" was now designated "attention deficit hyperactivity disorder" (ADHD). This change took place because attention deficit disorder with hyperactivity was more common and better defined than the syndrome without hyperactivity. In the DSM-III-R classification (APA, 1987), a single-item list of symptoms and a single cut-off score replaced the three DSM-III clusters, i.e., inattention, impulsivity, and hyperactivity, and the cut-off scores used individually for them in DSM-III. In DSM-III-R, the item list was based on empirically derived dimensions of child behavior drawn from behavior rating scales. The cut-off scores and the items were chosen following a large field trial conducted to evaluate their sensitivity, specificity, and distinguishing features. In DSM-III-R, it was emphasized that the symptoms were developmentally inappropriate to the child's mental age, and the coexistence of affective disorders with ADHD was no longer an exclusionary criteria for the diagnosis of ADHD. Finally, the category of "ADD without hyperactivity" was removed and a new category, "undifferentiated attention deficit disorder," was added to incorporate it and as a reminder that additional subtyping might be possible. ADHD was classified as part of a new grouping, the disruptive behavior disorders, along with oppositional defiant disorder and conduct disorder.

In DSM-IV (APA, 1994) the categorization has been further revised and refined. Three general designations have been introduced: attention deficit/hyperactivity disorder, predominantly inattentive type; attention deficit/hyperactivity disorder, predominantly hyperactive-impulsive type; and attention deficit/hyperactivity disorder, combined type. In addition there is a residual category attention-deficit/hyperactivity disorder not otherwise specified. The DSM-IV criteria are listed in Table 13–1.

Extended Definition of Attention Deficit Disorder: Executive Dysfunction

Although not included in the DSM-IV classification, Barkley (1990) has proposed a consensus definition of AD/HD that highlights the developmental nature of self-regulation. He emphasizes the issue of volition and provides an extended definition of attention deficit disorder. In this extended definition, a functional aspect is added by highlighting deficient rule-governed behavior and difficulties in maintaining work performance. Barkley's extended definition is as follows:

> Attention-deficit/hyperactivity disorder is a developmental disorder characterized by developmentally inappropriate degrees of inattention, overactivity, and impulsivity. These often arise in early childhood; are relatively chronic in nature; and are not readily accounted for on the basis of gross neurological, sensory, language, or motor impairment, mental retardation, or severe emotional disturbance. These difficulties are typically associated with deficits in rule governed behavior and in maintaining a consistent pattern of work performance over time.

Rule-governed behavior refers to the capacity for language, i.e., commands, directions, instructions, descriptions to act as "discriminative stimulus for behavior." Rules specify contingencies for action.

MOTIVATIONAL DEFICIT DISORDER: EXECUTIVE DYSFUNCTION

Barkley's (1990) extended definition suggests that AD/HD be viewed as a disorder in motivation rather than in attention and suggests that deficits in rule-governed behavior may account for many of the behaviors. In this view, AD/HD might stem from an insensitivity to environmental consequences, either reinforcement or punishment. A motivational model provides greater explanatory value to account for situational variability in attention and is consistent with recent neuroanatomic studies that suggest decreased activation of brain reward centers and associated cortico-limbic regulating circuits (Lou, Henriksen, and Bruhn, 1984; Lou et al., 1989). It is also consistent with neurotransmitter studies implicating dopamine pathways

Table 13–1. DSM-IV Criteria for Attention Deficit/Hyperactivity Disorder

A. Either (1) or (2):
   (1) six (or more) of the following symptoms of **inattention** have persisted for at least 6 months to a degree that is maladaptive and inconsistent with developmental level:

      Inattention
      (a) often fails to give close attention to details or makes careless mistakes in schoolwork, work, or other activities
      (b) often has difficulty sustaining attention in tasks or play activities
      (c) often does not seem to listen when spoken to directly
      (d) often does not follow through on instructions and fails to finish schoolwork, chores, or duties in the workplace (not due to oppositional behavior or failure to understand instructions)
      (e) often has difficulties organizing tasks and activities
      (f) often avoids, dislikes, or is reluctant to engage in tasks that require sustained mental effort (such as schoolwork or homework)
      (g) often loses things necessary for tasks or activities (e.g., toys, school assignments, pencils, books, or tools)
      (h) is often easily distracted by extraneous stimuli
      (i) is often forgetful in daily activities
   (2) six (or more) of the following symptoms of **hyperactivity-impulsivity** have persisted for at least 6 months to a degree that is maladaptive and inconsistent with developmental level:

      Hyperactivity
      (a) often fidgets with hands or feet or squirms in seat
      (b) often leaves seat in classroom or in other situations in which remaining seated is expected
      (c) often runs about or climbs excessively in situations where it is inappropriate (in adolescents or adults, may be limited to subjective feelings of restlessness)
      (d) often has difficulty playing or engaging in leisure activities quietly
      (e) is often "on the go" or often acts as if "driven by a motor"
      (f) often talks excessively

      Impulsivity
      (g) often blurts out answers before questions have been completed
      (h) often has difficulty awaiting turn
      (i) often interrupts or intrudes on others (e.g., butts into conversations or games)

B. Some hyperactive-impulsive or inattentive symptoms that caused impairment were present before age 7 years.

C. Some impairment from the symptoms is present in two or more settings (e.g., at school [or work] and at home).

D. There must be clear evidence of clinically significant impairment in social, academic, or occupational functioning.

E. The symptoms do not occur exclusively during the course of a Pervasive Developmental Disorder, Schizophrenia or other Psychotic Disorder, and are not better accounted for by another mental disorder (e.g., Mood Disorder, Anxiety Disorder, Dissociative Disorder, or a Personality Disorder).

Code based on type:

314.01 Attention-Deficit/Hyperactivity Disorder, Combined Type: If both Criteria A1 and A2 are met for the past 6 months

314.00 Attention-Deficit/Hyperactivity Disorder, Predominantly Inattentive Type: If Criterion A1 is met but Criterion A2 is not met for the past 6 months

314.01 Attention-Deficit/Hyperactivity Disorder, Predominantly Hyperactive-Impul sive Type: If Criterion A2 is met but Criterion A1 is not met for the past 6 months

Coding note: For individuals (especially adolescents and adults) who currently have symptoms that no longer meet full criteria, "In Partial Remission" should be specified.
From APA, 1994.

in regulating not only locomotor behavior but also learning based on incentives.

Another view consistent with deficits in rule-governed behavior, as described by Barkley, is that of Denckla (1989), who extends the definition further when she suggests that many children with ADHD have features of executive dysfunction. (Executive function is described in Chapter 3 on neuropsychological testing.) In keeping with this hypothesis, she has used neuropsychological tests to identify difficulty with planning and sequencing complex behaviors, paying attention to several features at once, capacity to grasp the gist of a complex situation, resistance to distraction and interference, inhibition of inappropriate response tendencies, and ability to maintain behavioral output over time. Particular problems are noted in organizing, planning, and managing time. This approach is described in detail in the section on etiology.

EPIDEMIOLOGY

Prevalence rates of ADHD in early studies ranged from less than 1% to more than 14% (Szatmari, 1992). This variability was most likely due to variations in the symptoms used to diagnose the disorder, the criteria used to define a case, the methods of data collection, and which respondents (i.e., parents, teachers) provided the information. Because of this variability, prevalence data from early epidemiologic studies have been difficult to interpret. However, with the publication of diagnostic criteria, first in DSM-III and then in DSM-III-R, greater consensus on diagnosis has been reached. Szatmari (1992) reviewed six epidemiologic studies of ADHD from several sites (United States, New Zealand, Puerto Rico, West Germany, and Canada) that used clear diagnostic criteria, structured interviews, and multistage cluster sampling of households to obtain a representative sample. Based on these studies, the prevalence rates for ADHD range from a low of 2.0% to a high of 6.3%. The disorder was found more commonly in boys than in girls and more often in lower socioeconomic settings. The rates were lower in adolescence, although the exact prevalence in adolescence remains to be clarified. ADD without hyperactivity may be more common in adolescence than in childhood; the Ontario Child Health Survey (Canada) found the rates were lower than in childhood, with a population prevalence of 1.4% for boys and 1.0% for girls.

There is a high co-occurrence between ADHD and other disruptive behavior disorders, particularly conduct disorder. In the Ontario Child Health Survey, (Szatmari, Offord, and Boyle, 1989), 42% of boys with ADDH, age 4 to 11, and 36% of girls with ADDH, age 4 to 11, had co-occurring conduct disorder with higher rates reported for adolescents. Anderson et al. (1987) (New Zealand) found 47% of children with ADD to have co-occurring diagnoses of either oppositional disorder or conduct disorder, and Bird et al. (1989) (Puerto Rico) found 53.6% with co-occurring disruptive behavior disorders. Moreover, overlap between ADDH and anxiety or emotional disorders occurs in between 17% to 26% of children, depending on the study (Anderson et al., 1987; Bird et al., 1989; Szatmari, Offord, and Boyle, 1989). In the Ontario Child Health Survey, children with pure ADDH had more developmental problems than those with pure conduct disorder. Those with conduct disorder came from more disadvantaged backgrounds and had a greater family history of aggressive behavior. Those with co-occurring disorders had higher rates of both developmental disorders and psychosocial problems (Szatmari, 1992) and had a worse prognosis.

Despite the widely different geographic population sample, sample size, age range studied, and differences in informants chosen, there was surprising agreement among these studies, suggesting the utility of using these estimates. Future epidemiologic studies need to consider the best way to combine data from several informants and to clarify whether behaviors can simply be pooled. Should each source, e.g., parent, teacher, contribute independently to the diagnosis, and should subthreshold diagnoses from one or two separate sources be considered together? There continues to be some uncertainty about the criteria of a case for epidemiologic purposes and how diagnostic criteria should be operationalized. Although additional work needs to be done, these studies provide the best estimates that are currently available.

Because of the discrepancy of diagnosis between the United States and England, a cross-national study was carried out. When similar criteria were used by specially trained research teams in both countries, interrated agreement was reached (Prendergast et al., 1988). It should be noted that in other countries the diagnosis has generally been made at the same rate as in the United States.

ETIOLOGY

Attention

It is unlikely that any one area or any one neurochemical system will be found to fully explain AD/HD because its symptoms involve various interrelated neuroanatomic and neurochemical systems. However, brain systems that may be involved in attention, inhibition, activity, and their control are the subject of ongoing investigation.

The attention systems are extensive and, therefore, vulnerable to damage and dysfunction. Attention is based on arousal; attention involves vigilance, a span of apprehension, perseverance to maintain it, and the capacity to resist distractions (Denckla, 1989). There are various aspects to attention including focusing, executing, sustaining, and shifting attention. The reticular activating system mediates the attentional state involved in the rapid modulation of information processing (brainstem and midbrain) as attention is channeled to higher levels of the nervous system. These attentional functions involve brain regions that are interconnected and organized into systems. Depending on the locus of the insult, various aspects of attention may be affected. The capacity to shift attention from one aspect of the environment to another is supported by the prefrontal cortex; focusing attention on environmental events is shared by the superior temporal and inferior parietal cortices as well as by the components of the corpus striatum, i.e., caudate putamen and globus pallidus. In addition, inferior parietal and corpus striatal regions are involved in motoric executive function. The hippocampus is involved in encoding stimuli that are involved in memory functions which may be required for some aspects of attention. Finally, sustaining attention involves rostral brain structures including the tectum, mesopontine reticular formation, and midline and reticular thalamic nuclei (Mirsky, 1987).

Denckla (1989) suggests that these various components of attention must be assessed to study the heterogeneity of ADHD. This might include study of the state/channel dimension (arousal), the dimension involving the right and left hemispheric contributions to attention (right hemispheric damage has greater effect than the left), the motivational aspects of attention (cingulate/limbic), the sensory-representational aspects (mainly posterior parietal cortex), and the motor-exploratory aspects that depend on the frontal lobe and its subcortical connections. The frontal lobe is central to attention, yet it is the last part of the brain to develop and has the longest period of vulnerability (Mesulam, 1985).

Frontal lobe involvement in AD/HD has been suggested by several authors, such as Chelune et al. (1986), who point out that prefrontal regions of the frontal lobes have reciprocal pathways with the reticular formation and those diencephalic structures which regulate arousal and the ability to inhibit responses to stimuli that are not task relevant. Lesions to these brain regions might decrease the modulation of impulsive behavior and goal-directed activity. Using the model of frontal lobe lesions, these authors found some support for the frontal lobe dysfunction hypothesis when they compared normal controls and children with hyperactivity, impulsivity, and inattention on a comprehensive neuropsychological test battery. Additional support for the involvement of the prefrontal system comes from Gorenstein, Mammato, and Sandy (1989), Everett et al. (1991), and Tannock et al. (1989). Heilman, Voeller, and Nadeau (1991) have reviewed syndromes involving abnormal mental awareness associated with the prefrontal, frontal, and striatal dysfunction. They suggest that abnormalities seen in these individuals resemble those documented in children with AD/HD. Overall, these investigators suggest that prefrontal and right frontal striate systems might be involved in children with AD/HD. Ongoing research focuses on how different aspects of the syndrome may be involved in brain systems that are interconnected into reciprocal modulating systems.

Executive Dysfunction Syndrome

Denckla (1989) suggests that many children with AD/HD have features of executive dysfunction. As noted earlier, these are characterized by difficulty in planning and sequencing complex behaviors, the capacity to pay attention to several components of a problem at once, the inhibition of inappropriate response tendencies, the ability to grasp the gist of a complex situation, resistance to distraction and interference, and the ability to sustain behavioral output for relatively long periods (Denckla, 1989; Struss and Benson, 1984). Children with executive dysfunction have difficulty organizing and managing time. These abilities depend on the integrity of the frontal lobes and their subcortical connections, including the basal ganglia, particularly, the striatum. Barkley's view that AD/HD is a disability involving rule-governed behavior is consistent with Denckla's neuropsychological interpretation.

The conceptualization of AD/HD as an executive function syndrome has the advantage of focusing specifically on brain regions that may be evaluated, using neuropsychological testing procedures. Dennis (1991) has suggested that frontal lobe systems are involved in the general areas of attention/inhibition, self-monitoring, and the regulation of social discourse. Problems in all three of these areas are commonly demonstrated in children with this disorder. The difficulties with attention and inhibition are clearly specified in the diagnostic criteria in versions of DSM-III. However, self-monitoring and the maintenance of rule-governed behavior are involved in attentional processes and inhibition and seem linked to Barkley's emphasis on a motivational deficit. Finally, problems in maintenance of social discourse have been highlighted when pragmatic language and narrative production have been assessed. Documentation of these deficits in executive function can be tested, as outlined in Chapter 3 on neuropsychology. Assessment of attention deficits and self-monitoring may be carried out, using the Test of Variables of Attention (TOVA), and narrative abilities may be assessed in children, using a story retelling task (Tannock, Purvis, and Schachar, 1993). Although no specific battery of tests is absolutely identified to demonstrate executive dysfunction, Denckla (1989) proposes a neuropsychological approach to evaluate the psychological or cognitive processes and establish how the mind is working. The test procedure utilizes systematic assessment of the executive function domain including, but not limited to, continuous performance tests. Using this approach, specific qualitative errors are detected that are pathognomonic if a deficiency in psychological processes involved in rule-governed performances are tested. One proposal for accomplishing this is the use of constructs of initiating (planning), sustaining (concentrating), inhibiting (self-monitoring), and shifting (cognitive flexibility) on a battery of tests. For example, a continuous performance test, such as the TOVA, measures concentration as does the Trails A/B Test. The Stroop Color Word Interference Test evaluates concentration, self-monitoring, and cognitive flexibility. Verbal fluency is useful in assessing all four of these constructs. From these tests, Denckla derives a neuropsychological equivalent of attention deficit disorder. A detail description of the analysis of a neuropsychological profile is provided at the end of Chapter 3.

Genetic Factors

Genetic factors have been implicated in AD/HD (Pauls, 1991). Although the type of genetic transmission is unknown, three lines of evidence support a role for genetic factors in some cases: family studies, twin studies, and adoption studies. Family studies are consistent with there being a genetic component for hyperactivity in that there is a higher rate of disorders in the families of children identified with AD/HD (Biederman et al., 1986). Biederman, Newcorn, and Sprich (1991) evaluated 73 males with ADD and 264 of their first-degree relatives along with 26 male pediatric normal controls and their 92 relatives. This study used structured interviews, age-corrected analyses of risks, and blinded interviewers and found evidence for familial transmission of both ADD and co-occurring mood disorders. The risk for ADD in relatives of identified children with ADD and identified children with both ADD and mood disorder was 27% and 22%, whereas the rate in the control population was 5%. The co-occurrence of mood disorder was thought to be related to nonfamilial stressful environmental circumstances. In extending these studies (Faraone et al., in press) to 140 identified children with AD/HD, 120 in a control group and 822 first-degree relatives, a segregation analysis suggests a familial distribution of AD/HD that might be attributed to a single major gene defect. These authors estimate that 46% of boys and 32% of girls who carry a putative AD/HD gene may actually develop AD/HD. The model also predicts that as many as 38% of the boys with AD/HD may not carry this putative gene. Therefore, authors also emphasize the importance of environmental factors as well as genetic ones.

Goodman and Stevenson (1989a, 1989b) carried out a well-designed study of 570 13-year-old twins. These authors concluded that genetic factors could account for approximately 50% of the variance in these studies. Although this twin study may not generalize fully to clinical groups because it included normal as well as deviant behaviors, it is the most comprehensive study to date. Goodman and Stevenson postulated that the high male to female ratio in ADHD might be due to a higher dose effect in girls; this hypothesis was not confirmed because the siblings of female twins with ADHD had the same prevalence of ADHD as that found in boys. There was evidence that boys as a group show greater inattentiveness and possibly greater hyperactivity when compared with girls.

Adoption studies have also been conducted to evaluate genetic factors in ADHD. Adoption studies provide a control for the similar rearing environments of monozygotic twins. Morrison and Stewart (1973) compared adoptive parents of children with ADHD with biological parents of other children with ADHD. These authors found that the adoptive parents and their biological relatives had lower levels of childhood hyperactivity; the adoptive parents showed low rates of pathological behavior (2.1%). Cadoret and Stewart (1991) collected data on the biological parents of adoptees from two adoption agencies in regard to both psychiatric and criminal histories. Two hundred eighty-three male adoptees and their adoptive parents were assessed with reference to their genetic background, environmental factors, and outcomes in relation to ADHD, aggression, and antisocial personality features. These authors concluded that there is a genetic component for ADHD but did not demonstrate a genetic component for aggression. This is consistent with other reports that aggression and hyperactivity are independent dimensions.

NEUROBIOLOGICAL STUDIES

Functional Brain-Imaging Studies

Functional brain-imaging techniques are being utilized to evaluate suspected neurophysiologic abnormalities in individuals with ADD. SPECT scanning with Xenon 133 (XE-133) has been utilized to study ADD in children and adolescents by Lou, Henriksen, and Bruhn (1984, 1990) and by Lou and colleagues (1989). The first two reports by these authors showed decreased striatal region cerebral blood flow (rCBF) in individuals with ADD. Blood flow was found to increase following treatment with methylphenidate. In the most recent study by these authors (Lou, Henriksen, and Bruhn, 1990), 9 subjects with ADD, 8 subjects with ADD and dysphasia, and 15 normal control subjects were evaluated. Regional cerebral blood flow was decreased bilaterally in the striatal region and increased in the occipital region in the ADD subjects.

PET scanning has been used by Zametkin et al. (1990) to evaluate whole brain and regional cerebral glucose metabolism in 25 adults with childhood onset ADD and age-matched controls. The adult subjects had lower global glucose metabolism and showed regional reductions in glucose metabolism primarily in the prefrontal and premotor cortex. Zametkin et al. (1993) also have investigated brain metabolism in 10 adolescent males with ADD who were compared with 10 adolescent male controls. The subjects with ADD had decreased metabolism in frontal, temporal, thalamic, and hippocampal areas. However, the overall reductions in blood glucose metabolism were minimal. Subsequently, females with ADD were studied and found to show a greater reduction in brain metabolism than males for both the adult and adolescent populations. These findings raise questions regarding the pathophysiology of ADD as a function of age and gender (Ernst et al., 1993).

Matochik et al. (1993) have suggested that single acute doses of dextroamphetamine, when compared to methylphenidate, may have different effects on cerebral metabolism in adults with ADD. These authors studied 13 subjects with dextroamphetamine and found increased metabolism in the anterior medial frontal, right posterior temporal, right thalamus, and right caudate regions. Decreases were noted in the right rolandic, left anterior frontal, and right anterior frontal regions when compared to the subjects' baseline. Fourteen subjects who were treated with methylphenidate had increased metabolism in the left posterior frontal and left parietal regions, and decreased metabolism in anterior medial frontal, left parietal, and left/occipital regions compared to their baseline measures. These findings indicate that stimulants may lead to widespread changes—both increases and decreases in brain metabolism.

NEUROCHEMICAL STUDIES

Neurochemical studies of systems that may be involved in AD/HD include neuroanatomical investigations of neurotransmitters thought to be involved, biochemical studies of neurotransmitters and their metabolites, and pharmacological investigations (Zametkin and Rapoport, 1987). Neuroanatomical studies involving neurotransmitters have been complicated because any particular brain region may involve several neurotransmitter systems and may receive projections from nuclei that use a variety of neurotransmitters. Consequently, neuroanatomical studies have not been conclusive. Another approach is the measurement of monoamines and their metabolites in urine, plasma, platelets, and/or cerebral spinal fluid in subjects with AD/HD and normal controls. Such studies are limited because peripheral measures of metabolites do not clearly reflect central nervous system neurotransmitter activity. Therefore, no consistent differences in any peripheral measures of monoamines and their metabolites have been identified when children with AD/HD have been compared to normal controls. The third approach evaluates the effect of particular psychopharmacological agents on one or more neurotransmitter systems and evaluates the clinical effects.

Several neurotransmitter hypotheses have been proposed to account for symptoms of AD/HD. These are discussed next.

Dopamine

The dopamine hypothesis has been proposed by several authors. Wender (1975) suggested that behavioral difficulties in affected children and adolescents following the encephalitis pandemic of 1918 might have been related to abnormalities in dopamine function linked to the infection. Subsequently, Shaywitz, Yager, and Klopper (1976) proposed that selective brain dopamine depletion in developing rats led to hyperactivity when they reached maturity. This was followed by investigations of cerebral spinal fluid and monoamine metabolites in children with AD/HD that suggested evidence of altered brain dopamine (Shaywitz, Cohen, and Bower, 1977); however, such changes were not confirmed by other investigators. The dopamine hypothesis has also been proposed by Roeltgen and Schneider (1991) based on studies of chronic low-dose MPTP (a neurotoxin) administration in nonhuman developing primates. Schneider and Kovelowski (1990) have also investigated the effects of low-dose MPTP in regard to cognitive deficits in monkeys without motor symptoms. Both groups of authors found that monkeys who were given this neurotoxin had caudate frontal dysfunction and cognitive difficulties consistent with those seen in children with AD/HD. Neurochemical studies on a pilot group of these monkeys have suggested abnormalities in dopamine and norepinephrine metabolism. Wong et al. (1993) have demonstrated that the dopamine transporter antagonist WIN 35,428 may be used as a PET marker for the dopmine transporter. Because methylphenidate is thought to activate dopamine neurons by decreasing reuptake of dopamine through action on the DA transporter, the use of this PET ligand is of interest for AD/HD. Stimulants also have dopamine-releasing effects that may be a factor in drug response. Dopamine systems are involved in the control of locomotion and seem crucial for positive and negative reinforcement.

Noradrenergic

The noradrenergic system has been considered to be involved in AD/HD primarily through pharmacological investigations. Dextroamphetamine is one of the most commonly used medications to treat AD/HD and has been shown to release epinephrine in the hippothalamus. During clinical investigations, dextroamphetamine as well as methylphenidate elevate urinary epinephrine excretion (Elia et al., 1990). In addition, clonidine and guanfacine, both alpha-adrenergic agonists, have been utilized in the treatment of ADHD (Hunt et al., 1984, Hunt et al., 1995). These authors have proposed that clonidine's and guanfacine's effects are mediated by direct stimulation of presynaptic alpha 2-adrenergic sites to decrease the release of norepinephrine; this leads to an increase in postsynaptic noradrenergic sensitivity. Moreover, antidepressants, such as desipramine, show moderate effectiveness and may involve the noradrenergic mechanism of action (Donnelly et al., 1986).

Other authors (McCraken, 1991) have suggested the involvement of both dopamine and norepinephrine systems. McCraken proposes that stimulant medication increases dopamine release and concurrently inhibits the noradrenergic locus coeruleus through adrenergic-mediated mechanisms. The locus coeruleus is involved in arousal activation and exploratory behavior and may play a central role in AD/HD. A defect in adrenergic inhibition of noradrenergic locus coeruleus can lead to a state of hypervigilance that may overlap with AD/HD symptoms (Castellanos and Rapoport, 1992).

Serotonin

There is less evidence for the involvement of serotonergic systems in AD/HD. Animals depleted of serotonin tend to show increased aggression along with hyperactivity. Still, some pharmacological agents that affect the serotonin system may be moderately effective in AD/HD. However, these medications are ordinarily prescribed for concurrent mood disorder rather than for AD/HD alone; their role in "pure" AD/HD requires further clarification. No clear pattern of change in platelet and blood 5-hydroxytryptophan have been demonstrated in AD/HD. When L-tryptophan, a serotonin precursor, was administered to children with AD/HD, no consistent behavioral changes were noted (Nemzer et al., 1986).

Interactive Effects

In addition, no significant differences in levels of dopamine-beta-hydroxylase, monoamine oxidase, and catechol-O-methyl-transferase have been demonstrated (Brown, Ebert, and Minichiello, 1985). Based on these various hypotheses, it seems most likely that several neurotransmitter systems are involved in AD/HD. The most effective drug treatment for these children involves medications that promote catecholamine utilization in the synapse through facilitating synthesis and release of catecholamines and through blocking reuptake. Currently, the dopamine-catecholamine hypothesis of AD/HD is the most parsimonious (Castellanos and Rapoport, 1992). Although difficult to confirm, both challenge studies and neurotransmitter and neurotransporter imaging studies may be pertinent in further evaluation of the neurochemical mechanisms involved.

In summary, progress is being made in understanding the neurobiology of AD/HD. Anatomically, the prefrontal and striate brain regions have been implicated in the condition. Neurotransmitters, particularly dopamine and norepinephrine, are thought to be involved. However, no one brain region or neurotransmitter dysfunction adequately explains the clinical presentation. It is currently assumed that the condition involves the interaction of various brain regions and several neurotransmitters. The distinction made in DSM-IV between predominant attention deficit disorder and predominant impulsivity-hyperactivity may lead to more specific hypotheses as to which of these clinical presentations involve which brain regions. The association of co-occurring conditions involving oppositional behavior, compulsive behavior, anxiety, or mood disorder may provide additional cues to neurotransmitter systems that may be involved.

SOCIAL COGNITIVE DOMAIN

Social cognition is important to consider in children with AD/HD because it is not only off-task behavior and distractibility but also social perception (interpreting nonverbal cues such as facial expression); role taking (taking another's point of view); social problem solving (generating alternative solutions); and social communication (social pragmatics, e.g., maintaining a conversation) that may be problematic for these children. Social cognition refers to the processing of information that culminates in accurate perception of the dispositions and intentions of others. Social cognition has an intimate tie to affective or emotional relations with others and has evolved in response to the demands of a complex social environment. The evolutionary basis of social cognition and the possibility of there being a social cognitive network in the brain has received new emphasis with the identification of feature recognition cells in the temporal lobe of the brain in primates (Desimone, 1991). The linkage of these cells to the prefrontal cortex suggests a selective response of single neurons or groups of neurons to social contact.

Even though the existence of a specific social cognitive network in the brain has not been demonstrated in humans, deficits in response inhibition have been suggested to be the result of dysfunction in the right fronto-striate system. In addition, social emotional learning disability (SELD) has been attributed to right hemispheric dysfunction. Therefore, inattention may extend beyond short attention span to social inattention, potentially as a "social" neglect syndrome.

Dysfunctional Affect Discrimination

Another aspect of the social deficit in AD/HD relates to affective discrimination. In normal development, a variety of affective responses are normally discriminated (Izard, 1991). These include joy, anger, fear, sadness, and disgust. Verbal labeling of the emotions is a task that follows a developmental sequence. It is proposed that affect discrimination may be dysfunctional in AD/HD.

A case report by Damasio, Tranel, and Damasio (1990) may be pertinent to the mechanism of frontal lobe dysfunction involved in emotional labeling. Damasio and colleagues described a patient with sociopathic behavior who failed to respond automatically to social stimuli following frontal lobe damage. They pointed out that following damage to the ventromedial frontal cortices, adults with previously normal personalities developed deficits in decision making and planning associated with abnormal social conduct. These authors propose that the defect is due to an inability to activate somatic states linked to punishment and reward. In this patient's previous experience, his somatic states were associated with social situations. In new situations, prior somatic states could be reactivated in connection with anticipated responses from others to provide contextually appropriate options to respond. However, following the frontal lobe damage, this ability seems to have been lost.

Damasio and colleagues argue that failure to activate somatic (bodily) states deprives an individual of an automatic device to signal the ultimately deleterious consequences of decisions. Longer term consequences may go unrecognized even though impulsive decisions might bring immediate reward. For example, normally, activation of somatic or bodily states might focus an individual's attention on the negative consequences of his choices based on past experiences. With this awareness, one might choose to inhibit behavior. Here, we are speaking of the experience of the body in the mind, commonly referred to as "gut feelings" about what action to take.

Clinically, the automatic response to social stimuli could be deficient in AD/HD. Children with AD/HD may not adequately discriminate bodily feeling states and/or may misperceive social situations. Alternatively, the child or adolescent might experience faulty, negative, or adversive bodily sensations and have difficulty in linking affect to cognition. The child might say to himself (and then to others to justify the behavior), that another child "looked at him the wrong way" to justify his fighting (Harris, 1994).

Narrative Production

Difficulties in organization are associated with executive dysfunction. Children with attention deficit disorders often have difficulty organizing their schoolwork and organizing their activities. This lack of organization may extend to individuals with AD/HD having difficulty in narrative production but not in narrative comprehension (Douglas and Benezra, 1990; Hamlett, Pellegrini and Connors, 1987; Tannock, Purvis and Schachar, 1993; Zentall, 1988). Assessing narrative production in AD/HD is necessary because narratives play a central role in social interactions and in academic activities. Narrative production involves storytelling and retelling, describing past experiences, and giving directions; narratives require comprehension and extended language production. To meet the listener's needs, an oral monologue is maintained while the listener remains relatively passive. Information must be presented by the speaker that is accurate, organized, and complete. Such narrative accounts require metacognitive functions or executive control of processes of on-line monitoring, planning, and organization in addition to linguistic ability (Tannock, Purvis, and Schachar, 1993).

Executive control allows the speaker to integrate and adapt to information from relevant sources that include the social context, the meaning of what is said, the content of what is said, and the characteristics of the speaker. Deficits in internal planning, organizing, and on-line monitoring have been reported in AD/HD. Such deficits are assessed through the use of a story retelling task to evaluate narrative abilities. Boys with AD/HD have been found to provide less information overall, to produce poorly organized stories, stories that are less cohesive, and stories that contain more inaccuracies. Consequently, their stories may be confusing and difficult to follow. Because organization and monitoring of information requires executive functioning, these deficits may reflect deficiencies in metacognitive processing.

Typically in the analysis of a story, sequence errors, misinterpretations, substitutions, ambiguous reference, and embellishment are evaluated. Tannock, Purvis, and Schachar (1993) assessed the narrative abilities in 30 boys with AD/HD and 30 normally developing boys who were matched for age and IQ. The authors evaluated whether or not the idea unit was retold in a different order than the original story, which affected the story theme (sequence error), whether the meaning of an action was incorrectly interpreted (misinterpretation), whether a word used for an object, character, or event in the original story was replaced with an inappropriate word that was not a synonym, whether ambiguous reference was present (a person is not linked to a specific character so its referent is ambiguous), and whether new events or characters are introduced that were not part of the original story event (embellishment). These authors confirmed previous research (O'Neill and Douglas, 1991; Zentall, 1988) suggesting that children with AD/HD did not differ in comprehension of narratives and had the ability to differentiate important and relevant information from nonessential detail. However, they also confirmed a narrative production deficit, as had been found in previous studies. These authors point out that those studies which have presented test stories through the auditory route are more likely to demonstrate the deficit. However, studies of narration where the provision of content support is offered by allowing a child to read along with the tester, using a copy of the test story, may not show differences between groups (O'Neill and Douglas, 1991). Overall, storytelling in the AD/HD group showed a higher frequency of sequence errors and cohesion errors that reflect a breakdown in the ability to globally organize a story's theme. Affected children also produced more local errors of information processing across story production. Although misinterpreted information and using inappropriate word substitutions could reflect problems in comprehension because there was no difference from controls on comprehension measures, these abnormalities may reflect a failure to monitor information resulting from deficits in executive control.

The interpretation of results of these narrative story findings must consider whether the problems are attributable to deficits in executive processes or language impairment, or both. Some children with AD/HD could show production deficits that could be quantitatively similar to that produced by others with language impairment, whereas their linguistic competence is better than those with a language disorder. Word substitutions, delays, and problems in cohesion may be associated with both language disorders (German and Simon, 1991) and deficits in executive processes. Most studies on narration have not assessed language abilities other than those involved in narratives. Although there is no specific evidence that children with AD/HD exhibit deficits in verbal memory span or memory capacity in itself (Weingartner et al., 1980), they may have co-occurring learning disorders. Children with this disorder comprise a heterogeneous group, and concurrent learning disabilities are present in 10% to 50% of them (Hinshaw, 1992). Still, Purvis, Schachar, and Tannock (in press) have suggested that the presence of learning disability leads to a different pattern of deficits than they found in children with the AD/HD diagnosis, using the narrative assessment method.

Stimulant medication, through its ability to enhance executive processes (Douglas et al., 1988), might improve narrative production. The effects of stimulant medication on improving narrative production, if confirmed, will provide an additional reason why children with AD/HD should be properly identified and treated pharmacologically.

INTERPERSONAL ASPECTS: SOCIAL BEHAVIOR

Whalen and Henker (1992) identified five aspects related to the interpersonal behavior of children with AD/HD: response patterns, style of approach, social information processing, peer appeal, and interpersonal impact of the disorder. These authors note that although a sample of children with AD/HD is necessarily heterogeneous and the children evaluated commonly have associated behavioral difficulties, these interpersonal patterns described are generally applicable if the child meets the diagnostic criteria for the disorder.

First, the individual response pattern tends to be one of an increased rate of social contact that heightens awareness of the child's presence by others. Excessive contact increases the likelihood of inappropriate interpersonal interactions that place the child at risk for being in conflict and being rejected. Whitehouse (1989) suggests that "hyper-reactivity" may be a useful term to describe their responses, which may be "too fast and too much" to environmental stimulation. The majority of children with AD/HD engage in socially objectionable acts, such as noncompliance, intrusiveness, rule breaking, bossiness, and disruptive behavior. In some instances, these behaviors seem intentional and, in others, this is not the case. In the intentional group, co-occurring diagnoses of AD/HD with either conduct disorder or oppositional defiant disorder may be found. For the nonvolitional group, there may be a high level of social interest, impulsive rather than planned social approaches, and/or an emotionally labile temperament. These children are action oriented and the effects of their behavior on others are largely inadvertent. With peers, they tend to be less likely to evaluate the social context when they enter a new group, to consider the social norms, or wait for an appropriate invitation to enter. Rather than wait, they may make demands and attempt to redirect or revise the rules of the group. Some children with AD/HD seem socially awkward rather than deliberately intrusive, and their responses may relate to problems in social perception (e.g., social-emotional learning disability) or immaturity. These characteristic responses, which are not interpersonally matched to ongoing events, may result in the individual's appearing insensitive to others' needs and not responsive to feedback from peers or adults.

An assessment procedure that includes evaluation of interpersonal social transactions may be more clinically useful than a more classical behavioral approach that involves monitoring frequency counts of excessive and deficit behaviors. One way of evaluating the social response pattern is to contrast communication patterns of two nonaffected boys to those of a nonaffected boy with a boy who has AD/HD. When compared to noninvolved age-mates, boys with a diagnosis of AD/HD are less socially aware. They seem less likely to watch peers, more likely to attempt contact and interrupt when peers are working independently, and more likely to respond to unauthorized questions when asked by teachers to work without talking (Cunningham, Siegel, and Offord, 1985). In addition, less joint activity and more aggression, lower rates of verbal reciprocity, and more social withdrawal following aggression have been noted among boys with AD/HD. Hubbard and Newcomb (1991) found that the nonaffected pairs of boys achieved the highest level of play, that is, rule-governed play, more rapidly than the pairs where one boy had AD/HD (within 3 minutes versus 17 minutes).

Prosocial behaviors may or may not be in the behavioral repertoire of children with AD/HD. Although inappropriate behavior is most commonly emphasized in research studies, there is no clear-cut evidence for deficiencies in prosocial behavior (Buhrmester et al., 1992). An evaluation of prosocial behavior and the identification of the presence or absence of prosocial dysfunction is crucial in treatment planning. Prosocial behaviors involve helping others, empathy toward others in distress, and capacity to maintain friendships. Prosocial behaviors are particularly important to evaluate with a co-occurring conduct disorder.

Problems in response pattern and dyadic communication may not be evident on first office visits, but rather become apparent as tasks are introduced a second and third time. Apparently normal responsiveness is also commonly seen on initial evaluation visits with professionals. Whalen and Henker (1992) speculate that there may be several reasons to account for the apparent worsening of behavior with repeated assessment. These include decreasing novelty and loss of interest, inability to sustain social attention, problems with goal orientation, or simply fatigue. During unstructured activities and free play, no differences in behavior may be noted between affected and nonaffected children. Differences become more apparent in situations where there are task demands and increasing constraints. This occurs particularly when certain rules must be followed or the task, such as a set of math problems, must be completed.

Second, the style of the child's approach to others has been studied. This involves assessment of the intensity of response, behavioral modulation of responses, and modulation of affect. Although children with AD/HD may know the appropriate social norms and may even have an adequate repertoire of interpersonal routines, the modulation of their responses and the timing of their interactions may be inappropriate. They may show more intense interactions that are forceful, vigorous, and loud. Henker, Astor-Dubin, and Varni (1986) evaluated perceived intensity in children with AD/HD and documented atypical levels of intensity not only in the classroom but also when the child was playing alone. These authors found that the child's intensity is decreased with stimulant medication. In addition, Whalen, Henker, and Dotemoto (1980) have documented that teachers may be more intense when interacting with children with AD/HD when compared with nonaffected children and that medication effects on the child may normalize the level of the adult's intensity, which suggests reciprocal influences.

The modulation of behavior as situational demands change has been documented by other investigators (Landau and Milich, 1988). These authors found that the communication patterns of nonaffected boys are more flexible than those of boys with ADHD in structured situations where roles must be reversed, such as in a task that involves the child's having to switch back and forth between talk show guest and host. Problems in role shifting were also documented by Whalen et al. (1979) in a simulated space flight communication task where boys took turns as mission control and astronaut. The messages given by the boys with AD/HD were more rigidly consistent across roles as they moved from one role to the other, suggesting a failure to modulate role requirements based on variations in task demands.

Dysregulation or modulation of affect is pertinent to style and intensity of interaction. Children with AD/HD are commonly thought to be emotionally labile and inappropriately responsive to both physical and social stimulation in social situations. Efforts are commonly made by teachers and parents to prevent affective arousal because arousal may build up rapidly and make it difficult to redirect the child. The emotionality of the child with AD/HD may lead to excessive enthusiasm or explosive, intrusive behavior. Dysregulation of affect may decrease interpersonal contact and further remove the child from involvement with peers. However, treatment with stimulant drugs may dampen the expression of affect, produce a decrease in affective communication between peers (Hubbard and Newcomb, 1991), lead to disengagement with others, and produce a mild dysphoria. Further investigation is needed to clarify the effects of drug treatment on mood in AD/HD and whether or not excessive mood changes are linked to a co-occurring affective disorder, rather than being medication effects.

Third, how the child processes social information has been evaluated. Because of the frequency of interpersonal difficulty, the cognitive basis of social dysfunction has been evaluated in regard to potential failures in recognizing social cues. However, there is no definitive evidence of problems in social cognition that involve the understanding of social rules and routines. Recent efforts have focused on evaluating attributional reasoning, the ways that children explain life events to themselves, in those with AD/HD. This includes assessment of whether or not the child infers hostile intent to ambiguous actions by peers, understands the assignment of responsibility for behavior, appreciates the extent of his own aggressiveness, and assumes blame for inappropriate behavior. Problems in social information processing that relate to inaccurate appraisals of others' intentions and inappropriate attributions regarding others' behavior should be identified. Such appraisals may influence ongoing interactions and color future expectations about others' behavior. Finally, children with AD/HD may have difficulty with general social competencies that relate to social problem-solving skills. Whalen and Henker (1992) find that there is variability among children with AD/HD regarding the extent of their noncompliance and aggression; in fact, there is a significant proportion of children with these diagnoses who have few externalizing difficulties. This is an area requiring further exploration and better defined measures to assess it.

Fourth, unpopularity with peers is an ongoing problem for children with AD/HD. Behavioral patterns of inattention and impulsivity apparently make independent contributions to peer rejection (Milich and Landau, 1989). Although both aggression and overactivity are related to rejection, hyperactivity has been found to be the more important determinant of low peer acceptance (Pope, Bierman, and Mumma, 1989). Whalen and Henker (1992) suggest that there are two subtypes of children with ADHD who are unpopular: the first are actively rejected by peers and the second, passively neglected. The actively rejected group rapidly reestablish their rejected status when they move into a new group setting. The passively neglected children, however, interact less frequently with peers and generally do not do things to offend others. Of the two groups, the rejected subgroup is least responsive to intervention and has the greatest risk at long-term follow-up. These authors suggest that those children diagnosed with DSM-III ADHD may be more often actively rejected, and those with the diagnosis of DSM-III ADD without hyperactivity are more often passively neglected. Although both groups have social impairment, the differences between them in peer status and in peer relationships may be factors in prognosis. With the recognition of ADD without hyperactivity and the need to subcategorize within the DSM-IV attention deficit/hyperactive-impulsive diagnostic grouping, peer relations must be considered as a factor in assessing outcome.

Fifth, the social impact of the behavior of children with AD/HD on others is a major concern. Overall, children with ADHD markedly impact their social environment. Because of these effects, the impact of the child's behavior on the environment is an important consideration in treatment planning. Not only does the child's level of distress and dysfunction need to be considered, but also the social response and disharmony that are produced by the child's behavior. Untreated children change teachers' behavior and change the overall atmosphere of a classroom (Whalen, Henker, and Dotemoto, 1980). Moreover, parents show increased levels of negative and controlling behaviors as they interact with untreated children with this disorder. The evidence is mixed in regard to effects of a child with ADHD on peers. In evaluating behavioral change, the assessment must also take into account changes in others' behavior toward the child as well as change in their own behavior. An adult's overreaction, lack of response, or constraint in relation to the child may increase or decrease the responsiveness of the child. Peer reactions may prevent or provoke behavioral escalation. Peer experiences over time may provide social learning opportunities or prevent them and, consequently, impact interpersonal competence.

EFFECT OF THE DISORDER ON OTHERS

The presence of prosocial behaviors, the capacity for psychological reflectivity, the ability to self-monitor, the ability to self-regulate, the capacity to identify and label affect, responsiveness to medication, and concurrent language and learning disabilities are all factors in the child that influence the family relationship. As the result of problems in social cognition and affect discrimination, the child may be unaware of the effect of his of her behavior on others. Children with attention deficit/hyperactivity-impulsivity disorder generally do not complain of a sense of psychological suffering or express conflict about their symptoms. This lack of awareness of the effect of one's behavior on others may lead to misunderstanding in the family and reduced self-esteem when others respond negatively toward them.

The family relationship is influenced not only by associated social emotional deficits but also by co-occurring diagnoses of oppositional disorder and/or conduct disorder (Munir, Biederman, and Knee, 1987). The co-occurrence of other disruptive behavior disorders and/or difficult temperament generally have a greater negative effect on others and lead to a worse prognosis (August and Stewart, 1983; Harris et al., 1984). The recognition and treatment of associated language and learning disabilities is of particular importance to prevent or reduce antisocial behavior (Harris, 1989; Satterfield, Satterfield, and Cantwell, 1981).

Problems with executive dysfunction that includes rule-governed behavior may interact with temperament and personality features associated with ADHD. These include low self-esteem, mood lability, low frustration tolerance, anhedonia (e.g., lack of pleasure in accomplishment or gratitude for gifts), and temper outbursts. These personality and temperament features predispose affected children to developing oppositional-defiant behavior and conduct problems. Through their interactions with peers, family members, and others, they may become demoralized or possibly clinically depressed based on the learned helplessness model of depression.

EFFECTS OF MEDICATION ON SOCIAL BEHAVIOR

With the institution of drug treatment, adults may respond more positively toward affected children when medication treatments are compared to placebo conditions. Studies of changes in peer behavior following the introduction of medication, however, are mixed. In one study (Whalen et al., 1989), improved peer evaluations were noted when stimulant medication and placebo were compared. However, the authors report that peer perceptions were not normalized. With improvement in overactivity, peers may be less controlling or dominating toward the child, but their responses are not necessarily more positive (Cunningham, Siegel, and Offord, 1985). Therefore, it is possible that despite a generally good response to medication, periodic behavioral outbursts or fluctuations in behavior during the day, depending on duration of action of medication, may maintain negative peer responses.

Medication may be effective in the improvement of undesirable interpersonal behaviors including aggression, social disruption, and noncompliance in school and may improve behavior in nonclassroom interpersonal activities, such as group games and team sports. Finally, with medication, the behavior and perceptions of adult caregivers toward the child's behavior may improve (Barkley, 1989) and, to a variable extent, peer status may improve. Because medication treatment fails to normalize the relationships, it is not an exclusive treatment for the various chronic problems that define this syndrome. Yet parent training programs, behavioral interventions, and psychosocial interventions alone (without medication) also show limited effectiveness. Despite this, an additional emphasis on social development in treatment is needed to define better outcome regardless of the intervention used.

DEVELOPMENTAL COURSE

Attention deficit/hyperactivity disorder (AD/HD) begins in infancy but is not ordinarily diagnosed then because the symptoms are nonspecific and may reflect a variety of disorders that occur later in life. Infants vary greatly in their level of activity. Individual differences in temperament in infants show limited stability; however, early recognition of symptoms may occur if careful assessment of activity is an aspect of a temperament measurement. Retrospective histories do include symptoms, such as irritability, feeding and sleep problems, irregular rhythms, tantrums, stereotypies, overactivity, and disorganization, that began in infancy. In the preschool child, behavior continues to be poorly differentiated; it can be difficult to distinguish AD/HD as a component in generally disruptive behavior at this age. Campbell (1985, 1987) and Campbell et al. (1986) followed up preschool children who were difficult to manage and found that about one third lost their symptoms in grade school, but the other two thirds had a later diagnosis of disruptive disorder (AD/HD, oppositional defiant disorder, conduct disorder, and others). Those whose symptoms had resolved by age 6 previously had similar symptoms of short attention span and overactivity when compared to the persistent group, although their symptoms were less severe, and interpersonal difficulty with peers as well as the severity of conduct problems were less. Overall, maternal reports were more reliable predictors of later behavior problems; behavior observed by the investigators did not specifically predict subsequent AD/HD. However, McGee et al. (1991) reported less difficulty making the diagnosis in the preschool years and identified 2% of a preschool sample as pervasively hyperactive, with persistent problems at follow-up 12 years later. Ross and Ross (1982) found that few preschool children presented with clinical symptoms, but those who do often have difficulty with peers and in preschool. However, because of the lack of specificity in the behavioral presentation, there is a risk of overdiagnosing AD/HD in the preschool years.

Most AD/HD research has been conducted with school-age children, aged 6 to 10 years, and it is in this group that the classical symptoms of attention deficit, impulsivity, distractibility, and overactivity have been most clearly identified. Even though the diagnosis of AD/HD is most commonly recognized in the early school years, when the child's prior development is reviewed, the onset is generally found to be before age 5 and may be as early as age 2 or younger. Although more common in boys, the disorder does occur in girls, who have been referred to as a silent minority with this disorder. (Berry, Shaywitz, and Shaywitz, 1985).

In adolescence, the tendency has been to underdiagnose AD/HD because it was initially believed the disorder is residual by this age. Yet longitudinal studies show that symptoms persist into adolescence, although they may have to be specifically sought out (Barkley et al., 1991; Klein and Mannuzza, 1991; Weiss and Hechtman, 1993) and that about 70% of adolescents who had AD/HD in childhood continue to have difficulty. In adolescence, attentional and impulsive problems are more apparent, and hyperactivity may be reduced. Associated problems, such as mood changes, poor motivation, and delinquent behavior, often become the focus of attention in adolescence so that the attention deficit and impulsive symptoms may not be sought out. The more severe problems with substance abuse and aggression may draw more attention from caregivers and teachers. Situational factors, such as multiple classes in high school and greater independence, may lead to less teacher surveillance for this disorder (Werry, 1992).

DIAGNOSTIC ASSESSMENT

The social/family/school context is basic to the diagnostic and assessment process. AD/HD is recognized in a family or at school. It is family members or teachers who recognize the condition and initiate referral. The DSM-IV criteria for the diagnosis of AD/HD are based on others' observations of the child. Both behavior rating scales and structured interviews rely on teacher ratings and the parental interview to confirm the diagnosis. Rating scales are particularly useful for parents to complete at the time of referral, or as part of the screening procedure, to allow them to designate the child's referral problem. Epidemiologic studies use parental ratings, such as the CBCL (Achenbach and Edelbrock, 1981), or teacher and parent ratings (Connors, 1985) to identify the externalizing symptoms of AD/HD and co-occurring behavioral disturbances. The teacher's report of behavior in the classroom (Connors, 1985) is often needed to confirm the diagnosis of AD/HD because behavioral problems are most apparent in a group setting. This is essential because children often will not show enough symptoms to make the diagnosis in a one-to-one office setting. Teachers benefit from their experience making age-related comparisons between children and their peers in the classroom. Teacher reports may document the effects of the child's behavior on others and responses to the child from peers.

Assessment of Family Functioning

The family assessment involves an evaluation of the interpersonal relationship between parent and child. Adversive/coercive interpersonal exchanges with parents are common as a consequence of the social, cognitive, and emotional recognition difficulties. The parent–child interaction may be marred by poor child compliance, time off task, negative responses to parent requests, poorly regulated rule-governed behavior, and less sustained attention to task. The child's negative response to requests leads to a vicious cycle of negativity with adversive and coercive interactions with the parent.

Specific family issues that must be considered in addressing the parent–child relationship include parental factors, such as psychosocial background, parental psychiatric and developmental diagnosis (antisocial behavior, depression, alcohol abuse, learning disability), parenting stress and the extent of parental acknowledgment of the child's disability, and parental motivation to participate in a multimodal treatment program. A description of parent–child interaction, ascertainment of parental psychological state, and evaluation of marital functioning are all recorded.

Social interactions between children with AD/HD and their parents have been shown to be different (more stressful and negative) when contrasted to families without an affected child (Breen and Barkley, 1988). Yet the sex of the affected child is not at issue; similar family effects are seen for both boys and girls (Breen and Barkley, 1988). Parents and siblings in families with a child with AD/HD themselves experience a higher rate of psychological distress. Mothers report lower levels of parenting self-esteem and higher levels of depression especially when the child with AD/HD is a preschool child (Barkley, 1990). There is an increased prevalence of antisocial behavior, depression, alcohol abuse, and learning disability in family members. This is especially the case in instances when AD/HD co-occurs with other disruptive behavior disorders (Barkley, 1990; Cantwell, 1972; Stewart, deBlois, and Cummings, 1980).

TREATMENT

Children with AD/HD have multiple difficulties involving social, emotional, and academic areas. Consequently, medication alone is not adequate to treat the multiple problems that most of these children present. Because of the complexity of their presentation, multimodal treatment interventions have been recommended by Satterfield, Satterfield, and Cantwell (1981). These authors evaluated 117 children who received stimulant medication. Of the total group, 41% received individual psychotherapy, 30% group therapy, and 41% educational therapy. Parents were seen for either individual counseling (57%), group counseling (30%), or family therapy (48%). The authors suggested that this comprehensive treatment approach had a better outcome than more traditional individual interventions. They found that, on follow-up (Satterfield, Satterfield, and Schell, 1987), delinquent behavior was reduced in those who received the multimodal approach compared to those who received drug treatment alone. The group who received only medication treatment had significantly more arrests and more institutional placement than the multimodal interventions group. These studies were not controlled or randomized but were sufficiently systematic that they have led to ongoing interest in the development of multimodal interventions. In North America, there is a six-site study sponsored by the National Institutes of Mental Health to evaluate multimodal treatment. More than 700 children with AD/HD will be treated in this study.

Multimodal treatment may include family systems approaches, focused interventions with the child, adversive/coercive behavioral intervention based on the Barkley model (Barkley, 1990), drug treatment, and selective couples' or individual parental treatment. The elements involved in a multimodal approach also include parent training and education, pharmacotherapy, individual therapy for the child, social skills groups, academic skills training and remediation, peer activity groups, and ongoing parent involvement. Combinations of these interventions are being compared with more conventional treatment in the study sites. In one program (Weiss and Hechtman, 1993), the multimodal treatment group receives the following: well-titrated stimulant medication, weekly social skills training and academic remediation, weekly parental counseling, and weekly individual therapy for the child. In addition, weekly interventions in the context of after-school programs are conducted twice a week for 1 year, and monthly "boosters" occur in the second year. In contrast, the conventional treatment group receives well-titrated stimulant medication, monthly meeting for medication monitoring, family support and counseling, crisis intervention, school consultation, and other interventions to deal with crises as necessary (maximum 6 to 8 sessions) A comprehensive formulation of the case is necessary before treatment planning.

For any family, multimodal treatment must be individualized. Parent education and training will assist in the acknowledgment of the disability and in improving parental self-esteem. Family therapy is an important aspect of treatment and is not included in the protocol just listed. However, the conduct of treatment in a family context is essential. A systematic multimodal approach should also incorporate, or make available, a family therapy component. In addition, parents may need individual therapy for themselves including pharmacotherapy for adult onset AD/HD or mood disorder. Where substance abuse is a problem, referral to Alcoholics Anonymous or an analogous group for the abuse of other substances is necessary.

Pharmacotherapy

Drug treatment is part of a multimodal approach. Pharmacological intervention affects the child in his relations with the family and school. Pharmacological intervention may lead to improvement in interpersonal compliance and a reduction of negative parent–child interactions (Schachar et al., 1987). But pharmacotherapy is only one aspect of a treatment and must be carried out in the context of other interventions. Combined drug treatment may be needed in some instances and includes augmentation of stimulant medication for co-occurring diagnoses, such as intermittent explosive behavior, aggressive displays, and depression. Drug treatment for this disorder is discussed in Chapter 20 on psychopharmacology.

Behavioral Approaches

The techniques of behavior modification may be applied in the treatment of AD/HD, although these approaches need to be combined with appropriate diagnosis and drug treatment (Christensen and Sprague, 1973; Gittelman et al., 1980). When used, operant conditioning approaches need to be carefully specified. Such approaches have been most useful for short-term reduction of off-task behavior. In any treatment package, behavior reduction strategies need to be balanced with strategies to enhance socially appropriate behavior. Reward-based approaches can be used to reduce overactivity and fidgetiness; however, the reduction of activity derived from behavioral interventions alone is generally not great enough to help with the child's adjustment, so its coordination with pharmacotherapy must be considered. The child needs to be taught specific positive skills of learning, particularly of social interaction. A focus on the establishment of prosocial behaviors in addition to reduction of disruptive behavior is essential to treatment (Barkley, 1990).

Cognitive behavior therapy has been utilized as a tool for teaching techniques of self-control and problem solving. In laboratory tests, cognitive behavioral approaches do improve impulsiveness. However, longer term effects and changes in real-life performance have not been clearly established. These approaches emphasize self-regulatory intervention, channeling behavioral excess, the fostering of a reflective approach, and the appreciation of situational social cues. These social cognitive strategies are essential in directly teaching social communicative behavior and affect labeling (Whalen, Henker, and Hinshaw, 1985).

Family Intervention

A family approach is essential and takes into account parental beliefs and attitudes, psychological distress, strategies for conflict resolution, and other family system issues. The depressed parent presents a particular dilemma. The depressed mother often rates her child as more defiant, may make more critical remarks, and may act more aggressively toward the child. Family intervention is critical because poor child management techniques (handling adversive/coercive interactions), parental psychopathology (especially maternal depression, paternal aggression, and antisocial behavior), and marital discord are more commonly found in families with an affected child than in controls and play an important role in behavioral outcome (August and Stewart, 1983). Often conjoint family therapy is indicated.

School-Based Intervention

Because failure in school is common, it is important that psychiatric liaison with schools and awareness of special education needs be highlighted in every psychiatric assessment. Furthermore, because of the negative feedback that these children receive, they often think of themselves as dumb or stupid and may require counseling to help them deal specifically with problems in self-esteem.

Specific intervention in the classroom is critical for long-term success. One well-developed program is the University of Washington PATHS (providing alternative thinking strategies) program. It uses educators and counselors to facilitate self-control, emotional awareness, and interpersonal problem-solving skills. Its goals are to enhance social competence and social understanding in the classroom. The children's language developmental level must be considered in implementing the curriculum.

Kusche and Greenberg (1991) and Cook, Greenberg, and Kusche (1991) used the PATHS program to investigate individual differences in emotional understanding and in children's behavioral responses. They utilized the curriculum for 69 children (Grades 1 through 4) in special needs classes who were randomly assigned to intervention and comparison groups by classroom and school. Intervention children used the PATHS 4 days a week for 7 months. At posttest, the intervention children showed significant improvement in frustration tolerance, improved assertive social skills, better task orientation, enhanced peer social skills, and improved emotional labeling. These findings suggest PATHS is effective for promoting adaptive classroom behavior and improving emotional understanding in special needs children.

The following specific goals are incorporated in the PATHS curriculum and serve as clear goals to address deficits in social cognition and affect regulation: (1) Increase self-control; the ability to stop and think before acting, especially when upset or coping with a conflict situation. This lesson also includes the recognition of upset feelings. (2) Teach attributional processes that lead to an appropriate sense of self-responsibility. (3) Enhance understanding of the vocabulary of logical reasoning and problem solving, e.g., "if . . . then" and "why . . . because." (4) Increase understanding and use of the vocabulary of emotions and emotional states; e.g., excited, disappointed, confused, guilty, etc. Increased use of verbal mediation. (5) Increase ability to recognize and interpret similarities and differences in the feelings, reactions, and points of view of self and others. (6) Increase recognition and understanding of how one's behavior affects others. (7) Increase knowledge of, and skill in, the steps of social problem solving: stopping and thinking, identifying problems and feelings, setting goals; generating alternative solutions, anticipating and evaluating consequences; planning, executing, and evaluating a course of action, trying again if the first solution fails. (8) Increase ability to apply social problem-solving skills to prevent, then resolve problems and conflicts in social interactions.

SUMMARY

The child with AD/HD has a disorder that requires comprehensive intervention. The child's difficulty in self-regulation and affect discrimination may adversely impact family functioning. Parental difficulties may compound the child's problems and increase the risk for co-occurring diagnoses. Treatment must involve family members in a multimodal treatment paradigm that may include individual, drug, behavioral, social cognitive, family, and school-based interventions. Practice parameters for the assessment and treatment of AD/HD have been developed by the American Academy of Child and Adolescent Psychiatry (AACAP, 1991).

REFERENCES

Achenbach, T.M., and Edelbrock, C.S. (1981). Behavioral problems and competencies reported by parents of normal and disturbed children aged four through sixteen. *Monographs of the Society for Research in Child Development,* 46:1–82.

American Academy of Child and Adolescent Psychiatry Work Group on Quality Issue. (1991). Practice parameters for the assessment and treatment of attention-deficit hyperactivity disorder. Journal of the American Academy of Child and Adolescent Psychiatry, 30:1–3.

American Psychiatric Association, Committee on Nomenclature and Statistics. (1952). *Diagnostic and statistical manual of mental disorders.* Author, Washington, DC.

American Psychiatric Association, Committee on Nomenclature and Statistics. (1968). *Diagnostic and statistical manual of mental disorders,* 2nd ed. Author, Washington, DC.

American Psychiatric Association, Committee on Nomenclature and Statistics. (1980). *Diagnostic and statistical manual of mental disorders,* 3rd ed. Author, Washington, DC.

American Psychiatric Association, Committee on Nomenclature and Statistics. (1987). *Diagnostic and statistical manual of mental disorders,* 3rd ed., revised. Author, Washington, DC.

American Psychiatric Association, Committee on Nomenclature and Statistics. (1994). *Diagnostic and statistical manual of mental disorders,* 4th ed. Author, Washington, DC.

Anderson, J.C., Williams, S., McGee, R., and Silva, P.A. (1987). DSM-III disorders in preadolescent children: Prevalence in a large sample from the general population. *Archives of General Psychiatry,* 44:69–76.

August, G.J., and Stewart, M.A. (1982). Is there a syndrome of pure hyperactivity? *British Journal of Psychiatry,* 140:305–311.

______, and ______. (1983). Family subtypes of childhood hyperactivity. *Journal of Nervous and Mental Disease,* 171:362–368.

Barkley, R.A. (1982). Specific guidelines for defining hyperactivity in children (attention deficit disorder with hyperactivity). In B. Lahey and A. Kazdin (eds.), *Advances in clinical child psychology,* Vol. 5, pp. 137–180. Plenum, New York.

______. (1989). Hyperactive boys and girls: Stimulant drug effects in mother–child interaction. *Journal of Child Psychology and Psychiatry,* 30:379–390.

______. (1990). *Attention deficit disorder: A handbook for diagnosis and treatment,* pp. 3–38 [history]; p. 47 [extended definition]. The Guilford Press, New York.

______, Fischer, M., Edelbrock, C., and Smallish, L. (1991). The adolescent outcome of hyperactive children diagnosed by research criteria: III. Mother-child interactions, family conflicts and maternal psychopathology. *Journal of Child Psychology and Psychiatry,* 32:233–255.

Bender, L. (1942). Postencephalitic behavior disorders in children. In J.N. Neal (ed.), *Encephalitis: A clinical study.* Grune & Stratton, New York.

Berry, C.A., Shaywitz, S.E., and Shaywitz, B.A. (1985). Girls with attention deficit disorder: A silent minority? A report on behavioral and cognitive characteristics. *Pediatrics,* 76:801–809.

Biederman, J., Munir, K., Knee, D., Habelow, W., Armentano, M., Autor, S., Hoge, S.K., and Waternaux, C. (1986). A family study of patients with attention deficit disorder and normal controls. *Journal of Psychiatric Research,* 20:263–274.

______, Newcorn, J., and Sprich, S. (1991). Comorbidity of attention deficit hyperactivity disorder with conduct, depressive, anxiety, and other disorders. *American Journal of Psychiatry,* 148:564–577.

Birch, H.G. (1964). *Brain damage in children: The biological and social aspects.* Williams & Wilkins, Baltimore.

Bird, H.R., Gould, M.S., Yager, T., Staghezza, B., and Canino, G. (1989). Risk factors for maladjustment in Puerto Rican children. *Journal of the American Academy of Child and Adolescent Psychiatry,* 28:847–850.

Bond, E.D., and Appel, K.E. (1931). *The treatment of behavior disorders following encephalitis.* Commonwealth Fund, New York.

Bradley, C. (1937). The behavior of children receiving benzedrine. *American Journal of Psychiatry,* 94:557–585.

Bradley, W., and Bowen, C. (1940). School performance of children receiving amphetamine (benzedrine) sulfate. *American Journal of Orthopsychiatry,* 10:782–788.

Breen, M.J., and Barkley, R. A. (1988). Child psychopathology and parenting stress in girls and boys having attention deficit disorder with hyperactivity. *Journal of Pediatric Psychology,* 13:265–280.

Brown, G.L., Ebert, M.H., and Minichiello, M.D. (1985). Biochemical and pharmacological aspects of attention deficit disorder. In L.M. Bloomingdale (ed.), *Attention deficit disorder: Identification, course and treatment rationale.* Spectrum, New York.

Buhrmester, D., Whalen, C.K., Henker, B., MacDonald, V., and Hinshaw, S.P. (1992). Prosocial behavior in hyperactive boys: Effect of stimulant medication and comparison with normal boys. *Journal of Abnormal Child Psychology,* 20:103–121.

Cadoret, R.J., and Stewart, M.A. (1991). An adoption study of attention deficit/hyperactivity/aggression and their relationship to adult antisocial personality. *Comprehensive Psychiatry,* 32:73–82.

Campbell, S.B. (1985). Hyperactivity in preschoolers: Correlates and prognostic implications. *Clinical Psychology Review,* 5:405–428.

______. (1987). Parent-referred problem three-year-olds: Developmental changes in symptoms. *Journal of Child Psychology and Psychiatry,* 28:835–845.

______, Breaux, A.M., Ewing, L.J., and Szumowski, E.K. (1986). Correlates and predictors of hyperactivity and aggression: A longitudinal study of parent-referred problem preschoolers. *Journal of Abnormal Child Psychology,* 14:217–234.

Cantwell, D. (1972). Psychiatric illness in the families of hyperactive children. *Archives of General Psychiatry,* 27:414–427.

Carlson, C. (1986). Attention deficit disorder without hyperactivity: A review of preliminary experimental evidence. In B. Lahey and A. Kazdin (eds.), *Advances in clinical child psychology,* Vol. 9, pp. 153–176. Plenum, New York.

Castellanos, F.X., and Rapoport, J.L. (1992). Etiology of attention-deficit hyperactivity disorder. *Child and Adolescent Psychiatric Clinics of North America,* 1:373–384.

Chelune, G.J., Ferguson, W., Koon, R., and Dickey, T.O. (1986). Frontal lobe disinhibition in attention deficit disorder. *Child Psychiatry and Human Development,* 16:221–234.

Chess, S. (1960). Diagnosis and treatment of the hyperactive child. *New York State Journal of Medicine,* 60:2379–2385.

Christensen, D., and Sprague, R. (1973). Reduction of hyperactive behavior by conditioning procedures alone and combined with methylphenidate Ritalin. *Behavior Research and Therapy,* 11:331–334.

Clements, S.D. (1966). *Task Force One: Minimal brain dysfunction in children: Terminology and identification.* Phase one of a three-year project. (NINDB Monograph No. 3). U.S. Department of Health, Education and Welfare, Washington, DC.

Connors, C.K. (1985). The Connors Rating Scales: Instruments for the assessment of childhood psychopathology. Children's Hospital National Medical Center, Washington, DC.

Cook, R.T., Greenberg, M.T., and Kusche, C.A. (March 1991). *The relationships between emotional understanding, intellectual functioning, and disruptive behavior problems in elementary school aged children.* Paper presented at the Annual Meeting of the Society for Research in Child Development, Seattle, WA.

Cunningham, C.E., Siegel, L.S., and Offord, D.R. (1985). A developmental dose- response analysis of the effects of methylphenidate on the peer interactions of attention deficit disordered boys. *Journal of Child Psychology and Psychiatry,* 26:955–971.

Damasio, A. R., Tranel, D., and Damasio, H. (1990). Individuals with sociopathic behavior caused by frontal damage fail to respond automatically to social stimuli. *Behavioural Brain Research,* 41:81–94.

Denckla, M.B. (1989). Executive function, the overlap between attention deficit hyperactivity disorder and learning disabilities. *International Pediatrics,* 4:155–160.

Dennis, M. (1991). Frontal lobe function in childhood and adolescence: A heuristic for assessing attention regulation, executive control, and the intentional states important for social discourse. *Developmental Neuropsychology,* 7:327–358.

Desimone, R. (1991). Face-selective cells in the temporal cortex of monkeys. *Journal of Cognitive Neuroscience,* 3:1–8.

Donnelly, M., Zametkin, A.J., Rapoport, J.L., Ismond, D.R., Weingartner, H., Lane, E., Oliver, J., Linnoila, M., and Potter, W.Z. (1986). Treatment of hyperactivity with desipramine: Plasma drug concentration, cardiovascular effects, plasma and urinary catecholamine levels and clinical response. *Clinical Pharmacology and Therapeutics,* 39:72–81.

Douglas, V.I. (1972). Stop, look, and listen: The problem of sustained attention and impulse control in hyperactive and normal children. *Canadian Journal of Behavioural Science,* 4:259–282.

______, Barr, R.G., Amin, K., O'Neill, M.E., and Britton, B.G. (1988). Dosage effects and individual responsivity to methylphenidate in attention deficit disorder. *Journal of Child Psychology and Psychiatry,* 29:453–475.

______, and Benezra, E. (1990). Supraspan verbal memory in attention deficit disorder with hyperactivity, normal and reading-disabled boys. *Journal of Abnormal Child Psychology,* 18:617–638.

Ebaugh, F.G. (1923). Neuropsychiatric sequelae of acute epidemic encephalitis in children. *American Journal of Diseases of Children,* 25:89–97.

Elia, J., Borcherding, B.G., Potter, W.Z., Mefford, I.N., Rapoport, J.L., and Keysor, C.S. (1990). Stimulant drug treatment of hyperactivity: Biochemical correlates. *Clinical Pharmacology and Therapeutics,* 48:57–66.

Ernst, M., Liebenauer, M.A., Matchik, J.A., Fitzgerald, G.A., Cohen, R.M., and Zametkin, A.J. (1993). *Reduced brain metabolism in hyperactive girls.* Abstract presentation at the annual meeting of American Academy of Child and Adolescent Psychiatry, San Diego, CA.

Everett, J., Thomas, J., Cote, F., Levesque, J., and Michaud, D. (1991). Cognitive effects of psychostimulant medication in hyperactive children. *Child Psychiatry and Human Development,* 22:79–87.

Faraone, S.V., Biederman, J., Chen, W.J., Krifcher, B., Keenan, K., Moore, C., Sprich, S., and Tsuang, M.T. (1992). Segregation analysis of attention deficit hyperactivity disorder. *Psychiatric Genetics,* 2:257–275.

German, D.J., and Simon, E. (1991). Analysis of children's word-finding skills in discourse. *Journal of Speech and Hearing Research,* 34:309–316.

Gittelman, R., Abikoff, H., Pollack, E., Klein, D.F., Katz, S., and Mattes, J. (1980). A controlled trial of behavior modification and methylphenidate. In C.K. Whalen and B. Henker (eds.), *Hyperactive children: The social ecology of identification and treatment.* Academic Press, New York.

Goodman, R., and Stevenson, J. (1989a). A twin study of hyperactivity: I. An examination of hyperactivity scores and categories derived from Rutter teacher and parent questionnaires. *Journal of Child Psychology and Psychiatry,* 30:671–689.

______, and ______. (1989b). A twin study of hyperactivity: II. The aetiological role of genes, family relationships and perinatal adversity. *Journal of Child Psychology and Psychiatry,* 30:691–709.

Gorenstein, E.E., Mammato, C.A., and Sandy, J.M. (1989). Performance of inattentive-overactive children on selected measures of prefrontal-type function. *Journal of Clinical Psychology,* 45:619–632.

Hamlett, K.W., Pellegrini, D.S., and Connors, C.K. (1987). An investigation of executive processes in the problem solving of attention deficit disorder-hyperactive children. *Journal of Pediatric Psychology,* 12:227–240.

Harris, J.C. (1989). Interrelationship of learning and emotional difficulty: Their genesis and treatment. In M.B. Denckla (ed.), *Attention-deficit disorder, hyperactivity, and learning disabilities: Current theory and practical approaches,* pp. 69–77. Ciba-Geigy Corporation, Summit, NJ.

______. (1994). The establishment of self-regulation and social understanding in children and adolescents with ADHD: Family factors. In A.J. Capute, P.J. Accardo, and B.K. Shapiro (eds.), *Learning disabilities spectrum: ADD, ADHD, and LD.* York Press, Baltimore.

______, King, S., Reifler, J., and Rosenberg, L. (1984). Comparison of behavioral and learning disabled children in special schools. *Journal of the American Academy of Child Psychiatry,* 23(4):431–437.

Heilman, K.M., Voeller, K.S., and Nadeau, S.E. (1991). A possible pathophysiologic substrate of attention deficit hyperactivity disorder. *Journal of Child Neurology,* 6(suppl.):S76–S81.

Henker, B., Astor-Dubin, L., and Varni, J. (1986). Psychostimulant medication and perceived intensity in hyperactivity children. *Journal of Abnormal Child Psychology,* 14:105–114.

Hinshaw, S.P. (1992). Externalizing behavior problems and academic underachievement in childhood and adolescence: Causal relationships and underlying mechanisms. *Psychological Bulletin,* 111:127–155.

Hoffmann, H. (1862). *Struwwelpeter,* p. 18. George Routledge & Sons, Philadelphia.

Hohman, L.B. (1922). Post-encephalitic behavior disorders in children. *Johns Hopkins Hospital Bulletin,* 33:372–375.

Hubbard, J.A., and Newcomb, A.F. (1991). Initial dyadic peer interaction of attention deficit-hyperactivity disorder and normal boys. *Journal of Abnormal Child Psychology,* 19:179–195.

Hunt, R.D., Arnsten, A.F.T, and Asbell, M. (1995). An open trial of guanfacine in the treatment of Attention Deficit Hyperactivity Disorder. *Journal of the American Academy of Child and Adolescent Psychiatry,* 34:50–54.

______, Cohen, D.J., Anderson, G., and Clark, L. (1984). Possible changes in noradrenergic receptor sensitivity following methylphenidate treatment: Growth hormone and MHPG response to clonidine challenge in children with attention deficit disorder and hyperactivity. *Life Sciences,* 35:885–897.

Ireland, W.H. (1877). *On idiocy and imbecility.* Churchill, London.

Izard, C. (1991). *The psychology of emotions.* Plenum, New York.

Kahn, E., and Cohen, L.H. (1934). Organic drivenness: A brainstem syndrome and an experience with case reports. *New England Journal of Medicine,* 210:748–756.

Kessler, J.W. (1980). History of minimal brain dysfunction. In H. Rie and E. Rie (eds.), *Handbook of minimal brain dysfunctions: A critical view,* pp. 18–52. John Wiley, New York.

Klein, R.G., and Mannuzza, S. (1991). Long-term outcome of hyperactive children: A review. *Journal of the American Academy of Child and Adolescent Pyschiatry,* 30:383–387.

Kusche, C.A., and Greenberg, M.T. (1991). *Teaching PATHS in your classroom: The PATHS Curriculum Instructional Manual (Special Needs Version).* University of Washington Press, Seattle.

Landau, S., and Milich, R. (1988). Social communication patterns of attention- deficit-disordered boys. *Journal of Abnormal Psychology,* 16:69–81.

Laufer, M., and Denhoff, E. (1957). Hyperkinetic behavior syndrome in children. *Journal of Pediatrics,* 50:463–474.

______, ______, E., and Solomons, G. (1957). Hyperkinetic impulse disorder in children's behavior problems. *Psychosomatic Medicine,* 19:38–49.

Levin, P.M. (1938). Restlessness in children. *Archives of Neurology and Psychiatry,* 39:764–770.

Loney, J. (1983). Research diagnostic criteria for childhood hyperactivity. In S.B. Guze, F.J. Earls, and J.E. Barrett (eds.), *Childhood psychopathology and development,* pp. 109–137. Raven Press, New York.

______, Langhorne, J., and Paternite, C. (1978). An empirical basis for subgrouping the hyperkinetic/minimal brain dysfunction syndrome. *Journal of Abnormal Psychology,* 87:431–441.

Lou, H.C., Henriksen, L., and Bruhn, P. (1984). Focal cerebral hypoperfusion in children with dysphasia and/or attention deficit disorder. *Archives of Neurology,* 41:825–829.

______, ______, and ______. (1990). Focal cerebral dysfunction in developmental learning disabilities. *Lancet,* 335:8–11.

______, ______, ______, Borner, H., and Nielsen, J.B. (1989). Striatal dysfunction in attention deficit and hyperkinetic disorder. *Archives of Neurology,* 46:48–52.

Matochik, J.A., Nordahl, T.E., Gross, M., Semple, W.E., King, A.C., Cohen, R.M., and Zametkin, A.J. (1993). Effects of acute stimulant medication on cerebral metabolism in adults with hyperactivity. *Neuropsychopharmacology,* 8:377–386.

McCraken, J. (1991). A two-part model of stimulant action on attention deficit hyperactivity disorder in children. *Journal of Neuropsychiatry,* 3:201–209.

McGee, R., Partridge, F., Williams, S., and Silva, P.A. (1991). A twelve-year follow-up of preschool hyperactive children. *Journal of the American Academy of Child and Adolescent Psychiatry,* 30:224–232.

Mesulam, M.M. (1985). Attention, confusional states, and neglect. In M.M. Mesulam (ed.), *Principles of behavioral neurology.* Davis, Philadelphia.

Milich, R., and Landau, S. (1989). The role of social status variables in differentiating subgroups of hyperactive children. In L.M. Bloomingdale, J.M. Swanson, and R. Klorman (eds.), *Attention deficit disorder: Current concepts and emerging trends in attentional and behavioral disorders of childhood,* Vol. 4, pp. 1–16. [Book supplement to] *Child Psychology and Psychiatry,* No. 6. Pergamon Press, New York.

______, Loney, J., and Landau, S. (1982). The independent dimensions of hyperactivity and aggression: A validation with playroom observation data. *Journal of Abnormal Psychology,* 91:183–198.

Mirsky, A. (1987). Behavioral and psychophysiological markers of disordered attention. *Environmental Health Perspectives,* 74:191–199.

Morrison, J.R., and Stewart, M.A. (1973). The psychiatric status of the legal families of adopted hyperactive children. *Archives of General Psychiatry,* 28:888–891.

Munir, K., Biederman, J., and Knee, D. (1987). Psychiatric co-morbidity in patients with attention deficit disorder: A controlled study. *Journal of the American Academy of Child and Adolescent Psychiatry,* 26:844–848.

Nemzer, E.D., Arnold, L.E., Votolato, N.A., and McConnell, H. (1986). Amino acid supplementation as therapy for attention deficit disorder. *Journal of the American Academy of Child and Adolescent Psychiatry,* 25:509–513.

O'Neill, M.E., and Douglas, V.I. (1991). Study strategies and story recall in attention deficit disorder, reading disabled, and normal boys. *Journal of Abnormal Psychology,* 19:671–692.

Pauls, D.L. (1991). Genetic factors in the expression of attention-deficit hyperactivity disorder. *Journal of Child and Adolescent Psychopharmacology,* 1:353–360.

Pope, A.W., Bierman, K.L., and Mumma, G.H. (1989). Relations between hyperactive and aggressive behavior and peer relations at three elementary grade levels. *Journal of Abnormal Child Psychology,* 17:253–267.

Porrino, L.J., Rapoport, J.L., Behar, D., Sceery, W., Ismond, D.R., and Bunney, W.E., Jr. (1983). A naturalistic assessment of the motor activity of hyperactive boys: I. A comparison with normal controls. *Archives of General Psychiatry,* 40:681–687.

Prendergast, M., Taylor, E., Rapoport, J.L., Bartko, J., Donnelly, M., Zametkin, A., Ahearn, M.D., Dunn, G., and Wieselberg, H.M. (1988). The diagnosis of childhood hyperactivity. A U.S.-U.K. cross-national study of DSM-III and ICD-9. *Journal of Child Psychology and Psychiatry,* 29:289–300.

Purvis, K.L., Schachar, R., and Tannock, R. (in press). Comparative analysis of narrative language abilities in boys with attention deficit hyperactivity disorder and learning disabilities. *Journal of Abnormal Child Psychology.*

Rapin, I. (1964). Brain damage in children. In J. Brennemann (ed.), *Practice of pediatrics,* Vol. 4. Prior, Hagerstown, MD.

Roeltgen, D., and Schneider, J.S. (1991). Chronic low-dose MPTP in non-human primates: A possible model for attention deficit disorder. *Journal of Child Neurology,* 6(suppl.):S82-S89.

Ross, D.M., and Ross, S.A. (1982). *Hyperactivity: Current issues, research and theory,* 2nd ed., John Wiley, New York.

Rutter, M. (1977). Brain damage syndromes in childhood: Concepts and findings. *Journal of Child Psychology and Psychiatry,* 18:1–21.

______. (1982). Syndromes attributed to "minimal brain dysfunction" in childhood. *American Journal of Psychiatry,* 139:21–33.

______, Graham, P., and Yule, W. (1970). A neuropsychiatric study in childhood. *Clinics in Developmental Medicine* 35/36. Heinemann Medical School Press, London.

Satterfield, J.H., Satterfield, B.T., and Cantwell, D.P. (1981). Three-year multimodality treatment study of 100 hyperactive boys. *Journal of Pediatrics,* 98:650–655.

______, ______, and Schell, A.E. (1987). Therapeutic interventions to prevent delinquency in hyperactive boys. *Journal of the American Academy of Child and Adolescent Psychiatry,* 26:56–64.

Schachar, R., Taylor, E., Wiselberg, M., Thorley, G., and Rutter, M. (1987). Changes in family function and relationships in children who respond to methylphenidate. *Journal of the American Academy of Child and Adolescent Psychiatry,* 26:728–732.

Schneider, J.S., and Kovelowski, C.J. (1990). Chronic exposure to low doses of MPTP: Cognitive deficits in motor asymptomatic monkeys. *Brain Research,* 519:122–128.

Sergeant, J. (1988). From DSM-III attentional deficit disorder to functional defects. In L. Bloomingdale and J. Sergeant (eds.), *Attention deficit disorder: Criteria, cognition, and intervention,* pp. 183–198. Pergamon Press, New York.

Shaywitz, B.A., Cohen, D.J., and Bower, M.B. (1977). CSF monoamine metabolites in children with minimal brain dysfunction: Evidence for alteration of brain dopamine. A preliminary report. *Journal of Pediatrics,* 90:671–677.

______, Yager, R.D., and Klopper, J.H. (1976). Selective brain dopamine depletion in developing rats. *Science,* 191:305–308.

Stewart, M.A., deBlois, C.S., and Cummings, C. (1980). Psychiatric disorder in the parents of hyperactive boys and those with conduct disorder. *Journal of Child Psychology and Psychiatry,* 21:283–292.

Still, G.F. (1902). The Coulstonian lectures on some

abnormal psychical conditions in children. *Lancet,* i:1008–1012, 1077–1082, 1163–1168.

Strauss, A.A., and Lehtinen, L. (1947). *Psychopathology and education of the brain-injured child.* Grune & Stratton, New York.

______, and Werner, W.H. (1943). Comparative psychopathology of the brain-injured child and traumatic brain-injured adult. *American Journal of Psychiatry,* 99:835.

Struss, D., and Benson, D.F. (1984). Cognition and memory. In E. Perecman (ed.), *The frontal lobes, revisited.* IRBN Press, New York.

Szatmari, P. (1992). The epidemiology of attention deficit-hyperactivity disorders. *Child and Adolescent Psychiatry Clinics,* 1:361–371.

______, Offord, D.R., and Boyle, M.H. (1989). Ontario child health study: Prevalence of attention deficit disorders with hyperactivity. *Journal of Child Psychology and Psychiatry,* 30:219–230.

Tannock, R., Purvis, K.L., and Schachar, R.J. (1993). Narrative abilities in children with attention deficit hyperactivity disorder and normal peers. *Journal of Abnormal Child Psychology,* 21:103–117.

______, Schachar, R.J., Carr, R.P., Chajczyk, D., and Logan, G.D. (1989). Effects of methylphenidate on inhibitory control in hyperactive children. *Journal of Abnormal Child Psychology,* 17:473–491.

Taylor, E.A. (1986). Childhood hyperactivity. *British Journal of Psychiatry,* 149:562–573.

______. (1988). Diagnosis of hyperactivity: A British perspective. In L. Bloomingdale and J. Sergeant (eds.), *Attention deficit disorder: Criteria, cognition, and intervention,* pp. 141–160. Pergamon Press, New York.

Tredgold, A.F. (1908). *Mental deficiency (amentia).* W. Wood, New York.

Weingartner, H., Rapoport, J.L., Buschbaum, M.S., Bunney, W.E., Ebert, M.H., Mikkelson, E.L., and Caine, E.D. (1980). Cognitive processes in normal and hyperactive children and their response to amphetamine treatment. *Journal of Abnormal Psychology,* 89:25–37.

Weiss, G., and Hechtman, L.T. (1993). *Hyperactive children grown up: ADHD in children, adolescents, and adults,* 2nd ed. The Guilford Press, New York.

Wender, P.H. (1971). *Minimal brain dysfunction in children.* Wiley, New York.

______. (1975). The minimal brain dysfunction syndrome. *Annual Review of Medicine,* 26:45.

Werry, J.S. (1992). Attention-deficit hyperactivity disorder: History, terminology, and manifestations at different ages. *Child and Adolescent Psychiatric Clinics of North America,* 1:297–310.

Whalen, C.K., and Henker, B. (1992). The social profile of attention-deficit hyperactivity disorder. *Child and Adolescent Psychiatric Clinics of North America,* 1:395–410.

______, ______, Buhrmester, D., Hinshaw, S.P., Huber, A., and Laski, K. (1989). Does stimulant medication improve the peer status of hyperactive children? *Journal of Consulting and Clinical Psychology,* 57:545–554.

______, ______, Collins, B.E., McAuliffe, S., and Vaux, A. (1979). Peer interaction in a structured communication task: Comparisons of normal and hyperactive boys and of methylphenidate (Ritalin) and placebo effects. *Child Development,* 50:388–401.

______, ______, and Dotemoto, S. (1980). Methylphenidate and hyperactivity: Effects on teacher behaviors. *Science,* 208:1280–1282.

______, ______, and Hinshaw, S. P. (1985). Cognitive behavioral therapies for hyperactive children: Premises, problems, and prospects. *Journal of Abnormal Child Psychology,* 13:391–410.

Whitehouse, D. (1989). 30 years of experience with attention-deficit disorder (ADD), hyperactivity, and the use of methylphenidate. In M.B. Denckla (ed.), *Attention deficit disorder, hyperactivity, and learning disabilities: Current theory and practical approaches.* CIBA-GEIGY Corporation, Summit, NJ.

Wong, D.F., Yung, B., Dannals, R.F., Shaya, E.K., Ravert, H.T., Chen, C.A., Chan, B., Folio, T., Scheffel, U., Ricaurte, G.A., Neumeyer, J.D., Wagner, H.N., and Kuhar, M.J. (1993). *In vivo* imaging of baboon and human dopamine transporters by positron emission tomography using [C^{11}]WIN 35,428. *Synapse,* 15(2):130–142.

Zametkin, A.J., Liebenauer, L.L., Fitzgerald, G.A., King, A.C., Minkunas, D.V., Herscovitch, P., Yamada, E.M., and Cohen, R.M. (1993). Brain metabolism in teenagers with attention deficit hyperactivity disorder. *Archives of General Psychiatry,* 50:333–340.

______, Nordahl, T.E., Gross, M., King, A.C., Semple, W.E., Rumsey, J., Hamburger, S., and Cohen, R.M. (1990). Cerebral glucose metabolism in adults with hyperactivity of childhood onset. *New England Journal of Medicine,* 323:1361–1366.

______, and Rapoport, J.L. (1987). Neurobiology of attention deficit disorder with hyperactivity: Where have we come in 50 years? *Journal of the American Academy of Child and Adolescent Psychiatry,* 26:676–686.

Zentall, S.S. (1988). Production deficiencies in elicited language but not in the spontaneous verbalizations of hyperactive children. *Journal of Abnormal Child Psychology,* 16:657–673.

CHAPTER 14

SCHIZOPHRENIA: A NEURODEVELOPMENTAL DISORDER

The recognition of psychoses with an onset in childhood began in 1874 with Maudsley's description of the "insanity of early life" in his textbook, *Physiology and Pathology of Mind.* His approach was developmental as he wrote,

> If the account of the gradual evolution of the mental faculties be correct, the insanity met within children must be of the simplest kind; where no mental faculty has been organized, no disorder of mind can well be manifest. . . . The extent of mental disorder possible is clearly limited by the extent of existence of mental faculty . . . the observed facts agree with theory; when a child is, by reason of bad descent or of baneful influences during uterine life, born with such an extreme degree of instability of nervous element. (Maudsley, 1977/1874).

He included monomania, cataleptoid insanity, mania, melancholia, and affective insanity among the seven categories of insanity of early life. Since Maudsley's time, the debate has continued about how to identify, categorize, and treat psychoses beginning in early life and about whether there should be a neurodevelopmental category of schizophrenia to designate its onset in childhood (Murray et al., 1992; Werry, 1992). In other disorders, such as Huntington's disease, differences in presenting signs and symptoms may be seen with juvenile onset, yet the genetic etiology may be the same for child and adult cases. The challenge is to recognize the earliest manifestations of a disorder during the developmental period and carefully monitor long-term outcome in individual cases and among family members. The earliest manifestations may provide clues as to the underlying neurobiological mechanisms. Moreover, information regarding the onset and clinical course is essential to classification.

This chapter reviews the history, epidemiology, definition and diagnostic criteria, natural history, etiology, neurochemistry, and treatment of early onset and very early onset schizophrenia and other psychotic conditions in childhood. It is proposed that childhood onset forms may be the most severe and present the earliest manifestation of the disease; however, long-term follow-up is needed to establish the course.

HISTORY

Maudsley's delineation of early onset insanity is a landmark and eventually led to the recognition of the childhood psychoses as legitimate topics for psychiatric inquiry. Maudsley was followed in 1883 by Spitzka (Kanner, 1973), who, in his *Treatment of Insanity,* discussed the infantile psychoses, which were considered to be rare and caused by heredity, fright, sudden changes of temperature, or masturbation. By the end of the 19th century four textbooks had appeared that dealt with this subject (Kanner, 1973). Concurrently, Kraepelin (1896/1971) was extracting catatonia, hebephrenia, simple deteriorating, and certain paranoid states from the generic terms "lunacy" or "insanity," and defining the unifying category "dementia praecox."

In 1906 De Santis (1906/1969) in Italy extended dementia praecox to children and introduced the category of dementia praecocissima, thereby emphasizing the early onset. He pointed out that not only children who are mentally retarded display "psychotic behavior," but others who are not also may show the early onset of psychosis. The term "dementia praecocissima" was eventually abandoned because it began to be used too broadly as a general designation for many etiologically unrelated disorders.

In 1911 Bleuler clustered psychoses into the "group of schizophrenias," noting at the time that "This concept may be only of temporary value inasmuch as it may later have to be reduced, in the same sense as the discoveries in bacteriology necessitated the subdivision of the pneumonias in terms of various etiological agents" [quoted by Kanner, 1973]. Bleuler wrote of adolescent and adult onset cases but did not discuss infantile or childhood onset.

In the 1930s the diagnosis of "infantile schizophrenia" was introduced by Potter (1933). He described loss of interest in the environment, disturbances of thought (blocking, condensation, perseveration, and incoherence), lack of emotional rapport, diminution and distortion of affect, and changes in mobility with a tendency to develop stereotypies.

Other early investigators began with Kraepelin's (1971) original categories and attempted to apply them directly to children but found there were differences in onset and clinical course; one group of affected children had an acute onset and another group had a more insidious one. Bender (1947) suggested three clinical types: the pseudodefective, the pseudoneurotic, and the pseudopsychopathic. She noted an inherited predisposition for schizophrenia, an early physiologic or organic crisis, clinical features that varied at different epochs in the individual's development, and a relationship to adaptive defenses and environmental factors. Her formulation avoided the functional/organic distinction and emphasized the psychobiological nature of the condition. Moreover, she emphasized long-term case follow-up (Bender, 1973).

By 1943 Kanner had identified the syndrome of infantile autism as a new grouping. Other categories, such as "symbiotic psychosis" (Mahler, 1952) and "organic" and "nonorganic types" of schizophrenia (Goldfarb, 1974), were introduced. Still others declined to discriminate types and used generic terms such as "the atypical child," one who showed signs of ego fragmentation that were intertwined with maternal psychopathology (Rank, 1949). Most emphasized variability in the developmental presentation and used the general category "childhood schizophrenia" for children with the onset of psychotic symptoms in childhood.

Eventually, the designation "childhood schizophrenia" also became overly inclusive as had dementia praecocissima before it, and was removed from the classification system with the introduction of DSM-III (APA, 1980). This change was based on the work of Kolvin (1971) and others who demonstrated the distinctiveness of the various psychoses with onset in childhood and similarity between child and adult schizophrenia. It is thought that research on adults is applicable to children by making appropriate developmental adjustments. In DSM-III "pervasive developmental disorder" was introduced to describe the onset of dysfunctional development and behavior in infancy and early childhood; separate categories were introduced for an early onset disorder beginning in the first 30 months of life—infantile autism—and a later onset condition, following a period of apparently normal development—childhood onset pervasive developmental disorder. This latter category included some children who in the past were diagnosed as childhood onset schizophrenia or symbiotic psychosis. For older children who were sufficiently verbal, the diagnosis of schizophrenia was suggested in DSM-III, utilizing the adult diagnostic criteria. In line with these changes in classification, the *Journal of Autism and Childhood Schizophrenia* became the *Journal of Autism and Developmental Disorders.* The pervasive developmental disorder category and the use of the same criteria for schizophrenia for children and adults introduced in DSM-III is maintained in DSM-IV (APA, 1994).

EPIDEMIOLOGY

In adult onset schizophrenia, the male to female sex ratio is equal. In early childhood onset cases the male to female ratio is about 2.5 to 1, but with adolescent onset, the male to female ratios become closer to 1 to 1 as seen in adulthood. Males have a worse outcome than females, exhibit more structural brain abnormalities, and have fewer affective symptoms than females (Castle and Murray, 1991).

Systematic epidemiologic data of prevalence in large-scale population-based samples, using standardized diagnostic criteria, is not available for very early onset schizophrenia (onset before age 13), which is quite rare. However, it is thought that childhood onset schizophrenia is less common than autistic disorder. Kolvin (1971) reports that autistic disorder occurs 1.4 times more frequently than schizophrenia in young children. Most studies of very early onset schizophrenia are based on clinic samples rather than community surveys so data from these sources may reflect referral bias.

Retrospective review of the time of symptom onset are complicated by the overinclusive use of the term "childhood schizophrenia" for all psychoses that presented in childhood prior to the publication of ICD-9 (WHO, 1977) and DSM-III. Future epidemiologic studies must clarify whether childhood onset and adolescent or adult onset cases are diagnostically the same, and if diagnostically the same, whether the presentation is sufficiently distinct in childhood to warrant a neurodevelopmental category. When the adult criteria are met in childhood, are some children who do have the diagnosis of schizophrenia excluded because the criteria do not encompass the developmental aspects of symptom presentation? (Werry, 1992). Moreover, are there additional symptoms in children that are not present in adults? To establish the validity of a neurodevelopmental category, one must consider the characteristic features, such as age of onset, natural history, and familial pattern, as well as prevalence, extent of impairment, premorbid personality, and predisposing factors.

An evaluation of studies of very early onset schizophrenia published since 1975, when adult criteria have been systematically applied to children and adolescents, suggests the diagnostic criteria used for adult cases, based on symptomatology, severity of functional disturbance, and duration of symptoms, can be reliably used for child and adolescent cases. Yet other early onset cases who are preverbal or mentally retarded or who have a different symptoms profile might be excluded. The primary diagnostic symptoms—hallucinations and delusions—are cognitive; other characteristics such as intellectual level, perceptual disturbances, or developmental disturbances in affective regulation might result in differences in symptom profiles in childhood.

There is a significant increase in the frequency of the diagnosis after age 11 to 12 years, but it is not clear whether this is related to the onset and stage of puberty. The prevalence rates increase and rise each year from age 13 onward. Werry (1992) has suggested that onset between age 13 and 18 be designated "early onset schizophrenia" and that "very early onset" be used for those under age 13 years. Positive symptoms may appear for the first time after the onset of puberty in children with premorbid personality features. Diagnosis in children over age 5 who are severely mentally retarded, autistic, or language disordered requires further study (Reid, 1989).

Epidemiologic studies have focused on time of birth and investigations of nonfamilial schizophrenics. Nonfamilial cases of schizophrenia largely account for findings of increased births in later winter and early spring. These patients are more likely to have a history of obstetrical complications than cases where there is a family history. The nonfamilial group is also likely to have smaller head circumference that is not related to obstetrical complications. Both the season of birth and the smaller head circumference have been accounted for by possible maternal virus infection. Following the influenza epidemic in Helsinki in 1957, there was almost a doubling of the births of individuals who later became schizophrenic (Mednick, et al., 1988). Earlier reports are consistent with influenza as a possible etiologic factor as are recent reports of prenatal exposure during the 1957 A2 influenza epidemic (Cooper, 1992). The introduction of the concept of neurodevelopmental schizophrenia as a distinguishable form of the illness is being evaluated epidemiologically. McCreadie et al. (1994) evaluated premorbid social adjustment, premorbid schizoid and schizotypal personality traits, and the obstetrical history of 40 schizophrenic patients and their 102 siblings using maternal interviews and patient symptom rating scales. They found significant correlations between premorbid functioning, age of illness onset, current symptoms, and premorbid intelligence in males. They did not demonstrate associations between family history of severe mental disorder and obstetrical complications. The authors focused on adolescent and young adult onset (mean age 23.8±5.9 years in males and 24.4±7.5 years in females). Similar studies should be conducted for very early onset schizophrenia that might be more likely to have a more clear cut neurodevelopmental basis.

DEFINITION AND DIAGNOSTIC CRITERIA

Schizophrenia is a syndrome and most probably includes several subtypes; the diagnosis is based on recognizable signs and symptoms. In the United States, Bleuler's emphasis on primary and secondary symptoms has largely been replaced by what are now termed negative and positive symptoms; heritability seems greatest for negative symptoms. Positive symptoms include hallucinations, delusions, and formal thought disorder; negative symptoms refer to the absence or diminution of behaviors, such as social withdrawal, loss of drive, poverty of speech, and flattening of affect. Crow (1980, 1985) originally used these terms in describing two main types of schizophrenia: Type I, or acute schizophrenia, with positive symptoms, and Type II, with negative symptoms, which follows a more chronic course. When compared with Kraepelin's (1896/1971) original dementia simplex cases, the childhood onset cases may be similar to simple schizophrenics and Crow's Type II schizophrenia. Negative symptoms have a poorer long-term outcome and may be caused by structural changes in the brain. Whether or not Type II schizophrenia always starts in childhood is not clearly known.

Because positive symptoms may be present in a substantial minority of patients with affective psychosis, course and outcome as well as the phenomenology of symptoms must be considered in diagnosing childhood cases. Moreover, it is possible that positive symptoms do not have predictive value. The DSM-IV (APA, 1994) criteria reflect the emphasis on positive and negative symptoms. The early Bleulerian terms maintained in DSM-III-R (APA, 1987), i.e., "loosening of associations" and "grossly inappropriate affect," are no longer included. In their place are "disorganized speech," which refers to frequent derailment or incoherent speech, and "negative symptoms," which consist of affective flattening, alogia, and avolition (Table 14–1).

In addition to these characteristic symptoms, adaptive failure in social and academic areas is required for the diagnosis. In children and adolescents, adaptive failure is indicated by deterioration in developmentally appropriate interpersonal and academic functioning that was achieved before the onset of symptoms. Moreover, there is a duration criteria that requires a symptomatic prodromal phase of at least 6 months. Schizoaffective disorder and mood disorder with psychotic features are exclusionary criteria, as are substance abuse and psychotic symptoms related to a general medical condition.

Cognitive and Intellectual Dysfunction

Family interview studies of a schizophrenia spectrum disorder suggest a predisposition toward cognitive dysfunction (Asarnow, Asarnow, and Strandburg, 1989) as a major vulnerability factor. In several studies, at least one third showed cognitive abnormalities (Aylward, Walker, and Bettes, 1984) and personality, and social dysfunction in childhood. These findings are more characteristic in males. Subtle cognitive dysfunction involving executive function and memory has been reported in the unaffected twin in sets of identical twins (Goldberg et al., 1992). In some studies, children who test in the mentally retarded range have not been included; in those where they have been included, IQ in the borderline to mildly retarded range has been found in 10% to 20% (Eggers, 1978; Green and Padron-Gayol, 1986; Werry, McClellan, and Chard, 1991). This finding is consistent with reports of lowered IQ in schizophrenic children and adolescents (Aylward, Walker, and Bettes, 1984). Mental retardation is considered a premorbid feature and not a secondary effect following the onset of schizophrenia.

Neuropsycholcgical Testing

Schizophrenic patients show impairment in neuropsychological functioning. These patterns

Table 14–1. DSM-IV Criteria for Schizophrenia

Schizophrenia

A. *Characteristic symptoms:* Two (or more) of the following, each present for a significant portion of time during a 1-month period (or less if successfully treated):
   (1) delusions
   (2) hallucinations
   (3) disorganized speech (e.g., frequent derailment or incoherence)
   (4) grossly disorganized or catatonic behavior
   (5) negative symptoms, i.e., affective flattening, alogia, or avolition.

Note: Only one Criterion A symptom is required if delusions are bizarre or hallucinations consist of a voice keeping up a running commentary on the person's behavior or thoughts, or two or more voices conversing with each other.

B. *Social/occupational dysfunction:* For a significant portion of the time since the onset of the disturbance, one or more major areas of functioning such as work, interpersonal relations, or self-care are markedly below the level achieved prior to the onset (or when the onset is in childhood or adolescence, failure to achieve expected level of interpersonal, academic, or occupational achievement).

C. *Duration:* Continuous signs of the disturbance persist for at least 6 months. This 6-month period must include at least 1 month of symptoms (or less if successfully treated) that meet Criterion A (i.e., active-phase symptoms), and may include periods of prodromal or residual symptoms. During these prodromal or residual periods, the signs of the disturbance may be manifested by only negative symptoms or two or more symptoms listed in Criterion A present in an attenuated form (e.g., odd beliefs, unusual perceptual experiences).

D. *Schizoaffective and Mood Disorder exclusion:* Schizoaffective Disorder and Mood Disorder with Psychotic Features have been ruled out because either: (1) no Major Depressive, Manic, or Mixed episodes have occurred concurrently with the active-phase symptoms; or (2) if mood episodes have occurred during active-phase symptoms, their total duration has been brief relative to the duration of the active and residual periods.

E. *Substance/general medical condition exclusion:* The disturbance is not due to the direct physiological effects of a substance (e.g., a drug of abuse, a medication) or a general medical condition.

F. *Relationship to a Pervasive Developmental Disorder:* If there is a history of Autistic Disorder or another Pervasive Developmental Disorder, the additional diagnosis of Schizophrenia is made only if prominent delusions or hallucinations are also present for at least a month (or less if successfully treated).

Schizophrenia Subtypes

The subtypes of Schizophrenia are defined by the predominant symptomatology at the time of evaluation.

295.30 Paranoid Type

A type of Schizophrenia in which the following criteria are met:

A. Preoccupation with one or more delusions or frequent auditory hallucinations.

B. None of the following is prominent: disorganized speech, disorganized or catatonic behavior, or flat or inappropriate affect.

295.10 Disorganized Type

A type of Schizophrenia in which the following criteria are met:

A. All of the following are prominent:
   (1) disorganized speech
   (2) disorganized behavior
   (3) flat or inappropriate affect

B. The criteria are not met for Catatonic type.

295.20 Catatonic Type

A type of Schizophrenia in which the clinical picture is dominated by at least two of the following:
   (1) motoric immobility as evidenced by catalepsy (including waxy flexibility) or stupor
   (2) excessive motor activity (that is apparently purposeless and not influenced by external stimuli)

(3) extreme negativism (an apparently motiveless resistance to all instructions or maintenance of a rigid posture against attempts to be moved) or mutism
(4) peculiarities of voluntary movement as evidenced by posturing (voluntary assumption of inappropriate or bizarre postures), stereotyped movements, prominent mannerisms, or prominent grimacing
(5) Echolalia or echopraxia

295.90 Undifferentiated Type
A type of Schizophrenia in which symptoms that meet Criterion A are present, but the criteria are not met for the Paranoid, Disorganized, or Catatonic Type.

295.60 Residual Type
A type of Schizophrenia in which the following criteria are met:
A. Absence of prominent delusions, hallucinations, disorganized speech, and grossly disorganized or catatonic behavior.
B. There is continuing evidence of the disturbance, as indicated by the presence of negative symptoms or two or more symptoms listed in Criterion A for Schizophrenia, present in an attenuated form (e.g., odd beliefs, unusual perceptual experiences).

Classification of Longitudinal Course for Schizophrenia

Episodic with Interepisode Residual Symptoms: when the course is characterized by episodes in which Criterion A for Schizophrenia is met and there are clinically significant residual symptoms between the episodes.
With Prominent Negative Symptoms can be added if prominent negative symptoms are present during these residual periods.

Episodic with No Interepisode Residual Symptoms: when the course is characterized by episodes in which Criterion A for Schizophrenia is met and there are no clinically significant residual symptoms between the episodes.

Continuous: when characteristic symptoms of Criterion A are met throughout all (or most) of the course.
With Prominent Negative Symptoms can be added if prominent negative symptoms are also present.

Single Episode in Partial Remission: when there has been a single episode in which Criterion A for Schizophrenia is met and some clinically significant residual symptoms remain.
With Prominent Negative Symptoms can be added if these residual symptoms include prominent negative symptoms.

Single Episode in Full Remission: when there has been a single episode in which Criterion A for Schizophrenia has been met and no clinically significant residual symptoms remain.

Other or Unspecified Pattern: if another or an unspecified course pattern has been present.

295.40 Schizophreniform Disorder
A. Criteria A, D, and E of Schizophrenia are met.
B. An episode of the disorder (including prodromal, active, and residual phases) lasts at least 1 month but less than 6 months. (When the diagnosis must be made without waiting for recovery, it should be qualified as "Provisional.") *Specify if:*

Without Good Prognostic Features
With Good Prognostic Features: as evidenced by two (or more) of the following:
(1) onset of prominent psychotic symptoms within 4 weeks of the first noticeable change in usual behavior or functioning
(2) confusion or perplexity at the height of the psychotic episode
(3) good premorbid social and occupational functioning
(4) absence of blunted or flat affect

From APA, 1994.

may vary by subgroup. Disturbances in attention, memory, executive functions, language, and motor functions have been demonstrated in adult studies. Attentional deficits involve the ability to flexibly distribute attention from one area to another and return to task following distractions. During periods of acute psychosis in patients with high positive symptom profiles, selective attention may be reduced; however, impaired selective attention is not a characteristic problem in general. In chronic schizophrenia, there may be memory problems with difficulty encoding information. This may be related to memory organizational deficits. Comparable deficits have been reported in word recall and design recall in chronic patients, implying bilateral involvement (Calev et al., 1987).

Executive functions involve the frontal lobes and include the initiation of responses to the environment, maintaining the response, and shifting to a new set of responses. Executive function testing has revealed problems in maintaining cognitive set, perseveration (poor mental flexibility), and self-monitoring. On the Wisconsin Card Sort, one test of executive function, difficulties have been demonstrated in these areas (Weinberger, 1988). One aspect of impaired self-monitoring relates to reports of hearing voices; the voices may be subvocalizations the patient does not recognize as his own. Although test findings may vary among the different subtypes of schizophrenia, the impairment seems to involve the frontal and temporal lobes as they relate to the limbic system. These findings may be used to target primary neuropsychological deficits for rehabilitation and psychopharmacological intervention. The target deficits are the processes that generate and coordinate mental activity. Evidence for brain dysfunction in early onset cases relates to developmental factors, such as lower IQ, language delays, and other developmental delays. Additional studies are needed for testing of young children and adolescents that utilize more refined neuropsychological tests.

Diagnostic Issues Related to Very Early and Early Onset

Schizophrenia was originally described narrowly as a severe condition that predominantly affected young men, with a male to female ratio of 3 to 1; the majority of cases having an onset by age 22 years (Kraepelin, 1896/1971). This male to female ratio is similar to that described for early onset neurodevelopmental schizophrenia (Castle and Murray, 1991; Murray, 1994). Subsequently, catatonia and paranoid deterioration were added as variants of schizophrenia and, with their inclusion, the sex distribution became more equal and the mean age of onset increased. The definition of schizophrenia was enlarged by Bleuler (1911/1950) and Schneider (1959) who based their diagnoses on the phenomenology of presenting symptoms rather than course and outcome.

A developmental approach must return to the more narrow definitions initially proposed, placing emphasis again on course and outcome. This approach suggests that congenital schizophrenia, or neurodevelopmental schizophrenia, is a consequence of aberrant brain development that begins during fetal and neonatal life. Patients with this disorder are expected to show structural brain changes and cognitive impairment, male predominance, early onset, and generally poor outcome, as did the original cases described by Kraepelin. Late adolescent and adult onset schizophrenia, however, may be more heterogeneous in their origins. An initial diagnosis of pervasive developmental disorder is commonly made for younger children who do not meet diagnostic criteria for positive symptoms of schizophrenia.

Because identification of the positive symptoms of schizophrenia depends on language development, the diagnosis cannot be made, using the current criteria, in children who are nonverbal, those who are too young to have language, and those with severe mental retardation and/or certain language disorders. Diagnosis also requires the maturation of logical thinking and the ability to be aware of the communicative needs of a listener. Most studies are consistent with the earliest age for diagnosis being 6 to 7 years; however, Caplan et al. (1989, 1990) identified positive symptoms as early as age 5, and there are case reports of symptom onset as early as age 3 (Russell, Bott, and Sammons, 1989). Therefore, it is premature to suggest a lower age limit for the diagnosis until such time as better diagnostic criteria are established for younger children.

The Thought Disorder Index provides one systematic approach to investigate thought disorder in school-age children and has been used to assess thought disorder in children age 5 to 16 years. Using this index the level of thought disorder in psychotic children and high-risk children was approximately three times that of normal children in one study (Arboleda and Holzman, 1985).

Studies of early onset schizophrenia (Werry, McClellan, and Chard, 1991) generally do not emphasize subtypes because the majority of younger children may belong to the "undifferentiated type" and show characteristics of several different subcategories. The subcategories of schizophrenia are paranoid, catatonic, disorganized, or a combination of these (undifferentiated). Yet there seems to be age-dependent variation in symptoms as children grow older (Asarnow, 1994; Bettes and Walker, 1987; Eggers, 1978; Russell, Bott, and Sammons, 1989; Watkins, Asarnow, and Tanguay, 1988; Werry, McClellan, and Chard, 1991). Well-formulated and consistently reported delusions are rare in early onset and, particularly, in very early onset forms. Hallucinations, disorganized thinking, and inappropriate affect may be characteristic of childhood onset after age 5 years, although there may be developmental differences in associated thought content (Caplan et al., 1990). Catatonic symptoms are less frequently reported in very early onset cases, and prevalence of catatonic symptoms in adults also is not clearly documented. Moreover, catatonic symptoms may be related to affective disorders. Thus undifferentiated forms and disorganized thinking may be characteristic for the younger children, and hallucinations and delusions more common with later onset.

It is not clear whether or not there is an increased prevalence in lower socioeconomic groups, although for adults there may be a downward drift in social class with increasing chronicity of schizophrenic symptomatology. Family studies have been confounded by later diagnoses of mood disorders in patients who were initially classified as schizophrenic. The subsequent recognition of mood disorders in index cases reflects the need for better delineation of diagnostic criteria for younger children. Even when initial diagnostic criteria are met, the initial diagnosis may not be accurate due to overlapping symptoms between schizophrenia and affective disorders with psychotic features and possibly personality disorder (Carlson, 1990; McClellan, Werry, and Ham, 1993).

NATURAL HISTORY

The extent of impairment is related to poor premorbid functioning, early onset of symptoms, and problems in acquiring cognitive skills. With the early onset of schizophrenia, there is a higher frequency of premorbid developmental disorder; rates of 54% to 90% have been reported, depending on the study; the earlier the onset, the more likely the developmental disorder. Premorbid schizoid or schizotypal personality features are commonly reported; the child is seen by others as odd, anxious, and socially isolated.

The onset of symptoms, especially in preschool children, tends to be insidious (Green and Padron-Gayol, 1986; Kolvin, 1971), but in adolescence, onset is more likely to be acute. With an earlier age of onset, the course may be more chronic; however, this is not always the case (Eggers, 1978). With adolescent onset, chronicity is reported in 83% of cases (Werry, McClellan, and Chard, 1991), which is slightly higher than the 75% occurrence of chronic cases reported in adult series (Westermeyer and Harrow, 1984).

Eggers (1978) reported information on 57 schizophrenic patients with onset between age 7 and age 13. The average length of follow-up is 15 years. Those cases with acute or relapsing episodes occurred more often than chronic cases. However, before age 11 acute cases were less frequent. Twenty percent showed complete recovery, 30% relatively good adjustment, 50% moderate or poor outcome. Premorbid personality development was of prognostic value, but family incidence of psychiatric disorders and poor family environment was not.

The lifetime risk for suicide in adults with schizophrenia is about 15% in the first 10 years after the onset of the illness. Werry (1992) suggests that the risk for suicide or accidental death may be 5% to 15% with the onset of illness in childhood.

ETIOLOGY

Neurodevelopmental

The issue of schizophrenia having a developmental onset is being reconsidered. Fish (1977), and before her Bender (1942, 1947), suggested an inherited neurointegrative defect in early onset schizophrenia and emphasized that although childhood onset schizophrenia seems to be on a continuum with adult schizophrenia, it represents the more severe neurobiological presentation. Increasingly, there is evidence of abnormal neurological development in infants who are later diagnosed as schizophrenic. Disorders in the development of speech, and maturation of language function and thought processing have been considered critical in the diagnosis of schizophrenia in childhood by many authors,beginning with the early descriptions of Potter (1933), Despert (1938), Bender (1942, 1947), and Kanner (1973).

Findings of brain abnormality have been interpreted as consistent with schizophrenia being a neurodevelopmental disorder (Murray et al., 1988; Weinberger, 1987) most likely involving the medial temporal lobe (Murray, Jones, and O'Callaghan, 1991; Roberts, 1991). It is important to establish the relationship of any abnormality of brain development to abnormalities in brain biochemistry. Murray et al. (1992) suggest that the neurodevelopmental form of schizophrenia is characterized by abnormalities that are present at birth but may not be recognized in early life. A neurodevelopmental form could result from a genetic defect that leads to decreased cortical volume and smaller temporal lobe structures. These might be visualized, using neuroimaging techniques. Moreover, postmortem studies suggest migration failure of cells in the entorhinal cortex (Jones and Murray, 1991). Still, it is possible that similar clinical and neuropathological findings may be the result of early environmental insults or a combination of genetic predisposition with environmental insults, among these being early brain injury and infections.

The evidence for a developmental origin, therefore, comes from neuropathological studies and from neuroimaging studies. Recent studies show loss of volume in brain regions along with the absence of fibrillary gliosis or of reactive astrocytes, which is suggestive of a developmental disturbance. Astrocytes are involved in axonal guidance and become mature in regard to the fibrillary reaction at about 6 months of gestation in the human fetus. A lack of gliosis reported in most studies suggests a fetal origin of brain abnormality; however, in some cases the abnormalities could arise at birth or even later deriving from an inflammatory neurodegenerative process. Support for a disturbance in neuronal migration also comes from the demonstration of cytoarchitectonic abnormalities in layer II of the limbic cortex with displacement of layer II cells into layer III (Jakob and Beckmann, 1986, 1989).

Genetic

The importance of a genetic contribution to schizophrenia is well recognized and dates back to proposals in Bleuler's original description. Genetic and possibly viral etiologies, or possibly the occurrence of a viral illness in a genetically predisposed individual, have been studied. Because such precise sequential steps underlie neuronal migration, synapse formation, and synapse reconstruction, genetic factors must be considered as involved in etiology during the developmental period (Bloom, 1993). For example, the premature switching off of genes responsible for certain trophic factors or their receptors may lead to structural changes. In a particular pedigree, the genome may fail to maintain the expression of genes required to complete the process of cortical neuronal migration. A variety of other factors, such as nutrition, toxins, or trauma, might interact in a genetically vulnerable person.

Genetic aspects are then the most commonly proposed etiologic factors in schizophrenia. Yet how genetic factors lead to vulnerability to schizophrenia remains unclarified. The nature and magnitude of genetic effects is the major issue. Questions about what is inherited, the mode of transmission, which genes might be involved, and what other variables influence predisposed individuals to becoming symptomatic continue to be the focus of investigations. Because schizophrenia is a complex disorder where the mode of transmission is unknown, penetrance may be incomplete, and the disorder might result from the interaction of a few major genes. It is thought that there is variable expressivity, diagnostic instability, and probable etiologic heterogeneity.

Because the etiology of schizophrenia and its subcategories is unknown, multifactorial as well as possible single-gene forms continue to be investigated. There may be risk factors that relate to cognitive dysfunction and to brain damage in later onset as well as in early onset cases; their specificity is being studied extensively. Schizophrenic patients have an increased risk of pre- or perinatal obstetrical complications and an increased risk of prematurity. There also may be an excessive number of minor physical anomalies that suggests abnormal fetal development (Waddington, O'Callaghan, and Larkin, 1990).

The mode of transmission for schizophrenia, then, remains to be determined. Genetic approaches focus on the study of both single-gene mutations that might be inherited in a Mendelian dominant, recessive, or sex-linked manner or through polygenic inheritance. Monogenic (single-gene) inheritance is more commonly associated with rare conditions, and because schizophrenia is relatively common, polygenic inheritance seems more likely. Polygenic inheritance involves multiple abnormal genes that might have interactive effects in contrast to a single gene producing large effects. An intermediate model referred to as a "oligogenic model" has been proposed. This is a polygenic model with "graduated locus effects" wherein a small number of genes may have a substantial effect on the final phenotypic expression. Moreover, these modes of genetic transmission may be part of a multifactorial transmission model that allows for the joint effects of a major gene or a few major genes, a polygenic background, and environmental influences.

Genes might code for neurochemical abnormalities, code for specific events in neurodevelopment, such as proliferation and neuronal migration, or control factors that relate to susceptibility (e.g., sensitivity of temporal lobe cells to anoxia or central nervous system viral infection).

One approach, the vulnerability-stress model (Zubin and Spring, 1977), postulates that actual onset depends on an interaction among biological, psychological, and environmental factors. The risk for schizophrenia in the general population is approximately 1%; however, high-risk family studies have consistently demonstrated an increased risk for schizophrenia in first-degree relatives. Estimates by Tsuang and Vandermey (1980), are shown in Table 14–2, namely parents, 4.4%; siblings, 8.5%; children of a schizophrenic person, 12.3%, both parents affected, 36.6%, and for identical twins, 57.7%.

But even well-designed family studies cannot fully distinguish between the genetic and environmental factors that lead to an increased prevalence of schizophrenia within families. As a result, twin and adoption studies have been carried out to identify genetic and environmental factors. Studies of large pedigrees and studies of schizophrenic twins indicate an increased prevalence in families where there is an early onset of schizophrenia; however, the samples are small and further work needs to be done on assessment methodology. The boundary of the disorder must be defined because a spectrum of symptoms are seen.

Table 14–2. Genetic Risk Factors in Schizophrenia

Relation	Risk %
First-degree relatives	
Parents	4.4
Brothers and sisters	8.5
Neither parent schizophrenic	8.2
One parent schizophrenic	13.8
Fraternal twins of opposite sex	5.6
Fraternal twins of same sex	12.0
Identical twins	57.7
Children	12.3
Both parents schizophrenic	36.6
Second-degree relatives	
Uncles and aunts	2.0
Nephews and nieces	2.2
Grandchildren	2.8
Half brothers/sisters	3.2
First cousins (third-degree relatives)	2.9
General population	0.86

Adapted from Tsuang and Vandermey, 1980.

The initial twin studies of schizophrenia were conducted in the 1920s; since then over 800 monozygotic twin pairs and 1,000 dizygotic twin pairs have been examined (Torrey, 1992). Studies of identical twins discordant for schizophrenia must take into account the greater likelihood of co-twin involvement if the index case is more severely ill (Suddath, Christison, and Torrey, 1990). Reveley et al. (1982), found that the schizophrenic member of co-twins had larger ventricles than the identical co-twin and the unaffected co-twin had larger ventricles than a normal control case.

Twin studies also have some limitations because environmental factors as well as genetic differences may influence relative risk for schizophrenia in twins. Moreover, the prenatal and postnatal environments of monozygotic and dizygotic twins may be different. To address these issues, adoption studies of monozygotic twins reared apart and adoptee studies have been conducted, using the adoptee family method.

Studies of monozygotic twins reared apart have shown high concordance for schizophrenia, providing further evidence of the genetic component. Kety, Rosenthal, and Wender (1978) found that schizophrenia and related disorders were more common in the biological relatives of 34 schizophrenic adoptees than in the biological relatives of matched control adoptees. Torrey (1992) reevaluated eight twin studies, which included 341 monozygotic twins and 723 dizygotic twins where representative samples and zygosity were carefully determined, and found the concordance rate for monozygotic twin pairs to be 28% and that of dizygotic twins to be 6%.

Communication deviance has been found in parents of affected children (Asarnow, Goldstein, and Ben-Meir, 1988). Family and adoption studies suggest that not only schizophrenia but also schizotypal and paranoid personality disorders are demonstrable in biological relatives of schizophrenic patients. These findings indicate the predisposition is not only to schizophrenia but also to a spectrum of disorders. Consequently, the genetic vulnerability may be to various components of the disorder, such as positive symptoms, negative symptoms, latent trait predisposition to both schizophrenia and eye movement dysfunction, and attentional and preattentional abnormalities (Kaufmann and Malaspina, 1991). High-risk offspring of schizophrenic parents must be evaluated for these potentially predisposing traits.

A variety of genetic research strategies, including segregation analysis, have been developed to evaluate these various modes of transmission. Although results are inconclusive, there is continuing interest in using linkage analysis to identify disease susceptibility markers. Genetic analysis is complex because half or more of monozygotic twin pairs are discordant for schizophrenia despite being genetically identical. Such differences have been attributed to incomplete penetrance, etiologic heterogeneity (with several genetic forms, some of which affect both members of twins), and possible environmental forms that interact with genetic predisposition. The genetic inheritance of schizophrenia receives further support in follow-up studies of the offspring of the nonschizophrenic co- twin. The offspring of both the nonschizophrenic and the schizophrenic twin may have the same increased risk for developing the disorder. This implies reduced penetrance as a factor in the discordance among monozygotic twins.

Another explanation for difference is that there may be an interaction among a few major genes. An individual may be at genetic risk at one specific locus but lack susceptibility at a second locus and, therefore, not express a disorder. Diagnostic assessment must be carefully considered because the gene conferring susceptibility to the disorder might produce several clinical manifestations. This applies not only to other diagnoses, such as schizotypal personality and paranoid presentations, but also to possible neurophysiological changes, such as eye movement dysfunction. Moreover, psychiatric manifestations of schizophrenia may vary within individuals over time. Finally, phenocopies of schizophrenia may occur; these cases might result from head injury or epilepsy occurring in susceptible individuals.

A number of specific genetic abnormalities have been evaluated in schizophrenia. The greatest interest has been in linkage studies involving autosomal chromosomes 2 and 5 and the X chromosome (Kaufmann and Malaspina, 1991; Malaspina et al., 1992). In addition, fragile sites have been reported on several chromosomes, including 3, 9, and 17. The fragile chromosome sites that have been suggested should be pursued in this regard. The finding of expansions of tandem repeats in chromosome regions in several disorders, such as the fragile X syndrome and Huntington's disease, could potentially be relevant to schizophrenia. In fragile X, females with schizophrenia spectrum and affective disorders have been suggested (Reiss et al., 1988). Yet despite extensive investigations of multiple family members, no conclusive results have been reached that firmly and specifically link any of these loci to schizophrenia. Early enthusiasm for linkage analysis on particular chromosomes has been followed by a failure to demonstrate linkage when additional families that were added to the original pedigree were examined. Overall, the factors that must interact to produce schizophrenia require considerable additional study. Future family studies might focus on the early neurodevelopmental forms of schizophrenia to clarify whether there is worsening of symptoms from one generation to the next.

Neuropathological Findings

Since the original description of schizophrenia, there has been considerable interest in demonstrating postmortem changes in cellular neuropathology in adult subjects. Yet findings have been so conflicting that schizophrenia was regarded as the "graveyard of neuropathology." However, Bogerts (1993) has reviewed 50 neuroanatomical postmortem studies that were published in the past 20 years and notes various subtle abnormalities in limbic structures and parts of the basal ganglia, thalamus, cortex, corpus callosum, and brainstem neurotransmitter systems. Many of these studies are based on small sample size, so conclusions remain preliminary. He suggests that the absence of normal cerebral asymmetry in a number of these cases, cytoarchitectonic abnormalities, and lack of gliosis in the limbic areas are suggestive of a disorder of prenatal brain development rather than a progressive degenerative brain disorder.

In the past several years, both structural and functional evidence suggesting underlying microscopic pathology in the frontal lobes of schizophrenic patients has been reported. Particular efforts have been made to correlate the severity of negative symptoms with brain changes.

Neuroimaging Findings

Evidence of brain abnormalities in schizophrenia has come from neuroimaging studies as well as from neuropathological investigations. Findings include increased ventricular size and a widening of the cortical sulci in CT studies (Owen, Lewis, and Murray, 1988). These findings have been corroborated through MRI studies (Levy et al., 1992; Suddath, Christison, and Torrey, 1990) where decreased volume of the temporal lobes, reduced brain weight, reduction in volume of medial temporal lobe structures (Brown et al., 1986), and bilateral reductions in volumes of the hippocampal formation and internal pallidum have been reported (Bogerts and Falkai, 1990). Other findings include reduced cortical gray matter and hypometabolism of part of the frontal lobes and parts of the basal ganglia that occurs independently from the effects of neuroleptic drugs. There continues to be argument about whether brain abnormalities are found in all types of schizophrenia.

The demonstration of static brain abnormalities on neuroimaging in schizophrenia is consistent with a neurodevelopmental hypothesis. CT scan abnormalities have been noted in young patients at the time of their initial presentation and seem to be nonprogressive. CT findings may also indicate premorbid psychopathology, e.g., marked ventricular dilatation has been noted before the development of frank psychotic symptoms in an adolescent case (O'Callaghan et al., 1988).

That there is substantial neuropathology in schizophrenia is no longer in doubt; however, which changes are reproducible signs of its basic pathology and which suggest causative, reactive, or maladaptive reactions to these cerebral changes is not clear.

Pandysmaturation (PDM)

The possibility of a genetically based neurointegrative defect in schizophrenia was initially proposed by Bender (1947) and later referred to as "pandysmaturation" by Fish (1977). Pandysmaturation (PDM) was introduced following a 1952 study of infants who were thought to be genetically vulnerable to develop schizophrenia later in life. Support for this hypothesis comes from findings of delayed development in schizophrenic infants and their performance on psychological evaluations. Pandysmaturation seems to have neurodevelopmental origins rather than being the result of obstetrical complications.

Careful study of infant development in children considered to be at risk for schizophrenia has led to continued interest in the pandysmaturation hypothesis (Fish et al., 1992; Weinberger, 1988). Fish et al. suggest a transient retardation in gross motor and/or visual-motor development, which is followed by a subsequent acceleration in the rate of development, then a return to more normal rates. In addition, this period of transient retardation is associated with an abnormal developmental profile where earlier psychological test items are failed, although more complex items requiring a higher level of performance are passed. Moreover, there may be an accompanying retardation in skeletal growth. The transient developmental lag is identified by this combination of abnormal developmental profiles along with a lag in skeletal growth. Anatomically, developmental hypoplasia of certain brain regions, particularly in the medial temporal lobe, is postulated in PDM.

The most characteristic feature of PDM is an innate dysregulation of normal neurological development involving the normal timing of developmental sequences and spatial organization. Affected children have periods when previously acquired abilities are lost.

Pandysmaturation may be recognized during the rapid period of brain growth during the first 2 years of life. With maturation of the nervous system, its expression varies with increasing age. In the older child, less specific developmental evidence of changes are found, such as problems with smooth-pursuit eye movements, subtle, nonlocalizing neurological signs, and abnormalities in attention and information processing. Moderate to severe social/affective symptoms begin between 3 and 6 years. This is followed by cognitive deficits and moderate to severe psychological symptoms by age 10, with the recognition of schizotypal disorders or schizophrenia during adolescence or early adulthood. Still, the developmental profile does not predict which children will become schizophrenic and which will show schizotypal symptoms. Pandysmaturation is highly correlated with a parental diagnosis of schizophrenia. Follow-up studies show that the role of obstetrical complications is nonspecific, even though such complications may precipitate or facilitate the expression of the disorder.

Additional support for a developmental abnormality in childhood onset schizophrenia includes increased prevalence of prematurity (McNeil, 1990) and an excess of minor physical anomalies (Waddington, O'Callaghan, and Larkin, 1990).

Synaptic Pruning and Cell Death

The onset of schizophrenia in adolescence (ages 13 to 18) may relate to lack of appropriate neurobiological integration that may be linked to faulty synaptic elimination and possibly cell death. Because the age of onset of schizophrenia is ordinarily in late adolescence and early adulthood, Feinberg (1982/1983) has proposed that an abnormality in programmed synaptic elimination during adolescence may account for this age of onset. The evidence for a reorganization in brain function in adolescence is supported by a substantial reduction in the amount of deep sleep that occurs over the stages of puberty, a fall in the rate of brain metabolism, and a decline in the latency of certain event-related potentials. In addition, the capacity for recovery of brain function after brain injury decreases, and adult formal operational thinking emerges. Concurrently, there is a reduction in cortical synaptic density in postmortem tissue (Huttenlocher, 1979) and reductions in D_1 and D_2 dopamine receptors. The changes in dopamine receptors during development has been shown by Seeman et al. (1987) in postmortem tissue and in living subjects by Wong et al. (1988).

Abnormal Neuronal Migration Cortical Areas

Support for a neurodevelopmental origin comes from the postmortem pathological findings being as severe early in the course of the illness as they are later in its course. This neurodevelopmental view of schizophrenia is based on various microscopic findings in postmortem tissue that include missing or abnormal size of neurons, abnormal patterns of myelination, and disoriented neurons. Akbarian et al. (1993a, 1993b) have moved beyond microscopic analysis and used immunohistochemistry to study cortical neurons rather than focus on cell size, myelination patterns, and neuronal density. These authors studied the enzyme NADPH diaphorase, which is found in a particular subset of neurons in the frontal lobe. These neurons are resistant to degeneration, possibly because NADPH-d may prevent cell death by the local release of nitric oxide. They found a significant reduction in NADPH-d immunoreactive neurons in the superficial white matter and in the cortical gray matter in the frontal lobes in 5 schizophrenic subjects. There was also a significant increase in the number of these NADPH-d neurons in the white matter 3 mm or more below the cortical gray matter. These findings are of interest in relationship to how the cortex may develop in neurodevelopmental schizophrenia.

Findings of abnormal cell migration with the absence of gliosis suggest a nondestructive lesion in the second or third trimester. These results could also be explained by a primary glial cell abnormality because these glial cells guide cortical cells to their final destinations. The finding of persistence of NADPH-d staining cells is of particular interest because one model of schizophrenia involves excitotoxicity, leading to excessive activation of NMDA and other excitatory amino acid neurotransmitters resulting in NO release; the released NO may mediate excitotoxicity.

At the neural tube stage, the embryonic central nervous system consists of a single layer of pseudostratified columnar epithelium, termed the "ventricular zone," which generates all of the neurons and glia of the adult brain. Shortly after the formation of the ventricular zone, a second embryonic layer, the marginal zone, appears at the outer surface of the developing brain. The marginal zone is relatively cell free, although it is the source of early afferent fibers that are destined for cortical precursor regions. Subsequently, an intermediate zone is produced between the marginal and ventricular zones as postmitotic neurons differentiate and leave the ventricular zone to migrate to their final destinations in the gray matter. During the migratory process, the cortical cells form into an inside-out laminar pattern, that is, the cells destined for the deeper layers of cortex migrate from the ventricular zone first; those cells that will move to more superficial locations migrate later. In humans, cortical neuronal genesis is thought to occur between embryonic days 4 and 125, during the first and early second trimester of pregnancy.

In the junctional region between the intermediate and marginal zones of developing cortex, the migrating neurons form the cortical plate, a transient structure. The cortical plate establishes the location for incoming fibers entering the cortical regions as well as the location of outgoing fibers of the earliest differentiating intrinsic cortical neurons. Moreover, at the interface between the intermediate zone and the ventricular zone, which is deeper in the brain, a new proliferative layer, the subventricular zone, is formed. The subventricular zone becomes the sole cellular proliferative area for subsequent brain organogenesis. In the region between the cortical plate and the subventricular zone, fibers entering and leaving the cortex eventually form cortical white matter.

Following migration and place specification, synaptogenesis occurs, leading to the production of excessive numbers of neurons and their connections. Redundant connections are eventually destroyed, and cell number is reduced through programmed cell death. This is followed by myelination and, finally, networks are functionally validated through adaptive experiences. Those neurons that do not make appropriate functional circuits will die so surviving neurons do not remain in isolation (Cowan et al., 1984).

The NADPH-d immunoreactive neurons are found in abundance in the cortical subplate layer. They ultimately migrate to upper cortical layers and should be among the last cells that pass through the cortical plate. The displacement of NADPH-d immunoreactive neurons from the superficial cortical white matter to the deeper subcortical white matter suggests either abnormal migration of this group of neurons or persistent survival within their layer of proliferation beyond that expected in the life cycle of the developing cortex. Akbarian et al.'s (1993a, 1993b) findings are compatible with a developmental disturbance where the normal pattern of programmed cell death is affected in some way, accompanied by a defect in the orderly, normal migration of neurons toward the cortical plate and may reflect a primary disturbance of the developmentally regulated cortical subplate. Changes in the distribution of these cells may have serious consequences for the establishment of normal patterns of cortical connections that might result in a breakdown of frontal lobe functioning in schizophrenia. The persistence of these neurons in an abnormal location suggests they may have established functional connections with surrogate targets; however, additional studies are needed to clarify what their appropriate innervation patterns should be.

Hippocampus

In the temporal lobe and hippocampal formation, these same authors found 4 of their 5 schizophrenic subjects had lower numbers of NADPH-d neurons in the hippocampal formation and in the neocortex of the lateral temporal lobe as well as a significant increase in cell number in the white matter of the lateral temporal lobe. Findings in these brain regions in addition to the cortex suggest a more global developmental defect. It is expected that if abnormal migrations may have occurred, they are most likely to have taken place in the middle to late part of the second trimester of pregnancy. The timing of these events requires further study. Investigations of other brain regions, such as the cerebellar cortex, where neuronal generation and migration continues later on into pregnancy, are needed to better define the time of migration. The misplaced NADPH-d neurons may be parts of dysfunctional circuits and poorly responsive to activity-dependent experiences. Given these findings, more extensive neuroanatomic analyses of the pathophysiology of schizophrenia are needed. Some developmental analyses have been conducted in children at high risk for schizophrenia, using Fish's pandysmaturation index (Fish et al., 1992). In addition, adults with an early onset of schizophrenia should be evaluated for signs of neurointegrative defects.

Cell migration in the hippocampus has also been considered by other authors. Synaptic formation in the human hippocampus is completed earlier than in other parts of the cortex, making the hippocampus more susceptible at an earlier stage to abnormalities in those processes of regression that shape the final neuronal circuitry (Rakic et al., 1986). Hippocampal development begins during the second month of uterine life. It continues through the third postnatal month. Studies of the time course of cell migration in the hippocampus (Rakic and Nowakowski, 1981) demonstrate that the deepest layer of the entorhinal cortex is the earliest structure that can be detected. Subsequently, cells in other parts of the hippocampal formation proliferate simultaneously but stop their proliferation at different times. Later, CA_2 is the first area that is differentiated and CA_1 and CA_4 follow. The dentate granule cells develop throughout the second half of gestation, continuing until the second postpartum month. These cells migrate from the medial wall of the lateral ventricle at approximately 15 mm per day for the hippocampus, 100 mm per day for the parahippocampal gyrus, and about 114 mm per day for the cortex. Because of these findings on migration, Jakob and Beckmann (1989) suggested that the cytoarchitectonic abnormalities demonstrated in the brains of schizophrenics are related to migrational arrest of cells during the second trimester.

Nongenetic Factors Influencing Development

Animal studies in mice by Conrad and Scheibel (1987) suggest that influenza may affect the hippocampus in ways that are reminiscent of those found in schizophrenia. These authors found pyramidal cell disorganization in the hippocampus similar to reports in schizophrenics.

NEUROCHEMISTRY IN SCHIZOPHRENIA

Because of the findings of dysplastic changes in the medial temporal lobe in neuroimaging and neuropathological studies, the relationship of abnormalities of brain development to brain biochemistry must be considered. Not only the neurochemical consequences of temporal lobe pathology but also the pharmacology of trophic factors that may be involved in aberrant development must be evaluated; both relate to the neuronal and neurochemical abnormalities seen in postmortem schizophrenic brains. Reynolds (1983) studied the medial temporal lobe and found increased dopamine in the left amygdala in brains of schizophrenic persons in keeping with the dopamine model of schizophrenia.

Others have studied nondopaminergic neurotransmitter systems within the medial temporal lobe, including the excitatory amino acids, the neuropeptides (particularly CCK), the PCP receptor system, and gamma-aminobutyric acid. The relationship between the glutamate system and the dopamine system has been investigated in the temporal lobe region where low concentrations of aspartate, a marker for glutamine terminals, has been reported. Detailed quantitative autoradiographic studies have shown bilateral loss of receptor binding by kainate localized to the CA_4/CA_3 region of the hippocampus and in the entorhinal cortex (Kerwin, Patel, and Meldrum, 1990). Subsequently, Harrison, McLaughlin, and Kerwin (1991) used *in situ* hybridization histochemistry to show that this loss of non-NMDA receptors is associated with a loss of the mRNA that encodes a region homologous to both kainate and quisqualate receptor genes. This suggests that the glutamate receptor abnormalities may be a product of altered gene expression.

Another approach to neurochemistry has focused on neuropeptides that may be co-localized with neurotransmitters. Cholecystokinin (CCK) is a neuroleptic-like substance biochemically and behaviorally and is highly concentrated in the hippocampus; postmortem studies of schizophrenic brains have shown that it is reduced in the hippocampus, temporal cortex, and the amygdala while cortical levels are unchanged (Crow et al., 1982). There is concomitant loss of CCK receptors in these brain regions that also may be involved in negative symptoms of schizophrenia.

GABA neurons in the temporal lobe have CCK as their co-localized peptide. They also possess excitatory amino acid receptors (Hendry et al., 1984). Simpson et al. (1989) found a loss of the GABA terminals bilaterally in the amygdala and hippocampus. Reynolds, Czudek, and Andrews (1990) found no changes in the amygdala but did find losses in the left hippocampus.

These findings provide evidence of a neurochemical abnormality in the temporal lobes in schizophrenia. Additional research is needed on the role of glutamate and cholecystokinin (CCK), and the interaction of these substances with phencyclidine and GABA-related systems. These systems may interact in the regulation of dopamine release, leading to secondarily increased activity of dopamine systems in schizophrenia. Finally, Akbarian et al. (1995) studied gene expression for glutamic acid decarboxylase (GAD) in postmortem brain tissue from 10 chronic schizophrenic patients. They found a pronounced decrease in GAD expression in GABA cortical neurons without significant cell loss in the dorsolateral prefrontal cortex (DLPFC).

Trophic Functions of Neurotransmitters

Vertebrate neurons rely on nerve growth factor and other trophic factors for survival. Prior to their functioning as neurotransmitters, excitatory neurotransmitters, CCK, and GABA influence neuronal development, connectivity, and polarity, and also promote or inhibit neurite outgrowth or retraction (Mattson, 1988).

Kerwin and Murray (1992) suggest that those neurotransmitter systems reported to be abnormal in the medial temporal lobe in schizophrenia (excitatory neurotransmitters and CCK) also play a role as trophic factors in hippocampal development; consequently, these systems must be considered in a neurodevelopmental hypothesis of schizophrenia.

A major component of a neurodevelopmental hypothesis is concerned with neuronal plasticity and how mature nerve cells interact with adverse external factors. Experience-dependent synaptic plasticity has been shown for NMDA receptors. These receptors are important in the synaptic remodeling processes, such as long-term potentiation in the hippocampus (Harris, Ganong, and Cotman, 1984) and visual-dependent plasticity of striate cortex (Bear et al., 1990). These findings have led to the proposal that glutamate systems play a major role in the maintenance and modulation of the cytoarchitecture of neuronal systems.

The cloning and sequencing of several glutamate receptor genes may also lead to better ways to study the trophic role of glutamate. There are four separate AMPA genes, and each has two isoforms. These eight entities have a very precise developmental pattern that is expressed. It may be possible to look for abnormal expression of developmental forms or the persistence of developmental forms in autopsy material as a method for investigating the role of glutamate genes in controlling hippocampal cell architecture. Another way that excitatory amino acids could be involved in the neurodevelopmental hypothesis involves their role in hypoxic neuronal damage. Excessive endogenous excitatory amino acid receptor activity mediates some negative consequences of ischemia; phencyclidine and MK801 can protect against this damage. Cerebral ischemia that is secondary to viral infection or birth complications could lead to neuronal loss that is mediated by glutamate receptors. Excitatory neurotransmitters might thus play a role in those developmental processes that might be negatively affected by hypoxia. This could be one mechanism for the interaction of genetic predisposition and obstetrical complications in the offspring of schizophrenics.

Cholecystokinin (CCK) and its receptors play a role in hippocampal development just as glutamate does. The laminar arrangement of CCK-containing cells may act to attract ingrowing afferents. An overexpression of CCK cells at the trophic stage of embryonic development might be related to subsequent overactivity of dopamine systems. This suggests the hypothesis that CCK- containing pathways from the temporal lobe interact with limbic dopamine systems to produce a hyperdopaminergic state (Roberts, 1991). Kerwin and Murray (1992) suggest that CCK abnormalities during embryonic development are widespread and could lead to a general decrease in cortical volume in schizophrenia. If this were the case, the generalized cortical changes may be related to negative symptoms, but hippocampal abnormalities may be more important in the generation of positive symptoms.

In summary, a common theme in schizophrenia research is that structural abnormalities in some schizophrenic patients are of developmental origin. Such schizophrenic patients may suffer neurodevelopmental lesions in fetal or neonatal life. This would suggest that the fault is in the genetic control of neurodevelopment. In other instances, early environmental hazards, such as maternal influenza or birth complications, might interact with mutant neurodevelopmental genes. Consequently, there may be migrational arrests. Neurotransmitters that have been consistently abnormal in postmortem studies of the temporal lobe may play an important role in the control of hippocampal development. No specific single mechanism has been reported to account for all these changes, but these neurotransmitter systems do play a major role as trophic factors in development. Further studies are necessary to investigate how CCK peptides and excitatory amino acid receptor genes might be involved in aberrant neurodevelopment.

Pharmacological Models: PCP Model

Considerable interest has focused on the phencyclidine (PCP) model of schizophrenia. Unlike amphetamine, PCP-induced psychoses produce both negative and positive schizophrenic-like symptoms, formal thought disorder, and neuropsychological deficits. When given to schizophrenic patients, the thought disorder may be exacerbated and hostility increased. (Neuropsychological tests in these patients demonstrated disturbances in attention, perception, and symbolic thinking.) PCP binds to a brain receptor located in the ion channel formed by the NMDA receptor complex. When PCP binds to its receptor, voltage-dependent NMDA channels are blocked and long-term potentiation (LTP) is inhibited, which leads to blockage of the effects of glutamate and inhibition of neurotransmission. PCP inhibits discriminative and associative learning. The PCP/NMDA system is located in hippocampus, frontal cortex, striatum and limbic system. The phencyclidine receptor site is involved in the modulation of the activated glutamatergic NMDA receptors.

TREATMENT

There is little specific research on the treatment of very early onset schizophrenia; however, it is generally assumed that similar mechanisms apply to child and adult cases. In children and adolescents, the treatment approach includes multiple treatment modalities. Pharmacological treatments must be targeted toward characteristic positive and negative symptoms. Psychosocial treatment addresses individual psychological and social needs of the particular child and family who must cope with the disorder. Moreover, treatment must be appropriate to the phase of illness and address illness onset, rehabilitation, and chronic management and provide ongoing monitoring of residual symptoms.

Psychosocial Treatments

Psychosocial treatments are critical in mitigating the disability and in the prevention of relapse. Family members must be well educated regarding the natural history of the disorder and its particular presentation in their child. The effective use of medication requires the institution of effective psychosocial interventions with active family involvement in medication management.

A comprehensive approach to childhood onset (very early onset) schizophrenia involves individual supportive therapy with the child, educational and supportive therapy with his or her parents, psychoeducational school programs, and an ongoing maintenance medication treatment. This combination of approaches is likely to decrease relapse rates in children. Specific efforts should be made to work with the child to help him or her understand the nature of the illness and to recognize early symptoms as they begin to emerge. Following the child's progress will include monitoring the use of drawings for younger children because disorganization and bizarreness in drawings may provide additional clues to deterioration. With the parents, a supportive and educational approach is essential to help them adapt and modulate their emotional responses to the child's condition. Highly expressed emotion shown in overprotectiveness or expressed criticism of the child may increase the risk of relapse. A sensitive approach with parents is essential because family interactions become increasingly complex as the family adapts to living with the child with schizophrenia. In adults, the relapse within the first year after diagnosis, on medication alone, has been reported as 30% to 50%, but when family treatment is combined with medications, the relapse rate may be as low as 12% (Goldstein, 1989). Family therapy should be combined with social skills training for the child and an intensive education about the illness. Family therapy interventions are focused toward helping family members establish a better understanding of the illness and its causes as well as strategies that may be utilized to deal with symptoms when they are expressed.

Special education services are an essential component of a comprehensive treatment program. Children and adolescents with schizophrenia tend to have difficulties in a normal classroom setting and may need a self-contained classroom with an individualized curriculum. This is particularly the case for younger children with developmental dysfunction who often have learning disorders as well as schizophrenia. If hospitalization is involved, a subsequent day treatment program that provides both educational and mental health services is often needed. A school psychoeducational program must include social skills training, vocational training, basic life skills training, and teach social problem-solving strategies. In addition, families should be engaged in the treatment process.

Long-term treatment requires a somewhat different focus than that for the initial, acute episode. Positive symptoms most likely will bring patients to the attention of mental health care staff, yet it is the negative symptoms—inattention, anergia, apathy, and lack of interest in interpersonal relationships—that tend to cause the greater long-term disability. Social work case management services may be crucial in organizing such therapeutic programs and for ensuring that the patient remains actively engaged in the treatment process. As the child matures, long-term planning is required to facilitate entry into adult services.

Pharmacotherapy

Drug treatment also must be coordinated with the natural history of the disorder and take into account its phases, i.e., prodromal, active, recuperative/recovery, and residual (Kane, 1987). The efficacy of treatment with neuroleptic medications for schizophrenic symptoms in adults has been demonstrated in more than 100 double-blind, randomly assigned, and control treatment studies (Davis, Comaty, and Janicak, 1987). There are few studies in adolescents and no long-term studies of neuroleptic effects in children. There is no evidence that pharmacotherapy is not effective in early onset schizophrenia (McClellan and Werry, 1992). Each of the neuroleptics has similar effects on positive symptoms; however, side effects do differ among drug groups, particularly in regard to atropinic and extrapyramidal effects, which may lead to differences in choice of medications. Higher dosages may be needed during the active phase of the illness than during phases of recovery or maintenance and for acute control of short-term exacerbation of behavioral dyscontrol. In considering medication response, children must be screened for both positive (hallucinations, delusions, thought disorder) and negative symptoms (social withdrawal, poverty of speech, and flattening of affect) and monitored accordingly. Although it was initially suggested that children with schizophrenia may respond poorly to neuroleptic medications, this may not be true with refinements in assessment procedures and the use of radioreceptor assays to measure blood levels. Children may require higher doses of medication because, in some instances, they may metabolize the medications more rapidly. Haloperidol is effective in acutely psychotic adolescents when compared to placebo, but again, long-term studies are needed (Pool et al., 1976). Even though comprehensive treatment studies require further evaluation, particularly for younger children, the use of neuroleptic medications is the current agreed-upon standard of care. Their effects are thought to result from the action of these drugs on the mesolimbic dopamine system. Neuroleptics do not change and may even worsen the negative symptoms, such as apathy and anergia (Andreasen et al., 1990). It may be because of effects on negative symptoms that neuroleptics have been reported to be less effective in children because younger children with severe developmental dysfunction may demonstrate negative symptom patterns.

The most serious problems with neuroleptic medication relate to lack of compliance with treatment. More severe drug-related effects, such as neuroleptic malignant syndrome, are rare; however, one must be on guard for their appearance. Routine monitoring for tardive dyskinesia is essential and, fortunately, it tends to be nonprogressive in the majority of patients. The long- term effects of early initiation of neuroleptic treatment in early childhood requires continuing study.

Medication side effects vary with the type of medication chosen. The drug effects that are most common are treatment-emergent effects that may result in extrapyramidal symptoms, including dystonias, akithesia, and pseudoparkinsonian symptoms due to dopaminergic effects on nigrostriatal pathways. The long-term effects of dopaminergic blockade may lead to tardive dyskinesia. In addition, dopamine effects on the tuberoinfundibular pathway produces effects on endocrine systems, such as elevated prolactin levels, which may lead to galactorrhea and menstrual disturbances in teenage girls. Other effects of dopamine antagonists are related to the individual drug's effects on adrenergic and cholinergic systems.

There is no evidence that a particular neuroleptic is superior to another in the treatment of schizophrenia. Drug choice is based on the spectrum of side effects, the history of medication response in the patient, and, to some extent, the history of medication response of similar medications in family members, the route of administration, the cost, and the availability of depot preparations. Those drugs that bind with greater specificity to the dopamine receptor are referred to as "high potency drugs" and tend to produce extrapyramidal effects, whereas other medications are viewed as "low potency," such as thioridazine, but may have more anticholinergic side effects, including sedation and possible effects on memory. Some side effects are more specific to a particular agent, such as effects on the lens of the eye with very high doses of thioridazine; other side effects, such as extrapyramidal symptoms, must be monitored with all of the neuroleptic drugs. Even though no evidence indicates that individual responses for the different medications vary, if there is lack of effect after at least 6 weeks of treatment with adequate doses, another neuroleptic may be considered. Considerable care must be taken in changing medications too quickly because longer term treatment may be needed in children before effects are demonstrated; on the other hand, dosing is of particular importance in childhood.

About 25% of adult and adolescent onset schizophrenic patients do not respond to neuroleptic drugs. Most commonly, this is the result of incorrect dosing and inadequate duration of treatment or poor compliance. However, some cases may be nonresponders, but before establishing that a patient does not respond, two or three different neuroleptics should be tried, with selections from different chemical classes. Drug-level monitoring may be useful to check both compliance and drug absorption. Even though therapeutic windows are not established for neuroleptic drugs, monitoring can establish that absorption is appropriate and levels are not too low or too high. If there continues to be a lack of response, drug-free periods should be utilized to reassess diagnoses, particularly in regard to partial response.

Depot preparations of neuroleptics tend to be used more commonly with adults, but also must be considered in adolescents and in some children where compliance with medication is a particular concern. Poor oral absorption is a factor in the use of depot preparations and monitoring absorption requires measuring serum blood levels. The depot neuroleptics are given at 2- to 4-week intervals by intramuscular injection. The dosage amounts and intervals vary depending on weight and previous drug response. Frequent reassessment is needed because the medications have a long half-life and accumulate in bodily fat stores. Doses may be lowered and intervals between injections lengthened when symptoms are adequately controlled because depot drug effects may last over several months. Due to concerns about long-term neuroleptic side effects in the developing organism and the lack of systematic trials, these medications generally are only considered for adolescents who have well-documented chronic psychotic symptoms and would rarely be used in the preadolescent population.

The long-term outcome is guarded for both

very early onset and early onset schizophrenia. Howells and Guirguis (1984) report that children diagnosed as schizophrenic retain most of the cardinal signs and symptoms into adulthood. Campbell et al. (1978) notes that these children remain aloof, lonely, and generally relate poorly to their families, often developing symbiotic relationships with others. This poor long-term outcome calls for continued research, focusing on the very early and early onset cases. An emphasis on the neurodevelopmental aspects of schizophrenia may lead to a better understanding of this tragic condition in both children and adults.

REFERENCES

Akbarian, S., Bunney, W.E., Jr., Potkin, S.G., Wigal, S.B., Hagman, J.O., Sandman, C.A., and Jones, E.G. (1993a). Altered distribution of nicotinamide-adenine dinucleotide phosphate-diaphorase cells in frontal lobe of schizophrenics implies disturbances of cortical development. *Archives of General Psychiatry,* 50:169–177.

______, Vinuela, A., Kim, J.J., Potkin, S.G., Bunney, W.E., Jr., and Jones, E.G. (1993b). Distorted distribution of nicotinamide-adenine dinucleotide phosphate-diaphorase neurons in temporal lobe of schizophrenics implies anomalous cortical development. *Archives of General Psychiatry,* 50:178–187.

______, Kim, J.J., Potkin, S.G., Hagman, J.D., Tafazzoli, A., Bunney, W.E., and Jones, E.G. (1995). Gene expression for glutamic acid decarboxylase is reduced without loss of neurons in prefrontal cortex of schizophrenics. *Archives of General Psychiatry,* 52:258–266.

American Psychiatric Association, Committee on Nomenclature and Statistics. (1980). *Diagnostic and statistical manual of mental disorders,* 3rd ed. Author, Washington, DC.

American Psychiatric Association, Committee on Nomenclature and Statistics. (1987). *Diagnostic and statistical manual of mental disorders,* 3rd ed, revised. Author, Washington, DC.

American Psychiatric Association, Committee on Nomenclature and Statistics. (1994). *Diagnostic and statistical manual of mental disorders,* 4th ed. Author, Washington, DC.

Andreasen, N.C., Falum, M., Swayze, V.W., Tyrrel, G., and Arndt, S. (1990). Positive and negative symptoms in schizophrenia. *Archives of General Psychiatry,* 47:615–621.

Arboleda, C., and Holzman, P. (1985). Thought disorder in children at risk for psychosis. *Archives of General Psychiatry,* 42:1004–1013.

Asarnow, J.R. (1994). Annotation: Childhood-onset schizophrenia. *Journal of Child Psychology and Psychiatry,* 35:1345–1371.

______, Goldstein, M.J., and Ben-Meir, S. (1988). Parental communication deviance in childhood onset schizophrenia spectrum and depressive disorders. *Journal of Child Psychology and Psychiatry,* 29:825–838.

Asarnow, R.F., Asarnow, J.R., and Strandburg, R. (1989). Schizophrenia: A developmental perspective. In D. Cicchetti (ed.), *Rochester symposium on developmental psychology,* pp. 189–220. Cambridge University Press, Cambridge.

Aylward, E., Walker, E., and Bettes, B. (1984). Intelligence in schizophrenia: Meta analysis of the research. *Schizophrenia Bulletin,* 10:430–459.

Bear, M.F., Kleinschmidt, A., Gu, Q., and Singer, W. (1990). Disruption of experience dependent synaptic modifications in striate cortex by infusion of an NMDA receptor antagonist. *Journal of Neuroscience,* 10:909–925.

Bender, L. (1942). Child schizophrenia. *Nervous Child,* 1:138–140.

______. (1947). Childhood schizophrenia: Clinical study of one hundred schizophrenic children. *American Journal of Orthopsychiatry,* 17:40–56.

______. (1973). The life course of children with schizophrenia. *American Journal of Psychiatry,* 130:783–786.

Bettes, B.A., and Walker, E. (1987). Positive and negative symptoms in psychotic and other psychiatrically disturbed children. *Journal of Child Psychology and Psychiatry,* 28:555–567.

Bleuler, E. (1950). *Dementia praecox or the group of schizophrenias.* (J. Zinkin, trans.). International Universities Press, New York. (Original work published 1911)

Bloom, F. (1993). Advancing a neurodevelopmental origin for schizophrenia. *Archives of General Psychiatry,* 50:224–227.

Bogerts, B. (1993). Recent advances in the neuropathology of schizophrenia. *Schizophrenia Bulletin,* 19:431–445.

______, and Falkai, P. (1990). Post-mortem volume measurements of limbic system and basal ganglia structures in chronic schizophrenics. Initial results from a new brain collection. *Schizophrenia Research,* 3:295–301.

Brown, R., Colter, N., Corsellis, J.A.N., Crow, T.J., Frith, C.D., Jagoe R., Johnstone, E.C., and Marsh, L. (1986). Post-mortem evidence of structural brain changes in schizophrenia: Differences in brain weight, temporal horn and parahippocampal gyrus compared with affective disorder. *Archives of General Psychiatry,* 43:36–42.

Calev, A., Kovin, Y.L., Kugelmass, S., and Leser, B. (1987). Performance of chronic schizophrenics on matched word and design recall tasks. *Biological Psychiatry,* 22:699–709.

Campbell, M., Hardesty, A.S., Breuer, H., and Polevoy, N. (1978). Childhood psychosis in perspective: A follow-up of 10 children. *Journal of the American Academy of Child Psychiatry,* 17:14–28.

Caplan, R., Guthrie, D., Fish, B., Tanguay, P.E., and David-Lando, G. (1989). The Kiddie Formal Thought Disorder Scale (K-FTDS). Clinical assessment, reliability, and validity. *Journal of the American Academy of Child Psychiatry,* 28:208–216.

______, Perdue, S., Tanguay, P.E., and Fish, B. (1990). Formal thought disorder in childhood onset schizophrenia and schizotypal personality disorder. *Journal of Child Psychology and Psychiatry,* 31:1103–1114.

Carlson, G.A. (1990). Child and adolescent mania: Diagnostic considerations. *Journal of Child Psychology and Psychology,* 31:331–342.

Castle, D., and Murray, R.M. (1991). The neurodevelopmental basis of sex differences in schizophrenia. *Psychological Medicine,* 21:565–575.

Conrad, A.J., and Scheibel, A.S. (1987). Schizophrenia and the hippocampus: The embryological hypothesis extended. *Schizophrenia Bulletin,* 13:577–587.

Cooper, S.J. (1992). Schizophrenia after prenatal exposure to 1957 A2 influenza epidemic. *British Journal of Psychiatry,* 161:394–396.

Cowan, W.M., Fawcett, J.W., O'Leary, D.D.M., and Stanfield, B.B. (1984). Regressive events in neurogenesis. *Science,* 224:1258–1266.

Crow, T.J. (1980). Positive and negative schizophrenic symptoms and the role of dopamine. *British Journal of Psychiatry,* 137:383–386.

______. (1985). The two-syndrome concept: Origins and current states. *Schizophrenia Bulletin,* 11:471–486.

______, Ferrier, I.N., Johnstone, E.C., Owens, D.G.C., Roberts, G.W., Lee, Y.C., Bloom, S.R., and Polak, J.M. (1982). Neuroendocrine aspects of schizophrenia. In G. Fink and L.J. Whalley (eds.), *Neuropeptides: Basic and clinical aspects,* pp. 222–239. Churchill Livingstone, Edinburgh.

Davis, J.M., Comaty, J.E., and Janicak, P.G. (1987). The psychological effects of antipsychotic drugs. In C.N. Stefanis and A.D. Rabavilas (eds.), *Schizophrenia, recent biosocial developments,* pp. 165–181. Human Sciences Press, New York.

De Santis, S. (1969). On some varieties of dementia praecox (M.L. Osborn, trans.). In J.G. Howells (ed.), *Modern perspectives in international child psychiatry,* pp. 540–609. Brunner/Mazel, New York. (Original work published 1906)

Despert, J.L. (1938). Schizophrenia in children. *Psychiatry Quarterly,* 12:366–371.

Eggers, C. (1978). Course and prognosis of childhood schizophrenia. *Journal of Autism and Childhood Schizophrenia,* 8:21–36.

Feinberg, I. (1982/1983). Schizophrenia: Caused by a fault in programmed synaptic elimination during adolescence. *Journal of Psychiatric Research,* 17:319–334.

Fish, B. (1977). Neurobiologic antecedents of schizophrenia in children: Evidence for an inherited, congenital neurointegrative defect. *Archives of General Psychiatry,* 34:1297–1313.

______, Marcus, J., Hans, S., Auerback, J.G., and Perdue, S. (1992). Infants at risk for schizophrenia: Sequelae of a genetic neurointegrative defect. *Archives of General Psychiatry,* 49:221–235.

Goldberg, T.E., Torrey, E.F., Gold, J.M., and Weinberger, D.R. (1992). Neuropsychological impairment in monozygotic twins discordant and concordant for schizophrenia. *Society for Neuroscience,* 18:911 (abstract 379.4).

Goldfarb, W. (1974). *Growth and change of schizophrenic children: Longitudinal study.* V.H. Winston & Sons, New York.

Goldstein, M.J. (1989). Psychosocial treatment of schizophrenia. In S.C. Schulz and C.A. Tamminga (eds.), *Schizophrenia: Scientific progress,* pp. 318–324. Oxford University Press, New York.

Green, W.H., and Padron-Gayol, M. (1986). Schizophrenic disorder in childhood: Its relationship to DSM-III criteria. In C. Shagass (ed.), *Biological psychiatry, 1985,* pp. 107–122. Elsevier, Amsterdam.

Harris, E.W., Ganong, A.H., and Cotman, C.W. (1984). Long term potentiation involves activation of N-methyl-D-aspartate receptors. *Brain Research,* 323:132–137.

Harrison, P.J., McLaughlin, D., and Kerwin, R.W. (1991). Decreased hippocampal expression of a glutamate receptor gene in schizophrenia. *Lancet,* 337:450–452.

Hendry, S.H.C., Jones, F.G., DeFelipe, J., Schmechel, D., Brandon, C., and Emson, P.C. (1984). Neuropeptide containing neurons of the cerebral cortex are also GABAergic. *Proceedings of the National Academy of Science USA,* 81:6526–6530.

Howells, J., and Guirguis, W. (1984). Childhood schizophrenia 20 Years later. *Archives of General Psychiatry,* 1:123–128.

Huttenlocher, P.R. (1979). Synaptic density in human frontal cortex: Developmental changes and the effects of aging. *Brain Research,* 163:195–205.

Jakob, H., and Beckmann, H. (1986). Prenatal developmental disturbances in the limbic allocortex in schizophrenics. *Journal of Neural Transmission,* 65:303–326.

______, and ______. (1989). Gross and histological criteria for developmental disorders in brains of schizophrenics. *Journal of the Royal Society of Medicine,* 82:466–469.

Jones, P., and Murray, R.M. (1991). Aberrant neurodevelopment as the expression of the schizophrenia genotype. In P. McGuffin and R.M. Murray (eds.), *The new genetics of mental illness,* pp. 112–129. Heinemann Medical Books, London.

Kane, J.M. (1987). Treatment of schizophrenia. *Schizophrenia Bulletin,* 13:171–186.

Kanner, L. (1973). Childhood psychosis: An historical overview. In L. Kanner (ed.), *Childhood psychosis: Initial studies and new insights.* V.H. Winston and Sons, New York.

Kaufmann, C.A., and Malaspina, D. (1991). Molecular genetics of schizophrenia. In J. Brosius and R. T. Fremeau, Jr., (eds.), *Molecular approaches to neuropsychiatric disease,* pp. 307–345. Academic Press, New York.

Kerwin, R.W., and Murray, R.H. (1992). A developmental perspective on the pathology and neurochemistry of the temporal lobe in schizophrenia. *Schizophrenia Research,* 7:1–12.

______, Patel, S., and Meldrum, B.S. (1990). Autoradiographic localisation of the glutamate receptor system in control and schizophrenic postmortem hippocampal formation. *Neuroscience,* 39:25–32.

Kety, S.S., Rosenthal, D., and Wender, P.H. (1978). Genetic relationships within the schizophrenia spectrum: Evidence from adoption studies. In R.L. Spitzer and D.F. Klein (eds.), *Critical issues in psychiatric diagnosis,* pp. 213–223. Raven Press, New York.

Kolvin, I. (1971). Studies in the childhood psychoses. *British Journal of Psychiatry,* 118:381–419.

Kraepelin, E. (1971). *Dementia praecox and paraphrenia.* (Translated by R. Mary Barclay). Robert E. Krieger, Huntington, N.Y. (Original work published 1896)

Levy, D.L., Bogerts, B., Degreef, G., Dorogusker, B., Waternaux, C., Ashtari, M., Jody, D., Geisler, S. and Lieberman, J.A. (1992). Normal eye tracking is associated with abnormal morphology of medial temporal lobe structures in schizophrenia. *Schizophrenia Research,* 8:1–10.

Mahler, M. (1952). On child psychosis and schizophrenia: Autistic and symbiotic infantile psychoses. In S. Harrison and J. McDermott (eds.), *Childhood psychopathology,* pp. 670–687. International Universities Press, New York.

Malaspina, D., Warburton, D., Amador, X., Harris, M., and Kaufmann, C.A. (1992). Association of schizophrenia and partial trisomy of chromosome 5P: A case report. *Schizophrenia Research,* 7:191–196.

Mattson, M.P. (1988). Neurotransmitters in the regulation of neuronal cytoarchitecture. *Brain Research Review,* 13:179–212.

Maudsley, H. (1977). *The physiology and pathology of the mind.* Greenwood Publishing Group, Westport, Conn. (Original work published 1874)

McClellan, J.M., and Werry, J.S. (1992). Schizophrenia. *Psychiatric Clinics of North America,* 15:131–148.

______, ______, and Ham, M. (1993). A follow-up study of early onset psychosis: Comparison between outcome diagnoses of schizophrenia, mood disorders, and personality disorders. *Journal of Autism and Developmental Disorders,* 23:243–262.

McCreadie, R.G., Connolly, M.A., Williamson, D.J., Athawes, R.W.B., and Tilak-Singh, D. (1994). The Nithsdale schizophrenia surveys. XII. 'Neurodevelopmental' Schizophrenia: A search for clinical correlates and putative etiological factors. *British Journal of Psychiatry,* 165:340–346.

McNeil, T.F. (1990, August). *Head circumference at birth in schizophrenic patients.* Paper presented at the World Psychiatric Association regional symposium, Oslo.

Mednick, S., Machon, R.A., Huttunen, M.O., and Bonett, D. (1988). Adult schizophrenia following prenatal exposure to an influenza epidemic. *Archives of General Psychiatry,* 45:189–192.

Murray, R.M. (1994). Neurodevelopmental schizophrenia: The rediscovery of dementia praecox. *British Journal of Psychiatry,* 165:6–12.

______, Jones, D., and O'Callaghan, E. (1991). Foetal brain development and later schizophrenia: The childhood environment and adult disease. *CIBA Foundation Symposium,* 156:155–163. [Discussion: 163–170].

______, Lewis, S.W., Owen, M.J., and Foerster, A. (1988). The neurodevelopmental origins of dementia praecox. In P. McGriffin and P. Bebbington (eds.), *Schizophrenia: The major issues,* pp. 90–107. Heinemann, London.

______, O'Callaghan, E.,Castle, D.J., and Lewis, S.W. (1992). A neurodevelopmental approach to the classification of schizophrenia. *Schizophrenia Bulletin,* 18:319–332.

O'Callaghan, E., Larkin, C., Redmond, O., Stack, J., Ennis, J.T., and Waddington, J.L. (1988). Early onset schizophrenia after teenage head injury. *British Journal of Psychiatry,* 153:394–396.

Owen, M.J., Lewis, S.W., and Murray, R.M. (1988). Obstetric complications and schizophrenia: A computed tomographic study. *Psychological Medicine,* 18:331–339.

Pool, D., Bloom, W., Mielke, D.H., Roniger, J.J., and Gallant, D.M. (1976). A controlled evaluation of loxitane in seventy-five adolescent schizophrenia patients. *Current Therapeutic Research, Clinical and Experimental,* 19:99–104.

Potter, H.W. (1933). Schizophrenia in children. *American Journal of Psychiatry,* 89:1253–1270.

Rakic, P., Bourgeois, J.P., Zecevic, N., Eckenhopp, M.E., and Goldman-Rakic, P.S. (1986). Isochronic overproduction of synapses in diverse regions of the primate cerebral cortex. *Science,* 232:232–235.

______, and Nowakowski, R.S. (1981). The time of origin of neurons in the hippocampal region of the rhesus monkey. *Journal of Comparative Neurology,* 196:99–128.

Rank, B. (1949). Adaptation of psychoanalytic techniques for the treatment of young children with atypical development. *American Journal of Orthopsychiatry,* 19:130–139.

Reid, A.H. (1989). Schizophrenia in mental retardation: Clinical features. *Research in Developmental Disabilities,* 10:241–249.

Reiss, A.L., Hagerman, R.J., Vinogradov, S., Abrams, M., and King, R.J. (1988). Psychiatric disability in female carriers of the fragile X chromosome. *Archives of General Psychiatry,* 45:25–30.

Reveley, A.M., Reveley, M.A., Clifford, C.A., and Murray, R.M. (1982). Cerebral ventricular size in twins concordant and discordant for schizophrenia. *Lancet,* i:540–541.

Reynolds, G.P. (1983). Increased concentrations and lateral asymmetry of amygdala dopamine in schizophrenia. *Nature,* 305:527–529.

______, Czudek, C., and Andrews, H.B. (1990). Deficit and hemispheric asymmetry of GABA uptake sites in the hippocampus in schizophrenia. *Nature,* 305:527–529.

Roberts, G.W. (1991). Schizophrenia: A neuropathological perspective. *British Journal of Psychiatry,* 158:8–17.

Russell, A.T., Bott, L., and Sammons, C. (1989). The phenomenology of schizophrenia occurring in childhood. *Journal of the American Academy of Child and Adolescent Psychiatry,* 28:399–407.

Schneider, K. (1959). *Clinical psychopathology* (M.W. Hamilton, trans.). Grune & Stratton, London.

Seeman, P., Bzowej, N.H., Guan, H-C., Bergeron, C., Becker, L.E., Reynolds, G.P., Bird, E.D., Riederer, P., Jellinger, K., Watanabe, S., and Tourtellote, W. (1987). Human brain dopamine receptors in children and aging adults. *Synapse,* 1:399–405.

Simpson, M.D.C., Slater, P., Deakin, J.T.W., Royston, M.C., and Skan, W.J. (1989). Reduced GABA uptake sites in the temporal lobe in schizophrenia. *Neuroscience Letters,* 107:211–215.

Suddath, R.I., Christison, G.W., and Torrey, E.F. (1990). Anatomical abnormalities in the brains of monozygotic twins discordant for schizophrenia. *New England Journal of Medicine,* 322:789–794.

Torrey, E.F. (1992). Are we overestimating the genetic contribution in schizophrenia? *Schizophrenia Bulletin,* 18:159–170.

Tsuang, M.T., and Vandermey, R. (1980). *Genes and the mind.* Oxford University Press, New York.

Waddington, J.L., O'Callaghan, E., and Larkin, C. (1990). Physical anomalies and neurodevelopmental abnormality in schizophrenia: New clinical correlates. *Schizophrenia Research,* 3:90.

Watkins, J.M., Asarnow, R.F., and Tanguay, P. (1988). Symptom development in childhood onset schizophrenia. *Journal of Child Psychology and Psychiatry,* 29:865–878.

Weinberger, D.R. (1987). Implications of normal brain development for the pathogenesis of schizophrenia. *Archives of General Psychiatry,* 44:660–667.

______. (1988). Schizophrenia and the frontal lobe. *Trends in Neuroscience,* 11:367–370.

Werry, J. (1992). Child and adolescent (early onset) schizophrenia: A review in light of DSM III-R. *Journal of Autism and Developmental Disorders,* 22:601–624.

______, McClellan, J.M., and Chard, L. (1991). Childhood and adolescent schizophrenia, bipolar and schizoaffective disorders: A clinical and outcome study. *Journal of the American Academy of Child and Adolescent Psychiatry,* 30:457–465.

Westermeyer, J.F., and Harrow, M. (1984). Prognosis and outcome using broad (DSM-II) and narrow (DSM-III) concepts of schizophrenia. *Schizophrenia Bulletin,* 10:624–637.

Wong, D.F., Bropussolle, E.P., Ward, G., Villemagne, V., Dannals, R.F., Links, J.M., Zacur, H.A., Harris, J., Naidu, S., Braestrup, C., Wagner, H.N., Jr., and Gjedde, A. (1988). *In vivo* measurement of dopamine receptors in human brain by positron emission tomography: Age and sex differences. *Annals of the New York Academy of Science,* 515:203–214.

World Health Organization (1977). *International classification of diseases,* 9th ed. Author, Geneva.

Zubin, J., and Spring, B. (1977). Vulnerability: A new view of schizophrenia. *Journal of Abnormal Psychology,* 86:103–126.

CHAPTER 15

TOURETTE'S DISORDER

Tic disorders have their onset during the developmental period and may be transient or chronic in nature. The best known of these conditions is Tourette's disorder, which involves both multiple motor and phonic tics. Although once considered rare and unusual, Tourette's disorder is now recognized as occurring more commonly and varying in severity from mild to severe. Although involuntary in their initiation, tic behaviors can be modified by psychological state. Because they are socially disruptive, tics may lead to problems in self-esteem, social acceptance, school performance, and family functioning. Tic disorders may be associated with disinhibited behavior or speech, distractibility, impulsivity, excessive motoric activity, and obsessive-compulsive symptoms.

This chapter reviews the history, epidemiology, diagnosis/natural history, associated features, differential diagnosis, etiology, neuroanatomic and neurophysiologic features, and treatment of Tourette's disorder.

HISTORY

Although designated the "Gilles de la Tourette syndrome," the first complete description of the disorder was provided in 1825 by Itard. However, the earliest case report may be one described in the United Kingdom in 1663 by Drage (Lees et al., 1984). Itard described a French noblewoman who developed symptoms of Tourette's disorder at the age of 7. During her lifetime, persistent body tics, barking vocalizations, and spontaneous utterances of obscenities developed. Because her vocalizations were socially unacceptable, she lived as a recluse until her death at age 85. Subsequently, in 1885, Georges Gilles de la Tourette reported on 9 cases of what has come to be known as Tourette's disorder. He highlighted a triad of multiple tics, involuntary movements, and echolalia and coprolalia (spontaneous utterance of obscenities). The movement disorder he described is not a startle reaction, but rather a spontaneous movement disorder characterized by both motor and vocal (phonic) tics. Between 1885 and 1965, Shapiro et al. (1988) found that only 50 additional cases were reported in the medical literature. Since that time, specific diagnostic criteria have been developed, leading to a considerable increase in case identification.

EPIDEMIOLOGY

Tourette's disorder has been reported in all racial and cultural groups, but tends to be more rare among African Americans. Although ethnic predominance has been reported in some studies, it has not been confirmed in others. Approximately 150,000 persons are affected in the United States. The syndrome occurs three to four times more commonly in males and is found in all social classes. Robertson, Trimble, and Lees (1988) found that 61% of 59 cases did not reach the same social class status as their parents, suggesting social underachievement. Shapiro and Shapiro (1982) note no evidence that parents' age at the onset of birth, birth order, birth weight, perinatal complications, parents' medical history, or the family medical history differentiate Tourette's disorder patients from the general population. Other studies (Lees et al., 1984) suggest a possible relationship to birth complications in some cases. Tourette's disorder occurs in severe and profoundly mentally retarded persons, but often is not recognized. Crews et al. (1993) provide guidelines for recognition in this population.

The exact prevalence is not known, but it is estimated to be about 0.5 in 1,000. However, this may be an underestimate because the disorder is now becoming more widely recognized and more often diagnosed. The apparent increase may be explained by the identification of patients with milder symptoms; the original emphasis was on the most severe and bizarre presentation. Burd et al. (1986) estimated the prevalence of Tourette's disorder in North Dakota to be 0.22 in 10,000 for women and 0.77 in 10,000 for men. The prevalence rate for girls was 1.0 in 10,000 and for boys 9.3 in 10,000. Children are 5 to 12 times more likely to be identified as having a tic disorder than adults, and as stated earlier, males are more commonly affected than females. The disparity between childhood prevalence and adult prevalence may be related to underdiagnosis in adults or possibly the reduction of symptoms by adulthood. Kurlan et al. (1986) suggest many cases are sufficiently mild that they do not come to medical attention. Caine et al. (1988) reported on the prevalence in schools in Monroe County, New York. Of 142,636 pupils enrolled and evaluated, 41 total cases (37, male; 4, female) were detected with a population prevalence of 28.7 in 100,000. Twenty of the identified cases had obsessive-compulsive symptoms, although only 3 were thought to have a disabling presentation. For the most part, the cases were mild and did not require treatment. Shapiro et al. (1988) suggest a lifetime prevalence in the range of 1 to 10 in 1,000.

DIAGNOSIS/NATURAL HISTORY

The age of symptom onset ranges from 2 to 15 years of age, although the mean age of symptom onset is around age 7. Symptoms have appeared in 96% of cases by age 11 (Robertson, 1989). The initial symptoms are usually tics involving the eyes (38% to 59%) that most commonly is manifested as eye blinking—36% in one study (Lees et al., 1984) and 48% in another study (Comings and Comings, 1985). Other presenting symptoms are tics of the head and face, and vocalizations—most commonly, throat clearing (Comings and Comings, 1985). The spontaneous utterance of obscenities (coprolalia) less commonly is a presenting symptom. If cumulative lifetime symptoms are considered, tics of the face are present in 94% to 97%; the head, neck and shoulder, 89% to 92%; upper arms, 51% to 81%; legs, 40% to 55%; and body, 41% to 54% (Robertson, 1989). Excessive licking and spitting also have been reported. The DSM-IV (APA, 1994) diagnostic criteria are listed in Table 15–1.

Although Tourette's disorder is referred to as a tic disorder, other movement symptoms are present. The most frequent of these are touching, hitting and striking, jumping, smelling objects, and a variety of disturbances in gait, such as retracing one's steps, twirling, and knee bending. The prevalence of these symptoms varies from one study to the next; in one study (Caine et al., 1988), 61% showed complex hand movements. Vocalizations usually start several years after the motor tics, with a mean

Table 15–1. DSM-IV Criteria for Tourette's Disorder

307.23 Tourette's Disorder

A. Both multiple motor and one or more vocal tics have been present at some time during the illness, although not necessarily concurrently. (*A tic* is a sudden, rapid, recurrent, nonrhythmic, stereotyped motor movement or vocalization.)
B. The tics occur many times a day (usually in bouts), nearly every day or intermittently throughout a period of more than 1 year; and during this period, there was never a tic-free period of more than 3 consecutive months.
C. The disturbance causes marked distress or significant impairment in social, occupational, or other important areas of functioning.
D. The onset is before age 18 years.
E. The disturbance is not due to the direct physiological effects of a substance (e.g., stimulants) or a general medical condition (e.g., Huntington's disease or postviral encephalitis).

From APA, 1994.

age of onset of about 11 years. Vocalizations include throat clearing, barking-like sounds, snorting, grunting, coughing, word accentuation, humming, clicking, emotional exclamations, as well as a variety of low-pitched and high-pitched inarticulate sounds.

The involuntary and inappropriate utterance of obscenities, or coprolalia, was reported originally by Gilles de la Tourette in 1885 and is often reported. Still, the frequency is variable from one study to the next; for example, Shapiro and Shapiro (1982) reported approximately 60%; Robertson, Trimble, and Lees (1988) found rates of only 30%. It should be noted that as milder cases of Tourette's disorder are reported, the prevalence of coprolalia has dropped into the 30% range. Coprolalia may be less common in children, but it does occur in those with the most severe symptoms. Robertson (1989) found that coprolalia had a mean age of onset of between 13 and 14 years and disappeared with age in approximately a third of her sample. In addition to coprolalia, copropraxia (involuntary obscene gestures) has also been reported, with rates up to 20% in some samples. Echolalia (the repeating back of sounds or words) also occurs, with a prevalence of 20% to 40%, and echopraxia (the repetition of other's movements) in 10% to 35%. Finally, Robertson identified palilalia (the repetition of the last word or phrase of a sentence) in 6% to 15% of affected individuals.

The motor tics and vocalizations may be exaggerated and become more intense with stress, anxiety, fatigue, or excitement. When concentrating on an interesting task, or when relaxed, however, motor symptoms may temporarily remit. Stress is commonly mentioned as a precipitating factor, and although no specific types of stress have been identified, some subjects have reported periods of chronic stress before symptom onset (Eisenberg, Ascher, and Kanner, 1959; Faux, 1966). Throughout a patient's lifetime, the appearance of new tics and the disappearance of old ones is reported. The long-term course has not been fully documented. In the first case described by Itard (1825), the patient's symptoms began at age 7 and continued until she died at age 85. There have been some reports of complete remission, but this is exceptional. More commonly, certain symptoms may remit. Patient reports of their experience of the illness (Bliss, 1980) are rare but are helpful in understanding their psychological experience and adaptation to the illness. The patient described by Bliss discusses how sensory stimuli precede movements or sounds, how new tics and vocalizations begin, and how he has sought to control his symptoms.

Although originally thought to be a lifelong condition, marked improvement or spontaneous remissions may occur without the use of medication (Singer and Walkup, 1991). Thirty to 40 percent of children may have remission of all tic symptoms by late adolescence and, in an additional 30%, considerable reductions are noted. The remainder will remain symptomatic into adulthood (Erenberg, Cruse, and Rothner, 1986). All stimulants, such as methylphenidate (Golden, 1977; Lowe et al., 1982), may precipitate or increase Tourette's disorder symptoms. Erenberg, Cruse, and Rothner (1986) found that 48 of 200 Tourette's disorder patients had received stimulant drugs; of these, 9 had been treated before the onset of tics, and stimulants had exacerbated tics in 11, although 26 reported no effect, and 2 stated the tics were decreased. Some behavioral improvement was noted in 22 of a methylphenidate-treated group.

Although it has been thought that movements disappear during sleep, this may not be the case (Incagnoli and Kane, 1983). Tics involving the eyes, face, and head may be persistent and refractory to treatment (Leckman and Cohen, 1983).

Behavioral Features

Obsessive-compulsive symptoms commonly are linked to Tourette's disorder and may be an integral part of the syndrome (Robertson, 1989). Hyperactivity, attention deficit disorder, and learning disabilities commonly occur and, in fact, may be the primary symptoms leading to referral. Self-injury also may occur (Eisenberg, Ascher, and Kanner, 1959; Eldridge et al., 1977) although the rates are variable, ranging from approximately 13% in some studies (Comings and Comings, 1987) to 53% in others (Moldofsky, Tullis, and Lamon, 1974). In addition, inappropriate sexual activity, exhibitionism, and antisocial behavior may be noted. Problems with aggression and associated disruptive behavior have been reported in up to 40%; such episodes may be associated with anger and violent outbursts (Comings and Comings, 1987). Despite these reports of aggression, few individuals with Tourette's disorder in the community show antisocial behavior; therefore, referral bias of the most severe cases to specialty clinics may account for the difference.

Attention deficit disorder is reported in approximately a third of the cases (Erenberg, Cruse, and Rothner, 1986). The latter authors reported difficulties in concentration and learning problems in approximately half of their sample. Yet behavioral symptoms of Tourette's disorder also wax and wane just as the motor and vocal symptoms do. Behavioral symptoms may persist after tics, both motor and phonic, have disappeared (Leckman and Cohen, 1983). Comings and Comings (1987) found attention deficit disorder, learning, school problems, sleep difficulties, affective disorder, and conduct disorder to co-occur. However, Pauls et al. (1988) did not find high rates of these disorders. Caine et al. (1988) reported coprolalia in 22% of patients, attention deficit disorder with hyperactivity in 27%, learning disabilities in 24%, and self-injurious behavior in 17%. These reported prevalences may reflect referral of children with severe problems to specialty clinics. It is noted that Tourette's disorder in larger epidemiological studies may be a milder disorder.

Sleep disorders are commonly associated with Tourette's disorder and include initial, middle, and delayed insomnia, nightmares, night terrors, sleepwalking, bed-wetting, bruxism, and sleep talking (Moldofsky, Tullis, and Lamon, 1974; Robertson, Trimble, and Lees, 1988). Sleep disorders are described in detail in Chapter 16.

Self-Injurious Behavior

Robertson, Trimble, and Lees (1989) suggest that self-injurious behavior is underreported in Tourette's disorder. They note that self-destructive behavior in these patients is correlated with obsessionality and hostility on rating scales. Those patients with self-injury tend to be at the most severe end of the spectrum. The types of self-injury reported in individuals with Tourette's disorder are not typically the same as those encountered with other self-injurious syndromes, such as Lesch-Nyhan disease. The topography of self-injury was more nonspecific and similar to that seen in more severely retarded individuals, although the Tourette's disorder patients were of average intelligence. These authors suggest that self-injurious behavior in individuals with Tourette's disorder might stem from self-destructive obsessions, for example, hitting the head in conjunction with a hand jerk. Other forms of self-injury are more complex and include pulling out teeth and eye poking. Rather than being a tic behavior, the self-injury seems heterogeneous and, in some instances, appears compulsive, whereas in others, it may be related to a "directed tic."

The topography of self-injury in 30 Tourette syndrome patients (Robertson, Trimble, and Lees, 1989) included head banging, body punching or slapping, head or face punching, hitting body on hard objects, poking sharp objects into the body, scratching parts of the body, and a variety of other forms. Trimble (1992) has noted tattooing in some individuals with Tourette's disorder and also coprographia. Overall, one third, or 30 of 90 patients referred, showed self-injurious behavior.

ASSOCIATED FEATURES

Psychiatric Symptoms

Early descriptions of associated psychiatric symptoms were those of Gilles de la Tourette (1899) who noted anxieties and phobias in his patients. However, with more comprehensive assessment, Shapiro and Shapiro (1982) have not found an association between Tourette's disorder and a specific psychiatric syndrome. They did note that a subgroup of patients may have particular difficulty with compulsive and ritualistic behavior. Corbett et al. (1969) reported more obsessional symptoms, habit disorders, and hypochondriasis. Other authors (Robertson, Trimble, and Lees, 1988) suggest that patients with Tourette's disorder are vulnerable to symptoms of depression and anxiety that may be related to the duration of the disorder or, potentially, to the social experience of having a stigmatizing disease.

Neurological Features

The majority of individuals with Tourette's disorder have subtle neurological deficits, although frank abnormalities may also be present.

Shapiro et al. (1988) reported them in 57%; most of this group had minor motor asymmetry, although 20% showed chorea or choreoathetoid movements. Other abnormalities included posturing, poor coordination, and asymmetrical reflexes. Other investigators have found only minor, nonspecific neurological abnormalities (Erenberg, Cruse, and Rothner, 1986; Robertson, Trimble, and Lees, 1988). However, chorea, dystonia, torticollis, dysphonia, and postural abnormalities and motor uncoordination are verified in the majority of reports.

DIFFERENTIAL DIAGNOSIS

The most common differential diagnosis is that of motor tics, which may begin between age 5 and 10. Such tics ordinarily spontaneously remit and usually improve with age. These conditions are referred to as "transient tic disorder" or "chronic motor tic disorder," as described in Tables 15–2 and 15–3.

A condition referred to as "acquired Tourettism" has been reported following short-term and long-term treatment with neuroleptics (Jeste et al., 1983; Klawans et al., 1978; Seeman, Patel, and Pyke, 1981). Symptoms identical to those of Tourette's disorder have been reported following acute or chronic cerebral insults, for example, following encephalitis or head trauma (Fahn, 1982; Sacks, 1982).

Sydenham's chorea is a movement disorder that occurs most often in females; 75% of the cases are associated with rheumatic fever. Swedo et al. (1993) reported on chorea manifested by gait disturbances and adventitious movements of the face, neck, trunk, and extremities. Obsessive-compulsive symptoms, increased emotional lability, and motor hyperactivity were also noted.

A variety of other movement disorders have been considered in the differential diagnosis, one of which is athetoid cerebral palsy, seen most commonly among mentally retarded individuals, having an age of onset between birth and 3 years and a static course. Another condition, dystonia musculorum deformans, might be considered. It presents with torsion dystonia generally involving the legs and is a progressive condition with rare remissions. Huntington's chorea ordinarily begins in the third to fifth decade of life, but rarely may begin in childhood. This syndrome is a progressive disorder associated with the eventual emergence of dementia.

Misdiagnoses of Tourette's disorder are common, occurring most often due to lack of familiarity with the disorder, the individual's

Table 15–2. DSM-IV Criteria for Transient Tic Disorder

307.21 Transient Tic Disorder

A. Single or multiple motor and/or vocal tics (i.e., sudden, rapid, recurrent, nonrhythmic, stereotyped motor movements or vocalizations).
B. The tics occur many times a day, nearly every day for at least 4 weeks, but for no longer than 12 consecutive months.
C. The disturbance causes marked distress or significant impairment in social, occupational, or other important areas of functioning.
D. The onset is before age 18 years.
E. The disturbance is not due to the direct physiological effects of a substance (e.g., stimulants) or a general medical condition (e.g., Huntington's disease or postviral encephalitis).
F. Criteria have never been met for Tourette's or Chronic Motor or Vocal Tic Disorder.

Specify if:
Single Episode or **Recurrent**

From APA, 1994.

Table 15–3. DSM-IV Criteria for Chronic Motor or Vocal Disorder

307.22 Chronic Motor or Vocal Tic Disorder

A. Single or multiple motor or vocal or motor tics (i.e., sudden, rapid, recurrent, nonrhythmic, stereotyped motor movements or vocalizations) but not both, have been present at some time during the illness.
B. The tics occur many times a day, nearly every day or intermittently throughout a period of more than 1 year; and during this period, there was never a tic-free period of more than 3 consecutive months.
C. The disturbance causes marked distress or significant impairment in social, occupational, or other important areas of functioning.
D. The onset is before age 18 years.
E. The disturbance is not due to the direct physiological effects of a substance (e.g., stimulants) or a general medical condition (e.g., Huntington's disease or postviral encephalitis).
F. Criteria have never been met for Tourette's Disorder.

From APA, 1994.

ability to suppress symptoms, and the persistent belief that coprolalia must be present to make the diagnosis.

ETIOLOGY

Genetic

Tourette's disorder is most likely inherited as an autosomal single dominant gene with incomplete penetrance and variable expression (Van de Wetering and Heutink, 1993), and may be present with mild to severe symptoms. The exact pathogenesis is not known. Linkage studies are under way to clarify the mode of inheritance. The goal of the linkage studies is to "link" a specific DNA sequence, with a known chromosomal localization, with the disease in affected family members. Differences in findings among genetic studies may be related to differences in the specific definition of the disorder used. The phenotype must be clearly defined and its expression is complicated by incomplete penetrance. Cases may be mild and go undetected when associated with behavioral symptoms, such as impulse control disorder, obsessive-compulsive symptoms, and AD/HD. Whether these associated behavioral symptoms are part of the phenotype remains to be established. Obsessive-compulsive disorder is frequently considered part of the phenotype (Singer and Walkup, 1991). Robertson, Trimble, and Lees (1989) reported on 90 cases and found a high incidence of depression, hostility, and obsessionality that were significantly associated with features of the syndrome, such as echophenomena, coprolalia, and a family history of tics or Tourette's disorder. However, Shapiro and Shapiro (1992) question this association and call for the development of specific criteria for classification of obsessive compulsive symptoms/obsessive compulsive disorder/Tourette's syndrome (OCS-OCD-TS), reliable and valid measures of OCS-OCD-TS, and blind evaluation and data analyses. Trimble (1992) notes that patients may describe the same subjective sensory experience with the onset of a tic or a compulsive act and emphasizes the importance of the clinical interview in the diagnosis. It is agreed that compulsive behaviors are associated; the major issue is how they may be best characterized to be useful in epidemiological surveys. Compulsive symptoms are commonly associated with disorders that involve the basal ganglia. However, the mechanism may prove to be more complicated than a single dominant gene so multifactorial inheritance must be considered.

The data suggesting genetic involvement comes from twin studies and family studies. Price et al. (1985) reported a large twin study that involved 43 pairs of same-sex twins in which at least one co-twin had Tourette's disorder. The concordance rates were 53% for monozygotic twin pairs and 8% for dizygotic pairs. When the criteria included any tics at all in co-twins, concordance rates rose to 77% and 23%, respectively. These authors concluded that although such concordances are consistent with genetic etiology, nongenetic factors may play a role in symptom expression. Leckman et al. (1987) reevaluated the data from this study and found that when twins were discordant, the unaffected co-twin had a higher birth weight. Possible nongenetic factors in symptom expression, then, might include prenatal events that stress the mother during pregnancy, drug treatment, or other events which might increase sensitivity to dopamine receptors.

In addition to twin studies, many family studies have been conducted which suggest that relatives of those affected may present with either the full syndrome or motor or vocal tics only. In some families, chronic multiple tics and Tourette's disorder are genetically related (Kidd, Prusoff, and Cohen, 1980; Pauls and Leckman, 1986). These extended family studies suggest an increased incidence of both simple and chronic tics and Tourette's disorder in relatives of affected patients.

NEUROANATOMICAL AND NEUROPHYSIOLOGIC FEATURES

The underlying pathophysiology and neuroanatomical location remains to be established. Computed tomographic (CT) and magnetic resonance imaging (MRI) in living subjects have only revealed isolated abnormalities or minor structural alterations. When CT scans were carried out in Tourette's disorder, Robertson, Trimble, and Lees (1988) found 71 of 73 individuals with Tourette's disorder had normal CT scans, although Caparulo et al.

(1981) reported some abnormalities, including mild ventricular dilatation, prominent sylvian fissures, or cortical sulci in 6 of 16 patients. Harcherik et al. (1985) compared CT scans in 19 patients with Tourette's disorder with individuals with other diagnoses, including autistic disorder, attention deficit disorder, and language disorder, as well as a control group. No significant differences were found among the groups in ventricular volume, ventricular asymmetries, or ventricle to brain ratios. Overall, 18 of 172 documented CT scans have been abnormal, but these abnormalities do not seem to be of etiologic significance (Robertson, 1989).

Abnormal EEGs have been reported with varying frequency, ranging from 12½% (Krumholz et al., 1983) to 37% (Robertson, Trimble, and Lees, 1988). EEG abnormalities are nonspecific and there are no reports of paroxysmal activity linked to the tics (Obeso, Rothwell, and Marsen, 1982). Although it has been suggested that those with more severe learning disabilities may have greater evidence of EEG abnormality, this has not been confirmed in a large sample.

There is also wide variation in abnormality in electromyelogram (EMG) patterns recorded from various muscle groups. More complex tics are associated with a greater variety of EMG patterns (Obeso, Rothwell, and Marsen, 1982). These investigators note that the buildup of a negative potential over the half second or so prior to EMG activation of an involved muscle group may represent changed activity in cortical neurons in preparation for movement. The normal premovement potential ordinarily associated with voluntarily initiated motor activity was not evident before spontaneous simple tics. Robertson (1989) suggests that simple tics, then, are not generated through normal cortical motor pathways which are involved in willed human movements.

No consistent abnormalities have been reported with visual- and sensory-evoked potentials (Krumholz et al., 1983). Event-related auditory evoked potentials showed no abnormalities in early and late components in one study (Van de Wetering et al., 1985); however, those components in the 90 to 280 millisecond range were affected, which may indicate specific attention deficits. Tolosa, Montserrat, and Bayes (1986) studied neuronal excitability during voluntary tic inhibition. These authors studied the effect of a conditioning stimulus on blink reflexes. Six patients were studied again during maximal voluntary tic suppression and found to show increased brainstem interneuron excitability that was reduced during voluntary tic inhibition.

Single photon emission tomography (SPECT) scanning and positron emission tomography (PET) have been used to evaluate Tourette's disorder by several groups of investigators. Chase et al. (1986) reported abnormalities in 5 patients, using 18-fluorodeoxyglucose. In evaluating 12 untreated individuals with Tourette's disorder, they found nonnormalized glucose utilization rates were approximately 15% below control values in the region of the frontal cingulate and possibly insular cortex and the inferior corpus striatum (p less than 0.01).

Routine postmortem examinations of patients with classical Tourette's disorder during their lifetime have revealed no specific abnormality (Richardson, 1982). However, Bonnet (1982) considered anatomical structures related to the vocalizations and movement symptoms, such as blinking and tics, and suggested that limbic forebrain structures, including the anterior cingulate cortex and nuclei that are interrelated to it, may be involved. Eldridge and Denckla (1987) have suggested a complex interaction between androgenic and immunologic factors that lead to susceptibility to those neurodevelopmental changes which lead to Tourette's disorder. These authors note that Balthasar (1957) found an increased number of neurons in the caudate and putamen consistent with immature neuronal pattern.

Neurochemical Basis

Although there is a lack of evidence for specific anatomical localization, neurochemical abnormalities have been proposed. The evidence for neurochemical abnormalities is based on response to specific medications, measurement of neurotransmitter metabolites in blood and cerebralspinal fluid, and on analysis of postmortem brain samples (Singer, 1992). Despite the fact that the neurochemical basis for Tourette's disorder has not yet been clarified, abnormalities involving the dopamine system have received the most support. However, Caine

(1985), in examining five possible chemical abnormalities, suggests an imbalance of central nervous system neurotransmitters. Evidence for dopamine involvement includes the response to dopamine antagonists and the exacerbation of symptoms with stimulant drugs, such as dextroamphetamine and methylphenidate. Moreover, the dopamine metabolite HVA has been found to be decreased in the cerebral spinal fluid in some affected persons. The potential role of the D_1 and D_2 dopamine receptors has been reviewed by Friedhoff (1986). Other investigators studying the relationships between neurotransmitter systems have suggested decreased activity of the endogenous opiate system (Gillman and Sandyk, 1985). Studies that strongly implicate other neurotransmitter systems, such as the noradrenergic, acetylcholine, and serotonin and GABA systems, have been equivocal.

Singer (1992) conducted a postmortem neurochemical study in Tourette's disorder and measured synaptic markers in several regions of the cortex and striatum. Reductions of cyclic AMP were found in all four cortical areas in 3 of 4 patients studied. In the striatum, binding of [^{3}H] mazindol, a marker for the dopamine transporter, was increased (37% increase in the caudate and 50% increase in the striatum). The reduction in cyclic AMP may be consistent with an abnormality in the interaction between the receptor recognition site and the second messenger cyclic AMP. A second messenger abnormality might explain alterations involving multiple neurotransmitter systems. Although a promising hypothesis, it requires more extensive verification. However, the additional finding of an increase in the presynaptic dopamine transporter suggests involvement of the dopamine system. Singer (1992) suggests that the transporter findings are consistent with dopamine hyperinnervation of the striatum. Additional studies are needed to confirm these findings in living subjects, using PET ligands for the dopamine transporter sites.

TREATMENT

The treatment of Tourette's disorder involves both psychosocial and pharmacological interventions; direct intervention with family members is critical. The type of intervention depends on the severity of symptoms. For all ages, comprehensive education about the disorder is essential. Educational interventions may be carried out through the use of booklets and direct instruction. For an individual who is mildly involved, making the diagnosis is itself important and education is particularly useful.

In the moderately and severely involved, one must also take into account other associated features, including attention deficit disorder, the obsessive-compulsive behavior, self-injury, and, in some instances, conduct disorder.

Pharmacotherapy

The primary treatment for motor and vocal symptoms of Tourette's disorder is pharmacotherapy. Dopamine antagonists are the most commonly used medication. Haloperidol was successfully introduced for treatment in 1961 (Seignot, 1961) and has been used extensively since that time. Shapiro and Shapiro (1982) report that 86% of patients show a response to haloperidol, although they found 14% discontinued the medication because of side effects. Among the most commonly reported side effects reported are sedation, dysphoric mood, and school refusal. Sedation generally resolves when doses are increased gradually. Effects on mood and phobic symptoms may respond to reduction in drug dose, although discontinuation and the use of alternative treatments may be needed.

Pimozide also may be effective and produces less sedation, although it has not demonstrated superiority over haloperidol (Colvin and Tankanow, 1985). It is generally considered as a second-line drug for patients who have not responded to haloperidol. No adverse cardiac effects have been reported for either medication (Fulop et al., 1987); however, the QTC interval may be significantly prolonged by pimozide, suggesting that EKG monitoring should be carried out. Sensitivity to dopamine antagonists may extend to long-term effects, such as tardive dyskinesia (Bruun, 1984; Caine and Polinski, 1981) particularly if there is a family history of movement disorder.

Clonidine has also been utilized in the treatment of Tourette's disorder (Cohen et al., 1980; Leckman et al., 1985), although the results are variable; reports of responses were 46% in one study and 47% in another. Bruun (1984) found that 15% of individuals treated responded best to a combination of clonidine and haloperidol when compared to haloperidol alone. However, Leckman et al. (1986) found that tics may worsen as clonidine is withdrawn. Other medications that have been utilized in treatment are fluphenazine (Singer, Gammon, and Quaskey, 1986), clomipramine (Ciprian, 1980), and clonazepam (Bruun, 1984; Merikangas et al., 1985).

Mesulam and Petersen (1987), in reviewing pharmacological treatment of 58 patients over an 8-year period, found that differences in response patterns to medication were common and treatment needed to be tailored to the individual. Overall, dopamine antagonists were the most commonly used form of treatment, but alternatives were often necessary and previously successful drugs sometimes lost their effectiveness, or side effects led to their discontinuation. These authors found that clonidine was inferior to dopamine antagonists for vocal and motor tics but found some role for obsessive-compulsive symptoms. No cases of tardive dyskinesia were reported in this series. Calcium channel blockers, such as verapamil (Walsh et al., 1986), have also been utilized.

Treatment of self-injury relates to both the severity of the Tourette's disorder symptoms and associated forms of psychopathology. Treatment of the Tourette's disorder features or the associated psychopathology might lead to a reduction or disappearance of self-injury. However, the self-injurious behavior may be targeted in itself as a specific syndrome, as described in Chapter 17 on self-injurious behavior. Behavioral techniques include tracking the behavior through self-recording, operant behavioral techniques, behavior reduction procedures, and various combinations of differential reinforcements of other behavior.

Psychological and Psychosocial Management

The mainstay of psychological treatment is supportive psychotherapy and disability counseling for both the affected individual and family. This is essential for both mild and severe presentations. The illness has a major impact on both the individual affected and relatives. Moreover, guidance to teachers is critical for school management (Stefl and Rubin, 1985).

Management in school is particularly important for children. Teachers should be notified regarding how to discuss Tourette's disorder in class. A comprehensive educational evaluation is essential, and adaptations may be needed to provide a longer time for testing so as to allow the child to complete examinations. Other approaches include the use of behavior therapy, which may be helpful as an adjunct to treatment but whose overall effectiveness has not been demonstrated. Behavioral programs have been utilized for the severe obsessive-compulsive behavior to help in the development of strategies to cope with these symptoms. Overall, supportive and psychoeducational approaches are recommended because psychological symptoms emerge as the individual tries to adapt to the illness. Psychodynamic psychotherapy is reserved for other psychological symptoms that may emerge in Tourette's disorder and is not treatment for the disorder in itself.

National associations for affected patients and family members play an important role in the dissemination of information and the provision of support. In the United States, the Tourette Syndrome Association was founded in 1972 and currently has chapters in most states. Similar associations exist in the United Kingdom and in the Netherlands as well as in other countries. The associations meet routinely and provide group support and information to patients, families, teachers, physicians, and others interested in the disorder as well as fund and stimulate research.

SUMMARY

Tourette's disorder has a higher prevalence than previously suspected and may involve a spectrum of difficulties, including chronic multiple tics, simple tics, AD/HD, and obsessional-compulsive symptoms. It occurs in all racial groups, although more commonly in males than females. The natural history of the symptoms is that of the waxing and waning of multiple motor and vocal tics; echophenomena and coprolalia are present in approximately a third of cases. Although the precise etiology is not known, presynaptic transporter and neurotransmitter abnormalities, particularly involving the dopamine system, are most commonly emphasized and the limbic forebrain structures, especially the cingulate gyrus and basal ganglia, are possible anatomical sites. Brain-imaging studies, both SPECT and PET scanning, may contribute to a better delineation of brain regions that are involved, and brain neurochemistry studies are ongoing. In regard to treatment, early identification and recognition of the spectrum of Tourette-related disorders is important, as is continuing research in both psychopharmacological and psychosocial interventions.

REFERENCES

American Psychiatric Association, Committee on Nomenclature and Statistics (1994). *Diagnostic and statistical manual of mental disorders,* 4th ed. Author, Washington, DC.

Balthasar, K. (1957). Uber das anatomische Substrat der generalisierten Tic-Krankheit (maladie des tics, Gilles de la Tourette): Entwicklungshemmung des Corpus striatum. *Archiv für Psychiatrie und Nervenkrankheiten (Berlin),* 195:531–549.

Bliss, J. (1980). Sensory experiences of Gilles de la Tourette syndrome. *Archives of General Psychiatry,* 37:1343–1347.

Bonnet, K.A. (1982). Neurobiological dissection of Tourette syndrome: A neurochemical focus on a human neuroanatomical model. In A.J. Friedhoff and T.N. Chase, (eds.), *Gilles de la Tourette Syndrome. Advances in neurology,* Vol. 35, pp. 433–436. Raven Press, New York.

Bruun, R.D. (1984). Gilles de la Tourette's disorder: An overview of clinical experience. *Journal of the American Academy of Child Psychiatry,* 23:126–133.

Burd, L., Kerbeshian, J., Wikenheiser, M., and Fisher, W. (1986). Prevalence of Gilles de la Tourette's disorder in North Dakota adults. *American Journal of Psychiatry,* 143:787–788.

Caine, E.D. (1985). Gilles de la Tourette's disorder: A review of clinical and research studies and consideration of future directions for investigation. *Archives of Neurology,* 42:393–397.

______, McBride, M.C., Chiverton, P., Bamford, K.A., and Rediess, S. (1988). Tourette syndrome in Monroe country school children. *Neurology,* 38:472–475.

______, and Polinsky, R.J. (1981). Tardive dyskinesia in persons with Gilles de la Tourette's disease. *Archives of Neurology,* 38:471–472.

Caparulo, B.K., Cohen, D.J., Rothman, S.L., Young, J.G., Katz, J.D., Shaywitz, S.E., and Shaywitz, B.A. (1981). Computed tomographic brain scanning in children with developmental neuropsychiatric disorders. *Journal of the American Academy of Child Psychiatry,* 20:338–357.

Chase, T.N., Geoffrey, V., Gillespie, M., and Burroughs, G.H. (1986). Structural and functional studies of Gilles de la Tourette syndrome. *Revue Neurologique (Paris),* 142:851–855.

Ciprian, J. (1980). Three cases of Gilles de la Tourette's disorder. Treatment with clomipramine: A preliminary report. *Journal of Orthomolecular Psychiatry,* 9:116–120.

Cohen, D.J., Detlor, J., Young, J.G., and Shaywitz, B.A. (1980). Clonidine ameliorates Gilles de la Tourette syndrome. *Archives of General Psychiatry,* 37:1350–1357.

Colvin, C.L., and Tankanow, R.M. (1985). Pimozide: Use in Tourette's syndrome. *Drug Intelligence and Clinical Pharmacy,* 19:421–424.

Comings, D.E., and Comings, B.G. (1985). Tourette syndrome: Clinical and psychological aspects of 250 cases. *American Journal of Human Genetics,* 37:435–450.

______, and ______. (1987). A controlled study of Tourette syndrome, I–VII. *American Journal of Human Genetics,* 41:701–866.

Corbett, J.A., Matthews, A.M., Connell, P.H., and Shapiro, D.A. (1969). Tics and Gilles de la Tourette's disorder: A follow-up study and critical review. *British Journal of Psychiatry,* 115:1229–1241.

Crews, W.D., Bonaventura, S., Hay, C.L., Steele, W.K., and Rowl, F.B. (1993). Gilles de la Tourette disorder among individuals with severe or profound mental retardation. *Mental Retardation,* 31:25–28.

Eisenberg, L., Ascher, E., and Kanner, L. (1959). A clinical study of Gilles de la Tourette's disease (maladie des tics) in children. *American Journal of Psychiatry,* 115:715–723.

Eldridge, R., and Denckla, M.B. (1987). The inheritance of Gilles de la Tourette's disorder. *New England Journal of Medicine,* 317:1346–1347.

______, Sweet, R., Lake, C.R., Ziegler, M., and Shapiro, A.K. (1977). Gilles de la Tourette's disorder: Clinical, genetic, psychologic, and biochemical aspects in 21 selected families. *Neurology,* 27:115–124.

Erenberg, G., Cruse, R.P., and Rothner, A.D. (1986). Tourette syndrome: An analysis of 200 pediatric and adolescent cases. *Cleveland Clinic Quarterly,* 53:127–131.

Fahn, S. (1982). A case of post-traumatic tic syndrome. In A.J. Friedhoff and T.N. Chase (eds.), *Gilles de la Tourette syndrome. Advances in neurology,* Vol. 35, pp. 349–350. Raven Press, New York.

Faux, E.J. (1966). Gilles de la Tourette syndrome, social psychiatric management. *Archives of General Psychiatry,* 14:139–142.

Friedhoff, A.J. (1986). Insights into the pathophysiology and pathogenesis of Gilles de la Tourette syndrome. *Revue Neurologique (Paris),* 142:860–864.

Fulop, G., Phillips, R.A., Shapiro, A.K., Gomes, J.A., Shapiro, E., and Nordlie, J.W. (1987). ECG changes during haloperidol and pimozide treatment of Tourette's disorder. *American Journal of Psychiatry,* 144:673–675.

Gilles de la Tourette, G. (1885). Etude sur une affection nerveuse caracterisée par de l'incoordination motrice accompagnée d'écholalie et de copralalie. *Archives of Neurology,* 9:19–42, 158–200.

______. La maladie des tics convulsifs. *La Semaine Médicale,* 19:153–156. (Original work published 1899)

Gillman, M.A., and Sandyk, R. (1985). Tourette syndrome and the opioid system. *Psychiatry Research,* 15:161–162.

Golden, G.S. (1977). The effect of central nervous system stimulants on Tourette syndrome. *Annals of Neurology,* 2:69–70.

Harcherik, D.F., Cohen, D.J., Ort, S., Paul, R., Shaywitz, B.A., Volkmar, F.R., Rothman, S.L.G., and Leckman, J.F. (1985). Computed tomographic brain scanning in four neuropsychiatric disorders of childhood. *American Journal of Psychiatry,* 142:731–734.

Incagnoli, T., and Kane, R. (1983). Developmental perspective of the Gilles de la Tourette syndrome. *Perceptual and Motor Skills,* 57:1271–1281.

Itard, J.M.G. (1825). Mémoire sur quelques fonctions involontaires des appareils de la locomotion de la préhension et de la voix. *Archives of General Medicine,* 8:385–407.

Jeste, D.V., Cutler, N.R., Kaufmann, C.A., and Karoum, F. (1983). Low-dose apomorphine and bromocriptine in neuroleptic-induced movement disorder. *Biological Psychiatry,* 18:1085–1091.

Kidd, K.K., Prusoff, B.A., and Cohen, D.J. (1980). Familial pattern of Gilles de la Tourette syndrome. *Archives of General Psychiatry,* 37:1336–1337.

Klawans, H.L., Falk, D.K., Nausieda, P.A., and Weiner, W.J. (1978). Gilles de la Tourette syndrome after long-term chlorpromazine therapy. *Neurology,* 28:1064–1066.

Krumholz, A., Singer, H.S., Niedermeyer, E., Burnite, R., and Harris, K. (1983). Electrophysiological studies in Tourette's disorder. *Annals of Neurology,* 14:638–641.

Kurlan, R., Behr, J., Medved, L., and Como, P. (1986). Familial Tourette's disorder: Report of a large pedigree and potential for linkage analysis. *Neurology,* 36:772–776.

Leckman, J.F., and Cohen, D.J. (1983). Recent advances in Gilles de la Tourette syndrome: Implications for clinical practice and future research. *Psychiatric Developments,* 3:301–316.

______, Detlor, J., Harcherik, D.F., Ort, S., Shaywitz, B.A., and Cohen, D.J. (1985). Short and long term treatment of Tourette's disorder with clonidine: A clinical perspective. *Neurology,* 35:343–351.

______, Ort, S., Caruso, K.A., Anderson, G.M., Riddle, M.A., and Cohen, D.J. (1986). Rebound phenomena in Tourette's disorder after abrupt withdrawal of clonidine. *Archives of General Psychiatry,* 43:1168–1176.

______, Price, R.A., Walkup, J.T., Ort, S., Pauls, P.L., and Cohen, D.J. (1987). Nongenetic factors in Gilles de la Tourette's disorder. *Archives of General Psychiatry,* 44:100.

Lees, A.J., Robertson, M., Trimble, M.R., and Murray, N.M. (1984). A clinical study of Gilles de la Tourette syndrome in the United Kingdom. *Journal of Neurology, Neurosurgery and Psychiatry,* 47:1–8.

Lowe, T.L., Cohen, D.J., Detlor, J., Kremenitzer, M.W., and Shaywitz, B.A. (1982). Stimulant medications precipitate Tourette's disorder. *Journal of the American Medical Association,* 247:1168–1169.

Merikangas, J.R., Merikangas, K.R., Kopp, U., and Hanin, I. (1985). Blood choline and response to clonazepam and haloperidol in Tourette's disorder. *Acta Psychiatrica Scandinavica,* 72:395–399.

Mesulam, M.M., and Petersen, R.C. (1987). Treatment of Gilles de la Tourette's disorder: Eight-year, practice-based experience in a predominantly adult population. *Neurology,* 37:1828–1833.

Moldofsky, H., Tullis, C., and Lamon, R. (1974). Multiple tic syndrome (Gilles de la Tourette's disorder). *Journal of Nervous and Mental Disease,* 15:282–292.

Obeso, J.A., Rothwell, J.C., and Marsen, C.D. (1982). The neurophysiology of Tourette syndrome. In A.J. Friedhoff and T.N. Chase, (eds.), *Gilles de la Tourette syndrome. Advances in neurology,* Vol. 35. Raven Press, New York.

Pauls, D.L., Cohen, D.J., Kidd, K.K., and Leckman, J.F. (1988). The Gilles de la Tourette syndrome [letter to the editor]. *American Journal of Human Genetics,* 43:206–209.

______, and Leckman, J.F. (1986). The inheritance of Gilles de la Tourette's disorder and associated behaviors. *New England Journal of Medicine,* 315:993–997.

Price, R.A., Kidd, K.K., Cohen, D.J., Pauls, D.L., and Leckman, J.F. (1985). A twin study of Tourette syndrome. *Archives of General Psychiatry,* 42:815–820.

Richardson, E.P. (1982). Neuropathological studies of Tourette syndrome. In A.J. Friedhoff and T.N. Chase (eds.), *Gilles de la Tourette syndrome. Advances in neurology,* Vol. 35, Raven Press, New York.

Robertson, M.M. (1989). The Gilles de la Tourette syndrome: The current status. *British Journal of Psychiatry,* 154:147–169.

______, Trimble, M.R., and Lees, A.J. (1988). The psychopathology of the Gilles de la Tourette syndrome: A phenomenological analysis. *British Journal of Psychiatry,* 152:383–390.

______, ______, and ______. (1989). Self-injurious behaviour and the Gilles de la Tourette syndrome. A clinical study and review of the literature. *Psychological Medicine,* 19:611–625.

Sacks, O.W. (1982). Acquired Tourettism in adult life. In A.J. Friedhoff and T.N. Chase (eds.), *Gilles de la Tourette syndrome. Advances in neurology,* Vol. 35. Raven Press, New York.

Seeman, M.V., Patel, J., and Pyke, J. (1981). Tardive dyskinesia with Tourette-like syndrome. *Journal of Clinical Psychiatry,* 42:357–358.

Seignot, M.J.N. (1961). Un cas de maladie des tics de Gilles de la Tourette gueri par le R.-1625. *Annales Médico-Psychologiques (Paris),* 119:578–579.

Shapiro, A.K., and Shapiro E. (1982). Tourette syndrome: History and present status. In A.J. Friedhoff and T.N. Chase (eds.), *Gilles de la Tourette syndrome. Advances in Neurology,* Vol. 35. Raven Press, New York.

______, and ______. (1992). Evaluation of the reported association of obsessive compulsive symptoms or disorder with Tourette's disorder. *Comprehensive Psychiatry,* 33:152–165.

______, ______, Young, J.G., and Feinberg, T.E. (1988). *Gilles de la Tourette syndrome,* 2nd ed. Raven Press, New York.

Singer, H.S. (1992). Neurochemical analysis of postmortem cortical and striatal brain tissue in patients with Tourette syndrome. *Advances in Neurology,* 58:135–144.

______, Gammon, K., and Quaskey, S. (1986). Haloperidol, fluphenazine and clonidine in Tourette syndrome: Controversies in treatment. *Pediatric Neuroscience,* 12:71–74.

______, and Walkup, J.T. (1991). Tourette syndrome and other tic disorders: Diagnosis, pathophysiology, and treatment. *Medicine,* 70:15–32.

Stefl, M.E., and Rubin, M. (1985). Tourette syndrome in the classroom: Special problems, special needs. *Journal of School Health,* 55:72–75.

Swedo, S.E., Leonard, H.L., Schapiro, M.B., Casey, B.J., Mannheim, G.B., Lenane, M.C., and Rettew, D.C. (1993). Sydenham's chorea: Physical and psychological symptoms of St. Vitus Dance. *Pediatrics,* 91:706–713.

Tolosa, E.S., Montserrat, L., and Bayes, A. (1986). Reduction of brainstem interneuron excitability during voluntary tic inhibition in Tourette's disorder. *Neurology,* 36(suppl. 1):118–119.

Trimble, M. (May 1992). *Gilles de la Tourette syndrome.* Presentation at the annual meeting of the American Psychiatric Association, Washington, DC.

Van de Wetering, B.J.M., and Heutink, P. (1993). The genetics of Gilles de la Tourette syndrome: A review. *Journal of Laboratory and Clinical Medicine,* 121:638–645.

______, Martens, C.M.C., Fortgens, C., Slaets, J.P.J., and Van Woerkom, T.C.A.M. (1985). Late components of the auditory evoked potentials in Gilles de la Tourette syndrome. *Clinics in Neurology and Neurosurgery,* 87:181–186.

Walsh, T.L., Lavenstein, B., Licamele, W.L., Bronheim, S., and Oleary, J. (1986). Calcium antagonists in the treatment of Tourette's disorder. *American Journal of Psychiatry,* 143:1467–1468.

CHAPTER 16

SLEEP DISORDERS

Sleep disturbances are commonly reported by the parents of children and adolescents with developmental neuropsychiatric disorders. The investigation of their sleep disturbances is important from both clinical and research perspectives. From a clinical standpoint, sleep disturbances may be a consequence of brain injury acquired during the perinatal period or subsequently, represent a maturational delay or deviation associated with a developmental disorder, be a consequence of stress or psychosocial events, be an intrinsic characteristic of a genetic syndrome, or be associated with a seizure disorder. Whatever the etiology, sleep disturbances are an important but frequently underemphasized characteristic of developmental disorders, and even when recognized may still go untreated.

The usual concern presented by parents is about irregular sleep habits, insufficient or too much sleep, problems at bedtime, poor sleep, waking during the night, nightmares, night terrors, sleepwalking, bed-wetting, and sleepiness during the day. Sleep problems also may be related to co-occurring disorders, such as epilepsy with nighttime seizures, or depressive disorders. In addition, injuries may occur during sleep, for example, during sleepwalking or other nighttime disorders.

Ordinarily, sleep problems are evaluated on an outpatient basis; however, more complicated cases may require inpatient sleep laboratory assessment. Recent developments in classification of sleep problems have provided new information about when these assessments should be carried out.

Stores (1992) suggests several questions that might be answered in regard to sleep disturbances. One question deals with the developmental delay hypothesis. Is the type and extent of sleep difficulty in children with mental retardation syndromes the same as those in normally developed children of comparable ages? If so, are similar treatments applicable to both groups? A question requiring continuing evaluation is an assessment of the specific factors that may be associated with a disabling condition which may contribute to the sleep problem. Can such factors be identified and be either avoided or compensated for? Both developmental and psychosocial factors may be involved in the genesis of sleep disorders. Attention to bedtime behavior may be positively reinforced, as has been demonstrated in behavior management programs for sleep disturbance. Just as younger children may be reinforced in their abnormal sleep patterns, so may disabled children who actually may be given additional attention because of the severity of their sleep difficulties. Does the stress of a disability and family relations affect the sleep disturbance? Finally, the relationship between sleep disturbance and daytime performance and cognitive functioning needs to be addressed.

In regard to research on sleep, studies of developmental disorders may shed light on the relationship of information processing in sleep to memory function, the ontogeny of dream production, and cognitive development. Treatment of sleep disturbance in developmental disorders requires both chronobiological techniques as well as the use of sleep medication.

This chapter outlines the development of the sleep cycle, reviews the prevalence of sleep disorders in mental retardation, outlines the DSM-IV classification of sleep disorders, discusses possible mechanisms of sleep disturbance (perinatal brain damage, abnormal sleep/wake rhythm, seizures, obstructive sleep apnea, sleep disturbance associated with particular syndromes), and considers treatment approaches.

DEVELOPMENT OF THE SLEEP CYCLE

The development of the sleep cycle is related to age. As children become older, there are decreases in total amount of sleep, total amount of rapid eye movement (REM) sleep, and total amount of deep (stage 3 and 4) sleep. In premature infants, sleep is marked by more wakefulness than in full-term infants and there is more irregularity and instability in the sleep/wake mechanism. In infancy, the amounts of active sleep or rapid eye movement (REM) sleep are substantially greater than they are later in life; almost half of the infant's sleep time in the first week of life is spent in REM sleep. Gradually, the rapid eye movement sleep, or REM, sleep cycles are shifted to the second half of the night.

The type of sleep disturbance bears some relation to age, thus separation anxiety at bedtime is an issue for toddlers, and in young preschool children, bedtime fears, nightmares, bed-wetting, and night terrors emerge. Because there are individual differences in sleep requirements and patterns among children, adherence to rigid sleep schedules may complicate bedtime difficulties and sleep problems. The older child gradually begins to show sleep patterns similar to those of adults, yet there are differences from adults in sleep patterns up through the adolescent years. Difficulty falling asleep, waking during the night, difficulty getting up in the morning, and daytime sleepiness are commonly reported in adolescence.

In the first year of life following the initial establishment of a full night's sleep pattern, a period of renewed wakefulness takes place at approximately 9 to 10 months of age followed by the reestablishment of a full night pattern. In toddlers, the major difficulties are in settling down to sleep and in nighttime waking. In the preschool child, problems include extensive bedtime routines and resistance to falling asleep. One study (Ferber, 1985) found that two thirds of normal 5-year-olds require more than 30 minutes to fall asleep. Similar problems are found in mentally retarded children and often in adolescents.

In the grade school years, parents often note restless sleep, which is increased in children with ear, nose, and throat symptoms. Children with emotional and behavioral difficulties have significantly higher numbers of sleep complaints than other children who are not disordered. Achenbach and Edelbrock (1981) found that clinically referred children had higher rates of nightmares, excessive tiredness, excessive sleep, difficulty with sleeping, and too little sleep compared to normal children. Simeon (1987) found, in a sample of 962 normal children and 103 child psychiatry patients, that sleep talking, difficulty falling asleep, night waking, and enuresis as well as overtiredness were three times higher in the psychiatric group than in the normal group. Poor or restless sleep was six times as frequent.

Sex differences were not noted between normal children, but there were large differences between male and females in the psychiatric population, with boys having more sleep talking, enuresis, early morning waking, and daytime naps. Girls reported more restless sleep, night waking, and poor sleep. Therefore, both normal and behaviorally disturbed children have a variety of sleep problems. Furthermore, there is an association between frequency of sleep problems and psychological and behavior disorders.

PREVALENCE OF SLEEP DISORDER IN MENTAL RETARDATION

Sleep disturbances have been found in several surveys of mixed groups of severely and profoundly retarded individuals. In one study 51% of 200 severely mentally retarded children under age 16 were described by their mothers as having difficulty settling down for bed at night (Stores, 1992). In this survey, 67% were found to awaken once or twice a week and disturbed their parents' sleep. Difficulties in settling down for bed persisted, and sleep problems continued in a number of cases when followed up 4 years later. In this study, a relationship was reported between mental impairment and the child's communication skills and their sleep difficulty. Daytime behavior problems also were noted and considered to be potentially related to sleep difficulty. These authors noted psychosocial problems that might interface with the sleep, such as marital difficulty, maternal irritability, and maternal stress.

In 1985 Bartlett, Rooney, and Spedding evaluated sleep questionnaires from parents of 214 severely mentally retarded children, ranging in age from 6 to 16 years. The problem areas inquired about included preparation for bedtime, settling down to sleep, nighttime waking, and morning routines. Eight percent of the children in this group had one or more sleep problems in the previous 7 days. Fifty-six percent had 1 to 4 difficulties, and 23% had 5 to 10 difficulties.

In 1986 Clements, Wing, and Dunn evaluated 155 severely mentally retarded children under age 16 in the Camberwell Burrough of London. Both sleep disturbances and limitation in the hours of sleep were included in a general developmental and behavioral questionnaire. Sleep problems were a particular problem in children under 5 and occurred in 56% of this group. However, difficulty with sleep continued to be a problem and also was found in 26% of the 10- to 15-year-old group. Overall, 34% of the children studied had some type of sleep problem. That substantial number of children continued to have sleep problems which persisted rather than resolved with development was an ongoing stress to the families. Moreover, sleep problems were strongly associated with daytime behavioral difficulties. The authors suggest that night waking, particularly in younger children, was associated with self-injurious behavior, and fewer hours of sleep was associated with attachment to routines.

CLASSIFICATION OF SLEEP DISORDERS

The classification system for sleep disorders deals with chronic disorders rather than transient disturbances that are part of everyday life. Sleep problems lasting a few nights following a particular psychosocial stressor are not diagnosed as sleep disorders. However, children who are symptomatic for more than a month are considered to be disordered and may require referral for further assessment, diagnosis, and treatment.

Problems in sleep may accompany both mental and physical disorders, particularly conditions involving changes in mood and those causing pain or discomfort. Sleep disturbances may occur at the beginning of an illness and can exacerbate other disorders. However, if the sleep disturbance is the predominant complaint, a sleep disorder is the primary diagnosis.

The type of sleep disturbance is classified according to the Diagnostic Classification of Sleep and Arousal Disorders (Association of Professional Sleep Societies, 1979) and the DSM-IV classification system (APA, 1994). The two major groups of sleep disorders are the dyssomnias and the parasomnias. In dyssomnia, the primary disturbance is in the quality, timing, or amount of sleep, whereas in parasomnia, the primary disturbance is an abnormal event that occurs during sleep. Other conditions, such as sleep apnea, which is associated with excessive daytime sleepiness, and narcolepsy, are classified as hypersomnias related to a known medical disorder. Nocturnal enuresis occurring in the first third of the night associated with sudden arousal from deep sleep may be regarded as a sleep disorder. A sleep disorder that occurs independently of known mental or physical conditions is considered a primary insomnia or hypersomnia.

DYSSOMNIAS

Dyssomnias are manifested by disturbances in the quality, amount, or timing of sleep. This category includes primary insomnia, primary hypersomnia, narcolepsy, breathing-related sleep disorder, circadian rhythm sleep disorder, and dyssomnia not otherwise specified. In insomnia, sleep is deficient in quality or in the amount necessary for normal active daytime functioning. In hypersomnia, the individual feels excessively sleepy during the daytime despite apparently normal sleep length. In the circadian rhythm sleep disorder (sleep/wake schedule disorders), the person's sleep and daytime waking pattern differs from an appropriate day/night routine for his environment.

Insomnia includes a complaint of difficulty in both initiating or maintaining sleep or not feeling rested after apparently normal sleep time. To make the diagnosis, the sleep problem must occur for at least a month, and lead to complaints of daytime fatigue or observations by others of symptoms related to sleep loss, such as irritability. Insomnia may be primary, related to a known organic factor, or related to a nonorganic mental disorder. The diagnostic criteria for primiary insomnia are shown in Table 16–1.

There is considerable variation in the amount of time it takes for a person to fall asleep or in the amount of sleep an individual requires to feel alert and rested. Ordinarily, sleep begins within 30 minutes after settling down in bed, although sleep length varies depending on age. Insomnia occurs more often following periods of stress and is related to behavioral or emotional symptoms. It may be complicated by treatment with pharmacological agents, such as sedatives or hypnotics; this is a particular concern when disabled persons are treated with these agents.

Childhood onset insomnia is rare in school-age children. When it occurs, sleep may be ill-defined and associated with an atypical EEG. In adolescents, the insomnia complaint may be difficulty in falling asleep or premature wakening. Insomnia may be linked to a delayed sleep phase syndrome where sleep onset difficulties are associated with difficulty waking in the morning. However, if the individual is allowed to continue to sleep, he will sleep a normal number of hours. Price et al. (1978) found that normal 11th- and 12th-grade students reported a 12.6% incidence of severe sleep disturbance. Those with the sleep problems also reported more tension, worries, moodiness, and difficulty with solving personal problems, as well as low self-esteem.

Table 16–1. DSM-IV Criteria for Primary Insomnia

307.42 Primary Insomnia

A. The predominant complaint is difficulty initiating or maintaining sleep, or nonrestorative sleep, for at least 1 month.

B. The sleep disturbance (or associated daytime fatigue) causes clinically significant distress or impairment in social, occupational, or other important areas of functioning.

C. The sleep disturbance does not occur exclusively during the course of a Narcolepsy, Breathing-Related Sleep Disorder, Circadian Rhythm Sleep Disorder, or a Parasomnia.

D. The disturbance does not occur exclusively during the course of another mental disorder (e.g., Major Depressive Disorder, Generalized Anxiety Disorder, a delirium).

E. The disturbance is not due to the direct physiological effects of a substance (e.g., a drug of abuse, a medication) or a general medical condition.

From APA, 1994.

Insomnia may occur in conjunction with a mental disorder, such as mood disorder, anxiety disorder, adjustment disorder with anxious or depressed mood, or in obsessive-compulsive personality. Moreover, insomnia may occur because of a known organic factor, such as pain or a specific medical condition, or as a side effect from the use of psychoactive drugs. Some physical disorders seem symptomatic only during sleep, as with sleep apnea, where waking respiration is usually normal. Drugs influencing sleep include amphetamines or other stimulants, serotonin reuptake inhibitors, corticosteroids, and bronchodilators. Alcohol and other substances may disturb sleep as well.

In primary insomnia, the individual will worry about not being able to fall asleep at night, and this may become a preoccupation. Such worries about falling asleep may increase arousal and complicate the sleep disturbance.

Hypersomnia Disorders

Children and adolescents with excessive daytime sleepiness or somnolence (EDS) often are considered inattentive or labeled as lazy or poor learners. Such symptoms usually result from disrupted nighttime sleep in conditions such as sleep apnea and narcolepsy. The onset of excessive daytime sleepiness ordinarily first occurs during adolescence. A careful past medical history and sleep history as well as physical examination are important in the diagnosis. The DSM-IV criteria for hypersomnia are shown in Table 16–2.

The diagnosis of hypersomnia includes the following features: The primary feature is

Table 16–2. DSM-IV Criteria for Primary Hypersomnia

307.44 Primary Hypersomnia

A. The predominant complaint is excessive sleepiness for at least 1 month (or less if recurrent) as evidenced by either prolonged sleep episodes or daytime sleep episodes that occur almost daily.
B. The excessive sleepiness causes clinically significant distress or impairment in social, occupational, or other important areas of functioning.
C. The excessive sleepiness is not better accounted for by insomnia and does not occur exclusively during the course of another Sleep Disorder (e.g., Narcolepsy, Breathing-Related Sleep Disorder, Circadian Rhythm Sleep Disorder, or a Parasomnia) and cannot be accounted for by an inadequate amount of sleep.
D. The disturbance does not occur exclusively during the course of another mental disorder.
E. The disturbance is not due to the direct physiological effects of a substance (e.g., a drug of abuse, a medication) or a general medical condition.

Specify if:

Recurrent: if there are periods of excessive sleepiness that last at least 3 days occurring several times a year for at least 2 years.

From APA, 1994.

either excessive daytime sleepiness or sleep attacks (not accounted for by an inadequate amount of sleep) or prolonged transition into a fully awake state when awakening (sleep drunkenness). The condition occurs every day for at least a month or episodically for longer periods of time and is severe enough to interfere with social activities, relationships, and school. Hypersomnia disorders may be primary or related to nonorganic mental factors, or to medical or neurological disorders. Daytime sleepiness is defined as falling asleep easily, often in 5 minutes or less, anytime during the day even after apparently normal or prolonged amounts of nighttime sleep. Falling asleep is unintentional; sleep attacks are discrete periods of sudden, irresistible sleep. The majority of cases of hypersomnia, or excessive daytime somnolence, are related to a known organic factor. About half of these are associated with sleep apnea, about 25% with narcolepsy, and 10% with sleep-related myoclonus.

The course is related to the presence of other associated physical or mental disorders or to the primary condition. Social and occupational impairment may be mild or severe. Individuals with these problems may become demoralized, and the complications of accidental injury may ensue because of the excessive sleepiness.

Hypersomnia may be related to another mental disorder, particularly mood disorders, such as depression; it is more characteristic of adolescent onset depression. In other mental disorders, such as somatoform disorder, personality disorder, or schizophrenia, hypersomnia is uncommon; in these conditions, daytime drowsiness is attributed to nonrestorative sleep.

Breathing-Related Sleep Disorder

Breathing-related sleep disorder can occur in children of any age, but the incidence increases with age and involves males more often than females. Predisposing factors include enlarged tonsils or adenoids, upper airway or maxillofacial abnormalities, hyperthyroidism, and obesity. Sleep apnea is associated with several mental retardation syndromes including Down syndrome, several mucopolysaccharidoses, and Prader-Willi syndrome. Sleep-disordered breathing may also be noted in Angelman syndrome. There is associated loud snoring followed by pauses in respiration and brief arousals that are often accompanied by restless movements. Associated symptoms include decreased school performance, excessive daytime sleepiness, reoccurrence of nocturnal enuresis, morning headaches, irritability, distractibility, attentional and memory problems, and changes in mood and personality. Changes in weight may occur, and if the condition is persistent, pulmonary hypertension may result. Sleep apnea's effect on intellectual functioning may be greater than in narcolepsy. Some children may be misdiagnosed as being intellectually limited. Unrecognized nighttime symptoms may, with time, become more apparent during the day, particularly if cardiovascular or pulmonary abnormalities develop. The criteria for this disorder are shown in Table 16–3.

The sudden infant death syndrome (SIDS) may be linked to sleep apnea in infants. SIDS is responsible for the death of 2 to 3 infants per 1,000 live births. It occurs more often in males. Children at risk include those who had prior intensive care and whose mothers are substance abusers. Near-miss SIDS is a heterogeneous disorder that is linked to various unrelated res-

Table 16–3. DSM-IV Criteria for Breathing-Related Sleep Disorder

780.59 Breathing-Related Sleep Disorder

A. Sleep disruption, leading to excessive sleepiness or insomnia, that is judged to be due to a sleep-related breathing condition (e.g., obstructive or central sleep apnea syndrome or central alveolar hypoventilation syndrome).
B. The disturbance is not better accounted for by another mental disorder and is not due to the direct physiological effects of a substance (e.g., a drug of abuse, a medication) or another general medical condition (other than a breathing-related disorder). **Coding note:** Also code sleep-related breathing disorder on Axis III.

From APA, 1994.

Chapter 16–4. DSM-IV Criteria for Narcolepsy

347 Narcolepsy

A. Irresistible attacks of refreshing sleep that occur daily over at least 3 months.
B. The presence of one or both of the following:
(1) cataplexy (i.e., brief episodes of sudden bilateral loss of muscle tone, most often in association with intense emotion).
(2) recurrent intrusions of elements of rapid eye movement (REM) sleep into the transition between sleep and wakefulness, as manifested by either hypnopompic or hypnagogic hallucinations or sleep paralysis at the beginning or end of sleep episodes.
C. The disturbance is not due to the direct physiological effects of a substance (e.g., a drug of abuse, a medication) or another general medical condition.

From APA, 1994.

piratory, cardiac, or sleep stage difficulties. Siblings of children with this disorder may have a three- to fourfold increase in the prevalence of SIDS. Because of concern about breathing-related problems at night it is recommended that infants not be allowed to sleep in the prone position.

Narcolepsy

Twenty percent of adult narcoleptics report the onset of daytime sleepiness before age 11. Children with narcolepsy are usually referred when teachers complain about napping during class at school. Unrecognized microsleep may occur in the classroom so others may be unaware the child is napping. Children with this disorder have been considered by teachers to be poorly motivated and sometimes thought to have attention deficit disorder or learning problems. In school, the child may become active or apparently overactive as he or she struggles to fight daytime sleepiness. Associated hypnogogic, auditory, or visual hallucinations are vivid, often frightening, and may not be reported to parents. Children with this condition may be fearful of going to bed because of their hallucinatory experiences when they fall asleep. Unlike seizure disorders, children who lose muscle tone with narcolepsy remain aware of their surroundings. The diagnostic criteria for narcolepsy are shown in Table 16–4.

Narcolepsy is associated with cataplexy (episodic loss of muscle tone initiated by strong emotions), hypnagogic or hypnopompic hallucinations, and sleep paralysis (inability to move while falling asleep or upon sudden wakening). Narcolepsy ordinarily begins around the time of puberty. Obstructive sleep apnea is seen primarily in infants, and in older children with large tonsils and adenoids. Both of these conditions are associated with hypersomnia.

Circadian Rhythm Sleep Disorders (Sleep/Wake Schedule Disorders)

In circadian rhythm sleep disorder, there is a lack of synchronization between normal sleep/wake schedules demanded by the external environment and the individual's internal circadian rhythm. This results in complaints of either insomnia or hypersomnia because the individual has difficulty in falling asleep until late at night and also has problems in waking the following day. Children with this condition may meet the diagnostic criteria for dyssomnias—either insomnia or hypersomnia disorder. The diagnostic criteria for circadian rhythm sleep disorder are shown in Table 16–5.

Delayed Sleep Phase Type

In delayed sleep phase type, there is a persistent pattern of late sleep onset and late awakening times, with an inability to fall asleep and awaken at a desired earlier time (APA, 1994). The onset of sleep is advanced or delayed in relation to sleep. If advanced cycles are evident, the individual may fall asleep early in the evening and wake up in the middle of the night.

Table 16–5. DSM-IV Criteria for Circadian Rhythm Sleep Disorder

307.45 Circadian Rhythm Sleep Disorder

A. A persistent or recurrent pattern of sleep disruption leading to excessive sleepiness or insomnia that is due to a mismatch between the sleep-wake schedule required by a person's environment and his or her circadian sleep-wake pattern.
B. The sleep disturbance causes clinically significant distress or impairment in social, occupational, or other important areas of functioning.
C. The disturbance does not occur exclusively during the course of another Sleep Disorder or other mental disorder.
D. The disturbance is not due to the direct physiological effects of a substance (e.g., a drug of abuse, a medication) or a general medical condition.

Specify type:

Delayed Sleep Phase Type: a persistent pattern of late sleep onset and late awakening times, with an inability to fall asleep and awaken at a desired earlier time.

Jet Lag Type: sleepiness and alertness that occur at an inappropriate time of day relative to local time, occurring after repeated travel across more than one time zone.

Shift Work Type: insomnia during the major sleep period or excessive sleepiness during the major wake period associated with night shift work or frequently changing shift work.

Unspecified Type

From APA, 1994.

In the delayed type, sleep occurs late in the evening or in the early morning, and waking occurs in the middle of the day. There is also a disorganized type where sleep is generally random in pattern, and there is no major daily sleep period. Finally, the frequently changing, or jet lag type, is the result of frequent changes in sleep and waking times, e.g., airline travel involving time zone changes.

A sleep phase disorder may be associated with nonspecific symptoms, such as lack of energy and irritability or malaise. Because circadian rhythm changes occur during adolescence, there may be an increased vulnerability to the delayed type during this age period. The disorganized type may occur at any age and is most common in developmentally disabled persons. Impairment in social function is primarily related to the time of day that the sleep disturbance occurs. The condition may be complicated by accidents because of lack of alertness. Essentially, there is a mismatch between normal sleep/wake schedule for a person's environment and his circadian sleep/wake pattern, resulting in complaints of either insomnia or hypersomnia. Circadian phase sleep disorder is a common concern when dealing with developmentally-disordered individuals, particularly in blind persons and in severely and profoundly mentally retarded persons.

PARASOMNIAS

The parasomnias are a group of conditions where an abnormal event occurs either during sleep or at the threshold between wakefulness and sleep. The parasomnias listed in the DSM-IV include sleep terror disorder, sleepwalking disorder, nightmare disorder, and parasomnia not otherwise specified. The primary complaint is the specific disturbance rather than sleepiness or excessive wakefulness. In a parasomnia such as night terror and sleepwalking, the parent complains about the event rather than the child. From the perspective of the sleep disorder classification, enuresis occurring during sleep in the first hours of the night may be a parasomnia. In some instances, nocturnal seizure disorders may mimic the symptoms of parasomnia, thus requiring an overnight polysomnogram to clarify whether or not the seizures are linked in to a particular sleep stage.

Sleep Terror Disorder (Pavor Nocturnus)

This is a condition that involves repeated episodes of abrupt wakening from sleep. It is often heralded with a scream. The episode ordinarily occurs during the first third of the night, with a rapid arousal from the first interval of nonrapid eye movement (NREM) sleep. The age of onset is ordinarily between 4 and 12 years. Sleep terror episodes are accompanied by EEG delta activity (sleep stages 3 and 4) and generally last 1 to 10 minutes. The diagnostic criteria are shown in Table 16–6.

In a typical episode, the child sits up abruptly in bed, appears frightened and demonstrates signs of intense anxiety, including dilated pupils, excessive perspiration, piloerection, rapid breathing and rapid pulse. He is generally unresponsive to the efforts of others to comfort him until the agitation and confusion subside as he gradually awakens. On the following morning, there is no memory of the episode and

Table 16–6. DSM-IV Criteria for Sleep Terror Disorder

307.46 Sleep Terror Disorder

A. Recurrent episodes of abrupt awakening from sleep, usually occurring during the first third of the major sleep episode and beginning with a panicky scream.
B. Intense fear and signs of autonomic arousal, such as tachycardia, rapid breathing, and sweating, during each episode.
C. Relative unresponsiveness to efforts of others to comfort the person during the episode.
D. No detailed dream is recalled, and there is amnesia for the episode.
E. The episodes cause clinically significant distress or impairment in social, occupational, or other important areas of functioning.
F. The disturbance is not due to the direct physiological effects of a substance (e.g., a drug of abuse, a medication) or a general medical condition.

From APA, 1994.

behavior may be back to his baseline. Occasionally, the individual will recount a sense of terror on being aroused from the night terror but mention only fragmentary mental images unlike the recall of a dream. Sleep terror episodes occur more often with fatigue and following stress.

Prior to a severe episode, EEG delta waves may be higher in amplitude than usual for that phase of sleep, and breathing and heart rate may be slower. Yet the episode itself may be accompanied by a twofold or fourfold increase in heart rate. There is no consistently associated psychopathology with night terrors in children. The course is variable, usually occurring in intervals of days or weeks, but episodes may occur on consecutive nights. The disorder gradually resolves during childhood and ordinarily disappears by early adolescence.

The primary impairment related to sleep terror disorder is related to the avoidance of situations when others might become aware of the disturbance. The child must be protected if he gets up during the episode to avoid accidental injury. The prevalence is estimated to be 1% to 4% for the full disorder, although a larger percentage of children may have isolated symptoms. It is a condition more common in males than in females. The disorder is more common among first-degree relatives of people with the disorder than in the general population.

Treatment consists primarily of education of the family regarding the nature of the sleep terror disorder. In those instances where night terrors occur quite frequently and are disruptive to family life, pharmacotherapy with diazepam or alprazolam may be indicated.

Sleepwalking Disorder

Sleepwalking repeated episodes consist of leaving bed and walking without being conscious of the episode or remembering it. It ordinarily occurs during the first third of the major sleep period, the period of NREM sleep. Sleepwalking lasts from a few minutes up to about half an hour. In a typical episode the child sits up, makes perseverative movements such as picking at a blanket, then proceeds to semipurposeful movements including walking, opening doors, eating, dressing, or going to the bathroom. An episode may terminate before sleepwalking is accomplished. The diagnostic criteria are shown in Table 16–7.

When observed, the sleepwalker has a blank facial expression, appears to stare, and is unresponsive to the efforts of others to communicate with him or efforts to influence the sleepwalking. Awakening is accomplished only with great difficulty. Coordination is poor during the episode; however, the individual apparently may see and walks around objects. Nonetheless, he may stumble or lose balance and be injured, particularly when taking a hazardous route. If walking terminates spontaneously, the sleepwalker may awaken but is disoriented. In other instances, the sleepwalker may return to bed without reaching consciousness or fall asleep in another place away from the bed and be surprised at finding himself there on waking.

On the EEG, slow waves may increase in amplitude in stage 4 sleep just preceding the episode. There is a flattening of the EEG indicating arousal that occurs before the episode itself. Ordinarily in sleepwalking, the high amplitude slow wave pattern gives way to a mixture of NREM stages and lower amplitude EEG activity. This condition is more likely to occur in individuals who are fatigued or have experienced stress during the previous day.

Aggression toward other persons or toward objects in the environment is infrequent during sleepwalking. The condition may be accompanied by sleep talking but, if so, articulation is poor. Sleepwalkers have an increased incidence of

Table 16–7. DSM-IV Criteria for Sleepwalking Disorder

307.46 Sleepwalking Disorder

A. Repeated episodes of arising from bed during sleep and walking about, usually occurring during the first third of the major sleep episode.
B. While sleepwalking, the person has a blank, staring face, is relatively unresponsive to the efforts of others to communicate with him or her, and can be awakened only with great difficulty.
C. On awakening (either from the sleepwalking episode or the next morning), the person has amnesia for the episode.
D. Within several minutes after awakening from the sleepwalking episode, there is no impairment of mental activity or behavior (although there may initially be a short period of confusion or disorientation).
E. The sleepwalking causes clinically significant distress or impairment in social, occupational, or other important areas of functioning.
F. The disturbance is not due to the direct physiological effects of a substance (e.g., a drug of abuse, a medication) or a general medical condition.

From APA, 1994.

other episodic disorders associated with NREM sleep, such as sleep terrors. No specific psychopathology, however, has been demonstrated in children and adolescents with this disorder.

The onset is ordinarily between age 6 and 12 years and ordinarily lasts several years. Usually symptoms have resolved by the end of the teens or in the early 20s. The primary impairment is the occurrence of injuries during an episode. Prevalence is estimated at 1% to 6%, but as many as 15% of children may have isolated episodes. It occurs more commonly in males than in females. It is also more common among first-degree biological relatives than in the general population.

Nightmares (Dream Anxiety Disorder)

Nightmares are frightening dreams that are frequently followed by awakening. Awake, the child or adolescent may be tearful or agitated and appear frightened and will generally seek comfort. Dream content can usually be recalled, particularly immediately after waking, by children with verbal abilities that are sufficient to allow them to describe their experiences. Because REM sleep occurs primarily in the second half of the night, nightmares occur during this period and are most frequent in the early morning hours. In REM sleep, there is tonic motor inhibition so a child does not appear agitated or talk during the nightmare. The distress related to nightmares becomes apparent only after the child is awakened. Nightmares occur with equal frequency in boys and girls; the peak age of their onset is between ages 3 and 5 (Terr, 1987). Nightmares are found in 25% to 50% of preschool children and continue to be experienced, but with less frequency, in older children, adolescents, and adults (Adair and Bauchner, 1993). It should be noted that based on behavior after awakening, nightmares may also occur in preverbal children and in children who are mentally retarded.

The dream is sometimes described by children as consisting of pictures they see at night. The dream is made up of vivid mental imagery that is usually visual but may contain auditory, olfactory, or tactile experiences as well. During dreaming, it is thought that daily experiences are incorporated into memory. Dreams consistently show a bizarre pattern but may have a simple narrative structure. In terms of dream content, Foulkes (1982) has studied the content of dreams in children at different ages. For example, animals are prominent in the nightmares of 4- to 5-year-olds.

Ordinarily, occasional nightmares are not a reason for concern; however, recurrent nightmares may reflect stressful daytime experiences and require exploration. The DSM-IV criteria for nightmare disorder are shown in Table 16–8.

Each of these sleep disorders may occur in mentally retarded and developmentally disordered persons. Common problems include lack of the establishment of a regular diurnal rhythm (circadian rhythm sleep disorder), dyssomnias (primary insomnia, difficulty falling asleep and remaining asleep), and primary hypersomnia (excessive sleepiness), sleep-related behavioral problems, parasomnias (nightmare disorder, sleep terror disorder, sleepwalking disorder, bruxism), sleep-related breathing problems (breathing-related sleep disorder), and sleep disorder related to another medical condition (e.g., epilepsy).

THE ONTOGENY OF SLEEP IN DEVELOPMENTAL DISORDERS

In investigating the sleep cycle in developmental disorders, three issues must be taken into

Table 16–8. DSM-IV Criteria for Nightmare Disorder

307.47 Nightmare Disorder

A. Repeated awakenings from the major sleep period or naps with detailed recall of extended and extremely frightening dreams, usually involving threats to survival, security, or self-esteem. The awakenings generally occur during the second half of the sleep period.
B. On awakening from the frightening dreams, the person rapidly becomes oriented and alert (in contrast to the confusion and disorientation seen in Sleep Terror Disorder and some forms of epilepsy).
C. The dream experience, or the sleep disturbance resulting from the awakening, causes clinically significant distress or impairment in social, occupational, or other important areas of functioning.
D. The nightmares do not occur exclusively during the course of another mental disorder (e.g., a delirium, Posttraumatic Stress Disorder) and are not due to the direct physiological effects of a substance (e.g., a drug of abuse, a medication) or a general medical condition.

From APA, 1994.

account: the time spent asleep, the distribution of sleep during the 24-hour period, and the depth of sleep—all of which vary considerably throughout the life cycle.

Animal studies have established the brain mechanisms involved in the establishment of circadian rhythms and the mechanisms for NREM and REM sleep. Brainstem nuclei have been linked to sleep, particularly the locus coeruleus for generation of the sleep stages and the suprachiasmatic nuclei for the establishment of circadian rhythms of sleep and wakefulness.

Sleep is one aspect of the 25-hour circadian sleep/wake cycle that is entrained to a 24-hour clock. Time cues related to bedtime and wake time, mealtime, and school schedules are all aspects of the circadian cycle. The circadian cycle and these time cues may be disrupted in developmental disorders. The sleep cycle is accompanied by particular hormonal rhythms that occur during sleep, such as the release of growth hormone, prolactin, and cortisol release that is coupled with sleep. Growth hormone is released shortly after entering into deep sleep, and prolactin reaches its peak between 5 and 7 A.M. Corticosteroid secretion is ordinarily initiated during the night but becomes desynchronized in sleep with changes in the sleep/wake schedule. When the sleep schedule changes, cortisol is initially released at the same time as before but gradually adjusts to the new cycle.

In preparation for extrauterine adaptation, the degree of maturation of the central nervous system is a critical factor in establishing the sleep/wake cycle. Following birth, the infant is exposed to numerous environmental influences, and to adapt, the infant must develop his own biological clock for sleep and waking. In children with brain impairment or mental retardation, the development of sleep/wake rhythm may be hindered.

In newborn infants, the circadian rhythm of sleep and wake develops gradually, with initial alternations of sleep and wake of several hours in duration. This 24-hour sleep/wake rhythm is only established 12 to 16 weeks after birth (Kleitman and Engelman, 1953; Meier-Koll et al., 1978). The establishment of the circadian rhythm of sleep and wakefulness occurs as the infant is entrained to the environmental cycle. Indicators of environmental time are called zeitgebers (*zeit,* meaning *time; geber,* meaning *giver*) (Aschoff, 1954). Those zeitgebers that are most important are the 24-hour environmental light/dark cycle (Czeisler et al., 1981), the timing of feeding (Goetz, Bishop, and Halberg, 1976), and social contacts (Vernikos-Danellis and Winget, 1979; Wever, 1979) with others. However, changes of temperature, relative humidity, and other physical influences that occur during the day may also affect the circadian cycle. Roffwarg, Muzio, and Dement (1966) studied the ontogenic development of the human sleep-dream cycle and suggested that REM sleep in early life may play a role in the development of the central nervous system.

Brain impairment or dysfunction in newborn infants may lead to delayed development, and appropriate links to environmental time may not develop. In some instances visual defects interfere with perception of visual stimuli and may affect the development of circadian rhythms. In addition, mentally retarded and brain-impaired children who lack effective social contact due to their disabilities may be delayed in the establishment of socially entrained rhythms. Social contacts may be lacking or inadequate because of the delayed development of mental functions.

Patients with central nervous system disorders often have disturbed sleep, sometimes exhibiting disordered sleep/wake rhythm, insomnia, and hypersomnia. These symptoms are attributed either to dysfunction or destruction of specific areas in the brain.

In brain-impaired neonates, the normal links between and the characteristic features of the different stages of sleep are not present. In REM, irregular respiration or heart rate, changes of EEG activity, and abolishment of electromyographic (EMG) activity may not occur simultaneously as expected in nonimpaired infants. Variables associated with NREM sleep also may not show systematic changes in brain-impaired infants.

Sleep Disorders of the Perinatal Period

In neonates, conditions such as asphyxia neonatorum, intraventricular hemorrhage, convulsions, and infections may profoundly affect brain maturational processes at a time before sleep/wake rhythms have been established. The same may be the case for infants with intrauterine growth retardation. Perinatal sleep disorders include abnormal sleep cyclic organization of REM and NREM sleep and lack of integration of motor, breathing, and brain activity. These symptoms are attributed either to dysfunction or destruction of specific brain areas involved in generating sleep and the sleep/wake rhythm.

A period of quiet sleep lasting longer than 30 minutes or a period of active sleep whose duration is longer than 60 minutes is considered a pathological cyclic organization (Dreyfus-Brisac and Monod, 1970). Waking time ordinarily increases after the acute stage of severe diseases. In less severe illness, cyclic organization may be disrupted, similar to that occurring in premature infants. Severe illness is ordinarily followed by an immediate period of reorganization.

Newborn babies with chromosomal anomalies with and without brain malformations may be poor sleepers (Monad and Guidasci, 1976). They frequently have a longer waking time than normal neonates, some have considerable difficulty settling for sleep, and others may have difficulty maintaining sleep. The cycling of active and quiet sleep in infancy, motility, respiration, and electromyogram (EMG), may be variable.

Despite the limited number of reports on sleep disorders in abnormal infants that review the establishment of ultradian and circadian rhythms, such problems are commonly reported by caregivers. Development of sleep/wake rhythm reflects an important central nervous system maturation process. The longitudinal observation of the sleep/wake rhythm in mentally retarded and brain-impaired children is important in the prognosis and evaluation of the effects of therapy.

An irregular sleep/wake rhythm is often observed in extensively brain-impaired children, and is usually caused by severe central nervous system disease that occurs in the perinatal period. When studying children with brain damage, the usual sleep classification is difficult to apply because sleep is dispersed over the 24-hour day without following the usual circadian pattern. Okawa and Sasaki (1987) have referred to this as "monostage" sleep. Other decerebrate children do have a day/night sleep cycle, but abnormalites occur in the amount and phasing of REM and NREM sleep. The sleep EEG may show abnormal patterning and lack sleep spindles; sharp waves over the vertex may make it difficult to distinguish between sleep and waking. The sleep/wake rhythm mechanism and that of the establishment of the sleep EEG are independent mechanisms; as noted earlier, the brainstem is important in the establishment of the sleep/wake rhythm.

SLEEP AND DEVELOPMENTAL DISORDERS

Studies of clinical sleep disorders are a neglected area but one of clinical significance. The problem in settling down at bedtime, nighttime waking, short sleep time, and daytime sleepiness are all problems commonly reported but often not taken seriously enough. The effect of sleep disturbances on the family is particularly important. Recognizing that sleep problems beginning in early life persist in a significant minority of disabled children when contrasted to normal children is a consideration when counseling parents and other caregivers. When sleep problems are not recognized and treated, other forms of sleep disturbance may occur, for example, circadian cycle disorders.

Studies of clinical sleep disorders in children and adolescents with developmental disability is an area of ongoing interest. Physiological studies in the sleep laboratory have shown general relationships between neuropathology and disordered sleep mechanisms, particularly those involving abnormal sleep spindle activity, REM sleep disturbances, and changes and reductions in the amount of non-REM sleep. Although physiological disturbances have not been clearly documented among the different mental retardation syndromes, some problems, such as obstructive sleep apnea, have been recognized as important in several disorders.

Sleep disorders in relation to central nervous system dysfunction or brain malformation have been reported in children with blindness, brain malformations, chromosomal abnormalities, and associated with developmental psychopathology. Among the latter are attention deficit disorder, Tourette's disorder, Down syndrome, Prader-Willi syndrome, mucopolysaccharidoses, tuberous sclerosis, phenylketonuria, bilirubinemia, Menkes' kinky hair disease, some forms of dwarfism, and some seizure disorders. In those conditions where there is a predisposition to clinical sleep disorder, such as obstructive sleep apnea in Down syndrome and in most forms of mucopolysaccharidoses, hypersomnolence in Prader-Willi syndrome, and difficulty settling down for sleep in autistic disorder, a review of sleep is an important aspect of the diagnostic assessment.

Effective treatments for sleep disorders are available to assist parents in working with their children. These include behavioral treatments (Howlin, 1984; Summers et al., 1992), pharmacological treatments, and physiological treatments. Behavioral treatments are helpful for establishing sleep routines. Pharmacological treatments are available for inducing and maintaining sleep. Physiological treatments are used for certain disorders such as sleep apnea.

The Blind Child

Human subjects isolated from environmental cues such as light, darkness, temperature, and humidity, develop patterns of sleep/wake rhythm, body temperature, and other biological rhythms that vary from the familiar 24-hour pattern. This free-running rhythm is close to 25 hours in duration and is considered to be the endogenous rhythm (Halberg et al., 1959). The light/dark cycle in the environment is one of the dominant synchronizers of the human circadian system (Czeisler et al., 1981). In blind subjects, sensitivity to light varies, and the subjects are reported to have a high incidence of sleep/wake disorders (Miles and Wilson, 1977). However, most blind subjects who live in a normal environment are able to be entrained to a 24-hour day by means of social contacts (Wever, 1979) or other scheduling, such as bedtime, waking times, and mealtimes. Mentally retarded children with blindness are vulnerable for problems in entrainment of the sleep/wake rhythm to a 24-hour cycle. This is a particular problem for those with severe or profound mental retardation.

Free-running rhythms and irregular sleep/wake rhythms in some blind children may be very strong, and attempts at entrainment to a 24-hour rhythm system, by either forced awakening or scheduled mealtimes, have been unsuccessful for the most part (Okawa et al., 1985). Sleep/wake disorders in blind children might be caused by either an insufficient perception of environmental zeitgebers due to blindness compounded by mental retardation, or an inadequate intrinsic capacity to reset the biological clock.

In animal experiments, Rusak (1977) found that after either enucleation of both eyes or transection of the optic nerves, entrainment to the light/dark cycle no longer occurred, and the rest/activity rhythm became free running in both the light/dark cycle and in contrast darkness. The free-running rhythm of blind mentally retarded children is similar to this situation. In rodents, when the suprachiasmatic nuclei were destroyed and visual connections were intact, some persistent clustering of daylight activity can be observed during the light period of the light/dark cycle. However, when the animals with destroyed suprachiasmatic nuclei were exposed to constant conditions, rest/activity rhythms totally disappeared, and a free-running rhythm was not apparent (Rusak, 1977). The suprachiasmatic nuclei are considered to be a biological clock and pacemaker of the free-running rhythm system. Blind mentally retarded children who show a persistent free-running rhythm do seem to have an intact pacemaker. The suprachiasmatic nuclei in the human brain have not been fully identified, and their function is not clearly understood.

Attention Deficit/Hyperactivity Disorder

Difficulty falling asleep, waking frequently during the night, and restless sleep are commonly reported in children with attention deficit/hyperactivity disorder (this disorder is described in Chapter 13). Kaplan et al. (1987) reviewed parent reports of sleep disturbance in 116 medication-free children with a DSM-III diagnosis of ADHD and 88 age-matched control subjects. Difficulty falling asleep, nighttime waking, early morning waking, and crying out during the night were significantly ($p<0.001$) more frequent. Greenhill et al. (1983) found that parents reported restless sleep in 57% of children with this diagnosis.

Even though parents' concerns about sleep disturbance are frequent, reports of disturbed sleep are difficult to demonstrate in the sleep laboratory. Despite parental reports of restlessness, Greenhill et al. (1983) did not find abnormal polysomnographic evidence of disrupted sleep. Busby, Firestone, and Pivik (1981) found a trend toward increased nighttime movement, but concluded that there was no overall evidence of marked sleep disturbance. However, when Busby and Pivik (1985) evaluated responses of children to auditory tones that were presented during sleep, they did find a slightly increased sensitivity to auditory stimuli during sleep in nonmedicated children with a diagnosis of attention deficit disorder. It may be necessary to use automated analyses of subtypes of EEG waves to detect subtle changes in sleep (Coble et al., 1984).

Initial insomnia may result from drug treatment using stimulant medication and require adjustments in dosage schedules and, in some instances, discontinuation of long-acting preparations. Yet some children may show less difficulty settling for sleep when they are given late afternoon doses or long-acting preparations, possibly related to better organization and cooperation with nighttime routines (Dahl and Puig-Antich, 1990). Delayed sleep onset with stimulant medication has been studied in the sleep laboratory. Polysomnographic studies have documented delayed sleep onset (average 15 to 20 minutes) and delayed REM latency (Chatoor et al., 1983; Greenhill et al., 1983; Haig, Schroeder, and Schroeder, 1974; Small, Hibi, and Feinberg, 1971).

Finally, sleep deprivation may be associated with inattention, overactivity, and aggressiveness. Dahl and Puig-Antich (1990) note that the treatment of sleep disturbance in children with attention deficit disorder may lead to significant improvement of their ADD and learning disablity symptoms. Additional studies are needed to provide better understanding of the relationship between sleep regulation and the neurobiology of attention deficit disorder.

Reading Disability

Mercier, Pivik, and Busby (1993) compared sleep patterns in reading-disabled (n = 24) and age-matched normal controls (n = 15) boys. Polysomnograms were conducted in the sleep laboratory for 4 consecutive nights (2 adaptation, 2 baseline). When the two groups were compared on baseline sleep measures, collapsing nights 3 and 4, the reading-disabled children showed significantly more stage 4 sleep, less rapid eye movement sleep, a longer REM onset latency period, and an extended initial non-REM cycle. The authors propose that chronic sleep deprivation and maturational delay might account for these variations in sleep architecture. They suggest that these factors, alone or together, might impair information processing and contribute to the cognitive deficits seen in children with reading disability. In support of the maturational hypothesis, the stage 4 percentages obtained for the children with reading disability are similar to those reported for 6- to 7-year-olds and higher than those found for 8- to 10-year-olds (Coble et al., 1987).

Future studies require better documentation of daytime sleepiness and napping behavior and the use of computerized analysis of EEG activity, which may provide more accurate quantification of slow wave activity. In addition, there are likely to be subtypes of reading disability that may account for the variability found among the reading-disabled subjects.

Tourette's Disorder

Sleep disorders are commonly associated with Tourette's disorder (Chapter 15) and also occur more frequently in family members of persons with Tourette's disorder (Nee et al., 1980). Studies of younger patients with Tourette's disorder have documented that tics may occur during all sleep stages (Barabas, Matthews, and Ferrari, 1984b; Glaze, Frost, and Jankovic, 1983). Sleep disturbances include initial, middle, and delayed insomnia, nightmares, night terrors, sleepwalking, bed-wetting, bruxism, and sleep talking (Moldofsky, Tullis, and Lamon, 1974; Robertson, Trimble, and Lees, 1988). Increased partial arousals out of deep sleep (stage 4) may be linked to night terrors, sleepwalking, and bed-wetting. Mendelson et al. (1980) suggested that patients with Tourette's disorder have a 30% decrease in sleep stages 3 and 4, yet others (Glaze, Jankovic, and Frost, 1983) reported an increase in these same sleep stages. Mendelson et al. (1980) also found that waking time was higher and that non-REM sleep was reduced in Tourette's disorder patients when contrasted to controls. Other authors (Barabas, Matthews, and Ferrari, 1984a, 1984b) have reported high rates of sleepwalking and night terrors (33%) in Tourette's disorder when contrasted to children with seizure disorders (3%) or learning disabilities (8%). These findings are consistent with Tourette's disorder being a disorder of arousal. Others (Erenberg, 1985) have not concurred with the hypothesis of an arousal disorder but did find an increased prevalence of nightmares and insomnia in 20% of the cases they studied. The average age of onset for the latter group is higher, which may explain the differences. It should be noted that arousal disorders tend to occur in younger children and disappear with maturation. However, physiological and neurophysiological testing (Bock and Goldberger, 1985) have not supported the arousal disorder hypothesis.

Allen et al. (1992) used a parent sleep questionnaire and collected data on boys aged 7 to 14 years with diagnoses of TD only (57), ADHD only (21), and TD and ADHD (89) who were compared to an age-matched control group. Significant sleep disturbance was found in 90% of those with combined TD and ADHD and 26% of those with TD only. The authors concluded that the sleep problems in the group with both diagnoses is consistent with an arousal disorder. Drake et al. (1992) recorded outpatient sleep in 20 patients (predominantly male, age range 10 to 36 years) with Tourette's disorder utilizing a 4-channel cassette EEG system. This approach allows recording to be conducted in the usual sleeping environment. Seven had chronic tics only, 8 had tics and attention deficit/hyperactivity disorder, and 5 had tics and obsessions and compulsions. Reduced sleep, decreased sleep efficiency, increased awakenings, and decreased slow wave sleep were confirmed. Increased nocturnal awakenings and movements were most apparent in those who had tics during sleep. Sleep fragmentation and the loss of slow wave sleep was most striking in those with attention deficit disorder, and sleep latency was increased, REM sleep reduced, and REM latency decreased in those with associated compulsions and obsessions. These findings suggest that the type of sleep disturbance may vary according to symptoms associated with Tourette's disorder. These authors suggest chronic tics that persist during sleep may cause awakenings, the co-occurrence of attention deficit disorder may be associated with a disorder of arousal and alertness, and obsessions and compulsions might be linked to the mechanism involving REM sleep.

Mental Retardation (Mixed Etiologies)

In children who are not mentally retarded, sleep variables such as total sleep time and the percentage of time spent in various sleep stages changes with increasing age. If we consider the developmental delay hypothesis of mental retardation, sleep characteristics should be similar to those of younger children rather than nonretarded children of their own age. However, when brain dysfunction is associated with mental retardation and involves brain areas involved with sleep organization, sleep disorders may be manifested differently. Sleep studies have been carried out in mentally retarded persons with specific etiologies and in those where the etiology is not known. A number of sleep parameters have been studied; for example, total sleep time is shorter in mentally retarded persons in contrast to that of nonretarded children.

Among the various sleep stages, REM sleep has been of particular interest in mental retardation syndromes. A relationship between the amount of REM sleep and levels of intelligence has been actively debated. Yet phylogenetic studies in animals have demonstrated that younger animals, in fact, have higher amounts of REM sleep than older animals. In the human neonate, the percentage of REM sleep is also high and declines with age. A higher percentage of REM sleep would seem to indicate immaturity of the brain. Therefore, it would also be expected the REM sleep percentage would be higher in mentally retarded persons than in the nonretarded persons; however, many studies indicate REM sleep time is reduced. The reason is unclear, although it has been suggested that any type of brain impairment might lead to a decrease in REM sleep.

REM sleep latency (the time interval between the onset of sleep and initiation of the first REM sleep period) varies considerably among individuals and is hypothesized to be an index of the maturation of cerebral function. Rapid eye movements during REM sleep have been intensively studied in regard to intelligence, especially the time intervals between eye movements. Both REM density and the amount of rapid eye movements have been reported to correlate with intelligence. In newborns, active sleep is the first phase of sleep but, by 3 months, quiet sleep is the first phase. Ellingson and Peters (1980a, 1980b) and Shibagaki and Kiyono (1983) have reported a possible relationship between the occurrence of the first NREM sleep onset and the maturation of the central nervous system in mentally retarded children.

Autistic Disorder

DeMyer (1979) reported that the majority of children with autistic disorder (49%) evaluated on a clinical research unit had sleep disturbance and about half had severe problems as contrasted to 3% of a normal control group. Severe problems occurred several times a month over a 6-month period. Problems of initiating (97%) and maintaining (72%) sleep were most commonly reported. Sleep in infancy was best, and sleep between ages 2 and 3 was the worst (48% of reports). Parents described irritability resulting from sleep loss. Sleep problems at home were confirmed during an inpatient stay on the clinical research unit. Wing (1966) also described irregular sleep/wake patterns in children with autistic disorder. A significantly high incidence of sleep disorders, such as irregular sleep/wake rhythm and short duration of the sleep period, was reported after an investigation of the early symptoms of autistic disorder, accomplished by a questionnaire (Hoshino et al., 1984; Inamura, 1984). Segawa (1985) reported on the sleep/wake rhythm in children with autistic disorder, using a day-by-day plotting method that involved observations made by the families. There was a marked irregularity in many children with autistic disorder, and a free-running rhythm was sometimes observed. Most sleep laboratory reports on the sleep of children with autistic disorder have focused on REM variables or the NREM/REM sleep cycle. Ornitz (1978) carried out a series of polygraphic studies of sleep in children with autistic disorder and compared them to controls. No specific differences were seen in the REM/NREM cycle. Onheiber et al. (1964) found no differences between those with autistic disorder and controls in regard to the amount of REM sleep. However, ratios of phasic and tonic REM have not been carefully delineated. These authors considered that a delay in maturation of EEG activity may suggest a dysfunction of central vestibular mechanisms. To answer this question, IQ-matched control groups are needed.

There have been discussions about the effect of lacking or inadequate social cues in regard to a disturbed circadian system or on the appearance of free-running rhythms, but to date how social contacts act as zeitgebers in relation to the biological clock is unknown. Segawa suggested that, in the brains of children with autistic disorder and children with Rett's syndrome, noradrenergic and dopaminergic neurons play an important role, functioning as modulators of the circadian system.

Down Syndrome

Sleep in Down syndrome (Chapter 10.4) has been investigated the most thoroughly. However, findings are inconsistent and vary from one child to the next and among children with Down syndrome at different IQ levels.

In infants with Down syndrome, sleep has been characterized by an increase in the waking state (Prechtl, Theorell, and Blair, 1973). Lower percentage of REM sleep, frequent body movements, and reduction in the period of transition from REM to NREM sleep have been reported (Goldie et al., 1968, Hamaguchi et al., 1989). In studies of children and adolescents with Down syndrome, total sleep time was longer than that of control nonretarded children in two studies (Clausen, Sersen, and Lidsky, 1977; Fukuma et al., 1974; Petre-Quadens, 1972). REM sleep density in persons with Down syndrome was significantly lower than in normal control groups (Clausen, Sersen, and Lidsky, 1977; Fukuma et al., 1974). Polysomnograms revealed poorly organized alpha activity, few sleep spindles, and atypical K-complexes. Sleep spindles increase rapidly in normal children under 2 years of age; the rate of increase slows between the ages of 2 and 3 years when the structure of spindles becomes steady. Because the increase of spindles may accompany brain development, abnormalities in Down syndrome could result from maturational delay.

Attempts to improve cognitive performance in Down syndrome have been carried out pharmacologically by administering 5-hydroxytryptophan (5HTP), a precursor of serotonin, based on reports of deficiences of serotonin in Down syndrome. Petre-Quadens and De Lee (1975) reported a temporary increase in the density of eye movements following 5HTP. Moreover, butoctamide hydrogen succinate has been reported by Gigli et al. (1987) to increase the amount of REM sleep in children with Down syndrome and to increase the frequency of eye movements following structured teaching. Like other attempts to use 5HTP to treat Down syndrome, these findings are inconclusive.

In his review of sleep studies in mental disability, Stores (1992) found a significantly higher proportion of children with Down syndrome had sleep problems and quotes a DHSS report (Cunningham et al., 1986) that documented marked problems in settling down at night (20%), waking at night (41%), and insistence on sleeping with parents (24%). Sleep problems were noted in Down syndrome children when compared to normals at all ages. These authors considered that the sleep behaviors were linked to family problems, which included poor parent–child relationships, stress related to disabilities, and disagreements between parents.

Stores (1992) also completed a questionnaire survey of sleep disorders of children with Down syndrome and found that all of the children with this disorder have frequently occurring sleep problems at a significantly higher rate than a control group. Boys were found to have more sleep difficulties than girls; frequent wakings, restless sleep, and snoring were prominent. This author found evidence of an association between severe sleep problems and disturbed daytime behavior, which included relationships between types of sleep disorder and behavioral disturbances. He suggested that restless sleep and snoring were linked to generalized disturbances of behavior during the day which, in this group, included irritability, overactivity, and stereotypies. Daytime behavioral difficulties related to sleep disturbances in Down syndrome may potentially be related to an increased rate of obstructive sleep apnea in Down syndrome (Silverman, 1988). Obstructive sleep apnea is associated with snoring, restlessness, changes in sleep posture, and bedwetting. Learning problems may follow daytime sleepiness. Stebbens et al. (1991) suggested that factors contributing to upper airway obstruction in Down syndrome include a large posteriorly placed tongue, enlarged tonsils and adenoids, hypotonia of the pharnygeal muscles, and possibly congenital narrowing of the upper airways.

Prader-Willi Syndrome

Prader-Willi syndrome, a condition characterized by neonatal hypotonia, mental retardation, obesity, hypogonadism, and short stature, is described in Chapter 10.1. A variety of sleep disorders have been reported in this syndrome. Their obesity and hypotonia place these patients at particular risk for sleep-disordered breathing (Friedman et al., 1984; Hertz et al., 1993; McCoy, Koopman, and Taussig, 1981; Orenstein et al., 1977, 1980). However, there is lack of agreement on whether or not sleep-disordered breathing is a significant problem for this population. Friedman et al. (1984) studied 9 cases referred from an obesity clinic and found evidence of respiratory disturbance in 8. This included obstructive sleep apnea in 4 cases, oxygen desaturation with loud snoring without apnea in 2 cases, and mild central apnea in 2 cases. However, Vela-Bueno et al. (1984) investigated 9 cases of Prader-Willi syndrome and reported only one case of sleep-disordered breathing, which was apparently a mild REM-related hypopnea. There is one study of the relationship between degree of obesity and the severity of the sleep-disordered breathing in children with the Prader-Willi syndrome. For adults, sleep-disordered breathing is more likely to occur in the more obese, and the severity of the sleep-disordered breathing is generally reduced by weight loss. Similar relationships have not been documented for children with the Prader-Willi syndrome; in particular, it has not been shown that weight loss will benefit these children with sleep-disordered breathing.

Daytime sleepiness is commonly reported by family members and may be secondary to another sleep disorder, such as sleep-disordered breathing, or it may represent a primary sleep disturbance. Greenswag (1987) found that sleepiness was a problem in 231 of 232 individuals with Prader-Willi syndrome. Clarke, Waters, and Corbett (1989) surveyed 64 cases and suggested this daytime sleep abnormality was not related to the degree of obesity. Sleepiness occurred when the individuals were not occupied, e.g., when watching television or traveling by car. An abnormality in sleep pattern characterized by sleep onset REM also has been reported (Vela-Bueno et al., 1984) that could be the result of a sleep disorder, such as narcolepsy or sleep-disordered breathing, or represent a primary circadian disturbance of REM sleep. In addition, these authors reported initial insomnia and increased nocturnal sleep duration. They concluded that hypothalamic dysfunction was the most likely cause of excessive daytime sleepiness. This interpretation was challenged by Spielman, Thorpy, and Sher (1985) who suggested shortened REM latency may result from chronic REM sleep deprivation due to sleep-related hypopnea.

The problem of daytime sleepiness has been reported as a clinical symptom but has not been objectively evaluated in this syndrome. Vela-Bueno et al. (1984) reported on parental observations of daytime sleepiness in 8 of their 9 cases. Their one case without excessive sleepiness could either represent error introduced by the subjective nature of the data or indicate daytime sleepiness is common but not a characteristic or primary symptom of the disorder. Objective assessment of the daytime sleepiness is needed to determine both prevalence and severity of the symptom and also to test for a possible secondary relationship to other features of the syndrome, such as obesity or sleep-disordered breathing.

There is lack of agreement regarding occurrence of sleep onset REM. Although this was reported in 5 of 9 cases by Vela-Bueno et al. (1984), Friedman et al. (1984) did not comment on sleep onset REM in the 9 patients they studied, presumably because this abnormality was not observed in their study. The 5 cases with sleep onset REM were aged 17 or younger and, except for excessive daytime sleepiness, did not have symptoms of narcolepsy. Neither of these investigators used daytime nap studies (Multiple Sleep Latency Test) to look for the sleep onset REM ordinarily seen in daytime nap studies of narcoleptics. However, Harris and Allen (1985) completed multiple sleep latency tests and found that daytime sleepiness persisted, although to a lesser degree.

Phenylketonuria

Petre-Quadens (1972) conducted polysomnograms in subjects with phenylketonuria (Chapter 11.3) and compared the data with those of normal subjects of the same age. These authors found that those with phenylketonuria showed a decreased percentage of active sleep and "indeterminate sleep." But Schulte et al. (1973) reported no significant differences in sleep stages between patients with the untreated condition, patients with the treated condition, and age-matched normal controls. However, increased spindle activity was found in cases of phenylketonuria.

Bilirubinemia

High levels of bilirubin may be associated with excessive drowsiness, poor feedings, and diffuse hypotonia. In a study of the sleep/wake rhythm of infants with a bilirubin level of 10 to 20 mg/dl, Prechtl, Theorell, and Blair (1973) found a reduced amount of time spent in the waking state compared to a control group. The duration of NREM sleep was in the normal range, but REM sleep periods were significantly prolonged. Jaundiced infants appeared very sleepy and spent longer periods in REM sleep. Their symptoms might be caused by the neurotoxic effects of bilirubin on systems linked to REM sleep.

Tuberous Sclerosis

Sleep problems are commonly reported in tuberous sclerosis (Chapter 10.7) Hunt (Hunt and Stores, 1994) carried out a mail questionnaire survey on a group of patients with tuberous sclerosis, which included 201 children, age range from 6 months to 16 years. Parents reported difficulties in settling down for bed in 68%, difficulty maintaining sleep with nighttime waking in 58%, and early morning waking in 57%. Over 90% of those individuals with tuberous sclerosis with mental retardation had sleep difficulties. Sleep problems were of particular concern in children who had uncontrolled seizures. Current seizure disorder and daytime behavioral problems were significantly associated with sleep disturbance. Families reported no clear-cut reduction in these various sleep problems with increasing age. In this disorder, there seems to be a strong relationship between sleep disturbance and seizures. Moreover, Curatolo, Cusmai, and Cortesi (1992) found that night waking problems in a series of children with tuberous sclerosis were associated with low cognitive functioning, seizures, and the extent of behavioral disturbance. Whether treatment of seizures leads to better nighttime sleep and subsequently improved behavior is not clear.

Lesch-Nyhan Disease

Children with Lesch-Nyhan disease (Chapter 11.1) have been reported to show more nighttime waking when compared to healthy controls (Mizuno et al., 1979). These authors investigated the relationship of self-injury to sleep stage and found that self-mutilation could occur in any sleep stage, although it was least common in deep stages 3 and 4 sleep. Other authors have reported night terrors in individuals with Lesch-Nyhan disease.

Joubert Syndrome

Joubert syndrome is a mental retardation syndrome with associated abnormal eye movements, ataxia, and agenesis of the cerebellar vermis. Episodes of tachypnea may occur during sleep. Bolthauser et al. (1980) suggested that the tachypneic spells occurred primarily in non-REM sleep and were associated with periods of apnea. These authors reported normal sleep structure.

Mucopolysaccharidoses

The mucopolysaccharidoses are a group of inborn errors of metabolism (see Chapter 11.6). In the mucopolysaccharidoses, glycosaminoglycans accumulate in various organs systemically and produce abnormalities of the central nervous system, soft tissues, and musculoskeletal systems. Obstructive airway disease, including breathing-related sleep disorders, is not uncommon (Shapiro, Strome, and Crocker, 1985). Mahowald et al. (1989) carried out sleep studies in children and adults with several mucopolysaccharidoses (Hurler, Hunter, or Morquio syndromes). Obstructive sleep apnea or severe hypercapnia was common and demonstrated to be worse during REM sleep. The cause may relate to skeletal malformations involving the cervical spine and thorax as well as the accumulation of metabolic products in soft tissues. In the Sanfilippo syndrome, obstructive sleep apnea is not an important feature, most likely because of the mildness of the somatic and skeletal problems, although other sleep problems may occur. The recognition of obstructive sleep apnea is important not only for medical reasons but also because of the daytime effects of sleep deprivation on behavior. Treatment of obstructive sleep apnea may utilize nocturnal oxygen administration or, in some instances, nasal continuous positive airway pressure. With the recent use of bone marrow transplantation as a way of reducing soft tissue hypertrophy, sleep apnea could potentially improve as well.

Menkes' Kinky Hair Disease

Menkes' kinky hair disease is characterized by kinky hair, convulsions, mental retardation, and low blood levels of copper and ceruloplasmin; the disease is thought to be the consequence of an inherited defect in copper absorption. The EEGs of these children show a spike wave complex, hysarrhythmia, or both (French, Sherard, and Lubell, 1972).

Hashimoto, Kawano, and Hiura (1982) studied an all-night polygraphic recording of a 5-month-old infant with Menkes' kinky hair disease and found increased waking periods, with frequent awakening every 60 to 120 minutes. They noted a marked decrease in quiet sleep and a marked increase in active and intermediate sleep. The infant appeared to have a circadian sleep/wake rhythm that was not fully developed. Neither insomnia nor sleep stages during the night improved after the administration of copper.

The sleep disturbances of the disease have been attributed to thalamic and hypothalamic disorders because the results of autopsy studies have shown marked degeneration of the thalamus (Aguilar et al. 1966; Hashimoto, Kawano, and Hiura, 1982; Iwata, Hirano, and French, 1980; Menkes, Alter, and Steigler, 1962), and laboratory studies have shown hypersecretion of thyrotropin-releasing hormone, follicle stimulating hormone, luteinizing hormone-releasing hormone, and luteinizing hormone (Hashimoto, Kawano, and Hiura, 1982).

Hypothyroidism (Cretinism)

In patients with hypothyroidism, there is a general decrease in the amplitude and frequency of the EEG pattern, a predominance of monomorphic theta activity, and a decrease in the frequency or disappearance of alpha waves (D'Avignon and Melin, 1949; Harris, Rovene, and Prior, 1965; Nieman, 1961). Schultz and co-workers (1968) studied hypothyroid infants by means of serial polygraphic recordings and observed the delay of sleep EEG development: The immature EEG pattern of trace alternans was still present at 11.5 weeks in hypothyroid infants, whereas normal infants did not show this pattern beyond 4 to 8 weeks of age. Either a delay in development or a decrease in the incidence of sleep spindles was evident in all hypothyroid infants. After thyroid therapy, some hypothyroid infants developed a normal number of spindles, but others continued to show fewer spindles than normal infants. Those infants who developed normal spindle activity tended to demonstrate normal developmental quotients at follow-up examination, whereas those who did not showed lower developmental quotients.

Sleep Disturbance in Seizure Disorders

Although there are a variety of seizure disorders and in mentally retarded persons the underlying cause, physiological type, and severity may vary, sleep disturbances commonly occur in disabled persons with seizures. For those sleep disturbances not directly attributable to a seizure disorder, physiological changes include increased wakefulness after sleep onset, reduction in REM sleep, and difficulty in classifying sleep epochs with increased shifting between one sleep stage and another and changes in duration of sleep stages when contrasted to normal subjects. Decreased time spent in non-REM sleep has also been noted. Seizures during sleep worsen sleep pathology. When seizures are particularly severe, it is difficult to characterize the sleep stage because of excessive slowing and the absence of physiological features, such as sleep spindles or K-complexes. In one study (Declerck et al., 1982), 23.5% were in this category. Changes in electrical activity during sleep may relate to night wakings. Night disturbances in behavior are common in children, and diagnostic confusion may arise regarding whether a sleep disorder, night time seizures, or both are present. In-home video and physiological monitoring can be helpful to resolve the diagnosis. (Stores, 1991).

Infantile Spasms

During infantile spasms, reductions in REM sleep and reduction in total sleep time have been reported (Hrachovy, Frost, and Kellaway, 1981). Because structures in the pons are important in the regulation of REM sleep, it has been suggested that dysfunction in infantile spasms occurs at the pontine level. In infantile spasms, REM sleep may become disorganized and treatment with ACTH may regularize REM activity, although findings have been inconsistent in this regard. Zaiwalla and Stores (1989) have reported preliminary findings of difficulty getting to sleep, restless sleep, nonrestorative sleep, frequent wakings, and daytime sleepiness by parents of a group of children with seizure disorders of mixed etiology. Those children with nonrestorative sleep had more subclinical arousals than a control group on polysomnography. Additional investigations are needed to clarify the effect of seizures on sleep, however, in those syndromes, such as tuberous sclerosis, where seizure disorders are common. An evaluation of nighttime seizures and appropriate medication adjustment is in order.

In addition to seizures, physical discomfort at night related to disabling conditions, such as muscle spasms in children with cerebral palsy, difficulty in changing posture in bed, bed-wetting, and skin irritations may all disrupt sleep. Consequently, the child's physical care and comfort are important issues to attend to in a sleep assessment.

SUMMARY

The sleep/wake rhythm is a circadian biological rhythm that provides for adaptation to the environment. Sleep disorders are one result of a disordered biological clock. Mentally retarded and brain-impaired children may lack the capability to adjust themselves to the environment and have sleep/wake rhythm disturbances.

The mechanisms that maintain the human biological clock have not yet been established. In chronobiological studies in animals, the hypothalamic area, including the suprachiasmatic nuclei, has been found to play an important role in regulating the clock mechanism. The same conclusion has not yet been reached for humans. Many mentally retarded or brain-impaired children who have sleep/wake disorders probably have malfunctions in specific parts of the brain that are directly responsible for those disorders. An understanding of the mechanisms of the human biological clock is indispensable for the treatment of mentally retarded or brain-impaired children. Investigations of disordered sleep/wake rhythm in relation to morphological and/or biochemical changes could provide important information toward such an understanding.

REFERENCES

Achenbach, T.M., and Edelbrock, C.S. (1981). Behavioral problems and competencies reported by parents of normal and disturbed children aged four through sixteen. *Monograph, Society for Research in Child Development,* 46:1.

Adair, R.H., and Bauchner, H. (1993, April). Sleep problems in children. *Current Problems in Pediatrics,* pp. 161–162.

Aguilar, M.J., Chadwick, D.V., Okuyama, K., and Kamoshita, S. (1966). Kinky hair disease: I. Clinical and pathological features. *Journal of Neuropathology and Experimental Neurology,* 25:507–522.

Allen, R.P., Singer, H.S., Brown, J.E., and Salam, M.M. (1992). Sleep problems in Tourette syndrome: A primary or unrelated problem. *Pediatric Neurology,* 8:275–280.

American Psychiatric Association, Committee on Nomenclature and Statistics. (1994). *Diagnostic and statistical manual of mental disorders,* 4th ed. Author, Washington, DC.

Aschoff, J. (1954). Zeitgeber der tierischen Tagesperiodik. *Naturwissenschaften,* 431:49–56.

Association of Professional Sleep Societies, Sleep Disorders Classification Committee. (1979). *Diagnostic classification of sleep and arousal disorders.* Author, Rochester, MN.

Barabas, G., Matthews, W.S., and Ferrari, M. (1984a). Somnambulism in children with Tourette syndrome. *Developmental Medicine and Child Neurology,* 26:457–460.

______, ______, and ______. (1984b). Disorders of arousal in Gilles de la Tourette's disorder. *Neurology,* 34:815–817.

Bartlett, L.B., Rooney, V., and Spedding, S. (1985). Nocturnal difficulties in a population of mentally handicapped children. *British Journal of Mental Subnormality,* 31:54–59.

Bock, R., and Goldberger, L. (1985). Tonic, phasic and cortical arousal in Gilles de la Tourette's disorder. *Journal of Neurology, Neurosurgery and Psychiatry,* 48:535–544.

Bolthauser, E., Herdan, M., Dumermuth, G., and Isler, W. (1980). Joubert syndrome: Clinical and polygraphic observations in a further case. *Neuropediatrics,* 12:181–191.

Busby, K., Firestone, P., and Pivik, R.T. (1981). Sleep patterns in hyperkinetic and normal children. *Sleep,* 4:366–383.

______, and Pivik, R.T. (1985). Auditory arousal thresholds during sleep in hyperkinetic children. *Sleep,* 8:332–341.

Chatoor, I., Wells, K.C., Conners, K.C., Seidel, W.T., and Shaw, D. (1983). The effects of nocturnally administered stimulant medication on EEG sleep and behavior in hyperactive children. *Journal of the American Academy of Child and Adolescent Psychiatry,* 22:337–342.

Clarke, D.J., Waters, J., and Corbett, J.A. (1989). Adults with Prader-Willi syndrome: Abnormalities of sleep and behaviour. *Journal of the Royal Society of Medicine,* 82:21–24.

Clausen, J., Sersen, E.A., and Lidsky, A. (1977).

Sleep patterns in mental retardation: Down's syndrome. *Electroencephalography and Clinical Neurophysiology,* 43:183–191.

Clements, J., Wing, L., and Dunn, G. (1986). Sleep problems in handicapped children: A preliminary study. *Journal of Child Psychology and Psychiatry,* 27:399–407.

Coble, P.A., Kupfer, D.J., Reynolds, C.F., and Houck, P. (1987). EEG sleep of healthy children 6 to 12 years of age. In C. Guilleminault (ed.), *Sleep and its disorders in children.* Raven Press, New York.

______, Taska, L.S., Kupfer, D.J., Kazdin, A.E., Unis, A., and French, N. (1984). EEG sleep `abnormalties' in preadolescent boys with a diagnosis of conduct disorder. *Journal of the American Academy of Child and Adolescent Psychiatry,* 23:438–447.

Cunningham, C., Sloper, T., Rangecroft, A., Knussen, C., Lennings, C., Dixon, I., and Reeves, D. (1986). *The effects of early intervention on the occurrence and nature of behaviour problems in children with Down's syndrome.* Final report to DHSS, Hester Adrian Research Centre, University of Manchester.

Curatolo, P., Cusmai, R., and Cortesi, F. (November 1991). *Sleep EEG findings and epilepsy in tuberous sclerosis: Relationship with psychiatric aspects.* Presentation to the Society for the Study of Behavioural Phenotypes, Welshpool, UK.

Czeisler, C.A., Richardson, G.S., Zimmerman, J.C., Moore-Ede, M.C., and Weitzman, E.D. (1981). Entrainment of human circadian rhythms by light dark cycles: A reassessment. *Photochemistry and Photobiology,* 34:239–247.

Dahl, R.E., and Puig-Antich, J. (1990). Sleep disturbances in child and adolescent psychiatric disorders. *Pediatrician,* 17:32–37.

D'Avignon, M., and Melin, K.A. (1949). The electroencephalogram in congenital hypothyrosis. *Acta Paediatrica (Uppsala),* 38:37–44.

Declerck, A.C., Wauquier, A., Sijben-Kiggen, R., and Martens, W. (1982). A normative study of sleep in different forms of epilepsy. In M.B. Sterman, M.N. Shouse, and P. Passouant (eds.), *Sleep and epilepsy.* Academic Press, New York.

DeMyer, M.K. (1979). *Parents and children in autism,* pp. 89–100. V.H. Winston & Sons, Washington, DC.

Drake, M.E., Hietter, S.A., Bogner, J.E., and Andrews, J.M. (1992). Cassette EEG sleep recordings in Gilles de la Tourette syndrome. *Clinical Electroencephalography,* 23:142–146.

Dreyfus-Brisac, C., and Monod, N. (1970). Sleep and brain malformation in abnormal newborn infants. *Neuropaediatrie,* 1:354–366.

Ellingson, R.J., and Peters, J.F. (1980a). Development of EEG and daytime sleep patterns in normal full-term infants during the first 3 months of life: Longitudinal observations. *Electroencephalography and Clinical Neurophysiology,* 49:112–124.

______, and ______. (1980b). Development of EEG and daytime sleep patterns in normal full-term infants during the first year of life: Longitudinal observations. *Electroencephalography and Clinical Neurophysiology,* 50:475–486.

Erenberg, G. (1985). Sleep disorders in Gilles de la Tourette's disorder. *Neurology,* 35:1397.

Ferber, R. (1985). *Solve your child's sleep problem.* Simon & Schuster, New York.

Foulkes, D. (1982). *Children's dreams: Longitudinal studies.* John Wiley, New York.

French, J.H., Sherard, E.S., and Lubell, H. (1972). Trichopoliodystrophy: I. Report of a case and biochemical studies. *Archives of Neurology,* 26:229–244.

Friedman, E., Ferber, R., Wharton, R., and Dietz, D. (1984). Sleep apnea in Prader Willi syndrome. *Sleep,* 13:142.

Fukuma, E., Umezawa, Y., Kobayashi, K., and Motoike, M. (1974). Polygraphic study on the nocturnal sleep of children with Down's syndrome and endogenous mental retardation. *Folia Psychiatrica Neurologica Japanica,* 28:333–345.

Gigli, G.L., Grubar, J.C., Colognola, R.M., Amata, M.T., Pollicina, C., Ferri, R., Musumeci, S.A., and Bergonzi, P. (1987). Butoctamide hydrogen succinate and intensive learning sessions: Effect on night sleep of Down's syndrome patients. *Sleep,* 10:563–569.

Glaze, D.G., Frost, J.D., and Jankovic, J. (1983). Sleep in Gilles de la Tourette syndrome: Disorder of arousal. *Neurology,* 33:586–592.

Goetz, F., Bishop, J., and Halberg, F. (1976). Timing of single daily meal influences relations among human circadian rhythms in urinary cyclic AMP and hemic glucagon, insulin and iron. *Experientia,* 32:1081–1084.

Goldie, L., Curtis, J.A.H., Svendsen, V., and Roberton, N.R.C. (1968). Abnormal sleep rhythms in mongol babies. *Lancet,* i:229–230.

Greenhill, L., Puig-Antich, J., Goetz, R., Hanlon, C., and Davies, M. (1983). Sleep architecture and REM sleep measures in prepubertal children with attention deficit disorder with hyperactivity. *Sleep,* 6:91–101.

Greenswag, L.R. (1987). Adults with Prader-Willi syndrome: A survey of 232 cases. *Developmental Medicine and Child Neurology,* 29:145–152.

Haig, J.R., Schroeder, C.S., and Schroeder, S.R. (1974). Effects of methylphenidate on hyperactive children's sleep. *Psychopharmacologia,* 37:185–188.

Halberg, F., Halberg, E., Barnum, C.P., and Bittner, J.J. (1959). Physiologic 24-hour periodicity in human beings and mice, the lightening regimen and daily routine. In R.B. Withrow (ed.), *Photoperiodism and related phenomena in plants and animals.* American Association for the Advancement of Science, Washington, DC. Publication 55:803–873.

Hamaguchi, H., Hashimoto, T., Mori, K., and Tayama, M. (1989). Sleep in the Down's syndrome. *Brain Development,* 11:399–406.

Harris, J.C., and Allen, R.P. (1985). Excessive daytime sleepiness in the Prader Willi syndrome: Sleep apnea or idiopathic hypersomnolence. *Proceedings of the American Academy of Child Psychiatry,* 1:27.

Harris, R., Rovene, M.D., and Prior, P.F. (1965). Electroencephalographic studies in infants and children with hypothyroidism. *Archives of Diseases in Childhood,* 40:612–617.

Hashimoto, T., Kawano, N., and Hiura, K. (1982). Sleep polygraphic studies of Menkes' kinky hair disease: Effect of copper administration. *Rinsho Noha,* 24:418–422. Quoted from Okawa, M., and Sasaki, H. (1987). Sleep disorders in mentally retarded and brain-impaired children. In C. Guilleminault (ed.), *Sleep and its disorders in children.* Raven Press, New York.

Hertz, G., Cataletto, M., Feinsilver, S.H., and Angulo, M. (1993). Sleep and breathing patterns in patients with Prader Willi syndrome (PWS): Effects of age and gender. *Sleep,* 16:366–371.

Hoshino, Y., Watanabe, H., Yashima, Y., Kaneko, M., and Kumashiro, H. (1984). An investigation on sleep disturbance of autistic children. *Folia Psychiatrica Neurologica Japanica,* 38:45–51.

Howlin, P. (1984). A brief report on the elimination of long term sleeping problems in a 6-year-old autistic boy. *Behavioural Psychotherapy,* 12:257–260.

Hrachovy, R.A., Frost, J.D., and Kellaway, P. (1981). Sleep characteristics in infantile spasms. *Neurology,* 31:688–694.

Hunt, A., and Stores (1994). Sleep disorder and epilepsy in children with tuberous sclerosis: A questionnaire-based study. *Developmental Medicine and Child Neurology,* 36:108–115.

Inamura, K. (1984). Sleep-wake patterns in autistic children. *Japanese Journal of Child and Adolescent Psychiatry,* 25:205–217.

Iwata, M., Hirano, A., and French, J.H. (1980). Degeneration of the thalamic nuclei in X-chromosome-linked copper malabsorption (Mendes' kinky hair disease). *Shinkei Kenkyu No Shinpo,* 24:304–314.

Kaplan, B.J., McNichol, J., Conte, R.A., and Moghadam, H.K. (1987). Sleep disturbance in preschool-aged hyperactive and nonhyperactive children. *Pediatrics,* 6:839–844.

Kleitman, N., and Engelman, T.G. (1953). Sleep characteristics of infants. *Journal of Applied Physiology,* 7:169–282.

Mahowald, M.W., Iber, C., Rosen, G.M., Krivitt, W., Ramsay, N.K.C., Kersey, J.H., Belani, K., and Whitley, C.B. (1989). Sleep disordered breathing in the mucopolysaccharidoses. *Sleep Research,* 18:348.

McCoy, K.S., Koopman, C.F., and Taussig, L.M. (1981). Sleep related breathing disorders. *American Journal of Otolaryngology,* 2:228–239.

Meier-Koll, A., Hall, U., Hellwing, U., Kott, G., and Meier-Koll, V. (1978). A biological oscillator system and the development of sleep-waking behavior during early infancy. *Chronobiologia,* 5:425–440.

Mendelson, W.B., Caine, E.D., Goyer, P., Ebert, M., and Gillin, J.C. (1980). Sleep in Gilles de la Tourette syndrome. *Biological Psychiatry,* 15:339–343.

Menkes, J.H., Alter, M., and Steigler, G.K. (1962). A sex-linked recessive disorder with retardation of growth, peculiar hair and focal cerebral and cerebellar degeneration. *Pediatrics,* 29:764–779.

Mercier, L., Pivik, R.T., and Busby, K. (1993). Sleep patterns in reading disabled children. *Sleep,* 16:207–215.

Miles, L.E., and Wilson, M.A. (1977). High incidence of cyclic sleep wake disorders in the blind. *Sleep Research,* 6:192.

Mizuno, T., Reiko Ohta, M.A., Kodama, K., Kitazumi, E., Mimejima, N., Takeishi, M., and Segawa, M. (1979). Self-mutilation and sleep stage in the Lesch-Nyhan syndrome. *Brain Development,* 2:121–125.

Moldofsky, H., Tullis, C., and Lamon, R. (1974). Multiple tic syndrome (Gilles de la Tourette's disorder). *Journal of Nervous and Mental Disease,* 15:282–292.

Monod, N., and Guidasci, S. (1976). Sleep and brain malformation in the neonatal period. *Neuropaediatrie,* 7:229–249.

Nee, L.E., Caine, N.D., Polinsky, R.J., Eldridge, R., and Ebert, M.H. (1980). Gilles de la Tourette syndrome. Clinical and family study of 50 cases. *Annals of Neurology,* 7:41–49.

Nieman, E.A. (1961). The electroencephalogram in congenital hypothyroidism: A study of 10 cases. *Journal of Neurology, Neurosurgury, and Psychiatry,* 24:50–57.

Okawa, M., Nanami, T., Wada, T., Shimizu, T., Sasaki, H., and Hishikawa, Y. (1985). Congenital blind children with circadian sleep-waking rhythm disorder. *Sleep Research,* 14:309.

______, and Sasaki, H. (1987). Sleep disorders in mentally retarded and brain-impaired children. In C. Guilleminault (ed.), *Sleep and its disorders in children.* Raven Press, New York.

Onheiber, P., White, P.T., DeMyer, M.K., and Ottinger, D.R. (1964). Sleep and dream patterns of child schizophrenics. *Archives of General Psychiatry,* 12:568–571.

Orenstein, D.M., Boat, T.F., Owens, R.P., Horowitz, J.G., Primiano, F.P., Jr., Germann, K., and Doershuk, C.F. (1980). The obesity hypoventilation syndrome in children with Prader-Willi syndrome: A possible role for familial decreased response to carbon dioxide. *Journal of Pediatrics,* 97:765–767.

______, ______, ______, Stern, R.C., Doershuk, C.F., and Light, M.S. (1977). Progesterone treatment of the obesity hypoventilation syndrome in a child. *Journal of Pediatrics,* 90:477–479.

Ornitz, E.M. (1978). Neurophysiologic studies. In M. Rutter and E. Schopler (eds.), *Autism: A reappraisal of concepts and treatment.* Plenum Press, New York.

Petre-Quadens, O. (1972). Sleep in mental retardation. In C.D. Clemente, D.P. Purpura, and F.E. Mayer (eds.), *Sleep and the maturing nervous system,* pp. 384–417. Academic Press, New York.

______, and De Lee, C. (1975). 5hydroxtryptophan and sleep in Down's syndrome. *Journal of the Neurological Sciences,* 26:443–453.

Prechtl, H.F.R., Theorell, K., and Blair, A.W. (1973). Behavioural state cycles in abnormal infants. *Developmental Medicine and Child Neurology,* 15:606–615.

Price, V.A., Coates, T.J., Thoresen, C.E., and Grinstead, O.A. (1978). Prevalence and correlates of poor sleep among adolescents. *American Journal of Diseases of Children,* 132:583–586.

Robertson, M.M., Trimble, M.R., and Lees, A.J. (1988). The psychopathology of the Gilles de la Tourette syndrome: A phenomenological analysis. *British Journal of Psychiatry,* 152:383–390.

Roffwarg, H.P., Muzio, J.N., and Dement, W.C. (1966). Ontogenic development of the human sleep-dream cycle: The prime role of dreaming sleep in early life may be in the development of the central nervous system. *Science,* 152:604–619.

Rusak, B. (1977). The role of the suprachiasmatic nuclei in the generation of circadian rhythms in the golden hamster, *Mesocricetus auratus. Journal of Comparative Physiology,* 118:145–164.

Schulte, F.J., Kaiser, H.J., Engelbart, S., Bell, E.F., Castell, R., and Lenard, H.G. (1973). Sleep patterns in hyperphenylalanaemia: A lesson on serotonin to be learned from phenylketonuria. *Pediatric Research,* 7:588–599.

Schultz, M., Schulte, F.J., Akiyama, Y., and Parmelee, A.H. (1968). Development of electroencephalographic sleep phenomena in hypothyroid infants. *Electroencephalography and Clinical Neurophysiology,* 25:351–358.

Segawa, M. (1985). Circadian rhythm in early infantile autism. *Shinkei Kenkyu No Shinpo,* 29:140–153.

Shapiro, J., Strome, M., and Crocker, A.C. (1985). Airway obstruction and sleep apnea in Hurler and Hunter syndromes. *Annals of Otology, Rhinology and Laryngology,* 94:458–461.

Shibagaki, M., and Kiyono, S. (1983). The first phase of nocturnal sleep in mentally retarded children. *Electroencephalography and Clinical Neurophysiology,* 55:286–289.

Silverman, M. (1988). Airway obstruction and sleep disruption in Down's syndrome. *British Medical Journal,* 296:1618–1619.

Simeon, J. (1987). Treatment of sleep disturbances in children: Recent advances. In J.D. Noshpitz (ed.), *Basic handbook of child psychiatry,* Vol. 5, pp. 470–478. Basic Books, New York.

Small, A. Hibi, S., and Feinberg, I. (1971). Effects of dextroamphetamine sulfate on EEG patterns of hyperactive children. *Archives of General Psychiatry,* 25:369–380.

Spielman, A.J., Thorpy, M.J., and Sher, A. (1985). [Letter]. *Archives of Neurology,* 42:110.

Stebbens, V.A., Dennis, J., Samuels, M.P., Croft, C.B., and Southall, D.P. (1991). Sleep-related upper airway obstruction in a cohort with Down's syndrome. *Archives of Diseases in Childhood,* 66:1333–1338.

Stores, G. (1991) Confusions concerning sleep disorders and the epilepsies in children and adolescents. *British Journal of Psychiatry* 158:1–7.

______, (1992). Sleep disorders. *Current Paediatrics,* 2:145–150.

Summers, J.S., Lynch, P.S., Harris, J.C., Burke, J.C., Allison, D.B., and Sandler, L. (1992). A combined behavioral/pharmacological treatment of sleep-wake schedule disorder in Angelman syndrome. *Journal of Developmental and Behavioral Pediatrics,* 13:284–287.

Terr, L. (1987). Nightmares in children. In C. Guilleminault (ed.), *Sleep and its disorders in children,* pp. 231–232. Raven Press, New York.

Vela-Bueno, A., Kales, A., Soldatos, C.R., Dobladez-Blanco, B., Compos-Castello, J., Espino-Hurtado, P., and Olivan-Palacios, J. (1984). Sleep in the Prader-Willi syndrome: Clinical and polygraphic findings. *Archives of Neurology,* 4:294–296.

Vernikos-Danellis, J., and Winget, C.M. (1979). The importance of light, postural and social cues in the regulation of the plasma cortisol rhythms in man. In A. Reinberg and F. Halberg (eds.), *Chronopharmacology,* pp. 101–106. Pergamon Press, New York.

Wever, R.A. (1979). *The circadian system of man: Results of experiments under temporal isolation.* Springer-Verlag, New York.

Wing, L. (1966). *Early childhood autism: Clinical, educational and social aspects.* Pergamon Press, New York.

Zaiwalla, Z., and Stores, G. (1989). Sleep and arousal disorders in children with epilepsy. *Sleep Research,* 18:129.

CHAPTER 17

DESTRUCTIVE BEHAVIOR: AGGRESSION AND SELF-INJURY

Destructive behavior that is manifested as injury to self, to others, or to property is a major problem in developmental neuropsychiatric disorders, particularly in mentally retarded persons. Among the manifestations of destructive behavior, aggression toward others and self-injurious behavior (SIB) are of particular concern for psychiatrists and other health professionals because of their severity, frequency, and resistance to treatment. Aggression and self-injury are the major behavior problems that result in the failure of community placement for children and adolescents with developmental disorders. In particular, self-injury poses serious therapeutic, economic, and ethical dilemmas for caregivers. Prevention of self-mutilation may require restraints that are morally unacceptable, or a density of staff supervision that hospitals or institutions have great difficulty in funding. Moreover, there is considerable controversy regarding treatment, particularly the use of aversive procedures. In a comprehensive treatment program for destructive behavior, the psychiatrist assumes a central role as the leader, or core member, of an interdisciplinary team that develops an integrated approach to treatment.

Until recently, the primary emphasis in studies of self-injury focused on environmental determinants; there is substantial data on the effects of environmental contingencies on SIB. Behavior modification treatment procedures have been the most commonly used forms of treatment of self-injurious behavior (Bachman, 1972; Frankel and Simmons, 1976; Johnson and Baumeister, 1978; Maisto, Baumeister, and Maisto, 1978; Picker, Poling, and Parker, 1979; Russo, Carr, and Lovaas, 1980; Schroeder et al., 1978). However, behavioral treatment techniques may not be successful in reducing self-injury, or if they are initially effective, then in maintaining the improvement in behavior. Carr (1977) has convincingly argued that self-injury is multiply determined. Neurobiological factors must be considered as well as environmental ones. Knowledge about the possible biological mechanisms involved in self-injury might be employed in conjunction with other treatment procedures for more effective treatment and to reduce the considerable cost involved in both initial treatment and generalization of treatment into a home or community setting.

In this chapter aggression and self-injury in mentally retarded persons are discussed in regard to prevalence, theoretical approaches to aggression, definition, classification, differential diagnosis, predisposing factors, etiologic models, conditions associated with self-injury, natural history, assessment, diagnostic formulation; selection of treatment, and medicolegal issues. The focus is primarily on self-injurious behavior.

PREVALENCE

Aggression

The reported prevalence rate of aggressive behavior in severely retarded persons has been quite variable because of lack of consistency in the definition of aggressive acts. Ross (1972) reported at least monthly aggressive acts toward persons and property in 27% of residents in state facilities for the mentally disabled in California. Other investigators have reported rates of 30% in public institutions and 16% in community facilities (Hill and Bruininks, 1984). Notably, aggressive behavior generally accounted for the majority of readmissions to these facilities, 42% and 38%, respectively. Treatment of aggressive behaviors is of particular importance because aggression may lead to reduced services and more restrictive programming (Mullick and Schroeder, 1980).

Self-Injurious Behavior

Stereotypy and self-injury may be seen in normally intelligent infants and in mentally retarded individuals; head banging is the most common typography (Abe, Oda, and Amatomi, 1984). De Lissovoy (1962) found the onset of head banging in children began at about 8 months of age and disappeared in their normally intelligent group by 36 months of age. Other stereotyped movements, such as self-rocking, began in early life before the onset of head banging. In two other studies involving nearly 2,000 children, the incidence of head banging was 3.6% to 6.5% and was more common in males than in females, the ratio being 3.5 to 1 (Kravitz et al., 1960). Ordinarily, head banging ceased to occur after 32 months of age. Kravitz et al. (1960) found self-injurious behavior in about 20% of the siblings of head bangers they studied, suggesting a familial pattern. The most common factor preceding the onset of head banging was the eruption of teeth—usually central and lateral incisors. In another study, 15 head bangers were compared to matched controls, and the only statistically significant difference between the two groups was that the head bangers had a higher prevalence of otitis media (De Lissovoy, 1963).

In developmentally disabled persons, Griffin et al. (1987) found a prevalence of self-injurious behavior among 2,663 mentally retarded, autistic, or multiply-disabled children and adolescents in a large community metropolitan school district. They found that 69 individuals (2.6%) had demonstrated self-injurious behavior during the 12 months chosen for the survey; 59% were male and 41% were female. The majority of this group, 83%, were severely or profoundly retarded. The mean age was 10.2 years and the majority (72%) self-injured every day. For those who were 14 years of age or above, the community prevalence was lower, a factor the authors attribute to residential placements for older individuals. The most common topographies were hand biting, head hitting, and head banging. Only one third of the sample were in treatment programs; 8.7% were receiving medications. Medical and psychiatric diagnoses were not provided by the authors.

In contrast to the community setting, self-injurious behavior has been reported in 10% to 17% of institutionalized retarded persons (Baumeister and Rollings, 1976; Schroeder et al., 1978); the lower the IQ, the higher the prevalence rate. Over a 3-year period, Schroeder et al. (1978) surveyed institutional settings and found that cases occurred most frequently in younger children who had associated severe language disabilities, visual impairments, or seizure disorders and who tested in the profoundly retarded range of mental retardation. Other investigators, such as Smeets (1971), also had come to the conclusion that severe mental retardation, accompanied by physiological abnormalities, led to a higher risk for self-injurious behavior in early childhood. The prevalence of the behavior has been reported to peak at adolescence in severely mentally retarded individuals.

In addition to occurring in a heterogeneous group of severely or profoundly mentally retarded individuals, self-injurious behavior is also associated with several specific syndromes which, although associated with mental retardation, show a range in level of intelligence—from severe mental retardation to the low normal range. These are: Lesch-Nyhan disease where self-biting occurs in the majority of cases, Rett's disorder where hand–mouth stereotypes with tissue involvement are characteristic, the fragile X syndrome where hand biting was found in 74% of 37 cases reported (Hagerman et al., 1986), the Cornelia de Lange syndrome, Tourette's disorder where one third of those who are severely involved are symptomatic, the Riley-Day syndrome, and congenital insensitivity to pain where self-injury is common, and although usually accidental, may come under operant control. The high frequency of self-injury is sufficiently characteristic in some of these disorders to be designated as a behavioral phenotype (Nyhan, 1972). In addition, in developmental disorders, such as pervasive developmental disorder, self-injurious behavior is commonly associated, particularly in lower functioning individuals.

THEORETICAL APPROACHES TO AGGRESSION

The traditional psychodynamic approach to aggression focuses on an aggressive drive (Freud, 1922). In self-psychology, the emphasis is on the response to perceived threats to the self. An ethological view addresses adaptation as it relates to those brain mechanisms involved in self-preservation. From a behavioral point, the focus is on the function of the behavior and on what maintains the behavior. The original drive theorist argued that frustration results in the blocking of goal-directed behavior and increases aggressive behavior. A drive theory approach to aggression suggests that aggression could be channeled into less harmful behaviors. Another view is that severe aggressive behavior can be channeled into more directed assertive behavior. Based on a misunderstanding of drive theory, it was suggested the aggressive drive could be reduced by giving it an outlet rather than understanding that aggression is not based on a hydraulic model, but more likely is part of a feedback mechanism involving maintenance of the self-system. Allowing permission to be aggressive generally maintains the behavior rather than reducing it; simple expression is not a cathartic solution for aggression. Behavioral approaches to aggression deal with establishing an interpersonal context for the behavior and considering events that shape and maintain aggressive behavior.

Behavioral Analytic View of Aggression

Rates of aggression may be altered when behavioral interventions are used to rearrange environmental events so that contingent consequences are delivered for aggressive behavior. However, contingency management of consequences may not be enough and antecedent events may also need to be considered. A behavioral analytical approach assumes the aggressive behavior is a learned response that can be affected by environmental events. These events are seen to control aggression because they serve as either antecedent or discriminative stimuli that reinforce the behavior. To understand what is meant by discriminative and by reinforcing stimuli, the approach of experimental analysis of behavior is used. Day (1991) described two types of aggression from a behavioral perspective, namely, elicited aggression that is brought about by antecedent conditions, such as aversive or painful stimulation or the removal or termination of reinforcement; and evoked aggression that is produced through consequent events, either positive reinforcement following an aggressive act, or the removal of negative reinforcement which is contingent on aggressive behavior.

In evaluating antecedent conditions, Carr and Newson (1985) found that rates of aggression were reliably higher under demand when contrasted to nondemand situations. Aggression was found to be highest when followed by social attention rather than removal of task demands.

DEFINITION

Aggressive Behavior

Definitions of an aggressive response differ based on the theoretical approach taken by the author and the target population being described (Fehrenbach and Thelan, 1982). The major considerations are the type or pattern of aggressive response and the intent of the individual. The establishment of intent is difficult, particularly in nonverbal mentally retarded persons, and intervention requires a functional analysis of behavior. Aggressive behavior refers to aggressive acts that have the potential for causing specific injury. An aggressive act may be defined in regard to the result—the infliction of pain on another person (Patterson, 1982)—either physical injury, or psychological injury from aggressive verbalization or threatening behavior. It may also be defined in regard to its object, whether it is directed toward a person or toward a physical object; this is the usual behavioral definition. What finally distinguishes aggressive behavior from nonaggressive behavior is not only the aggressive response itself but its frequency, severity, and the conditions under which aggression occurs. Therefore, a person who exhibits chronic aggression is often someone who destroys property or attempts to injure others in socially inappropriate settings over a long period of time (Day, 1991). Furthermore, because the environmental context is frequently important in establishing aggressive behavior, chronic aggression is considered to be present when the frequency of the behavior limits educational and habilitative activities.

Self-Injurious Behavior

The term "self-injurious behavior" or "SIB" is used when referring to developmentally disabled persons who harm themselves, and the term "deliberate self-harm syndrome" or "DSH" (Pattison and Kahan, 1983) has been proposed to describe self-aggression in individuals with major mental illness and personality disorder. SIB is one of the least understood and most difficult behavior problems to treat in the developmentally disabled population. It is characterized by multiple episodes of physically self-damaging acts.

CLASSIFICATION OF SELF-INJURIOUS BEHAVIOR

The DSM-IV (APA, 1994) classification of stereotypic movement disorder has been changed to allow specification of "with self-injurious behavior" if the behavior results in bodily damage that requires medical treatment or would result in bodily damage if protective measures were not used. The DSM-IV diagnostic criteria are shown in Table 17–1.

The exclusionary criteria "does not meet criteria for pervasive developmental disorder" (included in DSM-III-R) is eliminated in DSM-IV; in fact, self-injurious behavior is commonly a problem in pervasive developmental disorder. The previous designation "stereotypy habit" disorder was eliminated for several reasons. First, stereotypy does not predict self-injury and is not necessarily found in individuals who self-injure. Secondly, the term "habit disorder" is no longer in general use, although it was used in the early classifications in psychiatry. This disorder was the only one in DSM-III-R where the term "habit disorder" appeared. Finally, referral for treatment of stereotypy alone is uncommon; most referrals are for interventions for actual or threatened self-injury. Given the frequency of self-injury in severely retarded persons, a better designation than stereotypic movement disorder with self injurious behavior might simply be "self-injurious behavior disorder."

The essential features of the DSM-IV classification of stereotypic movement disorder are repetitive, seemingly driven, and nonfunctional motor behavior that may include hand shaking or waving, body rocking, head banging, mouthing of objects, self-biting, and picking at skin or bodily orifices. Common topographies include face or head hitting, incessant nose picking, hair pulling, eye and anus gouging, noncommunicative, repetitive vocalizations, breath holding, hyperventilation, and swallowing air (aerophagia). This diagnosis is only given when the disturbance either markedly interferes with normal activities or results in physical injury to the individual that requires medical treatment or

Table 17–1. DSM-IV Criteria for Stereotypic Movement Disorder

307.3 Stereotypic Movement Disorder

A. Repetitive, seemingly driven, and nonfunctional motor behavior (e.g., hand shaking or waving, body rocking, head banging, mouthing of objects, self-biting, picking at skin or bodily orifices, hitting own body).

B. The behavior markedly interferes with normal activities or results in self-inflicted bodily injury that requires medical treatment (or would result in an injury if preventive measures were not used).

C. If Mental Retardation is present, the stereotypic or self-injurious behavior is of sufficient severity to become a focus of treatment.

D. The behavior is not better accounted for by a compulsion (as in Obsessive-Compulsive Disorder), a tic (as in Tic Disorder), a stereotypy that is part of a Pervasive Developmental Disorder, or hair pulling (as in Trichotillomania).

E. The behavior is not due to the direct physiological effects of a substance or a general medical condition.

F. The behavior persists for 4 weeks or longer.

Specify if:

With Self-Injurious Behavior: if the behavior results in bodily damage that requires medical treatment (or would result in bodily damage if protective measures were not used).

From APA, 1994.

would result in injury if preventive measures were not used.

Intentionality is not included in the definition of stereotypic movement disorder as it was for stereotypy habit disorder in DSM-III-R (APA, 1987). In developing the DSM-IV criteria, how to judge intentionality became a major issue for severely mentally retarded persons. By definition, a stereotypy is a meaningless behavior; Hamilton (1985) defines it as a repetitive, nongoal-directed action carried out in a uniform way. Because ascribing intentionality is difficult, this requirement was removed from the criteria in DSM-IV. Some self-injury, for example in Lesch-Nyhan disease, seems not to be a learned behavior and has been described as a behavioral phenotype (Harris, 1987; Nyhan, 1972), yet once initiated, there may be a role for environmental contingencies in its maintenance. It is common for children with this disorder to insist on being restrained because they are unable to control their self-injury—their expressed intention being not to harm themselves.

The term "deliberate self-harm syndrome" (Pattison and Kahan, 1983) has been suggested for individuals with psychiatric disorders who deliberately intend to harm themselves. The proposed diagnostic criteria are shown in Table 17–2.

Pattison and Kahan suggested this term be added to the psychiatric classification to describe forms of deliberate self-harm that may occur associated with major mental illness and personality disorder. Most commonly, deliberate self-harm is linked to feelings of hopelessness or severe anxiety. In the deliberate self-harm syndrome, the individual intends self-harm and ordinarily uses a specific means to carry out the action, e.g., a weapon, such as a knife. Individuals who deliberately self-harm may be diagnosed with psychiatric disorders or may be intoxicated at the time of the behavior but generally do not have the intention of dying. Their clinical course is characterized by many episodes of physically self-damaging acts that are of low lethality. The question about motivation in the deliberate self-harm syndrome is an interesting one because these individuals often state they are deliberately trying to hurt themselves to reduce "tension" in contrast to those with the self-injurious behavior syndrome who are often nonverbal, appear out of control, and self-injure after the onset of a tantrum. Deliberate self-harm has only been described in verbal individuals. In mentally retarded persons, SIB may come under operant control, may be an extension of self-stimulation, but also may be associated with a concurrent mental illness.

Table 17–2. Criteria for Deliberate Self-Harm Syndrome

1. A sudden, irresistible impulse to harm oneself physically.
2. A psychological experience of existing in an intolerable, uncontrollable situation from which one cannot escape.
3. Mounting anxiety, agitation, and anger in response to the perceived situation.
4. Perceptual and cognitive constriction, resulting in a narrowed perspective of the situation and of alternatives to action.
5. Self-inflicted destruction or alteration of body tissues done in a private setting.
6. A rapid, temporary feeling of relief following the act of self- harm.

From Pattison and Kahan, 1983.

DIFFERENTIAL DIAGNOSIS

Self-injurious behaviors can be seen as associated features in various disorders. In such cases, the diagnosis of self-injurious behavior should not be made unless the self-injury leads to a substantial dysfunction and becomes the focus of treatment. When self-injurious behavior is diagnosed, any co-occurring mental disorder should be diagnosed as well. Normal self-stimulatory behaviors in young children, such as thumb sucking, rocking, and head banging, are usually self-limiting and rarely result in tissue damage requiring treatment. Self-stimulatory behaviors associated with blindness in persons not otherwise disabled (so-called blindisms, such as head rocking from side to side or light gazing) usually do not result in dysfunction or in self-injury. Behaviors seen in tic disorder are usually involuntary, nonrhythmic, rapid, exhibited in shorter bursts, and described by the individual as irresistible. Ordinarily, they do not result in self-injury. Factitious disorders are intentional and motivated by psychological need to assume a sick role and may involve deliberate self-harm. In obsessive-compulsive disorders, the person feels driven to perform the act in question (which usually is more complex and ritualistic) in order to prevent or reduce distress. Self-injury may be associated with some behaviors, such as repetitive hand washing. In mentally retarded persons, obsessions may not be elicited, but compulsions may be identified.

In trichotillomania, by definition, the topography (focus and location) of self-injury is limited to hair pulling. Self-mutilation (deliberate self-harm) associated with certain psychotic and personality disorders is premeditated, voluntary, intentional, sporadic, and has a meaning for the individual within the context of the underlying severe mental disorder (e.g., is the result of delusional thinking). Involuntary movements associated with neurological disorders usually follow a typical pattern, and the signs and symptoms of the neurological disorder are present and self-injury usually does not occur.

Stereotypic movement disorder associated with self-injurious behavior and the deliberate self-harm syndrome need to be considered phenomenologically as potentially distinct and distinguishable according to their association with other diagnoses. The topography (focus and location) of the self-injurious behaviors may be extremely varied from person to person and from one point in time to another, in the same person. In some persons with self-injury, self-restraining behaviors can be seen, such as holding hands inside shirts or in pockets. When this is prevented, self-injurious behaviors return; this behavior provides evidence for the intention to prevent self-injury. The psychiatric diagnosis in children and adolescents that is most commonly used with self-injurious behavior (SIB) is the Axis I diagnosis of pervasive developmental disorder: autistic disorder. Thus significant impairments in adaptive behavior, communicative language, and social withdrawal may be present. Self-injury may also occur in association with psychotic disorders and, in particular, self-mutilation (deliberate self-harm) may be linked to somatic delusions.

Signs of chronic tissue damage may be present, depending on the topography (location and focus) of the behaviors in question. These may include cuts, scratches, skin infection, bruises, alopecia areata, bite marks, rectal fissures, foreign bodies in bodily orifices and in gastrointestinal tract, retinal detachment, and abdominal distension (from aerophagia). In addition, if a syndrome associated with mental retardation is present, its signs and symptoms will be present as well. In addition to association with affective disorder and psychosis, self-injury may be associated with disruptive behavior disorders, such as oppositional defiant disorder and conduct disorder (Green, 1967). The Axis III diagnoses most often associated with self-injury are Lesch-Nyhan disease, Cornelia de Lange syndrome, congenital insensitivity to pain, fragile X syndrome, Rett's disorder, Tourette's disorder, and specific diagnostic etiologies of blindness, such as retrolental fibroplasia. Although the focus is generally on SIB in mentally retarded persons, deliberate self-harm does occur and should also be considered because it may be associated with a major psychiatric disorder.

PREDISPOSING FACTORS

Various factors have been hypothesized to underlie the self-injurious behavior. Environmental, psychosocial, and biological theories of causation have been proposed (see section on etiology). Mechanisms that have been implicated include dopaminergic supersensitivity, maintenance of physiological homeostasis through reduction of the level of arousal, reduction of dysphoria through release of endogenous opioids, escape/avoidance (from adversive situations), and self-stimulation. Most probably, these self-injurious behaviors do not represent a single homogeneous disorder and several factors might be involved in their pathogenesis (Szymanski, 1991). For instance, a person exhibiting self-injury, which was initiated by one mechanism, can learn it results in increased attention from the caregivers, and this learned experience might become the factor maintaining the self-injury. Self-injurious behavior is more common in nonstimulating institutional environments, where it may serve the adaptive function of attracting staff attention.

Mental retardation is probably the most important predisposing factor, the risk being higher the more severe the retardation, especially if it is associated with severe sensory deficits (blindness and deafness), pervasive developmental disorders, or painful physical illness in a nonverbal person. Self-injurious behaviors occur in certain mental retardation associated syndromes, such as fragile X, Rett, Cornelia de Lange, and Lesch-Nyhan disease.

ETIOLOGIC MODELS OF SELF-INJURY

Isolation Rearing

Nonhuman primates show considerable self-directed behavior, such as scratching and self-grooming. Other types of self-directed behavior are pathological and typically are seen in animals who experience privation or deprivation early in life, especially rearing apart (the deprivation syndrome). Self-directed behaviors include: (1) self-clasping; using hands or feet to grasp legs, arms, chest, or head; (2) self-orality involving digit sucking; (3) self-aggression consisting of biting, slapping, or hitting body parts; (4) rock/sway back and forth; and (5) saluting, which involves raising a hand to the ipsilateral eye like a salute, occasionally with the thumb pressure against the eyeball. These behaviors may be seen in combination, such as self-clasp with rocking. They have been noted with (1) fear or frustration; (2) when activities are thwarted or escape prevented; (3) apparent dissatisfaction; and (4) when an animal could not adapt to a new situation. Isolation results in limitation of motor activity, lack of parent and peer contact, impaired learning of social skills, and altered affective state.

These forms of self-stimulation and self-mutilation may be sequelae of isolation during sensitive developmental periods. Anderson and Chamove (1980) compared animals that received restricted rearing experience with a control group of feral and group-reared animals. At 5 years of age, the restriction-reared monkeys showed four times more self-aggression than social aggression; the control monkeys were never observed to be self-aggressive. Self-biting occurred in social contexts, such as displacement by a more dominant monkey during social aggression, and when startled by sudden movement of others. Self-biting was noted at less than 3 months, frequently in the context of digit sucking. Goosen and Ribbens (1980) reported self-aggression in individually housed, wild born, stump-tailed macaques that decreased in frequency with social pairings. These behaviors are reported in animals raised in captivity as opposed to feral animals transferred to a zoo. They have been noted in such diverse species as opossums, jackals, hyenas, marmosets, squirrel monkeys, and long-tail monkeys (Meyer-Holzapfel, 1968). Closer to humans is the substantial research that has been conducted with rhesus macaques (Jones and Barraclough, 1978). Isolation-reared males showed self-biting in 50% of the observed sessions, and isolation-reared females in 35%, but nondeprived animals showed virtually no self-injury (Sackett, 1968). An important aspect of the effects of isolation on the pathogenesis of self-injury is that the aberrant behavior may be increased when the organism is placed in a new environment or confronted with stress or novel stimuli (Hutt and Hutt, 1968). The effects of isolated rearing on self-stimulation and self-injury in humans has been suggested by reports of children reared in severely deprived and isolated situations (Davis, 1940, 1946; Freedman and Brown, 1968).

The factors related to the development of self-injury subsequent to isolation are found more often in the early developmental periods. For example, in one study, two groups of animals were reared under conditions that were identical with respect to physical restriction but differed in terms of the amount of visual stimuli, i.e., one group was housed outside and in view of other animals and activities. The visually isolated animals demonstrated greater stereotyped behavior (Mason, 1967). Mason provides two suggestions for the effects of developmental isolation on behavior: (1) the filial response or contact-seeking behavior with the mother to establish attachment which reduces arousal, and (2) exploratory behavior through social and motor play to increase stimulation or arousal. He suggests that behavior, such as a rocking stereotypy, may be a self-provision of passive movement stimulation ordinarily received from the parent and notes that infant monkeys raised with a mobile surrogate do not show rocking whereas those raised with a stationary surrogate do rock, indicating the importance of movement stimulation. Subsequently (Mason and Capitanio, 1988), he reported that experience with an animate surrogate (dog) leads to both attachment and increased environmental responsiveness. With regard to increased arousal, Mason suggests that primates who are deprived of general environmental stimulation have a motivational disturbance and become overwhelmed and hyperexcitable in new and novel situations. They are fearful or extremely aggressive; males may be sexually inadequate, and females, maternally inadequate.

The most severe forms of self-injury occur in animals that are the most agitated, and self-injury may lead to reduced agitation. This could be a homeostatic mechanism elicited in severely socially deprived environments (Jones, 1982). Another means of reducing arousal is autogrooming or allogrooming. Allogrooming leads to reduced arousal and because an isolated animal has no companion, it may groom itself, resulting in stereotypy and perhaps self-injury. Goosen and Ribbens (1980) found that self-injury may be preceded by autogrooming. Self-injury also may occur when fighting behavior is prevented. Stereotypy and self-injury might reduce other more aversive stimulation or indicate loss of control in a new and novel situation. Early experiences may result in behavioral sensitization and predispose to recurrence when there is exposure to a situation analogous to the original one. It has been hypothesized that children may have similar responses, beginning with stereotypies which may extend to self-injury. The arousal-increasing and arousal-decreasing hypotheses are of interest, although the evidence for them may be subject to a variety of interpretations. Additional research on rearing in physical and social isolation and studies on early infant stimulation and early attachment are needed for a better understanding of the biological factors involved in self-injury related to deprivation of early experience.

Neuromaturational Processes in Development

Neuromaturational and neuroanatomical changes may also be important in the occurrence of stereotypies and self-injury. Some authors have suggested the development of the cerebellum is of importance in relation to the emergence of self-stimulation, a finding of interest given the recent demonstration of cerebellum abnormalities in some autistic children (Courchesne et al., 1988). Furthermore, the onset of self-biting during a particular stage of development suggests a relationship to neuromaturational changes. For example, Iriki, Shuicki, and Nakamura (1988) have reported that different regions of the frontal lobe in a rodent are responsible for sucking and chewing. Chewing is a developmental acquisition requiring synaptic reorganization that ordinarily takes place around the time teeth erupt. The transition from finger sucking to biting may be a consequence of the maturational acquisition and exercise of chewing. Stimulation of the vestibular system by rocking, spinning, or other forms of body movement has been shown to influence motor development of normal and developmentally delayed children (Clark, Kreutzberg, and Chee, 1977) and may be a factor in children with abnormalities in this brain region. From these studies, stereotypy and self-injury might be a mentally subnormal individual's attempt at providing neurologically based self-stimulation. This stimulation may not only be reinforcing but necessary for neuronal development.

Opioid and Nonopioid Stress-Induced Analgesia

The identification of endogenous peptides with similar structure and function to morphine (Snyder, 1977) has opened new avenues for research on pain and pain-related behavior. Three genetically distinct families of opioid peptides have been identified in the central nervous system: endorphin/corticotrophins, enkephalins, and dynorphin/neoendorphins. The localization of their binding sites indicates that these peptides play an important role in the control of pain (Kuhar, Pert, and Snyder, 1973; Murrin, Coyle, and Kuhar, 1980). Infusions into the periaquaductal gray matter have been shown to decrease pain responsiveness (Hosobuchi, 1981). Increases in opioid peptide production and inhibition in pain responsiveness may accompany acutely stressful states, leading to insensitivity to pain, so-called stress-induced analgesia (SIA) in animals (Madden et al., 1977) and in humans (Willer, Dekers, and Cambier, 1981). Such effects are partially reversible with naloxone, an opiate antagonist whose administration has been associated with an increase in pain perception threshold (Buchsbaum, Davis, and Bunny, 1977). The administration of an enkephalinase inhibitor has been shown to potentiate stress-induced analgesia; this effect has also been blocked by naloxone. Both central and peripheral opioid mechanisms have been suggested for SIA (Kelly, 1982; Lewis et al., 1982). In addition, anatomical studies by Stuckey et al. (1989) have found decreased binding of mu (μ) opiate receptors in rat brain following inescapable shock.

The discovery of opioid receptors has led to investigations into opioid self-administration. Opiate receptors are densely distributed in brain regions associated with self-stimulatory behavior in animals, and opioid substances have been shown to have reinforcing properties for self-stimulation (Olds and Fobes, 1981). Animal studies with rhesus monkeys and rats have demonstrated that microinfusions of opioids (methionine enkephalin, morphine) into the ventral tegmentum, substantia nigra, or nucleus accumens facilitate self-stimulation, in some instances in a dose-related manner. Animals will bar-press for the delivery of enkephalin (Belluzzi and Stein, 1977), demonstrating their reinforcing properties. These findings regarding the opiate system have led to several hypotheses in regard to self-injury. First, repeated occurrence of SIB might lead to opioid-mediated stress-induced analgesia that may be associated with elevated levels of endogenous opioid peptides which inhibit pain. Secondly, it is possible that some individuals might engage in SIB as a means of self-administering opioid peptides. These hypotheses have been tested indirectly by administering naloxone or naltrexone and reported in a series of individual case reports (Bernstein et al., 1987; Davidson et al., 1983; Richardson and Zaleski, 1983); 4 subjects who were chronically self-injurious were described and 3 of these showed at least temporary decreases in SIB. The method of administration was intravenous, by slow intravenous drip, or orally, and results were attributed either to acute effects on opiate systems or receptor down regulation. The authors suggest that naloxone or naltrexone effects might have been due to either (1) reducing the pain threshold, therefore intensifying the normally painful effects of SIB, or (2) extinguishing the reinforcing effects of SIB. However, other authors (Szymanski et al., 1987) found no effects of naltrexone on SIB in two cases in a double-blind, placebo-controlled study utilizing a within-subject design.

The opiate system is not the only neurotransmitter system involved in SIA. Animal studies of foot shock stress produce potent analgesia in the rat; prolonged intermittent foot shock elicits analgesia medicated by opioid peptides, but brief continuous shock produces nonopioid analgesia as does the cold water swim test. Nonopioid SIA may involve histamine H2 receptors (Gogas and Hough, 1988). Furthermore, estrogen has been implicated in the modulation of stress-induced analgesia (Ryan and Maier, 1988). Therefore, in addition to neuronal opiate-induced analgesia, there are other categories of SIA, including neuronal nonopiate, humoral opiate, and humoral nonopiate forms. Furthermore, there are interactions between these neurotransmitter systems. For example, the dopamine system has been investigated in intracranial self-stimulation studies, and ascending dopaminergic fibers from the ventral tegmental area (VTA) have been implicated in "brain reward circuitry" (Olds and Fobes, 1981). Opioid peptides and dopamine are closely related to one another and found in similar brain regions. Enkephalins might influence self-stimulation indirectly via dopamine (DA) neurons that are thought to be presynaptically inhibited by enkephalin (Mulder et al., 1984; Pollard et al., 1978). Morphine alters the turnover of dopamine in the brain (Lal, 1975), and dopaminergic manipulations alter morphine analgesia. Intrastriatal enkephalins have been found to stimulate dopamine synthesis in the caudate nucleus by an action on opiate receptors localized on dopamine nerve terminals. Substantia nigra lesions have been shown to result in 40% to 50% reductions in opiate receptor density. These findings suggest that pharmacological studies must take into account the type of stress-induced analgesia as well as consider interactions among neurotransmitter systems when planning pharmacotherapy.

The identification of specific neurotransmitter abnormalities, such as those in patients who exhibit SIB, could provide evidence related to etiology and provide an experimental basis for future pharmacological intervention.

Altered Anatomy and Physiological State

Numerous surgical procedures have resulted in self-injury in animals, including lesions in the temporal lobe in macaques (Kluver and Bucy, 1939) and lesions in the spinal cord (bilateral cervicothoracic dorsal rhizotomy from C5 to T2) (Busbaur, 1974), sciatic nerve section, and sectioning of the middle of the lateral funiculus (Jones and Barraclough, 1978). A primary consideration is whether the surgery results in the complete elimination of sensory input (anesthesia) or alters input (paresthesia), possibly associated with constant irritation. Taub (1977; personal communication; Taub, Perrella, and Barro, 1973) found self-injury in sensory deafferentated monkeys whose sensory pathways have been disrupted, which suggests sensory isolation as a mechanism.

Other investigators have studied paresthesia in animals. For example, Innovar (fentanyl citrate/droperidol), a drug causing local irritation, has resulted in self-injury in animals. One possible explanation for these stereotypies and self-injury is that arousal is increased by local irritation and that stereotypies reduce arousal. Stereotypies and self-injury have been frequently noted under conditions of increased arousal suggesting (1) neurophysiological arousal causes increased stereotypies and self-injury, and (2) specific motor activity related to stereotyped and self-injurious behavior reduces arousal.

Drug-Induced Changes in Physiological State

Although drugs or surgical lesions involving the spinal cord or affecting the peripheral nervous system may lead to self-injury, centrally acting drugs that increase stereotypies and lead to self-injury in animals also may provide important information on mechanisms. These substances include alcohol (Charmove and Harlow, 1970); caffeine (Mueller et al., 1982; Peters, 1967); methylxanthine (Lloyd and Stone, 1981); clonidine (Bhattacharya et al., 1988; Katsuragi, Ushijima, and Furukawa, 1984; Mueller and Nyhan, 1982a); pemoline (Mueller, Hollingsworth, and Petit, 1986; Mueller and Nyhan, 1982b); and amphetamine (Randrup and Munkvad, 1967). Rylander (1971) has studied the relationship of amphetamine administration to stereotypies in humans in amphetamine addicts who show stereotyped movements. Amphetamine-induced stereotypies in animals are used to test neuroleptic drugs. High-dose pemoline has similar effects to amphetamine on self-injury and is blocked by the dopamine antagonist haloperidol. Low-dose pemoline has similar effects on adult and weaning rats and results in intermittent SIB and stereotypy; however, Mueller, Hollingsworth, and Petit (1986) suggest that although they occur together, there are distinct mechanisms for self-injury and stereotypy. O'Neil (1982) found that isolation-induced SIB and stereotypy were not different in their response to a drug treatment with imipramine. She investigated 8 rhesus monkeys and found a decrease in SIB duration and frequency of stereotypy with an increase in self-clasp, self-stimulation, and self-grooming with medication.

Rats and rabbits who were underfed and then received long-term administration of very high doses of caffeine or theophylline, methylpurine derivatives, eventually developed self-mutilating behavior. The ability of these purine derivatives to produce self-injury in animals is of interest. Purine derivatives are released from cells and influence neuronal activity as presynaptic modulators of neurotransmitter release and as regulators of receptor sensitivity (Kopin, 1981). Most of the purines affecting the central nervous system are related to adenine or guanine. Adenosine is synthesized from adenine and GMP derives from guanine. Behavioral stimulants, such as caffeine or theophylline, bind to adenosine receptors. Hypoxanthine interferes with the binding of diazepam to its receptor. Because caffeine also inhibits the binding of diazepam to its receptors, Kopin (1981) suggested a diazepam binding site may be involved in producing some of the behavioral manifestations of self-biting. He suggests that future studies of interactions between neurotransmitters and modulators that regulate brain function might have impact on developing a rational approach to chemotherapy.

Endogenous peptides, such as ACTH, also may produce stereotypies. Intraventricularly administered $ACTH_{1-24}$ in rats has been shown to produce excessive grooming (Gispen et al., 1976; Jolles, Rompa-Barendregt, and Gispen, 1979), and the dopaminergic system has been linked to the effects of ACTH on grooming (Cools, Wiegant, and Gispen, 1978). It is suggested that excessive grooming is a response that serves to decrease arousal of the organism following activation of the ACTH system

(Delius, Craig, and Chaudoir, 1976; Jolles, Rompa-Barendregt and Gispen, 1979). The response to the particular stimulus continues until the stimulus condition is altered. Once avoidance responding has stabilized, the pituitary-adrenal response to a previously arousing stimulus is attenuated (Hennessey and Levine, 1979). An inhibitory feedback effect on adrenocortical activity is exerted by the execution of species-specific behavior that either removes the external excitatory stimulus (escape, avoidance behavior, etc.) or mitigates the internal state (e.g., arousal stereotypy). A mentally retarded individual in an environment that makes excessive demands in novel situations where there is uncertainty and conflict may have no appropriate behavioral response to these situations (avoidance or escape). Under such conditions, stereotypies may serve as an effective means to reduce the level of arousal. Under these circumstances, self-injury may present as an extreme form of stereotyped behavior when the individual is stressed and highly aroused. Ordinarily, pain suppresses behavior; however, as previously described, stress-induced analgesia may occur, leading to a decrease in pain perception in these circumstances.

Behavioral Effects of Neurotoxic Lesions in the Developmental Period

Another approach to self-injury is through administration of neurotoxins during the developmental period followed by subsequent pharmacological challenge. Using this approach, a relationship between dopaminergic supersensitivity and self-injury has been demonstrated in experimental animals (Breese et al., 1984). Rats were given injections of 6-hydroxydopamine (6-OHDA) at 5 days of age to denervate basal ganglia regions unilaterally. These brain regions developed supersensitive dopamine receptors. Self-biting was seen in the lesioned animals when they were challenged as adults with a dopamine agonist; however, untreated adult rats did not show this behavior after being given the agonist. Similar studies in monkeys were carried out by Goldstein et al. (1985) to investigate the striatal dopamine regulation of motor activity. Goldstein studied the effects of dopamine agonists on monkeys who had unilateral denervated nigrostriatal systems for 10 to 14 years. L-dopa and apomorphine, dopamine agonists, elicited self-biting of the digits of the fingers contralateral to the lesion. This effect was blocked by a D_1 dopamine antagonist (SCH 23390) and by fluphenazine, a D_1/D_2 agonist, but was not blocked by a pure D_2 antagonist. The self-injury was elicited by dopamine antagonists whose effects are predominantly on the D_1 receptor and were blocked by a D_1 antagonist, suggesting a potential treatment for the self-injury.

Ungerstedt (1971) produced unilateral destruction of a dopamine pathway in the nigrostriatal system, resulting in postsynaptic supersensitivity following 6-hydroxydopamine injections and also reported self-injury. Another investigation involving the nigrostriatal system in self-biting was carried out by Baumeister and Frye (1985). Their work focuses on the mediation of dopamine-related stereotypy through striatal nigral GABAergic pathways. They injected muscimol, a GABA agonist that mimics the activity of GABA, into the substantia nigra in rats. When gnawing was prevented, self-biting was demonstrated in 42%, 69%, and 36% of animals when 10, 30, or 100 mg of the substance was injected. The administration of saline did not lead to self-biting. Bicuculline, a GABA antagonist, did not prevent this effect. Behaviors noted were stereotyped sniffing and head nodding. Here the administration of a GABA agonist into the substantia nigra led to self-biting. In each instance, biting behavior was produced by damage to the striatal nigral system. The mechanism is unclear and both studies require replication.

The emphasis in these studies on injury during the developmental period on later behavior is of considerable importance and may potentially suggest new approaches to treatment.

CONDITIONS ASSOCIATED WITH SELF-INJURY

Pervasive Developmental Disorders

Pervasive developmental disorders have commonly been associated with self-injurious behavior. In the first edition of DSM-III (APA, 1980), "childhood onset pervasive developmental disorder" included self-injury among its diagnostic characteristics. Although this condition is no longer included in the classification system, self-injury is a major consideration in individuals with pervasive developmental disorders and, in fact, pervasive developmental disorders may account for the majority of mentally retarded persons with severe self-injury. There is no specific topography of self-injury in this population; head banging, face hitting, self-biting, and other forms of self-injurious behavior are seen.

Bartak and Rutter (1976) compared a group of children with autistic disorder with IQs below 70 and above 70 on nonverbal scales. The two groups differed in their pattern of symptoms, although they were similar in meeting diagnostic criteria for an autistic disorder. However, the low IQ and high IQ groups differed substantially in that the lower IQ group had significantly more self-injury and stereotypies.

Based on his neurophysiological studies, Ornitz (1974) has suggested that there are problems in sensory modulation and motility in persons with autistic disorder. These potential problems in sensory modulation as well as deficits in metacognition and social perception may contribute to self-injury. Complex behavioral interactions require social communication skills that are lacking in persons with autistic disorder and may increase their vulnerability to aggression or self-injury when demands are placed on them. Moreover, persons with autistic disorder show a markedly restricted repertoire of activities and interests that include stereotyped and repetitive movements.

Lesch-Nyhan Disease

Lesch-Nyhan disease (Lesch and Nyhan, 1964; Nyhan, 1976), an inborn error of purine metabolism in which self-injury is a major behavioral manifestation, is described in Chapter 11.1. The full syndrome requires virtual absence of the enzyme. Other syndromes with partial hypoxanthine phosphoribosyltransferase (HPRT) deficiency are associated with gout without the neurological and behavioral symptoms, including self-injury.

The onset of self-injury may be as early as 1 year or rarely as late as the teens. Children demonstrate self-mutilation initially through self-biting, which is intense and causes tissue damage, often leading to amputation of fingers and loss of tissue around the lips (Lesch and Nyhan, 1964; Mizuno and Yugari, 1974). With increasing age, they also may self-mutilate by picking the skin with their fingers. The biting often results in extraction of primary teeth; severe self-injurious behavior may lead to institutional placement. In type, the behavior is different from that seen in other mental retardation syndromes of self-injury where self-hitting and head banging are the most common presentations. The self-injury occurs although all sensory modalities, including the pain sense, are intact. The self-injurious behavior often requires that the patient be restrained. Despite their dystonias, when restraints are removed, the child may appear terrified and quickly and accurately place a hand in the mouth. The child may ask for restraints to prevent elbow movement and when restraints are placed, he may become relaxed and more good humored (Nyhan, 1976). The dysarthric speech may result in interpersonal communication problems that cause frustration in social situations. Still, the higher functioning children can express themselves and participate in their treatment. Hemiballismic arm movements can also create difficulty because the raised arm is sometimes interpreted as a threatening gesture by others and may be socially reinforced, leading to hitting others.

Understanding the molecular disorder has led to effective drug treatment for those aspects of a disease that are related to uric acid accumulation and subsequent arthritic tophi, renal stones, and neuropathy. However, reduction in uric acid has not influenced the neurological and self-injurious behavior. In fact, some children have been diagnosed with HPRT deficiency and treated from birth for the elevation in uric acid with xanthine oxidase inhibitors, yet they still have behavioral and neurological symptoms despite never having had high levels of uric acid.

Because it is a condition where self-injury has been described as a behavioral phenotype in that it is uniquely present in all cases, Lesch-Nyhan disease has been investigated as a potential biological model for self-biting. Both anatomical and neurochemical studies have been undertaken in this condition and are described in Chapter 11.1. Brain-imaging studies suggest involvement of the dopamine system in Lesch-Nyhan disease (Harris, 1992). Early studies showing prophylactic effects of

L-5 hydroxytryptophan on self-mutilation were not confirmed (Mizuno and Yugari, 1975).

Cornelia de Lange Syndrome

Cornelia de Lange syndrome is described in Chapter 10.8. Self-injury in this syndrome includes face hitting, face picking, and lip biting, but no one specific pattern has been found nor is the behavior as intense as that found in Lesch-Nyhan disease (Shear et al., 1971; Singh and Pulman, 1979). In a review of 64 cases, Hawley, Jackson, and Kurnit (1985) found frequent tantrum behavior but do not indicate how often it was associated with self-injury. Although the self-injury may be treated using behavior therapy, no specific treatment in a series of cases of Cornelia de Lange individuals has been reported. In several cases, onset of self-injurious behavior coincided with the eruption of teeth. There is one case report (Fellow and Tennstedt, 1986) where insensitivity to pain was found, but other reports have not confirmed this finding. The relationship of self-injury to tantrums and biological factors related to delayed tooth eruption, chewing behavior, and pain sensitivity requires further evaluation. Furthermore, Greenberg and Coleman (1973) have reported low serotonin levels in whole blood in contrast to controls in 7 of 7 males and 2 of 4 females ranging in age from 10 to 30 years with the disorder, another finding that requires replication. The relationship of serotonin levels and self-injury requires continuing assessment.

Congenital Insensitivity to Pain

Congenital insensitivity to pain may occur as an autosomal recessive disorder. This condition has been associated with self-injury; however, the self-injury may be accidental and not follow a syndrome pattern. The following criteria are required for diagnosis: (1) pain sensation should be absent from birth; (2) the entire body should be affected; and (3) all other sensory modalities should be intact or minimally impaired and the tendon reflexes present. Mental retardation is seen in approximately one third of reported cases. Thrush (1973) reports chewing of the fingers and tongue in one child in a report involving 4 children in the same family with this disorder. Another child had a behavior disorder and took unnecessary risks that resulted in self-injury.

In several studies of patients with congenital insensitivity to pain, endogenous opiates have been strongly implicated. In one study, administration of naloxone dramatically reduced the pain threshold by 67% as measured by the nociceptive flexion reflex (Dehen et al., 1977). Dehen et al. (1986) subsequently reported that spontaneously elevated nociceptive (pain) threshold levels were markedly diminished after naloxone injections in 4 patients with congenital insensitivity to pain. Although cerebral spinal fluid (CSF) beta endorphin was either not elevated or was only slightly elevated in these patients, their clinical response to opioid antagonists suggests a possible treatment in some identified children with this disorder. Another study failed to replicate the antagonist effect of naloxone but noted elevated opioid levels in the CSF (Manfredi et al., 1981). By restoring the pain response with naloxone, accidental self-injury would be expected to be reduced.

Riley-Day Syndrome (Familial Dysautonomia)

The Riley-Day syndrome (Riley et al., 1949), or familial dysautonomia, is an identified autosomal recessive disorder with an estimated incidence of 1 in 10,000 to 1 in 20,000 that has been identified in over 200 families, almost all of whom are descendants of Ashkenazi Jews. Patients with Riley-Day syndrome have distinctive physical features and both neurological and physiological abnormalities; the most pertinent to self-injury are those associated with abnormal sensory nerves, nerve fibers, and autonomic nerve plexuses. Taste perception and discrimination are markedly deficient, and pain perception is reduced or absent (Riley et al., 1949). Studies of Riley-Day syndrome have shown decreases in dopamine-hydroxylase, the enzyme that converts dopamine to norepinephrine. This suggests the dopamine system might be involved in this disorder.

Rett's Disorder

Rett's disorder (Rett, 1966) is described in Chapter 9.3. In Rett's disorder, there is characteristic hand wringing and hand-to-mouth behavior. The diagnosis of Rett's disorder is based on a characteristic neurodevelopmental phenotype. A system for staging the progress of the condition is as follows (Naidu et al., 1986): In stage 1, a general slowing of development is noted, particularly in motor abilities; hypotonia is present. Developmental delay is insidious at onset and the initial symptoms may be vague. In the second stage, loss of acquired abilities is identified. It is during this stage that the characteristic hand wringing and hand-to-mouth movements begin. These stereotyped behaviors are important diagnostic clues in girls who have lost previously acquired purposeful hand skills and demonstrate this behavior to the exclusion of other types of hand use. During this phase of deterioration, autistic-like social withdrawal has been described along with hyperventilation, clumsy movements, and seizures. The autistic-like behaviors are most likely related to a developing encephalopathy, and the child may be misdiagnosed as having a pervasive developmental disorder. When autistic disorder is considered in girls, Rett's disorder must be ruled out. This stage is followed by a third stage where there is a plateau in symptomatology with no further loss of skills. The girls subsequently appear less autistic-like. Seizures are common, as is severe mental retardation and gait apraxia/ataxia. During the fourth stage, motor deterioration is noted with decreasing mobility, spasticity, scoliosis, muscle wasting, and vasomotor disturbances; social response and eye contact is improved. This is an important syndrome to recognize in girls because the hand-to-mouth movement may be reduced, but not eliminated, by behavioral intervention (Iwata et al., 1986). Differential reinforcement procedures combined with a response interruption technique have been used to reduce hand-to-mouth behavior. Because of involvement of the dopamine system reported from postmortem brain tissue of a patient with Rett syndrome and increased neurotransmitter metabolites (Riederer et al., 1985), positron emission tomography was carried out in a 25-year-old woman with Rett syndrome to assess D_2 dopamine receptor binding in the corpus striatum (Harris et al., 1986). Abnormalities were not identified in D_2 receptor binding. Future studies of the dopamine system in this disorder should address D_1 receptor binding because these receptors have been linked to self-biting in neonatal rats (Breese et al., 1984).

Tourette's Disorder

Tourette's disorder is described in Chapter 15. Self-injury may occur in this disorder (Eisenberg, Ascher, and Kanner, 1959; Eldridge et al., 1977) although the rates are variable, ranging from approximately 13% in some studies (Comings and Comings, 1985) to 53% in others (Moldofsky, Tullis, and Lamon, 1974). Problems with aggression and associated disruptive behavior have been reported in up to 40%; such episodes may be associated with anger and violent outbursts (Comings and Comings, 1987). Despite these reports of aggression, few individuals with Tourette's disorder in the community show antisocial behavior; therefore, referral bias of the most severe cases to specialty clinics may account for the difference.

Robertson, Trimble, and Lees (1989) suggest that self-injurious behavior is underreported in Tourette's disorder. They note that self-destructive behavior in these patients is correlated with obsessionality and hostility on rating scales. Those patients with self-injury tend to be at the most severe end of the spectrum. The types of self-injury reported in individuals with Tourette's disorder are not typically the same as those encountered with other self-injurious syndromes, such as Lesch-Nyhan disease. The topography of self-injury was more nonspecific and similar to that seen in more severely retarded individuals, although the Tourette's disorder patients were of average intelligence. These authors suggest that self- injurious behavior in individuals with Tourette's disorder might stem from self-destructive obsessions, for example, hitting the head in conjunction with a hand jerk. Other forms of self-injury are more complex and include pulling out teeth and eye poking. Rather than being a tic behavior, the self-injury seems heterogeneous and, in some instances, appears compulsive; in others, it may be related to a "directed tic."

The topography of self-injury in 30 Tourette's disorder patients (Robertson, Trimble, and Lees, 1989) included head banging, body punching or slapping, head or face punching, hitting body on hard objects, poking sharp objects into the body, scratching parts of the body, and a variety of other forms. Trimble (1992) has noted tatooing in some individuals with Tourette's disorder and also coprographia. Overall, one third, or 30 of 90 patients referred, showed self-injurious behavior.

Fragile X Syndrome

The fragile X syndrome is described in Chapter 10.3. It is associated with self-biting as well as autistic-like symptoms in some cases.

The behavioral features and the cognitive profile are features that are useful in identifying higher functioning individuals with fragile X syndrome. Behavioral features are helpful in diagnosis, especially for prepubertal males who may not show the classical physical features. There is a range of behavioral problems from difficulties in social communication with strangers to pervasive developmental disorder, autistic-like behavior, self-injury, and periodic violent outbursts of behavior. Hand flapping was noted in 66% of 50 males, hand biting in 74%, and unusual hand mannerisms in 88% (Hagerman et al., 1986). Most males with fragile X syndrome do not have a pervasive lack of relatedness to caregivers, so they do not meet the DSM-IV criteria for autistic disorder. Males with fragile X syndrome can be happy, likeable, and friendly. Currently, pervasive developmental disorder, not otherwise specified, rather than classic autistic disorder, would be the more common diagnosis. As indicated, the older category, childhood onset pervasive developmental disorder, includes oddities in motor movement, abnormalities of speech, self-mutilation, and hyper- or hyposensitivities to sensory stimuli among its characteristics, and this diagnosis might be applicable in some cases. A diagnosis of autistic disorder has been reported in 5% to 15% of males with the fragile X syndrome; however, these estimates depend on the criteria used for autistic disorder. Hand flapping, hand biting, perseverative speech, and poor eye contact in a child who is overactive and mentally retarded or learning disabled suggest the need for an evaluation for the fragile X syndrome as well.

Repetitive hand mannerisms may increase when the child is upset, angry, or frightened. Characteristics seen in children with autistic disorder, such as spinning, are also noted. These autistic-like behaviors may relate to problems in sensory integration. Reiss (1988) has reported reductions in the size of the cerebellar vermis in this disorder similar to those previously reported in autistic disorder (Courchesne et al., 1988). No specific neurotransmitter abnormalities have been identified in the fragile X syndrome.

NATURAL HISTORY

There is no typical age or pattern of onset of self-injurious behavior. The onset often follows a stressful environmental event. In nonverbal persons with a severe degree of retardation, it may be triggered by a painful physical condition, such as middle ear infection in young children. The self-injurious behaviors often peak in adolescence and then may gradually decline, but may also persist for years, especially in persons with severe/profound mental retardation. The focus of these behaviors often changes; e.g., a person may engage in hand biting that may then subside and head hitting may emerge. Quite commonly, an individual engages in a stereotypic behavior that usually does not result in self-injury (e.g., light head banging, skin picking), but at times the stereotypic behavior may progress in its intensity to the point that self-injury results.

The most serious complications are the result of tissue damage. In less severe cases, a chronic skin irritation or calluses from biting, pinching, scratching, or saliva smearing may be present. The serious complications include blindness (due to retinal detachment following eye gouging or hitting), intestinal obstruction (from pica—swallowing of solid objects), infections, and even death. If these behaviors are extreme and repulsive, there may be psychosocial complications due to the individual's exclusion from social and community activities.

CONDITIONS ASSOCIATED WITH AGGRESSIVE BEHAVIOR

Mutation in the Structural Gene for Monoamine Oxidase A

A major metabolic pathway involved in the degradation of dietary and neurotransmitter amines utilizes oxidative deamination by the monoamine oxidases, i.e., MAO-A and MAO-B. The genes for these monoamines are located at the p11.3 region of the X chromosome. Brunner et al. (1993) described a mutation in the MAO-A gene in a large Dutch kindred that is significantly linked with a clinical phenotype that consists of borderline mental retardation and abnormal behavior. There is characteristic aggressive and sometimes violent behavior that may be triggered by stress. In addition, other forms of antisocial behavior have been reported that includes attempted rape, arson, and exhibitionism. Twenty-four urine specimens in three patients indicated a severe disturbance in monoamine metabolism. Analysis of platelets shows normal MAO-B activity. Additional assessment of individuals in this kindred requires analysis and extensive neuropsychological and neuropsychiatry study to further define the clinical phenotype. Other than this one family there is a lack of consistent evidence of X-linkage in other types of impulsivity and aggression. Future studies to further characterize the role of MAO-A in behavior may benefit from studies of transgenic mice that express this deficit.

COMPREHENSIVE ASSESSMENT

The role of the psychiatrist in assessment is to diagnose and integrate the components of the interdisciplinary assessment because aggressive and self-injurious behavior is multiply determined. The psychiatrist may function as a primary mental health caregiver and core member of an interdisciplinary team, which he or she may or may not lead. In all instances, coordination with nonmedical professionals is essential.

The psychiatric assessment requires observations of and an interview with the patient, parent, or guardian and others who are directly involved with the patient's care. The interview with the patient may require augmented and alternative communication devices. In addition, neurodevelopmental/medical assessment (including syndrome identification); critical review of past psychological tests and cognitive profiles (the IQ alone is not sufficient); request of new tests as needed; psychosocial stressor evaluation (understanding of the disability by parent or guardian, effects of disability on caregivers, degree of restrictiveness of treatment, e.g., restraint use); and review of previous treatment (especially behavioral and pharmacological approaches) are included.

In conducting an examination, the following should be considered. From a neurobiological perspective, self-injurious behavior is multiply determined and involves maturational factors, current physiological state, past life experience, the social context of the behavior, and initiation into novel environmental settings. In both human and animal studies one must consider a severe form with sudden onset and a less severe form following stereotypy with regularly repeated injury. The social context must be considered because past social isolation may lead to increased vulnerability for future injury when stressed. In pervasive developmental disorder where there is deviant social development, the deficiency in bonding may enhance vulnerability to self-injury because of lack of response to social reinforcement. The role of depression and learned helplessness also should be considered.

The physiological state of the organism must also be taken into account. A state of agitation may accompany emotional lability, be a temperamental factor, an aspect of a mental disorder, or a consequence of environmental variables. Both surgical and neurochemical interventions show that abnormal neurological conditions, particularly those affecting sensory input, result in stereotypy and sometimes self-injury. Mentally subnormal individuals often have neurological abnormalities involving sensory systems, and excessive agitation may occur when conditions are perceived as confusing or threatening to them.

DIAGNOSTIC FORMULATION

The essential elements to any individual formulation is a description of the developmental level, current diagnoses, communication skills, associated disabilities (particularly sensory and motor), environmental contingencies as they relate to self-injury, and family and psychosocial circumstances. Discussion of co-occurring severe mental illness is particularly important.

SELECTION OF TREATMENT

The treatment plan is based on the case formulation and depends on the unique aspects of the individual case. The approach is pluralistic and may include individual, family, group, collaborative, behavioral, and pharmacological interventions. Most successful treatments involve multiple elements of therapy. Those that increase mastery and enhance behaviors by emphasizing communication skills and use augmented communication are of particular importance. Behavioral reduction procedures are reviewed in the NIH Consensus Development Conference on the Treatment of Destructive Behaviors in Persons with Developmental Disabilities (NIH, 1991). The consensus statement suggests the "behavioral reduction approaches should be selected for their rapid effectiveness only if the exigencies of the clinical situation require such restrictive interventions and only after appropriate review. These interventions should be used only in the context of a comprehensive and individualized behavioral enhancement treatment program."

Careful consideration must be given to the possible biological bases for self-injury, its association with organic brain conditions, and how biological factors relate to treatment approaches. Knowledge about the possible biological mechanisms involved in self-injury might be employed along with other treatment procedures for more effective management and to reduce the considerable cost involved in both initial treatment and generalization of treatment into a home or community setting. This is particularly important when considering psychopharmacological interventions.

In planning a program dealing with self-injury, it is important to consider the impairment in reciprocal social interactions and the subsequent development of social attachment. An essential component to treatment is the establishment of a program of functional language communication. Establishing social attention is extremely important because disabled persons with social deficits often do not respond spontaneously to language communication or initiate social interaction. Their lack of social awareness and the failure to establish attachment is a major factor in choosing therapeutic strategies. The individual with a pervasive developmental disorder may not show proximity-seeking behavior, and social interaction may seem unrewarding for them. Their impairments in communication and imaginative skills are critical elements to consider in program planning. Lower functioning individuals with pervasive developmental disorders, especially, do not initiate social communication spontaneously or respond to nonverbal cues, such as a frown from an adult or other gestures that ordinarily serve as a signal to end an activity. The stereotypies these children show may be used as reinforcers in working with the child. Ongoing involvement in treatment by family members, caregivers, and staff members is vital so the same approach is consistently applied across treatment settings.

In regard to behavioral interventions, Carr (1991) recommends that a high quality nonaversive intervention should include the following components: a systematic functional analysis or assessment, a multicomponent treatment intervention based on the results of the analysis or assessment, a concern for building functionally equivalent skills to replace problem behaviors, and a concern for altering living environments to promote lifestyle changes that minimize (that is, are not discriminative stimuli for) problem behaviors. Regular follow-up and case review is essential to monitor the emergence of social attachment and self-regulation, the appropriateness of behavioral interventions, and the effectiveness of pharmacological treatments.

MEDICOLEGAL ISSUES

Medicolegal issues are essential considerations for the treatment of self-injury. Informed consent by the parent or legal guardian is required for the initiation, implementation, and major changes in the treatment plan. State guidelines are of particular importance in monitoring the use of psychotropic drugs. The use of aversive interventions remains controversial; empirical, ethical, and legal considerations enter into their use (Gerhardt et al., 1991). An The NIH Consensus Development Conference mentioned earlier has provided recommendations regarding specific interventions for destructive behaviors.

SUMMARY

Self-injury is commonly observed in children less than 3 years of age and most often in persons with severe and profound mental retardation whose mental ages are in this age range. This suggests the potential importance of neuromaturational factors and perhaps also disrupted brain development.

Environmental experiences during sensitive phases of development have been implicated in self-injury in animals. Isolation, particularly from social contact with subsequent impairment in social skills, is one of the best documented examples of an environmental intervention occurring during a sensitive period.

Self-injury may follow increased arousal, leading to frustration and rage. Some forms of self-injury may involve exaggerations of the grooming mechanism and others may relate to averted fighting behavior.

Self-injury has been specifically associated with pervasive developmental disorder and with several mental retardation syndromes. This raises the question of whether self-injury is a learned response, the result of deviant development, or an ethologically derived pattern of behavior elicited in stressful circumstances. Involvement of catecholamine, indoleamine, and opioid neurotransmitter systems or their interaction has been proposed; however, no specific interaction leading to self-injury has been demonstrated.

A variety of centrally acting psychotropic drugs have been implicated in eliciting stereotypy and self-injury including subcutaneous amphetamine and intermittent dosages of pemoline. These effects are antagonized by dopamine antagonists. Other drugs produce paresthesias and provide a peripheral stimulus for arousal, perhaps leading to stereotypy and possibly self-injury.

Stereotypy and self-injury can result from administration of neurotoxins early in development, and anatomic lesions, such as sensory deafferentation, may result in self-injury.

Stress-induced analgesia may be a factor in eliciting or maintaining self-injury. Whether subjects stimulate to facilitate sensory input or to self-administer endogenous opioids is an open question, as is the issue of whether stress-induced analgesia is a secondary consequence of the behavior. Studies of stress-induced analgesia are complicated because there are both opioid and nonopioid forms of stress-induced analgesia.

In working with an individual, treatment considers each of these mechanisms in conjunction with the psychiatric diagnosis and findings from a comprehensive interdisciplinary assessment.

REFERENCES

Abe, K., Oda, N., and Amatomi, M. (1984). Natural history and predictive significance of head banging, headrolling, and breath holding spells. *Developmental Medicine Child Neurology,* 26:644–648.

American Psychiatric Association, Committee on Nomenclature and Statistics. (1980). Diagnostic and statistical manual of mental disorders, 3rd ed., Author, Washington, DC.

American Psychiatric Association, Committee on Nomenclature and Statistics. (1987). Diagnostic and statistical of mental disorders, 3rd ed., revised. Author, Washington, DC.

American Psychiatric Association, Committee on Nomenclature and Statistics. (1994). Diagnostic and statistical manual of mental disorders, 4th ed., Author, Washington, DC.

Anderson, J.R., and Chamove, A.S. (1980). Self-aggression and social aggression in laboratory reared macaques. *Journal of Abnormal Psychology,* 89:539–550.

Bachman, J.A. (1972). Self-injurious behavior: A behavioral analysis. *Journal of Abnormal Psychology,* 80:211–224.

Bartak, L., and Rutter, M. (1976). Differences between mentally retarded and normally intelligent autistic children. *Journal of Autism and Childhood Schizophrenia,* 6:109–120.

Baumeister, A., and Frye, G.D. (1985). The biochemical basis of the behavioral disorder in the Lesch-Nyhan syndrome. *Neuroscience and Biobehavioral Reviews,* 9:169–178.

_______, and Rollings, J.P. (1976). Self-injurious behavior. *International Review of Research in Mental Retardation,* 8:1.

Belluzzi, J.D., and Stein, L. (1977). Enkephalin may mediate euphoria and drive-reduction reward. *Nature,* 266:556–558.

Bernstein, G.A., Hughes, J.R., Mitchell, J.E,. and Thompson, T. (1987). Effects of narcotic antagonists on self-injurious behavior: A single case study. *Journal of the American Academy of Child and Adolescent Psychiatry,* 26:886–889.

Bhattacharya, S.K., Jaiswal, A.K., Mukhopadhyay, M., and Datla, K.P. (1988). Clonidine-induced automutilation in mice as a laboratory model for clinical self-injurious. *Journal Psychiatry Residency,* 22:43–50.

Breese, G.R, Baumeister, A.A., McCown, T.J., Emerick, S.G., Frye, G.D., Crotty, K., and Mueller, R.A. (1984). Behavioral differences between neonatal and adult 6-hydroxy-dopamine-treated rats to dopamine agonists: Relevance to neurological symptoms in clinical syndromes with reduced brain dopamine. *Journal of Pharmacology and Experimental Therapeutics,* 231:343–354.

Brunner, H.G., Nelen, M.R., van Zandvoort, P., Abeling, N.G.G.M., van Gennip, A.H., Wolters, E.C.,

Kuiper, M.A., Ropers, H.H., and van Oost, B.A. (1993). X-linked borderline mental retardation with prominent behavioral disturbance: Phenotype, genetic localization, and evidence for disturbed monoamine metabolism. *American Journal of Human Genetics,* 52:1032–1039.

Buchsbaum, M.S., Davis, G.C., and Bunny, W.G. (1977). Naloxone alters pain perception and somatosensory evoked potentials in normal subjects. *Nature,* 267:620–622.

Busbaur, A.I. (1974). Effects of central lesion on disorders produced by dorsal rhizotomy in rats. *Experimental Neurology,* 42:490–501.

Carr, E.G. (1977). The motivation of self-injurious behavior: A review of some hypotheses. *Psychological Bulletin,* 84:800–816.

______. (1991). Comment: Replacing factionalism with functionalism. *Journal of Autism and Developmental Disorders,* 21:277–278.

______, and Newson, C. (1985). Demand elicited tantrums, conceptualization and treatment. *Behavioral Modification,* 9:403–426.

Charmove, A.S., and Harlow, H.F. (1970). Exaggeration of self-aggression following alcohol ingestion in rhesus monkeys. *Journal of Abnormal Psychology,* 75:207–209.

Clark, D.L., Kreutzberg, J.R., and Chee, F.K.W. (1977). Vestibular stimulation influence on motor development in infants. *Science,* 196:1228–1229.

Comings, D.E., and Comings, B.G. (1985). Tourette syndrome: Clinical and psychological aspects of 250 cases. *American Journal of Human Genetics,* 37:435–450.

______, and ______. (1987). A controlled study of Tourette syndrome, I–VII. *American Journal of Human Genetics,* 41:701–866.

Cools, A.R., Wiegant, U.M., and Gispen, W.H. (1978). Distinct dopaminergic systems in ACTH induced grooming. *European Journal of Pharmacology,* 50:265–268.

Courchesne, E., Yeung-Courchesne, R., Press, G.A., Hesselink, J.R., and Jernigan, T.L. (1988). Hypoplasia of cerebellar vermal lobules VI and VII in autism. *New England Journal of Medicine,* 318:1349–1354.

Davidson, P.W., Klune, B.M., Carroll, M., and Rockowitz, R.J. (1983). Effects of naloxone on self-injurious behavior: A case study. *Applied Research in Mental Retardation,* 4:1–4.

Davis, K. (1940). Extreme isolation of a child. *American Journal of Sociology,* 45: 554–565.

______. (1946). Final note on a case of extreme isolation. *American Journal of Sociology,* 52:432–437.

Day, R.T. (1991). Treatment of aggression. *Advances in Mental Retardation and Developmental Disabilities,* 4:93–120.

Dehen, H., Amsallem, B., Colas-Linhart, N., and Cambier, J. (1986). Cerebrospinal fluid beta endorphin in congenital insensitivity to pain. *Review of Neurology (Paris),* 142:541–544.

______, Willer, J.C., Boureau, F., and Cambier, J. (1977). Congenital insensitivity to pain, and endogenous morphine-like substances. *Lancet,* ii: 293–294.

De Lissovoy, V. (1962). Head-banging in early childhood. *Child Development,* 33:43–56.

______. (1963). Head-banging in early childhood. A suggested cause. *Journal of Genetic Psychology,* 102:109–114.

Delius, J.D., Craig, B., and Chaudoir, C. (1976). Adrenocorticotropic hormone. Glucose displacement activities in pigeon. *Zeitschrift für Tierpsychologie,* 40:183–193.

Eisenberg, L., Ascher, E., and Kanner, L. (1959). A clinical study of Gilles de la Tourette's disease (maladie des tics) in children. *American Journal of Psychiatry,* 115:715–723.

Eldridge, R., Sweet, R., Lake, C.R., Ziegler, M., and Shapiro, A.K. (1977). Gilles de la Tourette's disorder: Clinical, genetic, psychologic, and biochemical aspects in 21 selected families. *Neurology,* 27:115–124.

Fehrenbach, P.A., and Thelen, M.H. (1982). Behavioral approaches to the treatment of aggressive disorders. *Behavioral Modification,* 6:465–497.

Fellow, P., and Tennstedt, A. (1986). Cornelia de Lange syndrome with analgesia. *Psychiatry, Neurology, Medicine, and Psychology,* 38:33–38.

Frankel, F., and Simmons, J.Q. (1976). Self-injurious behavior in schizophrenic and retarded children. *American Journal of Mental Deficiency,* 80:512–522.

Freedman, D.A., and Brown, S.L. (1968). On the role of coenesthetic stimulation in the development of psychic structure. *Psychoanalytic Quarterly,* 37:418–438.

Freud, S. (1922). *Beyond the pleasure principle.* Psychoanalytic Press, London.

Gerhardt, P., Holmes, D.L., Alessandri, M., and Goodman, M. (1991). Social policy in the use of aversive interventions: Empirical, ethical, and legal considerations. *Journal of Autism and Developmental Disorders,* 21:265–278.

Gispen, W.H., Wiegant, V.M., Grevan, H.M., and De Wied, D. (1976). The induction of excessive grooming in the rat by intraventricular application of peptides derived from ACTH: Structure-activity studies. *Life Sciences,* 17:645–652.

Gogas, K.R., and Hough, L.B. (1988). H2 receptor mediated stress induced analgesia is dependent on neither pituitary or adrenal activation. *Pharmacology, Biochemistry, and Behavior,* 30:791–94.

Goldstein, M., Anderson, L.T., Reuben, R., and Dancis, J. (1985). Self-mutilation in Lesch-Nyhan disease is caused by dopaminergic denervation. *Lancet,* i:338–339.

Goosen, C., and Ribbens, L.G. (1980). Autoaggression

and tactile communicationin pairs of adult stump tailed macaques. *Behavior,* 73:155–174.

Green, A.H. (1967). Self-mutilation in schizophrenic children. *Archives of General Psychiatry,* 17: 234–244.

Greenberg, A., and Coleman, M. (1973). Depressed whole blood serotonin levels associated with behavioral abnormalities in the de Lange syndrome. *Pediatrics,* 51:720–724.

Griffin, J.C., Ricketts, R.W., Williams, D.E., Locke, B.J., Altmeyer, B.K., and Stark, M.T. (1987). A community survey of self-injurious behavior among developmentally disabled children and adolescents. *Hospital and Community Psychiatry,* 38:959–963.

Hagerman, R.J., Jackson, A.W., Levitas, A., Rimland, B., and Braden, M. (1986). An analysis of autism in fifty males with fragile X syndrome. *American Journal of Medical Genetics,* 23:359–374.

Hamilton, M. (1985). *Fish's clinical psychopathology: Signs and symptoms in psychiatry.* John Wright and Sons, Ltd., Bristol, England.

Harris, J. C. (1987). Behavioral phenotypes in mental retardation syndromes. In R. Barrett and J. Matson (eds.), *Advances in developmental disorders,* Vol. 1, pp. 77–106. JAI Press, New York.

______. (1992). Neurobiological factors in self-injurious behavior. In J.K. Luiselli, J.L. Matson, and N.N. Singh (eds.), *Self-injurious behavior: Analysis, assessment and treatment,* pp. 59–92. Springer-Verlag, New York.

______, Wong, D.F., Wagner, H.N., Rett, A., Naidu, S., Dannals, R.F., Links, J.M., Batshaw, M.L., and Moser, H.W. (1986). Positron emission tomographic study of D_2 dopamine receptor binding and CSF biogenic animal metabolites in Rett syndrome. *American Journal of Medical Genetics,* 24:201–210.

Hawley, P.P., Jackson, L.G. and Kurnit, D.M. (1985). Sixty-four patients with Brachman de Lange syndrome: A survey. *American Journal of Medical Genetics,* 20:453–459.

Hennessey, J.W., and Levine, S. (1979). Stress, arousal, and the pituitary adrenal system: A psychoendocrine hypothesis. In J.M. Strague and A.N. Epstein (eds.), *Progress in psychobiology and physiological psychology,* Vol. 8. Academic Press, New York.

Hill, B.K., and Bruininks, R.H. (1984). Maladaptive behavior of mentally retarded individuals in residential facilities. *American Journal of Mental Deficiency,* 88:380–387.

Hosobuchi, Y. (1981). Periaqueductal gray stimulation in humans produces analgesia accompanied by elevation of beta-endorphin and ACTH in ventricular CSF. *Modern Problems in Pharmacopsychiatry,* 17:109–122.

Hutt, C., and Hutt, S.J. (1968). Stereotypies and their relation to arousal: A study of autistic children. In S.J. Hutt and C. Hutt (eds.), *Behavior studies in psychiatry.* Pergamon, London.

Iriki, A., Shuicki, N., and Nakamura, Y. (1988). Feeding behavior in mammals: Corticobulbar projection is reorganized during conversion from sucking to chewing. *Developmental Brain Research,* 44:189–196.

Iwata, B.A., Pace, G.M., Willis, K.D., Gamache, T.B., and Hyman, S.L. (1986). Operant studies of self-injurious hand biting in the Rett syndrome. *American Journal of Medical Genetics,* 24:157–166.

Johnson, W., and Baumeister, A. (1978). Self-injurious behavior: A review and analysis of methodological details of published studies. *Behavior Modification,* 2: 465–484.

Jolles, J., Rompa-Barendregt, J., and Gispen, W.H. (1979). ACTH-induced excessive grooming in the rat: The influence of environmental and motivational factors. *Hormones and Behavior,* 12:60–72.

Jones, I.H. (1982). Self-injury: Toward a biological basis. *Perspectives in Biology and Medicine,* 26:137–150.

______, and Barraclough, B.M. (1978). Auto-mutilation in animals and its relevance to self-injury in man. *Acta Psychiatrica Scandinavica,* 58:40–47.

Katsuragi, T.I., Ushijima, I., and Furukawa, T. (1984). The clonidine-induced self-injurious behavior of mice involves purinergic mechanisms. *Pharmacology, Biochemistry, and Behavior,* 20:943–946.

Kelly, D.D. (1982). The role of endorphins in stress-induced analgesia. *Annals of the New York Academy of Science,* 398:260–271.

Kluver, H., and Bucy, A.S. (1939). Preliminary analysis of functions of the temporal lobe in monkeys. *Archives of Neurology and Psychiatry,* 42:978–1000.

Kopin, I.J. (1981). Neurotransmitters and the Lesch-Nyhan syndrome. *New England Journal of Medicine,* 305:1148–1150.

Kravitz, H., Vin Rosenthal, Y., Teplitz, Z., Murphy, I., and Lesser, R. (1960). A study of headbanging in infants and children. *Diseases of the Nervous System,* 21:203–208.

Kuhar, M.J., Pert, C.B., and Snyder, S.H. (1973). Regional distribution of opiate receptor binding in the monkey and human brain. *Nature,* 245:447–450.

Lal, H. (1975). Narcotic dependence, narcotic action, and dopamine receptors. *Life Sciences,* 17:483–496.

Lesch, M., and Nyhan, W.L. (1964). A familial disorder of uric acid metabolism and central nervous system function. *American Journal of Medicine,* 36:561–570.

Lewis, J.W., Tordoff, M.G., Sherman, J.E., and Liebeskind, J.C. (1982). Adrenal medullary enkephalin-like peptides may mediate opioid stress analgesia. *Science,* 217:557–559.

Lloyd, H.G.E., and Stone, T.W. (1981). Chronic methylxanthine treatment in rats: A comparison of wistar and fischer 344 strains. *Pharmacology, Biochemistry, and Behavior,* 14:827–830.

Madden, J., Akil, H., Patrick, R.L., and Barchas, J.D. (1977). Stress-induced parallel changes in central opioid levels and pain responsiveness in the rat. *Nature,* 265:358–360.

Maisto, C.R., Baumeister, A.A., and Maisto, A.A. (1978). An analysis of variables related to self-injurious behavior among institutionalized retarded persons. *Journal of Mental Deficiency Research,* 22:27–36.

Manfredi, M., Bini, G., Cruccu, G., Accornero, N., Berardelli, A., and Medolago, L. (1981). Congenital absence of pain. *Archives of Neurology,* 38: 507–511.

Mason, W.A. (1967). Early social deprivation in nonhuman primates: Implications for human behavior. In D.C. Glass (ed.), *Environmental influences,* pp. 70–101. Rockefeller University Press, New York.

______, and Capitanio, J.P. (1988). Formation and expression of filial attachment in rhesus monkeys raised with living and inanimate mother substitutes. *Developmental Psychobiology,* 21:401–430.

Meyer-Holzapfel, M. (1968). Abnormal behavior in zoo animals. In F.W. Fox (ed.), *Abnormal behavior in animals,* pp. 476–503. W.B. Saunders, Philadelphia.

Mizuno, T., and Yugari, Y. (1974). Self-mutilation in the Lesch-Nyhan syndrome. *Lancet,* 1:761.

______, and ______. (1975). Prophylactic effect of L-5 hydroxytryptophan on self-mutilation in the Lesch-Nyhan syndrome. *Neuropaediatrie,* 6:13–23.

Moldofsky, H., Tullis, C., and Lamon, R. (1974). Multiple tic syndrome (Gilles de la Tourette's disorder). *Journal of Nervous and Mental Disease,* 15:282–292.

Muller, K., Hollingsworth, E., and Petit, H. (1986). Repeated pemoline produces self-injurious behavior in adult and weaning rats. *Pharmacology, Biochemistry, and Behavior,* 25:933–938.

______, and Nyhan, W.L. (1982a). Clonidine potentiates drug induced self- injurious behavior in rats. *Pharmacology, Biochemistry, and Behavior,* 18:891–894.

______, and ______. (1982b). Pharmacologic control of pemoline induced self-injurious behavior in rats. *Pharmacology, Biochemistry, and Behavior,* 16:957–963.

______, Saboda, R., Palmour, R., and Nyhan, W.L. (1982). Self-injurious behavior produced in rats by daily caffeine and continuous amphetamine. *Pharmacology, Biochemistry, and Behavior,* 17:613–617.

Mulder, A.H., Wardeh, G., Hogenboom, F., and Frakenhuyzen, A.L. (1984). Kappa and delta opiate receptor agonists differentially inhibit striatal dopamine and acetylcholine release. *Nature,* 308:278–280.

Mullick, J.A., and Schroeder, S.R. (1980). Research relating to management of antisocial behavior in mentally retarded persons. *The Psychological Record,* 30:397–417.

Murrin, L.C., Coyle, J.T., and Kuhar, M.J. (1980). Striatal opiate receptors: Pre- and postsynaptic localization. *Life Sciences,* 27:1175–1183.

Naidu, S., Murphy, M., Moser, H.W., and Rett, A. (1986). Rett syndrome: Natural history in 70 cases. *American Journal of Medical Genetics,* 24:61–72.

National Institutes of Health (1991, September). Consensus Development Conference on the Treatment of Destructive Behaviors in Persons with Developmental Disabilities. U.S. Department of Health and Human Services, Public Health Service. NIH Publication No. 91–2410, Washington, D.C.

Nyhan, W.L. (1972). Behavioral phenotypes in organic genetic disease. Presidential address to the Society for Pediatric Research, May l, 1971. *Pediatric Research*, 6:1–9.

______. (1976). Behavior in the Lesch-Nyhan syndrome. *Journal of Autism and Childhood Schizophrenia,* 6:235–252.

Olds, M.E., and Fobes, J.L. (1981). The central basis of motivation: Intracranial self-stimulation studies. *Annual Review of Psychology,* 32:523–594.

O'Neil, M.N. (1982). *Effects of an anti-depressant drug given to isolate primates who display self-injurious behaviors: A comparative study.* Unpublished doctoral dissertation, University of Wisconsin, Madison.

Ornitz, E.M. (1974). The modulation of sensory input and motor output in autistic children. *Journal of Autism and Childhood Schizophrenia,* 4:197–215.

Patterson, G.R. (1982). *Coercive family process: A social learning approach.* Oregon Social Learning Center, Portland.

Pattison, E.M., and Kahan, J. (1983). The deliberate self-harm syndrome. *American Journal of Psychiatry,* 140:867–872.

Peters, J.M. (1967). Caffeine induced hemorrhagic automutilation. *Archives Internationales de Pharmaco-dynamie et de Thérapie,* 169:139–146.

Picker, M., Poling, A., and Parker, A. (1979). A review of children's self-injurious behavior. *The Psychological Record,* 29:435–452.

Pollard, H., Llorens, C., Schwartz, J.C., Gros, C., and Dray, F. (1978). Localization of opiate receptors and enkephalins in the rat striatum with relation to the nigrostriatal dopaminergic system: Lesion studies. *Brain Research,* 151:392–398.

Randrup, A., and Munkvad, I. (1967). Stereotyped activities produced by amphetamines in several animal species and man. *Psychopharmacologia,* 11:300–310.

Reiss, A.L. (1988). Cerebellar hyperplasia and autism [Letter]. *New England Journal of Medicine,* 319:1152–1153.

Rett, A. (1966). Uber ein eigneartiges hirnatrophisches syndrom bei hyperammonamie im kindersaltger. *Weiner Medicinische Wochenschrift,* 116:723–726.

Richardson, J.S., and Zaleski, W.A. (1983). Naloxone and self-mutilation. *Biological Psychiatry,* 18:99–101.

Riederer, P., Brucke, T., Kienzl, E., Schnecker, K., Schay, V., Kruzik, P., Killian, W., and Rett, A. (1985). Neurochemistry of Rett syndrome. *Brain and Development,* 7:351–360.

Riley, C.M., Day, R.L., Greeley, D.M., and Langford, W.S. (1949). Central autonomic dysfunction with defective lacrimation. *Pediatrics,* 3:468–478.

Robertson, M.M., Trimble, M.R., and Lees, A.J. (1989). Self-injurious behaviour and the Gilles de la Tourette syndrome. A clinical study and review of the literature. *Psychological Medicine,* 19:611–625.

Ross, R.T. (1972). Behavioral correlates of levels of intelligence. *American Journal of Mental Deficiency,* 76:545–549.

Russo, D.C., Carr, E.G., and Lovaas, O.I. (1980). Self-injury in pediatric populations. In J. Ferguson and C.B. Taylor (eds.), *Comprehensive handbook of behavioral medicine,* Vol. 3, pp. 23–41. Spectrum Publications, Holliswood, NY.

Ryan, S.M., and Maier, S.F. (1988). The estrus cycle and estrogen modulate stress induced analgesia. *Behavioral Neuroscience,* 102:371–380.

Rylander, G. (1971). Stereotypy in man following amphetamine abuse. In S.B. deBaker (ed.), *The correlation of adverse effects in man with observations in animals,* Series no. 220, pp. 28–31. Excerpta Medica, International Congress, Amsterdam.

Sackett, G.P. (1968). Abnormal behavior in laboratory reared rhesus monkey. In F.W. Fox (ed.), *Abnormal behaviour in animals,* pp. 293–374. W.B. Saunders, Philadelphia.

Schroeder, S.R., Schroeder, C.S., Smith R., and Dalldorf, J. (1978). Prevalence of self-injurious behaviors in a large state facility for the retarded: A three-year follow-up study. *Journal of Autism and Childhood Schizophrenia,* 8:261–269.

Shear, C.S., Nyhan, W.L., Kirman, B.H., and Stern, J. (1971). Self-mutilative behavior as a feature of the de Lange syndrome. *Journal of Pediatrics,* 78:506–509.

Singh, N.N., and Pulman, R.M. (1979). Self injury in the de Lange syndrome. *Journal of Mental Deficiency Research,* 23:79–84.

Smeets, P.M. (1971). Some characteristics of mental defectives displaying self-mutilative behaviors. *Training School Bulletin (Vineland),* 68:131–135.

Snyder, S.H. (1977). Opiate receptors in the brain. *New England Journal of Medicine,* 296:266–271.

Stuckey, J., Marra, S., Minor, T., and Insel, T.R. (1989). Changes in mu opiate receptors following inescapable shock. *Brain Research,* 476:167–169.

Szymanski, L. (1991). The search for a single mechanism of self-injurious behavior. *Journal of child and adolescent psychopharmacology,* 1:315–317.

______, Kedesdy, J., Sulkes, S., and Cutler, A. (1987). Naltrexone in treatment of self-injurious behavior: A clinical study. *Research in Developmental Disabilites,* 8:179–190.

Taub, E. (1977). Movement in nonhuman primates deprived of somatosensory feedback. In J.F. Keogh (ed.), *Exercise and sports sciences reviews,* Vol. 4, pp. 335–376. Journal Publishing Affiliates, Santa Barbara, CA.

______, Perrella, P.N., and Barro, G. (1973). Behavioral development following forelimb deafferentation on the day of birth in monkeys with and without blinding. *Science,* 81:959–960.

Thrush, D.C. (1973). Congenital insensitivity to pain: A clinical, genetic, and neurophysiological study of four children from the same family. *Brain,* 96:369–386.

Trimble, M. (1992). *Gilles de la Tourette syndrome.* Presentation at the annual meeting of the American Psychiatric Association, Washington, DC.

Ungerstedt, U. (1971). Postsynaptic supersensitivity after 6-hydroxydopamine induced degeneration of the nigro-striatal dopamine system. *Acta Psychiatrica Scandinavica,* 367(suppl.):69–93.

Willer, J.P., Dekers, A., and Cambier, J. (1981). Stress induced analgesia in humans: Endogenous opioids and naloxone reversible suppression of pain reflexes. *Science,* 212:689–691.

PART V
TREATMENT OF DEVELOPMENTAL NEUROPSYCHIATRIC DISORDERS

Treatment for developmental neuropsychiatric disorders requires an understanding of the nature of the disorder, a comprehensive assessment, and the coordinated efforts of an interdisciplinary treatment team. Some aspects of treatment specific to the various disorders have been discussed in the preceding chapters. Part V focuses on several therapeutic categories and includes chapters on psychotherapy, behavior therapy, pharmacotherapy, and genetic counseling. The final chapter of this part also includes a discussion of gene therapy and potential counseling issues that may involved with these new technological advances in treatment.

Chapter 18, the first chapter in Part V, discusses psychotherapy with disabled persons. Psychotherapeutic interventions may involve the parent and other caregivers as well as the affected individual. Attachment theory is suggested as a basic model for psychotherapeutic intervention with developmentally disabled persons. The orientation of the psychotherapist, the impact of specific developmental disabilities on the conduct of psychotherapy, the adaptation of psychotherapeutic methods to the individual's needs, and the role of the family in treatment are discussed. Modifications in therapeutic techniques using augmented and alternative forms of communication are emphasized for the most severely disabled. Interpersonal treatments are generally recommended following a multidisciplinary diagnostic evaluation that takes into account the nature of the disabilities and how they may limit the individual's capacity to participate in treatment.

Chapter 19 reviews behavior therapy and includes a glossary of behavioral terminology at the end of the chapter. The behavior therapies are the most widely used and best studied treatment interventions for behavioral disturbances in persons with mental retardation and other developmental disorders. The principles of behavior therapy are emphasized rather than addressing behavioral treatments for specific disorders. The chapter emphasizes using applied behavior analysis, operant techniques, and functional communication methods to help severely developmentally disabled persons.

Chapter 20 provides an overview of pharmacotherapy and reviews the use of psychotropic drugs in individuals with developmental disorders. Mental retardation and other developmental disorders have multiple etiologies and there may be variability in susceptibility to mental disorders as well as in the metabolism of psychotropic drugs. Epidemiologic issues related to drug use, the methodology of drug studies, assessment and diagnostic considerations, and the basic categories of drugs utilized in treatment are discussed.

The final chapter in Part V, Chapter 21, discusses the definition of genetic counseling, the information presented at a genetic counseling session, counseling for specific syndromes, counseling for nonspecific syndromes, and preventive counseling. In addition, there is a detailed discussion of current developments in the treatment of genetic disorders. A table is included that outlines recent advances in gene therapy for disorders involving the brain.

CHAPTER 18

PSYCHOTHERAPY IN DEVELOPMENTAL DISORDERS

Psychotherapeutic interventions are an important component in the treatment of emotional and behavioral disturbances manifested by children and adolescents with developmental disorders. This is particularly true for those with milder degrees of cognitive impairment who can present their life story the most coherently. Mentally retarded and other developmentally disabled persons are exposed to a variety of psychosocial stressors that lead to internalized conflict and maladaptive behavior. Repeated failure, social rejection, frequent losses, and dependency on others often result in feelings of inferiority, ambivalence, anxiety, and anger. Family conflicts are also common, and there may be feelings of jealousy toward normally developing siblings and tension with parents regarding emancipation and independence. Such individuals are highly motivated to establish interpersonal relationships and frequently demonstrate a strong desire for enhancing their personal competence and gaining greater independence. Despite this, psychotherapeutic interventions tend to be underutilized for disabled persons, often because of misconceptions regarding their effectiveness (Gair, Hersch and Wiesenfeld, 1980). Yet mentally retarded and other developmentally disabled persons can be very good candidates for interpersonal psychotherapy. Experiences of psychological conflict commonly result in demoralization, dysphoria, and anxiety, all of which may be targeted for treatment.

Individuals with mild cognitive impairments have been shown to benefit from individual, family, and group psychotherapy. The general goals for the interpersonal treatment of developmentally disabled individuals are the same as those for nondisabled persons. Psychotherapeutic interventions focus on alleviating or reducing behavioral symptoms and subjective suffering, resolving internalized conflicts, improving self-esteem, and enhancing personal competence. Emphasis is placed on attaining the maximum possible psychosocial development and autonomy, depending on the disability, and in improving social and adaptive functioning. Psychotherapeutic endeavors with disabled persons are conducted in collaboration with family members, educators, and other caregivers. Such treatment is generally recommended following a multidisciplinary diagnostic evaluation that takes into account the nature of the disabilities and how they may limit the child's capacity to participate in treatment; this is particularly true for communication disorders.

This chapter discusses attachment theory as a basis for psychotherapy in developmental disorders, the orientation of the psychotherapist, the impact of specific developmental disabilities on the conduct of psychotherapy, an approach to psychotherapy, methods to adapt psychotherapeutic methods to the individual's needs, family intervention, crisis intervention and time-limited approaches, and outcome.

ATTACHMENT THEORY: A BASIS FOR PSYCHOTHERAPY IN DEVELOPMENTAL DISORDERS

Attachment theory provides a basis for and may underlie various forms of psychotherapy (Holmes, 1993). Attachment theory may be linked to the common factors in psychotherapy described by Frank (1973, 1986; Frank and Frank, 1991) that are key elements in the various forms of psychotherapy. These consist of a relationship, an explanation of current difficulties, and a method for understanding them. Attachment theory investigates secure and insecure parent–child bonding in early life and its consequences for later development. The application of assessments of secure and insecure bonding in the first years of life for the disabled person can provide potential guidelines to assess the capacity to form relationships in therapy.

Attachment theory may also provide a basis for developing psychotherapeutic approaches with developmentally disordered persons. From the perspective of ethology and the emergence of the self-system, attachment theory places its primary emphasis on interpersonal relationships between parent and offspring whose evolutionary function is the protection of the young from danger. The early relationship between parent and offspring has its basis in interpersonal feedback rather than simply in the early feeding relationship. The emergence of attachment leads to the "secure base" phenomenon so that early attachments are characterized by the seeking of physical proximity to the parent, which is activated by separation from the caregiver in infancy, and by threat, fatigue, or illness in the older child or adolescent. When in close proximity to the attachment figure, the individual feels safe and may engage in exploration of the environment. The extensiveness of exploration and the security of the attachment are reciprocally related.

Separation from the secure base leads to separation protest and intense, and often angry, efforts to reestablish reunion. With permanent separation or loss, the capacity to explore or feel secure is diminished. The "attachment dynamic" (Heard and Lake, 1986) begins in infancy and continues through childhood into adult life. In close proximity to the parent, the individual develops and maintains a map or "internal working model" of his or her world and representations of the location and the interactive patterns of potential attachment figures. Personal development proceeds and represents the movement from dependence to separateness, from immaturity to mature dependency, or to emotional autonomy (Holmes and Lindley, 1989).

Four typical patterns of attachment have been described (Main, 1990) based on the Strange Situation paradigm (Ainsworth, 1969), and may be considered as a basis for planning psychotherapy. To review, they are listed here along with the frequency in which they occur: secure attachment (65%) (separation protest, easy pacification on reunion, return to exploratory play); insecure-avoidant attachment (10%) (little protest on separation, wary on reunion, does not play freely); insecure-ambivalent attachment (15%) (protests at separation, cannot be pacified, clings, and pushes toys away); and insecure-disorganized attachment (4%) (freezes on separation, unable to sustain organized patterns of behavior). Moreover, patterns of maternal or caregiver behavior may be associated with these patterns of attachment. The caregiver of a securely attached child is responsive, attuned to the child, and playfully interacts with him when contrasted to the caregiver of an insecure infant or child. Mothers or caregivers of insecure-avoidant children provide functional support in that they may be efficient in feeding and cleaning the child but tend to play less with the infant or child and show little attention to the child's social cues for holding and attention. The mother or caregiver of an insecure-ambivalent child is inconsistent in her behavior, often intrudes when the child is engaged in an activity and at other times ignores his distress. Finally, following major maternal or caregiver failure, as is seen with abuse or gross neglect, an insecure-disorganized pattern is produced. Differences in attachment are not based specifically on temperament because mothers and fathers may classify attachment differently.

Attachment status tends to be stable if there are no major changes in the relationship with the caregiver over time. If there are major changes in life circumstances, however, the attachment pattern may change from secure to insecure. However, working with a caregiver whose infant or child is insecurely attached may lead to secure attachment status as the parent works through his or her own interpersonal conflicts. At school age, securely attached children tend to interact more fully with peers, whereas insecure-avoidant children tend to isolate themselves and may show unprovoked aggression. Insecure-ambivalent children tend to cling to teachers and are more passive in their play. Insecure-disorganized children generally have the most behavioral difficulties in the school setting.

The attachment status of older children has been investigated by using tasks that involve narrative production. Bretherton (1991) found that when using a picture completion task, securely attached children produced stories that resolved difficulty and offered happy endings to stories which began with unhappy separation situations. Insecurely attached children in the same study were generally unable to find ways to resolve problems in their story or to deal with separation themes adequately. Main (1991) studied narratives by asking 10- to 11-year-olds to give an autobiographical description of themselves. Children who, in the past, had been classified as securely attached were better able to tell a coherent story about their lives and to describe unpleasant experiences they had undergone. These children showed greater self-awareness and an ability to reflect on their own thought processes, that is, to use metacognitive monitoring.

Main (1990) also evaluated attachment phenomena in adults using an Adult Attachment Interview (AAI). Using this semistructured interview, individuals were asked about feelings regarding current and past attachments and separations and about their emotional responses to loss and difficult life experiences (Main, 1991). Secure adults gave a coherent account of their lives and demonstrated the capacity to describe stressful events in the past, such as a major parental separation, in a coherent nondetached way. Others, described as "insecure-dismissive," tended to be unable to remember details about the past, stating they had difficulty remembering or that "things were fine." An "insecure-enmeshed" group had difficulties describing past emotional experiences and presented tearful accounts or incoherent descriptions. Fonagy, Steele, and Steele (1993) used the Adult Attachment Interview with pregnant mothers and their partners, then subsequently used the Strange Situation paradigm to classify their infants at a year of age. Based on the maternal Adult Attachment Interview, the infant's attachment pattern was predicted with 70% accuracy. Correlations were found between securely attached mothers and securely attached infants and dismissive mothers and avoidant infants. Less consistency was found between enmeshed mothers and ambivalent infants.

Although these early reports of narrative production and autobiographical competence require replication, they do suggest that narrative accounts should be encouraged in assessment and might be considered in assessing developmentally disabled persons as well. Such an approach traces the line of attachment beginning with the mother's sense of security in pregnancy, then moves on to attachment status in the infant during the first year of life and beyond that, for both nondisabled and disabled children. The relationship between narrative, or autobiographical, capability in later childhood and adolescence and attachment and security deserves evaluation in disabled persons.

Holmes (1993) suggests that attachment theory is pertinent to the following aspects of psychotherapy: (1) the provision of a secure base in the therapeutic relationships; (2) the establishment of autobiographical competence; (3) the importance of affect and its processing as a central theme; (4) the role of cognition; (5) separation and loss; and (6) sexuality. Each of these aspects should be considered in working with developmentally disabled persons. The implementation of psychotherapy for disabled persons requires considerable flexibility and ingenuity on the part of the therapist due to the complexity of various disabling conditions.

Establishing a Secure Base

The provision of a secure base as a basis for attachment may be complicated for developmentally disordered persons. First, the parents' own sense of security and confidence in caregiving may be undermined by the nature of the disabling condition. The parents or caregivers need to work through and grieve the expected normal child and acknowledge the disability as a prerequisite to developing confidence in their own caregiving ability. Security of attachment has been shown to be linked to a confiding relationship between the primary caregiver and a spouse or significant other person. Cassidy (1988) found that single-parent mothers who formed a stable relationship with a male partner changed from insecure to secure bonding patterns with their infant. Murray and Cooper (in press) have demonstrated how brief therapy with mothers of insecure children may alter the child's attachment status as the mother improves in treatment. Similar studies need to be carried out in the parents of developmentally disabled children.

After working with a primary physician or therapist and an interdisciplinary team has established this sense of confidence, the parent must help facilitate preattachment behaviors in a child who may have limitations in communicative and motor behavior. Physical handling is particularly important because the inhibition of primitive reflexes (see Chapter 6 on cerebral palsy) through handling techniques that facilitate inhibition may be needed to reduce inappropriate vocalizations, such as high-pitched crying, and facilitate more normal affiliative ones. Experiences must be provided that allow the child to approach or move away from the parent. This might include help with scooting rather than crawling, and the use of motorized devices for children with cerebral palsy or other movement disorders.

Multiple caregivers are often involved with disabled infants and children so that consistency, reliability, and regularity of contact may require particular effort. Ainsworth (1969) identified maternal or caregiver responsiveness as a crucial element in a child's later attachment status. A responsive parent picks the infant up sooner than a nonresponsive one and is aware of the infant or child's emotional cues. Stern (1985), Brazelton and Cramer (1991), and other authors have observed mother–infant interactions and suggest that maternal attunement and the development of an "interactive envelope" are characteristic of successful mother–infant "conversations." Holmes (1993) suggests that the origins of metaphor, i.e., linking similar and dissimilar experiences, may emerge from Stern's descriptions of "cross-modal attunement." These early attunement experiences—linking physical contact with vocal utterances—are more difficult to accomplish in the disabled child and not only require the use of special handling techniques for the physically disabled but also increased vigilance by the parent to recognize the limited repertoire of social signals emitted from disabled infants.

Autobiographical Competence

Autobiographical competence, which should lead to a shared narrative between the therapist and the developmentally disabled person, is complicated by potential difficulties in the individual's initiating communication and the frequent need for specific devices, such as communication boards, speech synthesizers, and tape recorders. Helping nonverbal individuals to use signs to initiate communication with others may be their first opportunity for self-expression. Once communication is established, security may be enhanced by the mastery which comes from understanding that one's actions may have an effect on the environment. The use of simple signs, such as the sign for "go" to indicate a request for assistance in moving from one place to another, or the sign for "more" to request more food, or the sign for "toilet" to indicate the need for assistance in toileting, provide means of demonstrating competence (self-efficacy) in dealing with the environment. For higher functioning individuals who use language, criteria are being developed to assess narratives for coherence and capacity to present a meaningful story in describing experiences of loss and emotional discomfort. "Secure-attachment" stories have not been evaluated in disabled individuals but may be assessed just as they are for nondisabled persons. Both mental age and chronological age must be taken into account in estimating the capacity for autobiographical memory. Moreover, the relationship of autobiographical competency to metacognition, using the theory of mind paradigm, must be considered in individuals with pervasive developmental disorder.

Regulation of Affect

The processing of affect and the regulation of affect is a particularly important aspect of attachment theory as it applies to the developmentally disabled. In attachment theory, unmodulated emotional expression may be related to patterns of insecure attachment, either avoidant or ambivalent. Nonverbal, physically disabled infants struggling with unmanageable, undifferentiated feelings, such as rage, terror, or extreme excitement, require a responsive caregiver to help transform this distress into more manageable emotions through attunement and facilitation of some means to take action. Moreover, the modulation of affect, with the therapist's assistance, may allow such undifferentiated emotions to be expressed. Modulation of affective expression through feedback is an important element in a secure attachment and should be linked to narrative competence as words and signs are produced to identify, discriminate, and label emotions.

The attachment model emphasizes awareness of interpersonal interaction rather than intrapersonal development. An interpersonal focus is important for disabled persons because patterns of secure and insecure attachment can be directly perceived by observing separation and reunion behavior and, in doing so, the interpersonal context specified. An overall goal is to establish emotion regulation that involves personal identification, discrimination, and direct expression of emotion. Uncertain responses from caregivers may lead to insecure-avoidant patterns where there is fear of intimacy, or insecure-ambivalent patterns where there is fear of abandonment. The pattern of attachment and the extent of affect regulation have been studied in disabled persons, using modifications of the Strange Situation paradigm.

Cognitive Development

Cognitive development is linked to attachment theory in that individuals develop an internal map, or internal working models. These internal working models are schemata in which self and others are represented. The cognitive contribution takes into account Vygotsky's zone of proximal development (Rogoff, 1990). It is at this interface that growth and development occur. If the zone of proximal development is securely established, then the opportunity for the child to utilize cognition from cognitive exchanges with the adult at his or her level of understanding may be enhanced. Therapeutic companionship is an important ingredient for cognitive understanding to develop. Cognitive schemata may be linked to affective states and overt behavior. Due to the degree of their mental retardation, developmentally disabled individuals may have difficulty internalizing working models so that autobiographical competence must be judged in the context of cognitive development. It will need to be clarified whether or not the age that children develop autobiographical memories is entirely mental-age dependent or is related to both mental age and chronological age, i.e., duration of life experiences. For children with pervasive developmental disorders, metacognitive abilities will need to be considered, using the theory of mind framework, in treatment planning. For the latter group, the development of social cognition may be critical in establishing internal working models. Metacognitive monitoring is an aspect of secure attachment in older individuals and requires contributions of both intellectual and social cognitive awareness.

The response of the disabled individual to experiences of separation and loss and its impact on attachment needs to be taken into account. The cognitively disabled individual may be unable to mobilize an intense protest at the time of separation or to demonstrate the intense reunion experience seen in nondisabled individuals. A child with cerebral palsy will have difficulty in approaching, and nonverbal children may show nonverbal means of pleasure in reunion with a parent. The emotions related to grief may be less intense in more mentally retarded persons so that bereavement counseling requires great sensitivity. Moreover, how internal working models are linked to bereavement in the developmentally disabled must also be taken into account. In addition, the expression of loss and how it is affectively modulated may be influenced by the disabling condition. Finally, the effects of loss of the therapist as the child moves from one setting to the other and grows older needs to be considered.

Attachment and Sexuality

Attachment theory distinguishes between sexual and attachment dynamics. Therefore, sexuality in infancy and early childhood is viewed as a function of both the parent and the infant or young child's contribution to the attachment relationship. Holmes (1993) and Erikson (1993) suggest that the ethological evidence points to the presence of altruistic behavior and incest avoidance when interpersonal bonding is secure. Heightened sexuality, inappropriately sexualized relationships, or abusive relationships between parent and child lead to insecure attachment. Yet interpersonal differences in regard to sibling rivalry, sharing, and envy do arise within the attachment bond and may require intervention.

Attachment Theory and Psychotherapy

In the individual therapy situation, the affective interactions between the therapist and the individual in treatment involves modeling as well as interpersonal modulation of affect. Attachment theory may be utilized as a means of understanding the difficulty that those who are abused find in separating themselves from an abuser. Because attachment behavior is activated by threat, the attached tend to cling to the attachment figure when threatened. If the attachment figure is the perpetrator of abuse, either aggressive or sexual, then a cycle is established that is difficult for the victim to resolve. In these circumstances, pathology in the attachment bond emerges so that activation of both separation and threat lead to feelings of panic and may enhance clinging. Secure attachment may be an important element in protecting a disabled person from abuse. Establishing or reestablishing a secure attachment is a goal for an abused person.

In group therapy, attachment theory is also applicable. Companionable interactions occur in the group so that the group serves as a secure base from which those involved may explore their feelings, their relationships with one another, their relationship with the therapist, and their past experiences (Sigman, 1985).

In family therapy, the child plays an important part in the regulation of attachment relationships. The child or adolescent may serve as a buffer between parents who have difficulty achieving intimacy and yet are unable to separate (Holmes, 1993). When potential separation occurs between the parents, the child may become more symptomatic and show increased behavioral difficulty. However, the child may be drawn into parental conflicts if the parents have difficulty tolerating intimacy between one another and the child may, in that instance, be more demanding of attention. Attachment theory suggests that attachment patterns are transmitted via family scripts that may be similar to internal working models and individual scripts. These scripts have been proposed as being common to the family. Such scripts may prohibit certain topics from being discussed within the family or maintain particular power relationships.

In summary, attachment theory emphasizes secure bonding and the coherence of the family group as essential to the "fitness function" of the individual. In this sense, psychotherapy may be conceived as a means of regulating an individual's relationship within the family group and in the wider community. Children with developmental disorders strain the cohesiveness of the family group. An appreciation of the natural history of specific developmental disorders in regard to unique features in facilitating the establishment of an attachment bond is essential in treatment planning.

ORIENTATION OF THE PSYCHOTHERAPIST

The psychotherapist working with a disabled individual must openly accept the disabled individual as a person and develop a sense of respect for his individuality. A developmental orientation is needed which applies the results from cognitive, language, and other evaluations to treatment sessions that are designed to facilitate socialization and mastery of developmental challenges. The therapist must appreciate the individual's relative strengths and take satisfaction in small increments of change. He or she must be prepared to accept the degree of dependency that may emerge during therapy while concurrently providing praise and reassurance as a means to facilitate independence. In the treatment setting itself, the therapist sets structure, give specific suggestions, and provides direction. In so doing, an accepting and receptive attitude is needed to help the individual improve his communicative expression. If inappropriate manifestations of aggression occur during sessions, an attitude that allows for nonpunitive intervention is required.

The therapist should be familiar with the physical and behavioral characteristics associated with particular syndromes and must be comfortable in sharing information and utilizing information provided by other professionals in regard to the particular disorder. Finally, the therapist must come to appreciate and empathize with the difficulties that parents experience in raising a child or adolescent with a disability and be able to offer practical advice and direction to them.

IMPACT OF DEVELOPMENTAL DISABILITIES

The most important issue in establishing a psychotherapeutic relationship with a disabled person is an appreciation of the extent of the communication disorder and how to compensate for the lack of communication skills in the receptive, expressive, and pragmatic language domains. Facilitating communication is the starting point of therapy so that recognition, labeling, discriminating, and describing the various emotions becomes possible. Perceptual difficulties in understanding social cues, limited ability to assume social roles, and limited appreciation of the intentions of others all complicate this process.

Such problems are linked to executive dysfunction in self-monitoring, abstracting, and understanding the subtleties of social communication with peers and caregivers. Because of these potential cognitive and affective limitations, the repertoire of social behaviors may be reduced. Limitations in communication become most apparent when the disabled person is stressed, at which time emotion dysregulation may lead to reduced impulse control and aggressive behavior. Moreover, communication problems may arise in abstracting and generalizing better self-awareness and behavioral gains to new settings. Communicative approaches used in treatment include, but are not restricted to, the use of both verbal and nonverbal methods (signing, communication boards, and speech synthesizers).

In addition to the communication problems, limitations in life experience influence the psychotherapeutic relationship. The therapist must take into account possible lack of basic social understanding based on limited life experiences. Parental or caregiver overprotection may be an important factor in limiting life experience (Levy, 1943). The overprotective parent or caregiver may restrict social contact with peers and activities outside the home and in the community. Such caregivers tend to infantilize the child or adolescent by making limited demands on him to master age-appropriate tasks. Besides this, life experiences may be restricted in other ways, such as placement in self-contained classrooms or being separated from peers in other settings. Time in school tends to be very structured and involves extensive behavior management programs that may allow little free time for recreation and informal activity with peers. This lack of support for normalized activity may extend to an absence of long-term planning for adaptation in other areas. Developmental issues, such as sexuality, vocational training, and assistance in independent living, may not be adequately addressed.

Mentally retarded and developmentally disabled children and adolescents may be teased or stigmatized because of their disability and ignored or excluded from normative peer activities. Such stigmatization is traumatic and may become a source of psychological stress. Reiss and Benson (1984) emphasize how stigmatization brought about through labeling, segregation, peer rejection and ridicule, restricted opportunities, as well as exploitation and repeated failure in developmental tasks, impact on self-esteem.

In summary, the impact of the developmental disorder may lead to psychological problems in disabled persons. These may occur as a consequence of poor communication skills, poor self-monitoring, distorted social perception, lack of life experiences, and traumatic life experiences leading to poor self- esteem, loneliness, compensatory denial of being disabled, and increased dependency.

APPROACH TO PSYCHOTHERAPY

The overall psychotherapeutic goal is to improve adaptive functioning and help the individual master developmental tasks, avoid stigmatization, increase resiliency to cope with psychosocial stressors, and prevent the emergence of symptoms during development as new capacities emerge. Information provided by the family and other caregivers is a critical component in approaching psychotherapy because disabled persons may often be unable to provide essential background and ongoing descriptions about their life experiences.

In conducting psychotherapy with disabled persons, the psychotherapist must address the same basic issues in the initiation of treatment as with nondisabled persons. Making therapeutic contact requires considerable initial effort, but is critical because establishing rapport is basic to enhancing motivation to change. As the psychotherapeutic process unfolds, additional diagnostic information may become available regarding the extent of communication deficits, response to psychosocial stressors, and co-occurring behavior and psychiatric disorders. Because this is often the case, the first part of treatment also serves as an extended evaluation that may be utilized to develop a more comprehensive and realistic case formulation.

The psychotherapy includes an educational component that teaches new adaptive skills. In working with the parents or caregivers, one goal is to evaluate child/adolescent rearing techniques and teach them, if necessary. Ongoing work with family members and caregivers is essential because they will be able to provide confirmatory information on progress the referred patient may not be able to supply. Because the child or adolescent may not report significant life events and previous traumas, family members or other caregivers must be relied on to provide this information as well as to report new family problems that may adversely affect the disabled person. The parents or caregivers also play a critical role in ongoing day-to-day guidance and in identifying additional resources. Psychotherapeutic endeavors do not only involve parents and other caregivers; the therapy must be coordinated with educational, communication science, occupational therapy, behavior therapy, medical and social services, and other professionals who may be involved. For those persons who are placed in group homes or residential settings, staff should be actively involved in developing the psychotherapeutic goals. Contact must be maintained with agencies who are involved with the child or adolescent.

An optimal treatment program uses multiple modalities of treatment. Any intervention must be consistently applied across various settings; staff and family members need to assist in generalizing therapy to maintain gains across these settings. This applies particularly to the teaching of social skills with family members, teachers, and peers. Because information derived in one setting may require a change of program in others, communication across settings is vital. When new information comes up during psychotherapy that is pertinent to another treatment setting, it is essential there be a format for it to be conveyed. Finally, the psychotherapist should be prepared for long-term continuous treatment involvement with periodic frequent visits and less frequent sessions as symptomatic improvement becomes apparent.

ADAPTING PSYCHOTHERAPEUTIC METHODS

There are many challenges in adapting psychotherapeutic methods to the treatment of a disabled person. Yet Hurley (1989) reports that developmentally disabled individuals respond positively to psychotherapy and recommends six adaptations to psychotherapeutic techniques that are derived from multiple published reports. Although these adaptations are based largely on case reports, they do provide reasonable general guidelines for clinical practice. Such adaptations include matching the technique to the child or adolescent's cognitive and developmental level, a directive approach, flexibility in the choice of methods, involvement of family and staff, recognition of interpersonal distortions and biases, and helping the person to acknowledge the extent of his disability. Each of these adaptations is discussed separately.

First, the therapeutic intervention must be matched to the patient's cognitive and developmental level as well as the type of disabling condition. This requires using syntactically simple language geared to the child or adolescent's developmental level and offering concrete examples in a context the person can understand. The therapist must check frequently to see if the patient has understood what has been said and repeat concepts from one session to the next until they are grasped (Hurley and Hurley,

1986). In older mentally retarded persons, Hurley and Hurley (1987) recommend carefully building the relationship as one would in therapy with younger nondisabled children. Initial sessions may be used to help the patient discriminate and describe feelings before working to link feelings and situations.

Second, a directive approach is needed to keep the focus of the therapeutic interactions on pertinent issues. In the first session, the reason for the referral is identified, a concrete explanation is given of what therapy is, how often it will take place, and what will occur in each session. The therapist must be very specific in explaining the rules and structure for each therapy session, set firm but appropriate limits for aggressive, destructive and excessively affectionate behavior and, in speaking with the child or adolescent, ask for minute particulars in the child's description of events that have taken place and the child's responses to them. The therapist may specifically recommend alternative means of coping with stressors and alternative interpretations of life events. The individual is encouraged to express curiosity and ask questions because, in the past, he may not have been encouraged or provided an opportunity to do so. When the person in therapy asks specific questions, the therapist must consider answering them directly rather than looking for fantasy material that may underlie them. Giving appropriate feedback for effective behavior and providing reassurance when the child or adolescent reports successes is crucial. Acknowledging the child or adolescent's potential doubt about dealing with tasks and problems and letting him know that, in general, people are not always sure how to accomplish a task may be useful. Moreover, frequently asking him about alternative strategies to master a problem is a way to facilitate personal problem-solving ability and rational thinking.

Third, flexibility is needed so a range of techniques can be employed. Alternative approaches are often necessary when treatment is not progressing adequately. In making treatment choices, the child's cognitive, communicative, and affective developmental level are considered in choosing particular verbal and play techniques. Play techniques (Chess, 1962; Leland and Smith, 1965) must be adapted to the child or adolescent's mental age; drawings, music, and puppets are commonly employed. In regard to the therapy sessions themselves, the length and frequency of the sessions should be based on the patient's ability to tolerate the designated length of time for the session and to use it effectively (Stavrakaki and Klein, 1986). More frequent and short sessions may be necessary for disabled persons. In crisis situations, it is particularly important to maintain continuity and establish a time perspective.

Fourth, throughout treatment, the family and caretaking staff must be utilized to furnish information, function as co-therapists when needed, and provide support. Working with the patient in isolation may be futile (Hurley, 1989) because disabled individuals are so dependent on others for care. Therapy is like that for younger persons who cannot make all their own decisions and depend on caregivers (Menolascino, Gilson, and Levitas, 1986). Moreover, family members need support in accepting and adjusting to the disability. Still, confidentiality is also required to maintain trust with the patient. Excessive involvement by the therapist may make the therapy more difficult and may potentially reduce the patient's confidence in the therapeutic process (Szymanski, 1980). Yet the patient should be encouraged to view himself as an important source of information.

Fifth, interpersonal distortions, biases, and overprotection on the part of the therapist may emerge in working with disabled persons in the same way they do with persons who are not disabled. Important interpersonal issues include the therapist's attitude toward the individual and possible discomfort the therapist may feel in the presence of a disabled person. Devaluing or minimizing a retarded or disabled person's individuality may occur in subtle ways. It is a necessary adaptation for the therapist to acknowledge the reality, chronicity, and permanence of the patient's limitations. Recognizing and treating the child or adolescent at his own developmental level and acknowledging and encouraging mastery of his particular life experiences are important to avoid infantilizing the patient and increasing his dependency. The therapist should be aware that he, himself, may harbor wishes to rescue the disabled person, develop an overprotective attitude, and be reluctant to set adequate limits (Jakab, 1982; Szymanski, 1980). It is essential that the therapist not overemphasize the individual's symptoms but address his independence and individual accomplishments.

From the child or adolescent's point of view, dependency is a major concern so he may become quite dependent on the therapist. In doing so, the therapist may be idealized or considered as a parent (Szymanski, 1980). This occurs most commonly when the therapist is the first person the individual can openly confide in without being treated as if he were younger than his age. Levitas and Gilson (1987) point out that such idealization is not necessarily abnormal and may be similar to that seen in normally developing children. However, the person being treated may distort the interpersonal relationship (parataxic distortion) by projecting fears or actual previous experiences of rejection or maltreatment onto the therapist. There may be the expectation that the therapist, as others have, will impose severe prohibitions on him or her. Finally, the disabled person may develop romantic fantasies in regard to the therapist. Higher functioning, especially mildly retarded persons, are very aware of negative interpersonal responses to them (Reiss and Benson, 1984). Like other disabled persons, a developmentally disabled person suffers when realizing he is different and is stigmatized as a member of a devalued group.

Sixth, the issue of the specific disability itself must also be addressed. The developmentally disabled, especially mentally retarded persons, have commonly not been targeted as a group who can benefit from disability counseling (Hurley, 1989). Yet specific problems arise in disability counseling because the individual may not clearly understand the nature of his disability. This is particularly true with mental retardation where limitations in cognitive ability themselves restrict insight and reasoning about the nature of the disability. However, an accurate understanding of the disability is a necessary preparatory step in beginning therapy. A mentally retarded person may have no initial awareness of what "retarded" means although he is sensitive to being labeled "retarded" (Szymanski and Rosefsky, 1980). Such anxiety may be relieved by explaining that mental retardation refers to slowed development in some areas but that there may be strengths in other areas. However it is carried out, the explanation needs to be concrete and at the individual's developmental level. In discussing the specific disability, the disabled person may be asked if he understands the diagnostic label, why he is in special classes, and how his development differs from that of a sibling.

Concurrent with disability counseling, the therapist provides ability counseling by helping children or adolescents put their overall disability into perspective (Hurley, 1989). They might be taught they have value as human beings that is separate and distinct from their identifying themselves as a disabled persons; that they are unique as people and their abilities are important. In addition, Hurley suggests the use of the principles of rational-emotive therapy developed for use with nondisabled children, for mentally retarded adolescents, and adults (Ellis and Bernard, 1983). The therapist may need to confront children or adolescents in working with their possible unwillingness to acknowledge or accept the limitations of mental retardation or other disabilities. In doing so, the therapist must be careful not to overidentify with their patients' awareness of stigmatization and even shame as they acknowledge their disabilities. Care must be taken if the therapist feels he is "attacking" the patient's self-esteem when asking directly about limitations (Feinstein, 1993).

Smith, McKinnon, and Kessler (1976) emphasize the "stickiness of development" and plateau effects that reflect continued concerns about mastery of early development tasks. They note the rigidity in doing things in exactly the same way and limited anticipatory fantasies, i.e., make-believe identities about what their future might hold for them.

School programs, particularly extensive and continuous systematic behavioral training to increase compliance, may limit children's or adolescents' views of themselves as able to initiate activity on their own. Because this is the case, the therapist must continually work to help disabled persons function autonomously and make choices. Often disabled individuals are not aware they have choices; this must be recognized and remedied. Developmentally, disabled individuals function lower than their chronological age in specific skill areas, yet they may strive to master developmental tasks of nondisabled peers who are their same chronological age and become frustrated.

Encouraging autonomy also has risks because the individual may be impulsive and, because of cognitive limitations, make choices that could be dangerous. Because of these risks, the context outside of the therapy session in which the child or adolescent might make decisions must be carefully understood. In developing choices, training in appropriate social assertiveness is also quite important.

Self-Understanding

In psychotherapy, the capacity for self-understanding is linked to the cognitive stage of development. Some higher functioning mentally retarded and developmentally disabled children and adolescents may benefit from interpretation of their behavior and may show some self-understanding (Feinstein, 1993). With younger children, drawings and pictures may be very useful to facilitate this understanding. Self-observation may develop in some adolescents, most commonly those in the mild to borderline range of intelligence. With ongoing therapy, the higher functioning group may develop some self-monitoring and provide introspective responses to the therapist about their behavior. The disabled person may identify with the therapist's being supportive and acknowledge his observations as helpful. Others may identify with the verbal process of therapy itself, may model the therapist's approach to them, and internalize thinking about behavior and feelings, for example, by remembering the therapist's statement "How are you feeling now?" and asking it of themselves through using self-talk when stressed. Identifying with and internalizing the therapist's approach may facilitate self-evaluation if the disabled person reflects on the "here and now" and identifies and discriminates feeling states before acting.

In considering disabled persons' ability to respond and utilize interpretations about their behavior, the cognitive and linguistic ability to talk about past events and utilize autobiographical memory is critical. One must clarify whether or not these individuals have reached the stage of development where theory of mind, that is, the ability to anticipate the intentions and desires of others and act based on these anticipations and awarenesses, is present. In assessing this kind of awareness, the therapist might ask questions, such as "What might have you been feeling when she did that?" Those individuals who tend to benefit most from therapy have the ability to recognize the similarity of their current life situations with life events they have experienced in the past at other times in their lives. This self-understanding may lead them to make different choices based on recognition of past maladaptive patterns of behavior.

The individual must be prepared for an interpretation of feelings that may be out of his current awareness. Those individuals who are eager to comply and please the therapist may feel anxious if feelings they consider unacceptable are attributed to them. In psychotherapeutic work, the therapist might use figurines in play to clarify the child or adolescent's understanding of emotion by asking questions, such as "I can't see any feelings in the soldier's face when the man knocked him over, but maybe he was having some secret feelings." One might then add, "But maybe the soldier had a secret feeling of being angry or scared but thought he shouldn't tell anyone about it. What do you think?" Moreover, individuals may require specific education to learn how to acknowledge and interpret feelings. They might be told they are not alone in how they feel; that many people become angry or become jealous of their siblings; or that many people may have bad feelings toward others even though they love them.

Working with Younger Children

Both chronological age and mental age are important in choosing psychotherapeutic approaches. Younger children show more problems with self-monitoring, and their emotions are generally less differentiated. In such children, anxiety may lead to excessive and unfocused activity. Undifferentiated emotions may be associated with outbursts of undirected aggressive behavior because the individual may lack an understanding of the conventional means of expressing them. Such social skills deficits are generally more prominent in younger children. To deal with these problems, special care is needed in preparation for the therapy session. In setting up a therapy session, planning is needed to establish structure. The therapist must clarify the time of the session, what will be done, what specific activities will be carried out, why talking is important in therapy, what the rules are in terms of the individual's behavior during the session, and what the therapist will do. Materials should be chosen that the individual can use for mastery in imaginative activities (play) which helps to modulate emotional arousal. In the sessions themselves, the development of a relationship with the therapist as a means to foster social development is crucial. To facilitate this, therapists sometimes describe themselves as a particular kind of friend or a special friend who helps with problems.

In addition to individual and family interventions, both activity and interpersonal group therapy may be combined with individual therapy to enhance peer social development and to provide an opportunity for direct observation of how the child responds to a peer.

Working with Adolescents

In the adolescent group, just as with younger developmentally disabled children, specific structure, support, assurance, and guidance are necessary in organizing sessions. The general goals of treatment are to improve emotion differentiation, develop better emotion regulation, increase social skills, enhance social perspective taking, and establish the capacity to generalize behavior beyond the therapy session. Sessions also emphasize helping the adolescent to improve social interactions and to deal with conflicts in interpersonal relationships with parents and peers. To meet these goals, a determination of his capacity for self-examination must be carefully evaluated.

Because the capacity for self-awareness and self-monitoring is greater with adolescents, the sessions can be more specifically focused. Conflicts related to dependency and autonomy and other issues related to developmental tasks are addressed. Problems of self-esteem are elicited and efforts to enhance self-esteem are begun. An important focus of therapy with adolescents is to establish a reality-based sense of identity and to provide a forum for them to discuss life choices in regard to future plans. Moreover, support is provided for them to face their own lack of self-acceptance of their disability and possible embarrassment about being disabled. Finally, a safe haven is provided to discuss confidential topics, such as sexuality.

Group therapy is a particularly useful approach for the adolescent age group, more so than for younger children. In group therapy, there is an opportunity to practice social skills directly and learn how to develop supportive relationships. The adolescent age group may feel more comfortable discussing peer-related topics in a group setting with others of their own age group who have similar disabilities. In the group, the therapist actively facilitates these interactions and provides structure to keep the focus on the topic at hand. The support and reassurance of group members may be needed to help individuals verbalize their concerns. In the sessions themselves, specific topic areas will arise that may be further pursued in individual treatment sessions.

FAMILY INTERVENTION

The therapeutic endeavor may work best when individual and family therapy are combined to allow consistency in management across settings. The family commonly serves as a therapeutic source for change and provides opportunities to consolidate new skills. In doing so, parents may ask for advice in parenting as therapy progresses. Treatment of the disabled person may also lead to positive parenting skills and improved relationships with the disabled person's siblings.

In working with developmentally disabled children, the family and other caregivers require direct support. For the family, the issues that are most pertinent arise at the time of the initial diagnosis and during phases of adaptation when feelings are mixed and, if not addressed, may lead to chronic sorrow. Kanner (1953, p. 75) eloquently presented the parents' view:

> Whenever parents are given an opportunity to express themselves, they invariably air their emotional involvements in the form of questions, utterances of guilt, open and sometimes impatient rebellion against destiny, stories of frantic search for causes, pathetic accounts of matrimonial dissensions about the child's condition, regret about the course that has been taken so far, anxious appraisals of the child's future, and tearful pleas for reassurance.

Questions commonly asked by parents are shown in Table 18–1.

Families need support in identifying resources and specific guidance in management and support techniques. Advocacy by the therapist in helping families with educational programs and social agencies is essential.

Commonly, a family may become dysfunctional in coping with a disabled family member, and marital discord may result from conflicts over raising a developmentally disabled child. A pattern of maternal overinvolvement and paternal withdrawal from the therapy may occur and needs to be addressed at the onset of treatment. If this occurs, couples therapy with both parents may be necessary, or a parent may need to be seen individually to work through his or her bereavement. The disabled person may become a source of displacement and scapegoating for other family issues.

Table 18–1. Questions Commonly Asked by Parents Concerning a Child with Mental Retardation

What is the cause of our child's retardation?
Have we personally contributed to his condition?
Why did this have to happen to us?
What about heredity?
Is it safe to have another child?
Is there any danger that our normal children's offspring might be similarly affected?
How is his (or her) presence in the home likely to affect our normal children?
How shall we explain him (or her) to our normal children?
How shall we explain him (or her) to our friends and neighbors?
Is there anything that we can do to brighten him (or her) up?
Is there an operation which might help?
Is there any drug which might help?
Will our child *ever* talk?
What will our child be like when he (or she) grows up?
Can we expect graduation from high school? From elementary school?
Would you advise a private tutor?
Should we keep our child at home or place him (or her) in a residential school?
What specific school do you recommend?
If a residential school, how long will our child have to remain there?
Will our child become alienated from us if placed in a residential school?
Will our child ever be mature enough to marry?
Do you think that our child should be sterilized and, if so, at what age?

From Kanner, 1953.

Richmond (1972) has outlined several psychological processes in parents in adapting to the disabled child. He suggests phases of denial, projection, guilt, and dependency that must be worked through. Futterman (1975) has expanded this model further when dealing with the anticipated loss of a terminally ill child, but his approach is also applicable to the disabled person. In the case of the disabled person, the loss is that of the expected normal child which may be sequentially experienced at each stage of the life cycle. This author focused on the phases of parental anticipatory mourning when faced with loss and identified five processes: acknowledgment, grieving, reconciliation, memorialization, and detachment. These were particularly associated with adaptational processes that focused on the maintenance of confidence. Adaptational processes included search for factual information about the illness and participation in the physical care of the child. They noted the importance of balancing several contrasting perspectives, e.g., acknowledgment and hope, maintenance of everyday activities and grief, confidence and doubt. Interventions are aimed at understanding these processes and in helping the individual to be able to experience, express, and work through his or her loss.

Family interview sessions may involve the developmentally disabled person, and when they do, family interactional patterns can be observed as they may offer an additional source for diagnostic information. The family sessions also may provide specific information for individual treatment of the child or for parent guidance. Family therapy may be of particular use for adolescents because it provides an avenue to support new capabilities for independent functioning. It may lead to better family negotiating styles if there is conflict between the adolescent and the parent. It also may foster assertiveness in the adolescent and the family and may lead to better relationships with siblings who are often stressed when a child in the family has a developmental disorder.

CRISIS INTERVENTION AND TIME-LIMITED APPROACHES

When a crisis occurs, a spectrum of interventions may be utilized. Psychiatric emergency services are used for those whose adaptive capacities have already broken down; crisis support for those with limited coping capacities in danger of decompensating and with a history of poor adaptation; and crisis intervention for those in danger of decompensating, but who have sufficient coping ability and a past history of good adaptive functioning.

Crisis Intervention

The most common interventions following initial counseling about the disabling condition are crisis intervention and short-term treatment approaches. Major family crises may develop with the birth of a disabled child or when a child has a severe illness. Critical times for disabled and chronically ill children include (1) the establishment of a diagnosis and the discussion of its implications; (2) living with the child at home and participating in the specific management program; (3) time of school entry; (4) entry into adolescence; (5) dealing with loss of function and deterioration; and (6) leaving school and entry into the workplace, supportive employment, or an adult activity or training center; and (7) future family planning. Anticipatory guidance can be particularly helpful.

Crisis intervention is an approach taken for the treatment of acute psychological decompensation. The intervention attempts to maximize the individual's potential for psychological growth and maturation as the crisis is mastered, and in this way mastery of the situation has a potentially protective effect for coping with future crises—a strengthening or steeling effect. However, failure in coping, particularly in regard to catastrophic events, may have a sensitizing effect. Crisis intervention provides a conceptual framework to approach these situations.

In crisis management, the first stage is to determine the degree of decompensation. Secondly, the nature of the stressor or stressors is established. The intensity of the crisis, the individual's adaptive behavioral reserves, and previous ability to cope are noted. A psychiatric diagnosis, psychodynamic formulation, and a formulation of the current crisis that emphasizes the previous psychological equilibrium in the family, the critical events precipitating the crisis, and how the crisis is manifest in the individual are established.

Clarification and cognitive appraisal of the situation inducing the crisis, encouraging appropriate emotional expression, recognizing willingness to be helped, and mobilizing coping resources are emphasized. The task is to redefine the critical incident and to mobilize resources. The steps are to review the event and identify the tasks to be mastered.

Questions to consider in assessment are as follows: (1) What is the crisis? (2) Who does it affect? (3) Why is it disorganizing? (4) What were the prior resources for coping before the crisis? (5) What are the unspoken issues? (6) What strengths can be mobilized? (7) How can the individual be mobilized in his own behalf? (8) What tasks need to be performed for resolution of the crisis? (9) What specific help is needed? (10) How can gains be consolidated? (11) Does any family member have a preexisting psychiatric disorder, and is it being treated? It is often the case that crisis occurs in the most poorly organized families and those with preexisting disorders.

The principles of crisis intervention follow from the concepts of crisis theory although there is disagreement in regard to specific methods. However, there is agreement that it is a short-term approach.

Techniques

The therapist and the person in crisis agree on the issues that led to the crisis; the identified patient is actively involved rather than only a recipient of support. The length is from 1 or 2 sessions to several interviews over one to two months. Following the establishment of a therapeutic alliance, the sequence of events that have led to the crisis are reviewed and the maladaptive responses are identified. Interventions should not arouse resistance or exacerbate conflicts that will lead to further decompensation. Intervention is terminated when the crisis is resolved and the identified patient understands the steps that led to the crisis and its resolution.

Crisis intervention includes aspects of both anticipatory guidance and preventive intervention. Anticipatory guidance is the approach taken when a crisis can be predicted. Preventive intervention is a method of guidance for parents and children during the crisis itself. This approach recognizes the patient's increasing dependency and provides continuing support during the crisis. Help is provided by facilitating communication among family members and by discussion of their concerns and their plans for coping. During these discussions, the physician may point out that negative feelings are normal, sympathize with the family's frustration, and encourage the sharing of tasks among family members because fatigue may develop if one person takes on the major burden of care. Interview sessions should focus on present problems rather than emphasize discussion of past failures. Identification of the psychological needs of each family member and the development of confiding relationships among family members is essential in preventive intervention.

With the disabled or chronically ill child, the family's coping often depends on the support that family members can offer one another. It is the therapist's first responsibility to convene a support group at the time of diagnosis. Individuals in crisis show signs of stress that elicit care from others, be they relatives, friends, neighbors, or professionals. If this does not occur spontaneously, it is appropriate for the professionals involved to arrange active support. Depending on the circumstances, the first step is to counsel both parents together, rather than either parent alone, and then to assist the family in finding and utilizing local resources including extended family members, recognized parent support groups for the given condition, community agencies, and religious organizations.

Time-Limited Interventions

Time-limited treatments are commonly employed. Time-limited therapy initially establishes a positive therapeutic alliance. Emphasis is placed on clarifying internal feeling states and interpersonal difficulties. Limit setting, encouragement, reassurance, and direction may be offered. In some instances, a set number of sessions is recommended; in others, a set termination date without a set number of sessions is established, or it is agreed there will be a time limit, but the specific number of sessions is not established in advance and a specific date is not set. Children and mentally retarded adolescents may not have a fully developed sense of time, so aids may be necessary to help them appreciate the time-limited nature of treatment.

Assessment for Time-Limited Intervention

Approaches to brief therapy begin with an initial assessment of the entire family, the formulation of dynamic focal hypotheses, selection of the specific goals for treatment (MacLean, MacIntosh, and Taylor, 1982), and identification of who will participate in the treatment. Goals are chosen based on current specific target symptoms, behaviors, and attitudes that are addressed as "here and now" problems. How these foci are approached will depend on the model utilized, be it a brief supportive or dynamic intervention (Sifneos, 1989), focused time-limited therapy (Proskaer, 1969, 1971), short-term group therapy (Fine et al., 1989; Paramenter, Smith, and Cecic, 1987), or focal individual or family treatment (Bentovim and Kinston, 1978; Kinston and Bentovim, 1978; Lesse and Dare, 1975; Rosenthal, 1982; Selinger and Barcai, 1981). Aspects of the family system that are most in need of change and most amenable to treatment must be addressed. Who is engaged in treatment will vary from family to family.

The factor that is reported to correlate best with improvement is motivation for change; this may be more important than the severity of symptoms. This motivation may override chronicity and pervasiveness of symptoms. Recent onset is not necessarily correlated with good outcome (Malan, 1979).

For adults, a past history of meaningful, confiding relationships is an important ingredient in successful short-term intervention. Selection criteria for children and mildly mentally retarded adolescents include evidence of an intact and supportive family and evidence of motivation to change within the family system (Schulman, DeLafuente, and Suran, 1977). Psychotherapy is presented as a joint venture between therapist and patient. There must be agreed-upon goals.

Some indications for focused therapy in childhood include school refusal, adjustment disorder, mild dysthymic disorder, anxiety states, unresolved grief (complicated bereavement), less severe antisocial disorder (antisocial tendency), parent–child conflicts often associated with oppositional behavior, marital discord or pending divorce, and management of learning problems with associated inadequacy and low self-esteem (Leaverton, Rupp, and Poff, 1977; Wilson and Herzog, 1983).

A central focus is chosen and issues in regard to termination as an experience of eventual separation and loss are considered from the onset. The use of drawings and stories may be helpful in establishing a treatment focus (Proskaer, 1969). For mildly cognitively impaired individuals, asking about three wishes for things they would like to change in their lives, e.g., at school, at home, and in themselves, can also be utilized to elicit areas the child wishes changed, which may serve as a focus for short-term intervention. As termination nears, the child or adolescent may elaborate on imagined self-defeating interpersonal consequences following the end of treatment. The meaning of termination may be distorted in terms of the child or adolescent's negative self-esteem. A therapist must concurrently deal with the child or adolescent's discomfort about the approaching termination (Lester, 1968, 1975, 1986; Madger, 1980; McDermott and Char, 1984).

Establishing Contact

A rapid establishment of rapport is necessary to establish a therapeutic alliance in short-term therapy. In children, the use of special techniques to establish contact and choose a treatment focus is often necessary (Kestenbaum, 1985). This entails various uses of the imagination, including the use of drawings, stories, and other imaginal techniques. Winnicott described the "squiggle game" in *Therapeutic Consultations in Child Psychiatry* as a means of establishing contact with the child and exploring psychodynamic issues. It can also serve to help define a focus for treatment. Fantasies about the therapist as a helpful or nonhelpful person are elicited in early sessions. As Frank (1974) has noted, expectancy and belief in the therapist play an important role in any therapeutic endeavor. The child's own experience of the session and how he or she makes use of it outside the session is the important thing. The child surprises himself as he proceeds to complete drawings and sees his situation in a new way. Winnicott (1970) looked for what use the child made of any new understandings about himself that arose in the treatment session. Whether his parents were able to provide a normally expectable supportive environment that could facilitate therapy and lead to internalization of positive supportive inner figures was an important goal. Using imaginal techniques, a determination is then made to establish if the child could proceed with a time-limited approach or requires longer term intervention (management or long-term therapy). The parents' ability to make the necessary nurturant environmental provision can also be assessed by observing their responses to the child's drawings. Parental confidence in the therapist is necessary. Contraindications include adverse environmental factors and inability of the parent to "meet" the child psychologically and support the necessary changes in the child that are expected in treatment. Generally, a mental age of about 7 years is necessary for the introduction of the squiggle game. However, drawings may be used in therapy for some individuals whose mental age is less than 7 years.

Another means of making contact with the child, gathering information related to psychotherapeutic conflicts, and finding themes for short-term treatment is through the use of the mutual storytelling technique (Gardner, 1971). Like the squiggle game, the mutual storytelling technique may be used to facilitate therapeutic communication in those individuals with mild cognitive impairment.

For nonverbal severely mentally retarded persons and other nonverbal disabled persons with severe communication impairment, the use of various communication devices is necessary to facilitate interpersonal contact (Nuffield, 1986). These approaches are referred to as Augmentative and Alternative Communication (AAC) strategies. The therapist must become familiar with the use of signs and picture aids as well as speech synthesizers and other means of facilitating language in working with nonverbal persons. Rutter (1985) has outlined an approach to therapy for persons with autistic disorder that is applicable to other developmentally disabled persons. The goal is to facilitate communication for the nonverbal individual. Biklen (1990) has introduced a method of facilitated communication. This approach has been successfully used in some persons with cerebral palsy and other developmental disorders. It is largely based on Crossley's proposal that facilitated communication training helps the communicator overcome neuromotor difficulties by teaching hand skills needed to use communication aids. A series of steps are involved in facilitated communication. The disabled person types with one index finger, first with hand-over-hand or hand-at-the-wrist support by the facilitator and subsequently independently or with just a touch to the elbow or shoulder. Gradually, the patient progresses from structured activities to open-ended conversational text (Biklen et al., 1992). It has been hypothesized that the facilitated communication approach enhances attunement between the disabled person and facilitator. Such emotional support may assist in the initiation of communication and allow "functional selection skills" (Crossley and Remington-Gurney, 1992) to be expressed. Commonly, problems in initiating communication involve poor eye–hand communication, impulsivity, perseveration, and lack of confidence. In some instances, these might be linked to executive dysfunction in initiating activities and in motoric planning.

Unfortunately, excessive claims for this approach have been made by some practitioners and false expectations have been raised about the extent of the disabled person's abilities. Its strengths lie in the approach itself, which emphasizes sensitivity to the needs of a disabled person. Its weakness is in the difficulty clarifying that the communication is coming directly from the disabled person and not an interpretation by the facilitator of the disabled person's intentions and thoughts (Silliman, 1992). Therefore, caution is necessary in the utilization of this method until more evidence is available as to its efficacy for specific disorders.

OUTCOME

MacLean, MacIntosh, and Taylor (1982) found that favorable outcome in time-limited interventions depended on (1) warmth between family members; (2) a positive feeling of hope on the part of the therapist toward the family; (3) ability of the family to engage themselves as active agents and their recognition of the time-limited nature of the treatment; and (4) ability to define a clear treatment focus. This might be antisocial behavior to gain attention, projection of anger onto a child by a parent who identified him or her with a spouse or sibling, displacement of anger between parents onto a child or adolescent who is disabled; (5) ability to choose a functional unit for treatment—the person or persons most strategic to treat; (6) assignment of one therapist to the case rather than splitting the case between two; and (7) acknowledgment that the time frame will be recognized and adhered to. However, a family might return later with a different presentation or with different goals.

Richmond (1972) suggests that global goals for successful therapy include the establishment of a confiding relationship within the family and the capacity to plan for both the nondisabled and disabled child or adolescent's future. Kanner (1953) noted that mature acknowledgment of a disability is accompanied by an assignment of the child to a rightful place in the family in keeping with his or her unique strengths and weaknesses.

There has been considerable interest in outcome research regarding time-limited psychotherapy (Koss and Butcher, 1986; Koss, Butcher, and Strupp, 1986; Leventhal and Weinberger, 1975; Shaffer, 1984). Outcome research is needed for psychotherapeutic approaches to disabled persons. Focal time-limited therapy has been found to be an efficient and effective approach for nonmentally retarded persons and their families. Koss and Butcher (1986) in an extensive review conclude that studies comparing brief with unlimited therapy show essentially no difference in results. Still, there is a need for more sophisticated research designs with clearer specification of patients studied, particularly for disabled individuals. Shaffer (1984) emphasizes that such studies should assess therapy with the child and not the parent or caregiver alone. However, for disabling conditions, time-limited therapy with the family can be very effective. Future research requires that rather than ask whether time-limited therapy works for disabled persons and their families, investigators must answer the question: For whom and for what kind of problems is time-limited therapy effective?

REFERENCES

Ainsworth, M. (1969). Object relations, dependency and attachment: A theoretical review of the mother-infant relationship. *Child Development,* 40:969–1025.

Bentovim A., and Kinston W. (1978). Brief focal family therapy when the child is the referred patient: I. Clinical. *Journal of Child Psychology and Psychiatry,* 19:119–143.

Biklen, D. (1990). Communication unbound: Autism and praxis. *Harvard Educational Review,* 60:291–314.

______, Morton, M.W., Gold, D., Berrigan, C., and Swaminathan, S. (1992). Facilitated communication: Implications for individuals with autism. *Topics in Language Disorders,* 12:1–28.

Brazelton, T., and Cramer, B. (1991). Roots and growing points of attachment theory. In C.M. Parkes, J. Stevenson-Hinde, and P. Marris (eds.), *Attachment across the life cycle.* Routledge, London.

Bretherton, I. (1991). Roots and growing points of attachment theory. In C.M. Parkes, J. Stevenson-Hinde, and P. Marris (eds.), *Attachment across the life cycle.* Routledge, London.

Cassidy, J. (1988). The self as related to child-mother attachment at six. *Child Development,* 59:121–134.

Chess, S. (1962). Psychiatric treatment of the mentally retarded child with behavior problems. *American Journal of Orthopsychiatry,* 32:863–869.

Crossley, R., and Remington-Gurney, J. (1992). Getting the words out: Facilitated communication training. *Topics in Language Disorders,* 12:29–45.

Ellis, A., and Bernard, M.E. (1983). *Rational-emotive approaches to the problems of childhood.* Plenum Press, New York.

Erikson, M. (1993). Rethinking Oedipus: An evolutionary perspective on incest avoidance. *American Journal of Psychiatry,* 150:411–416.

Feinstein, C.B. (1993, October). Psychotherapeutic approaches for mentally retarded children, adolescents, and their family. In L. Szymanski, C. Feinstein, and J. Harris (eds.), *Mental retardation and psychotherapy: The new definitions, assessment, and treatment,* pp. 1–10. Institute, American Academy of Child and Adolescent Psychiatry, San Antonio, TX.

Fine, S., Gilbert, M., Schmidt, L., Haley, G., Maxwell A., and Forth, A. (1989). Short term group therapy with depressed adolescent outpatients. *Canadian Journal of Psychiatry,* 34:971–1002.

Fonagy, P., Steele, M., and Steele, H. (1991). Maternal representations of attachment during pregnancy predict the organization of infant-mother attachment at one year of age. *Child Development,* 62:891–905.

Frank, J. D. (1973). *Persuasion and healing: A comparative study of psychotherapy,* Revised ed. Johns Hopkins University Press, Baltimore.

______. (1974). Psychotherapy: The restoration of morale. *American Journal of Psychiatry,* 131:271–274.

______. (1986). Psychotherapy: The transformation of meanings. *Journal of the Royal Society of Medicine,* 79:341–346.

______, and Frank, J.B. (1991). *Persuasion and healing: A comparative study of psychotherapy,* 3rd ed. Johns Hopkins University Press, Baltimore.

Futterman, E.H. (1975). Studies of family adaptational responses to a specific threat. *Explorations in child psychiatry,* pp. 287–301. Plenum Press, New York.

Gair, D., Hersch, C., and Wiesenfeld, M. (1980). Successful psychotherapy of severe emotional disturbance in a young retarded boy. *Journal of the American Academy of Child Psychiatry,* 19:257–269.

Gardner, R.A. (1971). *Therapeutic communication with children: The mutual story telling technique.* Science House, New York.

Heard, D., and Lake, B. (1986). The attachment dynamic in adult life. *British Journal of Psychiatry,* 149:430–438.

Holmes, J. (1993). Attachment theory: A biological basis for psychotherapy? *British Journal of Psychiatry,* 163:430–438.

______, and Lindley, R. (1989). *The values of psychotherapy.* Oxford University Press, London.

Hurley, A.D. (1989). Individual psychotherapy with mentally retarded individuals: A review and call for research. *Research in Developmental Disabilities,* 10:261–275.

______, and Hurley, F.J. (1986). Counseling and psychotherapy with mentally retarded clients: I. The initial interview. *Psychiatric Aspects of Mental Retardation Reviews,* 5:22–26.

______, and ______. (1987). Counseling and psychotherapy with mentally retarded clients: II. Establishing a relationship. *Psychiatric Aspects of Mental Retardation Reviews,* 6:15–20.

Jakab, I. (1982). Psychiatric disorders in mental retardation: Recognition, diagnosis, and treatment. In K. Jakab (ed.), *Mental retardation,* pp. 270–322. Kargan, New York.

Kanner, L. (1953). Parents' feelings about retarded children. *American Journal of Mental Deficiency,* 57:375–383.

Kestenbaum, C.J. (1985). The creative process in child psychotherapy. *American Journal of Psychotherapy,* 39:479–489.

Kinston, W., and Bentovim, A. (1978). Brief focal family therapy when the child is the referred patient: II. Methodology and results. *Journal of Child Psychology and Psychiatry,* 19:119–143.

Koss, M., and Butcher, J.N. (1986). Research on brief psychotherapy. In *Handbook of psychotherapy and behavior change,* 3rd ed. John Wiley, New York.

______, ______, and Strupp, H. (1986). Brief psychotherapy methods in clinical research. *Journal of Consulting and Clinical Psychology,* 54:60–67.

Leaverton, D.R., Rupp, J.W., and Poff, M.G. (1977). Brief therapy for monocular hysterical blindness in childhood. *Child Psychiatry and Human Development,* 74:254–263.

Leland, H., and Smith, D.E. (1965). *Play therapy with mentally subnormal children.* Grune & Stratton, New York.

Lesse, S., and Dare C. (1975). A classification of interventions in child and conjoint family therapy. *Psychotherapy and Psychosomatics,* 25:116–125.

Lester, E.P. (1968). Brief psychotherapies in child psychiatry. *Canadian Journal of Psychiatry.* 13:301–309.

______. (1975). Language behaviour and child psychotherapy. *Canadian Journal of Psychiatry;* 20:175–181.

______. (1986). On transference: Developmental and clinical considerations. *Canadian Journal of Psychiatry.* 31:146–153.

Leventhal, T., and Weinberger, G. (1975). Evaluation of a large scale brief therapy program for children. *American Journal of Orthopsychiatry,* 45:119–132.

Levitas, A., and Gilson, S. (1987). Transference, countertransference, and resistance. *National Association for the Dually Diagnosed Newsletter,* 1L:2–7.

Levy, D.M. (1943). *Maternal overprotection.* Columbia University Press, New York.

MacLean, G., MacIntosh, B.A., and Taylor, E. (1982). A clinical approach to brief dynamic psychotherapies in child psychiatry. *Canadian Journal of Psychiatry.* 27:11–38.

Madger, D. (1980). The wizard of oz: A parable of brief psychotherapy. *Canadian Journal of Psychiatry.* 25:564–567.

Main, M. (1990). *A typology of human attachment organization with discourse, drawings, and interviews.* Cambridge University Press, New York.

______. (1991). Metacognitive knowledge, metacognitive monitoring, and singular (coherent) vs. multiple (incoherent) models of attachment: Findings and direction for future research. In C.M. Parkes, J. Stevenson-Hinde, and P. Marris (eds.), *Attachment across the life cycle.* Routledge, London.

Malan, D.H. (1979). *Individual psychotherapy and the science of psychodynamics,* 2nd ed. Butterworth, London.

McDermott, J.F., and Char, W.F. (1984). Stage related models of psychotherapy with children. *Journal of the American Academy of Child and Adolescent Psychiatry,* 23:537–543.

Menolascino, F.J., Gilson, S.F., and Levitas, A. (1986). Issues in the treatment of mentally retarded patients in the community mental health system. *Community Mental Health Journal,* 22:314–327.

Murray, L., and Cooper, P. (in press). Clinical applications of attachment theory and research: Change in infant attachment with brief psychotherapy. *Journal of Child Psychology and Psychiatry.*

Nuffield, E. (1986). Counselling and psychotherapy. In R. Barrett (ed.), *Severe behavior disorders in the mentally retarded: Nondrug approaches to treatment,* pp. 207–234. Plenum Press, New York.

Parmenter, G., Smith, J.C., and Cecic, N.A. (1987). Parallel and conjoint short term group therapy for school age children and their parents: A model. *International Journal of Group Psychotherapy,* 37:239–254.

Proskaer, S. (1969). Some technical issues in time limited psychotherapy with children. *Journal of the American Academy of Child and Adolescent Psychiatry,* 8:154–159.

______. (1971). Focused time limited therapy with children. *Journal of the American Academy of Child and Adolescent Psychiatry,* 10:619–639.

Reiss, S., and Benson, B. (1984). Awareness of negative social conditions among mentally retarded, emotionally disturbed outpatients. *American Journal of Psychiatry,* 141:1.

Richmond, J.B. (1972). The family and the handicapped child. *Clinical Proceedings of the Children's Hospital National Medical Center,* 8:156–164.

Rogoff, B. (1990). *Apprenticeship in thinking: Cognitive development in social context,* New York, Oxford University Press, pp. 137–150.

Rosenthal, P.A. (1982). Short term family therapy and pathological grief resolution with children and adolescents. *Family Process,* 19:15–19.

Rutter, M. (1985). The treatment of autistic children. *Journal of Child Psychology and Psychiatry,* 26:193–214.

Schulman, J.L., DeLafuente, M.E., and Suran, B.G. (1977). An indicator for brief psychotherapy: The fork in the road phenomenon. *Bulletin of the Meninger Clinic,* 41:553–562.

Selinger, D., and Barcai, A. (1981). Brief family therapy may lead to deep personality change. *American Journal of Psychotherapy,* 31:302–309.

Shaffer, D. (1984). Notes on psychotherapy research among children and adolescents. *Journal of the American Academy of Child and Adolescent Psychiatry,* 23:552–561.

Sifneos, P.E. (1989). Brief dynamic and crisis therapy. In H.I. Kaplan and B.J. Sadock (eds.), *The comprehensive textbook of psychiatry,* 5th ed., pp. 1562–1567. Williams & Wilkins, Baltimore.

Sigman, M. (1985). Individual and group psychotherapy with mentally retarded adolescents. In M. Sigman (ed.), *Children with emotional disorders and developmental disabilities,* pp. 259–275. Grune & Stratton, Orlando.

Silliman, R.R. (1992). Three perspectives on facilitated communication: Unexpected literacy, clever Hans, or enigma? *Topics in Language Disorders,* 12:60–68.

Smith, S., McKinnon, R., and Kessler, J. (1976). Psychotherapy with mentally retarded children. *The Psychoanalytic Study of the Child,* 31:493–314. Yale University Press, New Haven.

Stavrakaki, C., and Klein J. (1986). Psychotherapies with the mentally retarded. *Psychiatric Clinics of North America,* 9:733–743.

Stern, D. (1985). *The interpersonal world of the infant.* Basic Books, New York.

Szymanski, L. (1980). Individual psychotherapy with retarded persons. In L.S. Szymanski and P.E. Tanguay (eds.), *Emotional disorders of mentally retarded persons: Assessment, treatment, and consultation,* pp. 131–148. University Park Press, Baltimore.

______, and Rosefsky, Q.B. (1980). Group psychotherapy with retarded persons. In L.S. Szymanski and P.E. Tanguay (eds.), *Emotional disorders of mentally retarded persons: Assessment, treatment, and consultation,* pp. 173–194. University Park Press, Baltimore.

Wilson, P., and Herzog, L. (1983). Individual and group psychotherapy. In M . Rutter and L. Herzov (eds.), *Child psychiatry: Modern approaches.* Blackwell, London.

Winnicott, D.W. (1970). *Therapeutic consultations in child psychiatry.* Basic Books, New York.

CHAPTER 19

BEHAVIOR THERAPY

The behavior therapies are the most widely used and best studied treatment interventions for behavioral disturbances manifested by persons with mental retardation and other developmental disorders. The terms "behavior modification," "contingency management," and "applied behavior analysis," are included as components. As an approach, behavior therapy deals with the technology of behavior change (Jansen, 1980). Although behavioral procedures are based on the principles of learning theory and are effective for maladaptive patterns of behavior that are the result of faulty learning, they also may be effective for emotional and behavioral symptoms which result primarily from pathophysiological disorders. Behavioral treatments have been developed for enhancing adaptive, socially desirable behavior, reducing maladaptive behavior, and acquiring habilitative skills. For the behaviorist, behavior refers to anything a person does, thinks, or feels (overtly or covertly) that can be counted or measured.

Behavioral approaches have been applied to children with a variety of developmental disabilities including mental retardation, autistic disorder, and other pervasive developmental disorders, academic skills disorders, language and speech disorders, disruptive behavior disorders (attention deficit disorder, oppositional defiant disorder), anxiety disorders, eating disorders, tic disorders, elimination disorders, stereotypic movement disorders, schizophrenia, mood disorders, substance abuse, somatoform disorders, and sleep disorders. In this chapter, the principles of behavior therapy are emphasized rather than addressing behavioral treatments for each of these problems. The application of the various methods and the choice of procedures must be decided by the primary therapist generally working along with a behavioral psychologist. The emphasis here is on the use of applied behavior analysis, using operant techniques and functional communication methods with severely developmentally disabled persons. Because of the severity of behavior difficulty in these individuals, the reduction of undesirable behavior has received more emphasis than the development of new behaviors. The behavioral difficulties most commonly addressed in developmentally disabled individuals are aggressive behavior and property destruction, noncompliance, pica, regurgitation and rumination, tantrums, screaming and crying, self-injurious behavior, and stereotyped behavior (Johnson and Baumeister, 1981).

This chapter provides an historical background and definition of behavior therapy, offers an orientation for the therapist in working with the disabled person, and then discusses applied behavior analysis, behavior management techniques, behavior enhancement; behavior reduction approaches, functional assessment, and future directions.

HISTORY

Behaviorism was initially introduced as a technique by John Watson (1924) and explored as an approach in greater detail by B. F. Skinner (1953, 1974). The principles of behavior therapy and a variety of behavioral techniques were developed during the first part of the twentieth century before the Second World War. However, it was not until the late 1940s and 1950s that behavioral approaches were recognized as therapies distinct from the psychodynamic treatment models. Early behavioral approaches based on animal experimentation were subsequently adapted to human subjects where the problems presented were far more complex, leading to an increase in the scope and definition of behavior therapy. Initial applications used classical or respondent conditioning paradigms introduced by Pavlov, or operant conditioning and reinforcement procedures suggested by Skinner (1938). One of the first operant behavioral interventions for the mentally retarded person was that of Fuller in 1949. This author used sugar milk as a reward to teach a profoundly retarded 18-year-old to raise his arm. The author suggested that a range of adaptive responses might be conditioned in individuals who previously were thought unable to learn. Later, in the 1950s and 1960s, there was an extensive development of clinical approaches of behavior therapy to work with mentally retarded individuals, particularly in institutional settings. Behavior therapists worked with direct care staff, initially to develop programs for activities of daily living, such as toilet training (Ellis, 1963) and self-feeding (Bensberg, 1965). The positive results from these early interventions that aided mentally retarded persons in participating in school and vocational training programs were followed by interventions for difficult behavior. The most severe behavioral problems—assaultive and destructive behavior (Hamilton, Stephens, and Allen, 1967) and self-injury (Tate and Baroff, 1966)—began to be addressed. Wolpe's (1958) psychotherapy by reciprocal inhibition and Ullman and Krasner (1965) case studies on behavior modification brought these approaches to a wider audience.

Operant approaches were most commonly used and continued to evolve and now include functional communication training, which views behavioral responses as aberrant forms of communication. Functional communication takes into account the importance of severe communication impairments in children and adolescents with mental retardation who may not be able to make their needs known through the usual socially appropriate types of communication. It involves efforts to teach children self-direction to access reinforcement through communication (Carr and Durand, 1985). How internal complex events, such as thinking, could fit into a behavioral model was subsequently approached through the introduction of cognitive behavioral approaches. With this development, behavioral approaches included not only principles derived from animal learning and conditioning but also those derived from social and cognitive psychology. Ellis (1962) introduced rational emotive therapy, and Beck (1976), cognitive therapy.

DEFINITION

Behavior therapy has been defined as follows (Werry and Wollersheim, 1989 p.1): "Those treatments that utilize the principles and terms of learning theory and allied aspects of experimental psychology and that are committed to explicit specification of treatment procedures and goals and to the objective evaluation of therapeutic outcomes." Behavior therapy incorporates approaches ranging from procedures that focus only on overt behavior (behavior modification) to cognitive behavioral approaches which emphasize internal processes.

ORIENTATION OF THE THERAPIST

A sensitive orientation toward the person that emerges from attachment theory should be maintained in conducting behavioral interventions. This is particularly important in dealing with severely mentally retarded and autistic persons. Menolascino and McGee (1983) have emphasized the importance of moving from personal disconnectedness in applying behavioral techniques to human engagement. They recommend an approach to the person that emphasizes social attachment. McGee (1988) emphasizes that intervention techniques should serve to make mutual relationships possible. How a technique is delivered can be critical to its success, so the emotional posture of the caregiver toward the individual must be considered. McGee identifies three problematic postures: the overprotective posture, the authoritarian posture, and the mechanistic posture. The overprotective posture makes few demands and although it may be benevolent, without demands the individual will not grow. An authoritarian posture may lead to behavior reduction or suppression without the establishment of an interpersonal attachment. Finally, a mechanistic posture may emphasize conformity to routines without providing the personal contact needed to establish meaningful interpersonal attachment. A corrective to these postures is an approach to the person that focuses on engagement, with the goal of establishing attachment. This has been referred to as the gentle teaching paradigm. In gentle teaching, a warm, nonjudgmental attitude is maintained so, in interacting, the disabled person is taught that human presence signifies safety, consistency, and positive interaction or reward. This orientation is maintained while ignoring inappropriate behavior, interrupting it, redirecting the person, and finally, rewarding appropriate behavior.

APPLIED BEHAVIOR ANALYSIS

Applied behavior analysis emphasizes environmental influences on behavior and utilizes within-subjects' experimental designs to clarify which environmental interventions are most effective in producing behavior change (Kazdin, 1982). Applied behavior analysis makes the assumption that behavior is a function of current and past antecedents and consequences. Such behaviors may increase with either positive or negative reinforcement. Behavior that occurs more often under one set of environmental circumstances rather than another that precedes it is said to be under antecedent or stimulus control. Behavior that increases or decreases in frequency in relation to events that follow the targeted behavior is said to be under consequent control. Technically, the emphasis is placed on accurately defining the problem behaviors and identifying specific antecedents and consequences. Identification of the problem areas is accomplished through the use of interviews with caregivers and direct observation in conjunction with the use of behavior checklists and rating scales.

Rating scales used with mentally retarded persons have been reviewed by Aman (1991) and are discussed in Chapter 5 on mental retardation. The Reiss Screen for Maladaptive Behavior is one of the best overall screening instruments. The Strohmer-Prout Rating Scale is recommended for those persons functioning in the borderline to mild range of mental retardation, and the Aberrant Behavior Checklist for those functioning in the moderate to severe range of mental retardation. Although several rating scales diagnose specific psychiatric conditions, none are adequately validated; psychiatric diagnosis is ordinarily based on modifications of DSM-IV (APA, 1994) criteria. In general, rating scales are most useful for externalizing behaviors, such as aggression and self-injury, and less so for depression and anxiety.

Direct observation is more commonly used for applied behavior analysis by behavioral psychologists. When used diagnostically, conditions are established so that the diagnostic symptoms are most likely to occur and behaviors are systematically observed and recorded. Direct observation is often combined with single-case experimental designs to evaluate externalizing behaviors. In these paradigms, the methodology is generally referred to as functional analysis. Its focus is on identifying behavior consequences or outcomes that affect the frequency of behavior, i.e., its probability of occurring. The variables hypothesized to affect an individual's behavior are identified and manipulated, using single-case experimental design procedures to systematically test the extent to which these variables affected the targeted behavior.

In behavior analysis, the time and the conditions present at the onset of the behavior problem are identified, and each problem is listed in regard to its current frequency, duration, and intensity. The behavior is categorized according to whether it is situation specific or pervasive. Behavior problems are evaluated in regard to the time and the circumstances when they are most likely and least likely to take place. Antecedents and consequences for the target behavior are identified and previous management strategies discussed in regard to the particular methods used and their effectiveness. Family members are asked to specify their own goals for treatment and their motivation and willingness to participate in a contingency management program.

After completing the assessment and identifying target behaviors, behavior problems are prioritized in regard to their severity, the amount of effort, and the extent of training that may be needed by parents or caregivers to manage identified behaviors. Dangerous or destructive behaviors that require immediate attention or those that can be approached quickly through positive reinforcement methods may be targeted initially. Other behavior problems that are pervasive and difficult to change may not be targeted until the caregivers feel competent and have been successful in implementing strategies for less intense behavior problems or have successfully addressed the more dangerous ones.

The procedures introduced will range from informal recommendations in behavior management to intensive skills training. Specific contingency management procedures are presented along with their rationale, and brief written protocols are provided. Specific assignments are directly given to the caregivers and/or the identified person with behavior difficulties to track the target behavior and implement specific interventions. Behavior management programs need to be supported over time with continuous reevaluation because such time- and labor-intensive interventions are difficult to maintain without monitoring and support.

BEHAVIOR MANAGEMENT TECHNIQUES

Behavioral approaches are often grouped into those designed to enhance adaptive behavior and those designed to reduce maladaptive behavior. They are generally designated as behavior enhancement and behavior reduction strategies. Behavior enhancement procedures are preferable because they are directed toward a reduction of undesirable behaviors by promoting adaptive means to master problems. Enhancement is accomplished by increasing the probability that socially desirable behaviors will occur. Enhancement of adaptive behaviors will ultimately replace problem behaviors by strengthening desirable behaviors that compete with maladaptive ones. Behavior reduction procedures directly suppress maladaptive behaviors by consequating their occurrence with undesirable responses.

Environmental interventions recommended by applied behavior analysts are most commonly based on positive reinforcement, negative reinforcement, and punishment procedures. Specific behavioral terminology is included in the glossary at the end of the chapter.

Reinforcement

Reinforcement refers to an increase in the frequency of a response if it is immediately followed by certain consequences. The consequence that follows behavior must be contingent on the behavior itself; a contingent event that increases the frequency of behavior is referred to as a reinforcer. Two kinds of reinforcers are described, namely, positive and negative reinforcers, and both increase the frequency of response. Positive reinforcers can be distinguished from rewards in that a positive reinforcer is simply defined by its effect on behavior. If an event follows a behavior and the frequency of the behavior increases, that event is a positive reinforcer. Any event which does not increase behavior that follows is not a positive reinforcer. Rewards, on the contrary, are defined as something given or received in return for some activity or achievement of a goal but may not necessarily increase the probability of a behavior occurring.

Positive Reinforcement

With positive reinforcement, the presentation of an object or event, referred to as the reinforcer, following a behavior by the individual leads to an increase in the rate or the probability of that behavior occurring in the future. Generally, positive reinforcement procedures are used to increase rates of prosocial behavior. Premack (1965) found that if the opportunity to perform a behavior with a more probable response was made contingent on performing a behavior with a less probable response, the frequency of the latter would increase. Therefore, behaviors with a relatively high probability of occurring in an individual serve as reinforcers for lower probability behavior. Premack's observations led to the Premack principle, which says that of any pair of responses or activities in which an individual engages, the more frequent one can be used to reinforce the less frequent one. Therefore, a higher probability behavior may be used to reinforce a lower probability one. The determination of high or low frequency behaviors simply requires observing which behaviors an individual engages in when left to perform freely. Positive reinforcers may include social approval (praise, smiles, gestures of approval); permission to carry out activities (viewing television, extended play); preferred objects (toys, certificates of accomplishment, money); and things to eat (fruit, candy, etc.). Reinforcers, such as praise, smiles, money, or food, are delivered immediately after a response. However, for certain syndromes, for example, in autistic disorder where reinforcers may be difficult to identify, preferred activities might include being allowed to carry out certain autistic stereotypies for a limited time. In identifying positive reinforcers, an event that may be a positive reinforcer for one individual may not be so for another. Moreover, an event may be a reinforcer for one person in some circumstances and at some times but not under other circumstances or at other times. Consequently, careful assessment is needed to clarify what is reinforcing for a particular individual and under what circumstances.

Shaping Behavior

Commonly, desired behaviors may not be in the child's repertoire. If so, there is no opportunity to differentially reinforce behavior. To establish appropriate behavior, shaping procedures may be introduced. Shaping refers to reinforcing successive approximations of a desired behavior. Shaping may involve repeated prompting or guidance procedures, such as leading the child through the behavioral response. As the desired skill is shaped, the structure and involvement of the therapist is gradually reduced or faded; the independent demonstration of the new behavior is the expected result.

Imitation and Instruction

New behavior may also be taught through imitation by demonstrating the behavior to the person or by instructing the person on how to carry it out. With imitation, the behavior is demonstrated and the person is differentially reinforced, using shaping procedures to establish the behavior. With instruction, the therapist or caregiver describes what is to be done and then asks the individual to follow up on the request. Acknowledgment is provided for successful completion of the task.

Negative Reinforcement

Negative reinforcement refers to an increase in the frequency of a response that is brought about by removing a negative reinforcer immediately after the response is performed. A negative reinforcer or event, when withdrawn, contingent on demonstrating the response, increases the probability of the response recurring. An event is a negative reinforcer only if its removal after the response increases the frequency of performance of that response. An undesirable event may be aversive for one individual but not for another. Moreover, an event may be a negative reinforcer for an individual at one time but not at another. The negative reinforcer, just as the positive one, is defined solely by the effect it has on behavior (Kazdin, 1984). Like positive reinforcement, negative reinforcement always leads to an increase in behavior. Negative reinforcement processes also, just as positive reinforcement processes, may increase undesirable as well as desirable behaviors. For example, a child whining may be a negative reinforcer for the parent who picks the child up to terminate the behavior and yet, at the same time, may increase its frequency by attending to it. Negative reinforcement does require an aversive event that is presented to an individual before he responds, such as noise, isolation, or other events which can be removed or reduced immediately after the child does respond. Negative reinforcement occurs at those times when an individual escapes from an aversive event; escape from aversive events is strongly negatively reinforcing. Negative reinforcement is not commonly used to enhance behavior but, when used, an individual is allowed to avoid a predetermined punishment by engaging in an appropriate behavior.

Extinction

Extinction refers to withholding reinforcement from a previously reinforced response. When reinforcement is withheld, a response undergoes extinction and eventually decreases until it drops to its prereinforcement level or is eliminated. The most common example of extinction is planned ignoring of a child's inappropriate behavior. Ignoring may decrease the rate of those problem behaviors that are maintained by positive reinforcement, for example, attention to disruptive behavior or to inappropriate demands. Using extinction, the caregiver withholds positive reinforcement after an inappropriate behavior occurs. The positive reinforcer, in this instance prior attention to inappropriate behavior, is then withheld. Unfortunately, simply ignoring behavior takes considerable time to be effective in reducing it. Ignoring frequently produces a transient increase in the intensity and frequency of problem behaviors (extinction burst) before there is a subsequent reduction in behavior. It requires persistence to continue to ignore the behavior until it is eliminated. During extinction, spontaneous reappearance of the undesirable behavior may take place as the child tests to see whether or not the caregiver will again provide contingent attention to a problem behavior.

BEHAVIOR ENHANCEMENT APPROACHES

Differential Reinforcement

Behavior enhancement procedures are often grouped into several types of differential reinforcement strategies. Differential reinforcement refers to reinforcing a response in the presence of one stimulus and extinguishing a response in the presence of other stimuli. Positive reinforcement and extinction procedures are commonly used together because the inappropriate behavior targeted for change may occur along with acceptable behaviors that require continued positive reinforcement. The goal is to reinforce appropriate behavior while at the same time withholding reinforcement for inappropriate behavior. Using differential reinforcement, the caregiver might show gestures of approval for sharing but ignore aggressive behavior when the child refuses to share. For change to occur, differential reinforcement techniques must be applied by caregivers in each of the settings where the child demonstrates the inappropriate behavior. Differential reinforcement, rather than simple extinction, has the advantage that it helps the child distinguish which behaviors are appropriate and which are inappropriate.

Four types of differential reinforcement have been described based on principles of positive reinforcement (Johnson and Baumeister, 1981): differential reinforcement of appropriate or alternative behaviors (DRA), differential reinforcement of incompatible behaviors (DRI), differential reinforcement of other behaviors (DRO), and differential reinforcement of low rates of behavior (DRL). Each of these approaches involves positive reinforcement, but they differ in regard to the behaviors targeted for reinforcement. With the exception of DRL, none of these approaches directly consequate the aberrant behavior targeted for reduction.

Differential reinforcement of appropriate behavior (DRA), or compatible behavior (DRC), applies the reinforcement contingency to a specific response. The therapeutic goal is to achieve a higher proportion of that response, such as toy play or attention to task, which leads secondarily to a reduction in aberrant behavior. Unlike a differential reinforcement of other behaviors (DRO), the focus is on a specific response rather than nonspecific reinforcement. The response chosen is one that is already in the individual's behavioral repertoire and is most likely to be learned quickly.

Differential reinforcement of incompatible behavior (DRI) differs from DRA in that the performance of a response selected for reinforcement precludes a display of the targeted aberrant behavior. DRI involves the direct reinforcement of preselected adaptive behavior that competes with and eventually replaces the target behavior. For example, head hitting was reduced in one study when subjects were reinforced for holding a ball and passing it back and forth because this activity is incompatible with the hitting. Another example is shaking another person's hand rather than slapping one's head.

Differential reinforcement of other behavior (DRO) is one of the most popular positive reinforcement strategies for decreasing aberrant behavior. With DRO, the individual is reinforced for not exhibiting the target behavior. DRO refers to any procedure where positive reinforcement is supplied contingent on time periods when the aberrant behavior is not displayed. Some have referred to DRO as omission training. In some instances, it may be difficult to find periods when there is no occurrence of aberrant behavior to reinforce. When using DRO, a reinforcer is delivered if the target behavior has not occurred at the end of a clearly specified period of time. The time interval is established through a baseline assessment of the frequency of the target behavior. The interval should be long enough to require effort but short enough to encourage success. If the aberrant behavior does occur, the DRO time interval is restarted. This interval may be of fixed duration or varied duration. It may be gradually increased in length, perhaps beginning with short periods of several seconds and moving on to periods of several hours without aberrant responding. Like DRI, DRO has an advantage in that the aberrant behavior which is targeted for reduction cannot be an adventitious reinforcer because any aberrant response leads to a cancellation of the reinforcement. Overall, DRO is useful in that it provides reinforcement for refraining from abnormal or deviant behavior and, when successful, the frequency of the target behavior decreases as more adaptive, competing behaviors that are reinforced increase. A DRO procedure requires that reinforcement be delivered contingent on the absence of a behavior during the prescribed interval (e.g., absence of aggression) but not on the occurrence of a particular behavior. As such, it must be kept in mind that it may function as a response cost (described later) because reinforcement is delayed.

The fourth positive reinforcement approach, differential reinforcement of low rates of behavior (DRL), is used less frequently than the others. This method involves presenting a reinforcer contingent on occurrences of the aberrant behavior that is targeted for behavior reduction. The individual learns that display of the aberrant behavior will be followed by reinforcement. When this learning has taken place, the contingency schedule is changed so the behavior must be displayed in increasing lower rates to receive reinforcement. A dilemma with using this approach is that there may be ethical problems in directly reinforcing behavior that is maladaptive. An alternative is to choose a maladaptive behavior that occurs at a high rate. A predetermined frequency of the target behavior is chosen (lower than base line). This frequency is progressively lowered until the target behavior is eliminated.

Among these approaches, differential reinforcement of incompatible behaviors (DRI) seems to be the most efficacious. However, a shortcoming for all of these approaches is that if the reinforcers which have been used for treatment become unavailable, the undesired response may return (lack of generalization). This problem may be addressed by initially identifying reinforcers that naturally occur in the environment rather than introducing new ones which may be difficult to continue. In choosing one positive reinforcer, the therapist must also be sure to take the reinforcer's strength into account. Reinforcers may also be linked to neutral objects, such as tokens, which then become conditioned reinforcers.

BEHAVIOR REDUCTION APPROACHES

Behavior reduction procedures involve the introduction of an undesirable circumstance contingent on the occurrence of the target behaviors.

Punishment

Punishment approaches include contingent withdrawal procedures, such as time-out and response cost. Punishment in behavioral psychology does not refer to the common use of the word as a penalty imposed for a particular act. Instead, punishment refers to the presentation of a nonpreferred aversive stimulus or the removal of a positive event following the response that leads to a decrease in the frequency of the response (Kazdin, 1984). This definition includes the requirement that the frequency of the response is decreased following the intervention. Punishment does not necessarily entail pain or any physical coercion. It is not retribution for misbehavior but rather a technical term defined entirely by the effect of the prescribed action on behavior. Punishment may occur when a nonpreferred stimulus or activity or aversive event is presented after a response (Type I), for example, being reprimanded after engaging in a particular behavior or accidentally being burned after touching a hot stove. Another type of punishment is the removal of a reinforcer, a preferred stimulus or activity, after a response (Type II), for example, losing privileges for misbehaving. In this instance, some positive event is taken away after the response is performed. Another example is a loss of television privileges if a child did not dress himself in a timely fashion. With punishment, an action is taken following a behavior which results in a decrease in the rate or probability that behavior will occur under similar circumstances in the future.

The use of punishment techniques tends to be avoided in behavior therapy because there are many reinforcement-based procedures that are effective, making it unnecessary. Moreover, not only may punishment result in negative side effects, but it may also be misused. When punishment procedures are used, they are ordinarily implemented together with positive reinforcement procedures, thereby providing differential consequences for appropriate versus inappropriate behavior. Punishment procedures ordinarily are introduced only after positive reinforcement has not been effective.

The most common form of punishment is contingent negative verbal statements. For example, warnings and reprimands are given following misbehavior. However, such statements may have inconsistent effects, particularly when used with children with developmental disorders who may not fully understand. The manner in which verbal disapprovals are given, particularly voice tone, may determine their effectiveness. A quiet, private reprimand may be more useful than a loud one said in front of others. Moreover, misbehavior may only be suppressed. In some instances, punishments may serve as reinforcers and a means of negative attention and increase the rate of behavior— the opposite of the effect intended. Overall, punishment procedures tend to suppress behavior and, although used commonly, are best avoided or used only when other means of behavior reduction are exhausted.

One type of punishment procedure that is controversial is contingent stimulation. Examples of punishment using contingent stimulation include spraying lemon juice or water mist or using aromatic ammonia following self-injury. In rare instances, mild shock has been used, but this approach is no longer common and should be avoided. It was used in the past when the child placed himself at risk of injury or permanent impairment. Because of the controversy over the use of contingent stimulation, particularly shock, it is being increasingly regulated or banned. For example, in the state of Maryland, such procedures may only be used to terminate maladaptive behavior that poses an immediate threat to the safety or well-being of the client or others (Maryland State Department of Health and Hygiene, 1994). Any form of punishment procedure should be reviewed and approved by an impartial human rights committee. However, it is generally best simply to avoid contingent stimulation.

Time-Out

Time-out refers to removal of access to positive reinforcement. In a time-out, the child is not permitted to engage in certain preferred activities. Time-out should be consistently applied, of brief duration, and used sparingly; lengthy time-outs may lose their effectiveness. Time-out is most effective if applied for a limited number of problem behaviors at any point in time. As those problem behaviors are resolved, new behaviors may be targeted for treatment. Common examples of time-out are brief corner or chair time-out, partial removal from preferred activities with contingent observation from the side lines, and passively precluding the child from having an opportunity to receive reinforcement. The usefulness of time-out requires that all positive reinforcers which support the problem behavior are not available. Time-out is useful only when the child is removed from time-in (preferred activity). If a child is removed from the classroom because of misbehavior, this may not constitute a true time-out procedure because the child is allowed to escape or avoid school experiences that he may identify as aversive.

Time-out may be difficult to apply because it removes the child from reinforcement and may lead to resentment toward the caregiver. Time-out should be used sparingly because, during the time-out period, the child is not getting positive reinforcement. If not well administered, time-out may inadvertently provide negative attention for problem behaviors. This occurs most commonly if the child puts up considerable resistance to the procedure with either a physical or verbal struggle. Because the usual goal of behavior management is to help the child acquire or develop skills, time-out is used primarily when inappropriate behavior significantly interferes with learning or participation in a group.

Time-out differs from exclusion and physical restraint, which is used, in some circumstances, to protect peers and staff from the child's behavior — most commonly, aggressive behavior. It differs from these procedures in that it is systematically applied and of clearly defined duration. A variety of time-out procedures have been applied to reduce inappropriate behavior. Johnson and Baumeister (1981) refer to Schroeder and describe several time-out procedures, i.e., contingent observation, withdrawal time-out, and exclusion time-out. Contingent observation involves ignoring the individual for a period of time following the targeted behavior, for example, the caregiver averts gaze from the individual's face temporarily. Another approach is facial screening, which is a form of time-out similar to contingent observation and is applied by temporarily covering the individual's eyes and face following the inappropriate response. Withdrawal time-out occurs when the caregiver discontinues interacting with the individual and temporarily leaves the treatment setting following the inappropriate behavior. Exclusion time-out occurs in the treatment setting when the individual is temporarily prevented from participating in certain activities contingent on displaying designated target behaviors. When exclusion involves physical restraint, the time-out method is termed "contingent restraint." Seclusion refers to temporary removal to a separate setting where reinforcement is not available.

In establishing time-out programs, whether or not a verbal explanation for the time-out is given depends on the value of the explanation for the individual. Prior warnings or signals may be given indicating time-out will be implemented if the inappropriate behavior appears or if it continues. It is generally best for the individual to follow verbal instructions to go to a time-out area rather than being physically removed. The location for time-out may be one of isolation or nonisolation from the group. Nonisolation allows the individual to remain in the treatment setting and to witness peers receiving reinforcement he is missing as well as to observe ongoing activities and instruction. However, nonisolated time-out does provide increased opportunity for others to reinforce inappropriate behavior adventitiously.

The termination of the time-out may or may not be contingent on the individual's behavior during time-out. Time-out may end when the undesirable behavior is absent for a minimum period of time. A minimum time-out duration may be set with provision for an extension until the targeted behavior is terminated, or time-out periods may be fixed with fixed duration extensions if undesirable behavior occurs (White, Neilson, and Johnson, 1972). Time-out is generally most effective when the child or adolescent is removed from an environment rich in rewards. It is used most commonly for tantrums, aggressive behavior, or mild behavior problems.

Response Cost

Response cost involves the loss of a positive reinforcer or the introduction of a penalty when the child behaves inappropriately (Kazdin, 1984). Most commonly, response cost involves the loss of a positive reinforcer, such as a privilege, or a penalty that requires some work or effort. To fully participate in a response cost procedure, individuals who are cognitively limited may need help in learning the relationships between what they do and what happens as a result. With response cost, there is no required time restriction for available reinforcement, as is the case with time-out. When a penalty is imposed, there is no fixed period of time during which positive reinforcers are unavailable. Psychological association of the cost with the inappropriate behavior is established in advance and applied immediately in a consistent manner. Response cost is commonly applied along with positive reinforcement through specific protocols involving point systems or token economies. In these instances, points or tokens are provided for appropriate behavior and taken away for problem behaviors. Response cost, like other punishment procedures, may lead to resentment, aggression, or avoidance. However, it is easily implemented and may lead to rapid reductions in problem behavior if sensitively applied.

Overcorrection

Overcorrection is a punishment procedure that involves a penalty for inappropriate behavior.

Overcorrection procedure commonly involves a combination of activities and is best considered as a pair of general rationales rather than a specific technique. With overcorrection, there are two components— restitution and positive practice. If a behavior is destructive or disrupts the environment, the offender must first restore, i.e., correct damage caused by the inappropriate behavior. This rationale is referred to as restitution overcorrection (Foxx and Azrin, 1972). The second rationale is referred to as positive practice. In positive practice, the individual must perform a series of unreinforced behavior that is similar to, but specifically incompatible with, or more appropriate than, the inappropriate target behavior. With positive practice, the child or adolescent exhibits an acceptable alternative behavior. To be effective, an overcorrection procedure must include both components, and the components must be directly related to the problem behavior. Overcorrection procedures are applied immediately after the inappropriate behavior and preferred activities are withheld until the required activity is completed. In applying overcorrection procedures, graduated guidance where the individual is systematically led through the required practice procedure may be necessary. Physical prompts may be used to perform the required procedure and, as compliance increases, the physical prompts are faded, leaving only verbal direction to complete the task.

In general, clinical research studies have supported the short-term efficacy of behavior reduction procedures in suppressing maladaptive behaviors, at least under certain circumstances. However, the stability and generalization of these effects have not been firmly established. The most intrusive procedures typically have been reserved for addressing the most dangerous behaviors (e.g., serious aggression and self-injury).

Punishment procedures have been sharply criticized because of potential and real abuses and have become the source of considerable controversy. Many states have enacted regulations that either ban or seriously restrict their implementation. These regulations stem from ethical concerns and the fact that punishment alone suppresses behavior; punishment procedures by definition do not teach problem-solving skills or enhance adaptive responses to stress. Punishment cannot be endorsed in the absence of appropriate habilitative training and a positive behavior enhancement program. In 1989 the National Institutes of Heath sponsored a Consensus Development Conference on The Treatment of Destructive Behaviors in Persons with Developmental Disabilities. A panel of nationally recognized experts in the field of developmental disabilities reviewed the available research and heard testimony from investigators and clinicians working with severe behavioral disorders. Among the summary recommendations of the panel were the following:

1. Most successful approaches to treatment are likely to involve multiple elements of therapy (behavioral and psychopharmacologic), environmental change, and education.
2. Treatment methods may require techniques for enhancing desired behaviors; for producing changes in social, physical, and educational environments; and for reducing or eliminating destructive behaviors.
3. Treatments should be based on an analysis of medical and psychiatric conditions, environmental situations, consequences, and skill deficits. In the application of any of these treatments, an essential step involves a functional analysis of existing behavioral patterns.
4. Behavior reduction procedures should be selected for their rapid effectiveness *only* if the exigencies of the clinical situation require such restrictive interventions and *only* after appropriate review. These interventions should *only* be used in the context of a comprehensive treatment package. (NIH, 1991)

Combined Behavioral Treatment

Any of the behavioral methods described may be combined because combined treatments are generally needed to overcome drawbacks of particular techniques. In some instances, punishment may decrease one inappropriate behavior, but another behavior may appear. To avoid this, punishment might be combined with differential reinforcement of incompatible behavior so a desired alternative response is systematically reinforced positively rather than a second inappropriate one occurring as a response to the punishment.

Certain combinations are more common than others. Most combination approaches involve positive reinforcement as one component. For example, extinction is commonly involved in positive reinforcement strategies in the sense that the targeted inappropriate behavior is ignored while positive reinforcement is occurring. Another combination might be positive reinforcement along with a time-out procedure. An advantage to combining positive reinforcement and time-out in a group setting is that an effective intervention with one child can positively influence the behavior of peers in the same setting. Positive reinforcement has been used in combination with aversive stimulation and overcorrection procedures although, as noted, aversives should be avoided whenever possible.

Treatment Approach

Johnson and Baumeister (1981) suggest the following progression for behaviors that do not pose a threat of serious physical harm to others: An initial period of systematic observation is conducted to identify naturally occurring contingencies which affect the identified behaviors. The first intervention approach is positive reinforcement, most commonly a DRI procedure. Naturally occurring reinforcers are utilized, if possible. When other contingencies that influence the target behavior are introduced, they should be controlled to the degree possible. If this initial approach is not effective, manipulating the type, size, and schedule of reinforcement and the extent of deprivation is the next step. If the program continues to be ineffective, time-out may be added to the positive reinforcement procedure, and the time and length of the time-out may be manipulated. If the behavioral difficulty still continues, it may be necessary to replace time-out with overcorrection and, only as a last resort and after human subject review, to use contingent stimulation.

FUNCTIONAL ASSESSMENT

Functional assessment is an approach to behavior management that is increasingly utilized for severe behavior problems. There are two general types of functional assessment of behavior. The first type consists of a series of experimental conditions that are established to be analogous to the natural contingencies in the environment. This is referred to as an analogue, or functional assessment. The second type evaluates the variation in rates of behavior in objectively established events that occur in the individual's daily routine. This second approach is referred to as an ecological, or structural assessment procedure. The first approach is described in greater detail here.

In the functional assessment, the behavioral therapist manipulates both antecedents and/or consequences which may be associated with the target behavior. Data are taken across conditions and examined to clarify if the rates of behavior are reliably higher when the conditions are compared.

Iwata et al. (1982) utilized functional assessment and followed up on Carr's (1977) findings that self-injurious behavior is a multiply-controlled operant in that no single form of treatment may be consistently effective in the heterogeneous groups of children and adolescents who share this behavior. They utilized a functional analysis to determine the multiple conditions that maintained self-injurious behavior. In their analogue situations, three hypotheses are tested: The first is that self-injury is maintained by contingent social attention (positive reinforcement). The second is that self-injury is maintained by negative reinforcement expressed as escape from or avoidance of nonpreferred tasks. The third is that self-injury is a form of self-stimulation which provides internal reinforcement. However, self-injury occurs in relation to a combination or none of these hypotheses.

To test these hypotheses, these authors developed four different conditions to assess individuals with self-injurious behavior: social disapproval, academic demand, unstructured play, and an alone condition. In each setting, data were collected to establish the conditions that might be related to self-injurious behavior. First, in the social disapproval condition, the experimenter and subject enter a therapy room with a variety of toys available and within easy reach. The child is instructed to play with the toys while the experimenter sits by and reads a book or magazine. Attention is given to the subject contingent on episodes of self-injury and socially disapproving statements, such as "Don't do that!" are made, paired with brief, nonpunitive contact, such as a hand on the shoulder. All other responses are ignored. The social disapproval situation was included because self-injury often produces emotional responses and attention from caregivers whereas other behavior may be ignored. This condition was designed so statements of concern and social disapproval could be paired with nonpunitive physical contact contingent upon self-injury. Disapproval might maintain the behavior by inadvertently introducing positive reinforcement.

The second situation is that of academic demand where educational activities are appropriately selected based on a special education evaluation or derived from an individualized education program provided by the individual school. Educational tasks include stacking wooden blocks, putting pieces in a puzzle, threading plastic beads on a string, grasping small desired objects, or other tasks. The tasks chosen are difficult for the subject to perform even with physical guidance. Verbal instruction is given to carry out the task and 5 seconds are allowed to initiate a response. If there is failure to initiate a response, an instruction is repeated, and the correct response is modeled. If the child still is unable to initiate and complete the task, physical guidance is provided. Social praise is offered at the completion of the task whether or not modeling or guidance are necessary. If self-injury occurs at any time during the demand session, the trial is immediately terminated and the experimenter turns away from the subject for 30 seconds. The academic demand situation was developed to assess whether or not self-injury was maintained through negative reinforcement as a consequence of avoiding or escaping a demand situation.

The third condition involves unstructured play. In this instance, the therapist and the subject are in the same room, but no educational task is presented although an assortment of toys are easily available. The therapist maintains close contact with the individual and allows him to engage in spontaneous isolated or cooperative toy play and to move around the room. Periodically, toys are presented without making demands. Social praise and brief physical contact are offered contingent on appropriate behavior, that is, the absence of self-injury at least once every 30 seconds. If self-injury occurs, it is ignored unless its severity reaches a point where the session must be terminated. This condition acts as a control procedure for the presence of an experimenter, for the availability of potentially stimulating materials, for the absence of demands, and for the delivery of social approval for appropriate behavior, and the lack of approval for self-injury. Moreover, this condition is thought to function as an "enriched environment" where the child's attention could be drawn to play materials so that little self-injury would be expected.

The final condition is the alone condition where the child is in the therapy room alone and does not have access to toys or other materials that might serve as sources of stimulation. In this condition, the environment is impoverished in regard to both social and physical stimulation. This condition was introduced based on the assumption that self-stimulatory behavior may occur through self-produced reinforcement when external sensory or interpersonal stimulation is not available. Self-injury might be maintained in this way when there is lack of environmental stimulation. Therefore, one might find higher levels of self-injury in settings where minimal amounts of stimulation are provided by the environment.

Iwata et al. (1982) utilized these four conditions until apparent stability in the level of self-injury could be observed, unstable responding persisted in all four conditions for 5 days, or until 12 days of sessions could be completed. Using this paradigm, the occurrence of self-injury was found to vary considerably both between and within subjects. However, in their initial study, 6 of 9 subjects showed high levels of self-injury within one of the four conditions, thus providing some empirical evidence that self-injury may emerge from different sources of reinforcement, as proposed by Carr (1977). Four of 9 subjects showed the highest self-injury in an alone condition, 2 during the academic demand condition, and 1 subject showed higher levels of self-injury in the social disapproval condition. The authors expressed surprise that only 1 subject showed increased rates in the social disapproval condition because it has been commonly believed that social disapproval might well be the most important factor in reinforcing self-injury. Moreover, the identification of social disapproval as an important reinforcer would have allowed traditional behavioral approaches, such as extinction, time-out, and differential reinforcement of incompatible or other behavior, to be applied.

Three of the 9 subjects showed undifferentiated patterns or high levels of self-injury across all four of the conditions. Self-injury in this group might represent a response that serves multiple functions, such as providing stimulation when stimulation is lacking in the environment, gaining attention from others, and terminating undesirable demands. For this group, the need for different treatments applied to the same individual, alone or in combination, might be required. Overall, these authors provide a methodology for examining the multiple effects of the environment on the occurrence of self-injury. Such approaches that provide systematic assessment of behavior in defined conditions may contribute to a better understanding of the application of behavior management techniques. Yet it must be continually kept in mind that behavioral approaches are best provided in the context of a comprehensive treatment program which includes communication training, therapies specific to the child's disability, and, in some instances, pharmacotherapy.

Ongoing Behavior Management

For the execution of the behavioral plan, parents, teachers, and other caregivers must be willing to carry out the program in natural settings. Training for behavior management involves verbal instruction, modeling, rehearsal of the behavioral methods by the caregiver, and feedback (Parrish, 1993). Assessment of behavior must continue throughout all phases of treatment. Both the caregiver and, if possible, the child or adolescent are asked to track target behaviors as behavioral interventions are introduced and practiced. Family or caregiver contact is maintained by office visits and telephone contacts in between. Written records are reviewed at agreed-upon intervals in conjunction with verbal reports during telephone monitoring sessions. Based on this information, behavioral procedures are revised.

In summary, the overall goals of behavior management techniques with developmentally disabled individuals are to increase prosocial skills and reduce inappropriate behavior. Although the initial referral is generally for inappropriate behavior, behavior analysis gradually shifts to teaching the caregiver, the child or adolescent, and teachers and other professionals new skills (Parrish, 1993). The function of the child's behavior is carefully assessed because inappropriate behavior may be designed to get certain things that are desired or to escape or avoid things the individual does not want to do. An effective behavioral approach teaches the child or adolescent to achieve his own aims through more appropriate and acceptable behavior. As the program continues, the parents, caregiver, and teachers may learn better ways to guide the child or adolescent to behave more appropriately to facilitate interpersonal growth. A systematic approach to behavior analysis may prevent recurrences of inappropriate behavior and provide consistent support along with an orientation to behavior management that may be adapted if other problematic behaviors develop later. A successful program involves careful identification and analysis of the conditions under which inappropriate behavior occurs along with a carefully designed contingency management program that leads to replacement of inappropriate behavior with more adaptive responses. In this way, behavioral excesses and deficits in adaptive behavior may be systematically approached and successfully resolved.

FUTURE DIRECTIONS

Little systematic research has been conducted that identifies the specific behavioral interventions which are most efficacious for particular maladaptive behaviors. Most studies involve single-case designs with small sample sizes and rarely report clinical variables that might affect treatment outcome (e.g., clinical psychiatric syndromes and disorders, family history, psychosocial circumstances). Reviews and meta-analyses that include large numbers of studies allow for some support for these procedures. Positive behavioral interventions appear most efficacious for the treatment of affective symptoms (e.g., depression, anxiety) and social skills deficits; punishment procedures (e.g., extinction, disapproval, time-out, overcorrection), for destructive behaviors (e.g., aggression, self-injurious behavior). Stereotypic behaviors, psychophysiologic symptoms, and noncompliance are the most responsive to behavioral treatment (65% to 75% success rate); destructive behaviors are intermediate (45% to 65% success rate), and inappropriate social interactions are the least responsive (35% to 40% success rate) (Bregman and Harris, 1995).

REFERENCES

Aman, M.G. (1991). *Assessing psychopathology and behavioral problems in persons with mental retardation: A review of available instruments.* (DHHS Publication No. [ADM] 91–1712). U.S. Department of Health and Human Resources, Rockville, MD.

American Psychiatric Association, Committee on Nomenclature and Statistics (1994). *Diagnostic and statistical manual of mental disorders,* 4th ed. Author, Washington, DC.

Beck, A.T. (1976). *Cognitive therapy and emotional disorders.* International Universities Press, New York.

Bensberg, E.J. (1965). *Teaching the mentally retarded.* Southern Regional Education Board, Atlanta, GA.

Bregman, J., and Harris, J. (1995). Mental retardation. In H. Kaplan and B. Sadock (eds.), *Comprehensive textbook of psychiatry,* 6th ed. Williams and Wilkins, Baltimore, MD.

Carr, E.G. (1977). The motivation of self-injurious behavior. A review of some hypotheses. *Psychological Bulletin,* 34:800–816.

______, and Durand, V.M. (1985). Reducing behavior problems through functional communication training. *Journal of Applied Behavioral Analysis,* 18:111–126.

Ellis, A. (1962). *Reason and emotion in psychotherapy.* Stuart, New York.

______. (1963). Toilet training in the severely defective patient: An S-R reinforcement analysis. *American Journal of Mental Deficiency,* 68:98–103.

Foxx, R.M., and Azrin, N.H. (1972). Restitution: A method of eliminating aggressive-disruptive behavior of retarded and brain damaged patients. *Behavior Research and Therapy,* 10:15–27.

Fuller, P. (1949). Operant conditioning of a vegetative human organism. *American Journal of Psychology,* 62:587–590.

Hamilton, J., Stephens, L., and Allen, P. (1967). Controlling aggressive and destructive behavior in severely retarded institutionalized residents. *American Journal of Mental Deficiency,* 71:825–856.

Iwata, B.A., Dorsey, M., Slifer, K., Bauman, K., and Richman, G. (1982). Toward a functional analysis of self-injury. *Analysis and Intervention in Developmental Disabilities,* 3:1–20.

Jansen, P.E. (1980). Basic principles of behavior therapy with retarded persons. In L.S. Szymanski and P.E. Tanguay (eds.), *Emotional disorders of mentally retarded persons,* pp. 223–240. University Park Press, Baltimore, MD.

Johnson, W.L., and Baumeister, A.A. (1981). Behavioral techniques for decreasing aberrant behaviors of retarded and autistic persons. In M. Hersen, R.M. Eisler, and P.M. Miller (eds.), *Progress in behavioral modification,* Vol. 12, pp. 119–159. Academic Press, New York.

Kazdin, A.E. (1982). *Single-case research designs: Methods for clinical and applied settings.* Oxford University Press, New York.

______. (1984). *Behavior modification in applied settings.* Dorsey Press, Homewood, IL.

Maryland State Department of Health and Mental Hygiene (1994). Title 7: Developmental Disabilities Law, Subtitle 10: Rights of Individuals. Health General Article 7–1002, (B. Policy of State, No. 4) Annotated Code of Maryland.

McGee, J.J. (1988). Issues related to applied behavioral analysis. In J.A. Stark, F.J. Menolascino, M.H. Albarelli, and V.C. Gray (eds.), *Mental retardation and mental health: Classification, diagnosis, treatment, services,* pp. 203–212. Springer-Verlag, New York.

Menolascino, F.J., and McGee, J.J. (1983). Persons with severe mental retardation and behavioral challenges: From disconnectedness to human engagement. *Journal of Psychiatric Treatment and Evaluation,* 5(2 & 3):187–193.

National Institutes of Health (1991, September). Consensus Development Conference on the Treatment of Destructive Behaviors in Persons with Developmental Disabilities. U.S. Department of Health and Human Services, Public Health Service, NIH Publication No. 91–2410, Washington, DC.

Parrish, J.M. (1993). Behavior management in the child with developmental disabilities. *Pediatric Clinics of North America,* 40:617–628.

Premack, D. (1965). Reinforcement theory. In D. Levine (ed.), *Nebraska Symposium on Motivation,* pp. 123–180. University of Nebraska, Lincoln.

Skinner, B.F. (1938). *The behavior of organisms.* Appleton-Century-Crofts, New York.

______. (1953). *Science and human behavior.* Macmillan, New York.

______. (1974). *About behaviorism.* Knopf, New York.

Tate, B.G., and Baroff, G.S. (1966). Aversive control of self-injurious behavior in a psychotic boy. *Behavioral Research and Therapy,* 4:281–287.

Ullman, L.P., and Krasner, L. (1965). *Case studies in behavior modification.* Holt, Rinehart and Winston, New York.

Watson, J.B. (1924). *Behaviorism.* University of Chicago Press, Chicago.

Werry, J.S., and Wollersheim, J.P. (1989). Behavior therapy with children and adolescents: A twenty-year overview. *Journal of the American Academy of Child and Adolescent Psychiatry,* 28:1–18.

White, G.D., Neilson, G., and Johnson, S.M. (1972). Timeout duration and the suppression of deviant behavior in children. *Journal of Applied Behavioral Analysis,* 5:111–120.

Wolpe, J. (1958). *Psychotherapy by reciprocal inhibition.* Stanford University Press, Stanford, CA.

BEHAVIORAL GLOSSARY

aversive event Stimulus that suppresses a behavior it follows, or increases a behavior, resulting in termination of an aversive event. A noxious or unpleasant stimulus.

baseline Frequency at which a behavior is performed before the initiation of a behavior therapy program. The baseline is used to evaluate the effects of the behavioral program. Also termed the *free operant rate* of the behavior.

behavior Any observable and measurable response or act of an individual. Categories of behavior include operants, respondents, and coverants.

classical (or respondent) conditioning Type of learning in which a conditioned stimulus (CS) is paired with an unconditioned stimulus (UCS), which already automatically elicits an unlearned, reflexive response. After repeated pairings of the conditioned stimulus with the unconditioned stimulus, the conditioned stimulus alone will elicit a reflexlike response. In classical conditioning, new stimuli gain the power to elicit respondent behavior. Also termed *Pavlovian conditioning.*

conditioned response Reflexlike response elicited by a conditioned stimulus (CS) alone, in the absence of the unconditioned stimulus. The conditioned response (CR) resembles, but is not identical to, the unconditioned response.

conditioned stimulus Previously neutral stimulus which, through repeated associations with an unconditioned stimulus, can eventually elicit a reflexlike response.

consequence control Change in behavior reliably produced by a change in the stimulus that follows the behavior.

contingency Relationship between a behavior (the response to be changed) and the events (consequences) that follow the behavior. Sometimes events that precede the behavior are also specified by a contingency. An if . . . then relationship between events or stimuli.

differential reinforcement Reinforcing a response in the presence of one discriminative stimulus and simultaneously extinguishing the response in the presence of other stimuli.

differential reinforcement of alternative behavior (DRA) Behavioral treatment procedure involving the delivery of positive reinforcement only after the client has displayed an appropriate target behavior.

differential reinforcement of other behavior (DRO) Delivery of a reinforcer after any response except the target response. The individual is reinforced for not performing the target response. All behaviors other than the target response are reinforced.

direct observation procedures Set of assessment methods that focus on operationally defining and measuring the frequency, duration, and/or severity of observable behavior.

discrimination Responding differently in the presence of different cues or antecedent events.

discriminative stimulus Antecedent event or stimulus that signals a certain response will be reinforced.

escape Performance of a behavior that terminates an aversive event. Escape behavior is maintained by negative reinforcement.

extinction Procedure in which the reinforcer is no longer delivered for a previously learned response.

fading Gradual removal of discriminative stimuli, including prompts like instructions or physical guidance.

functional analysis The goal of functional analysis is to determine whether (and which) specific environmental outcomes or consequences of the behavior affect its frequency (Does the behavior occur because it results in adult attention?). With this methodology, variables hypothesized to affect behavior are directly manipulated under analogue conditions using single-case designs. When a functional analysis indicates one or more specific environmental consequences are reinforcing the behavior, an individually tailored intervention can be developed in which these consequences are used to reinforce appropriate behavior in place of the destructive behavior.

incompatible behavior Behavior that cannot be performed at the same time as, or that interferes with, another behavior.

intermittent reinforcement Schedule of reinforcement in which a response is not reinforced every time it is performed.

naturally occurring reinforcers Reinforcing events in the environment that are not introduced, but are usually available as part of the setting. Attention, praise, completion of an activity, and mastery of a task are naturally occurring reinforcers.

negative reinforcement Increase in the frequency of a response, which is followed by the termination or removal of an aversive event. Escape and avoidance behaviors are maintained by negative reinforcement.

observational learning Learning by observing another individual (a model) engage in a behavior. To learn from a model, the observer need not necessarily perform the behavior or receive direct consequences for his performance.

operant behavior Emitted behavior that is controlled by its consequences; voluntary behavior. The term *operant* is derived from the observation that specifiable groups of responses operate on the environment to produce consequences for the person.

operant conditioning Type of learning in which behaviors are altered primarily by regulating the consequences that follow time. The frequency of operant behaviors may be increased or decreased, depending on the consequences they produce.

positive reinforcement Increase in the frequency of a response that is followed by a rewarding stimulus or event.

Premack principle Principle stating that for any pair of responses or activities in which an individual freely engages, the more frequently performed one can be used to reinforce the less frequent one.

primary reinforcer Reinforcing event that does not depend on learning to achieve its reinforcing properties. Food, water, sleep, and sex are examples of primary reinforcers.

prompt Antecedent event that helps initiate a response. Instructions, gestures, physical guidance, and modeling cues can serve as prompts with retarded persons.

punishment Change in the consequence of a maladaptive target behavior that reliably produces a decrease in the behavior. Punishment may involve the withdrawal of a positive reinforcer (e.g., time-out from attention, loss of allowance) or the presentation of a negative reinforcer (e.g., hands-down, verbal reprimand). The consequence change is considered punishment if, and only if, it results in a reliable decrease in the maladaptive target behavior.

reinforcement Increase in the strength or frequency of a response when the response is immediately followed by a particular consequence. The consequence can be either the presentation of a positive reinforcer or the removal of a negative reinforcer.

respondent behavior Behavior that is elicited or automatically controlled by antecedent stimuli. The connection between unconditioned respondents and the antecedent events that control them is unlearned. Respondents may come under the control of otherwise neutral stimuli through classical or Pavlovian conditioning.

response cost Punishment procedure in which a positive reinforcer is lost, or some penalty is invoked, contingent on the occurrence of an undesirable behavior. Unlike **timeout**, there is no specified time limit to the withdrawal of the reinforcer. Loss of a token in token economies represents a common form of response cost.

response generalization Reinforcement of a particular target response, which increases the probability of occurrence of other responses that are similar to the target response or belong to the same response class.

satiation Providing an excessive amount of a reinforcer. A loss of reinforcing effectiveness that occurs after a large amount of the reinforcer has been delivered.

shaping Developing a new behavior by reinforcing successive approximations toward the terminal response.

single-case designs Set of experimental procedures that involve repeated measurement of the dependent variable under experimental and control conditions with a single case. The experimental and control conditions are manipulated such that a single subject serves as his or her own control. Examples include reversal designs (ABAB), multiple-baseline designs, and multielement designs.

social reinforcers Reinforcers that result from interpersonal interactions. Examples include attention, praise, approval, smiles, and physical contact.

stimulus Measurable event that may have an effect on the behavior of an individual.

stimulus control Presence of a particular antecedent stimulus serves as an occasion for a particular response to occur. A response is performed while in the presence of a stimulus, but not in its absence.

stimulus generalization Transfer of a learned response to situations or stimulus conditions other than those in which learning has taken place. The learned behavior generalizes to other environments.

successive approximations Responses that increasingly resemble the terminal behavior being shaped.

target behavior Behavior to be altered or focused on during behavior therapy program. The behavior subjected to baseline assessment.

time-out Time-out from positive reinforcement. A mild punishment technique where an individual is removed from the opportunity to earn positive reinforcement, contingent on the occurrence of disruptive behavior. Time-out is typically used for relatively brief, fixed time periods.

token economy Closed-ended system, governed by rules that specify behaviors to be reinforced, numbers of tokens to be provided for each behavior, and exchange rates of tokens for backup reinforcers.

token reinforcement Process whereby a desired behavior is immediately followed by the presentation of a generalized conditioned reinforcer (token). Tokens are later exchanged for a variety of backup reinforcers.

Adapted from Jansen, 1980.

CHAPTER 20

PSYCHOPHARMACOLOGICAL INTERVENTIONS

Mentally retarded and other developmentally disabled persons are at increased risk for psychiatric and behavioral disorders that may respond to psychopharmacological intervention. As a group, they are more vulnerable to environmental stresses and psychologically less able to adapt to physiologically mediated shifts in internal state. Psychotropic medication is used for the treatment of either recognized psychiatric disorders or specific behavioral symptoms.

Because mental retardation and other developmental disorders have multiple etiologies, there may be variability in susceptibility to mental disorders and in the metabolism of psychotropic drugs among the known syndromes. When used judiciously with careful attention to diagnoses and the risks and benefits of treatment, psychotropic drugs may have favorable effects in facilitating changes in behavior, cognition, mood, and socialization (Rivinus et al., 1989). Successful intervention may allow family members and other caregivers to become more hopeful and optimistic about outcome and change their behavior toward the individual being treated. However, there are ethical dilemmas in drug use related to informed consent, individual rights, the interface of drug treatment with other interventions, polypharmacy, and untoward side effects of drugs.

This chapter reviews the history of the use of pharmacotherapy for individuals with developmental disorders, epidemiological issues related to drug use, methodology of drug studies, specific issues in psychopharmacology, assessment, ethical and legal issues related to drug use, and the categories of drugs used.

HISTORY

Pharmacotherapy for emotional and behavioral disorders in children and adolescents began in the 1930s. The earliest effective drug treatment for disturbances in behavior was probably the use of benzedrine for disruptive behavior by Charles Bradley (Bradley, 1937). The next major group of medications, the antipsychotics or neuroleptics, were introduced in the 1950s. Their use was soon extended to treatment of mentally retarded persons with disruptive behavior in institutional settings where neuroleptics became the most commonly used drugs for behavior management in the control of aggressive and destructive behavior (Aman and Singh, 1991).

Surveys indicated that between one third and one half of mentally retarded individuals residing in institutions and one fourth to one third residing in community settings received some type of psychotropic drug. Significant interinstitutional and interagency differences were noted in prescribing patterns, with a range from under 10% to more than 75% for individuals who were similar in demographic and clinical characteristics. Neuroleptics were found to be prescribed most often, and antidepressants and stimulants were prescribed less commonly.

Inappropriate prescribing (Bates, Smelzer, and Arnoczky, 1986) and lack of clarity regarding the indications for drug treatment led to excessive prescription in the past for "behavioral symptoms" in children and adolescents who lacked an adequate interdisciplinary program. Because of the frequent use, the prescription of neuroleptics for the management of disruptive behavior became controversial, particularly their use for "chemical restraint." In some instances, class action suits were filed which specified that habilitation plans must include appropriate psychiatric diagnoses and careful monitoring of pharmacotherapy. Following a long period of distrust and challenge in the courts that involved a series of medicolegal initiatives, there has been a renewed interest in the use of psychotropic medications to treat behavioral and emotional disturbances in disabled persons (Aman, 1983). This interest follows an increased awareness that mentally retarded and other developmentally disabled persons may show a full spectrum of mental disorders that respond to psychotropic drugs (Corbett, 1979; Lund, 1985; Reid, 1982). For younger individuals, medication treatment involves family members and caregivers and must be carefully coordinated with other multidisciplinary programmatic interventions. Renewed interest in drug treatment for developmentally disabled persons has resulted in substantial refinement of clinical pharmacological practices. Psychiatrists are increasingly involved in making an appropriate psychiatric diagnosis and implementing psychotropic drug treatment and in overseeing the discontinuation of inappropriate drug regimens. As increasing concern has mounted about untoward drug effects, particularly the risk for tardive dyskinesia, newer psychotropic agents have been introduced.

Psychotropic drugs are currently prescribed both for behavioral symptoms and for psychiatric disorders in mentally retarded persons with developmental disorders. It is particularly important to separate dual diagnosis (the co-occurrence of psychiatric disorder and developmental disorder) from behavioral problems that are frequently encountered in developmentally disabled persons. Drug use may be adjunctive to overall management or essential when major psychiatric disorders occur. Regular standardized evaluation to assess drug use is needed to evaluate toxicity and the effect on overall adaptation because these agents are being used to bring about cognitive, behavioral, or affective changes leading to increased socialization. The anticipated outcome is that the disabled person will become more socially available to the family and staff members. The risk-benefit ratio must be carefully evaluated because behavioral toxicity is an ongoing risk that requires careful titration of drugs and their possible discontinuation.

Earlier studies focused on a variety of problem behaviors including aggressiveness, hyperactivity, destructive behavior, and self-injury. In the past, subject selection in research studies included a heterogeneous group of cases, but experimental design has improved in recent years. The current pattern is to use drugs utilized in adult disorders, such as neuroleptics, antidepressants, and lithium, for diagnoses of major mental illnesses in mentally retarded persons or for certain maladaptive behaviors. Treatment may be prescribed for major psychiatric disorders, acquired neurological conditions, and specific behavioral syndromes.

EPIDEMIOLOGY

Aman and Singh (1988) provided a comprehensive review of 30 drug surveys, primarily conducted in large residential facilities (state institutions for mentally retarded persons). Typically, 20% to 50% of residents in these settings were receiving psychotropic drugs and between 25% and 45% were taking anticonvulsants. Psychotropic drugs were used more commonly in older individuals, and anticonvulsant use was greatest in severely mentally retarded persons. Psychotropic drug use is less common in children with diagnoses of epilepsy or cerebral palsy.

The rates of psychotropic drug use in community residence settings was less (10% to 20%) than in public residential settings. Drug use in community settings requires careful monitoring. Dura, Aman, and Mulick (1988) found that psychotropic drug use was least (1%) in an Intermediate Care Facility for Mentally Retarded Persons (ICF/MR) setting for nonambulatory severely and profoundly mentally retarded children and adolescents. Anticonvulsant (67% to 71%) and muscle relaxant drug (11%) prescription was much higher than in surveys with ambulatory populations. The use of laxatives in this population was almost universal (99%).

In the past, thioridazine, chlorpromazine, and haloperidol accounted for a majority of drug prescriptions in state institutional settings. With advances in psychopharmacology, a greater variety of medications are currently used in community settings. Neuroleptics are now used less commonly in both settings and stimulants, anxiolytics, antidepressants, and anticonvulsants are used more often.

Surveys of drug use in both community and residential settings have focused on the total population of mentally retarded persons and have not adequately addressed diagnosis, drug metabolism, and the type of medication used among different populations, e.g., Down syndrome, Cornelia de Lange syndrome, fragile X syndrome.

METHODOLOGY OF DRUG STUDIES

The quality of drug studies with mentally retarded persons has generally been poor, making them difficult to interpret. Studies carried out in the era before 1975 generally lacked a number of basic methodological controls, as summarized by Sprague and Werry (1971). Since 1975, a greater number of studies have followed these methodological requirements and provide better data. Still, rational psychopharmacological treatment for mentally retarded individuals continues to be seriously restricted by a limited scientific database. There are relatively few methodologically sound studies that employ appropriate control groups. Rather, the literature is dominated by single-case reports and nonblind open trials that do not yield sufficient information for truly informed medication decisions. These clinical reports suffer from a number of methodological problems including reporting bias (underreporting of negative findings), retrospective, anecdotal data, lack of reliability testing, and the frequent concurrent use of other psychotropic medications (which are often changed during the course of the trial). There continue to be very few studies that include the appropriate guidelines for clinical trials, namely, random assignment of an adequate number of subjects to treatment conditions, double-blind, placebo-controlled procedures, treatment phases of adequate length, and valid and reliable methods for assessment at baseline and throughout the study.

Sprague and Werry (1971) suggest the following as basic to reviewing drug studies: (1) use of a suitable control group; (2) random assignment of subjects to treatment; (3) use of placebos and blind evaluations to minimize bias; (4) measures of the effect of drugs under standardized conditions; (5) appropriate statistical strategies; and (6) standardized doses. Moreover, when conducting drug studies, other drug treatments, if possible, should be discontinued. In addition, newer drug treatments should be compared with an alternative therapy, such as behavior therapy; or, in some instances, it may be more appropriate to establish a baseline with behavioral measures, add drug therapy, and reverse the drug while continuing the same behavioral program.

Because averaged group data is difficult to apply to individual subjects with a variety of developmental disorders, single-subject research designs have been developed. These approaches provide an alternative to the group design and are carried out in conjunction with comprehensive behavior analysis. Single-subject methodology uses within-subjects' evaluations and provides for intensive study of drug effects on a single person in a treatment setting, using controlled conditions. Moreover, this approach can address drug/psychosocial intervention. Operationalized diagnoses of disorders and behavioral target symptoms are established; the behavior is described, graphed, and then quantitatively recorded to evaluate drug efficacy. Barlow and Hersen (1984) have reviewed several experimental designs that may be used for single-subject drug studies. Among these are variants of withdrawal designs, multiple baseline designs, and alternating treatment designs.

Despite concerns about the individual applicability of group studies, both group and single-subject designs are needed for research. Group designs may be particularly helpful when specific disorders are targeted in known mental retardation syndromes or in other developmental disorders. For example, the prevalence of depression in Down syndrome may be increased; if so, group pharmacological studies on large numbers of Down individuals would be the most useful. However, single-subject designs make an important contribution when evaluating drug use for maladaptive behavior where specific psychiatric diagnosis is more difficult to establish. In addition, single-subject methods may contribute to assessment of major mental illness, particularly in severely and profoundly mentally retarded persons. Currently, the availability of a diversity of experimental designs provides a means to resolve complex issues of pharmacology in mentally retarded individuals. Therefore, both group and single-subject approaches are relevant. Regardless of the design chosen, parents and caretakers should be fully informed and engaged in the treatment of their family member.

SPECIFIC ISSUES IN PSYCHOPHARMACOLOGY

Aman and Singh (1991) suggest seven issues that are pertinent to psychopharmacological studies with developmental disorders: co-occurring diagnoses, dosage effects, limited number of studies examining learning, predictors of drug response, historic emphasis on institutional populations, paucity of follow-up studies, and physiologic risk.

Importance of Diagnosis

The development of a classification system of maladaptive behaviors and operational criteria for psychiatric disorders in developmentally disordered persons is needed so that drug studies can be conducted based on diagnoses and specific behavioral profiles rather than on isolated behavioral symptoms (Werry, 1988). Few research studies for mentally retarded persons have been carried out with individuals who have specific psychiatric or behavioral diagnoses. Reid (1982) has emphasized the difficulty in making accurate psychiatric diagnoses, particularly among severely and profoundly retarded persons. Communication disabilities make it difficult to assess certain symptoms, such as hallucinations, delusions, and changes in affect. Moreover, abnormal behaviors, such as stereotypies and echolalia that commonly occur in mentally retarded persons, may not in themselves be targets for drug treatment even though these symptoms are abnormal in individuals who do not have mental retardation syndromes.

Drug Dosage

Dosages of drugs have generally been individualized for each person being treated based on behavior improvement. Yet the use of titration to establish the effective dose presents difficulties in that there may be problems in establishing reliability regarding the end point or optimal dose. Consequently, doses of the same drug might vary considerably from one individual to the next. Moreover, drug-level information may not be used or may not be available, yet it is essential in any titration approach. When drugs are titrated against a criterion of behavior improvement, considerable care must be taken to clarify which behaviors are to be emphasized and what the expected response will be. An alternative is to look more carefully at the effects of various doses of the drug that are standardized by body weight and body surface area and to measure blood levels. In children with attention deficit disorder, stimulant medications may have complex effects, affecting different classes of behavior at different doses; for example, attention may improve with a lower dose of stimulant whereas impulsivity and hyperactivity may improve when doses are higher. Singh and Aman (1981) studied a low standard dose of thioridazine used for maladaptive behavior and contrasted it with previous treatment based on titration. These authors found that the standardized dose of thioridazine resulted in a therapeutic effect that was just as great as the titrated doses used. These were, on average, double the standardized dose.

Prediction of Outcome

Little attention has been paid to subject characteristics that may influence outcome. Cognitive level, behavioral profile, extent and type of brain damage and neurological dysfunction, and specific syndrome designation have been only rarely considered in regard to predictability of response. Although the effects of psychotropic drugs on neurotransmitters are frequently described in efforts to understand the mechanism of drug action, there have been few attempts to formulate treatment based on the possibility of particular neurotransmitter abnormalities related to specific syndromes. However, this approach has been taken in a few genetic syndromes, such as Down syndrome and Lesch-Nyhan disease. Bazelon et al. (1967) pursued a serotonin hypothesis for hypotonia in Down syndrome and administered 5-hydroxytryptophan to 14 infants with Down syndrome. Her initial report suggested improvement in muscle tone, but this was not validated in subsequent studies (Pueschel et al., 1980). The serotonin hypothesis for self-injury in Lesch-Nyhan disease has also been pursued, using treatment with 5-hydroxytryptophan. Initial reports (Mizuno and Yugari, 1975) suggested the drug relieved self-injury but did not affect choreoathetoid movement disorder in 4 cases. Nyhan et al. (1980) also reported a reduction in self-injury in 9 male patients, but this effect diminished over time. Other investigators have not demonstrated a therapeutic effect. Harris (1988) suggested a differential response of depression in Down syndrome to amitriptyline versus nortriptyline, using a serotonergic model of depression in Down syndrome. Another neurotransmitter-based approach is the use of naltrexone to treat self-injury in severely retarded persons but, in this instance, it is not specific to a particular syndrome.

In future studies, attention to basic subject characteristics is necessary to understand the nature of the drug response in the variety of developmental disorders. This is particularly the case when behavioral phenotypes, such as self-injury in Lesch-Nyhan disease, are addressed.

Emphasis on Studies in Institutional Settings

The majority of drug treatment studies for mentally retarded persons have been carried out in institutionalized populations, although the majority of mentally retarded persons are in community settings and receive pharmacotherapy outside of an institution. The emphasis on normalization and deinstitutionalization has resulted in fewer institutional placements. Although individuals who remain in the institutional setting may be the most severely involved and will continue to require pharmacotherapeutic interventions, they represent a minority of mentally retarded persons. It is essential that pharmacological research focus on community settings and take into account the greater variety of medications now being used. Community-based research has the advantage of the development of individualized programs based on normalization principles. Because program goals are normally well defined and behavioral goals are clearly specified, drug research can proceed more systematically than in the past.

Investigations of Cognitive Effects

Although mental retardation is a cognitive disorder and is primarily a disorder of learning, cognitive effects and educational performance have rarely been used as variables to evaluate drug outcome (Aman, 1984; Sprague and Werry, 1971). The IQ score has not commonly been used as a measure of learning in outcome studies. It has been demonstrated the IQ is not sensitive to drug manipulation either in mentally retarded or other clinical populations. More specific cognitive indices need to be considered. Aman (1991) suggests that the acquisition of a conditioned response, the use of operant paradigms to assess behavioral effects of drugs, assessment of effects on discrimination learning, effects on attention, and effects on short-term memory and on incidental learning be considered. Such studies might compare pharmacological interventions alone, behavioral interventions alone, and their combinations, to assess independent and interactive effects on learning and behavior (Fisher, Piazza, and Page, 1989).

Follow-up Studies

There are a limited number of long-term follow-up studies of psychoactive drug use in mentally retarded persons despite the fact that these medications have been prescribed for many years. Long-term effects might parallel those seen during short-term treatment, but this is not necessarily the case. One approach to study the effects of long-term treatment has focused on discontinuing medication and observing the outcome. Moore (1960) evaluated learning in a group of female residents who had been treated with long-term chlorpromazine. After discontinuing treatment, there were significant improvements in performance on the Stanford Achievement Test when compared to a group who continued on chlorpromazine. Others have found similar improvements when thioridazine was discontinued following long-term treatment (McAndrew, Case, and Treffert, 1972). Harris et al. (1982) used a radio-receptor assay and demonstrated that long-term thioridazine could be reduced or eliminated based on blood level findings. Other authors have reduced doses of neuroleptics that had been used long-term and found no effects on maladaptive or social behaviors (Millichamp and Singh, 1987). In some instances, the introduction of behavior management techniques has been successful in maintaining behavior improvement off medication when long-term drug treatment was discontinued. Guidelines are now in place in institutional settings and community programs for careful monitoring of medications that provide an opportunity to assess long-term effects when medications are discontinued. Regular monitoring of drug effects over time after the original target symptoms are resolved is essential.

An important issue is to clarify which individuals benefit from long-term maintenance medication. For those mentally retarded persons with major mental illnesses, medication may need to be continued for longer periods of time for long-term maintenance. In this instance, follow-up studies are crucial to clarify the ongoing need for treatment for diagnosed major mental illnesses.

Long-Term Behavioral Toxicity

Some drug effects, such as those on the gastrointestinal system, may subside as the individual adapts to pharmacotherapy. Other side effects may respond to treatment, as is the case with extrapyramidal effects. However, longer term effects on cognition, growth, and organ systems, such as the endocrine system, bear monitoring. Some anticonvulsant drugs may potentially have long-term effects on cognition. Long-term neuroleptic use places the individual at ongoing risk for tardive dyskinesia. Drug outcome studies are needed to identify which persons are most at risk for long-term complications, to clarify what those risks are, and to find the safest and lowest doses of medications and the best types of drugs to use in developing appropriate treatment.

When evaluating specific behaviors, the diagnosis must be taken into account. Mood disorder, brief reactive psychosis, and disruptive behavior disorder are among the most common disorders requiring drug prescription. For the major mental disorders, i.e., major depressive disorder, schizophrenia, modified diagnostic criteria may be required. Aggressive behavior, self-injury, and compulsions may be symptomatic of a major mental disorder that must be ruled out before instituting symptomatic treatment for target behaviors.

ASSESSMENT

The clinical interview (McHugh and Slavney, 1983) is ordinarily the principal means for psychiatric assessment. Ordinarily, a face-to-face meeting with an individual is used to determine whether drug treatment has been effective. Yet reliance on the clinical interview may not be possible with the mentally retarded or pervasively developmentally disordered person. Impairments in communication skills, reduced social skills, and deficits in abstract thinking make the clinical interview less adequate for assessment. Consequently, observations by others play an important role in decisions about drug treatment. Behaviorally based diagnostic and treatment evaluation methodologies that utilize repeated assessments by direct caregivers are necessary.

The evaluation of a person with mental retardation or a developmental disorder for pharmacotherapy begins with a comprehensive multidisciplinary evaluation. A major problem in the choice of psychopharmacological agents is establishing the correct diagnosis of a mental disorder. In addition to the clinical interview that involves the referred person and appropriate informants, behavior ratings are essential. Aman (1991) made a review of available assessment instruments in a report prepared for the National Institutes of Mental Health. His recommended instruments for assessment include the Reiss Screen for Maladaptive Behavior (screening), the AAMR Adaptive Behavior Scales (adaptive behavior), and the Aberrant Behavior Checklist (broad behavioral dimensions). The Clinical Interview Schedule and the Diagnostic Assessment of the Severely Handicapped are recommended for psychiatric diagnosis. Most of these interviews and rating scales rely on reports from parents, staff, and other informants. Rating scales completed by others are most useful for externalizing behaviors as contrasted to internalizing behaviors. Rating scales, interviews, and self-reports for anxiety, depression, obsessions, and thought disorder in mentally retarded and developmentally disabled persons are not well standardized.

Several special features must be considered in the assessment of disabled persons (Sovner, 1986). The first is that cognitive deterioration may occur with stress and lead to regression in adaptive functioning. The second is lack of reliability in reporting symptoms. This refers to limited capacity to identify internal feeling states and communicate them to caregivers. Diagnostically, important information may be difficult to elicit or may not be elicited from the person being treated regarding his behavior, feeling states, or mood so assessment must be based on the longitudinal collection of behavioral data. In addition, the disabled person may not be able to provide information about hallucinations and delusions; this is particularly true for those testing in the severe or profound range of mental retardation (Corbett, 1979; Reid, 1972). Without adequate communication skills, such symptoms cannot be confirmed. A third issue is that premorbid maladaptive behavior patterns may increase in frequency with the onset of a psychiatric disorder so that an increase in rates of baseline behavior is observed. Although increases in baseline rates of behavior are most commonly due to nonspecific stress, the exacerbation of preexisting behaviors can be an important diagnostic issue in clarifying the onset of a mental disorder. A fourth issue referred to by Sovner is "psychosocial masking" where the symptoms presented may be influenced by limited life experience and limited expectations from others. Moreover, older mentally retarded persons may describe symptoms, such as delusional perceptions and fears, in language similar to that used by children. Thus the assessment process must take into account the limited life experience and cognitive state of the individual.

Assessment procedures consider the co-occurrence of a behavior or psychiatric disorder and a developmental disability (dual diagnoses), the particular syndrome, past drug history, the presence of substance abuse, and the need for emergency pharmacotherapy.

The first step in assessment is to differentiate psychiatric symptoms from maladaptive behaviors that may be characteristic features of a developmental disorder to establish a diagnosis. Overall, treatment is not directed at behavioral symptoms per se, but rather addresses an underlying condition or pathophysiologic process. In evaluating the individual, maladaptive behaviors may be the outcome of operant conditioning and must be differentiated from behavioral symptoms related to a psychiatric disorder. For example, self-injury may serve behaviorally as an escape behavior from tasks or as a form of stimulation in a low-stimulus environment, and hyperactivity may be related to a diagnosis of bipolar disorder. To complete the assessment, the psychiatrist must differentiate behavior that is normal for the particular developmental disorder or even for that particular individual from abnormal behavior. In addition, exaggerated responses to stress may lead to behavioral decompensation and cognitive disintegration that results in misdiagnosis (Sovner, 1986). With sufficient stress, behavior may appear bizarre and disorganized; however, rather than being a specific sign of psychiatric disorder, such behavior may represent an adjustment disorder or a nonspecific stress response without specific diagnostic significance. Persons with autistic disorder and other pervasive developmental disorders who demonstrate atypical behavior may develop superimposed psychiatric disorders that must be differentiated from the behavioral patterns associated with the disorder. A second step in assessment is that diagnostic criteria must take into account the severity of the developmental disorder, particularly the extent of mental retardation.

Finally, the assessment for use of medications in emergency situations should be based on the diagnosis and type of symptom presentation. Because psychotropic medications are prescribed for specific reasons, the term "chemical restraint" should be avoided. P.R.N. prescription for emergency medication is generally unwise because such prescribing patterns may lead to excessive drug use.

Persons with mental retardation who are treated with psychotropic agents often have associated medical conditions that will influence the choice of medications used in the treatment of mental disorders. The drugs used for treatment may have adverse effects on cognitive and motor performance. Behavioral monitoring during the initiation of the drug trial, at its discontinuation, and long-term use are essential. Various rating scales for movement disorders are available and should be routinely employed. Among the areas that must be considered are effects of drugs on cognitive and motor performance, treatment emergent effects, effects of discontinuation of medication, and tardive dyskinesia.

ETHICAL AND LEGAL ISSUES RELATED TO DRUG USE

The most basic consideration is that the mentally retarded or developmentally disabled person be regularly evaluated after medications are prescribed. Regulations and laws regarding the use of psychotropic drugs vary considerably among the states. Some states have no specific laws or regulations but, in others, the regulations are very specific. It is essential to become aware of these laws and regulations. In some states, the guardian's consent is sufficient for drug prescription. In other states, separate court permission is required for administration of medication to incompetent adults except in emergency situations. Ethical issues relate to consent, individual rights, polypharmacy, and the monitoring of use in community facilities. Ethical and legal issues are discussed in Chapter 22.

SPECIFIC MEDICATION USE

A glossary of psychoactive drugs, showing the generic and trade names, is included as an appendix to this chapter.

NEUROLEPTIC MEDICATIONS

Maladaptive Behavior (Aggression, Self-injury, Stereotypy, Hyperkinesis)

The neuroleptics are most commonly prescribed for aggressive, destructive, self-injurious, hyperactive, and inappropriate social behavior in mentally retarded persons. The neuroleptics used include phenothiazines (e.g., thioridazine, chlorpromazine), butyrophenones (e.g., haloperidol), the thioxanthenes (e.g., thiothixine), and molindone. Among these, thioridazine and chlorpromazine were the most commonly used in the past, but haloperidol is now the most frequently prescribed.

Chlorpromazine

Early uncontrolled pharmacological studies with chlorpromazine suggested effectiveness in reducing disruptive behaviors in mentally retarded persons (Freeman, 1970; Lipman et al., 1978). Well-controlled pharmacological studies have questioned these earlier findings and suggest that although chlorpromazine may decrease aggression in some individuals (Marholin, Touchette, and Stewart, 1979; Schroeder, 1988), appropriate behaviors may worsen. Aman, White, and Field (1984) reported reduction in stereotyped movements with chlorpromazine, but noted sedation and reduced performance on an operant conditioning task. Based on these studies, the overall efficacy of chlorpromazine in treating inappropriate and maladaptive behaviors is not clear. Because of its sedative effects and the development of newer neuroleptic agents, it is rarely used.

Thioridazine

In 1980 Aman and Singh reviewed 24 studies of the use of thioridazine in childhood disorders. Six studies met methodological criteria for scientific validity. These studies, for the most part, relied on global impressions of change, but when specific behaviors were studied, improvements were noted in hyperactivity, aggression, eating behavior, and stereotypies. Subsequent reports indicated reduction in stereotypical behavior, hyperactivity, and bizarre behavior in severely and profoundly retarded individuals when lower doses (2.5 mg/kg) were prescribed. This low-dose range was found to be as effective in controlling stereotypies as were higher doses. However, Harris et al. (1982), using a radio-receptor assay, found a tenfold variation in blood level of neuroleptic activity at a dose of 2.0 mg/kg of thioridazine. Because of variability in blood level and metabolism, specific guidelines for dosing remain difficult to establish. Jakab

(1984) evaluated 10 individuals with mental retardation before and after thioridazine administration. Interval recording of behavioral symptoms showed reductions of inappropriate behavior following medication treatment. Aman and White (1988) used two doses and found that the higher of the two doses (1.25 versus 2.5 mg/kg per day) showed greater reductions in hyperactivity and self-injury but also were associated with increased lethargy. Schroeder and Gualtieri (1985) evaluated 23 individuals, most of whom were involved in a drug reversal design and were receiving thioridazine. When medication was discontinued, 9 subjects showed tardive dyskinesia and 6 showed exacerbation of behavioral symptoms, requiring reinstitution of the drug treatment. Staff ratings of abnormal behavior increased, particularly following abrupt drug withdrawal; these ratings tended to go along with ratings of tardive dyskinesia. Although direct observations of behavior have not shown consistent drug effects, thioridazine shows more evidence of an effect on maladaptive behavior than does chlorpromazine.

Haloperidol

Haloperidol is a member of the butyrophenone group of neuroleptic medications and is less sedative than thioridazine and chlorpromazine. Haloperidol also has been used to treat hyperactive, aggressive, hostile, and impulsive behaviors in mentally retarded persons (Sprague and Baxley, 1978). Establishment of efficacy is problematic because of the lack of adequately controlled studies; however, haloperidol may be superior to the phenothiazines (Burk and Menolascino, 1968; Le Vann, 1971) for treatment of hyperactive, aggressive, and stereotyped behavior. Other investigators (Vaisanen et al., 1981) have shown no difference between haloperidol and thioridazine for treatment of aggressive behavior, self-injury, and stereotypies.

Other Neuroleptics

The neuroleptic drugs have various effects on dopamine receptors; e.g., haloperidol is primarily a D_2 antagonist and thiothixine is a mixed D_1/D_2 antagonist. In addition to these drugs, D_1 dopamine antagonists also have been used to target maladaptive behavior in mentally retarded persons. Although not currently available, these medications are promising because they may produce fewer long-term side effects. Albert et al. (1977) reported that SCH-12679, a benzazepine D_1 dopamine antagonist, was effective in the management of aggressive individuals with mental retardation. Subsequently, Elie et al. (1980) compared SCH-12679 with thioridazine in aggressive individuals with mental retardation. Subjects were adult male and female severely mentally retarded individuals (IQ<40). Thirty-three adult men and 18 adult women were selected from 253 aggressive mentally retarded persons. Inclusion criteria were aggressive behavior that was not manageable without physical restraints or confinement. Individuals with diagnoses of schizophrenia or who had metabolic, renal, cardiac, or hepatic abnormalities were excluded.

A Target Symptom Aggressivity Scale (TSA) was used to evaluate drug effects of SCH-12679. Prior to drug treatment, all medications other than anticonvulsants were discontinued and replaced with chlorpromazine, 100 mg. t.i.d. After 3 weeks on this medication, the chlorpromazine was discontinued and aggressive behavior was rated. The trial involved comparison of SCH-12679, thioridazine, or placebo; the medication was determined by separate random allocations, using a double-blind procedure. During the second week of treatment, the total aggression score significantly decreased in the SCH-12679 group; neither thioridazine nor a placebo led to improved behavior. On the Target Symptom Aggressivity Scale, SCH-12679 reduced agitation and hyperactivity; subjects taking thioridazine demonstrated increased anger, violence, and provocativeness. On the Clinical Global Impression Checklist, SCH-12679 also had a greater effect in reducing the severity of aggression. However, side effects, including sedation, gastrointestinal disturbance, and anorexia, were more frequent in the SCH-12679 group. Despite this, the risk-benefit ratio was rated as higher than for thioridazine. For those individuals with seizures, no increase was noted in frequency during the test period. Weight remained stable, and there were no significant effects on hematologic studies, blood chemistry, urinalysis, and electrocardiogram. Although improvement was demonstrated in behavior, SCH-12679 was not marketed because of questions about the benefit-to-risk ratio and possible animal toxicity. Currently, other D_1 antagonists are being evaluated for their effects on schizophrenia and may become available for testing for aggressive behavior management in mentally retarded persons.

Risperidone is another drug that may potentially be helpful in the management of aggressive behavior in mentally retarded persons. Resperidone is a combined serotonin-dopamine antagonist. One double-blind, placebo-controlled crossover trial was conducted to evaluate its efficacy in treating mentally retarded individuals with persistent behavioral disturbance. Vanden Borre et al. (1993) compared resperidone with placebo and administered it as an add-on treatment to existing medication in 30 mentally retarded individuals. It was found to be significantly superior to placebo when ratings using the Aberrant Behavior Checklist and the Clinical Global Impression Checklist were reviewed. No differences were found between resperidone and placebo on an Extrapyramidal Symptom Rating Scale. Sedation, drowsiness, and dizziness were the most frequently reported drug side effects. The authors conclude that continuing assessment of the effects of resperidone, both as add-on therapy and as single treatment, is needed.

In summary, interpretation of drug studies with mentally retarded individuals is complicated by the multiplicity of syndromes and, frequently, by associated brain dysfunction. Despite this, neuroleptics do have some effect on decreasing inappropriate behavior. Specifically, neuroleptics have been reported to reduce maladaptive behavior and stereotypical behavior in mentally retarded individuals (Hollis, 1968; Singh and Aman, 1981). However, continued investigation is necessary to clarify the effects of neuroleptics on behavior. In some individuals, stereotypical behavior is suppressed and secondary to this, adaptive behaviors may be indirectly increased. However, because there are studies that suggest worsening of behavior as well, careful monitoring is essential. Stereotypies have also been reported to be decreased in individuals with autistic disorder with neuroleptics (Anderson et al., 1984). In those individuals with high rates of stereotypies, some positive effects also may be a consequence of reducing them.

The Use of Neuroleptics in Major Psychiatric Disorders

Early studies with neuroleptics focused on maladaptive behavior and frequently did not clarify a specific psychiatric diagnosis. However, neuroleptics are commonly prescribed for major psychiatric disorders in mentally retarded persons. Menolascino et al. (1985) compared thioridazine and thiothixene in mentally retarded and nonretarded individuals with a diagnosis of schizophrenia. Both drugs produced improvement in target symptoms; however, no placebo control group was available for comparison. A more rapid response was observed with thiothixene than thioridazine in the mentally retarded group.

Effects on Cognition

Although there is limited data on cognitive effects, both enhancement and interference with performance have been reported with neuroleptics. Most of the studies that showed interference with learning have involved chlorpromazine, one of the more sedative medications. Haloperidol is relatively nonsedative and several studies have suggested that learning might be enhanced when it was administered. Clarifying the effects of neuroleptic drugs on cognition is complicated, and the answer may depend on the drug studied, the dose, the type of problem targeted, and the specific syndrome.

Side Effects

Neuroleptic drugs produce side effects that are wide ranging and may be severe. These include anticholinergic effects, such as dry mouth, constipation, urinary retention, reduced gastric motility, mental confusion, blurred vision, and tachycardia. Other effects include alpha-adrenergic blockade, which involves postural hypotension, flushing of skin, and mydriasis. Drug effects related to the dopamine system include akathisia, acute dystonia, and tardive dyskinesia. Moreover, weight gain, photosensitivity, especially from chlorpromazine, and agranulocytosis may occur; therefore, careful monitoring is needed. Finally, alertness may decrease because of the sedative nature of many neuroleptic medications.

Tardive dyskinesia is a drug-induced movement disorder characterized by repetitive involuntary rhythmical movements of the face, mouth, and extremities. It may be masked by ongoing neuroleptic treatment. The incidence is difficult to establish in mentally retarded persons, but it is thought to be high. Golden (1988) concluded that 20% to 45% of mentally retarded persons taking neuroleptics will experience the onset or enhancement of dyskinetic symptoms during withdrawal of medication. Ongoing observation is necessary to establish whether or not tardive dyskinesia is present. Tardive dyskinesia is an important consideration when long-term drug treatment is recommended because it interferes with adaptive behavior. Continuous monitoring is needed using various movement rating scales, such as the Abnormal Involuntary Movement Scale (AIMS).

PSYCHOSTIMULANTS

The psychostimulant drugs, dextroamphetamine (Dexedrine), methylphenidate (Ritalin), and magnesium pemoline (Cylert), are considered to be drugs of choice in attention deficit/hyperactivity disorder in children of normal intelligence. In children with AD/HD, these medications improve attention span, reduce impulsivity, reduce activity level, increase behavioral compliance, improve cooperativeness with peers, and improve focus on learning tasks. However, academic achievement has not been shown to clearly improve as a result of stimulant treatment (Aman, 1980; Gittelman, 1983). The effects of these medications are not paradoxical because normal children and adults show improvements—although less striking ones—in their motor and cognitive performance (Rapoport et al., 1978; Werry and Aman, 1984) when they are administered.

Stimulant medication has been used less frequently in mentally retarded persons and, in fact, in a large number of control studies, mental retardation has been an exclusionary factor to participate in clinical trials with stimulants. Early surveys of the use of stimulant medication in residential settings for mentally retarded persons found 2% to 3% of institutional residents were taking these medications (Cohen and Sprague, 1977; Lipman, 1970). Community surveys (Gadow and Kalachnik, 1981) of use in mentally retarded persons documented a prevalence of 3.4% stimulant medication use. Reviews of the effectiveness of stimulant medication in mentally retarded persons suggests that the early studies focused primarily on severely and profoundly retarded persons with a wide variety of behavioral difficulties that included, but were not limited to, hyperactivity. The majority of these studies did not document statistically significant improvement in behavior; Aman (1982) found a possible increase in stereotypies.

However, studies that have included high-functioning mentally retarded children in the moderate to mild range with better target symptom identification have responded (Blacklidge and Ekblad, 1971; Varley and Trupin, 1982). Aman et al. (1991) evaluated methylphenidate in children with a range of IQs from untestable to 90. Significant clinical improvement was noted in some, but primarily in those with higher cognitive function (IQ 46 or higher). These findings have suggested a relationship between the effectiveness of stimulants and cognitive level. A subsequent double-blind crossover study of methylphenidate (0.4 mg/kg) in 28 nonautistic mentally retarded children with ADHD (Aman et al., 1993) failed to show a significantly better clinical response for subjects with higher mental ages; however, those with IQs greater than 45 responded better than those with IQ less than 45. Case selection is a major determinant of effectiveness; profound and severely retarded individuals who are carefully selected may respond to stimulants alone or in combination with other medications, such as clonidine.

Several arguments have been raised about why mentally retarded individuals may not respond well to stimulant medication. Aman (1982) has suggested that stimulants may cause an increased focusing of attention and that severely retarded persons have overly focused attention as it is, so their attention span may not improve. Others (Evans, Gualtieri, and Hicks, 1986) suggest that because stimulants may have effects on frontal lobe systems, intact frontal lobe systems are necessary for an adequate response. Chandler, Gualtieri, and Fahs (1988) postulate that cortical hypoplasia is a common neuropathological finding in mentally retarded persons and may be a factor in the lack of response. These hypotheses regarding the mechanism of action remain speculative because the mechanism for hyperactivity may be different from that of attention deficit. In the DSM-IV (APA, 1994) classification, attention deficit and impulsivity/hyperactivity are listed as possible subtypes. It may be that distractibility may be linked to stimulus-boundness, possibly involving the locus coeruleus, and that other mechanisms may be involved besides those proposed by these authors. Aman and Singh (1988) found improvement on an automated test of memory and attention span with methylphenidate and reductions in out-of-seat activity in a group of mildly retarded children with hyperactivity. The effects of stimulants on learning in mentally retarded populations require continued evaluation, although with functional rises in cognition, positive effects of stimulants on learning may be more evident. Lower doses of psychostimulants have been shown to lead to improvements in attention span and higher doses for reductions in hyperactivity.

Side Effects

The most common side effects of psychostimulants are decreased appetite, weight loss, decreased growth velocity, insomnia, abdominal pain, and headaches (Cantwell and Carlson, 1978). Less commonly, drowsiness, dysphoria, increased talkativeness, and dizziness are reported. Toxic psychoses have been occasionally reported with methylphenidate, but are rare (Bloom et al., 1988; Lucas and Weiss, 1971). Decreased growth velocity is of concern, but with appropriate medication management, growth suppression tends to be temporary (Roche et al., 1979).

ANTIDEPRESSANT DRUGS AND MOOD STABILIZERS

The tricyclic and tetracyclic antidepressants and the monoamine oxidase inhibitors (MAOIs) make up the major subgroups of antidepressant drugs. In the past, in institutional settings, antidepressants were used rarely and accounted for about 1% to 4% of drug prescriptions. In community settings, rates were similar, with 1% to 6% receiving these medications (Intagliata and Rinck, 1985; Martin and Agran, 1985). The tricyclic antidepressants, including imipramine, desipramine, and nortriptyline, are the primary drugs that have been evaluated. MAOIs are rarely used, largely because of concerns about side effects. There are few reports of their effects on problem behaviors in mentally retarded persons, and these studies indicate a lack of effectiveness (Heaton-Ward, 1962). Field et al. (1986), in a control single-subject study, evaluated the effects of imipramine in a moderately retarded woman with depressive symptoms. When contrasted with placebo, imipramine resulted in increased food intake, decreased screaming and crying, and stabilized sleep. Harris (1988) evaluated the effects of amitriptyline in the treatment of depression in Down syndrome and reported positive outcome in 5 individuals, all of whom showed increased appetite, increased interest in activities, improved sleep, and reduction in separation anxiety following drug treatment. In both instances, when used to treat a major mental disorder, e.g., depression, tricyclic antidepressants were found to be effective. But, when Aman et al. (1986b) used imipramine (3 mg/kg) in 10 institutionalized profoundly retarded adults with maladaptive behavior, there was a significant behavioral deterioration, with increased irritability, lethargy/social withdrawal, and hyperactivity, on the Aberrant Behavior Checklist (Aman and Singh, 1986; Marshburn and Aman, 1992).

In addition, antidepressants are used commonly for the treatment of enuresis; their effects are symptomatic rather than curative. However, this indication must be viewed with caution in developmentally disabled persons where Blackwell and Currah (1973) found a less favorable response based on a review of 7 studies.

The antidepressant drugs are most likely underutilized in mentally retarded persons because of difficulties establishing the diagnosis of a mood disorder. Yet mentally retarded persons in all IQ ranges experience the full range of mood disorders and are responsive to these medications.

Mood Stabilizers

Mood stabilizers have not been widely used with mentally retarded persons in either community or residential settings, and prevalence rates are commonly less than 1% (Hill, Balow, and Bruininks, 1985; Intagliata and Rinck, 1985). Among the mood stabilizers, lithium carbonate has received the most attention for treatment of behavioral disorders. It is the medication most commonly used for bipolar or recurrent unipolar depression in mentally retarded persons. However, carbamazepine and sodium valproate are increasingly recognized as important adjuncts for specific treatment and for mood stabilization. Several studies have demonstrated the effectiveness of these medications in controlled trials (Naylor et al., 1974; Rivinus and Harmatz, 1979), although the effects are modest in degree. Bipolar disorder may be atypical in mentally retarded persons or in others with developmental disorders, and rapid cycling may occur. In such instances, carbamazepine may be a more effective drug treatment than lithium carbonate.

In addition to mood disorders, mood stabilizers are commonly used for chronic hyperactivity, aggressiveness, and self-injurious behavior. A number of case studies have provided suggestive evidence for the efficacy of lithium carbonate in the management of these behaviors (Goetzl, Grunberg, and Berkowitz, 1977; Sovner and Hurley, 1981). Several clinical trials, most of which were uncontrolled, have also shown drug-related improvements, primarily in increased adaptability, reduced aggressiveness, and reductions in restlessness, self-injury, and motor activity. A five-center evaluation of the effects of lithium on aggression in severely mentally retarded adults has been completed (Aman and Singh, 1988). In this study, 16 of 22 patients (73%) who received lithium carbonate showed reductions in aggression, 4 showed no change, and 2 showed increased aggression. The best responders were those who had a high initial level of aggressive behavior. This study has methodological difficulties because different raters were used, and the subjects concurrently took other medications. These studies with lithium suggest its possible usefulness in controlling and reducing aggressive and assaultive behaviors in some mentally retarded persons, although specific guidelines for selecting cases are unclear.

Cognitive Effects

Studies of the effects of antidepressants and mood stabilizers on cognition in mentally retarded persons are needed. Lithium carbonate may result in some depression of cognition on certain tests (Platt et al., 1981). Clarification of possible cognitive effects is particularly important for mentally retarded individuals.

Side Effects

Antidepressant drugs generally have anticholinergic side effects. Common difficulties include postural hypotension, tachycardia, and changes in cardiac conduction. These effects may be sufficiently severe to lead to the medication being discontinued. Mood stabilizers such as lithium carbonate may have major effects on the central nervous system and produce a confusional state when blood levels are elevated (Chandler, Gualtieri, and Fahs, 1988). With lithium toxicity, sluggishness, tremor, ataxia, coma, and electrolyte changes may occur as well as seizure disorder. Less severe side effects may be present at therapeutic levels and include gastrointestinal symptoms, such as nausea, anorexia, cramping, and diarrhea. Careful monitoring of thyroid function and renal function is particularly important in mentally retarded as well as mentally disabled persons who are taking this medication. In some syndromes, such as Down syndrome, where thyroid dysfunction is associated, thyroid status must be carefully monitored.

Anticonvulsants

Anticonvulsant drugs may be useful in the treatment of mood disorders and in behavior management for mentally retarded, developmentally disabled persons, although these medications are most commonly prescribed for use in seizure disorders. Moreover, some medications in this group may have effects on behavior and cognition when prescribed primarily for seizure control. Yet other anticonvulsants may cause toxic reactions that mimic neurological disease; such toxicity may be difficult to detect in severely and profoundly mentally retarded individuals.

In institutional settings for mentally retarded

persons, anticonvulsants make up approximately 35% of drug prescriptions, which parallels the prevalence of convulsive disorders in this group (Gadow, 1979; Jasper, Ward, and Pope, 1969). Anticonvulsants require continuous review because they may be administered for many years or even throughout life. Subtle changes in behavior may occur associated with their use that may be overlooked (Stores, 1988).

With carbamazepine (Tegretol), there is little or no evidence of drug-related deterioration in psychomotor performance. Cognitive enhancement has been noted in some patients who have been treated with this medication, although such changes must be evaluated in the context of the reduction of prior medications that may be more sedating (Aman, 1984).

Anticonvulsants must be monitored carefully because of possible behavioral, cognitive, and motor effects in children and adolescents receiving these medications long term for seizure disorders. Phenobarbital, phenytoin, and primidone have, in some cases, been associated with psychomotor deterioration, particularly with high drug concentrations. Such changes have been evaluated, using IQ tests, specialized tests of learning and cognitive style, rating scales, and neuropsychological tests as well as clinical judgment. Some studies, however, indicate improvements, especially in low doses, on these tests, so a dose effect must be considered. Combinations of medications may have greater behavioral effect and must be carefully monitored. Evaluation of long-term effects of anticonvulsants is complex because it is possible that some behavioral changes noted represented neurological deterioration over time.

The relationship of blood level and behavior has been evaluated by several investigators (Trimble and Corbett, 1980). These authors found a positive relationship between blood level of phenobarbital, primidone, and phenytoin and teachers' rating of conduct problems. Moreover, those children showing the most substantial drops in intelligence had higher blood levels of phenytoin and primidone than children without such losses. Phenobarbital has been linked to overactivity (Ounsted, 1955; Schain, 1979). Forty-two percent of children treated with phenobarbital developed a behavioral disturbance compared to 18% who received no treatment in one study (Wolf and Forsythe, 1978). Because of the risk of increased hyperactivity and possibly aggressive behavior in some mentally retarded individuals, phenobarbital should be monitored for its behavioral effects as well as the anticonvulsant ones.

Specific toxic effects of anticonvulsants may be problematic in mentally retarded and other developmentally disabled persons. Symptoms of intoxication include mental confusion, ataxia, lethargy, and slurred speech. The lack of recognition of toxicity is of particular concern in children and adolescents who may not be able to report on their own behavior. Logan and Freeman (1969) suggest that careful monitoring is needed because, in some individuals, toxicity might occur on low doses, toxic symptoms might be confused with a coexisting neurological disorder, and classic symptoms of toxicity might be more difficult to detect in younger individuals and those who are low functioning. Because of possible toxicity, drug monitoring is crucial, particularly in community and institutional settings for low-functioning persons. Aman et al. (1986a) found 28% of a random sample of mentally retarded individuals taking phenytoin had blood levels above the therapeutic range, as did 16% of those taking carbamazepine. The risk-benefit ratio must be carefully considered because, in some instances, considerable adjustments in medication use are made to manage seizure disorders.

Because of concerns about effects on cognition and behavior, it is important to aim toward the use of one drug or the smallest number of agents to achieve seizure control. In addition, it is often possible to discontinue anticonvulsants when patients have been seizure free for specific time periods. However, if seizure medications are discontinued, mentally retarded persons must be monitored carefully for recurrence of symptoms because of the complexity of their disorders.

Phenytoin (Dilantin)

An early focus on the use of anticonvulsants for behavior management was based on the belief that disturbances in behavior might be aspects of underlying subthreshold convulsive disorders. Initial studies in behavior treatment focused on the effects of phenytoin (Dilantin) and suggested major effects on behavior. These early studies were frequently uncontrolled (Aman, 1983; Conners and Werry, 1979); later, well-controlled investigations (Conners et al., 1971) did not establish benefit from phenytoin treatment of behavioral disorders.

Carbamazepine (Tegretol)

In nonmentally retarded subjects, there is considerable evidence that carbamazepine is effective for bipolar disorder and leads to mood stabilization (Post and Uhde, 1986). Remschmidt (1976) evaluated 28 studies of carbamazepine in nonepileptic children with behavior disorders. In 7 well-controlled studies, evidence of significant improvement was demonstrated in 3. Effects on activity level were prominently mentioned. Reid, Naylor, and Kay (1981) carried out a double-blind, placebo-controlled crossover study of carbamazepine in 12 severely and profoundly retarded overactive adults. During a 7-month trial, those individuals who were overactive showed reductions in rate, particularly if the overactivity was accompanied by an elevation in mood. Responses were less clear when overactivity occurred in the context of multiple behavioral problems. No relationship was found between response to carbamazepine and presence or absence of seizure disorder. Effects were moderate but significant in the majority; 2 individuals who showed improvement were able to leave a ward setting and attend a training center. Because of difficulties in the diagnosis of mood disorder in severely mentally retarded individuals, subjects in this group should be carefully evaluated for mood disorder.

Sodium Valproate

Sodium valproate has been evaluated in several studies and found to have minimal adverse effects; possible deterioration in behavior in some individuals has been suggested when higher doses are used (Aman et al., 1987; Trimble and Thompson, 1984).

ANXIOLYTIC MEDICATIONS

Surveys of institutionalized populations have revealed that anxiolytic agents, such as diazepam and chlordiazepoxide, have been used relatively commonly in the past. Rates ranging from 13% to 18% (Hill, Balow, and Bruininks, 1985; Intagliata and Rinck, 1985) have been reported. In community settings, the rates range from 2% to 12%. In the Intagliata and Rinck study (1985) anxiolytics were being used to treat a variety of difficulties, including overactivity, agitation, and disruptive behavior as well as anxiety. Rather than focusing on anxiety, studies on the use of anxiolytic agents have focused on their effects on disruptive behavior. In controlled studies (LaVeck and Buckley, 1961; Walters, Singh, and Beale, 1977), some worsening in target symptoms has been reported. There is little evidence that anxiolytic drugs, specifically benzodiazepines, reduce specific problem behaviors in mentally retarded individuals. Moreover, careful studies of the cognitive effects of these drugs in mentally retarded persons are not available.

B-ADRENERGIC BLOCKERS

Propranolol

Propranolol has been targeted for sudden aggressive behavior in mentally retarded individuals. Ratey et al. (1986) studied propranolol in 19 individuals selected for aggression, assaultiveness, agitation, and self-injury. The majority were reported as either markedly or moderately improved using this medication. However, the study was uncontrolled and did not include placebo, double-blind procedures or standardized measures of outcome to clarify change. Control studies are needed to clarify positive or adverse effects of this medication.

OPIATE ANTAGONISTS

Naloxone and Naltrexone

Opiate antagonists have been used in a number of case studies for treatment of individuals with high rates of self-injurious behavior. The rationale for their use is based on the hypothesis that some individuals have abnormally high levels of endogenous opioids and, therefore, may have abnormally high thresholds of pain. Another hypothesis is that some developmentally disabled persons may deliberately engage in self-injurious behavior to cause the release of endorphins that may have reinforcing properties (Sokol and Campbell, 1988). This has led to the use of naloxone and naltrexone to treat self-injurious behavior in mentally retarded persons. In some studies, a reduction in self-injury has been found (Herman et al., 1987; Richardson and Zaleski, 1983; Sandman et al., 1983). Other studies have shown no change (Beckwith, Couk, and Schumacher, 1986; Davidson et al., 1983). Such studies are complicated by the heterogeneity of the population and the possibility of stress-induced analgesia, as described in Chapter 17 on self-injurious behavior.

SUMMARY

Considerable progress has been made in the psychopharmacological treatment of behavioral and psychiatric problems in persons with developmental disorders. Psychopharmacological research continues to introduce new hypotheses and, as new drugs become available for treatment, these hypotheses are being explored. Improved scientific methodology in the testing of new drugs allows better empirical validation or refutation of hypotheses. The rigorous application of experimental design in the evaluation of drug efficacy is taking place. When appropriately applied, improved research may lead to less polypharmacy and a more rational approach to treatment.

REFERENCES

Albert, J., Elie, R., Cooper, S.F., Clermont, A., and Langlois, Y. (1977). Efficacy of SCH-12679 in the management of aggressive mental retardates. *Current Therapeutic Research,* 21:789–795.

Aman, M.G. (1980). Psychotropic drugs and learning problems: A selective review. *Journal of Learning Disabilities,* 13:87–96.

______. (1982). Stimulant drug effects in developmental disorders and hyperactivity: Toward a resolution of disparate findings. *Journal of Autism and Developmental Disorders,* 12:385–398.

______. (1983). Psychoactive drugs in mental retardation. In J.L. Matson and F. Andrasik (eds.), *Treatment issues and innovations in mental retardation,* pp. 455–513. Plenum Press, New York.

______. (1984). Drugs and learning in mentally retarded persons. In G.D. Burrows and J.S. Werry (eds.), *Advances in human psychopharmacology,* Vol. 3, pp. 121–163. JAI Press, Greenwich, CT.

______. (1991). *Assessing psychopathology and behavior problems in persons with mental retardation: A review of available instruments.* (DHHS Publication No. [ADM] 91–1712). U.S. Department of Health and Human Services, Rockville, MD.

______, and Singh, N.N. (1980). The usefulness of thioridazine for treating childhood disorders. Fact or folklore? *American Journal of Mental Deficiency,* 84:331–33.

______, and ______. (1986). *Aberrant behavior checklist: Manual.* Slosson, East Aurora, NY.

______, and ______. (1988). *Psychopharmacology of the developmental disabilities.* Springer-Verlag, New York.

______, and ______. (1991). Pharmacological intervention. In J.L. Matson and J.H. Mulick (eds.), *Handbook of mental retardation,* 2nd ed., pp. 347–352. Pergamon Press, New York.

______, and ______, (1988). Thioridazine dose effects with reference to stereotypic behavior in mentally retarded residents. *Journal of Autism and Developmental Disabilities,* 18:355–366.

______, White, A.J., and Field, C.J. (1984). Chlorpromazine effects on stereotypic and conditioned behavior—a pilot study. *Journal of Mental Deficiency Research,* 28:253–260.

______, Kern, R.A., McGhee, D.E., and Arnold, L.E. (1993). Fenfluramine and methylphenidate in children with mental retardation and ADHD: Clinical and side effects. *Journal of the American Academy of Child and Adolescent Psychiatry,* 32:851–859.

______, Marks, R.E., Turbott, S.H., Wilsher, C.P., and Merry, S.N. (1991). The clinical effects of methylphenidate and thioridazine in intellectually subaverage children. *Journal of the American Academy of Child and Adolescent Psychiatry,* 30:246–256.

______, Paxton, J.W., Field, C.J., and Foote, S.E. (1986a). Survey of drug concentrations in retarded patients receiving anticonvulsant medication. *American Journal of Mental Deficiency,* 90:643–650.

______, Werry, J.S., Paxton, J.W., and Turbott, S.H. (1987). Effect of sodium valproate on psychomotor performance in children as a function of dose, fluctuations in concentration, and diagnosis. *Epilepsia,* 28:115–124.

______, White, A.J., Vaithianathan, C., and Teehan,

C.J. (1986b). Preliminary study of imipramine in profoundly retarded residents. *Journal of Autism and Developmental Disorders,* 16:263–273.

American Psychiatric Association, Committee on Nomenclature and Statistics. (1994). *Diagnostic and statistical manual of mental disorders,* 4th ed. Author, Washington, DC.

Anderson, L.T., Campbell, M., Grega, D.M., Perry, R., Small, A.M., and Green W.H. (1984). Haloperidol in the treatment of infantile autism: Effects on learning and behavioral symptoms. *American Journal of Psychiatry,* 141:1195–1202.

Barlow, D.H., and Hersen, M. (1984). *Single-case experimental designs,* 2nd ed. Pergamon Press, Elmsford, NY.

Bates, W.J., Smelzer, D.J., and Arnoczky, S.M. (1986). Appropriate and inappropriate use of psychotropic medications for institutionalized mentally retarded persons. *American Journal of Mental Deficiency,* 90:363–370.

Bazelon, M., Paine, R.S., Cowie, V.A., Hunt, O., Houck, J.C., and Mahanand, D. (1967). Reversal of hypotonia in infants with Dow 's syndrome by administration of 5-hydroxytryptophan. *Lancet,* i:1130–1133.

Beckwith, B.E., Couk, D.I., and Schumacher, K. (1986). Failure of naloxone to reduce self-injurious behavior in two developmentally disabled females. *Applied Research in Mental Retardation,* 7:183–188.

Blacklidge, V.Y., and Ekblad, R.L. (1971). The effectiveness of methylphenidate hydrochloride (Ritalin) on learning and behavior in public school educable mentally retarded children. *Pediatrics,* 47:923–926.

Blackwell, B., and Currah, J. (1973). The psychopharmacology of nocturnal enuresis. In I. Kolvin, R. McKeith, and S. Meadow (eds.), *Bladder control and enuresis.* Heineman, London.

Bloom, A.S., Russell, L.J., Weisshopf, B., and Blackerby, J.L. (1988). Methylphenidate-induced delusional disorder in a child with attention deficit disorder with hyperactivity. *Journal of the American Academy of Child and Adolescent Psychiatry,* 27:248–251.

Bradley, C. (1937). The behavior of children receiving benzedrine. *American Journal of Psychiatry,* 94:577–585.

Burk, H.W., and Menolascino, F.J. (1968). Haloperidol in emotionally disturbed mentally retarded individuals. *American Journal of Psychiatry,* 124:1589–1591.

Cantwell, D.P., and Carlson, G.A. (1978). Stimulants. In J.S. Werry (ed.), *Pediatric psychopharmacology: The use of behavior modifying drugs in children,* pp. 171–217. Brunner/Mazel, New York.

Chandler, M., Gualtieri, C.T., and Fahs, J.J. (1988). Other psychotropic drugs: Stimulants, antidepressants, the anxiolytics, and lithium carbonate. In M.G. Aman and N.N. Singh (eds.), *Psychopharmacology of the developmental disabilities,* pp. 119–145. Springer-Verlag, New York.

Cohen, M.N., and Sprague, R.L. (1977, March). *Survey of drug usage in two midwestern institutions for the retarded.* Paper presented at the Gatlinburg Conference on Research in Mental Retardation, Gatlinburg, TN.

Conners, C.K., Kramer, R., Rothschild, G.H., Schwartz, L., and Stone, A. (1971). Treatment of young delinquent boys with diphenylhydantoin sodium and methylphenidate. *Archives of General Psychiatry,* 24:156–160.

______, and Werry, J.S. (1979). Pharmacotherapy of psychopathology in children. In H.C. Quay and J.S. Werry (eds.), *Psychopathological disorders of childhood,* pp. 336–386. John Wiley, New York.

Corbett, J. (1979). Psychiatric morbidity and mental retardation. In F.E. James and R.P. Snaith (eds.), *Psychiatric illness and mental handicap,* pp. 11–25. Gaskell Press, London.

Davidson, P.W., Kleene, B.M., Carroll, M., and Rockwitz, R.J. (1983). Effects of naloxone on self-injurious behavior: A case study. *Applied Research in Mental Retardation,* 4:1–4.

Dura, J.R., Aman, M.G., and Mulick, J.A. (1988). Medication use in an ICF/MR for nonambulatory severely and profoundly mentally retarded children. *Journal of the Multihandicapped Person,* 1:155–160.

Elie, R., Langlois, Y., Cooper, S.F., Gravel, G., and Albert, J. (1980). Comparison of SCH-12679 and thioridazine in aggressive mental retardates. *Canadian Journal of Psychiatry,* 25:484–491.

Evans, R.W., Gualtieri, C.T., and Hicks, R.E. (1986). Neuropathic substrate for stimulant drug effects in hyperactive children. *Clinical Neuropharmacology,* 9:264–281.

Field, C.J., Aman, M.G., White, A.J., and Vaithianathan, C. (1986). A single-subject study of imipramine in a mentally retarded woman with depressive symptoms. *Journal of Mental Deficiency Research,* 30:191–198.

Fisher, W., Piazza, C., and Page, T. (1989). Assessing the independent and interactive effects of behavioral and pharmacologic interventions in a dually diagnosed child. *Journal of Behavior Therapy and Experimental Psychiatry,* 20:241–250.

Freeman, K.D. (1970). Psychopharmacology and the

retarded child. In F.J. Menolascino (ed.), *Psychiatric approaches to mental retardation,* pp. 294–368. Basic Books, New York.

Gadow, K.D. (1979). *Children on medication: A primer for school personnel.* Council for Exceptional Children, Reston, VA.

______, and Kalachnik, J. (1981). Prevalence and pattern of drug treatment for behavior and seizure disorders of TMR students. *American Journal of Mental Deficiency,* 85:588–595.

Gittelman, R. (1983). Treatment of reading disorders. In M. Rutter (ed.), *Developmental neuropsychiatry,* pp. 520–541. The Guilford Press, New York.

Goetzl, J., Grunberg, F., and Berkowitz, B. (1977). Lithium carbonate in the management of hyperactive aggressive behavior of the mentally retarded. *Comprehensive Psychiatry,* 18:599–606.

Golden, G.S. (1988). Tardive dyskinesia and developmental disabilities. In M.G. Aman and N.N. Singh (eds.), *Psychopharmacology of the developmental disabilities,* pp. 197–215. Springer-Verlag, New York.

Harris, J. (1988). Psychological adaptation and psychiatric disorders in adolescents and young adults with Down syndrome. In S. Pueschel (ed.), *The young person with Down syndrome: Transition from adolescence to adulthood.* P.H. Brookes, Baltimore.

______, Tune, L.E., Kurtz, M., and Coyle, J.T. (1982). Neuroleptic serum levels in mentally retarded boys taking thioridazine. *Psychopharmacology Bulletin,* 18:65–66.

Heaton-Ward, W.A. (1962). Inference and suggestion in a clinical trial (Niamid in mongolism). *Journal of Mental Science,* 108:865–870.

Herman, B.H., Hammock, M.K., Arthur-Smith, A., Egan, J., Chatoor, I., Werner, A., and Zelnik, N. (1987). Naltrexone decreases self-injurious behavior. *Annals of Neurology,* 22:550–552.

Hill, B.K., Balow, E.A., and Bruininks, R.H. (1985). A national survey of prescribed drugs in institutions and community residential facilities for mentally retarded people. *Psychopharmacology Bulletin,* 21:279–284.

Hollis, J.H. (1968). Direct measurement of differential behavioral effect. *Science,* 159:1487–1489.

Intagliata, J., and Rinck, C. (1985). Psychoactive drug use in public and community residential facilities for mentally retarded persons. *Psychopharmacology Bulletin,* 21:268–278.

Jakab, I. (1984). Short-term effect of thioridazine tablets versus suspension on emotionally disturbed/retarded children. *Journal of Clinical Psychopharmacology,* 4:210–215.

Jasper, H.H., Ward, A.A., and Pope, A. (eds.). (1969). *Basic mechanisms of the epilepsies.* Little, Brown, Boston.

LaVeck, G.D., and Buckley, P. (1961). The use of psychopharmacologic agents in retarded children with behavioral disorders. *Journal of Chronic Diseases,* 13:174–183.

Le Vann, L. (1971). Clinical comparison of haloperidol with chlorpromazine in mentally retarded children. *American Journal of Mental Deficiency,* 75:719–723.

Lipman, R.S. (1970). The use of psychopharmacological agents in residential facilities for the retarded. In F.J. Menolascino (ed.), *Psychiatric approaches to mental retardation.* Basic Books, New York.

______, DiMascio, A., Reatig, N., and Kirson, T. (1978). Psychotropic drugs and mentally retarded children. In M.A. Lipton, A. DiMascio, and K.F. Killam (eds.), *Psychopharmacology: A generation of progress,* pp. 1437–1449. Raven Press, New York.

Logan, W.J., and Freeman, J.M. (1969). Pseudodegenerative disease due to diphenylhydantoin intoxication. *Archives of Neurology,* 21:631–637.

Lucas, A., and Weiss, M. (1971). Methylphenidate hallucinosis. *Journal of the American Medical Association,* 217:1079–1081.

Lund, J. (1985). The prevalence of psychiatric morbidity in mentally retarded adults. *Acta Psychiatrica Scandinavica,* 72:563–570.

Marholin, D., Touchette, P.E., and Stewart, R.M. (1979). Withdrawal of chronic chlorpromazine medication: An experimental analysis. *Journal of Applied Behavior Analysis,* 12:159–171.

Marshburn, E.C., and Aman, M.G. (1992). Factor validity and norms for the Aberrant Behavior Checklist in a community sample of children with mental retardation. *Journal of Autism and Developmental Disorders,* 22:357–373.

Martin, J.E., and Agran, M. (1985). Psychotropic and anticonvulsant drug use by mentally retarded adults across community residential and vocational placements. *Applied Research in Mental Retardation,* 6:33–49.

McAndrew, J.B., Case, Q., and Treffert, D.A. (1972). Effects of prolonged phenothiazine intake on psychotic and other hospitalized children. *Journal of Autism and Childhood Schizophrenia,* 2:75–91.

McHugh, P.R., and Slavney, P.R. (1983). *The perspective of psychiatry.* Johns Hopkins University Press, Baltimore, MD.

Menolascino, F.J., Ruedrich, S.L., Golden, C.J., and Wilson, T.E. (1985). Diagnosis and pharmacotherapy of schizophrenia in the retarded. *Psychopharmacology Bulletin,* 21:316–322.

Millichamp, C.J., and Singh, N.N. (1987). The effects of intermittent drug therapy on stereotypy and collateral behaviors of mentally retarded persons. *Research in Developmental Disabilities,* 8:213–227.

Mizuno, T., and Yugari, Y. (1975). Prophylactic effect of L-5-hydroxytryptophan on self-mutilation in the Lesch-Nyhan syndrome. *Neuropaediatrie,* 6:13–23.

Moore, J.W. (1960). The effects of a tranquilizer (Thorazine) on the intelligence and achievement of educable mentally retarded women. *Dissertation Abstracts,* 20:3200.

Naylor, G.J., Donald, J.M., LePoidevin, D., and Reid, A.H. (1974). A double-blind trial of long-term lithium therapy in mental defectives. *British Journal of Psychiatry,* 124:52–57.

Nyhan, W.L., Johnson, H.G., Kaufman, I.A., and Jones, K.L. (1980). Serotonergic approaches to the modification of behavior in the Lesch-Nyhan syndrome. *Applied Research in Mental Retardation,* 1:25–40.

Ounsted, C. (1955). The hyperkinetic syndrome in epileptic children. *Lancet,* ii:303–311.

Platt, J.E., Campbell, M., Green, W.H., Perry, R., and Cohen, I.L. (1981). Effects of lithium carbonate and haloperidol on cognition in aggressive hospitalized school-age children. *Journal of Clinical Psychopharmacology,* 1:8–13.

Post, R.M., and Uhde, T.W. (1986). Anticonvulsants in non-epileptic psychosis. In M.R. Trimble and T.G. Bolwig (eds.), *Aspects of epilepsy and psychiatry,* pp. 177–212. John Wiley, New York.

Pueschel, S.M., Reed, R.B., Cronk, C.E., and Goldstein, B.I. (1980). 5-hydroxytryptophan and pyridoxine. Their effects in young children with Down's syndrome. *American Journal of Diseases of Childhood,* 134:838–844.

Rapoport, J.L., Buchsbaum, M.S., Zahn, T.P., Wemgartner, H., Ludlow, C., and Mikkelsen, E.J. (1978). Dextroamphetamine: Cognitive and behavioral effects in normal prepubertal boys. *Science,* 199:560–563.

Ratey, J.J., Mikkelsen, E., Smith, G.B., Upadhyaya, A., Zuckerman, H.S., Marello, D., Sorgi, P., Polakoff, S., and Bemporad, J. (1986). Beta blockers in the severely and profoundly mentally retarded. *Journal of Clinical Psychopharmacology,* 6:103–107.

Reid, A.H. (1972). Psychoses in adult mental defectives: II. Schizophrenic and paranoid psychoses. *British Journal of Psychiatry,* 120:213–218.

______. (1982). *The psychiatry of mental handicap.* Blackwell Scientific Publications, Oxford, UK.

______, Naylor, G.J., and Kay, D.S.G. (1981). A double-blind, placebo controlled, crossover trial of carbamazepine in overactive, severely mentally handicapped patients. *Psychological Medicine,* 11:109–113.

Remschmidt, H. (1976). The psychotropic effect of carbamazepine in nonepileptic patients, with particular reference to problems posed by clinical studies in children with behavioural disorders. In W. Birkmayer (ed.), *Epileptic seizures, behaviour, pain,* pp. 253–258. Hans Huber Publishers, Bern, Switzerland.

Richardson, J.S., and Zaleski, N.A. (1983). Naloxone and self-mutilation. *Biological Psychiatry,* 18:99–101.

Rivinus, T.M., Grofer, L.M., Feinstein, C., and Barrett, R.P. (1989). Psychopharmacology in the mentally retarded individual: New approaches, new directions. *Journal of the Multihandicapped Person,* 2:1–23.

______, and Harmatz, J.S. (1979). Diagnosis and lithium treatment of affective disorder in the retarded. Five case studies. *American Journal of Psychiatry,* 136:551–554.

Roche, A.F., Lipman, R.S., Overall, J.E., and Hung, W. (1979). The effects of stimulant medication on the growth of hyperkinetic children. *Pediatrics,* 63:847–850.

Sandman, C.A., Datta, P.C., Barron, J., Hoehler, F.K., Williams, C., and Swanson, J.M. (1983). Naloxone attenuates self-abusive behavior in developmentally disabled clients. *Applied Research in Mental Retardation,* 4:5–11.

Schain, R.J. (1979). Problems with the use of conventional anticonvulsant drugs in mentally retarded individuals. *Brain and Development,* 1:77–82.

Schroeder, S.R. (1988). Neuroleptic medications for persons with developmental disabilities. In M.G. Aman and N.N. Singh (eds.), *Psychopharmacology of the developmental disabilities,* pp. 82–100. Springer-Verlag, New York.

______, and Gualtieri, C.T. (1985). Behavioral interactions induced by chronic neuroleptic therapy with persons with mental retardation. *Psychopharmacology Bulletin,* 21:323–326.

Singh, N.N., and Aman, M.G. (1981). Effects of thioridazine dosage on the behavior of severely mentally retarded persons. *American Journal of Mental Deficiency,* 85:580–587.

Sokol, M.S., and Campbell, M. (1988). Novel psychoactive agents in the treatment of developmental disorders. In M.G. Aman and N.N. Singh (eds.), *Psychopharmacology of the developmental disabilities,* pp. 146–167. Springer-Verlag, New York.

Sovner, R. (1986). Limiting factors in the use of DSM-III criteria with mentally ill/mentally retarded persons. *Psychopharmacology Bulletin,* 22:1055–1059.

______, and Hurley, A.D. (1981). The management of chronic behavior disorders in mentally retarded adults with lithium carbonate. *Journal of Nervous and Mental Disease,* 169:191–195.

Sprague, R.L., and Baxley, G.B. (1978). Drugs for behavior management, with comment on some legal aspects. *Mental Retardation and Developmental Disabilities,* 10:92–129.

______, and Werry, J.S. (1971). Methodology of psychopharmacological studies with the retarded. In N.R. Ellis (ed.), *International review of research in mental retardation,* Vol. 5, pp. 147–219. Academic Press, New York.

Stores, G. (1988). Antiepileptic drugs. In M.G. Aman and N.N. Singh (eds.), *Psychopharmacology of the developmental disabilities,* pp. 101–118. Springer-Verlag, New York.

Trimble, M.R., and Corbett, J.A. (1980). Behavioural and cognitive disturbances in epileptic children. *Irish Medical Journal,* 73:21–28.

______, and Thompson, P.J. (1984). Sodium valproate and cognitive function. *Epilepsia,* 25(suppl.):S60–S64.

Vaisanen, K., Viukari, M., Rimon, R., and Raisanen, P. (1981). Haloperidol, thioridazine and placebo in mentally subnormal patients—serum levels and clinical effects. *Acta Psychiatrica Scandinavica,* 63:262–271.

Vanden Borre, R., Vermote, R., Buttiens, M., Thiry, P., Dierick, G., Geutjens, J., Sieben, G., and Heylen, S. (1993). Resperidone as add-on therapy in behavioural disturbances in mental retardation: A double-blind placebo-controlled crossover study. *Acta Psychiatrica Scandinavica,* 87:167–171.

Varley, C.K., and Trupin, E.W. (1982). Double-blind administration of methylphenidate to mentally retarded children with attention deficit disorder: A preliminary study. *American Journal of Mental Deficiency,* 86:560–566.

Walters, A., Singh, N., and Beale, I.L. (1977). Effects of lorazepam on hyperactivity in retarded children. *New Zealand Medical Journal,* 86:473–475.

Werry, J.S. (1988). Conclusions. In M.G. Aman and N.N. Singh (eds.), *Psychopharmacology of the developmental disabilities,* pp. 239–245. Springer-Verlag, New York.

______, and Aman, M.G. (1984). Methylphenidate in hyperactive and enuretic children. In B. Shopsin and L. Greenhill (eds.), *The psychobiology of childhood: Profile of current issues,* pp. 183–195. Spectrum Publications, Jamaica, NY.

Wolf, S.M., and Forsythe, A. (1978). Behavior disturbance, phenobarbital, and febrile seizures. *Pediatrics,* 61:728–731.

GLOSSARY OF PSYCHOACTIVE DRUGS
Generic Names and Trade Names

DRUG AND CLASS	TRADE NAME(S)
NEUROLEPTICS (Antipsychotics, "Major tranquilizers")	
Phenothiazines	
chlorpromazine	Largactil, Thorazine
fluphenazine	Prolixin
mesoridazine	Serentii
peracetazine	Quide
pericyazine	Neulactil
perphenazine	Trilafon
prochlorperazine	Compazine
promazine	Sparine
thioridazine	Mellaril
trifluoperazine	Stelazine
Thioxanthenes	
chlorprothixene	Tarctan, Tarasan
thiothixene	Navane
Butyrophenones	
haloperidol	Haldol, Serenace
pipamperon	Dipiperon
Diphenylbutylpiperidine	
pimozide	Orap

(continued)

DRUG AND CLASS	TRADE NAME(S)
Benzisoxazoles	
risperidone	Risperdal
Rauwolfia Alkaloids	
reserpine	Rauloydin, Reserpoid, Sandril
ANTICONVULSANTS	
carbamazepine	Tegretol
clonazepam	Clonopin
diazepam[1]	Valium
ethosuximide	Zarontin
lorazepam[1]	Ativan
phenobarbital (phenobarbitone)	Luminal, Gardenal
phenytoin (diphenylhydantoin, DPH)	Dilantin
primidone	Mysoline
sodium valproate	Depakene, Epilim
sulthiame	Ospolot
SEDATIVE-HYPNOTICS	
Antihistamines	
dyphenhydramine	Benadryl
hydroxyzine	Atarax
promethazine[2]	Phenergan
trimeprazine	Temaril, Vallergan
Benzodiazepines ("Minor Tranquilizers")	
alprazolam[1]	Xanax
diazepam[1]	Valium
chlordiazepoxide	Libriium
flurazepam	Dalmane
lorazepam	Ativan
oxazepam	Serax
prazepam	Verstran
temazepam	Restoril
triazolam	Halcion
Other	
chloral hydrate	Noctec
meprobamate	Equanil, Miltown
secobarbital	Seconal
ANTIDEPRESSANT/ANTIMANIC DRUGS	
Tricyclic Antidepressants	
amitriptyline	Elavil, Amitril, Endep
desipramine	Norpramin, Pertofrane
doxepin	Sinequan, Adapin
imipramine	Tofranil, Janimine, Dumex
notriptyline	Arentyl, Nortab, Pamelor
Phenylethylamine bicyclic antidepressant	
venlafaxine	Effexor
Monoamine Oxidase Inhibitors (MAOIs)	
isocarboxazid	Marplan
phenelzine	Nardil
tranylcypromine	Parnate

DRUG AND CLASS	TRADE NAME(S)
Atypical Antidepressants	
alprazolam[1]	Xanax
amoxapine	Asendin
maprotiline	Ludiomil
nomifensine	Merital
bupropion	Wellbutrin
Antimanic Drugs	
lithium carbonate	Eskalith, Lithane, Lithobid
Serotonin Reuptake Inhibitors	
fluoxetine	Prozac
sertraline	Zoloft
paroxetine	Paxil
CNS STIMULANTS	
amphetamine sulfate	Benzedrine
deanol (2-dimethylaminoethanol)	Deaner
dextroamphetamine (d-amphetamine)	Dexedrine
levoamphetamine (l-amphetamine)	Cydril
methylphenidate	Ritalin
pemoline	Cylert
ANTIPARKINSON DRUGS[3]	
benztropine mesylate	Cogentin
diphenhydramine hydrochloride	Benadryl
trihexyphenidyl hydrochloride	Artane
MISCELLANEOUS	
Clonidine HCl (alpha adrenergic blocker)	Catapres, Combipres
fenfluramine (serotonin depleter)	Pondimin, Ponderax
5-hydroxytryptamine (serotonin)	—
naloxone (endorphin antagonist)	Narcan
naltrexone (endorphin antagonist)	Trexan
propranolol (beta adrenergic blocker)	Inderal
glutamic acid amino acid)	Prostate, Selerex
essential fatty acid supplement (oleic/erucic acid combination)	—

[1]Belongs to more than one clinical group.

[2]Actually a phenothiazine but listed here because it is commonly used as an hypnotic in children.

[3]Not ordinarily used as psychotropic drugs but are used to counter extrapyramidal side effects of neuroleptic drugs.

CHAPTER 21

COUNSELING AND TREATMENT OF GENETIC DISEASES

The exact number of genetic diseases is unknown; however, it is thought that genetic factors play a role in all major illnesses. Approximately 4,000 genetic diseases have been identified that involve single-gene loci; therefore, about 4% of the 100,000 genes are currently known to be involved in diseases. Yet the number is much greater than this because this estimate does not include diseases that may involve multifactorial inheritance, such as schizophrenia. Of the recognized diseases, biochemical data are available for approximately 500. The gene mutation is known and the gene product has been identified for about 150 human genetic diseases, which is about 4% of the known genetic diseases.

Genetic disease can be treated at many levels—at the mutant gene or distant from it. The treatment approaches that have been introduced include metabolic treatment, enzyme replacement treatment, somatic cell or germ-line treatment, and intrauterine treatment. With these developments, metabolic, biochemical, and gene therapy for human genetic diseases is increasingly becoming a reality. Still, both genetic and environmental factors must be considered in planning treatment of genetic diseases; this is particularly the case for multifactorial disorders.

New knowledge about genetic disorders provides challenges not only in developing treatments but also in counseling affected patients and their families. Because genetic disease recurs within families, genetic counseling, unlike other disease-oriented counseling, focuses not only on the identified patient but also on present and future members of a patient's family. In the past, genetic counseling was ordinarily provided by the patient's general physician as an essential aspect of case management. However, with growing knowledge about genetic diseases and increasing sophistication in the laboratory tests available to diagnose them, specialty genetics clinics are increasingly involved as referral sites for individuals with genetic disorders or with family histories of a genetic disorder.

Genetic counseling begins with the establishment of the diagnosis and then applies genetic principles in working with families. Most commonly, in developmental neuropsychiatric disorders the persons seeking genetic counseling are the parents of a child who has a genetic disorder. Genetic counseling entails not only a careful and comprehensive description of the disorder and provision of data to those involved about its recurrence, but also considers psychological issues that may influence the family and individual decisions. Besides the concerns of the individual child and family about the disease, there are more general ethical considerations dealing with confidentiality, informed consent, and standards of care as they relate to different disorders. Other considerations focus on working with asymptomatic individuals who have disorders that may be diagnosed early in the developmental period, but for whom no treatment is available. Moreover, there are also legal issues about wrongful life when appropriate genetic counseling is not given or when errors occur in testing for genetic disorders.

This chapter reviews both genetic counseling and genetic interventions. It discusses the definition of genetic counseling, the information presented at a genetic counseling session, counseling for specific syndromes, counseling for nonspecific syndromes, and prevention counseling. The last section provides background information on the treatment of genetic disorders.

DEFINITION

The American Society of Human Genetics offers the following definition of genetic counseling:

> A communication process which deals with human problems associated with the occurrence or the risk of occurrence of a genetic disorder in a family. This process involves an attempt by one or more appropriately trained persons to help the individual or family to (1) comprehend the medical facts, including the diagnosis, natural history of the disorder and probable course of the disorder, and available management; (2) appreciate the way heredity contributes to the disorder and the risk of recurrence in specified relatives; (3) understand the alternatives for dealing with the risk of recurrence; (4) choose the course of action which seems to them appropriate in view of their risk, their family goals, and their ethical and religious standards, and to act in accordance with that decision; and (5) to make the best possible adjustment to the disorder in an affected family member and/or to the risk of recurrence of that disorder. (Epstein et al., 1975, pp. 240–241)

Effective genetic counseling requires an accurate diagnosis and proper application of the principles of human genetics and statistics. It also involves an appreciation of the psychological facts as they relate to an affected individual and family members, that is, the meaning they place on the statistical information provided to them (Leonard, Chase, and Childs, 1972).

GENETIC COUNSELING

The most common situations that require genetic counseling are single-gene disorders (known or suspected), multifactorial disorders (known or suspected), chromosomal disorders diagnosed in a child, the consultand, or a family member, and an abnormal trait or carrier state that has been identified or suspected through genetic screening, prenatal diagnosis, consanguinity, teratogen exposure, or through repeated pregnancy loss or infertility (Thompson, McInnes, and Willard, 1991).

Genetic counseling requires considerable preparation and follow-up. The first phase includes clarification of the reason for referral, a comprehensive collection of family history information and, if requested, clinical examination and laboratory tests of relatives of the index case. Once the diagnosis is established, then an estimate of current risks is discussed with family members and the individual affected, based on the diagnosis, on specific test results, and on analyses of the family pedigree.

The genetic counseling itself emphasizes a careful description of the nature and consequences of the identified disorder, the recurrence risk to family members, means available to modify those consequences, means of prevention of recurrence, and forms of therapy available for treatment to reduce morbidity or to treat the identified condition.

Many genetic disorders require the involvement of a multidisciplinary team and often include management by clinical specialists with a variety of backgrounds. Continuing clinical management is essential with particular attention paid to intercurrent illnesses that may have a greater psychological impact on the family who is caring for a disabled child. Often repeated office visits and discussions of the genetic implications are necessary because the family who has not acknowledged or adapted to the disabling condition may deny the existence of the disorder, blame themselves, project blame on others— becoming excessively dependent or, in some instances, develop a psychiatric disorder. The emergence of a psychiatric disorder, such as an adjustment disorder or a depressive disorder, may not only negatively influence family relationships but may also be associated with increased risk-taking behavior. An important aspect of preventive intervention is the provision of interpersonal support through family organizations that bring together families of children with the same disorders.

Information Presented in a Counseling Session

Because most parents and many relatives of children with genetic disorders express concern about the etiology of the condition and may be anxious about recurrence risks, genetic counseling should be made available to any family members who request it, and families should be alerted to concerns of other family members. Misinterpretations of the information about genetic disorders is common and ranges from irrational fears of being punished for past wrongdoing to aggressive and inappropriate expressions of anger directed toward the affected individual or his parents. In counseling it is essential that family members understand that biological processes, such as cell division, cell differentiation, and pattern formation during embryogenesis, are prone to error.

The genetic counseling session generally begins by allowing the parent or affected individual to express their specific concerns and ask questions. Their current level of understanding about the condition should be ascertained at the beginning of the session so misinformation can be more clearly addressed as the counseling session proceeds. The first information given to the family or affected individual emphasizes the specific manifestations and natural history of a disorder. Quite commonly, the family's first questions deal with long-term outcome, complications, treatment, and quality of life. These questions need to be addressed in a meaningful way because the type of disorder must be acknowledged by the consultand before the risks for future children, or even grandchildren, are discussed. Following clarification of the nature of the disorder, recommendations for future management are introduced. These emphasize the role of the various team members in care and the availability of members of the treatment team to respond to questions that may arise and to provide treatment when necessary. It is important for the family to understand they may have difficulties not only in understanding the illness itself but in coping with feelings that arise toward themselves, toward the affected individual, toward other family members, and toward society as a result of the disorder.

After discussing the known facts about how the disorder was caused, the recurrence risks are addressed. Ordinarily, counseling should involve both parents in this discussion so one parent does not become the messenger who notifies the spouse about the complexities of a genetic disorder. Finally, reproductive options are reviewed. Family members may choose various options including ignoring the risk altogether, limiting family size, opting for prenatal diagnosis, using artificial insemination, considering *in vitro* fertilization with a donor egg, and/or adopting other children. Reproductive options are of particular concern for siblings who are carriers of the disease gene but are currently unaffected. Considerable sensitivity is needed in discussing and making clear the choices that relate to sibling carrier status. This has been a particular concern in adrenoleukodystrophy, as described in Chapter 11.5.

At the end of the initial counseling session, the family is advised that counseling is an ongoing process, and it is expected they will have additional questions in the future. Follow-up after the counseling session is particularly important to clarify questions that arise after the initial session. Time must be provided for the involved family members to reflect on the information presented to them and review it with other family members. An audiotape or videotape of the proceedings and a specific written summary of the major points covered during the counseling session is helpful. Arrangements also may need to be made for further evaluation and management for the affected individual and for relatives who may be at risk.

Genetic counseling generally is focused on an identified genetic syndrome. However, genetic counseling may also be requested when questions arise about the cause, clinical features, or recurrence risk for nonsyndromic and even nonfamilial abnormalities. Certain conditions, such as gestational substance abuse, may lead to behavioral difficulties (e.g., fetal alcohol syndrome) that require counseling about manifestations just as is the case for a clearly known genetic disorder.

Counseling for Specific Syndromes

When known Mendelian syndromes are involved, the theoretical probabilities of transmission of genes through families, adjusted with information about penetrance and expressivity, is directly provided. Such genetic counseling may be complicated due to the absence of empirical data on expressivity and penetrance in gene carriers. In dominantly expressed genetic syndromes that have variable expression or incomplete penetrance, each gene carrier has a 50% chance of passing the gene on to each child. However, the chance the affected child will have the syndrome is less than 50%. The higher the penetrance, the less likely it is an unaffected individual carries the gene. The lower the penetrance, the less likely it is the individual will express the gene if it is transmitted. Counselors must keep in mind that, for many conditions, accurate data may not be available because the more severely affected individuals with a disorder come to medical attention first and tend to be studied before less severely affected individuals. Because this is the case, some risk figures based on published reports may overestimate the true prevalence for a gene carrier to be severely affected due to this ascertainment bias. Moreover, published reports that rely only on the history provided by relatives rather than on personal examination of relatives may be inaccurate (Aylsworth, 1992).

Particular dilemmas may emerge in those families where teratogens or gestational drug use has resulted in a birth defect or a behavioral syndrome. Discussions about recurrence risks in these instances hinge on the likelihood of exposure to the teratogen or substance in the future. There is currently no clear-cut and reliable way to identify the genetic factors that may influence or regulate maternal or fetal susceptibility to teratogens or ingested substances.

When syndromes of unknown origin present, counseling is particularly difficult due to the probable heterogeneous etiology for such phenotypes. Even though such conditions may occur sporadically, it must be kept in mind that eventually some familial causes may be found; therefore, it may not be possible to separate out specific syndromes of known cause. When the child is born with a severe genetic syndrome involving the nervous system, for example severe microcephaly, even though the disorder appears sporadic, there may be an unknown but increased empiric risk.

Counseling for Nonsyndromic Conditions

Birth defects not associated with specific syndromes may have many causes, including a combination of both environmental and genetic factors. Moreover, the genetic contribution may involve one or more genes. For such conditions, the hypothetical models proposed are multifactorial-threshold inheritance, polygenetic inheritance, and, in some instances, major single-gene inheritance with incomplete penetrance. Even though the abnormality may simply be the result of chance, genetic counseling still must consider an empirical risk of recurrence. Such empirical risks are essentially guesses about average risks in heterogeneous populations (Aylsworth, 1992). For example, an empiric average risk of 4% recurrence does not mean everyone is at 4% risk. For a small number of individuals, the risk might be 25%, and for the rest, the risk might be negligible or less than 4%. Rather than discuss an empiric risk of 4% derived from heterogeneous group data, it may be best to simply state that the risk is unknown but there is an observed recurrence rate for couples in a particular age range; in this example, the risk might be negligible or might be as high as 25% or more.

An average recurrence risk is an estimate of the relative likelihood the couple has a high risk rather than a low or negligible one. In this instance, one is counseling for uncertainty—uncertainty that must be acknowledged. Moreover, observed recurrence rates may vary depending on the family history and may be increased if there are several affected close relatives. The possibility of a major single gene that predisposes carriers becomes more likely as more family members are identified who are affected. For example, if two first-degree relatives are affected, e.g., siblings or a parent and a child, the rate for subsequent siblings may be increased perhaps into the 5% to 15% range. However, when more than two family members are affected, the occurrence rate may be higher, perhaps 30%. Therefore, the risk may change if additional family members are subsequently identified. Such findings complicate the use of recurrence risk data in counseling. When a family has one severely disordered child, care is essential in counseling that the birth is a chance occurrence because for severe malformations, there is frequently an empiric risk of recurrence. Moreover, families who have the same past history regarding the occurrence of a genetic disorder will have different genetic backgrounds; therefore, they may have different recurrence risks in the future.

PREVENTION OF RECURRENCE

Because a major goal of genetic counseling is to provide information that may prevent recurrence of the specific disorder, the genetic counselor should be aware of the various options for prevention.

Prenatal diagnosis is an approach that may be suitable for many families, but it is not a universal solution. In some instances, prenatal diagnosis is not feasible; in others, it is not an acceptable alternative for the family. The laboratory assessment in prenatal diagnosis includes biochemical analysis, or DNA analysis. With prenatal diagnosis, couples who have a family history of a genetic disorder may be reassured they are not at risk if the test is negative. If the test is positive, then counseling is needed regarding preventive measures. Moreover, knowledge about the disorder may discourage individuals from seeking further testing.

If the couple has no plans to have additional children, the use of contraception or sterilization may be chosen and information provided about contraception or sterilization procedures and associated risks. If the couple desires children, adoption may be a possibility. Unfortunately, the number of children available for adoption is limited. Moreover, obtaining information regarding the genetic background of children who are placed for adoption may be difficult. If a father has a gene for an autosomal dominant or an X-linked disorder or a heritable chromosome defect, then artificial insemination may be considered. Artificial insemination may also be an option if both parents are carriers of an autosomal recessive disorder. When it is used, genetic counseling and carefully conducted genetic tests of the sperm donor are an important part of the evaluation process. Another approach is the use of the polymerase chain reaction (PCR) for DNA analysis of embryos and subsequent implantation. This procedure is experimental, but in the future, for some parents, a decision not to implant an embryo found to be abnormal through this testing method may be more acceptable than an abortion at a later stage of their pregnancy.

In those instances where pregnancy termination is decided on, genetic counseling should be available regarding the various clinical procedures. Psychological counseling services should be available following termination of pregnancy.

Genetic Counseling and Prenatal Diagnosis

The following issues are generally covered in genetic counseling prior to prenatal diagnosis: the risk the fetus will be affected, the nature and probable consequences of an identified problem, the risk and the limitations of the testing procedures, the time required before a report can be prepared, and the potential need for a second procedure if the first is inconclusive or fails.

Prenatal diagnosis is most commonly recommended for late maternal age and is carried out in up to half of pregnant women over age 35 in North America and western Europe. A physician is generally considered negligent if prenatal diagnosis is not suggested to older mothers. Prenatal diagnosis is limited to determining whether the fetus has, or is likely to have, a disorder in those families where there is a positive family history. The guidelines for prenatal diagnosis by amniocentesis or chorionic villus sampling must balance the risk that the fetus is abnormal with the risk of the procedure itself. Both amniocentesis and chorionic villus sampling are associated with a small risk of fetal loss.

Guidelines for prenatal diagnosis include (1) advanced maternal age (generally at least 35 years of age at the expected date of confinement; (2) a previous child with a *de nova* or known chromosomal anomaly; (3) presence of a structural chromosomal anomaly in one of the parents; (4) a family history of a genetic defect that may be diagnosed or ruled out through biochemical or DNA analysis (disorders in this category are usually caused by single-gene defects and have risks of 25% to 50% in siblings of affected children); and (5) a family history of an X-linked disorder for which there is no specific prenatal diagnostic test. In this last instance, fetal sex determination might be considered in the decision, made with the genetic counselor, about either terminating or continuing the pregnancy.

One method used in prenatal diagnosis is DNA analysis to identify closely linked markers—hopefully markers that flank the suspected gene. As a method, it is indirect but it works well if certain requirements can be met. These include (1) close linkage between the mutation and the marker so a recombination event is unlikely; (2) crucial family members are available for the study and are heterozygous for the marker in addition to being heterozygous for the mutation; (3) the linkage phase can be reasonably inferred or is known; and (4) no recombination has occurred between the markers being followed and the disease gene itself. A second method is direct detection of the mutation, using the gene, cDNA, or synthetic probes, to detect the mutation in genomic DNA. These direct methods are rapid and accurate.

TREATMENT OF GENETIC DISEASES

When prevention of genetic disease is not feasible, then treatment must be considered. Metabolic, biochemical, and gene therapy approaches for human genetic diseases are considerations for some disorders. Treatments include metabolic treatment, enzyme replacement, and somatic cell or germ-line treatment. In many instances, these treatments are experimental in nature. Ongoing family support and professional counseling is particularly important for those families who elect to participate in experimental treatments.

The treatment of genetic disorders is undergoing significant change as new technologies are being developed. At present, treatments include dietary exclusion of deleterious substrates, the promotion of alternate metabolic pathways to remove toxic metabolites, gene product replacement (e.g., an exogenous hormone), bone marrow transplantation, and gene transfer therapy. With the present state of knowledge in regard to gene delivery to the brain using virus vectors, experimental studies to better understand the function of neural proteins and the control of neural genes can now be carried out.

Metabolic treatments and treatment at the protein level are described in the following section. Gene therapy is described in a separate section.

Metabolic Treatments

Currently, the most successful interventions are at the level of the metabolic abnormality. Metabolic treatments most commonly involve dietary interventions to compensate for enzymatic defects. Dietary treatment is introduced after the diagnosis is established and generally before symptom onset. For example, dietary approaches, which are essentially environmental interventions, have been applied in phenylketonuria and in adrenoleukodystrophy. In the case of phenylketonuria, early dietary treatment can be effective for peripheral and central aspects of the disease and has been successful in preventing mental retardation and neurological dysfunction. However, although it was initially thought the dietary treatment for phenylketonuria could be stopped before school entry, this is no longer certain. Learning problems and hyperactivity have been reported in school-age children with phenylketonuria; therefore, the dietary treatment may be necessary for longer than originally proposed. Despite years of investigation, the mechanism involved in the impairment of brain development for phenylketonuria is still poorly understood.

In adrenoleukodystrophy (ALD), the blood-brain barrier may be an important consideration in carrying out dietary treatments. In ALD, the brain does not myelinate appropriately due to the accumulation of long-chain fatty acids. A dietary treatment has been proposed that uses a combination of two preparations, one, oleic and the other, erucic acid. The early introduction of this dietary treatment has led to normalization of long-chain fatty acids in the blood, but long-term clinical effects of the diet are uncertain. When the diet is introduced in asymptomatic individuals, despite the fact that no clinical changes are evident, brain changes may show progression when monitored with MRI. Continuing research in ALD is needed to determine the best means to correct the genetic defect. Dietary treatment alone does not appear to be an adequate approach for this condition.

In addition to dietary restrictions, other metabolic approaches involve avoidance of substances that may interact with a deficiency; this is the case in G6PD deficiency. In congenital hypothyroidism, the replacement of a necessary substance, thyroid hormone, is involved. In other instances, metabolic diversion is used in which alternative metabolic pathways are utilized to reduce the concentration of a harmful metabolite. Finally, for some conditions, inhibition by enzymes that modify metabolic abnormalities and depletion of an abnormal metabolite by direct removal of the abnormal compound from the body are options.

Treatment at the Protein Level

In a genetic disorder, if a mutant protein has any remaining function, it may be possible to increase its stability by enhancing the residual function of the molecule. For example, 50% of patients with homocystinuria due to cystathionine synthase deficiency respond to high doses of pyridoxine (vitamin B6) with a substantial reduction or complete disappearance of homocystine from the plasma (Thompson, McInnes, and Willard, 1991). Another approach is protein replacement of an extracellular protein (e.g., Factor VIII deficiency) or intracellular replacement of an intracellular enzyme (e.g., adenosine deaminase deficiency).

Finally, the replacement of intracellular proteins has been attempted by targeting enzymes. In Gaucher's disease, the most common lysosomal storage disorder, the enzyme glucocerebrosidase has been replaced. This is an example of targeting a protein to a specific type of cell and to an intracellular address, i.e., the macrophage and the lysosome. For Gaucher's disease, this involves the intravenous infusion of glucocerebrosidase, the missing enzyme. Although such enzyme replacement therapy has been effective in Gaucher's disease (Type I), it has not been successful in Types II and III where there is brain involvement. The poor response may be due to blood-brain barrier considerations. When used, the long-term effectiveness of this approach for Gaucher's disease is not clear; however, it does represent a feasible strategy of directing an intracellular enzyme to its physiological site of action. Enzyme replacement approaches also are being developed for other lysosomal disorders.

In other diseases, it may be possible, using the cloned gene, to produce large amounts of protein in culture. The structure of such proteins could be modified as necessary for specific cellular and intracellular targets. However, for neurological diseases, the blood-brain barrier entry will be a major complication.

GENE THERAPY

Genetic Intervention

It is anticipated that human genetic disease and possibly some degenerative diseases may be correctable at the genetic level. The concepts involved in gene therapy were initially presented during the 1960s and early 1970s when it was proposed that foreign genes could correct genetic defects and disease phenotypes in mammalian cells *in vitro* (Friedmann, 1992; Friedmann and Roblin, 1972). The development of recombinant DNA techniques has resulted in the availability of cloned genes and with the introduction of retroviral vectors and other gene transfer methods, phenotype correction *in vitro* and *in vivo* has been demonstrated (Horellou et al., 1993). These findings make gene therapy an accepted approach and have led to applications for studies with human subjects. Although gene therapy is still in its infancy, it is now comprehensible and acceptable in principle. A substantial effort is being made to turn the concept into a clinical reality, particularly for children affected with genetic disorders.

The term "gene therapy" is generally used to refer to the correction of genetic diseases by the replacement of the defective gene *in vivo* with normal DNA to reverse the genetic defect or to transplant cells that have been genetically engineered to express molecules missing in particular diseases (Anderson, 1984). A number of techniques are available for inserting specific genes into either a living organism or into cells maintained in culture. However, because molecular genetic techniques of gene therapy may be utilized for nongenetic as well as genetic disease, the term "gene therapy" requires a more comprehensive definition and has been used to refer to the use of molecular genetic techniques in general as they apply to the treatment of disease (Jinnah, Gage, and Friedmann, 1993). An optimal gene therapy would correct genetic disease by targeting the genetic mutation responsible for the disease in all cells of the body. However, it also may be possible to correct the disease phenotype without correcting all the mutant gene cells in the body by targeting specific diseased tissues or organs.

An important gene therapy approach involves inserting an additional copy of a normal gene, a transgene, that is directed to a defect caused by mutant genes in diseased cells. Many studies have documented the possibility of introducing additional copies of normal genes into cells that function to complement the function of the defective mutant gene.

In gene therapy, the first step is to establish the molecular basis of a disorder. The next step after identification of the genes involved is sequencing them, determining the normal and mutated gene products, and eventually, to develop therapies. In experimental cell culture models and in experimental animal models of human disease, techniques of gene therapy have been applied for treatment with some success. For example, cells in culture that have the mutation for Lesch-Nyhan disease have had the mutation corrected by insertion of the normal HPRT gene (Miller et al., 1983). In transgenic animals lacking myelin basic protein gene, (e.g., Schiverer mice), the defect has been corrected by the insertion of human myelin basic protein gene into single-cell Schiverer mouse embryos.

MODIFICATIONS OF THE SOMATIC GENOME

Gene Transfer Therapy

In gene transfer, the delivery of the normal gene to appropriate somatic cells (as opposed to germ-line cells) is required. It is generally undesirable to alter the germ line of the patient treated for a genetic disease. There is concern that efforts to integrate a normal copy of a gene into the germ line (or into a fertilized egg) could carry a risk for a new mutation. Germ-line gene therapy has been used for genetic correction in a dwarf line of mice deficient in growth hormone. The rat growth hormone gene was introduced into single-cell dwarf mice embryos. This resulted in high levels of rat growth hormone and gigantic mice (Hammer, Palmiter, and Brinster, 1984). This study points out the ongoing problem of regulation of gene expression in the implementation of these approaches.

A transfer gene consists of a cDNA under the control of a promoter. Optimally, regulatory elements are chosen so the gene is transcribed into target cells at adequate levels and, if necessary, it can respond to regulatory signals.

Transplantation

Because transplanted cells retain the donor genotype, transplantation is a form of gene transfer therapy because it results in a modification of the somatic genome. However, the genome of the recipient remains unchanged in all other cell lines. Transplantation may be used to provide the genes for a protein that is defective or absent. Bone marrow transplantation is one of the most common forms and is an example of somatic cell gene therapy. Bone marrow cells are easily accessible and bone marrow cells divide so that donor DNA can be inserted and readily returned to the host. The perivascular microglial cells are of marrow origin, and this may be a factor in the effects of bone marrow transplantation in some storage diseases (Thompson, McInnes, and Willard, 1991). The mononuclear-phagocyte system in most tissues is derived from bone marrow cells (Parkman, 1986); therefore, after transplantation, this system is of donor origin.

Although bone marrow transplantation has been used in nonstorage diseases, such as β-thalassemia, its most pertinent use for developmental disorders is for lysosomal storage diseases. Bone marrow transplantations potentially may correct lysosomal storage in a variety of tissues and, in some instances, even the brain. Transplanted cells are a source of lysosomal enzymes that may be transferred to other cells via the extracellular fluid. Because bone marrow cells make up about 10% of the body's total cell mass, the quantity of enzyme involved is considerable. Bone marrow transplantation reduces the liver, spleen, and sometimes heart involvement in storage diseases, such as Hurler disease and Gaucher's disease, although the effects on the brain are unclear. Bone marrow transplantation may be useful in the juvenile or adult forms of metachromatic leukodystrophy if carried out before signs of central nervous system involvement occur (Krivit et al., 1990). It has been proposed that donor macrophages traverse the blood-brain barrier and are transformed into microglial cells which provide for appropriate metabolism and produce secreted enzymes that can be incorporated into lysosomes of neighboring cells. It takes about a year from the time of transplantation for donor cells to become effective (Kolodny, 1993).

In somatic cell therapy, fibroblasts with the neural gene are utilized and placed into cells in culture. The procedure is to insert human cDNA into the cells. Retroviral vectors also may be used. They can be inserted into cells because they contain reverse transcriptase. These approaches have been applied *in vitro* where a transmissible retrovirus was utilized that expresses human hypoxanthine HPRT for Lesch-Nyhan disease. Somatic cell therapy has been attempted in Duchenne muscular dystrophy, in Lesch-Nyhan disease, and in Gaucher's disease.

Bone marrow transplantations have been used in particular syndromes, such as Lesch-Nyhan disease and Hurler-Scheie disease. In Lesch-Nyhan disease, enyzme changes were noted in peripheral blood cells but effects were not seen in other cell lines. No improvement was noted in the compulsive behavior disorder or in the motoric symptoms in LND following the procedure. In Hurler-Scheie disease, bone marrow transplantation was successful in improving manifestations in peripheral tissues, and modest changes in cognitive development were also noted. In addition, these techniques also have been applied in the intrauterine treatment of Hurler disease. Normal development has been reported during the first year of life in a patient with this disorder who participated in such transplanation (Shull et al., 1987).

Mortality following bone marrow transplantation is significant, and the morbidity from graft-versus-host disease is as high as 20%. Problems with histoincompatibility are being addressed through the development of genetically modified autologous bone marrow cells.

ISSUES CONCERNING GENETIC INTERVENTION FOR DISORDERS INVOLVING THE BRAIN

A number of factors must be taken into account when applying gene therapy. Among these are the age of the affected individual, the gene or gene product to be introduced, the type and location of the cells identified for genetic modification, the amount of transgene expression needed for correction, and the method of introduction of transgenes (Jinnah, Gage, and Friedmann, 1993). Particular problems do arise for diseases involving the nervous system because of difficulties involved with crossing the blood-brain barrier. A comparison of methods for genetic intervention is shown in Table 21–1.

First, the age of the subject is an important consideration because many nervous system diseases are associated with developmental processes or with irreversible neurodegeneration. Phenylketonuria is the best known developmental disease where treatment must be initiated within the first few months of life. But timing is also crucial in considering other disorders, such as Lesch-Nyhan disease. Other conditions, such as adrenoleukodystrophy, have their onset later in childhood.

Second, various approaches may be taken in introducing the gene or gene product. In applying gene therapy to neurological disorders, ordinarily the mutant gene must be identified and replaced with a functional copy. However, this may not always be necessary because in dominant neurological diseases, which result from "gain of function mutations," genetic mutations may not be corrected by the introduction of additional copies of a normal gene. In Huntington's disease, the following might be considered: correction of the mutant gene directly, prevention of expression of the mutant gene, and introduction of a second gene that masks the functional consequences of the dominant mutation (Jinnah, Gage, and Friedmann, 1993).

Gene therapy also could be applied to neurological diseases with nongenetic origin. For example, although the degeneration of dopamine neurons in the substantia nigra in 1-methyl-4-phenyl-1,2,3,6-tetrahydropyridine (MPTP) toxicity is nongenetic, it may be possible to control symptoms by introducing genes or cells that express tyrosine hydroxylase to regain dopamine function. This approach has been taken in a rat model of Parkinson's disease where fibroblasts genetically modified to produce L-dopa have been introduced into the rat striatum (Wolff et al., 1989).

Third, the identification of the type and location of the cells targeted for genetic manipulation must be considered. For those diseases involving metabolic processes, it may be necessary to introduce genetic material throughout the nervous system; in others, it may be necessary to target only a restricted subpopulation of neurons in a specific brain region. For those disorders involving specific brain regions, genetically modified cells, or gene vectors, might be placed in one or more specific brain regions by surgical injection. However, for

Table 21–1. Comparison of Methods for Genetic Intervention in the Brain

Retrovirus vectors
Advantages. Useful for cell marking/lineage analysis and ablation of brain tumors.
Disadvantages. Only infect dividing cells, variable expression of foreign genes, maximum titres approximately 10^6PFU/ml, can accommodate only 6 to 8 kb of foreign DNA.

Herpes virus vectors
Advantages. Broad host and cell-type range, episomal (no possibility of insertional activation of host genes), stable expression, easy genetic manipulation, can accommodate up to 15 kb of foreign DNA.
Disadvantages. Maximum possible titres approximately 10^7PFU/ml (difficult to saturate a brain region with recombinant vector), occasional cytotoxicity, long-term safety unknown.

Adenovirus vectors
Advantages. Broad host and cell-type range, growth to high titres, purification by density gradients possible, episomal (no possibility of insertional activation of host genes), high level of expression of foreign genes.
Disadvantages. Stability of expression unknown, can accommodate only 6 to 8 kb of foreign DNA at present, genetic manipulation is unwieldy due to required recombination step for producing viral particles, long-term safety unknown.

Transgenic animals
Advantages. Consistent and precise propagation of phenotype by breeding facilitates experimentation, easy to evaluate developmental (especially prenatal) consequences of genetic intervention.
Disadvantages. Targeted expression only achieved through manipulation of expression control elements, cannot be used as models for gene therapy.

Grafting of genetically modified cells
Advantages. Easy to manipulate genetically, transfected cells made and analyzed *in vitro* can be used directly without transfer of foreign gene to a new vector, lack of cytotoxicity, circumvention of immunity problems if host cells used.
Disadvantages. Risk of tumor formation if cell lines are used, stability of expression difficult to achieve, may interfere with endogenous circuitry.

DNA-liposome complexes
Advantages. Biologically safe, easy to manipulate genetically, unmodified plasmid vectors without eukaryotic replicans can be used, virtually no size limitations, relatively stable expression, probably extrachromosomal.
Disadvantages. Cytotoxicity of cationic lipids, low efficiency of transfection.

RNA and antisense oligonucleotides
Advantages. Biologically safe, synthesis is straightforward, no viral vector intermediate required, no size limitations on gene from which RNA is synthesized.
Disadvantages. Effects are acute, necessitating repeated introduction of the nucleic acid, efficiency of introduction into cells is unknown, may only be effective when a very small cell population is targeted.

From Neve, 1993.

some disorders, genes must be delivered to widespread regions of the nervous system, possibly through the use of endothelial cells of the vascular system that may be genetically manipulated. Another approach could be to introduce catabolic enzymes into endothelial cells with the goal of degrading toxic substances produced by the brain. Gene transfer vectors might be introduced into the cerebral spinal fluid and thereby transduce ependymal cells that line the ventricles. However, the degree of diffusion of a gene vector or gene vector products into the brain itself, or the diffusion of toxic products from the brain substance to the ependymal cells may limit this approach. An additional approach might involve the use of bone marrow stem cells because these cells give rise to macrophages which, in certain conditions, can migrate to the brain. Whether or not macrophages can enter the brain in sufficient numbers for successful transplantation continues to be investigated.

The use of nonneural cells, such as bone marrow stem cells, for the delivery of the transgene is feasible but has some limitations. Such nonneural cells would be limited to the production of substances that diffuse from them, such as neurotransmitter precursors or neurotrophic factors. However, if needed precursors were manufactured, these cells might function as "biological minipumps" (Jinnah, Gage, and Friedmann, 1993). Still, nonneural cells would probably not be useful in situations that involve interactions between neurons, as in synaptic transmission, or for the glial cell–neuronal interactions that occur with myelination. Nonneural cells would not be expected to be effective in disorders that required restoration of a specific genetic function within a group of specific neurons. However, nonneural cells might be used to degrade neurotoxic substances that accumulate as a consequence of a genetic defect by functioning to degrade toxic wastes. Although fetal or neonatal neurons or glial cells have been suggested for replacement therapy, there is limited availability of such cells, and ethical issues are associated with obtaining fetal material. Moreover, fetal cells have a short life span in culture and have limited ability to survive and function when they are introduced into the nervous system. An alternative to fetal cells is the use of immortalized neuronal or glial cells for genetic interventions. However, when considering this alternative, the use of tumorigenic cell lines, considerable caution is necessary.

A fourth issue involves the extent of transgene expression required to restore function. To restore gene function, many metabolic diseases do not require complete restoration of gene function. For example, in Lesch-Nyhan disease, the complete neurobehavioral phenotype is not seen unless the activity of HPRT is reduced to less than 1% to 1.6% of normal. It may be possible to control the behavioral phenotype in Lesch-Nyhan disease by replacing about 2% of normal brain HPRT activity. In another disorder, phenylketonuria, it is estimated the restitution of less than 10% of normal phenylalanine hydroxylase activity would be adequate to render affected patients clinically normal. Findings in these disorders suggest the potential to correct neurological abnormalities by restoring a relatively small percentage of the total gene product involved.

Introduction of a Transgene

The direct injection of foreign DNA or RNA into an affected area is not an effective means to correct a genetic defect; however, transgenes (cloned foreign genes) that have been incorporated into a viral vector may be utilized. Such viral vectors express the foreign gene. Among the viral vectors used for gene delivery to the brain are retrovirus, herpes virus, and adenovirus.

Retrovirus

The retroviruses have been actively studied because their life cycle and molecular structure are well understood. These viruses infect a wide variety of cell types, and they are very efficient in infecting most cells. Special characteristics of each of them are useful in different experimental and therapeutic paradigms. However, the retrovirus vectors have not been demonstrated to be effective in gene delivery into the adult brain because they can only integrate into the genome of dividing cells, and most normal cells in the brain are postmitotic and not dividing. In addition, retrovirus particles are unstable *in vivo* so it is difficult to reach high enough virus titers for the inoculation. However, the ability to enter dividing cells selectively makes the retroviruses important potential vectors for the delivery of killer genes to tumor cells in the brain (Mann, Mulligan, and Baltimore, 1983).

Herpes Virus

The use of replication-defective herpes simplex virus (HSV 1) represents an advance in solving the cell division problem. Two varieties of herpes virus vectors have been developed to deliver genes to the central nervous system. Both of these may be relatively nonpathogenic to the brain because toxic genes have been "knocked out" in this herpes vector. Herpes virus can mediate transgene expression into a number of different cell types including neurons and glia. One advantage of such recombinant herpes vectors is that, unlike most of the other methods of gene transfer, the transgenes carried by herpes virus vectors will infect nondividing cells with high efficiency so that direct gene delivery is possible into quiescent cells *in situ*. They ordinarily do not integrate into host DNA sequences but rather the HSV provirus remains as an episome in the infected cell nucleus (Breakefield and DeLuca, 1991). A second advantage is that they may go into a latent state and establish long-term infection in neurons. This could potentially mediate stable transgene expression for many years. However, cell infection with the wild type of herpes virus can result in a toxic lytic response. Efforts are ongoing to remove the toxic lytic effect by deleting nonessential immediate-early and viron-component genes (Svendsen, 1993). A third advantage is the ability to carry relatively large fragments of DNA. Disadvantages include possible cytotoxicity and lack of information about long-term safety.

Adenovirus

The adenoviruses are becoming more important because of the large number of cells they can label and because of their low pathogenicity. Like herpes virus, adenoviruses infect nondividing cells. Adenoviruses have been utilized in cystic fibrosis in the airway epithelium. A number of studies are being carried out to explore their use for gene delivery to other cell types. Replication-defective adenovirus vectors are generally safe, because the virus is commonly found in humans and usually causes benign symptoms, such as the common cold. Because adenoviruses do not normally enter the brain, more information needs to be gathered about how neural factors and viral genes might interface.

Drawbacks to the adenovirus vector system comes from instability of transgene expression since expression may last up to months but not for years. Moreover, a strong immune response to the virus can prevent blood-borne vectors from reaching their destination and might cause an immune reaction against a recipient cell. In addition, direct inoculation of an adenovirus vector into the brain could possibly lead to toxic consequences. For example, a replication-competent adenovirus might be generated by combining with endogenous adenovirus sequences in the host cell genome. This might occur during propagation of the vector in culture or following inoculation into the brain. Adenovirus infections of the brain have also been reported. The establishment of recombinant replication-competent viruses may be a risk not only to the organism being treated but to the population in general. In addition, even replication-defective adenoviruses can kill cells if they are taken in large enough quantities, and neurons are not replaceable.

SUMMARY: GENE THERAPY

In regard to actual treatment, with the current state of knowledge gene therapy could cause damage to the brain and delivery at present can only be directed to many cells for a short period of time and to a few cells over a longer time frame. Those diseases that might be considered for gene therapy include genetic disorders, traumatic injury or stroke, neurodegenerative diseases, and brain tumors. With brain injury, delivery might reduce subsequent tissue damage that might be mediated by adenovirus vectors directed to ependymal cells. For the more progressive neurodegenerative diseases, such as Huntington's disease, one might produce stable delivery of potent-protective neurotrophic factors through the use of herpes virus latency in a few neurons. Each of the viral vectors might be used to deliver toxic genes to tumor cells in the brain. Despite the current limitations of these approaches, these viruses do carry the necessary features encoded in DNA sequences that might be combined to create synthetic vectors which are safer and more effective.

Although the full therapeutic potential, the benefits, and the drawbacks are still being assessed, gene therapy may improve and, in some conditions, normalize the life of children affected with genetic diseases. Future developments in genetic technology will assuredly result in the elimination of disease and improvement in the lives of children with genetic disorders and their families.

THE SCOPE OF GENETIC COUNSELING IN THE FUTURE

The scope of genetic counseling will increase as the knowledge base in medical genetics becomes more extensive. Increasingly, as genetic counseling enters into medical practice, its scientific basis must be understood as well as the limitations and knowledge it is based on. The use of molecular genetics to determine recurrence risks is an important consideration because many disease genes may be detected directly in carriers and affected persons, using DNA analysis. Application of molecular genetic techniques is essential because determination of the presence or absence of a particular gene occurs with essentially 100% accuracy.

Future research in genetic counseling will be influenced by advances in molecular neurobiology and in the treatment of genetic diseases. Genetic counseling will continue to be difficult because both pathogenic and etiologic heterogeneity must be considered. The recurrence risk of a disorder is based on a combination of the theoretical risk assessment and empirical data that has been published. Because of the uncertainty involved, genetic counseling is often a stressful experience for families due to continuing gaps in available data and the uncertainty involved in their interpretation. In conducting genetic counseling, family members and affected patients (to the degree possible) need to understand the assumptions on which the genetic counseling is based and the limitations involved in these estimates.

The social impact of genetic research and technology raises bioethical issues that must take into account not only the scientific evidence but also basic human values and beliefs. The International League of Societies for Persons with Mental Handicap (the League) (1994) has suggested that certain ethical guidelines be applied to ensure that the rights and integrity of people with disabilities are protected. The League suggests that the following principles be applied: justice, nondiscrimination, diversity and autonomy, and informed decision making. These principles and their application are discussed in their 1994 issue paper "Just Technology? From Principles to Practice in Bio-ethical Issues." The principles affirm the right to medical treatment, nondirective and nondiscriminatory counseling, legal protections, and employment and health coverage regardless of genetic make-up.

REFERENCES

Anderson, F. (1984). Prospects of human gene therapy. *Science,* 226:401–409.

Aylworth, A.S. (1992). Genetic counseling for patients with birth defects. *Pediatric Clinics of North America,* 39:229–253.

Breakefield, X.O., and DeLuca, N.A. (1991). Herpes simplex virus for gene delivery to neurons. *New Biology,* 3:203–208.

Epstein, C.J., Childs, B., Fraser, F.C., McKusick, V.A., Miller, J.R., Motulsky, A.G., Rivas, M., Thompson, M.W., Shaw, M.W., and Sly, W.S., (1975). Genetic counseling. *American Journal of Human Genetics,* 27:240–242.

Friedmann, T. (1992). A brief history of gene therapy. *Nature Genetics,* 2:93–98.

______, and Roblin, R. (1972). Gene therapy for human genetic disease? *Science,* 175:949–955.

Hammer, R.E., Palmiter, R., and Brinster, R.L. (1984). Partial correction of murine hereditary growth disorder by germ line incorporation of a new gene. *Nature,* 311:65–67.

Horellou, P., Lundberg, C., Robert, J.J., Bjorklund, A., and Mallet, J. (1993). Gene transfer *in situ* and in cells for intracerebral transplantation. *Seminars in the Neurosciences,* 5:453–459.

International League of Societies for Persons with Mental Handicap (1994). *From principles to practice in bio-ethical issues.* Roeher Institute, York University, North York, Ontario, pp. 23–41.

Jinnah, H.A., Gage, F.H., and Friedmann, I. (1993). Gene therapy and neurologic disease. In R. Rosenberg, S.B. Prusiner, S. DiMauro, R.L. Barchi, and L.M. Kunkel (eds.), *The molecular and genetic basis of neurological disease,* pp. 969–976. Butterworth-Heinemann, Boston, MA.

Kolodny, E.H. (1993). Metachromatic leukodystrophy and multiple sulfatase deficiency: Sulfatide lipidosis. In R.N. Rosenberg, S.B. Prusiner, S. DiMauro, R.L. Barchi, and L.M. Kunkel (eds.), *The molecular and genetic basis of neurological disease,* pp. 497–503. Butterworth-Heinemann, Boston, MA.

Krivit, W., Shapiro, E., Kennedy, W., Lipton, W., Lockman, L., Smith, S., Summers, C.G., Wenger, D.A., Tsai, M.Y., Ramsay, N.K.C., Kersey, J.H., Yao, J.K., and Kaye, E. (1990). Treatment of late infantile metachromatic leukodystrophy by bone marrow transplantation. *New England Journal of Medicine,* 322:28–32.

Leonard, C.O., Chase, G.A., and Childs, B. (1972). Genetic counseling: A consumer's view. *New England Journal of Medicine,* 287:433–439.

Mann, R., Mulligan, R.C., and Baltimore, D. (1983). Construction of a retrovirus packaging mutant and its use to produce helper-free defective retrovirus. *Cell,* 33:153–159.

Miller, A.D., Jolly, D.J., Friedmann, T., and Verma, I.M. (1983). A transmissible retrovirus expressing HGPRT. *Proceedings of the National Academy of Sciences, USA,* 80:4709–4713.

Neve, R.L. (1993). Adenovirus vectors enter the brain. *Trends in Neurosciences,* 16:251–253.

Parkman, R. (1986). The application of bone marrow transplantation to the treatment of genetic diseases. *Science,* 232:1373–1378.

Shull, R.M., Hastings, N.E., Selcer, R.R., Jones, J.B., Smith, J.R., Cullen, W.C., and Constantopoulos, G. (1987). Bone marrow transplantation in canine mucopolysaccharidosis I. *Journal of Clinical Investigation,* 79:435–443.

Svendsen, C. (1993). Gene therapy: A hard graft for neuroscientists. *Trends in Neuroscience,* 16:333–334.

Thompson, M.W., McGinnes, R.R., and Willard, H.F. (1991). *Genetics in medicine.* W.B. Saunders, Philadelphia.

Wolff, J.A., Fisher, L.J., Xu, L., Jinnah, H.A., Langlais, P.J., Iuvone, P.M., O'Malley, K.L., Rosenberg, M.B., Shimohama, S., Friedmann, T., and Gage, F.H. (1989). Grafting fibroblasts genetically modified to produce L-dopa in a rat model of Parkinson's disease. *Proceedings of the National Academy of Sciences, USA,* 86:9011–9014.

PART VI

LEGAL ASPECTS

CHAPTER 22

PUBLIC LAW AND THE RIGHTS OF THE DISABLED

The assessment and treatment of developmentally disabled persons requires not only an understanding of the nature of the disorder and the establishment of an individualized treatment program, but also recognition of ethical issues related to care and the individual's legal rights. During the past 20 years, ethical issues have been increasingly acknowledged and legal rights have been clarified in a series of landmark federal court decisions. The court decisions have established the right to habilitation, standards of care in institutional settings, and guidelines for the use of psychotropic drugs, among others. Although court decisions have primarily focused on mental retardation, they also are applicable to nonretarded persons with developmental disorders. Decisions take into account that it is a basic right of developmentally disabled persons to be responsible for themselves and to be held accountable for their behavior (Szymanski and Crocker, 1989). Ethical issues arise in assuring how this basic right is expressed.

This chapter considers the legal rights of the disabled, normalization, competency, legal issues in the use of psychotropic drugs and aversive interventions, and ethical concerns in working with developmentally disabled persons.

LEGAL RIGHTS OF MENTALLY RETARDED PERSONS

In 1972 the General Assembly of the United Nations reported the "Declaration on the Rights of Mentally Retarded Persons." This declaration stated that "the mentally retarded person has, to the maximum degree of feasibility, the same rights as other human beings . . . [including] a right to proper medical care." In 1975 the "Declaration on the Rights of Disabled Persons" was proclaimed. The U.N. General Assembly stated that persons with disabilities have an "inherent right to respect for their human dignity . . . [and] the same civil . . . rights as other human beings. . . . Disabled persons shall be able to avail themselves to qualified legal aid when such aid proves indispensable for the protection of their persons. . . ."

Landmark legal decisions that are pertinent to the rights of mentally retarded persons are shown in Table 22–1.

NORMALIZATION

Mentally retarded and developmentally disabled persons should be considered as individuals with their own unique needs and have the right to live in the most appropriate and least restrictive environment. "Normalization" is the term that has been used to highlight the importance of "making available to all mentally retarded people patterns of life and conditions of everyday living which are as close as possible to the norms and patterns of the mainstream of society" (Nirje, 1969). The focus on normalization originated in Scandinavia in the 1960s and was propagated and publicized in the

Table 22–1. Landmark Legal Decisions Regarding Care in State and Community Facilities

Wyatt v. Stickney (1972)	An Alabama case that established the right of institutionalized mentally retarded persons to appropriate habilitation. Minimal standards were set for medical care and privacy. The indiscriminate use of psychotropic medications, the use of aversive punishment procedures, and institutionalization of mildly retarded persons were prohibited.
New York Association for Retarded Children v. Rockefeller (1972)	A New York case that established minimal standards of care.
Souter v. Brennan (1973)	Prohibited involuntary unpaid labor by residents of institutions.
Donaldson v. O'Connor (1974, 1975)	Established the right to treat persons committed to mental hospitals as well as their right to remain in community settings if they could do so safely, by themselves, or with community support.
Wyatt v. Aderholt (1982)	Imposed strict restrictions on sterilization.
Youngberg v. Romeo (Pennhurst I, 1982)	This Pennsylvania case recognized that persons civilly confined in state institutions have specific constitutional rights that include reasonable safety, freedom from undue restraints, and appropriate training to enable them to exercise their rights.
Pennhurst v. Halderman (Pennhurst II, 1984)	This Pennsylvania case provided limitations on earlier interpretations and established rights of those with mental retardation regarding the least restrictive settings for care.

United States through the writings of both Wolfensberger (1972) and Nirje (1969). The goal has been to facilitate the adaptation of the mentally retarded person by providing supports that are culturally as normative as possible. This approach led to community care for mentally retarded persons and individualized free and appropriate educational programs and other specific services. It has served as a philosophical basis for deinstitutionalization.

Normative does not mean mentally retarded persons should be forced into everyday situations that are not appropriate for their abilities and their needs. The emphasis is on addressing social and emotional needs, as well as teaching specific skills. One of those needs may be provision of the opportunity for contact with disabled peers as part of their programming. Furthermore, in considering normalization, it is important to take into account the individual strengths, deficiencies, and the unique circumstances of their lives rather than applying a generic program for all mentally retarded persons. Age-appropriate expectations need to be taken into account with a focus on how these can be best achieved. Nirje's guidelines for normalization are outlined in Table 22–2.

The supportive employment initiative, which moves mentally retarded persons into the community with job coaches, has demonstrated that with adequate structure and support for a mentally retarded person, real jobs in the community can be accomplished.

COMPETENCY

Competency for the mentally retarded person refers to competency to manage one's own affairs, to physically care for one's self, and to care for others (parenting). Basic legal competency includes the ability to be a competent witness and the ability to stand trial as a person responsible for one's own actions (Smith and Kunjukrishnan, 1986).

The essential elements used to assess competency include an evaluation of the following: (1) the ability to understand information presented in regard to the consequences of a decision that is made; (2) the ability to weigh alternatives before making decisions; (3) the manner in which the decision is made (considering the alternatives and expressing a preference); and (4) the nature and degree of commitment to the final decision. A competent decision requires comprehension of the issue to be resolved, autonomy in decision making, a rational process of reasoning, an awareness of the future consequences of the decision, and the

Table 22–2. GUIDELINES FOR NORMALIZATION

1. Normalization means a normal rhythm of the day for the retarded.
2. Normalization implies a normal routine of life, i.e., not always structured.
3. Normalization means to experience the normal rhythm of the year with holidays and family days of personal significance.
4. Normalization means an opportunity to undergo normal developmental experiences of the life cycle, i.e., experiences and opportunities should be consistent with the appropriate life cycle whenever possible; adjustments and special provisions should be made for the mentally retarded adult and elderly.
5. Normalization means that choices, wishes, and desires of the mentally retarded themselves have to be taken into consideration as frequently as possible and respected.
6. Normalization means living in a world with both sexes.
7. Normalization means normal economic standards for the mentally retarded.
8. Normalization means that the standards of the physical facility should be the same as those regularly applied in society to the same kind of facilities for ordinary citizens.

From Nirje, 1969.

capacity to use judgment to make choices despite the uncertainty of the outcome. In legal decisions, the accused mentally retarded or developmentally disabled person should not be allowed to waive a competency examination. All parties involved in the competency process have the duty to raise the issue of competency, if there is any doubt (*Pate v. Robinson,* 383 U.S. 375, 1966).

Partial Competency/Guardianship

The mentally retarded person may be partially competent in that he can conduct some affairs but not others. There may be difficulty in managing financial matters, but competency in handling other affairs (Kapp, 1981; Mesibov, Conover, and Sauer, 1980). In such instances, a guardian is appointed to decide only financial matters. The assignment of the guardian may be based on the extent of mental retardation because mildly and moderately retarded individuals will have different degrees of understanding regarding their affairs. The decision should be based on adaptive functioning and not on IQ scores alone. Severely and profoundly mentally retarded persons may need the assignment of a long-term guardian.

Parental Competency

The issue of parental competence is a major consideration for the adult mentally retarded person. Mental retardation, per se, is not automatically considered evidence for lack of competency in child care; however, it is increasingly evident that successful parenting by a mentally retarded person is difficult, particularly in the care of children beyond infancy. Although adults who are mentally retarded may be overrepresented among neglectful parents, they are not necessarily abusing parents. The parents' capacity to care for a child on a day-to-day basis, to set appropriate limits on a child's behavior, and to make future plans for the child requires scrutiny (Feldman, 1986). Children of mentally retarded parents are also at risk for mental retardation, but a substantial number, 60% to 70% in one study (Accardo and Whitman, 1990), were not mentally retarded.

Factual evidence of competence is necessary for mild or moderately retarded parents; however, if the parent is severely or profoundly retarded, the child ordinarily will require placement outside the home. Considerable efforts are necessary to teach parenting skills to mild and moderately mentally retarded adults. Such teaching may occur either through group or individual instruction; the additional provision of ongoing home support services is also often necessary. In some instances, the parent and child may be jointly placed in a foster home so that foster parents can assume overall responsibility for the child's care, although the natural parent will assist them. Parenting by a mentally retarded person is of special concern when there are multiple children in the home and when the mentally retarded person has older children who test in the normal range of intelligence.

An assessment of parental competency requires a careful review of the individual's personal history and evaluation of their child or children (Whitman and Accardo, 1990). If homemakers are placed in the home to assist the mentally retarded person in child care, how the homemaker was perceived and what was observed in the home may be included in the assessment. It is important to verify whether or not a homemaker who was placed to help with the children of a mentally retarded adult is aware of the characteristic features of mental retardation. In addition, verification is needed regarding the degree of sensitivity shown by the homemaker to the mentally retarded parent and the homemaker's ability to facilitate the efforts of a mentally retarded person in child care.

Mentally retarded parents may be familiar with how to provide physical care, but may have difficulty in making judgments when unexpected situations or illnesses emerge. The mentally retarded parents' ability to understand the context of the child's misbehavior and respond to the child's unique needs is a major consideration in assessment. Can the parent differentiate a child's behavior that is a developmentally appropriate expression of independence from a defiant challenge to the adult's authority? Some mentally retarded parents will be able to provide appropriate physical care and nurturance to an infant, yet may have more difficulty with an older child, particularly an adolescent who demands more independence. In assessing the family system, the evaluator must take into account what alternatives are available within the family system for other family members to assist the disabled parent in child care. The overall assessment must consider whether it is in the child's best interest to be placed outside the home at an early age rather than later in life when parents' caregiving abilities may be more strained.

In an assessment of parenting, the legal system has generally emphasized three skills as essential: the expression of love and affection, the capacity to perform household tasks, and the capability to attend to the child's physical needs. Some courts have added a fourth factor, that of stimulating the child intellectually, if the parents are mentally retarded ("Retarded Parents in Neglect Proceedings," 1979).

An interest is shared by both parent and child in maintaining a family unit (Marafino, 1990). However, when termination of parental rights must be considered, the most common determining standards are the parent fitness standard and the child's best interest standard. The parent fitness standard is based on the common law presumption that parents act in their child's best interest; it emphasizes a parent's fundamental right to custody. The child's best interest standard focuses on the child's needs. A parent fitness standard is supported by several Supreme Court decisions (e.g., *Meyer v. Nebraska,* 1923; *Ginsberg v. New York,* 1968; *Santosky v. Kramer,* 1982) and emphasizes termination of parental rights only if there is proven unfitness; state statutes establish factors to be considered in fitness. The best interest standard, however, considers parental fitness but does not view it as the sole determining factor. Adopting the best interest standard allows greater flexibility; however, it may be difficult to apply because it is difficult to gauge a child's physical and emotional needs. Moreover, this standard requires consistent application. Some states use both standards; others have a parent fitness hearing first that is followed by a second best interest hearing. The best interest standard may potentially serve the interests of the parent, child, and state; however, guidelines need to be clearly specified and incorporated into legislation (*In re* J.J.B., 1987) to make it workable.

Temporary removal of custody from a parent with mental retardation and nonconsensual adoption are options if a parent is deemed unfit. In some instances, the court has ruled that incompetence to rear children cannot be necessarily inferred from the fact of general mental or legal incapacity (*Price v. Price,* 1979; Brakel, Parry, and Weiner, 1985). However, in other instances (*In re* C.L.M., 1981), evidence for a mother's general incapacity supported a change in custody based on the potential for neglect or harm in her home. Nonconsensual adoptions have been allowed where the parent has a mental disability and is not capable of giving valid legal consent for the adoption of the children. Brakel, Parry, and Weiner (1985) suggest that statutes should clearly distinguish between the situations where valid consent is the issue and others where the issue is termination of rights rather than consent. For termination of rights, parental fitness is the issue rather than consent. These authors define termination of rights and nonconsensual adoption as being separate issues. In the case of adoption, parents may want to give consent but may be mentally incapable of doing so. If they cannot give consent, they should be adjudicated incompetent to decide. When consent is not the issue, as in termination hearings, a finding of incapacity is not necessary.

When termination is considered, procedural safeguards are necessary for the mentally retarded parent. In addition to the mental retardation, other extenuating circumstances must be considered. The nature, extent, and success of support systems are taken into account. The same factors should be considered in cases involving parents who have mental retardation as are considered in families where there is no mental retardation. Evidence of harm to the child as well as proof of deficiencies in childrearing practices are the relevant considerations. IQ scores, in themselves, should not be the determining factor; adaptive functioning must also be considered. If there are parenting deficiencies, then the least restrictive alternative should be considered and, only at this point, should the nature and degree of parental mental retardation be introduced. If it is deemed the family unit can be preserved if appropriate services are offered, then they should be provided, and the child should remain with the parent. A reasonable opportunity should be provided to assist the parent in acquiring and maintaining those parenting skills necessary to provide adequate care for their child.

LEGAL COMPETENCY

Competency to Stand Trial

Competency to stand trial refers to the ability to comprehend the nature and quality of legal proceedings, and to advise legal counsel in the preparation and implementation of one's own defense. Individuals accused of a crime cannot be tried for that crime unless they understand both the charge made against them and the consequences if they are convicted. Furthermore, individuals must be able to aid a lawyer in their own defense. Because mentally retarded persons may have difficulties in each of these situations because of limited ability to understand the charges and limited ability to understand their consequences, legal counsel is essential. Furthermore, reduced intelligence, lack of life experience, inadequate education, a tendency to show overcompliance to please others, or a fear of authorities may be factors.

In most states, a defendant in a criminal trial who is thought to be incompetent is committed to a mental hospital for further assessment. If found incompetent, he will stay in the hospital for some time and then be released or committed on civil grounds. There is the expectation that the nonretarded individual may become competent at a later date when his illness is resolved. However, the acquisition of later competence is more complicated when considering mentally retarded persons. Mentally retarded persons sometimes have been committed to institutions for life when accused of offenses that are legally considered minor. If the mentally retarded person had been tried for such offenses instead and convicted, he may not have been incarcerated at all because the offense was minor. In the Supreme Court case of *Jackson v. Indiana* (406-US715, 1971), it was ruled that an incompetent offender could be committed to a hospital only for a reasonable period of time, after which he would be released or committed under a civil statute. The court noted that due process requires that the nature and duration of commitment bear a relationship to the purpose for the commitment. If individuals are committed because of their incapacity to proceed to trial, they cannot be held for more than a reasonable time to determine if there is substantial probability they would obtain the competence in the foreseeable future. If the retarded person cannot achieve capacity, the state must institute civil commitment proceedings, as would be the case for other citizens, or release him. However, if it is thought the individual will be able to stand trial at a future date, then continuing commitment may be justified, as long as there is evidence that progress is being made toward accomplishing certain agreed-upon goals.

Competency to Testify

In some circumstances, a mentally retarded person may be asked to testify for the prosecution in a criminal case. The defense may argue that the mentally retarded individual is not competent to be a witness and raise questions about his reliability. Because a witness is not specifically disqualified because he is mentally retarded, an individual assessment of competency may be needed. When carrying this out, the prospective witness must be capable of understanding that he may be punished for not telling the truth. He must also be able to demonstrate the ability to recall and report past events accurately. Consequently, the assessment must include an evaluation of language and memory capabilities, personal understanding of the meaning of the alleged crime, the pressures exerted by others on him, and the capacity to differentiate reality from fantasy. A final determination of credibility of the retarded witness will be up to the court and jury. The evaluation of a potentially mentally retarded witness should include whether or not there is a past history of compulsive reporting of fantasy stories about the issue in question. Furthermore, the impact of the testimony itself on the retarded person must be considered. This is particularly true of testimony directed against a family member or guardian who has a supervisory role for the mentally retarded person.

Criminal Liability

In criminal proceedings, mental retardation may be a mitigating circumstance that may lead to a reduction in the offender's personal culpability and moral blameworthiness for the act committed. The majority of individuals who are mentally retarded are not prone to criminal or violent behavior. Still, those who have multiple risk factors and have demonstrated violent behavior in the past require monitoring. One author (Lewis et al., 1988) reported that among 14 juveniles condemned to death in four states, 1 had an IQ score in the 60s and 5 were in the 70s. All of these individuals had a history of head trauma in childhood and 9 of the 14 had prior hospitalizations. Twelve of the group had histories of abuse in childhood. The majority had severe deficiencies in abstract reasoning. In the past, chromosomal anomalies such as the XYY syndrome have been linked to antisocial behavior. However, further investigation has not demonstrated specific antisocial behavior in XYY syndrome (Freyne and O'Connor, 1992; Schiavi et al., 1984; Theilgaard, 1984).

Due to misconceptions about what constitutes antisocial behavior, individuals with mental retardation may become involved in the criminal justice system through misunderstandings. When this occurs, they may be at risk of being treated unfairly (McAfee and Gural, 1988). The current evidence is that moderately and mildly mentally retarded persons may have a higher likelihood for being arrested for criminal behavior, especially minor delinquent behavior. The crimes that involve them tend to be based on impulsive acts rather than being intentionally planned. One study (Harris, 1992) suggested that difficulties in the inhibition of impulses was a more important consideration in arrests than having had prior fantasies about an aggressive act.

Rather than a specific cause for criminal behavior, mental retardation and its associated disabilities should be considered risk factors for legal difficulty. It is not the mental retardation per se, but the high rate of associated behavioral and emotional problems in mentally retarded persons that is of particular concern. The likelihood of emotional and behavioral problems is enhanced by experiences of frequent psychosocial adversity and by concurrent sensory nervous dysfunction. The increased prevalence of a coexisting mental disorder further increases the vulnerability of a mentally retarded person to act antisocially.

The issue of stigma must be considered as a risk factor because being different from average and being retarded are characteristics that influence attitudes toward retarded persons in the community. Often, the mentally retarded person is the first one in the neighborhood suspected of delinquency because of these attitudes.

Confessions

Clinically, the mentally retarded person should be considered a normalized individual with limited learning capacity. Competency must be considered in regard to the reliability of a confession to a crime made by a mentally retarded person (Praiss, 1989). The mentally retarded defendant who has pleaded guilty may be referred to a psychiatrist to determine whether he is competent to confess. A mentally retarded person may insist he is guilty and should be in prison. In some instances, the individual may be responding to the attention accorded to him at the time of his examination and hope such recognition might elevate his standing in the community.

Criminal confessions in response to questioning while in custody cannot be used in evidence unless the defendant voluntarily, knowingly, and intelligently waives Miranda rights. These rights ensure that a person, when taken into custody, is informed of the Fifth Amendment right to remain silent and to have counsel retained or appointed before an admissible confession can be obtained. Because of adaptive problems and intellectual limitations, care is needed in interpreting whether a waiver of Miranda rights is valid for a mentally retarded person. Due to their special needs, counsel should be brought in as early as the precustodial stage. With early access to an attorney and with a familiar person present, the mentally retarded person's waiver of Miranda rights is best protected and more likely to be voluntary.

Insanity Defense

An insanity defense traditionally is based on there being a mental disease or mental defect, i.e., mental retardation. Therefore, mental retardation can be used as a basis for the insanity defense. The culpability of persons with mental retardation can be considered to be reduced so that mental retardation would be considered a mitigating circumstance. Mental disorders and mental retardation are both considered in decisions regarding an insanity defense. The distinction between them is clearly made in international classifications of disorders and diseases. Yet this distinction may be blurred in court cases because cases brought for criminal action may involve both mental retardation and a mental disorder. Both should be considered in an assessment process.

Culpability refers to the capacity of the accused to distinguish between right and wrong. The legal standard that is applied most often is the McNaghten rule, which requires a lack of knowledge of the nature and wrongfulness of the committed act in order to be found not responsible.

The American Law Institute has suggested the following modification of the McNaghten rule: "A person is not responsible for criminal conduct if at the time of such conduct, as a result of mental disease or defect, he lacks substantial capacity either to appreciate the criminality (wrongfulness) of his conduct or to conform his conduct to the requirements of the law." The new wording substitutes the word "appreciate," which suggests both emotional and cognitive awareness, for "know." Knowing an act is wrong may indicate only surface knowledge of its wrongfulness without a full appreciation of why it is wrong. A mentally retarded person may know an act is wrong but, because of excessive impulsiveness, enhanced susceptibility, or acquiescence to authority, may have difficulty conforming his conduct to the law.

Responsibility in Capital Crimes/Murder

The Supreme Court has found that mental retardation must be considered a mitigating circumstance in capital crimes. Yet the Court has not ruled out the possibility that a mentally retarded person could be given the death penalty. When retarded persons are involved in capital crimes, they usually function in the mild to moderate range of mental retardation. In the *Penry v. Lynaugh* case (109S CT, 1934, 1989), it was concluded the death penalty would not be applied to severely mentally retarded persons. Still, a number of states do have statutes that permit the death penalty for all mentally retarded persons. An evaluation of the specific profile on psychological tests and formal assessment of adaptive function is needed to establish the degree of mental retardation.

The American Association on Mental Retardation (AAMR) position is that no mentally retarded person should be sentenced to death or executed (MPDLR, 1989). The AAMR suggests that such executions serve no purpose penologically, are disproportionate to the retarded person's culpability, do not consider degree of moral blameworthiness in a mentally retarded person, and are a cruel and unusual punishment.

RIGHTS OF THE INCOMPETENT

Mentally retarded persons may be judged mentally incompetent from birth; if so, the protection of their constitutional rights is an ongoing concern throughout their lifetime. For such persons, ethical issues are often raised in regard to procreation, sterilization, rights in regard to involuntary institutionalization, and the right of others to initiate medical intervention on their behalf or to terminate various forms of life support. Because mentally incompetent developmentally disabled individuals are unable to exercise their rights, procedural safeguards are necessary to protect them. The preservation of developmentally disabled persons' autonomy despite their incompetency is often a major challenge from a legal perspective.

Incompetent mentally retarded persons cannot voluntarily consent in regard to decisions about their well-being, nor can they adequately attend to their societal affairs. Decisions that others must make for them include (1) choice to undergo or terminate life-sustaining treatment; (2) the right to reproduce and give birth to children; and (3) the right to community placement rather than institutionalization. Although these rights are constitutionally protected, the right of self-determination must be exercised by another person—a parent or guardian appointed by the state through the courts to represent the disabled person. Two approaches have generally been taken in regard to the rights of incompetent mentally retarded persons. The first is the best interest test and the other, the substituted judgment test. The best interest test focuses primarily on the needs of the incompetent person. The expressed desires or intentions of the mentally retarded person are considered; however, they may be disregarded depending on the circumstances. Using the substituted judgment test, the court renders the decision for the developmentally disabled person. In doing so, the court considers the decision the person might render if he were competent. Questions have been raised about relying entirely on the substituted judgment test because it could lead to excessive involvement by the courts in matters that could be handled more personally and expeditiously by an appointed guardian or family member. However, the best interest procedure may lead to greater accountability; it also avoids the abstractions that are inherent problems when the court makes assumptions about how a person who has never been competent would make a decision.

Procedural safeguards available to protect the rights of incompetent individuals include (1) the appointment of a guardian *ad litem;* (2) an adversarial hearing; and (3) limits on control by the court. This final safeguard takes into consideration whether the judge has the expertise to resolve the problems that have arisen.

Guardian *ad litem*

The guardian *ad litem* is appointed to represent an incompetent person and may be appointed by the court following a legal statute or on a motion to the court. The guardian is responsible for defending the rights of the incompetent person and representing his best interest. In some instances, the guardian may help resolve differences between medical and legal issues.

Adversarial Hearing

In certain situations, a mandatory due process hearing may be required to decide specific issues, such as sterilization. Due process procedures must be followed in the hearing and include (1) the opportunity to be heard; (2) the opportunity to question and cross-examine witnesses; and (3) the right to offer evidence. These hearings are most commonly held when there is a question in regard to whether the family is acting in the best interest of their mentally retarded family member to protect his constitutional rights. However, in some instances, placement decisions have been made without adversarial hearings. For example, in *Parham v. J.R.* (442 U.S. 584, 602, 1979), the Supreme Court upheld a Georgia law that permitted the parents of a mentally retarded child to commit their child to a treatment program on their petition along with the recommendations of psychiatrists, but without a formal hearing. In this case, the court found that the commitment was purely medical and suggested a hearing process could "exacerbate whatever tensions already exist between child and parent."

The Role of the Court

A judge must consider all circumstances when determining the rights of an incompetent person and those of his family members. Family stability is a consideration when reviewing the constitutional rights of a disabled person. In some instances, the family might not be able to control a very aggressive child. Another family might not be able to provide for basic physical needs, such as dressing, toileting, and transporting their mentally retarded adolescent or young adult family member. The court would need to balance the constitutional interest of the child to remain in the family and the reasonable request from a family who report they cannot properly care for the disabled child in the home.

Sterilization/Antilibidinal Drugs/Sexual Expression

From a legal point of view, the major issues related to sexuality have to do with the rights of the individual regarding sterilization (*In re* Grady: 170 NJ Super 98, 405A 2d 851, 1979), sexual expression, and the use of antilibidinal drugs to decrease sexual arousal (Clarke, 1989). Sterilization comes up most frequently for female mentally retarded persons, and antilibidinal drug use for males. Indications for sterilization need to be carefully discussed with individuals and their families and types of birth control that are available reviewed. Pharmacological agents, such as Provera, have been used to reduce libido in mentally retarded individuals just as they have been with nonretarded persons. Particular care is needed to guard the rights of the retarded when antilibidinal medications are considered. Authors working in this area have suggested that small reductions in sexual drive may be adequate to enable an individual to avoid acting on sexual impulses that would lead to unacceptable behavior. Antilibidinal drug treatment reduces the intensity of the sexual drive but will not alter the direction of the drive. When antilibidinal drugs are considered, they are not administered in isolation but in conjunction with active psychotherapy or behavior management programs.

In regard to sterilization in mental retardation, standards have been recommended by the Mental Health Law Project (Abrams, Parker, and Weisberg, 1988) that include (1) representation by a disinterested guardian *ad litem;* (2) independent evaluation of the individual; and (3) the finding that the individual is not capable of and not able to develop the capacity to make an informed judgment. In addition, the individual must be capable of procreation and likely to engage in sexual activity, but found to be permanently incapable of caring for a child. Moreover, there must be no alternatives to sterilization. The major concerns in sterilization assessment are to protect the individual's rights and to follow due process procedures.

Stereotyping of sexual behavior in mentally retarded persons is common (Abrams, Parker, and Weisberg, 1988; Szymanski and Crocker, 1989). They may be considered as sexually inhibited or immature with sexual interests that correspond to their mental age or even thought to be asexual without sexual interest or needs. They alternatively may be thought to be sexually uninhibited. Based on concerns about uninhibited or indiscriminate sexual behavior, concerns about increased reproduction, and concerns about the heritability of mental retardation, sterilization of mentally retarded persons was routinely practiced in the past, and some states continue to have such legislation. In some instances, involuntary sterilization (Dickens, 1982) has been practiced and marriages between mentally retarded persons have been prohibited. Based on these considerations, a mentally retarded person might be denied the opportunity to socialize or develop an intimate relationship with someone of the opposite sex.

Sexual interest generally becomes apparent after puberty. However, there may be delays in puberty in mentally retarded persons, secondary to the etiology of the particular syndrome. Moreover, sexual interest may vary according to intelligence level. Regardless of the age of their pubertal onset, most severely and profoundly retarded individuals may show little sexual interest toward others. But mildly retarded individuals and many moderately retarded individuals may have normal pubertal development, show appropriate sexual interests, and establish sexual identities.

When the expression of their sexual interest is prohibited or denied, sexual activity may occur as a response—often as a way of demonstrating self-importance. Sexual behavior may also be aimed at attempts to gain acceptance from others. Just as with peer groups for nonmentally retarded individuals, sexual status may be important for mentally retarded persons. Encouraging relationships with others and teaching appropriate social skills are essential to developing appropriate self-esteem. Social skills should be emphasized prior to focusing specifically on instruction about sexual activity.

Mentally retarded persons, especially women, are at risk of sexual exploitation. Knowledge of sexuality is often not well developed because the usual sources of information may not be available to them. Sex education in the schools, peer groups where interpersonal issues are discussed, and printed reading material may be limited or unavailable. Mildly and moderately retarded adolescents often lack the most basic information on sexual anatomy, venereal disease, and contraceptive issues. Generally, knowledge of sexuality is related to life experience and opportunity rather than level of intelligence. Family members may be reluctant to review or discuss sexual matters with their retarded children or young adults but should be encouraged to do so.

A minority of mentally retarded individuals may come into conflict with the legal system as a result of socially unacceptable sexual behavior. Although early studies of criminality did report increased sexual offenses among the mentally retarded, these findings are questionable on methodological grounds. With a developmentally appropriate comprehensive program that includes sex education, issues of sexuality can be dealt with effectively and problems in sexual behavior are not expected.

PSYCHOACTIVE DRUG USE: LEGAL CONSIDERATIONS

During the past two decades, courts have developed rules and standards for regulating psychoactive drug use in developmentally disabled persons, particularly in institutional environments. Although there is consensus among jurisdictions in the various states that high professional standards are mandated in the monitoring of drug use, there are substantial differences concerning the circumstances under which psychotropic medications may be administered throughout the United States (Beyer, 1988).

In the early 1970s, the rights of persons with disabilities were widely proclaimed by national and international organizations. U.S. courts began to establish legal rights that were enforceable for mentally retarded persons in the community and within the walls of hospitals, state schools, and developmental programs (Beyer, 1988). Before this, the rights of the individual had not been specifically monitored on entry into a hospital or state facility in the belief the law should not interfere with the clinical relationship following hospital admission. This extension of legal protection into the mental retardation facility was occasioned by the frequent use of psychotropic drugs in those settings.

For large numbers of residents in the 1950s and 1960s, the use of psychotropic drugs for restraint in the absence of a comprehensive treatment program was an early issue. The availability of psychotropic medications had led to a reduction in the use and need for physical restraints, so they were commonly prescribed. However, as Brakel and Rock (1971, pp. 160–161) noted, "The line between physical restraint by mechanical device and by drugs may be a thin one . . . the latter may be as open to abuse as the former." The widespread use of psychoactive drugs in understaffed institutions for both mentally ill and mentally retarded individuals for purposes of restraint led to court involvement (*Halderman v. Pennhurst,* 1977; *Wyatt v. Stickney,* 1972). Questions were raised about these medications being used as substitutes for habilitative programs rather than for their expected use to treat a mental disorder or to prevent harm to oneself or others in emergency situations. The former use was considered a violation of individual rights and led to court orders and consent decrees. For example, *Wyatt v. Stickney* (1972) mandated that "Medications shall not be used as punishment, for the convenience of staff, as a substitute for a habilitation program or in quantities that interfere with the resident's habilitation program." Still, the courts have not held that the use of psychotropic drugs for restraint is never justified. The right or duty of staff members in state facilities to restrain individuals when necessary to prevent them from harming themselves or others was affirmed by the U.S. Supreme Court in its 1982 *Youngberg v. Romeo* decision, which is described in detail later in this chapter. The court did acknowledge the legitimate use of some restraint but found a resident has a constitutional right to be free of "unreasonable" restraints. Guidelines for the use of restraint recommended that, in a particular situation, the first priority is to consider whether any restraint is needed, and if so, whether the restraint used might be a psychotropic drug. In the past, restraints have been justified either as a way to protect society or through the state's *parens patriae* power (paternalistic power) to care for those individuals who are incapable of caring for themselves. There are differences among the states on how restraints are authorized, and guidelines are provided for their use. The American Psychiatric Task Force (1985) on the Psychiatric Uses of Seclusion and Restraint reported that in 23 states, indications for seclusion or restraint were to prevent harm to the patient or other persons. However, eight state regulations also included the prevention of substantial property damage, and two state regulations addressed disruption of the treatment environment as indications for the use of seclusion or restraint.

In general, two legal principles have been offered in regard to restraint. The first is that the use of restraints may be legally justified only in an "emergency situation that might occur when there is a serious threat of extreme violence, personal injury, or attempted suicide," but not as a routine convenience for custodial care. The second principle is that of the "least restrictive alternative." The latter principle offers guidance for actions taken in emergency situations. It requires that the steps undertaken in an emergency to avoid potential harm be the least intrusive and the least restrictive of an individual's liberty. Moreover, those steps chosen must be tailored to the circumstances. Essentially, emergency restraint may be used when it appears likely an individual will injure himself or another, damage the property of another, and where the emergency drug treatment is the only reasonable and practical mode of restraint. In other instances, the emergency drug may be used to preserve the person's life or health, to prevent permanent or severe injury, or to prevent great pain and suffering.

Less restrictive alternatives to restraint include various forms of psychotherapy, special educational training, and behavior modification approaches. The relationship of emergency pharmacotherapy or "chemical restraints" to mechanical restraints, involuntary commitment, or punishment procedures, such as time-out, is frequently debated. In some instances, the use of emergency medication for treatment is viewed by a state as less restrictive than seclusion, but in other states, "chemical restraints" may be considered more restrictive than seclusion or physical restraints (Wexler, 1982).

The use of psychotropic drugs is best considered as focused on target symptoms, and the term "emergency pharmacotherapy" is preferred to "chemical restraint." If an individual becomes aggressive, consideration should be given to the reason for the aggressive behavior, particularly whether or not it is related to delusional processes, is a stress response in a brain-injured person, or is related to difficulty in affect modulation in a severely retarded person. The diagnosis of psychophysiologic disturbance should be the deciding factor in the choice of medications and how they are used for emergency pharmacotherapy. In the choice of medication, the issue of the effectiveness of the medication is an important consideration. Because these medications are used for treatment of mental disorders, it is important to consider that many jurisdictions in the United States do recognize general rights to treatment or habilitation based on the state or the federal constitution or on state statutes.

As noted Chapter 20 on pharmacotherapy, the efficacy of psychotropic medications in treating mental disorders in individuals with mental retardation or developmental disorders is undergoing careful scrutiny. Neuroleptic medications, such as chlorpromazine and thioridazine, have been approved by the Food and Drug Administration (FDA) for use in persons who demonstrate "severe behavior problems." The FDA notes that "substantial evidence" does exist regarding their effectiveness for affected mentally retarded persons (Plotkin and Gill, 1979, p. 654). The FDA decision in approving these drugs for these indications has been questioned based on the scientific rigor of the studies used to establish the approved indication. Such questions regarding efficacy will be resolved when more data is available on management of disruptive behavior in specific syndromes.

Standards for Psychotropic Drug Administration

Standards for the administration of psychotropic drugs in institutions for mentally retarded persons have been offered through various U.S. court rulings. In a landmark decision by Judge Frank Johnson in 1972 in *Wyatt v. Stickney,* the federal court in Alabama held that the U.S. Constitution, at a minimum, requires the following:

> A. No medication shall be administered unless on the written order of a physician.
> B. Notation of each individual's medication shall be kept on his medical record . . . At least weekly, the attending physician shall review the drug regimen for each resident under his care . . . .
> C. Residents shall have a right to be free from unnecessary or excessive medication.
> D. . . . Medication shall not be used as punishment, for the convenience of the staff, as a substitute for a habilitation program, or in quantities that interfere with the resident's habilitation program.
> E. Pharmacy services at the institution shall be directed by a professionally competent pharmacist, licensed in the State of Alabama. Such pharmacist shall be a graduate of a School of Pharmacy accredited by the American Council on Pharmacological Education . . .

Subsequent cases have elaborated on these standards. In the *Halderman v. Pennhurst* case (1977), a class action suit was brought on behalf of residents of the Pennhurst State School in Pennsylvania. The federal district court ruled that "chemical restraints may be administered only upon the order of a physician." The administrators of the state school were asked by the court to ensure that only appropriately trained staff be allowed to administer drugs to residents. Monthly reviews by a physician were required, and training programs were required for staff who administered the drugs. Other states have expanded the Wyatt rules and also include monitoring the use of restraints and psychotropic medications and reduction of their utilization as soon as clinically possible. In *Connecticut Association for Retarded Citizens v. Thorne* (1983), it was required that, except in emergencies, restraints and/or psychotropic medication be employed only in conjunction with a written comprehensive behavior treatment plan that included six specific criteria outlined by the court. Medication levels were to be reviewed monthly by a pharmacist and team nurses and quarterly by an interdisciplinary team. Moreover, medications were to be administered only by nurses or other personnel licensed in the state.

The judicial decisions have made it clear that monitoring is essential to establish the effectiveness of the medication and its continuation. The 1977 Consent Decree in *Welsch v. Dirkswager* on behalf of mentally retarded residents in a Minnesota state hospital required that major tranquilizers for controlling behavior be used only if records, which are based on direct staff observation, are consistently maintained with the frequency and according to procedures specified in the medical record. Medications must not be used unless the determination to prescribe or continue is based on evaluation of the efficacy of the medication in controlling or modifying the specified maladaptive behavior. This consent decree provided for a qualified physician to analyze periodically the files of residents to verify compliance.

The courts have become involved with the use of psychotropic drugs in regard to side effects as well as in reference to restraint. Several court cases have addressed the efficacy of these medications in regard to their effects on the individual's ability to think, speak, ambulate, or learn (Plotkin and Gill, 1979, p. 662). Others (Gutheil and Appelbaum, 1983, p. 88) have argued that negative effects of medication have been emphasized too often and that a more balanced view is required. Particular concerns have been raised about side effects of medications, particularly that of tardive dyskinesia. Standards of care in regard to the prevention of tardive dyskinesia have been recommended, primarily based on monitoring and establishing the recognition of early symptoms. The practice of polypharmacy, the administration of multiple drugs to the same patient, must be considered in developing a care plan.

For the most part, in questions of drug use, courts have deferred to medical professionals. In the U.S. Supreme Court decision *Youngberg v. Romeo,* in 1982, the mother of a profoundly retarded 30-year-old man, who was involuntarily confined to Pennsylvania's Pennhurst School, had charged he was being improperly shackled and denied adequate protection and appropriate treatment. The Supreme Court held that individuals had the right to adequate food, shelter, clothing, and medical care, to safe conditions, freedom from unreasonable restraint, and at least minimal training in caring for themselves. The Court held that constitutional due process is satisfied when restraints are used on involuntarily confined mentally retarded persons in accordance with appropriate "professional judgment." The Court noted that a decision regarding restraints "if made by a professional, is presumably valid; liability may be imposed only when the decision by the professional is such a substantial departure from accepted professional judgment, practice or standards, to demonstrate that the person responsible did not base the decision on such judgment." The Court also noted that it was not appropriate for the Court to specify which of several professionally acceptable choices should be made. These findings supported the importance of carefully documenting and sensitively applying procedures, and using good professional judgment in regard to restraint. The Romeo opinion did not address drug use directly, but the language described is relevant because the decision does focus on the reasonableness of the use of restraints (Beyer, 1988).

The Issue of Consent

Consent to take medication should be informed, voluntarily, and competent. The courts have been active in establishing standards for the administration of psychotropic medication to institutionalized mentally retarded persons but have given little attention to determining how legal privacy rights and consent requirements apply. A person who receives medication for therapeutic purposes has a right to receive information about risks, potential benefits, and possible alternatives. These issues have been addressed primarily for the mentally ill, but alternative means in applying them have been required in mentally retarded persons who were deemed incompetent. Even for a competent individual, giving voluntary consent for placement in special education settings or in institutional environments is difficult to achieve. Currently, decisions in regard to the right to refusal of medication apply to psychiatric patients and have not been extended specifically to those with mental retardation disorders. However, the refusal issue also may be pertinent to an individual who tests in the mental retardation range and has a psychiatric disorder but refuses treatment for the psychiatric disorder.

Because of the difficulty in establishing consent, proxy decision making must be considered. If individuals are not competent and must receive psychoactive drugs, court determination must be made of their competence, and if they are not competent to make a decision, a proxy decision must be made. Competence requires an understanding of the nature and the consequences of the decision to take, or not to take, medication and the availability of relevant information to reach a rational choice. If an individual is competent, then the person's choice must be respected, as is the case for those who are not developmentally disabled. If an individual competently refuses to take a psychoactive medication that is recommended and the drug is not administered, it is still possible for that medication to be used in an emergency situation for emergency pharmacotherapy.

For the incompetent individual, a surrogate must make the decision regarding drug treatment. There has been considerable debate about who the proxy decision maker should be and how to establish the standards that should be used in making the decision. The most common situation is one where the court appoints a legal guardian who is empowered to make decisions on behalf of the "ward." In certain jurisdictions, the courts have found that psychoactive drugs are an "extraordinary" medical treatment that is too risky or intrusive for a legal guardian to agree to on behalf of another person. In Massachusetts, the court has ruled that the psychoactive drugs may not be administered to an incompetent person in a nonemergency situation in either an institution setting or in the community unless authorized by the court (*Guardianship of Roe, 1981; Rogers v. Commissioner of Mental Health, 1983).* This court ruled that "because incompetent persons cannot meaningfully consent to medical treatment, a substituted judgment by a judge should be undertaken for the incompetent patient even if the patient accepts a medical treatment." This decision only applies to functionally incompetent residents of mental retardation facilities. In making the substituted judgment, the court considers factors that might help it know what the values and preferences are of the incompetent person. The court must take into account the individual's religious beliefs, if known, and the effect they might have on the decision, the impact of the decision on the individual's family, the probability of side effects, the prognosis with and without treatment, and any other relevant factors. The Massachusetts model has been criticized because it is time consuming, expensive, and may be cumbersome. Critics have raised issues in regard to the ruling because it potentially limits the appropriate use of neuroleptic medications and the role of the family as the "bonded guardian" whose relationship was established with the individual before placement outside the home, and who might serve the person's "best interests" (Gutheil and Appelbaum, 1985).

With no definitive law in regard to right to refusal, relying on the best interest test, using the consent of the guardian, family member, or treating physician is the most common means for making a decision. However, substituted judgment is used in some jurisdictions. Beyer (1988) suggests four general principles for regulating administration of psychoactive drugs when there are questions of competence: (1) Psychoactive medication must be subject to controls that are at least as stringent as those used for mechanical restraints and seclusion. (2) Before psychoactive medications are used for therapeutic intervention, there needs to be clear evidence a particular drug is likely to be effective and the benefits are likely to outweigh the risks. Benefits are most clear cut in mentally retarded individuals with specific psychiatric disorders, such as schizophrenia. (The risk-benefit issue comes up most commonly when long-term neuroleptic medication is used for disruptive behavior without a specific diagnosis.) (3) When administering psychotropic medications to incompetent individuals when an appropriate indication is established, a well-considered decision-making process, decision maker, and standard for monitoring must be established. Because multiple caregivers may be involved, information should be gathered from those caregivers and involved members of a multidisciplinary team who are familiar with the individual being treated. A balance needs to be established between the decisions being made by individuals who are involved in clinical treatment and the need for legal safeguards. Whether the decision is made utilizing the substituted judgment or the best interest standards, it should be individualized based on the capacities of the individual involved. Beyer (1988) suggests that if the individual involved has possessed, or currently possesses, the capacity to understand and form an opinion regarding treatment, then the substituted judgment process should be considered. If the individual has never had the capacity to understand the issues around drug treatment, it might be best to acknowledge it is not possible to determine what that person would do if competent. He or she has never been competent, so a conscientious approach might utilize the best interest standard, deciding what society would consider best for the individual in these specific circumstances. (4) An effective monitoring and review mechanism must be developed to assure the use of the drugs conforms to high standards, such as those established in the Wyatt case and other cases that have followed it.

SUMMARY

Institutionalized mentally retarded individuals and those in community settings have made considerable advances during the past 30 years in gaining legal recognition for their rights. Although additional work is needed to develop standards that serve the best interests of the individual, there have been major gains in this area. The United Nations Declaration on the Rights of Disabled Persons remains an essential reminder and guide for future progress.

REFERENCES

Abrams, P.R., Parker, T., and Weisberg, S.R. (1988). Sexual expression of mentally retarded people: Educational and legal implications. *American Journal on Mental Retardation,* 93:328–334.

Accardo, P.J. and Whitman, B.Y. (1990). Children of mentally retarded parents. *American Journal of Diseases of Childhood,* 144:69–70.

American Psychiatric Association Task Force. (1985). *Seclusion and restraint, the pychiatric uses: Report of the American Psychiatric Association Task Force on the psychiatric uses of seclusion and restraint.* Author, Washington, DC.

Beyer, H.A. (1988). Litigation and the use of psychoactive drugs. In M.G. Aman and N.N. Singh (eds), *Psychopharmacology of the developmental disabilities,* pp. 29–57. Springer-Verlag, New York.

Brakel, S., and Rock, R. (eds.). (1971). *The mentally*

disabled and the law, revised ed. University of Chicago Press, Chicago.

______, Parry, F., and Weiner, B. (1985). *The mentally disabled and the law,* 3rd ed., pp. 516, 517, 520, 544–546. American Bar Association, Chicago.

Clarke, D.J. (1989). Antilibidinal drugs and mental retardation: A review. *Medicine, Science and the Law,* 29:136–146.

Connecticut Association for Retarded Citizens v. Thorne, Civil No. H-78–653 (U.S.D.C., D. Conn., consent decree, Nov. 7, 1983), at 10.

Dickens, B.M. (1982). Retardation and sterilization. *International Journal of Law and Psychiatry,* 5:529–318.

Feldman, M.A. (1986). Research on parenting mentally retarded persons. *Psychiatric Clinics of North America,* 9:777–796.

Freyne, A., and O'Connor, A. (1992). XYY genotype and crime: 2 cases. *Medicine, Science and the Law,* 32:261–263.

Ginsberg v. New York, 390 U.S. 629 (1968).

Guardianship of Roe, 383 Mass. 415 (1981).

Gutheil, T.G., and Appelbaum, P. (1983). "Mind control," "synthetic sanity," "artificial competence," and genuine confusion: Legally relevant effects of antipsychotic medication. *Hofstra Law Review,* 12:77–120.

______, and ______. (1985). The substituted judgment approach: Its difficulties and paradoxes in mental health settings. *Law, Medicine & Health Care,* 13:61–64.

Halderman v. Pennhurst, 446 F. Supp. 1295, 1307–08 (E.D. Pa. 1977).

Harris, J. (1992). Legal aspects of mental retardation. In D.H. Schetky and E.P. Benedeck (eds.), *Clinical handbook of child psychiatry and the law,* pp. 265–291. Williams and Wilkins, Baltimore.

In re C.L.M., 625 S.W.2d 613 (Mo. 1981).

In re Grady, 170 NJ Super 98, 405A 2d 851, 1979.

Jackson v. Indiana, 406 U.S. 715, 1971.

Kapp, M.B. (1981). Protecting the personal funds of the mentally retarded: New federal regulations. *Hospital and Community Psychiatry,* 32:567–571.

Lewis, D.O., Pincus, J.H., Bard, B., Richardson, E., Prichep, L.S., Feldman, M., and Yeager, C. (1988). Neuropsychiatric, psychoeducational, and family characteristics of 14 juveniles condemned to death in the United States. *American Journal of Psychiatry,* 145:584–589.

Malone, R. (1992, October). *State regulations and psychotropic drug use.* Summary prepared for the American Academy of Child and Adolescent Psychiatry Committee on Mental Retardation and Developmental Disabilities. (Unpublished)

Marafino, K. (1990). Parental rights of persons with mental retardation. In B.Y. Whitman and P.J. Accardo (eds.), *When a parent is mentally retarded,* pp. 163–189. Paul H. Brookes, Baltimore.

McAfee, J.K., and Gural, M. (1988). Individuals with mental retardation and the criminal justice system: The view from states' attorneys general. *Mental Retardation,* 26:5–12.

MPDLR. (1989). U.S. Supreme Court remands execution of man with mental retardation. *Medical and Physical Disability Law Reporter,* 13:334–338.

Mesibov, G.B., Conover, B.S., and Sauer, W.G. (1980). Limited guardianship laws and developmentally disabled adults: Needs and obstacles. *Mental Retardation,* 18:221–226.

Meyer v. Nebraska, 262 U.S. 390 (1923).

In re J.J.B. (1987). Minnesota adopts a best interests standard in parental rights termination proceedings. *Minnesota Law Review,* 71:1263–1292.

Nirje, B. (1969). A Scandinavian visitor looks at U.S. institutions. In W. Wolfensberger and R. Kugel (eds.), *Changing patterns in residential services for the mentally retarded,* pp. 51–58. President's Committee on Mental Retardation, Washington, DC.

Parham v. J.R., 442 U.S. 584, 602 (1979).

Pate v. Robinson, 383 U.S. 375, 1966.

Penry v. Lynaugh, 109S CT, 1934, 1989.

Plotkin, R., and Gill, K.R. (1979). Invisible manacles: Drugging mentally retarded people. *Stanford Law Review,* 31:637–678.

Praiss, D.M. (1989). Constitutional protection of confessions made by mentally retarded defendants. *American Journal of Law and Medicine,* 14:431–465.

Price v. Price, 255 S.E. 2d 652 (N.C. Ct. App. 1979).

Retarded parents in neglect proceedings: The erroneous assumption of parental inadequacy. (1979). *Stanford Law Review,* 31:785–788, 790–795, 797, 798, 801.

Rogers v. Commissioner of Mental Health, 390 Mass. 489, at 509 (1983).

Santosky v. Kramer, 455 U.S. 745, 747, 748, 753, 765, 769 (1982).

Schiavi, R.C., Theilgaard, A., Owen, D.R., and White, D. (1984). Sex chromosomes, hormones, and aggressivity. *Archives of General Psychiatry,* 41:93–99.

Smith, S.M., and Kunjukrishnan, R. (1986). Medicolegal aspects of mental retardation. *Psychiatric Clinics of North America,* 9:699–712.

Szymanski, L., and Crocker, A. (1989). Mental retardation. In H.I. Kaplan and B.J. Sadock (eds.), *Comprehensive textbook of psychiatry,* 4th ed., pp. 1728–1771. Williams and Wilkins, Baltimore.

Theilgaard, A. (1984). A psychological study of the

personalities of XYY and XXY men. *Acta Psychiatrica Scandinavica, Supplementum,* 315:1–133.

United Nations. (1972). *Resolution of the General Assembly.* January 21, 1972, Agenda Item #12 [A/Res/2856(XXVI)].

______. (1975). *Resolution of the General Assembly,* December 9, 1975 [A/10284/Add.1(XXX)].

Welsch v. Dirkswager, No. 4–72 Civil 451 (U.S.D.C., D. Minn., consent decree, Dec. 1977), at 17.

Wexler, D.B. (1982). Seclusion and restraint: Lessons from law, psychiatry, and psychology. *International Journal of Law and Psychiatry,* 5:285–294.

Whitman, B.Y., and Accardo, P.J. (1990). *When a parent is mentally retarded,* pp. 3–10. Paul H. Brookes, Baltimore.

Wolfensberger, W. (1972). *The principle of normalization in human services.* National Institution on Mental Retardation, Toronto, Ontario.

Wyatt v. Stickney, 344 F. Supp. 373, 344 F. Supp. 387 (M.D. Ala. 1972) aff'd sub nom. Wyatt v. Aderholt, 503 F2d 1305 (5th Cir 1974).

Youngberg v. Romeo, 102 S.Ct. 2452 (1982).

APPENDIX

STATE REGULATIONS REGARDING PSYCHOTROPIC DRUG USE

Malone (1992) has evaluated state regulations and found the following conditions have been recommended among the various states in regard to the use of psychotropic medications:

1. Approval by the interdisciplinary team is necessary.
2. A behavioral program must be in place.
3. There is a plan or attempt to reduce or discontinue the medication once begun.
4. The rules do not apply if treating a specific major psychiatric disorder.
5. Psychotropic drugs cannot be used for convenience.
6. Psychotropic drugs cannot be used as discipline.
7. Psychotropic drugs cannot be used in place of a comprehensive program.
8. The least restrictive treatment must be tried first.
9. Exceptions are made for emergency treatment.
10. Approval must be gained from a Human Rights Committee.
11. Various limits are placed on prescription of medication.
12. There are rules in place for monitoring effects.
13. There are rules in place for monitoring side effects.
14. Consent is needed.
15. There is a periodic review of medication.
16. The behavior to be treated must be clearly specified.
17. Laboratory tests must be used as appropriate for the medication use.
18. Rules are in place regarding medication doses given on an "as needed" basis.
19. No standing orders for the use of psychotropic medications are to be used.

CREDITS

The author is indebted to the following for permission to reproduce copyrighted material.

Figure 2–1 reprinted by permission of the author and publisher from MW Thompson et al., Patterns of single-gene inheritance. *Genetics in Medicine,* 5th edition. Philadelphia: W. B. Saunders Company. Copyright © 1991.

Table 3–1 reprinted by permission of the publisher from BF Pennington, *Diagnosing Learning Disorders.* New York: Guilford Press. Copyright © 1991.

Table 3–2 reprinted by permission of the author and publisher, adapted from SS Sparrow and AS Carter, Mental retardation: Current issues related to assessment. *Handbook of Neuropsychology,* Vol. 6, *Child Neuropsychology.* (I Rapin and SJ Segalowitz, eds). Amsterdam: Elsevier Science Publishers B.V. Copyright © 1992.

Tables 3–3 and 3–4 reprinted by permission of the author from MB Denckla, Neurodevelopmental Pathways to Learning Disabilities, P50 HD 25806, a grant from NINCDS, National Institutes of Health, Bethesda, MD., 1993.

Tables 4–1, 4–2, 4–3, 4–4, 4–5, 4–6 reprinted by permission of the author and publisher, adapted from JG Young et al., Advances in research techniques. *Child and Adolescent Psychiatry: A Comprehensive Textbook.* (M Lewis, ed). Baltimore: Williams & Wilkins. Copyright © 1991.

Table 4–7 reprinted by permission of the publisher from MR Stytz and O Frieder, Three-dimensional medical imaging modalities: An overview. *Critical Reviews in Biomedical Engineering* 18:1–25. Copyright © 1990 by CRC Press, Inc.

Table 4–8 reprinted by permission of the author and publisher, adapted from JG Young et al., Advances in research techniques. *Child and Adolescent Psychiatry: A Comprehensive Textbook.* (M Lewis, ed). Baltimore: Williams & Wilkins.

Figures 4–1 and 4–2 from MR Stytz and O Frieder, Three-dimensional medical imaging modalities: An overview. *Critical Reviews in Biomedical Engineering* 18:1–25. Copyright © 1990. Reprinted by permission of CRC Press, Boca Raton, Florida.

Figure 4–3 reprinted by permission of the publisher from SC Bushong, *Magnetic Resonance Imaging: Physical and Biological Principles.* St. Louis: Mosby Yearbook, Inc. Copyright © 1988.

Figure 4–4 from MR Stytz and O Frieder, Three-dimensional medical imaging modalities: An overview. *Critical Reviews in Biomedical Engineering* 18:1–25. Copyright © 1990. Reprinted by permission of CRC Press, Boca Raton, Florida.

Figure 4–5 reprinted by permission of the publisher from G Sedvall et al., Imaging of neurotransmitter receptors in the living human brain. *Archives of General Psychiatry* 43:995–1005. Copyright © 1986, American Medical Association.

Chapter 4 Glossary reprinted by permission of the publisher from SC Bushong, *Magnetic Resonance Imaging: Physical and Biological Principles.* St. Louis: Mosby Yearbook, Inc. Copyright © 1988.

Introduction to Part II: Table II–1 reprinted by permission of the author from *ICD-10 Classification of Mental and Behavioural Disorders: Clinical Descriptions and Diagnostic Guidelines.* Geneva: World Health Organization. Copyright © 1992.

Introduction to Part II: Table II–2 reprinted by permission of the author from *Diagnostic and Statistical Manual of Mental Disorders,* 4th edition. Washington DC: American Psychiatric Association. Copyright © 1994.

Table 5–1 reprinted by permission of the author from *Diagnostic and Statistical Manual of Mental Disorders,* 4th edition. Washington DC: American Psychiatric Association. Copyright © 1994.

Table 5–3 reprinted by permission of the author from *Mental Retardation: Definition, Classification, and Systems.* Washington DC: American Association on Mental Retardation. Copyright © 1992.

Table 5–4 reprinted by permission of the author, adapted from *Mental Retardation: Definition, Classification, and Systems.* Washington DC: American Association on Mental Retardation. Copyright © 1992.

Table 5–5 reprinted by permission of the author and publisher, adapted from MG Aman, Review and evaluation of instruments for assessing emotional and behavioural disorders. *Australia and New Zealand Journal of Developmental Disabilities* 17:127–145. Copyright © 1991 by the University of Newcastle, New South Wales, Australia.

Table 6–1 reprinted by permission of the author and publisher from K Nelson and J Ellenberg: Epidemiology of cerebral palsy. *Advances in Neurology* 19:421. Copyright © 1978 by Raven Press.

Figures 6–1 and 6–2 reprinted by permission of the author and publisher from AJ Capute and PJ Accardo, Cerebral palsy: The spectrum of motor dysfunction. *Developmental Disabilities in Infancy and Childhood.* (AJ Capute and PJ Accardo, eds). Brookes Publishing Co., P.O. Box 10624, Baltimore, MD 21285–0614. Copyright © 1991.

Chapter 6, page 140, Christy Brown, "Come Softly to My Wake" reprinted by permission of Secker and Warburg from Christy Brown, *Collected Poems,* Minerva, London, 1990. "Inheritance" by Christy Brown reprinted by permission of Secker and Warburg.

Figure 6–3 reprinted by permission of the author and publisher from HT Chugani, Functional brain imaging in pediatrics. *Pediatric Clinics of North America* 39:4. Copyright © 1992 by W.B. Saunders Company.

Table 7.1–1 reprinted by permission of the author from *Diagnostic and Statistical Manual of Mental Disorders,* 4th edition. Washington DC: American Psychiatric Association. Copyright © 1994.

Figure 7.1–1 Copyright © 1991 by The New York Times Company. Reprinted by permission.

Table 7.3–1 reprinted by permission of the author from *Diagnostic and Statistical Manual of Mental Disorders,* 4th edition. Washington DC: American Psychiatric Association. Copyright © 1994.

Table 7.4–1 reprinted by permission of the author from *Diagnostic and Statistical Manual of Mental Disorders,* 4th edition. Washington DC: American Psychiatric Association. Copyright © 1994.

Table 9.1–1 reprinted by permission of the author from *Diagnostic and Statistical Manual of Mental Disorders,* 4th edition. Washington DC: American Psychiatric Association. Copyright © 1994.

Figure 9.1–1 reprinted by permission of the author and publisher from SJ Rogers and BF Pennington, A theoretical approach to the deficits in infantile autism. *Development and Psychopathology,* Vol. 3. New York: Cambridge University Press. Copyright © 1991.

Table 9.2–1 reprinted by permission of the author from *Diagnostic and Statistical Manual of Mental Disorders,* 4th edition. Washington DC: American Psychiatric Association. Copyright © 1994.

Table 9.3–1 reprinted by permission of the publisher from Rett Syndrome Diagnostic Criteria Work Group: Diagnostic Criteria for Rett Syndrome. *Annals of Neurology* 23:425–428. Copyright © 1988 by Little, Brown & Co. Medical Journals.

Table 9.3–2 reprinted by permission of the author from *Diagnostic and Statistical Manual of Mental Disorders,* 4th edition. Washington DC: American Psychiatric Association. Copyright © 1994.

Figure 9.3–1 reprinted by permission of the author. Copyright © Kerr, 1988.

Table 9.4–1 reprinted by permission of the author from *Diagnostic and Statistical Manual of Mental Disorders,* 4th edition. Washington DC: American Psychiatric Association. Copyright © 1994.

Table 10.3–1 reprinted by permission of the publisher from JC Tarleton and RA Saul, Molecular genetic advances in fragile X syndrome. *Journal of Pediatrics* 122:169–185. Copyright © 1993 by Mosby Yearbook, Inc.

Figure 10.4–1 from RM Hodapp and E Zigler, Applying the developmental perspective to individuals with Down syndrome. *Children with Down Syndrome: A Developmental Perspective.* (D Cicchetti and M. Beeghly, eds). Copyright © Cambridge University Press 1990. Reprinted with the permission of Cambridge University Press.

Table 10.7–1 reprinted by permission of the publisher from ES Roach et al., Report of the Diagnostic Criteria Committee of the National Tuberous Sclerosis Association. *Journal of Child Neurology* 7:221–224. Copyright © 1992 by Decker Periodicals, Inc.

Table 10.8–1 reprinted by permission of the author from JM Berg et al., *The deLange Syndrome.* Copyright © 1970. (Out of print)

Table 11.1–1 reprinted by permission of the author and publisher from L Anderson and M Ernst, Self-Injury in Lesch-Nyhan disease. *Journal of Autism and Developmental Disorders* 24:67–81. Copyright © by Plenum Publishing Corporation 1994.

Figure 11.1–1 reprinted by permission of the author and publisher from T Page and WL Nyhan, The spectrum of HPRT deficiency: An update. *Advances in Experimental Medicine & Biology* 253A:129–132. Copyright © 1989 by Plenum Publishing Co.

Figure 11.1–2 reprinted from *Brain Research Bulletin,* Vol. 25, HA Jinnah et al., Animal models of Lesch-Nyhan syndrome, pp. 467–475, Copyright © 1990, with kind permission from Pergamon Press, Ltd, Headington Hill Hall, Oxford OX3 OBW, UK.

Figure 11.1–3 reprinted from *Brain Research Bulletin,* Vol. 25, HA Jinnah et al., Animal models of Lesch-Nyhan syndrome, pp. 467–475, Copyright © 1990, with kind permission from Pergamon Press, Ltd, Headington Hill Hall, Oxford OX3 OBW, UK.

Table 11.2–1 reprinted by permission of Wiley-Liss, a Division of John Wiley & Sons, Inc., modified from CV Dilts et al., Hypothesis for development of a behavioral phenotype in Williams Syndrome. *American Journal of Medical Genetics* Supplement 6:126–131. Copyright © 1990.

Figures 11.2–1 and 11.2–2 reprinted by permission of the author and publisher from U Bellugi et al., Language, cognition, and brain organization in a neurodevelopmental disorder. *Developmental Behavioral Neuroscience, The Minnesota Symposia on Child Psychology,* Vol. 24. (MR Gunnar and CA Nelson, eds). Copyright © 1992 by Lawrence Erlbaum Associates, Inc.

Table 12.1–1 reproduced by permission of *Pediatrics,* Vol. 91, page 1004, copyright 1993, from American Academy of Pediatrics Committee on Substance Abuse and Committee on Children with Disabilities: Fetal alcohol syndrome and fetal alcohol effects.

Table 13–1 reprinted by permission of the author from *Diagnostic and Statistical Manual of Mental Disorders,* 4th edition. Washington DC: American Psychiatric Association. Copyright © 1994.

Table 14–1 reprinted by permission of the author from *Diagnostic and Statistical Manual of Mental Disorders,* 4th edition. Washington DC: American Psychiatric Association. Copyright © 1994.

Table 14–2 reprinted by permission of Oxford University Press, adapted from MT Tsuang and R Vandermey, *Genes and the Mind.* Copyright © 1980.

Tables 15–1 through 15–3 reprinted by permission of the author from *Diagnostic and Statistical Manual of Mental Disorders.* 4th edition. Washington DC: American Psychiatric Association. Copyright © 1994.

Tables 16–1 through 16–8 reprinted by permission of the author from *Diagnostic and Statistical Manual of Mental Disorders,* 4th edition. Washington DC: American Psychiatric Association. Copyright © 1994.

Table 17–1 reprinted by permission of the author from *Diagnostic and Statistical Manual of Mental Disorders,* 4th edition. Washington DC: American Psychiatric Association. Copyright © 1994.

Table 17–2 reprinted by permission of the author and publisher from EM Pattison and J Kahan, The deliberate self-harm syndrome. *American Journal of Psychiatry* 140:867–872, 1983. Copyright © 1983, the American Psychiatric Association. Reprinted by permission.

Table 18–1 reprinted by permission of the publisher from L Kanner, Parents' feelings about retarded children. *American Journal of Mental Deficiency* 57:375–383. Copyright © 1953 by the American Association on Mental Retardation.

Chapter 19 Glossary reprinted by permission of the publisher, adapted from PE Jansen, Basic principles of behavior therapy with retarded persons. *Emotional Disorders of Mentally Retarded Persons.* (LS Szymanski and PE Tanguay, eds). Austin: Pro-Ed Journals. Copyright © 1980.

Table 21–1 reprinted by permission of the author and publisher from RL Neve, Adenovirus vectors enter the brain. *Trends in Neurosciences* 16:251–253. Copyright © 1993 by Elsevier Science Publishing Company.

INDEX